ICD-10-PCS Code Book

Professional Edition

2024

Anne B. Casto, RHIA, CCS

Consulting Editor

AHIMA
American Health Information
Management Association®

Copyright © 2024 by the American Health Information Management Association. All rights reserved. Except as permitted under the Copyright Act of 1976, no part of this publication may be reproduced, stored in a retrieval system, or transmitted, in any form or by any means, electronic, photocopying, recording, or otherwise, without the prior written permission of the AHIMA, 233 North Michigan Avenue, 21st Floor, Chicago, Illinois, 60601-5809 (https://www.ahima .org/education-events/education-by-product/books/textbook-resources/reprint-permissions/).

ISBN: 978-1-58426-949-6
eISBN: 978-1-58426-950-2
AHIMA Product No.: AC222223

AHIMA Staff:
Sarah Cybulski, MA, Production Development Editor
Christine Scheid, Content Development Manager
Megan Grennan, Director, Content Production and AHIMA Press
James Pinnick, Vice President, Content and Learning Solutions

Cover image: © fatmayilmaz: iStock. Laurie Entringer

Limit of Liability/Disclaimer of Warranty: This book is sold, as is, without warranty of any kind, either express or implied. While every precaution has been taken in the preparation of this book, the publisher and author assume no responsibility for errors or omissions. Neither is any liability assumed for damages resulting from the use of the information or instructions contained herein. It is further stated that the publisher and author are not responsible for any damage or loss to your data or your equipment that results directly or indirectly from your use of this book.

The Centers for Medicare and Medicaid Services (CMS) and the National Center for Health Statistics (NCHS), two departments within the US Federal Government's Department of Health and Human Services (HHS) provide the *International Classification of Diseases, Tenth Revision, Clinical Modification* (ICD-10-CM) for coding and reporting. ICD-10-CM is the US modification to the World Health Organization's (WHO) International Classification of Diseases, Tenth Revision (ICD-10).

Coding Clinic for ICD-10-CM and ICD-10-PCS is a publication of the American Hospital Association (AHA).

Unless otherwise noted, art pieces were created by Jason Isley and Cognition Studio, Inc, and are all copyright of the American Health Information Management Association.

The websites listed in this book were current and valid as of the date of publication. However, webpage addresses and the information on them may change at any time. The user is encouraged to perform his or her own general web searches to locate any site addresses listed here that are no longer valid.

All copyrights and trademarks mentioned in this book are the possession of their respective owners. AHIMA makes no claim of ownership by mentioning products that contain such marks.

For more information about AHIMA Press publications, including updates, visit https://www.ahima.org/education-events/ education-by-product/books/

American Health Information Management Association
233 North Michigan Avenue, 21st Floor
Chicago, Illinois 60601-5809
ahima.org

Contents

About the Consulting Editor	iv
Acknowledgments	iv

Introduction ... **v**
ICD-10-PCS Overview ... v
ICD-10-PCS Code Structure ... vii
ICD-10-PCS Organization and Official Conventions ... ix
AHA *Coding Clinic* for ICD-10-CM and ICD-10-PCS ... xi
ICD-10-PCS Official Guidelines for Coding
and Reporting, 2024 ... xii

Index ... **1**

Medical and Surgical ... **92**
Central Nervous System and
Cranial Nerves (001–00X) ... 103
Peripheral Nervous System (012–01X) ... 117
Heart and Great Vessels (021–02Y) ... 127
Upper Arteries (031–03W) ... 146
Lower Arteries (041–04W) ... 162
Upper Veins (051–05W) ... 179
Lower Veins (061–06W) ... 190
Lymphatic and Hemic System (072–07Y) ... 202
Eye (080–08X) ... 213
Ear, Nose, Sinus (090–09W) ... 226
Respiratory System (0B1–0BY) ... 241
Mouth and Throat (0C0–0CX) ... 258
Gastrointestinal System (0D1–0DY) ... 271
Hepatobiliary System and Pancreas (0F1–0FY) ... 295
Endocrine System (0G2–0GW) ... 308
Skin and Breast (0H0–0HX) ... 315
Subcutaneous Tissue and Fascia (0J0–0JX) ... 331
Muscles (0K2–0KX) ... 345
Tendons (0L2–0LX) ... 358
Bursae and Ligaments (0M2–0MX) ... 370
Head and Facial Bones (0N2–0NW) ... 383
Upper Bones (0P2–0PW) ... 394
Lower Bones (0Q2–0QW) ... 409
Upper Joints (0R2–0RW) ... 422
Lower Joints (0S2–0SW) ... 437
Urinary System (0T1–0TY) ... 457
Female Reproductive System (0U1–0UY) ... 472
Male Reproductive System (0V1–0VY) ... 487

Anatomical Regions, General (0W0–0WY)	500
Anatomical Regions, Upper Extremities (0X0–0XY)	511
Anatomical Regions, Lower Extremities (0Y0–0YW)	518

Obstetrics ... **524**

Placement ... **530**

Administration ... **539**

Measurement and Monitoring ... **557**

**Extracorporeal or Systemic Assistance and
Performance** ... **563**

Extracorporeal or Systemic Therapies ... **566**

Osteopathic ... **569**

Other Procedures ... **571**

Chiropractic ... **574**

Imaging ... **576**

Nuclear Medicine ... **612**

Radiation Therapy ... **624**

**Physical Rehabilitation and Diagnostic
Audiology** ... **643**

Mental Health ... **658**

Substance Abuse ... **662**

New Technology ... **665**

Appendix A: Root Operations Definitions ... **682**

Appendix B: Type and Qualifier Definitions ... **686**

Appendix C: Approach Definitions ... **694**

Appendix D: Medical and Surgical Body Parts ... **696**

**Appendix E: Medical and Surgical Device Table
(Device Key) and Device Aggregation Table** ... **709**

Appendix F: Substance Qualifier Table (Key) ... **718**

Online Appendix:

Appendix G: New ICD-10-PCS Codes FY2024 ... **721**

iii

About the Consulting Editor

Anne B. Casto, RHIA, CCS, is the president of Casto Consulting, LLC. Casto Consulting, LLC is a consulting firm that provides services to hospitals and other healthcare stakeholders primarily in the areas of reimbursement and coding. Casto Consulting, LLC specializes in linking coding and billing practices to positive revenue cycle outcomes. Additionally, the firm provides guidance to consulting firms, healthcare organizations and healthcare insurers regarding reimbursement methodologies and Medicare regulations.

Additionally, Ms. Casto is a lecturer in the HIMS department at The Ohio State University, School of Health and Rehabilitation Sciences. Over the past 20 years, Ms. Casto has taught numerous courses in the areas of healthcare reimbursement, coding, healthcare data trending, and coding analytics.

Prior to her current roles, Ms. Casto was the vice president of clinical information for Cleverley & Associates where she worked very closely with APC regulations and guidelines, preparing hospitals for the implementation of the Medicare OPPS. Ms. Casto was also the clinical information product manager for CHIPS/Ingenix. She joined CHIPS/Ingenix in 1998 and spent the majority of her time developing coding compliance products for the inpatient and outpatient settings.

Ms. Casto has been responsible for inpatient and outpatient coding activities in several large hospitals including Mt. Sinai Medical Center (NYC), Beth Israel Medical Center (NYC), and The Ohio State University. She worked extensively with CMI, quality measures, physician documentation, and coding accuracy efforts at these facilities.

Ms. Casto received her degree in Health Information Management at The Ohio State University in 1995. She received her Certified Coding Specialist credential in 1998 from the American Health Information Management Association. In 2009 Ms. Casto received her ICD-10-CM/PCS Trainer certificate from AHIMA. Ms. Casto is the author of an AHIMA-published textbook entitled *Principles of Healthcare Reimbursement*. Additionally, Ms. Casto was a contributing author to the published AHIMA books: *Severity DRGs and Reimbursement; A MS-DRG Primer* and *Effective Management of Coding Services*.

Ms. Casto received the AHIMA Legacy Award, part of the FORE Triumph Awards, in 2007 which honors a significant contribution to the knowledge base of the HIM field through an insightful publication. Additionally, Ms. Casto was honored with the Ohio Health Information Management Association's Distinguished Member Award in 2008 and the Ohio Health Information Management Association's Professional Achievement Award in 2011.

Acknowledgments

Many thanks to my family for their support during this project. Thanks to Dr. Susan White, The Ohio State University; your data manipulation skills are second to none. I thank the reviewers for their thoughtful comments and suggestions. Many thanks to Linda Hyde, RHIA, and Angela Comfort, MBA, RHIA, CDIP, CCS, CCS-P, CICA, for their very thorough technical review of the book.

Introduction

ICD-10-PCS Overview

The *International Classification of Diseases, Tenth Revision, Procedure Coding System* (ICD-10-PCS) was created to accompany the World Health Organization's (WHO) ICD-10 diagnosis classification. This coding system was developed to replace ICD-9-CM procedure codes for reporting inpatient procedures. ICD-10-PCS was designed to enable each code to have a standard structure and be very descriptive, and yet flexible enough to accommodate future needs.

History of ICD-10-PCS

The WHO has maintained the International Classification of Diseases (ICD) for recording cause of death since 1893. It has updated the ICD periodically to reflect new discoveries in epidemiology and changes in medical understanding of disease. The International Classification of Diseases Tenth Revision (ICD-10), published in 1992, is the latest revision of the ICD. The WHO authorized the National Center for Health Statistics (NCHS) to develop a clinical modification of ICD-10 for use in the United States. This version of ICD-10 is called ICD-10-CM, and is intended to replace the previous US clinical modification, ICD-9-CM, that had been in use since 1979. ICD-9-CM contains a procedure classification; ICD-10-CM does not.

The Centers for Medicare and Medicaid Services (CMS), the agency responsible for maintaining the inpatient procedure code set in the United States, contracted with 3M Health Information Systems in 1993 to design and then develop a procedure classification system to replace Volume 3 of ICD-9-CM. ICD-10-PCS is the result. ICD-10-PCS was initially released in 1998. It has been updated annually since that time.

ICD-10-PCS Design

ICD-10-PCS is fundamentally different from previous procedure classification systems in its structure, organization, and capabilities. It was designed and developed to adhere to recommendations made by the National Committee on Vital and Health Statistics (NCVHS). It also incorporates input from a wide range of organizations, individual physicians, healthcare professionals, and researchers. Several structural attributes were recommended for a new procedure coding system. These attributes include a multiaxial structure, completeness, and expandability.

Multiaxial Structure

The key attribute that provides the framework for all other structural attributes is multiaxial code structure. *Multiaxial code structure* makes it possible for the ICD-10-PCS to be complete, expandable, and provide a high degree of flexibility and functionality.

ICD-10-PCS codes are composed of seven characters. Each character represents a category of information that can be specified about the procedure performed. A character defines both the category of information and its physical position in the code. A character's position can be understood as a semi-independent axis of classification that allows different specific values to be inserted into that space, and whose physical position remains stable. Within a defined code range, a character retains the general meaning that it confers on any value in that position.

Completeness

Completeness is considered a key structural attribute for a new procedure coding system. The specific recommendation for completeness included that a unique code be available for each significant procedure, that each code retain its unique definition, and that codes that have been deleted are not reused.

In ICD-10-PCS, a unique code is constructed for every significantly different procedure. Within each section, a character defines a consistent component of a code, and contains all applicable values for that character. The values define individual expressions (Open, Percutaneous) of the character's general meaning (approach) that are then used to construct unique procedure codes. Because all approaches by which a procedure is performed are assigned a separate approach value, every procedure which uses a different approach will have its own unique code. This is true of the other characters as well. The same procedure performed on a different body part has its own unique code; the same procedure performed using a different device has its own unique code, and so on.

v

Because ICD-10-PCS codes are constructed of individual values rather than lists of fixed codes and text descriptions, the unique, stable definition of a code in the system is retained. New values may be added to the system to represent a specific new approach or device or qualifier, but whole codes by design cannot be given new meanings and reused.

Expandability

Expandability was also recommended as a key structural attribute. The specific recommendation for expandability included that the system be capable of accommodating new procedures and technology and that these new codes could be added to the system without disrupting the existing structure.

ICD-10-PCS is designed to be easily updated as new codes are required for new procedures and new techniques. Changes to ICD-10-PCS can all be made within the existing structure because whole codes are not added. Instead, a new value for a character can be added to the system as needed. Likewise, an existing value for a character can be added to a table(s) in the system.

ICD-10-PCS Additional Characteristics

ICD-10-PCS possesses several additional characteristics in response to government and industry recommendations. These characteristics are

- Standardized terminology within the coding system
- Standardized level of specificity
- No diagnostic information
- No explicit "not otherwise specified" (NOS) code options
- Limited use of "not elsewhere classified" (NEC) code options

Standardized Terminology

Words commonly used in clinical vocabularies may have multiple meanings. This can cause confusion and result in inaccurate data. ICD-10-PCS is standardized and self-contained. Characters and values used in the system are defined in the system. For example, the word *excision* is used to describe a wide variety of surgical procedures. In ICD-10-PCS, the word *excision* describes a single, precise surgical objective, defined as "cutting out or off, without replacement, a portion of a body part."

No Eponyms or Common Procedure Names

The terminology used in ICD-10-PCS is standardized to provide precise and stable definitions of all procedures performed. This standardized terminology is used in all ICD-10-PCS code descriptions. As a result, ICD-10-PCS code descriptions do not include eponyms or common procedure names.

In ICD-10-PCS, physicians' names are not included in a code description, nor are procedures identified by common terms or acronyms such as appendectomy or CABG. Instead, such procedures are coded to the root operation that accurately identifies the objective of the procedure.

ICD-10-PCS assigns procedure codes according to the root operation that matches the objective of the procedure. By relying on the universal objectives defined in root operations rather than eponyms or specific procedure titles that change or become obsolete, ICD-10-PCS preserves the capacity to define past, present, and future procedures accurately using stable terminology in the form of characters and values.

No Combination Codes

With rare exceptions, ICD-10-PCS does not define multiple procedures with one code. This is to preserve standardized terminology and consistency across the system. A procedure that meets the reporting criteria for a separate procedure is coded separately in ICD-10-PCS. This allows the system to respond to changes in technology and medical practice with the maximum degree of stability and flexibility.

Standardized Level of Specificity

ICD-10-PCS provides a standardized level of specificity for each code, so each code represents a single procedure variation. In general, ICD-10-PCS code descriptions are much more specific than previous procedure classification systems but sometimes an ICD-10-PCS code description is actually less specific. ICD-10-PCS provides a standardized level of specificity that can be predicted across the system.

Diagnosis Information Excluded

Another key feature of ICD-10-PCS is that information pertaining to a diagnosis is excluded from the code descriptions. Adding diagnosis information limits the flexibility and functionality of a procedure coding system. It has the effect of placing a code "off limits" because the diagnosis in the medical record does not match the diagnosis in the procedure code description. The code cannot be used even though the procedural part of the code description precisely matches the procedure performed. Diagnosis information is not contained in any ICD-10-PCS code. The diagnosis codes, not the procedure codes, will specify the reason the procedure is performed.

Not Otherwise Specified (NOS) Code Options Restricted

The standardized level of specificity designed into ICD-10-PCS restricts the use of broadly applicable NOS or unspecified code options in the system. A minimal level of specificity is required to construct a valid code.

Limited Not Elsewhere Classified (NEC) Code Options

NEC options are provided in ICD-10-PCS, but only for specific, limited use. In the Medical and Surgical section, two significant NEC options are the root operation value Q, Repair, and the device value Y, Other Device. The root operation Repair is a true NEC value. It is used only when the procedure performed is not one of the other root operations in the Medical and Surgical section. Other Device, on the other hand, is intended to be used to temporarily define new devices that do not have a specific value assigned, until one can be added to the system. No categories of medical or surgical devices are permanently classified to Other Device.

ICD-10-PCS Code Structure

Undergirding ICD-10-PCS is a logical, consistent structure that informs the system as a whole, down to the level of a single code. This means the process of constructing codes in ICD-10-PCS is also logical and consistent: the spaces of the code, called *characters* are filled with individual letters and numbers, called *values*.

Characters

All codes in ICD-10-PCS are seven characters long. Each character in the seven-character code represents an aspect of the procedure. The following are two examples of the code structure: one from the Medical and Surgical section and one from the Ancillary section.

Medical and Surgical Code Structure

Character 1	Character 2	Character 3	Character 4	Character 5	Character 6	Character 7
Section	Body System	Operation	Body Part	Approach	Device	Qualifier

Imaging Section Code Structure

Character 1	Character 2	Character 3	Character 4	Character 5	Character 6	Character 7
Section	Body System	Type	Body Part	Contrast	Qualifier	Qualifier

An ICD-10-PCS code is best understood as the result of a process rather than as an isolated, fixed quantity. The process consists of assigning values from among the valid choices for that part of the system, according to the rules governing the construction of codes.

Values

One of 34 possible values can be assigned to each character in a code: the numbers 0 through 9 and the alphabet (except the letters I and O, because they are easily confused with the numbers 1 and 0). A finished code looks like this: 02103D4.

This code is derived by choosing a specific value for each of the seven characters. Based on details about the procedure performed, values for each character specifying the section, body system, root operation, body part, approach, device, and qualifier are assigned. Because the definition of each character is a function of its physical position in the code, the same value placed in a different position in the code means something different. The value 0 in the first character means something different than 0 in the second character, or 0 in the third character, and so on.

Code Structure Example

The following example defines each character using the code 0LB50ZZ, Excision of right lower arm and wrist tendon, Open approach. This example comes from the Medical and Surgical section of ICD-10-PCS.

Character 1: Section

The first character in the code determines the broad procedure category, or section, where the code is found. In this example, the section is Medical and Surgical. 0 is the value that represents Medical and Surgical in the first character.

Character 1	Character 2	Character 3	Character 4	Character 5	Character 6	Character 7
Section	Body System	Root Operation	Body Part	Approach	Device	Qualifier
0						

Character 2: Body System

The second character defines the body system—the general physiological system or anatomical region involved. Examples of body systems include Lower Arteries, Central Nervous System, and Respiratory System. In this example, the body system is Tendons, represented by the value L.

Character 1	Character 2	Character 3	Character 4	Character 5	Character 6	Character 7
Section	Body System	Root Operation	Body Part	Approach	Device	Qualifier
0	L					

Character 3: Root Operation

The third character defines the root operation, or the objective of the procedure. Some examples of root operations are Bypass, Drainage, and Reattachment. In this example code, the root operation is Excision. When used in the third character of the code, the value B represents Excision.

Character 1	Character 2	Character 3	Character 4	Character 5	Character 6	Character 7
Section	Body System	Root Operation	Body Part	Approach	Device	Qualifier
0	L	B				

Character 4: Body Part

The fourth character defines the body part or specific anatomical site where the procedure was performed. The body system (second character) provides only a general indication of the procedure site. The body part and body system values together provide a precise description of the procedure site. Examples of body parts are Kidney, Tonsils, and Thymus. In this example, the body part value is 5, Lower Arm and Wrist, Right. When the second character is L, the value 5 when used in the fourth character of the code represents the right lower arm and wrist tendon.

Character 1	Character 2	Character 3	Character 4	Character 5	Character 6	Character 7
Section	Body System	Root Operation	Body Part	Approach	Device	Qualifier
0	L	B	5			

Character 5: Approach

The fifth character defines the approach, or the technique used to reach the procedure site. Seven different approach values are used in the Medical and Surgical section to define the approach. Examples of approaches include Open and Percutaneous Endoscopic. In this example code, the approach is Open and is represented by the value 0.

Character 1	Character 2	Character 3	Character 4	Character 5	Character 6	Character 7
Section	Body System	Root Operation	Body Part	Approach	Device	Qualifier
0	L	B	5	0		

Character 6: Device

Depending on the procedure performed, there may be a device left in place at the end of the procedure. The sixth character defines the device. Device values fall into four basic categories:

- Grafts and Prostheses
- Implants
- Simple or Mechanical Appliances
- Electronic Appliances

In this example, there is no device used in the procedure. The value Z is used to represent No Device, as shown here:

Character 1	Character 2	Character 3	Character 4	Character 5	Character 6	Character 7
Section	Body System	Operation	Body Part	Approach	Device	Qualifier
0	L	B	5	0	Z	

Character 7: Qualifier

The seventh character defines a qualifier for the code. A qualifier specifies an additional attribute of the procedure, if applicable. Examples of qualifiers include Diagnostic and Stereotactic. Qualifier choices vary depending on the previous values selected. In this example, there is no specific qualifier applicable to this procedure, so the value is No Qualifier, represented by the letter Z.

Character 1	Character 2	Character 3	Character 4	Character 5	Character 6	Character 7
Section	Body System	Operation	Body Part	Approach	Device	Qualifier
0	L	B	5	0	Z	Z

0LB50ZZ is the complete specification of the procedure "Excision of right lower arm and wrist tendon, open approach."

ICD-10-PCS Organization and Official Conventions

The *ICD-10-PCS Code Book, Professional Edition,* 2024 is based on the official *International Classification of Diseases, Tenth Revision, Procedure Coding System,* issued by the US Department of Health and Human Services (HHS) and CMS. This book is consistent with the content of the government's version of ICD-10-PCS and follows the official conventions.

Index

The Alphabetic Index is provided to assist the user with locating the appropriate table to construct procedure codes. Each table contains all the information required to construct valid procedure codes. Coders should not code from the PCS Index alone; the PCS code tables should always be consulted before assigning a PCS procedure code.

Main Terms

Main terms in the Alphabetic Index reflect the root operations, third character, of procedures. The Index includes not only root operation terms, but also other common procedural terms, anatomical sites, and device terms. The main terms are listed alphabetically. After the coder has located the correct main term and subterm in the Alphabetic Index, he or she is provided with the first three to four digits of the procedure code. The coder should then move to the Tables section of the code book and locate the appropriate table to complete the code construction. Even if the entire seven-digit code is provided in the Index, the coder should still reference the Tables to ensure the correct PCS code has been constructed.

See Reference

Common procedure terms are often listed with the *see* reference. The coder is instructed to follow the reference provided in order to locate the appropriate table to construct the code. For example, the *see* reference is present for the main term Colectomy. The Index excerpt is as follows:

Colectomy

see Excision, Gastrointestinal System 0DB

see Resection, Gastrointestinal System 0DT

ix

In this example, the coder should review the definition of the root operations Excision and Resection to determine which is consistent with the medical record documentation. The coder should then proceed to the corresponding table as suggested by the *see* reference.

Use Reference

Anatomical site terms and device terms are often listed with the *use* reference. The coder is instructed to follow the reference provided in order to locate the appropriate main term for the procedure in question. For example, the *use* reference is present for the main term Inferior rectus muscle. The Index excerpt is as follows:

Inferior rectus muscle

use Muscle, Extraocular, Left

use Muscle, Extraocular, Right

In this example, the coder should identify the root operation for the procedure, and then look for the subterm that identifies the body part indicated in the *use* reference. For example, the procedure is excision of the inferior rectus muscle. The coder would locate the main term Excision. The Index excerpt is as follows:

Excision

Muscle

Extraocular

Left 08BM

Right 08BL

In this example, the coder knows that the Code Table 08B is the correct table because the previous review of the *use* reference identified that the inferior rectus muscle is an extraocular muscle. The coder can now proceed to the 08B Table to finish constructing the PCS code.

In addition to the *use* reference, the coder may also consult appendix D for Body Part Table or appendix E for the Device Table.

Code Tables

ICD-10-PCS contains 17 sections of Code Tables, represented by the numbers 0 through 9 and the letters B through D, F through H, and X. The Tables are organized by general type of procedure. The three main sections of tables include:

1. **Medical and Surgical section**
   - Medical and Surgical (first character 0)

2. **Medical and Surgical Related sections**
   - Obstetrics (first character 1)
   - Placement (first character 2)
   - Administration (first character 3)
   - Measurement and Monitoring (first character 4)
   - Extracorporeal or Systemic Assistance and Performance (first character 5)
   - Extracorporeal or Systemic Therapies (first character 6)
   - Osteopathic (first character 7)
   - Other Procedures (first character 8)
   - Chiropractic (first character 9)

3. **Ancillary sections**
   - Imaging (first character B)
   - Nuclear Medicine (first character C)
   - Radiation Therapy (first character D)
   - Physical Rehabilitation and Diagnostic Audiology (first character F)
   - Mental Health (first character G)
   - Substance Abuse (first character H)
   - New Technology (first character X)

Each code table is defined by the first three characters of the PCS code. Each of these characters is displayed above the table. The table consists of all the options for characters 4 through 7. The root operation or root type, character 3, is present along with its official definition. Table 097 is provided here as an example of the table structure.

0   **Medical and Surgical**

9   **Ear, Nose, Sinus**

7   **Dilation: Expanding an orifice or the lumen of a tubular body part**

Body Part Character 4	Approach Character 5	Device Character 6	Qualifier Character 7
F Eustachian Tube, Right **G** Eustachian Tube, Left	**0** Open **7** Via Natural or Artificial Opening **8** Via Natural or Artificial Opening Endoscopic	**D** Intraluminal Device **Z** No Device	**Z** No Qualifier
F Eustachian Tube, Right **G** Eustachian Tube, Left	**3** Percutaneous **4** Percutaneous Endoscopic	**Z** No Device	**Z** No Qualifier

There can be multiple rows within the table for the first three characters, so the coder must carefully review all the applicable rows. Additionally, a table may cover multiple pages. Therefore, the coder must continue to review the code table options until the end of the table is reached to ensure the correct PCS code has been constructed.

AHA *Coding Clinic* for ICD-10-CM and ICD-10-PCS

The American Hospital Association began publishing coding guidance for ICD-10-CM and ICD-10-PCS in the fourth quarter of 2012. In this code book we identify procedure codes that are discussed in the *Coding Clinic* guidance fourth quarter 2012 through second quarter 2023. In the Medical and Surgical section, after each body system table section, there is an AHA *Coding Clinic* section that lists the references. For all other sections of the code book, the AHA *Coding Clinic* section follows the Tables section. In the AHA *Coding Clinic* section, the PCS codes included in AHA *Coding Clinic* guidance are listed with a sky blue note that alerts the coder to review the AHA *Coding Clinic* prior to assignment of the code to ensure appropriate and accurate reporting. The quarter of publication, year and page number(s) are provided in the note.

AHA CC: 4Q; 2012; pg#-pg#

AHA Coding Clinic Crosswalk for Deleted Codes

Deleted Code	Coding Clinic Reference	Replacement Code
047K3Z6	4Q, 2016, 88-89	047K3ZZ
04CK3Z6	4Q, 2016, 88-89	04CK3ZZ
04V03E6	4Q, 2016, 91-92	04V03EZ
04V03F6	4Q, 2016, 92-94	04V03FZ
0B5S0ZZ	2Q, 2016, 17-18	See 0B5T0ZZ
0BQR0ZZ	2Q, 2016, 22-23	See 0BQT0ZZ
0BQR4ZZ	3Q, 2014, 28	See 0BQT4ZZ
0BQS0ZZ	2Q, 2016, 22-23	See 0BQT0ZZ
0BQS4ZZ	3Q, 2014, 28	See 0BQT4ZZ
0NQS0ZZ	3Q, 2016, 29-30	See 0NQR0ZZ
0NSS04Z	3Q, 2014, 23-24	See 0NSR04Z
0NSS0ZZ	1Q, 2017, 20-21	See 0NSR0ZZ
0NR80JZ	3Q, 2017, 17	See 0NR70JZ

ICD-10-PCS Coding Guidelines

The ICD-10-PCS Coding Guidelines are presented here in the introduction and throughout this manual. Within the manual, the Medical and Surgical Section Guidelines are presented after the Introduction of the Medical and Surgical section. The Obstetric Section Guidelines are presented after the Introduction of the Obstetrics section. Lastly, the New Technology Guidelines are presented after the Introduction of the New Technology section.

ICD-10-PCS Official Guidelines for Coding and Reporting, 2024

The Centers for Medicare and Medicaid Services (CMS) and the National Center for Health Statistics (NCHS), two departments within the US federal government's Department of Health and Human Services (DHHS) provide the following guidelines for coding and reporting using the International Classification of Diseases, 10th Revision, Procedure Coding System (ICD-10-PCS). These guidelines should be used as a companion document to the official version of the ICD-10-PCS as published on the CMS website. The ICD-10-PCS is a procedure classification published by the United States for classifying procedures performed in hospital inpatient health care settings.

These guidelines have been approved by the four organizations that make up the Cooperating Parties for the ICD-10-PCS: the American Hospital Association (AHA), the American Health Information Management Association (AHIMA), CMS, and NCHS.

These guidelines are a set of rules that have been developed to accompany and complement the official conventions and instructions provided within the ICD-10-PCS itself. They are intended to provide direction that is applicable in most circumstances. However, there may be unique circumstances where exceptions are applied. The instructions and conventions of the classification take precedence over guidelines. These guidelines are based on the coding and sequencing instructions in the Tables, Index, and Definitions of ICD-10-PCS, but provide additional instruction. Adherence to these guidelines when assigning ICD-10-PCS procedure codes is required under the Health Insurance Portability and Accountability Act (HIPAA). The procedure codes have been adopted under HIPAA for hospital inpatient healthcare settings. A joint effort between the healthcare provider and the coder is essential to achieve complete and accurate documentation, code assignment, and reporting of diagnoses and procedures. These guidelines have been developed to assist both the healthcare provider and the coder in identifying those procedures that are to be reported. The importance of consistent, complete documentation in the medical record cannot be overemphasized. Without such documentation, accurate coding cannot be achieved.

Conventions

A1. ICD-10-PCS codes are composed of seven characters. Each character is an axis of classification that specifies information about the procedure performed. Within a defined code range, a character specifies the same type of information in that axis of classification.

Example: The fifth axis of classification specifies the approach in sections 0 through 4 and 7 through 9 of the system.

A2. One of 34 possible values can be assigned to each axis of classification in the seven-character code: they are the numbers 0 through 9 and the alphabet (except the letters I and O because they are easily confused with the numbers 1 and 0). The number of unique values used in an axis of classification differs as needed.

Example: Where the fifth axis of classification specifies the approach, seven different approach values are currently used to specify the approach.

A3. The valid values for an axis of classification can be added to as needed.

Example: If a significantly distinct type of device is used in a new procedure, a new device value can be added to the system.

A4. As with words in their context, the meaning of any single value is a combination of its axis of classification and any preceding values on which it may be dependent.

Example: The meaning of a body part value in the Medical and Surgical section is always dependent on the body system value. The body part value 0 in the Central Nervous body system specifies Brain and the body part value 0 in the Peripheral Nervous body system specifies Cervical Plexus.

A5. As the system is expanded to become increasingly detailed, over time more values will depend on preceding values for their meaning.

Example: In the Lower Joints body system, the device value 3 in the root operation Insertion specifies Infusion Device and the device value 3 in the root operation Replacement specifies Ceramic Synthetic Substitute.

A6. The purpose of the Alphabetic Index is to locate the appropriate table that contains all information necessary to construct a procedure code. The PCS Tables should always be consulted to find the most appropriate valid code.

A7. It is not required to consult the Index first before proceeding to the Tables to complete the code. A valid code may be chosen directly from the Tables.

A8. All seven characters must be specified to be a valid code. If the documentation is incomplete for coding purposes, the physician should be queried for the necessary information.

A9. Within a PCS Table, valid codes include all combinations of choices in characters 4 through 7 contained in the same row of the table. In the example below, 0JHT3VZ is a valid code, and 0JHW3VZ is *not* a valid code.

Section:	0	Medical and Surgical
Body System:	J	Subcutaneous Tissue and Fascia
Operation:	H	Insertion: Putting in a nonbiological appliance that monitors, assists, performs, or prevents a physiological function but does not physically take the place of a body part

Body Part (4th)	Approach (5th)	Device (6th)	Qualifier (7th)
S Subcutaneous Tissue and Fascia, Head and Neck **V** Subcutaneous Tissue and Fascia, Upper Extremity **W** Subcutaneous Tissue and Fascia, Lower Extremity	**0** Open **3** Percutaneous	**1** Radioactive Element **3** Infusion Device **Y** Other Device	**Z** No Qualifier
T Subcutaneous Tissue and Fascia, Trunk	**0** Open **3** Percutaneous	**1** Radioactive Element **3** Infusion Device **V** Infusion Pump **Y** Other Device	**Z** No Qualifier

A10. "And," when used in a code description, means "and/or," except when used to describe a combination of multiple body parts for which separate values exist for each body part (e.g., Skin and Subcutaneous Tissue used as a qualifier, where there are separate body part values for "Skin" and "Subcutaneous Tissue").

Example: Lower Arm and Wrist Muscle means lower arm and/or wrist muscle.

A11. Many of the terms used to construct PCS codes are defined within the system. It is the coder's responsibility to determine what the documentation in the medical record equates to in the PCS definitions. The physician is not expected to use the terms used in PCS code descriptions, nor is the coder required to query the physician when the correlation between the documentation and the defined PCS terms is clear.

Example: When the physician documents "partial resection" the coder can independently correlate "partial resection" to the root operation Excision without querying the physician for clarification.

Medical and Surgical Section Guidelines (section 0)

B2. Body System
General guidelines
B2.1a

The procedure codes in Anatomical Regions, General, Anatomical Regions, Upper Extremities and Anatomical Regions, Lower Extremities can be used when the procedure is performed on an anatomical region rather than a specific body part, or on the rare occasion when no information is available to support assignment of a code to a specific body part.

Examples: Chest tube drainage of the pleural cavity is coded to the root operation Drainage found in the body system Anatomical Regions, General. Suture repair of the abdominal wall is coded to the root operation Repair in the body system Anatomical Regions, General. Amputation of the foot is coded to the root operation Detachment in the body system Anatomical Regions, Lower Extremities.

B2.1b

Where the general body part values "upper" and "lower" are provided as an option in the Upper Arteries, Lower Arteries, Upper Veins, Lower Veins, Muscles and Tendons body systems, "upper" or "lower "specifies body parts located above or below the diaphragm respectively.

Example: Vein body parts above the diaphragm are found in the Upper Veins body system; vein body parts below the diaphragm are found in the Lower Veins body system.

B3. Root Operation
General guidelines
B3.1a

In order to determine the appropriate root operation, the full definition of the root operation as contained in the PCS Tables must be applied.

B3.1b

Components of a procedure specified in the root operation definition or explanation as integral to that root operation are not coded separately. Procedural steps necessary to reach the operative site and close the operative site, including anastomosis of a tubular body part, are also not coded separately.

Example: Resection of a joint as part of a joint replacement procedure is included in the root operation definition of Replacement and is not coded separately. Laparotomy performed to reach the site of an open liver biopsy is not coded separately. In a resection of sigmoid colon with anastomosis of descending colon to rectum, the anastomosis is not coded separately.

Multiple procedures
B3.2

During the same operative episode, multiple procedures are coded if:

a. The same root operation is performed on different body parts as defined by distinct values of the body part character.

   Examples: Diagnostic excision of liver and pancreas are coded separately. Excision of lesion in the ascending colon and excision of lesion in the transverse colon are coded separately.

b. The same root operation is repeated in multiple body parts, and those body parts are separate and distinct body parts classified to a single ICD-10-PCS body part value.

   Examples: Excision of the sartorius muscle and excision of the gracilis muscle are both included in the upper leg muscle body part value, and multiple procedures are coded. Extraction of multiple toenails are coded separately.

c. Multiple root operations with distinct objectives are performed on the same body part.

   Example: Destruction of sigmoid lesion and bypass of sigmoid colon are coded separately.

d. The intended root operation is attempted using one approach but is converted to a different approach.

   Example: Laparoscopic cholecystectomy converted to an open cholecystectomy is coded as percutaneous endoscopic Inspection and open Resection.

Discontinued or incomplete procedures
B3.3

If the intended procedure is discontinued or otherwise not completed, code the procedure to the root operation performed. If a procedure is discontinued before any other root operation is performed, code the root operation Inspection of the body part or anatomical region inspected.

Example: A planned aortic valve replacement procedure is discontinued after the initial thoracotomy and before any incision is made in the heart muscle, when the patient becomes hemodynamically unstable. This procedure is coded as an open Inspection of the mediastinum.

Biopsy procedures
B3.4a

Biopsy procedures are coded using the root operations Excision, Extraction, or Drainage and the qualifier Diagnostic. *Examples:* Fine needle aspiration biopsy of fluid in the lung is coded to the root operation Drainage with the qualifier Diagnostic. Biopsy of bone marrow is coded to the root operation Extraction with the qualifier Diagnostic. Lymph node sampling for biopsy is coded to the root operation Excision with the qualifier Diagnostic.

Biopsy followed by more definitive treatment
B3.4b

If a diagnostic Excision, Extraction, or Drainage procedure (biopsy) is followed by a more definitive procedure, such as Destruction, Excision or Resection at the same procedure site, both the biopsy and the more definitive treatment are coded.

Example: Biopsy of breast followed by partial mastectomy at the same procedure site, both the biopsy and the partial mastectomy procedure are coded.

Overlapping body layers
B3.5

If root operations Excision, Extraction, Repair or Inspection are performed on overlapping layers of the musculoskeletal system, the body part specifying the deepest layer is coded.

Example: Excisional debridement that includes skin and subcutaneous tissue and muscle is coded to the muscle body part.

Bypass procedures
B3.6a

Bypass procedures are coded by identifying the body part bypassed "from" and the body part bypassed "to." The fourth character body part specifies the body part bypassed from, and the qualifier specifies the body part bypassed to.

Example: Bypass from stomach to jejunum, stomach is the body part and jejunum is the qualifier.

B3.6b

Coronary artery bypass procedures are coded differently than other bypass procedures as described in the previous guideline. Rather than identifying the body part bypassed from, the body part identifies the number of coronary artery sites bypassed to, and the qualifier specifies the vessel bypassed from.

Example: Aortocoronary artery bypass of the left anterior descending coronary artery and the obtuse marginal coronary artery is classified in the body part axis of classification as two coronary arteries and the qualifier specifies the aorta as the body part bypassed from.

B3.6c

If multiple coronary arteries are bypassed, a separate procedure is coded for each coronary artery that uses a different device and/or qualifier.

Example: Aortocoronary artery bypass and internal mammary coronary artery bypass are coded separately.

Control vs. more definitive root operations
B3.7

The root operation Control is defined as, "Stopping, or attempting to stop, postprocedural or other acute bleeding." Control is the root operation coded when the procedure performed to achieve hemostasis, beyond what would be considered integral to a procedure, utilizes techniques (e.g. cautery, application of substances or pressure, suturing or ligation or clipping of bleeding points at the site) that are not described by a more specific root operation definition, such as Bypass, Detachment, Excision, Extraction, Reposition, Replacement, or Resection. If a more specific root operation definition applies to the procedure performed, then the more specific root operation is coded instead of Control.

Examples: Silver nitrate cautery to treat acute nasal bleeding is coded to the root operation Control. Liquid embolization of the right internal iliac artery to treat acute hematoma by stopping blood flow is coded to the root operation Occlusion. Suctioning of residual blood to achieve hemostasis during a transbronchial cryobiopsy is considered integral to the cryobiopsy procedure and is not coded separately.

Excision vs. Resection
B3.8

PCS contains specific body parts for anatomical subdivisions of a body part, such as lobes of the lungs or liver and regions of the intestine. Resection of the specific body part is coded whenever all of the body part is cut out or off, rather than coding Excision of a less specific body part.

Example: Left upper lung lobectomy is coded to Resection of Upper Lung Lobe, Left rather than Excision of Lung, Left.

Excision for graft
B3.9

If an autograft is obtained from a different procedure site in order to complete the objective of the procedure, a separate procedure is coded, except when the seventh character qualifier value in the ICD-10-PCS table fully specifies the site from which the autograft was obtained.

Examples: Coronary bypass with excision of saphenous vein graft, excision of saphenous vein is coded separately. Replacement of breast with autologous deep inferior epigastric artery perforator (DIEP) flap, excision of the DIEP flap is not coded separately. The seventh character qualifier value Deep Inferior Epigastric Artery Perforator Flap in the Replacement table fully specifies the site of the autograft harvest.

Fusion procedures of the spine
B3.10a

The body part coded for a spinal vertebral joint(s) rendered immobile by a spinal fusion procedure is classified by the level of the spine (e.g. thoracic). There are distinct body part values for a single vertebral joint and for multiple vertebral joints at each spinal level.

Example: Body part values specify Lumbar Vertebral Joint, Lumbar Vertebral Joints, 2 or More and Lumbosacral Vertebral Joint.

B3.10b

If multiple vertebral joints are fused, a separate procedure is coded for each vertebral joint that uses a different device and/or qualifier.

Example: Fusion of lumbar vertebral joint, posterior approach, anterior column and fusion of lumbar vertebral joint, posterior approach, posterior column are coded separately.

B3.10c

Combinations of devices and materials are often used on a vertebral joint to render the joint immobile. When combinations of devices are used on the same vertebral joint, the device value coded for the procedure is as follows:

- If an interbody fusion device is used to render the joint immobile (containing bone graft or bone graft substitute), the procedure is coded with the device value Interbody Fusion Device
- If bone graft is the *only* device used to render the joint immobile, the procedure is coded with the device value Nonautologous Tissue Substitute or Autologous Tissue Substitute
- If a mixture of autologous and nonautologous bone graft (with or without biological or synthetic extenders or binders) is used to render the joint immobile, code the procedure with the device value Autologous Tissue Substitute

Examples: Fusion of a vertebral joint using a cage style interbody fusion device containing morsellized bone graft is coded to the device Interbody Fusion Device. Fusion of a vertebral joint using a bone dowel interbody fusion device made of cadaver bone and packed with a mixture of local morsellized bone and demineralized bone matrix is coded to the device Interbody Fusion Device. Fusion of a vertebral joint using both autologous bone graft and bone bank bone graft is coded to the device Autologous Tissue Substitute.

Inspection procedures
B3.11a

Inspection of a body part(s) performed in order to achieve the objective of a procedure is not coded separately.

Example: Fiberoptic bronchoscopy performed for irrigation of bronchus, only the irrigation procedure is coded.

B3.11b

If multiple tubular body parts are inspected, the most distal body part (the body part furthest from the starting point of the inspection) is coded. If multiple non-tubular body parts in a region are inspected, the body part that specifies the entire area inspected is coded.

Examples: Cystoureteroscopy with inspection of bladder and ureters is coded to the ureter body part value. Exploratory laparotomy with general inspection of abdominal contents is coded to the peritoneal cavity body part value.

B3.11c

When both an Inspection procedure and another procedure are performed on the same body part during the same episode, if the Inspection procedure is performed using a different approach than the other procedure, the Inspection procedure is coded separately.

Example: Endoscopic Inspection of the duodenum is coded separately when open Excision of the duodenum is performed during the same procedural episode.

Occlusion vs. Restriction for vessel embolization procedures
B3.12

If the objective of an embolization procedure is to completely close a vessel, the root operation Occlusion is coded. If the objective of an embolization procedure is to narrow the lumen of a vessel, the root operation Restriction is coded.

Examples: Tumor embolization is coded to the root operation Occlusion, because the objective of the procedure is to cut off the blood supply to the vessel. Embolization of a cerebral aneurysm is coded to the root operation Restriction, because the objective of the procedure is not to close off the vessel entirely, but to narrow the lumen of the vessel at the site of the aneurysm where it is abnormally wide.

Release procedures
B3.13

In the root operation Release, the body part value coded is the body part being freed and not the tissue being manipulated or cut to free the body part.

Example: Lysis of intestinal adhesions is coded to the specific intestine body part value.

Release vs. Division

B3.14

If the sole objective of the procedure is freeing a body part without cutting the body part, the root operation is Release. If the sole objective of the procedure is separating or transecting a body part, the root operation is Division.

Examples: Freeing a nerve root from surrounding scar tissue to relieve pain is coded to the root operation Release. Severing a nerve root to relieve pain is coded to the root operation Division.

Reposition for fracture treatment

B3.15

Reduction of a displaced fracture is coded to the root operation Reposition and the application of a cast or splint in conjunction with the Reposition procedure is not coded separately. Treatment of a nondisplaced fracture is coded to the procedure performed.

Examples: Casting of a nondisplaced fracture is coded to the root operation Immobilization in the Placement section.

Putting a pin in a nondisplaced fracture is coded to the root operation Insertion.

Transplantation vs. Administration

B3.16

Putting in a mature and functioning living body part taken from another individual or animal is coded to the root operation Transplantation. Putting in autologous or nonautologous cells is coded to the Administration section.

Example: Putting in autologous or nonautologous bone marrow, pancreatic islet cells or stem cells is coded to the Administration section.

Transfer procedures using multiple tissue layers

B3.17

The root operation Transfer contains qualifiers that can be used to specify when a transfer flap is composed of more than one tissue layer, such as a musculocutaneous flap. For procedures involving transfer of multiple tissue layers including skin, subcutaneous tissue, fascia or muscle, the procedure is coded to the body part value that describes the deepest tissue layer in the flap, and the qualifier can be used to describe the other tissue layer(s) in the transfer flap.

Example: A musculocutaneous flap transfer is coded to the appropriate body part value in the body system Muscles, and the qualifier is used to describe the additional tissue layer(s) in the transfer flap.

Excision/Resection followed by replacement

B3.18

If an Excision or Resection of a body part is followed by a Replacement procedure, code both procedures to identify each distinct objective, except when the Excision or Resection is considered integral and preparatory for the Replacement procedure.

Examples: Mastectomy followed by reconstruction, both Resection and Replacement of the breast are coded to fully capture the distinct objectives of the procedures performed. Maxillectomy with obturator reconstruction, both Excision and Replacement of the maxilla are coded to fully capture the distinct objectives of the procedures performed. Excisional debridement of tendon with skin graft, both the Excision of the tendon and the Replacement of the skin with a graft are coded to fully capture the distinct objectives of the procedures performed. Esophagectomy followed by reconstruction with colonic interposition, both the Resection and the Transfer of the large intestine to function as the esophagus are coded to fully capture the distinct objectives of the procedures performed.

Examples: Resection of a joint as part of a joint replacement procedure is considered integral and preparatory for the Replacement of the joint and the Resection is not coded separately. Resection of a valve as part of a valve replacement procedure is considered integral and preparatory for the valve Replacement and the Resection is not coded separately.

Detachment procedures of extremities

B3.19

The root operation Detachment contains qualifiers that can be used to specify the level where the extremity was amputated. These qualifiers are dependent on the body part value in the "upper extremities" and "lower extremities" body systems. For procedures involving detachment of all or part of the upper or lower extremities, the procedure is coded to the body part value that describes the site of the detachment.

Example: An amputation at the proximal portion of the shaft of the tibia and fibula is coded to the Lower leg body part value in the body system Anatomical Regions, Lower Extremities, and the qualifier High is used to specify the level where the extremity was detached.

The following definitions were developed for the Detachment qualifiers.

Body Part	Qualifier	Definition
Upper arm and upper leg	1	High: Amputation at the proximal portion of the shaft of the humerus or femur
	2	Mid: Amputation at the middle portion of the shaft of the humerus or femur
	3	Low: Amputation at the distal portion of the shaft of the humerus or femur
Lower arm and lower leg	1	High: Amputation at the proximal portion of the shaft of the radius/ulna or tibia/fibula
	2	Mid: Amputation at the middle portion of the shaft of the radius/ulna or tibia/fibula
	3	Low: Amputation at the distal portion of the shaft of the radius/ulna or tibia/fibula
Hand and Foot	0	Complete*
	4	Complete 1st Ray
	5	Complete 2nd Ray
	6	Complete 3rd Ray
	7	Complete 4th Ray
	8	Complete 5th Ray
	9	Partial 1st Ray
	B	Partial 2nd Ray
	C	Partial 3rd Ray
	D	Partial 4th Ray
	F	Partial 5th Ray
Thumb, finger, or toe	0	Complete: Amputation at the metacarpophalangeal/metatarsal-phalangeal joint
	1	High: Amputation anywhere along the proximal phalanx
	2	Mid: Amputation through the proximal interphalangeal joint or anywhere along the middle phalanx
	3	Low: Amputation through the distal interphalangeal joint or anywhere along the distal phalanx

*When coding amputation of Hand and Foot, the following definitions are followed:
 -Complete: Amputation through the carpometacarpal joint of the hand, or through the tarsal-metatarsal joint of the foot.
 -Partial: Amputation anywhere along the shaft or head of the metacarpal bone of the hand, or of the metatarsal bone of the foot.

B4. Body Part
General guidelines
B4.1a

If a procedure is performed on a portion of a body part that does not have a separate body part value, code the body part value corresponding to the whole body part.

Example: A procedure performed on the alveolar process of the mandible is coded to the mandible body part.

B4.1b

If the prefix "peri" is combined with a body part to identify the site of the procedure, and the site of the procedure is not further specified, then the procedure is coded to the body part named. This guideline applies only when a more specific body part value is not available.

Examples: A procedure site identified as perirenal is coded to the kidney body part when the site of the procedure is not further specified. A procedure site described in the documentation as peri-urethral, and the documentation also indicates that it is the vulvar tissue and not the urethral tissue that is the site of the procedure, then the procedure is coded to the vulva body part. A procedure site documented as involving the periosteum is coded to the corresponding bone body part.

B4.1c

If a single vascular procedure is performed on a continuous section of an arterial or venous body part, code the body part value corresponding to the anatomically most proximal (closest to the heart) portion of the arterial or venous body part.

Examples: A procedure performed on a continuous section of artery from the femoral artery to the external iliac artery with the point of entry at the femoral artery is coded to the external iliac body part. A procedure performed on a continuous section of artery from the femoral artery to the external iliac artery with the point of entry at the external iliac artery is also coded to the external iliac artery body part.

Branches of body parts
B4.2

Where a specific branch of a body part does not have its own body part value in PCS, the body part is typically coded to the closest proximal branch that has a specific body part value. In the cardiovascular body systems, if a general body part is available in the correct root operation table, and coding to a proximal branch would require assigning a code in a different body system, the procedure is coded using the general body part value.

Examples: A procedure performed on the mandibular branch of the trigeminal nerve is coded to the trigeminal nerve body part value. Occlusion of the bronchial artery is coded to the body part value Upper Artery in the body system Upper Arteries, and not to the body part value Thoracic Aorta, Descending in the body system Heart and Great Vessels.

Bilateral body part values
B4.3

Bilateral body part values are available for a limited number of body parts. If the identical procedure is performed on contralateral body parts, and a bilateral body part value exists for that body part, a single procedure is coded using the bilateral body part value. If no bilateral body part value exists, each procedure is coded separately using the appropriate body part value.

Example: The identical procedure performed on both fallopian tubes is coded once using the body part value Fallopian Tube, Bilateral. The identical procedure performed on both knee joints is coded twice using the body part values Knee Joint, Right and Knee Joint, Left.

Coronary arteries
B4.4

The coronary arteries are classified as a single body part that is further specified by number of arteries treated. One procedure code specifying multiple arteries is used when the same procedure is performed, including the same device and qualifier values.

Examples: Angioplasty of two distinct coronary arteries with placement of two stents is coded as Dilation of Coronary Artery, Two Arteries, with Two Intraluminal Devices. Angioplasty of two distinct coronary arteries, one with stent placed and one without, is coded separately as Dilation of Coronary Artery, One Artery with Intraluminal Device, and Dilation of Coronary Artery, One Artery with no device.

Tendons, ligaments, bursae and fascia near a joint
B4.5

Procedures performed on tendons, ligaments, bursae and fascia supporting a joint are coded to the body part in the respective body system that is the focus of the procedure. Procedures performed on joint structures themselves are coded to the body part in the joint body systems.

Example: Repair of the anterior cruciate ligament of the knee is coded to the knee bursa and ligament body part in the Bursae and Ligaments body system. Knee arthroscopy with shaving of articular cartilage is coded to the knee joint body part in the Lower Joints body system.

Skin, subcutaneous tissue and fascia overlying a joint
B4.6

If a procedure is performed on the skin, subcutaneous tissue or fascia overlying a joint, the procedure is coded to the following body part:

- Shoulder is coded to Upper Arm
- Elbow is coded to Lower Arm
- Wrist is coded to Lower Arm
- Hip is coded to Upper Leg

- Knee is coded to Lower Leg
- Ankle is coded to Foot

Fingers and toes
B4.7

If a body system does not contain a separate body part value for fingers, procedures performed on the fingers are coded to the body part value for the hand. If a body system does not contain a separate body part value for toes, procedures performed on the toes are coded to the body part value for the foot.

Example: Excision of finger muscle is coded to one of the hand muscle body part values in the Muscles body system.

Upper and lower intestinal tract
B4.8

In the Gastrointestinal body system, the general body part values Upper Intestinal Tract and Lower Intestinal Tract are provided as an option for the root operations such as Change, Insertion, Inspection, Removal and Revision. Upper Intestinal Tract includes the portion of the gastrointestinal tract from the esophagus down to and including the duodenum, and Lower Intestinal Tract includes the portion of the gastrointestinal tract from the jejunum down to and including the rectum and anus.

Example: In the root operation Change table, change of a device in the jejunum is coded using the body part Lower Intestinal Tract.

B5. Approach
Open approach with percutaneous endoscopic assistance
B5.2a

Procedures performed using the open approach with percutaneous endoscopic assistance are coded to the approach Open.

Example: Laparoscopic-assisted sigmoidectomy is coded to the approach Open.

Percutaneous endoscopic approach with hand-assistance or extension of incision
B5.2b

Procedures performed using the percutaneous endoscopic approach with hand-assistance, or, with incision or extension of an incision to assist in the removal of all or a portion of a body part, or to anastomose a tubular body part with or without the temporary exteriorization of a body structure, are coded to the approach value Percutaneous Endoscopic.

Examples: Hand-assisted laparoscopic sigmoid colon resection with exteriorization of a segment of the colon for removal of specimen with return of colon back into abdominal cavity is coded to the approach value percutaneous endoscopic. Laparoscopic sigmoid colectomy with extension of stapling port for removal of specimen and direct anastomosis is coded to the approach value Percutaneous Endoscopic. Laparoscopic nephrectomy with midline incision for removing the resected kidney is coded to the approach value Percutaneous Endoscopic. Robotic-assisted laparoscopic prostatectomy with extension of incision for removal of the resected prostate is coded to the approach value Percutaneous Endoscopic.

External approach
B5.3a

Procedures performed within an orifice on structures that are visible without the aid of any instrumentation are coded to the approach External.

Example: Resection of tonsils is coded to the approach External.

B5.3b

Procedures performed indirectly by the application of external force through the intervening body layers are coded to the approach External.

Example: Closed reduction of fracture is coded to the approach External.

Percutaneous procedure via device
B5.4

Procedures performed percutaneously via a device placed for the procedure are coded to the approach Percutaneous.

Example: Fragmentation of kidney stone performed via percutaneous nephrostomy is coded to the approach Percutaneous.

B6. Device
General guidelines
B6.1a

A device is coded only if a device remains after the procedure is completed. If no device remains, the device value No Device is coded. In limited root operations, the classification provides the qualifier values Temporary and Intraoperative, for specific procedures involving clinically significant devices, where the purpose of the device is to be utilized for a brief duration during the procedure or current inpatient stay. If a device that is intended to remain after the procedure is completed requires removal before the end of the operative episode in which it was inserted, both the insertion and removal of the device should be coded.

B6.1b

Materials such as sutures, ligatures, radiological markers and temporary post-operative wound drains are considered integral to the performance of a procedure and are not coded as devices.

B6.1c

Procedures performed on a device only and not on a body part are specified in the root operations Change, Irrigation, Removal and Revision, and are coded to the procedure performed.

Example: Irrigation of percutaneous nephrostomy tube is coded to the root operation Irrigation of indwelling device in the Administration section.

Drainage device
B6.2

A separate procedure to put in a drainage device is coded to the root operation Drainage with the device value Drainage Device.

Obstetric Section Guidelines (section 1)

C. Obstetrics Section
Products of conception
C1

Procedures performed on the products of conception are coded to the Obstetrics section. Procedures performed on the pregnant female other than the products of conception are coded to the appropriate root operation in the Medical and Surgical section.

Example: Amniocentesis is coded to the products of conception body part in the Obstetrics section. Repair of obstetric urethral laceration is coded to the urethra body part in the Medical and Surgical section.

Procedures following delivery or abortion
C2

Procedures performed following a delivery or abortion for curettage of the endometrium or evacuation of retained products of conception are all coded in the Obstetrics section, to the root operation Extraction and the body part Products of Conception, Retained. Diagnostic or therapeutic dilation and curettage performed during times other than the postpartum or post-abortion period are all coded in the Medical and Surgical section, to the root operation Extraction and the body part Endometrium.

Radiation Therapy Section Guidelines (section D)

D. Radiation Therapy Section
Brachytherapy
D1.a

Brachytherapy is coded to the modality Brachytherapy in the Radiation Therapy section. When a radioactive brachytherapy source is left in the body at the end of the procedure, it is coded separately to the root operation Insertion with the device value Radioactive Element.

Example: Brachytherapy with implantation of a low dose rate brachytherapy source left in the body at the end of the procedure is coded to the applicable treatment site in section D, Radiation Therapy, with the modality Brachytherapy, the modality qualifier value, Low Dose Rate, and the applicable isotope value and qualifier value. The implantation of the brachytherapy source is coded separately to the device value Radioactive Element in the appropriate Insertion table of the Medical and Surgical section. The Radiation Therapy section code identifies the specific modality and isotope of the brachytherapy, and the root operation Insertion code identifies the implantation of the brachytherapy source that remain in the body at the end of the procedure.

Exception: Implantation of Cesium-131 brachytherapy seeds embedded in a collagen matrix to the treatment site after resection of brain tumor is coded to the root operation Insertion with the device value Radioactive Element, Cesium-131 Collagen Implant. The procedure is coded to the root operation Insertion only, because the device value identifies both the implantation of the radioactive element and a specific brachytherapy isotope that is not included in the Radiation Therapy section tables.

D1.b

A separate procedure to place a temporary applicator for delivering the brachytherapy is coded to the root operation Insertion and the device value Other Device.

Examples: Intrauterine brachytherapy applicator placed as a separate procedure from the brachytherapy procedure is coded to Insertion of Other Device, and the brachytherapy is coded separately using the modality Brachytherapy in the Radiation Therapy section. Intrauterine brachytherapy applicator placed concomitantly with delivery of the brachytherapy dose is coded with a single code using the modality Brachytherapy in the Radiation Therapy section.

New Technology Section Guidelines (section X)

E. New Technology Section

General guidelines

E1.a

Section X codes fully represent the specific procedure described in the code title, and do not require any additional codes from other sections of ICD-10-PCS. When section X contains a code title which describes a specific new technology procedure, and it is the only procedure performed, only the section X code is reported for the procedure. There is no need to report an additional code in another section of ICD-10-PCS.

Example: XW043A6 Introduction of Cefiderocol Anti-infective into Central Vein, Percutaneous Approach, New Technology Group 6, can be coded to indicate that Cefiderocol Anti-infective was administered via a central vein. A separate code from table 3E0 in the Administration section of ICD-10-PCS is not coded in addition to this code.

E1.b

When multiple procedures are performed, New Technology section X codes are coded following the multiple procedures guideline.

Examples: Dual filter cerebral embolic filtration used during transcatheter aortic valve replacement (TAVR), X2A5312 Cerebral Embolic Filtration, Dual Filter in Innominate Artery and Left Common Carotid Artery, Percutaneous Approach, New Technology Group 2, is coded for the cerebral embolic filtration, along with an ICD-10-PCS code for the TAVR procedure. An extracorporeal flow reversal circuit for embolic neuroprotection placed during a transcarotid arterial revascularization procedure, a code from table X2A, Assistance of the Cardiovascular System is coded for the use of the extracoporeal flow reversal circuit, along with an ICD-10-PCS code for the transcarotid arterial revascularization procedure.

F. Selection of Principal Procedure

The following instructions should be applied in the selection of principal procedure and clarification on the importance of the relation to the principal diagnosis when more than one procedure is performed:

1. Procedure performed for definitive treatment of both principal diagnosis and secondary diagnosis

   a. Sequence procedure performed for definitive treatment most related to principal diagnosis as principal procedure.

2. Procedure performed for definitive treatment and diagnostic procedures performed for both principal diagnosis and secondary diagnosis

   a. Sequence procedure performed for definitive treatment most related to principal diagnosis as principal procedure

3. A diagnostic procedure was performed for the principal diagnosis and a procedure is performed for definitive treatment of a secondary diagnosis.

   a. Sequence diagnostic procedure as principal procedure, since the procedure most related to the principal diagnosis takes precedence.

4. No procedures performed that are related to principal diagnosis; procedures performed for definitive treatment and diagnostic procedures were performed for secondary diagnosis

   a. Sequence procedure performed for definitive treatment of secondary diagnosis as principal procedure, since there are no procedures (definitive or nondefinitive treatment) related to principal diagnosis.

Index

3

3f (Aortic) Bioprosthesis valve
use Zooplastic Tissue in Heart and
Great Vessels

A

Abdominal aortic plexus
use Nerve, Abdominal Sympathetic
Abdominal cavity *use* Peritoneal Cavity
Abdominal esophagus
use Esophagus, Lower
Abdominohysterectomy
see Resection, Uterus 0UT9
Abdominoplasty
see Alteration, Abdominal Wall 0W0F
see Repair, Abdominal Wall 0WQF
see Supplement, Abdominal Wall
0WUF
Abductor hallucis muscle
use Muscle, Foot, Left
use Muscle, Foot, Right
ABECMA®
use Idecabtagene Vicleucel
Immunotherapy
AbioCor® Total Replacement Heart
use Synthetic Substitute
Ablation
see Control bleeding in
see Destruction
Abortion
Abortifacient 10A07ZX
Laminaria 10A07ZW
Products of Conception 10A0
Vacuum 10A07Z6
Abrasion
see Extraction
Absolute Pro Vascular (OTW)
Self-Expanding Stent System
use Intraluminal Device
Accelerate Pheno Test™ BC
XXE5XN6
Accessory cephalic vein
use Vein, Cephalic, Left
use Vein, Cephalic, Right
Accessory obturator nerve
use Nerve, Lumbar Plexus
Accessory phrenic nerve
use Nerve, Phrenic
Accessory spleen
use Spleen
Acculink (RX) Carotid Stent System
use Intraluminal Device
Acellular Hydrated Dermis
use Nonautologous Tissue Substitute
Acetabular cup
use Liner in Lower Joints
Acetabulectomy
see Excision, Lower Bones 0QB
see Resection, Lower Bones 0QT
Acetabulofemoral joint
use Joint, Hip, Left
use Joint, Hip, Right
Acetabuloplasty
see Repair, Lower Bones 0QQ
see Replacement, Lower Bones 0QR
see Supplement, Lower Bones 0QU
Achilles tendon
use Tendon, Lower Leg, Left
use Tendon, Lower Leg, Right
Achillorrhaphy
see Repair, Tendons 0LQ
Achillotenotomy, achillotomy
see Division, Tendons 0L8
see Drainage, Tendons 0L9

Acoustic Pulse Thrombolysis
see Fragmentation, Artery
Acromioclavicular ligament
use Bursa and Ligament, Shoulder,
Left
use Bursa and Ligament, Shoulder,
Right
Acromion (process)
use Scapula, Left
use Scapula, Right
Acromionectomy
see Excision, Upper Joints 0RB
see Resection, Upper Joints 0RT
Acromioplasty
see Repair, Upper Joints 0RQ
see Replacement, Upper Joints
0RR
see Supplement, Upper Joints
0RU
ACTEMRA® *use* Tocilizumab
Activa PC neurostimulator
use Stimulator Generator, Multiple
Array in 0JH
Activa RC neurostimulator
use Stimulator Generator, Multiple
Array Rechargeable in 0JH
Activa SC neurostimulator
use Stimulator Generator, Single
Array in 0JH
Activities of Daily Living Assessment
F02
Activities of Daily Living Treatment
F08
ACUITY™ Steerable Lead
use Cardiac Lead, Defibrillator in 02H
use Cardiac Lead, Pacemaker
in 02H
Acupuncture
Breast
Anesthesia 8E0H300
No Qualifier 8E0H30Z
Integumentary System
Anesthesia 8E0H300
No Qualifier 8E0H30Z
Adductor brevis muscle
use Muscle, Upper Leg, Left
use Muscle, Upper Leg, Right
Adductor hallucis muscle
use Muscle, Foot, Left
use Muscle, Foot, Right
Adductor longus muscle
use Muscle, Upper Leg, Left
use Muscle, Upper Leg, Right
Adductor magnus muscle
use Muscle, Upper Leg, Left
use Muscle, Upper Leg, Right
Adenohypophysis
use Gland, Pituitary
Adenoidectomy
see Excision, Adenoids 0CBQ
see Resection, Adenoids 0CTQ
Adenoidotomy
see Drainage, Adenoids 0C9Q
Adhesiolysis
see Release
Administration
Blood products
see Transfusion
Other substance
see Introduction of substance in
or on
Adrenalectomy
see Excision, Endocrine System 0GB
see Resection, Endocrine System 0GT
Adrenalorrhaphy
see Repair, Endocrine System 0GQ

Adrenalotomy
see Drainage, Endocrine System 0G9
Advancement
see Reposition
see Transfer
Advisa (MRI)
use Pacemaker, Dual Chamber in 0JH
afami-cel *use* Afamitresgene
Autoleucel Immunotherapy
Afamitresgene Autoleucel
Immunotherapy XW0
AFX® Endovascular AAA System
use Intraluminal Device
Aidoc Briefcase for PE (pulmonary
embolism) XXE3X27
AIGISRx Antibacterial Envelope
use Anti-Infective Envelope
Alar ligament of axis
use Bursa and Ligament, Head and
Neck
Alfapump® system
use Other Device
Alfieri Stitch Valvuloplasty
see Restriction, Valve, Mitral 02VG
Alimentation
see Introduction of substance in or on
ALPPS (Associating liver partition
and portal vein ligation)
see Division, Hepatobiliary System
and Pancreas 0F8
see Resection, Hepatobiliary System
and Pancreas 0FT
Alteration
Abdominal Wall 0W0F
Ankle Region
Left 0Y0L
Right 0Y0K
Arm
Lower
Left 0X0F
Right 0X0D
Upper
Left 0X09
Right 0X08
Axilla
Left 0X05
Right 0X04
Back
Lower 0W0L
Upper 0W0K
Breast
Bilateral 0H0V
Left 0H0U
Right 0H0T
Buttock
Left 0Y01
Right 0Y00
Chest Wall 0W08
Ear
Bilateral 0902
Left 0901
Right 0900
Elbow Region
Left 0X0C
Right 0X0B
Extremity
Lower
Left 0Y0B
Right 0Y09
Upper
Left 0X07
Right 0X06
Eyelid
Lower
Left 080R
Right 080Q

Alteration (continued)
Eyelid (continued)
Upper
Left 080P
Right 080N
Face 0W02
Head 0W00
Jaw
Lower 0W05
Upper 0W04
Knee Region
Left 0Y0G
Right 0Y0F
Leg
Lower
Left 0Y0J
Right 0Y0H
Upper
Left 0Y0D
Right 0Y0C
Lip
Lower 0C01X
Upper 0C00X
Nasal Mucosa and Soft Tissue 090K
Neck 0W06
Perineum
Female 0W0N
Male 0W0M
Shoulder Region
Left 0X03
Right 0X02
Subcutaneous Tissue and Fascia
Abdomen 0J08
Back 0J07
Buttock 0J09
Chest 0J06
Face 0J01
Lower Arm
Left 0J0H
Right 0J0G
Lower Leg
Left 0J0P
Right 0J0N
Neck
Left 0J05
Right 0J04
Upper Arm
Left 0J0F
Right 0J0D
Upper Leg
Left 0J0M
Right 0J0L
Wrist Region
Left 0X0H
Right 0X0G
Alveolar process of mandible
use Mandible
Alveolar process of maxilla
use Maxilla
Alveolectomy
see Excision, Head and Facial
Bones 0NB
see Resection, Head and Facial
Bones 0NT
Alveoloplasty
see Repair, Head and Facial Bones
0NQ
see Replacement, Head and Facial
Bones 0NR
see Supplement, Head and Facial
Bones 0NU
Alveolotomy
see Division, Head and Facial
Bones 0N8
see Drainage, Head and Facial
Bones 0N9

3f (Aortic) Bioprosthesis valve–Alveolotomy

1

Ambulatory cardiac monitoring
4A12X45
Amivantamab Monoclonal Antibody
XW0
Amniocentesis
see Drainage, Products of
Conception 10Q0
Amnioinfusion
see Introduction of substance in or
on, Products of Conception 3E0E
Amnioscopy 10J08ZZ
Amniotomy
see Drainage, Products of
Conception 10Q0
AMPLATZER® Muscular VSD
Occluder
use Synthetic Substitute
Amputation
see Detachment
AMS 800® Urinary Control System
use Artificial Sphincter in Urinary
System
Anacaulase-bcdb XW0
Anal orifice
use Anus
Analog radiography
see Plain Radiography
Anastomosis
see Bypass
Anatomical snuffbox
use Muscle, Lower Arm and Wrist,
Left
use Muscle, Lower Arm and Wrist,
Right
Andexanet Alfa, Factor Xa Inhibitor
Reversal Agent
use Coagulation Factor Xa,
Inactivated
Andexxa
use Coagulation Factor Xa,
Inactivated
AneuRx® AAA Advantage®
use Intraluminal Device
Angiectomy
see Excision, Heart and Great
Vessels 02B
see Excision, Upper Arteries 03B
see Excision, Lower Arteries 04B
see Excision, Upper Veins 05B
see Excision, Lower Veins 06B
Angiocardiography
Combined right and left heart
see Fluoroscopy, Heart, Right and
Left B216
Left Heart
see Fluoroscopy, Heart, Left B215
Right Heart
see Fluoroscopy, Heart, Right B214
SPY system intravascular
fluorescence
see Monitoring, Physiological
Systems 4A1
Angiography
see Computerized Tomography (CT
Scan), Artery
see Fluoroscopy, Artery
see Magnetic Resonance Imaging
(MRI), Artery
see Plain Radiography, Artery
Angioplasty
see Dilation, Heart and Great
Vessels 027
see Repair, Heart and Great Vessels
02Q
see Replacement, Heart and Great
Vessels 02R
see Dilation, Upper Arteries 037
see Repair, Upper Arteries 03Q
see Replacement, Upper Arteries 03R
see Dilation, Lower Arteries 047
see Repair, Lower Arteries 04Q
see Replacement, Lower Arteries 04R

Angioplasty *(continued)*
see Supplement, Heart and Great
Vessels 02U
see Supplement, Upper Arteries 03U
see Supplement, Lower Arteries 04U
Angiorrhaphy
see Repair, Heart and Great Vessels
02Q
see Repair, Upper Arteries 03Q
see Repair, Lower Arteries 04Q
Angioscopy
02JY4ZZ
03JY4ZZ
04JY4ZZ
Angiotensin II
use Vasopressor
Angiotripsy
see Occlusion, Upper Arteries 03L
see Occlusion, Lower Arteries 04L
Angular artery
use Artery, Face
Angular vein
use Vein, Face, Left
use Vein, Face, Right
Ankle Truss System™ (ATS)
use Internal Fixation Device,
Open-truss Design in New
Technology
Annular ligament
use Bursa and Ligament, Elbow, Left
use Bursa and Ligament, Elbow, Right
Annuloplasty
see Repair, Heart and Great Vessels
02Q
see Supplement, Heart and Great
Vessels 02U
Annuloplasty ring
use Synthetic Substitute
Anoplasty
see Repair, Anus 0DQQ
see Supplement, Anus 0DUQ
Anorectal junction
use Rectum
Anoscopy 0DJD8ZZ
Ansa cervicalis
use Nerve, Cervical Plexus
Antabuse therapy HZ93ZZZ
Antebrachial fascia
use Subcutaneous Tissue and Fascia,
Lower Arm, Left
use Subcutaneous Tissue and Fascia,
Lower Arm, Right
Anterior (pectoral) lymph node
use Lymphatic, Axillary, Left
use Lymphatic, Axillary, Right
Anterior cerebral artery
use Artery, Intracranial
Anterior cerebral vein
use Vein, Intracranial
Anterior choroidal artery
use Artery, Intracranial
Anterior circumflex humeral artery
use Artery, Axillary, Left
use Artery, Axillary, Right
Anterior communicating artery
use Artery, Intracranial
Anterior cruciate ligament (ACL)
use Bursa and Ligament, Knee, Left
use Bursa and Ligament, Knee, Right
Anterior crural nerve
use Nerve, Femoral
Anterior facial vein
use Vein, Face, Left
use Vein, Face, Right
Anterior intercostal artery
use Artery, Internal Mammary, Left
use Artery, Internal Mammary, Right
Anterior interosseous nerve
use Nerve, Median
Anterior lateral malleolar artery
use Artery, Anterior Tibial, Left
use Artery, Anterior Tibial, Right

Anterior lingual gland
use Gland, Minor Salivary
Anterior medial malleolar artery
use Artery, Anterior Tibial, Left
use Artery, Anterior Tibial, Right
Anterior spinal artery
use Artery, Vertebral, Left
use Artery, Vertebral, Right
Anterior tibial recurrent artery
use Artery, Anterior Tibial, Left
use Artery, Anterior Tibial, Right
Anterior ulnar recurrent artery
use Artery, Ulnar, Left
use Artery, Ulnar, Right
Anterior vagal trunk
use Nerve, Vagus
Anterior vertebral muscle
use Muscle, Neck, Left
use Muscle, Neck, Right
Anti-SARS-CoV-2 hyperimmune
globulin
use Hyperimmune Globulin
Antibacterial Envelope (TYRX)
(AIGISRx)
use Anti-Infective Envelope
Antibiotic-eluting Bone Void Filler
XW0V0P7
Antigen-free air conditioning
see Atmospheric Control,
Physiological Systems 6A0
Antihelix
use Ear, External, Bilateral
use Ear, External, Left
use Ear, External, Right
Antimicrobial envelope
use Anti-Infective Envelope
Antitragus
use Ear, External, Bilateral
use Ear, External, Left
use Ear, External, Right
Antrostomy
see Drainage, Ear, Nose, Sinus 099
Antrotomy
see Drainage, Ear, Nose, Sinus 099
Antrum of Highmore
use Sinus, Maxillary, Left
use Sinus, Maxillary, Right
Aortic annulus
use Valve, Aortic
Aortic arch
use Thoracic Aorta, Ascending/Arch
Aortic intercostal artery
use Upper Artery
Aortix™ System *use* Short-term
External Heart Assist System in
Heart and Great Vessels
Aortography
see Plain Radiography, Upper
Arteries B30
see Fluoroscopy, Upper Arteries B31
see Plain Radiography, Lower
Arteries B40
see Fluoroscopy, Lower Arteries
B41
Aortoplasty
see Repair, Aorta, Thoracic,
Descending 02QW
see Repair, Aorta, Thoracic,
Ascending/Arch 02QX
see Replacement, Aorta, Thoracic,
Descending 02RW
see Replacement, Aorta, Thoracic,
Ascending/Arch 02RX
see Supplement, Aorta, Thoracic,
Descending 02UW
see Supplement, Aorta, Thoracic,
Ascending/Arch 02UX
see Repair, Aorta, Abdominal 04Q0
see Replacement, Aorta,
Abdominal 04R0
see Supplement, Aorta, Abdominal
04U0

Apalutamide Antineoplastic
XW0DXJ5
Apical (subclavicular) lymph node
use Lymphatic, Axillary, Left
use Lymphatic, Axillary, Right
ApiFix® Minimally Invasive
Deformity Correction (MID-C)
System
use Posterior (Dynamic)
Distraction Device in New
Technology
Apneustic center *use* Pons
Appendectomy
see Excision, Appendix 0DBJ
see Resection, Appendix 0DTJ
Appendiceal orifice *use* Appendix
Appendicolysis
see Release, Appendix 0DNJ
Appendicotomy
see Drainage, Appendix 0D9J
Application
see Introduction of substance in
or on
aprevo™
use Interbody Fusion Device,
Custom-Made Anatomically
Designed in New Technology
Aquablation therapy, prostate
0V508ZZ
Aquapheresis 6A550Z3
Aqueduct of Sylvius
use Cerebral Ventricle
Aqueous humour
use Anterior Chamber, Left
use Anterior Chamber, Right
Arachnoid mater, intracranial
use Cerebral Meninges
Arachnoid mater, spinal
use Spinal Meninges
Arcuate artery
use Artery, Foot, Left
use Artery, Foot, Right
Areola
use Nipple, Left
use Nipple, Right
AROM (artificial rupture of
membranes) 10907ZC
Arterial canal (duct)
use Artery, Pulmonary, Left
Arterial pulse tracing
see Measurement, Arterial 4A03
Arteriectomy
see Excision, Heart and Great
Vessels 02B
see Excision, Upper Arteries 03B
see Excision, Lower Arteries 04B
Arteriography
see Plain Radiography, Heart B20
see Fluoroscopy, Heart B21
see Plain Radiography, Upper
Arteries B30
see Fluoroscopy, Upper Arteries B31
see Plain Radiography, Lower
Arteries B40
see Fluoroscopy, Lower Arteries B41
Arterioplasty
see Repair, Heart and Great Vessels
02Q
see Replacement, Heart and Great
Vessels 02R
see Repair, Upper Arteries 03Q
see Replacement, Upper Arteries
03R
see Repair, Lower Arteries 04Q
see Replacement, Lower Arteries
04R
see Supplement, Upper Arteries
03U
see Supplement, Lower Arteries
04U
see Supplement, Heart and Great
Vessels 02U

Arteriorrhaphy
see Repair, Heart and Great Vessels 02Q
see Repair, Upper Arteries 03Q
see Repair, Lower Arteries 04Q
Arterioscopy
see Inspection, Artery, Lower 04JY
see Inspection, Artery, Upper 03JY
see Inspection, Great Vessel 02JY
Arteriovenous Fistula, Extraluminal Support Device, Supplement X2U
Arthrectomy
see Excision, Upper Joints 0RB
see Resection, Upper Joints 0RT
see Excision, Lower Joints 0SB
see Resection, Lower Joints 0ST
Arthrocentesis
see Drainage, Upper Joints 0R9
see Drainage, Lower Joints 0S9
Arthrodesis
see Fusion, Upper Joints 0RG
see Fusion, Lower Joints 0SG
Arthrography
see Plain Radiography, Skull and Facial Bones BN0
see Plain Radiography, Non-Axial Upper Bones BP0
see Plain Radiography, Non-Axial Lower Bones BQ0
Arthrolysis
see Release, Upper Joints 0RN
see Release, Lower Joints 0SN
Arthropexy
see Repair, Upper Joints 0RQ
see Reposition, Upper Joints 0RS
see Repair, Lower Joints 0SQ
see Reposition, Lower Joints 0SS
Arthroplasty
see Repair, Upper Joints 0RQ
see Replacement, Upper Joints 0RR
see Repair, Lower Joints 0SQ
see Replacement, Lower Joints 0SR
see Supplement, Lower Joints 0SU
see Supplement, Upper Joints 0RU
Arthroplasty, radial head
see Replacement, Radius, Left 0PRJ
see Replacement, Radius, Right 0PRH
Arthroscopy
see Inspection, Upper Joints 0RJ
see Inspection, Lower Joints 0SJ
Arthrotomy
see Drainage, Upper Joints 0R9
see Drainage, Lower Joints 0S9
Articulating Spacer (Antibiotic)
use Articulating Spacer in Lower Joints
Artificial anal sphincter (AAS)
use Artificial Sphincter in Gastrointestinal System
Artificial bowel sphincter (neosphincter)
use Artificial Sphincter in Gastrointestinal System
Artificial Sphincter
Insertion of device in
Anus 0DHQ
Bladder 0THB
Bladder Neck 0THC
Urethra 0THD
Removal of device from
Anus 0DPQ
Bladder 0TPB
Urethra 0TPD
Revision of device in
Anus 0DWQ
Bladder 0TWB
Urethra 0TWD
Artificial urinary sphincter (AUS)
use Artificial Sphincter in Urinary System

Aryepiglottic fold
use Larynx
Arytenoid cartilage
use Larynx
Arytenoid muscle
use Muscle, Neck, Left
use Muscle, Neck, Right
Arytenoidectomy
see Excision, Larynx 0CBS
Arytenoidopexy
see Repair, Larynx 0CQS
Ascenda Intrathecal Catheter
use Infusion Device
Ascending aorta
use Thoracic Aorta, Ascending/Arch
Ascending palatine artery
use Artery, Face
Ascending pharyngeal artery
use Artery, External Carotid, Left
use Artery, External Carotid, Right
aScope™ Duodeno
see New Technology, Hepatobiliary System and Pancreas XFJ
Aspiration, fine needle
Fluid or gas
see Drainage
Tissue biopsy
see Excision
see Extraction
Assessment
Activities of daily living
see Activities of Daily Living Assessment, Rehabilitation F02
Hearing
see Hearing Assessment, Diagnostic Audiology F13
Hearing aid
see Hearing Aid Assessment, Diagnostic Audiology F14
Intravascular perfusion, using indocyanine green (ICG) dye
see Monitoring, Physiological Systems 4A1
Motor function
see Motor Function Assessment, Rehabilitation F01
Nerve function
see Motor Function Assessment, Rehabilitation F01
Speech
see Speech Assessment, Rehabilitation F00
Vestibular
see Vestibular Assessment, Diagnostic Audiology F15
Vocational
see Activities of Daily Living Treatment, Rehabilitation F08
Assistance
Cardiac
Continuous
Output
Balloon Pump 5A02210
Impeller Pump 5A0221D
Other Pump 5A02216
Pulsatile Compression 5A02215
Oxygenation, Supersaturated 5A0222C
Intermittent
Balloon Pump 5A02110
Impeller Pump 5A0211D
Other Pump 5A02116
Circulatory
Continuous, Oxygenation, Hyperbaric 5A05221
Intermittent, Oxygenation, Hyperbaric 5A05121
Respiratory
8-24 Consecutive Hours, Ventilation, Intubated Prone Positioning 5A09C5K

Assistance *(continued)*
Respiratory *(continued)*
24-96 Consecutive Hours
Continuous Negative Airway Pressure 5A09459
Continuous Positive Airway Pressure 5A09457
High Nasal Flow/Velocity 5A0945A
Intermittent Negative Airway Pressure 5A0945B
Intermittent Positive Airway Pressure 5A09458
No Qualifier 5A0945Z
Continuous, Filtration 5A0920Z
Greater than 24 Consecutive Hours, Ventilation, Intubated Prone Positioning 5A09D5K
Greater than 96 Consecutive Hours
Continuous Negative Airway Pressure 5A09559
Continuous Positive Airway Pressure 5A09557
High Nasal Flow/Velocity 5A0955A
Intermittent Negative Airway Pressure 5A0955B
Intermittent Positive Airway Pressure 5A09558
No Qualifier 5A0955Z
Less than 8 Consecutive Hours, Ventilation, Intubated Prone Positioning 5A09B5K
Less than 24 Consecutive Hours
Continuous Negative Airway Pressure 5A09359
Continuous Positive Airway Pressure 5A09357
High Nasal Flow/Velocity 5A0935A
Intermittent Negative Airway Pressure 5A0935B
Intermittent Positive Airway Pressure 5A09358
No Qualifier 5A0935Z
Associating liver partition and portal vein ligation (ALPPS)
see Division, Hepatobiliary System and Pancreas 0F8
see Resection, Hepatobiliary System and Pancreas 0FT
Assurant (Cobalt) stent
use Intraluminal Device
Atezolizumab Antineoplastic XW0
Atherectomy
see Extirpation, Heart and Great Vessels 02C
see Extirpation, Upper Arteries 03C
see Extirpation, Lower Arteries 04C
Atlantoaxial joint
use Joint, Cervical Vertebral
Atmospheric Control 6A0Z
AtriClip LAA Exclusion System
use Extraluminal Device
Atrioseptoplasty
see Repair, Heart and Great Vessels 02Q
see Replacement, Heart and Great Vessels 02R
see Supplement, Heart and Great Vessels 02U
Atrioventricular node
use Conduction Mechanism
Atrium dextrum cordis
use Atrium, Right
Atrium pulmonale
use Atrium, Left
Attain Ability® lead
use Cardiac Lead, Pacemaker in 02H
use Cardiac Lead, Defibrillator in 02H

Attain StarFix® (OTW) lead
use Cardiac Lead, Defibrillator in 02H
use Cardiac Lead, Pacemaker in 02H
Audiology, diagnostic
see Hearing Assessment, Diagnostic Audiology F13
see Hearing Aid Assessment, Diagnostic Audiology F14
see Vestibular Assessment, Diagnostic Audiology F15
Audiometry
see Hearing Assessment, Diagnostic Audiology F13
Auditory tube
use Eustachian Tube, Left
use Eustachian Tube, Right
Auerbach's (myenteric) plexus
use Nerve, Abdominal Sympathetic
Auricle
use Ear, External, Bilateral
use Ear, External, Left
use Ear, External, Right
Auricularis muscle
use Muscle, Head
Autograft
use Autologous Tissue Substitute
AutoLITT® System *see* Destruction
Autologous artery graft
use Autologous Arterial Tissue in Heart and Great Vessels
use Autologous Arterial Tissue in Lower Arteries
use Autologous Arterial Tissue in Lower Veins
use Autologous Arterial Tissue in Upper Arteries
use Autologous Arterial Tissue in Upper Veins
Autologous vein graft
use Autologous Venous Tissue in Heart and Great Vessels
use Autologous Venous Tissue in Lower Arteries
use Autologous Venous Tissue in Lower Veins
use Autologous Venous Tissue in Upper Arteries
use Autologous Venous Tissue in Upper Veins
Automated Chest Compression (ACC) 5A1221J
AutoPulse® Resuscitation System 5A1221J
Autotransfusion
see Transfusion
Autotransplant
Adrenal tissue
see Reposition, Endocrine System 0GS
Kidney
see Reposition, Urinary System 0TS
Pancreatic tissue
see Reposition, Pancreas 0FSG
Parathyroid tissue
see Reposition, Endocrine System 0GS
Thyroid tissue
see Reposition, Endocrine System 0GS
Tooth
see Reattachment, Mouth and Throat 0CM
Aveir™ AR, as dual chamber
use Intracardiac Pacemaker, Dual-Chamber in New Technology
Aveir™ DR, as dual chamber
use Intracardiac Pacemaker, Dual-Chamber in New Technology
Aveir™ VR, as single chamber
use Intracardiac Pacemaker in Heart and Great Vessels

Avulsion
see Extraction
AVYCAZ® (ceftazidime-avibactam)
use Other Anti-infective
Axial Lumbar Interbody Fusion System
use Interbody Fusion Device in Lower Joints
AxiaLIF® System
use Interbody Fusion Device in Lower Joints
Axicabtagene Ciloeucel
use Axicabtagene Ciloleucel Immunotherapy
Axicabtagene Ciloleucel Immunotherapy XW0
Axillary fascia
use Subcutaneous Tissue and Fascia, Upper Arm, Left
use Subcutaneous Tissue and Fascia, Upper Arm, Right
Axillary nerve
use Nerve, Brachial Plexus
AZEDRA®
use Iobenguane I-131 Antineoplastic

B

BAK/C® Interbody Cervical Fusion System
use Interbody Fusion Device in Upper Joints
BAL (bronchial alveolar lavage), diagnostic
see Drainage, Respiratory System 0B9
Balanoplasty
see Repair, Penis 0VQS
see Supplement, Penis 0VUS
Balloon atrial septostomy (BAS) 02163Z7
Balloon Pump
Continuous, Output 5A02210
Intermittent, Output 5A02110
Bandage, Elastic
see Compression
Banding
see Occlusion
see Restriction
Banding, esophageal varices
see Occlusion, Vein, Esophageal 06L3
Banding, laparoscopic (adjustable) gastric
Initial procedure 0DV64CZ
Surgical correction
see Revision of device in, Stomach 0DW6
Bard® Composix® (E/X)(LP) mesh
use Synthetic Substitute
Bard® Composix® Kugel® patch
use Synthetic Substitute
Bard® Dulex™ mesh
use Synthetic Substitute
Bard® Ventralex™ hernia patch
use Synthetic Substitute
Barium swallow
see Fluoroscopy, Gastrointestinal System BD1
Baroreflex Activation Therapy® (BAT®)
Stimulator Generator in Subcutaneous Tissue and Fascia
use Stimulator Lead in Upper Arteries
Barricaid® Annular Closure Device (ACD)
use Synthetic Substitute
Bartholin's (greater vestibular) gland
use Gland, Vestibular
Basal (internal) cerebral vein
use Vein, Intracranial

Basal metabolic rate (BMR)
see Measurement, Physiological Systems 4A0Z
Basal nuclei
use Basal Ganglia
Base of Tongue
use Pharynx
Basilar artery
use Artery, Intracranial
Basis pontis
use Pons
Beam Radiation
Abdomen DW03
Intraoperative DW033Z0
Adrenal Gland DG02
Intraoperative DG023Z0
Bile Ducts DF02
Intraoperative DF023Z0
Bladder DT02
Intraoperative DT023Z0
Bone
Intraoperative DP0C3Z0
Other DP0C
Bone Marrow D700
Intraoperative D7003Z0
Brain D000
Intraoperative D0003Z0
Brain Stem D001
Intraoperative D0013Z0
Breast
Left DM00
Intraoperative DM003Z0
Right DM01
Intraoperative DM013Z0
Bronchus DB01
Intraoperative DB013Z0
Cervix DU01
Intraoperative DU013Z0
Chest DW02
Intraoperative DW023Z0
Chest Wall DB07
Intraoperative DB073Z0
Colon DD05
Intraoperative DD053Z0
Diaphragm DB08
Intraoperative DB083Z0
Duodenum DD02
Intraoperative DD023Z0
Ear D900
Intraoperative D9003Z0
Esophagus DD00
Intraoperative DD003Z0
Eye D800
Intraoperative D8003Z0
Femur DP09
Intraoperative DP093Z0
Fibula DP0B
Intraoperative DP0B3Z0
Gallbladder DF01
Intraoperative DF013Z0
Gland
Adrenal DG02
Intraoperative DG023Z0
Parathyroid DG04
Intraoperative DG043Z0
Pituitary DG00
Intraoperative DG003Z0
Thyroid DG05
Intraoperative DG053Z0
Glands
Intraoperative D9063Z0
Salivary D906
Head and Neck DW01
Intraoperative DW013Z0
Hemibody DW04
Intraoperative DW043Z0
Humerus DP06
Intraoperative DP063Z0
Hypopharynx D903
Intraoperative D9033Z0
Ileum DD04
Intraoperative DD043Z0

Beam Radiation (continued)
Jejunum DD03
Intraoperative DD033Z0
Kidney DT00
Intraoperative DT003Z0
Larynx D90B
Intraoperative D90B3Z0
Liver DF00
Intraoperative DF003Z0
Lung DB02
Intraoperative DB023Z0
Lymphatics
Abdomen D706
Intraoperative D7063Z0
Axillary D704
Intraoperative D7043Z0
Inguinal D708
Intraoperative D7083Z0
Neck D703
Intraoperative D7033Z0
Pelvis D707
Intraoperative D7073Z0
Thorax D705
Intraoperative D7053Z0
Mandible DP03
Intraoperative DP033Z0
Maxilla DP02
Intraoperative DP023Z0
Mediastinum DB06
Intraoperative DB063Z0
Mouth D904
Intraoperative D9043Z0
Nasopharynx D90D
Intraoperative D90D3Z0
Neck and Head DW01
Intraoperative DW013Z0
Nerve
Intraoperative D0073Z0
Peripheral D007
Nose D901
Intraoperative D9013Z0
Oropharynx D90F
Intraoperative D90F3Z0
Ovary DU00
Intraoperative DU003Z0
Palate
Hard D908
Intraoperative D9083Z0
Soft D909
Intraoperative D9093Z0
Pancreas DF03
Intraoperative DF033Z0
Parathyroid Gland DG04
Intraoperative DG043Z0
Pelvic Bones DP08
Intraoperative DP083Z0
Pelvic Region DW06
Intraoperative DW063Z0
Pineal Body DG01
Intraoperative DG013Z0
Pituitary Gland DG00
Intraoperative DG003Z0
Pleura DB05
Intraoperative DB053Z0
Prostate DV00
Intraoperative DV003Z0
Radius DP07
Intraoperative DP073Z0
Rectum DD07
Intraoperative DD073Z0
Rib DP05
Intraoperative DP053Z0
Sinuses D907
Intraoperative D9073Z0
Skin
Abdomen DH08
Intraoperative DH083Z0
Arm DH04
Intraoperative DH043Z0
Back DH07
Intraoperative DH073Z0
Buttock DH09
Intraoperative DH093Z0

Beam Radiation (continued)
Skin (continued)
Chest DH06
Intraoperative DH063Z0
Face DH02
Intraoperative DH023Z0
Leg DH0B
Intraoperative DH0B3Z0
Neck DH03
Intraoperative DH033Z0
Skull DP00
Intraoperative DP003Z0
Spinal Cord D006
Intraoperative D0063Z0
Spleen D702
Intraoperative D7023Z0
Sternum DP04
Intraoperative DP043Z0
Stomach DD01
Intraoperative DD013Z0
Testis DV01
Intraoperative DV013Z0
Thymus D701
Intraoperative D7013Z0
Thyroid Gland DG05
Intraoperative DG053Z0
Tibia DP0B
Intraoperative DP0B3Z0
Tongue D905
Intraoperative D9053Z0
Trachea DB00
Intraoperative DB003Z0
Ulna DP07
Intraoperative DP073Z0
Ureter DT01
Intraoperative DT013Z0
Urethra DT03
Intraoperative DT033Z0
Uterus DU02
Intraoperative DU023Z0
Whole Body DW05
Intraoperative DW053Z0
Bedside swallow F00ZJWZ
Berlin Heart Ventricular Assist Device
use Implantable Heart Assist System in Heart and Great Vessels
beti-cel use Betibeglogene Autotemcel
Betibeglogene Autotemcel XW1
Bezlotoxumab Infusion see Introduction with qualifier Other Therapeutic Monoclonal Antibody
Biceps brachii muscle
use Muscle, Upper Arm, Left
use Muscle, Upper Arm, Right
Biceps femoris muscle
use Muscle, Upper Leg, Left
use Muscle, Upper Leg, Right
Bicipital aponeurosis
use Subcutaneous Tissue and Fascia, Lower Arm, Left
use Subcutaneous Tissue and Fascia, Lower Arm, Right
Bicuspid valve
use Valve, Mitral
Bili light therapy
see Phototherapy, Skin 6A60
Bioactive embolization coil(s)
use Intraluminal Device, Bioactive in Upper Arteries
Bioengineered Allogeneic Construct, Skin XHRPXF7
Biofeedback GZC9ZZZ
BioFire® FilmArray® Pneumonia Panel XXEBXQ6
Biopsy
see Drainage with qualifier Diagnostic
see Excision with qualifier Diagnostic
see Extraction with qualifier Diagnostic
BiPAP
see Assistance, Respiratory v5A09

Bisection
see Division
Biventricular external heart assist system
use Short-term External Heart Assist System in Heart and Great Vessels
Blepharectomy
see Excision, Eye 08B
see Resection, Eye 08T
Blepharoplasty
see Repair, Eye 08Q
see Replacement, Eye 08R
see Reposition, Eye 08S
see Supplement, Eye 08U
Blepharorrhaphy
see Repair, Eye 08Q
Blepharotomy
see Drainage, Eye 089
Blinatumomab
use Other Antineoplastic
BLINCYTO® (blinatumomab)
use Other Antineoplastic
Block, Nerve, anesthetic injection 3E0T3BZ
Blood glucose monitoring system
use Monitoring Device
Blood pressure
see Measurement, Arterial 4A03
BMR (basal metabolic rate)
see Measurement, Physiological Systems 4A0Z
Body of femur
use Femoral Shaft, Left
use Femoral Shaft, Right
Body of fibula
use Fibula, Left
use Fibula, Right
Bone anchored hearing device
use Hearing Device, Bone Conduction in 09H
use Hearing Device in Head and Facial Bones
Bone bank bone graft
use Nonautologous Tissue Substitute
Bone Growth Stimulator
Insertion of device in
Bone
Facial 0NHW
Lower 0QHY
Nasal 0NHB
Upper 0PHY
Skull 0NH0
Removal of device from
Bone
Facial 0NPW
Lower 0QPY
Nasal 0NPB
Upper 0PPY
Skull 0NP0
Revision of device in
Bone
Facial 0NWW
Lower 0QWY
Nasal 0NWB
Upper 0PWY
Skull 0NW0
Bone marrow transplant
see Transfusion, Circulatory 302
Bone morphogenetic protein 2 (BMP 2)
use Recombinant Bone Morphogenetic Protein
Bone screw (interlocking)(lag) (pedicle)(recessed)
use Internal Fixation Device in Head and Facial Bones
use Internal Fixation Device in Lower Bones
use Internal Fixation Device in Upper Bones

Bony labyrinth
use Ear, Inner, Left
use Ear, Inner, Right
Bony orbit
use Orbit, Left
use Orbit, Right
Bony vestibule
use Ear, Inner, Left
use Ear, Inner, Right
Botallo's duct
use Artery, Pulmonary, Left
Bovine pericardial valve
use Zooplastic Tissue in Heart and Great Vessels
Bovine pericardium graft
use Zooplastic Tissue in Heart and Great Vessels
BP (blood pressure)
see Measurement, Arterial 4A03
Brachial (lateral) lymph node
use Lymphatic, Axillary, Left
use Lymphatic, Axillary, Right
Brachialis muscle
use Muscle, Upper Arm, Left
use Muscle, Upper Arm, Right
Brachiocephalic artery
use Artery, Innominate
Brachiocephalic trunk
use Artery, Innominate
Brachiocephalic vein
use Vein, Innominate, Left
use Vein, Innominate, Right
Brachioradialis muscle
use Muscle, Lower Arm and Wrist, Left
use Muscle, Lower Arm and Wrist, Right
Brachytherapy
Abdomen DW13
Adrenal Gland DG12
Back
Lower DW1L
Upper DW1K
Bile Ducts DF12
Bladder DT12
Bone Marrow D710
Brain D010
Brain Stem D011
Breast
Left DM10
Right DM11
Bronchus DB11
Cervix DU11
Chest DW12
Chest Wall DB17
Colon DD15
Cranial Cavity DW10
Diaphragm DB18
Duodenum DD12
Ear D910
Esophagus DD10
Extremity
Lower DW1Y
Upper DW1X
Eye D810
Gastrointestinal Tract DW1P
Gallbladder DF11
Genitourinary Tract DW1R
Gland
Adrenal DG12
Parathyroid DG14
Pituitary DG10
Thyroid DG15
Glands, Salivary D916
Head and Neck DW11
Hypopharynx D913
Ileum DD14
Jejunum DD13
Kidney DT10
Larynx D91B
Liver DF10
Lung DB12

Brachytherapy *(continued)*
Lymphatics
Abdomen D716
Axillary D714
Inguinal D718
Neck D713
Pelvis D717
Thorax D715
Mediastinum DB16
Mouth D914
Nasopharynx D91D
Neck and Head DW11
Nerve, Peripheral D017
Nose D911
Oropharynx D91F
Ovary DU10
Palate
Hard D918
Soft D919
Pancreas DF13
Parathyroid Gland DG14
Pelvic Region DW16
Pineal Body DG11
Pituitary Gland DG10
Pleura DB15
Prostate DV10
Rectum DD17
Respiratory Tract DW1Q
Sinuses D917
Spinal Cord D016
Spleen D712
Stomach DD11
Testis DV11
Thymus D711
Thyroid Gland DG15
Tongue D915
Trachea DB10
Ureter DT11
Urethra DT13
Uterus DU12
Brachytherapy, CivaSheet®
see Brachytherapy with qualifier Unidirectional Source
see Insertion with device Radioactive Element
Brachytherapy seeds
use Radioactive Element
Brain Electrical Activity
Computer-aided Detection and Notification XX20X89
Computer-aided Semiologic Analysis XXE0X48
Breast procedures, skin only
use Skin, Chest
Brexanolone XW0
Brexucabtagene Autoleucel
use Brexucabtagene Autoleucel Immunotherapy
Brexucabtagene Autoleucel Immunotherapy XW0
Breyanzi® *use* Lisocabtagene Maraleucel Immunotherapy
Broad Consortium Microbiota-based Live Biotherapeutic Suspension XW0H7X8
Broad ligament
use Uterine Supporting Structure
Bromelain-enriched Proteolytic Enzyme *use* Anacaulase-bcdb
Bronchial artery
use Upper Artery
Bronchography
see Fluoroscopy, Respiratory System BB1
see Plain Radiography, Respiratory System BB0
Bronchoplasty
see Repair, Respiratory System 0BQ
see Supplement, Respiratory System 0BU
Bronchorrhaphy
see Repair, Respiratory System 0BQ

Bronchoscopy 0BJ08ZZ
Bronchotomy
see Drainage, Respiratory System 0B9
Bronchus Intermedius
use Main Bronchus, Right
BRYAN® Cervical Disc System
use Synthetic Substitute
Buccal gland
use Buccal Mucosa
Buccinator lymph node
use Lymphatic, Head
Buccinator muscle
use Muscle, Facial
Buckling, scleral with implant
see Supplement, Eye 08U
Bulbospongiosus muscle
use Muscle, Perineum
Bulbourethral (Cowper's) gland
use Urethra
Bundle of His
use Conduction Mechanism
Bundle of Kent
use Conduction Mechanism
Bunionectomy
see Excision, Lower Bones 0QB
Bursectomy
see Excision, Bursae and Ligaments 0MB
see Resection, Bursae and Ligaments 0MT
Bursocentesis
see Drainage, Bursae and Ligaments 0M9
Bursography
see Plain Radiography, Non-Axial Upper Bones BP0
see Plain Radiography, Non-Axial Lower Bones BQ0
Bursotomy
see Division, Bursae and Ligaments 0M8
see Drainage, Bursae and Ligaments 0M9
BVS 5000 Ventricular Assist Device
use Short-term External Heart Assist System in Heart and Great Vessels
Bypass
Anterior Chamber
Left 08133
Right 08123
Aorta
Abdominal 0410
Thoracic
Ascending/Arch 021X
Descending 021W
Artery
Anterior Tibial
Left 041Q
Right 041P
Axillary
Left 03160
Right 03150
Brachial
Left 0318
Right 0317
Common Carotid
Left 031J0
Right 031H0
Common Iliac
Left 041D
Right 041C
Coronary
Four or More Arteries 0213
One Artery 0210
Three Arteries 0212
Two Arteries 0211
External Carotid
Left 031N0
Right 031M0

Bisection–Bypass

5

Bypass *(continued)*
  Artery *(continued)*
    External Iliac
      Left 041J
      Right 041H
    Femoral
      Left 041L
      Right 041K
    Foot
      Left 041W
      Right 041V
    Hepatic 0413
    Innominate 03120
    Internal Carotid
      Left 031L0
      Right 031K0
    Internal Iliac
      Left 041F
      Right 041E
    Intracranial 031G0
    Peroneal
      Left 041U
      Right 041T
    Popliteal
      Left 041N
      Right 041M
    Posterior Tibial
      Left 041S
      Right 041R
    Pulmonary
      Left 021R
      Right 021Q
    Pulmonary Trunk 021P
    Radial
      Left 031C
      Right 031B
    Splenic 0414
    Subclavian
      Left 03140
      Right 03130
    Temporal
      Left 031T0
      Right 031S0
    Ulnar
      Left 031A
      Right 0319
  Atrium
    Left 0217
    Right 0216
  Bladder 0T1B
  Cavity, Cranial 0W110J
  Cecum 0D1H
  Cerebral Ventricle 0016
  Colon
    Ascending 0D1K
    Descending 0D1M
    Sigmoid 0D1N
    Transverse 0D1L
  Conduit through Femoral Vein to
    Popliteal Artery X2K
  Conduit through Femoral Vein to
    Superficial Femoral Artery X2K
  Duct
    Common Bile 0F19
    Cystic 0F18
    Hepatic
      Common 0F17
      Left 0F16
      Right 0F15
    Lacrimal
      Left 081Y
      Right 081X
    Pancreatic 0F1D
      Accessory 0F1F
  Duodenum 0D19
  Ear
    Left 091E0
    Right 091D0
  Esophagus 0D15
    Lower 0D13
    Middle 0D12
    Upper 0D11

Bypass *(continued)*
  Fallopian Tube
    Left 0U16
    Right 0U15
  Gallbladder 0F14
  Ileum 0D1B
  Intestine
    Large 0D1E
    Small 0D18
  Jejunum 0D1A
  Kidney Pelvis
    Left 0T14
    Right 0T13
  Pancreas 0F1G
  Pelvic Cavity 0W1J
  Peritoneal Cavity 0W1G
  Pleural Cavity
    Left 0W1B
    Right 0W19
  Spinal Canal 001U
  Stomach 0D16
  Trachea 0B11
  Ureter
    Left 0T17
    Right 0T16
  Ureters, Bilateral 0T18
  Vas Deferens
    Bilateral 0V1Q
    Left 0V1P
    Right 0V1N
  Vein
    Axillary
      Left 0518
      Right 0517
    Azygos 0510
    Basilic
      Left 051C
      Right 051B
    Brachial
      Left 051A
      Right 0519
    Cephalic
      Left 051F
      Right 051D
    Colic 0617
    Common Iliac
      Left 061D
      Right 061C
    Esophageal 0613
    External Iliac
      Left 061G
      Right 061F
    External Jugular
      Left 051Q
      Right 051P
    Face
      Left 051V
      Right 051T
    Femoral
      Left 061N
      Right 061M
    Foot
      Left 061V
      Right 061T
    Gastric 0612
    Hand
      Left 051H
      Right 051G
    Hemiazygos 0511
    Hepatic 0614
    Hypogastric
      Left 061J
      Right 061H
    Inferior Mesenteric 0616
    Innominate
      Left 0514
      Right 0513
    Internal Jugular
      Left 051N
      Right 051M
    Intracranial 051L
    Portal 0618

Bypass *(continued)*
  Vein *(continued)*
    Renal
      Left 061B
      Right 0619
    Saphenous
      Left 061Q
      Right 061P
    Splenic 0611
    Subclavian
      Left 0516
      Right 0515
    Superior Mesenteric 0615
    Vertebral
      Left 051S
      Right 051R
    Vena Cava
      Inferior 0610
      Superior 021V
    Ventricle
      Left 021L
      Right 021K
Bypass, cardiopulmonary 5A1221Z

C

Caesarean section
  see Extraction, Products of
    Conception 10D0
Calcaneocuboid joint
  use Joint, Tarsal, Left
  use Joint, Tarsal, Right
Calcaneocuboid ligament
  use Bursa and Ligament, Foot, Left
  use Bursa and Ligament, Foot, Right
Calcaneofibular ligament
  use Bursa and Ligament, Ankle, Left
  use Bursa and Ligament, Ankle, Right
Calcaneus
  use Tarsal, Left
  use Tarsal, Right
Cannulation
  see Bypass
  see Dilation
  see Drainage
  see Irrigation
Canthorrhaphy
  see Repair, Eye 08Q
Canthotomy
  see Release, Eye 08N
Canturio™ te (Tibial Extension) *use*
  Tibial Extension with Motion
  Sensors in New Technology
Capitate bone
  use Carpal, Left
  use Carpal, Right
Caplacizumab XW0
Capsulectomy, lens
  see Excision, Eye 08B
Capsulorrhaphy, joint
  see Repair, Lower Joints 0SQ
  see Repair, Upper Joints 0RQ
Caption Guidance system
  X2JAX47
Cardia
  use Esophagogastric Junction
Cardiac contractility modulation
  lead
  use Cardiac Lead in Heart and Great
  Vessels
Cardiac event recorder
  use Monitoring Device
Cardiac Lead
  Defibrillator
    Atrium
      Left 02H7
      Right 02H6
    Pericardium 02HN
    Vein, Coronary 02H4
    Ventricle
      Left 02HL
      Right 02HK

Cardiac Lead *(continued)*
  Insertion of device in
    Atrium
      Left 02H7Z
      Right 02H6
    Pericardium 02HN
    Vein, Coronary 02H4
    Ventricle
      Left 02HL
      Right 02HK
  Pacemaker
    Atrium
      Left 02H7
      Right 02H6
    Pericardium 02HN
    Vein, Coronary 02H4
    Ventricle
      Left 02HL
      Right 02HK
  Removal of device from, Heart
    02PA
  Revision of device in, Heart 02WA
Cardiac plexus
  use Nerve, Thoracic Sympathetic
Cardiac Resynchronization
  Defibrillator Pulse Generator
  Abdomen 0JH8
  Chest 0JH6
Cardiac Resynchronization
  Pacemaker Pulse Generator
  Abdomen 0JH8
  Chest 0JH6
Cardiac resynchronization therapy
  (CRT) lead
  use Cardiac Lead, Defibrillator in
    02H
  use Cardiac Lead, Pacemaker in 02H
Cardiac Rhythm Related Device
  Insertion of device in
    Abdomen 0JH8
    Chest 0JH6
  Removal of device from,
    Subcutaneous Tissue and Fascia,
    Trunk 0JPT
  Revision of device in, Subcutaneous
    Tissue and Fascia, Trunk 0JWT
Cardiocentesis
  see Drainage, Pericardial Cavity
    0W9D
Cardioesophageal junction
  use Esophagogastric Junction
Cardiolysis
  see Release, Heart and Great Vessels
    02N
CardioMEMS® pressure sensor
  use Monitoring Device, Pressure
    Sensor in 02H
Cardiomyotomy
  see Division, Esophagogastric
    Junction 0D84
Cardioplegia
  see Introduction of substance in or
    on, Heart 3E08
Cardiorrhaphy
  see Repair, Heart and Great
    Vessels 02Q
Cardioversion 5A2204Z
Caregiver training F0FZ
Carmat total artificial heart (TAH)
  use Biologic with Synthetic
    Substitute, Autoregulated
    Electrohydraulic in 02R
Caroticotympanic artery
  use Artery, Internal Carotid, Left
  use Artery, Internal Carotid, Right
Carotid (artery) sinus
  (baroreceptor) lead
  use Stimulator Lead in Upper Arteries
Carotid glomus
  use Carotid Bodies, Bilateral
  use Carotid Body, Left
  use Carotid Body, Right

Carotid sinus
  use Artery, Internal Carotid, Left
  use Artery, Internal Carotid, Right
Carotid sinus nerve
  use Nerve, Glossopharyngeal
Carotid WALLSTENT® Monorail® Endoprosthesis
  use Intraluminal Device
Carpectomy
  see Excision, Upper Bones 0PB
  see Resection, Upper Bones 0PT
Carpometacarpal ligament
  use Bursa and Ligament, Hand, Left
  use Bursa and Ligament, Hand, Right
CARVYKTI™ *use* Ciltacabtagene Autoleucel
Casirivimab (REGN10933) and Imdevimab (REGN10987)
  use REGN-COV2 Monoclonal Antibody
Casting
  see Immobilization
CAT scan
  see Computerized Tomography (CT Scan)
Catheterization
  see Dilation
  see Drainage
  Heart
    see Measurement, Cardiac 4A02
  see Irrigation
  see Insertion of device in
  Umbilical vein, for infusion 06H033T
Cauda equina
  use Spinal Cord, Lumbar
Cauterization
  see Destruction
  see Repair
Cavernous plexus
  use Nerve, Head and Neck Sympathetic
Cavoatrial junction *use* Superior Vena Cava
CBMA (Concentrated Bone Marrow Aspirate)
  use Other Substance
CBMA (Concentrated Bone Marrow Aspirate) injection,
  see Introduction of substance in or on, Muscle 3E02
Cecectomy
  see Excision, Cecum 0DBH
  see Resection, Cecum 0DTH
Cecocolostomy
  see Bypass, Gastrointestinal System 0D1
  see Drainage, Gastrointestinal System 0D9
Cecopexy
  see Repair, Cecum 0DQH
  see Reposition, Cecum 0DSH
Cecoplication
  see Restriction, Cecum 0DVH
Cecorrhaphy
  see Repair, Cecum 0DQH
Cecostomy
  see Bypass, Cecum 0D1H
  see Drainage, Cecum 0D9H
Cecotomy
  see Drainage, Cecum 0D9H
Cefiderocol Anti-Infective XW0
Ceftazidime-avibactam
  use Other Anti-infective
Ceftolozane/Tazobactam Anti-Infective XW0
Celiac (solar) plexus
  use Nerve, Abdominal Sympathetic
Celiac ganglion
  use Nerve, Abdominal Sympathetic
Celiac lymph node
  use Lymphatic, Aortic

Celiac trunk
  use Artery, Celiac
Central axillary lymph node
  use Lymphatic, Axillary, Left
  use Lymphatic, Axillary, Right
Central venous pressure
  see Measurement, Venous 4A04
Centrimag® Blood Pump
  use Short-term External Heart Assist System in Heart and Great Vessels
Cephalogram BN00ZZZ
CERAMENT® G
  use Antibiotic-eluting Bone Void Filler
Ceramic on ceramic bearing surface
  use Synthetic Substitute, Ceramic in 0SR
Cerclage
  see Restriction
Cerebral aqueduct (Sylvius)
  use Cerebral Ventricle
Cerebral Embolic Filtration
  Dual Filter X2A5312
  Extracorporeal Flow Reversal Circuit X2A
  Single Deflection Filter X2A6325
Cerebrum
  use Brain
Ceribell® Monitor XX20X89
Cervical esophagus
  use Esophagus, Upper
Cervical facet joint
  use Joint, Cervical Vertebral
  use Joint, Cervical Vertebral, 2 or more
Cervical ganglion
  use Nerve, Head and Neck Sympathetic
Cervical interspinous ligament
  use Bursa and Ligament, Head and Neck
Cervical intertransverse ligament
  use Bursa and Ligament, Head and Neck
Cervical ligamentum flavum
  use Bursa and Ligament, Head and Neck
Cervical lymph node
  use Lymphatic, Neck, Left
  use Lymphatic, Neck, Right
Cervicectomy
  see Excision, Cervix 0UBC
  see Resection, Cervix 0UTC
Cervicothoracic facet joint
  use Joint, Cervicothoracic Vertebral
Cesarean section
  see Extraction, Products of Conception 10D0
Cesium-131 Collagen Implant
  use Radioactive Element, Cesium-131 Collagen Implant in 00H
Change device in
  Abdominal Wall 0W2FX
  Back
    Lower 0W2LX
    Upper 0W2KX
  Bladder 0T2BX
  Bone
    Facial 0N2WX
    Lower 0Q2YX
    Nasal 0N2BX
    Upper 0P2YX
  Bone Marrow 072TX
  Brain 0020X
  Breast
    Left 0H2UX
    Right 0H2TX
  Bursa and Ligament
    Lower 0M2YX
    Upper 0M2XX
  Cavity, Cranial 0W21X
  Chest Wall 0W28X

Change device in *(continued)*
  Cisterna Chyli 072LX
  Diaphragm 0B2TX
  Duct
    Hepatobiliary 0F2BX
    Pancreatic 0F2DX
  Ear
    Left 092JX
    Right 092HX
  Epididymis and Spermatic Cord 0V2MX
  Extremity
    Lower
      Left 0Y2BX
      Right 0Y29X
    Upper
      Left 0X27X
      Right 0X26X
  Eye
    Left 0821X
    Right 0820X
  Face 0W22X
  Fallopian Tube 0U28X
  Gallbladder 0F24X
  Gland
    Adrenal 0G25X
    Endocrine 0G2SX
    Pituitary 0G20X
    Salivary 0C2AX
  Head 0W20X
  Intestinal Tract
    Lower Intestinal Tract 0D2DXUZ
    Upper Intestinal Tract 0D20XUZ
  Jaw
    Lower 0W25X
    Upper 0W24X
  Joint
    Lower 0S2YX
    Upper 0R2YX
  Kidney 0T25X
  Larynx 0C2SX
  Liver 0F20X
  Lung
    Left 0B2LX
    Right 0B2KX
  Lymphatic 072NX
    Thoracic Duct 072KX
  Mediastinum 0W2CX
  Mesentery 0D2VX
  Mouth and Throat 0C2YX
  Muscle
    Lower 0K2YX
    Upper 0K2XX
  Nasal Mucosa and Soft Tissue 092KX
  Neck 0W26X
  Nerve
    Cranial 002EX
    Peripheral 012YX
  Omentum 0D2UX
  Ovary 0U23X
  Pancreas 0F2GX
  Parathyroid Gland 0G2RX
  Pelvic Cavity 0W2JX
  Penis 0V2SX
  Pericardial Cavity 0W2DX
  Perineum
    Female 0W2NX
    Male 0W2MX
  Peritoneal Cavity 0W2GX
  Peritoneum 0D2WX
  Pineal Body 0G21X
  Pleura 0B2QX
  Pleural Cavity
    Left 0W2BX
    Right 0W29X
  Products of Conception 10207
  Prostate and Seminal Vesicles 0V24X
  Retroperitoneum 0W2HX
  Scrotum and Tunica Vaginalis 0V28X
  Sinus 092YX

Change device in *(continued)*
  Skin 0H2PX
  Skull 0N20X
  Spinal Canal 002UX
  Spleen 072PX
  Subcutaneous Tissue and Fascia
    Head and Neck 0J2SX
    Lower Extremity 0J2WX
    Trunk 0J2TX
    Upper Extremity 0J2VX
  Tendon
    Lower 0L2YX
    Upper 0L2XX
  Testis 0V2DX
  Thymus 072MX
  Thyroid Gland 0G2KX
  Trachea 0B21
  Tracheobronchial Tree 0B20X
  Ureter 0T29X
  Urethra 0T2DX
  Uterus and Cervix 0U2DXHZ
  Vagina and Cul-de-sac 0U2HXGZ
  Vas Deferens 0V2RX
  Vulva 0U2MX
Change device in or on
  Abdominal Wall 2W03X
  Anorectal 2Y03X5Z
  Arm
    Lower
      Left 2W0DX
      Right 2W0CX
    Upper
      Left 2W0BX
      Right 2W0AX
  Back 2W05X
  Chest Wall 2W04X
  Ear 2Y02X5Z
  Extremity
    Lower
      Left 2W0MX
      Right 2W0LX
    Upper
      Left 2W09X
      Right 2W08X
  Face 2W01X
  Finger
    Left 2W0KX
    Right 2W0JX
  Foot
    Left 2W0TX
    Right 2W0SX
  Genital Tract, Female 2Y04X5Z
  Hand
    Left 2W0FX
    Right 2W0EX
  Head 2W00X
  Inguinal Region
    Left 2W07X
    Right 2W06X
  Leg
    Lower
      Left 2W0RX
      Right 2W0QX
    Upper
      Left 2W0PX
      Right 2W0NX
  Mouth and Pharynx 2Y00X5Z
  Nasal 2Y01X5Z
  Neck 2W02X
  Thumb
    Left 2W0HX
    Right 2W0GX
  Toe
    Left 2W0VX
    Right 2W0UX
  Urethra 2Y05X5Z
Chemoembolization
  see Introduction of substance in or on
Chemosurgery, Skin 3E00XTZ
Chemothalamectomy
  see Destruction, Thalamus 0059

Chemotherapy, Infusion for cancer
see Introduction of substance in or on
Chest compression (CPR), external
Manual 5A12012
Mechanical 5A1221J
Chest x-ray
see Plain Radiography, Chest BW03
Chin *use* Subcutaneous Tissue and
Fascia, Face
Chiropractic Manipulation
Abdomen 9WB9X
Cervical 9WB1X
Extremities
Lower 9WB6X
Upper 9WB7X
Head 9WB0X
Lumbar 9WB3X
Pelvis 9WB5X
Rib Cage 9WB8X
Sacrum 9WB4X
Thoracic 9WB2X
Choana
use Nasopharynx
Cholangiogram
see Plain Radiography,
Hepatobiliary System and
Pancreas BF0
see Fluoroscopy, Hepatobiliary
System and Pancreas BF1
Cholecystectomy
see Excision, Gallbladder 0FB4
see Resection, Gallbladder 0FT4
Cholecystojejunostomy
see Bypass, Hepatobiliary System
and Pancreas 0F1
see Drainage, Hepatobiliary System
and Pancreas 0F9
Cholecystopexy
see Repair, Gallbladder 0FQ4
see Reposition, Gallbladder 0FS4
Cholecystoscopy 0FJ44ZZ
Cholecystostomy
see Drainage, Gallbladder 0F94
see Bypass, Gallbladder 0F14
Cholecystotomy
see Drainage, Gallbladder 0F94
Choledochectomy
see Excision, Hepatobiliary System
and Pancreas 0FB
see Resection, Hepatobiliary System
and Pancreas 0FT
Choledocholithotomy
see Extirpation, Duct, Common Bile
0FC9
Choledochoplasty
see Repair, Hepatobiliary System
and Pancreas 0FQ
see Replacement, Hepatobiliary
System and Pancreas 0FR
see Supplement, Hepatobiliary
System and Pancreas 0FU
Choledochoscopy 0FJB8ZZ
Choledochotomy
see Drainage, Hepatobiliary System
and Pancreas 0F9
Cholelithotomy
see Extirpation, Hepatobiliary
System and Pancreas 0FC
Chondrectomy
see Excision, Lower Joints 0SB
see Excision, Upper Joints 0RB
Knee
see Excision, Lower Joints 0SB
Semilunar cartilage
see Excision, Lower Joints 0SB
Chondroglossus muscle
use Muscle, Tongue, Palate, Pharynx
Chorda tympani
use Nerve, Facial
Chordotomy
see Division, Central Nervous
System and Cranial Nerves 008

Choroid plexus
use Cerebral Ventricle
Choroidectomy
see Excision, Eye 08B
see Resection, Eye 08T
Ciliary body
use Eye, Left
use Eye, Right
Ciliary ganglion
use Nerve, Head and Neck
Sympathetic
cilta-cel *use* Ciltacabtagene Autoleucel
Ciltacabtagene Autoleucel XW0
Circle of Willis
use Artery, Intracranial
Circumcision 0VTTXZZ
Circumflex iliac artery
use Artery, Femoral, Left
use Artery, Femoral, Right
CivaSheet®
use Radioactive Element
CivaSheet® Brachytherapy
see Brachytherapy with qualifier
Unidirectional Source
see Insertion with device
Radioactive Element
**Clamp and rod internal fixation
system (CRIF)**
use Internal Fixation Device in
Lower Bones
use Internal Fixation Device in Upper
Bones
Clamping
see Occlusion
Claustrum
use Basal Ganglia
Claviculectomy
see Excision, Upper Bones 0PB
see Resection, Upper Bones 0PT
Claviculotomy
see Division, Upper Bones 0P8
see Drainage, Upper Bones 0P9
Clipping, aneurysm
see Occlusion using Extraluminal
Device
see Restriction using Extraluminal
Device
Clitorectomy, clitoridectomy
see Excision, Clitoris 0UBJ
see Resection, Clitoris 0UTJ
Clolar
use Clofarabine
Closure
see Occlusion
see Repair
Clysis
see Introduction of substance in or on
Coagulation
see Destruction
Coagulation Factor Xa, Inactivated
XW0
**Coagulation Factor Xa,
(Recombinant) Inactivated**
use Coagulation Factor Xa,
Inactivated
**COALESCE® radiolucent interbody
fusion device**
use Interbody Fusion Device in
Lower Joints
use Interbody Fusion Device in
Upper Joints
CoAxia NeuroFlo catheter
use Intraluminal Device
**Cobalt/chromium head and
polyethylene socket**
use Synthetic Substitute, Metal on
Polyethylene in 0SR
Cobalt/chromium head and socket
use Synthetic Substitute, Metal in
0SR
Coccygeal body
use Coccygeal Glomus

Coccygeus muscle
use Muscle, Trunk, Left
use Muscle, Trunk, Right
Cochlea
use Ear, Inner, Left
use Ear, Inner, Right
**Cochlear implant (CI), multiple
channel (electrode)**
use Hearing Device, Multiple Channel
Cochlear Prosthesis in 09H
**Cochlear implant (CI), single
channel (electrode)**
use Hearing Device, Single Channel
Cochlear Prosthesis in 09H
Cochlear Implant Treatment F0BZ0
Cochlear nerve
use Nerve, Acoustic
COGNIS® CRT-D
use Cardiac Resynchronization
Defibrillator Pulse Generator
in 0JH
**COHERE® radiolucent interbody
fusion device**
use Interbody Fusion Device, in
Lower Joints
use Interbody Fusion Device in
Upper Joints
Colectomy
see Excision, Gastrointestinal
System 0DB
see Resection, Gastrointestinal
System 0DT
Collapse
see Occlusion
Collection from
Breast, Breast Milk 8E0HX62
Indwelling Device
Circulatory System
Blood 8C02X6K
Other Fluid 8C02X6L
Nervous System
Cerebrospinal Fluid 8C01X6J
Other Fluid 8C01X6L
Integumentary System, Breast Milk
8E0HX62
Reproductive System, Male, Sperm
8E0VX63
Colocentesis
see Drainage, Gastrointestinal
System 0D9
Colofixation
see Repair, Gastrointestinal System
0DQ
see Reposition, Gastrointestinal
System 0DS
Cololysis
see Release, Gastrointestinal System
0DN
Colonic Z-Stent®
use Intraluminal Device
Colonoscopy 0DJD8ZZ
Colopexy
see Repair, Gastrointestinal System
0DQ
see Reposition, Gastrointestinal
System 0DS
Coloplication
see Restriction, Gastrointestinal
System 0DV
Coloproctectomy
see Excision, Gastrointestinal
System 0DB
see Resection, Gastrointestinal
System 0DT
Coloproctostomy
see Bypass, Gastrointestinal
System 0D1
see Drainage, Gastrointestinal
System 0D9
Colopuncture
see Drainage, Gastrointestinal
System 0D9

Colorrhaphy
see Repair, Gastrointestinal System
0DQ
Colostomy
see Bypass, Gastrointestinal System
0D1
see Drainage, Gastrointestinal
System 0D9
Colpectomy
see Excision, Vagina 0UBG
see Resection, Vagina 0UTG
Colpocentesis
see Drainage, Vagina 0U9G
Colpopexy
see Repair, Vagina 0UQG
see Reposition, Vagina 0USG
Colpoplasty
see Repair, Vagina 0UQG
see Supplement, Vagina 0UUG
Colporrhaphy
see Repair, Vagina 0UQG
Colposcopy 0UJH8ZZ
Columella
use Nasal Mucosa and Soft Tissue
COMIRNATY®
use COVID-19 Vaccine
use COVID-19 Vaccine Booster
use COVID-19 Vaccine Dose 1
use COVID-19 Vaccine Dose 2
use COVID-19 Vaccine Dose 3
Common digital vein
use Vein, Foot, Left
use Vein, Foot, Right
Common facial vein
use Vein, Face, Left
use Vein, Face, Right
Common fibular nerve
use Nerve, Peroneal
Common hepatic artery
use Artery, Hepatic
Common iliac (subaortic) lymph node
use Lymphatic, Pelvis
Common interosseous artery
use Artery, Ulnar, Left
use Artery, Ulnar, Right
Common peroneal nerve
use Nerve, Peroneal
Complete (SE) stent
use Intraluminal Device
Compression
see Restriction
Abdominal Wall 2W13X
Arm
Lower
Left 2W1DX
Right 2W1CX
Upper
Left 2W1BX
Right 2W1AX
Back 2W15X
Chest Wall 2W14X
Extremity
Lower
Left 2W1MX
Right 2W1LX
Upper
Left 2W19X
Right 2W18X
Face 2W11X
Finger
Left 2W1KX
Right 2W1JX
Foot
Left 2W1TX
Right 2W1SX
Hand
Left 2W1FX
Right 2W1EX
Head 2W10X
Inguinal Region
Left 2W17X
Right 2W16X

Compression *(continued)*
Leg
  Lower
    Left 2W1RX
    Right 2W1QX
  Upper
    Left 2W1PX
    Right 2W1NX
Neck 2W12X
Thumb
  Left 2W1HX
  Right 2W1GX
Toe
  Left 2W1VX
  Right 2W1UX
Computer-aided Assessment
Cardiac Output XXE2X19
Intracranial Vascular Activity
  XXE0X07
Computer-aided Guidance,
  Transthoracic
  Echocardiography X2JAX47
Computer-aided Mechanical
  Aspiration X2C
Computer-aided Triage and
  Notification, Pulmonary Artery
  Flow XXE3X27
Computer-aided Valve Modeling
  and Notification, Coronary
  Artery Flow XXE3X68
Computer-assisted Intermittent
  Aspiration
  see New Technology,
    Cardiovascular System X2C
Computer-assisted Transcranial
  Magnetic Stimulation X0Z0X18
Computer Assisted Procedure
Extremity
  Lower
    No Qualifier 8E0YXBZ
    With Computerized
      Tomography 8E0YXBG
    With Fluoroscopy 8E0YXBF
    With Magnetic Resonance
      Imaging 8E0YXBH
  Upper
    No Qualifier 8E0XXBZ
    With Computerized
      Tomography 8E0XXBG
    With Fluoroscopy 8E0XXBF
    With Magnetic Resonance
      Imaging 8E0XXBH
Head and Neck Region
  No Qualifier 8E09XBZ
  With Computerized Tomography
    8E09XBG
  With Fluoroscopy 8E09XBF
  With Magnetic Resonance
    Imaging 8E09XBH
Trunk Region
  No Qualifier 8E0WXBZ
  With Computerized Tomography
    8E0WXBG
  With Fluoroscopy 8E0WXBF
  With Magnetic Resonance
    Imaging 8E0WXBH
Computerized Tomography (CT Scan)
Abdomen BW20
  Chest and Pelvis BW25
Abdomen and Chest BW24
Abdomen and Pelvis BW21
Airway, Trachea BB2F
Ankle
  Left BQ2H
  Right BQ2G
Aorta
  Abdominal B420
    Intravascular Optical
      Coherence B420Z2Z
  Thoracic B320
    Intravascular Optical
      Coherence B320Z2Z

Computerized Tomography (CT Scan) *(continued)*
Arm
  Left BP2F
  Right BP2E
Artery
  Celiac B421
    Intravascular Optical
      Coherence B421Z2Z
  Common Carotid
    Bilateral B325
    Intravascular Optical
      Coherence B325Z2Z
  Coronary
    Bypass Graft
      Multiple B223
      Intravascular Optical
        Coherence B223Z2Z
    Multiple B221
      Intravascular Optical
        Coherence B221Z2Z
  Internal Carotid
    Bilateral B328
    Intravascular Optical
      Coherence B328Z2Z
  Intracranial B32R
    Intravascular Optical
      Coherence B32RZ2Z
  Lower Extremity
    Bilateral B42H
      Intravascular Optical
        Coherence B42HZ2Z
    Left B42G
      Intravascular Optical
        Coherence B42GZ2Z
    Right B42F
      Intravascular Optical
        Coherence B42FZ2Z
  Pelvic B42C
    Intravascular Optical
      Coherence B42CZ2Z
  Pulmonary
    Left B32T
      Intravascular Optical
        Coherence B32TZ2Z
    Right B32S
      Intravascular Optical
        Coherence B32SZ2Z
  Renal
    Bilateral B428
      Intravascular Optical
        Coherence B428Z2Z
    Transplant B42M
      Intravascular Optical
        Coherence
          B42MZ2Z
  Superior Mesenteric B424
    Intravascular Optical
      Coherence B424Z2Z
  Vertebral
    Bilateral B32G
    Intravascular Optical
      Coherence B32GZ2Z
Bladder BT20
Bone
  Facial BN25
  Temporal BN2F
Brain B020
Calcaneus
  Left BQ2K
  Right BQ2J
Cerebral Ventricle B028
Chest, Abdomen and Pelvis
  BW25
Chest and Abdomen BW24
Cisterna B027
Clavicle
  Left BP25
  Right BP24
Coccyx BR2F
Colon BD24
Ear B920

Computerized Tomography (CT Scan) *(continued)*
Elbow
  Left BP2H
  Right BP2G
Extremity
  Lower
    Left BQ2S
    Right BQ2R
  Upper
    Bilateral BP2V
    Left BP2U
    Right BP2T
Eye
  Bilateral B827
  Left B826
  Right B825
Femur
  Left BQ24
  Right BQ23
Fibula
  Left BQ2C
  Right BQ2B
Finger
  Left BP2S
  Right BP2R
Foot
  Left BQ2M
  Right BQ2L
Forearm
  Left BP2K
  Right BP2J
Gland
  Adrenal, Bilateral BG22
  Parathyroid BG23
  Parotid, Bilateral B926
  Salivary, Bilateral B92D
  Submandibular, Bilateral
    B929
  Thyroid BG24
Hand
  Left BP2P
  Right BP2N
Hands and Wrists, Bilateral BP2Q
Head BW28
Head and Neck BW29
Heart
  Intravascular Optical Coherence
    B226Z2Z
  Right and Left B226
Hepatobiliary System, All BF2C
Hip
  Left BQ21
  Right BQ20
Humerus
  Left BP2B
  Right BP2A
Intracranial Sinus B522
  Intravascular Optical Coherence
    B522Z2Z
Joint
  Acromioclavicular, Bilateral
    BP23
  Finger
    Left BP2DZZZ
    Right BP2CZZZ
  Foot
    Left BQ2Y
    Right BQ2X
  Hand
    Left BP2DZZZ
    Right BP2CZZZ
  Sacroiliac BR2D
  Sternoclavicular
    Bilateral BP22
    Left BP21
    Right BP20
  Temporomandibular, Bilateral
    BN29
  Toe
    Left BQ2Y
    Right BQ2X

Computerized Tomography (CT Scan) *(continued)*
Kidney
  Bilateral BT23
  Left BT22
  Right BT21
  Transplant BT29
Knee
  Left BQ28
  Right BQ27
Larynx B92J
Leg
  Left BQ2F
  Right BQ2D
Liver BF25
Liver and Spleen BF26
Lung, Bilateral BB24
Mandible BN26
Nasopharynx B92F
Neck BW2F
Neck and Head BW29
Orbit, Bilateral BN23
Oropharynx B92F
Pancreas BF27
Patella
  Left BQ2W
  Right BQ2V
Pelvic Region BW2G
Pelvis BR2C
  Chest and Abdomen BW25
Pelvis and Abdomen BW21
Pituitary Gland B029
Prostate BV23
Ribs
  Left BP2Y
  Right BP2X
Sacrum BR2F
Scapula
  Left BP27
  Right BP26
Sella Turcica B029
Shoulder
  Left BP29
  Right BP28
Sinus
  Intracranial B522
    Intravascular Optical
      Coherence B522Z2Z
  Paranasal B922
Skull BN20
Spinal Cord B02B
Spine
  Cervical BR20
  Lumbar BR29
  Thoracic BR27
Spleen and Liver BF26
Thorax BP2W
Tibia
  Left BQ2C
  Right BQ2B
Toe
  Left BQ2Q
  Right BQ2P
Trachea BB2F
Tracheobronchial Tree
  Bilateral BB29
  Left BB28
  Right BB27
Vein
  Pelvic (Iliac)
    Left B52G
      Intravascular Optical
        Coherence B52GZ2Z
    Right B52F
      Intravascular Optical
        Coherence B52FZ2Z
  Pelvic (Iliac) Bilateral B52H
    Intravascular Optical
      Coherence B52HZ2Z
  Portal B52T
    Intravascular Optical
      Coherence B52TZ2Z

Computerized Tomography (CT Scan) *(continued)*
Vein *(continued)*
  Pulmonary
    Bilateral B52S
      Intravascular Optical
        Coherence B52SZ2Z
    Left B52R
      Intravascular Optical
        Coherence B52RZ2Z
    Right B52Q
      Intravascular Optical
        Coherence B52QZ2Z
  Renal
    Bilateral B52L
      Intravascular Optical
        Coherence B52LZ2Z
    Left B52K
      Intravascular Optical
        Coherence B52KZ2Z
    Right B52J
      Intravascular Optical
        Coherence B52JZ2Z
  Spanchnic B52T
    Intravascular Optical
      Coherence B52TZ2Z
  Vena Cava
    Inferior B529
      Intravascular Optical
        Coherence B529Z2Z
    Superior B528
      Intravascular Optical
        Coherence B528Z2Z
  Ventricle, Cerebral B028
  Wrist
    Left BP2M
    Right BP2L

Concerto II CRT-D
use Cardiac Resynchronization
  Defibrillator Pulse Generator in
  0JH

Condylectomy
see Excision, Head and Facial
  Bones 0NB
see Excision, Lower Bones 0QB
see Excision, Upper Bones 0PB

Conduit through Femoral Vein to
  Popliteal Artery, Bypass X2K

Conduit through Femoral Vein to
  Superficial Femoral Artery,
  Bypass X2K

Conduit to Short-term External Heart
  Assist System, Insertion X2H

Condyloid process
use Mandible, Left
use Mandible, Right

Condylotomy
see Division, Head and Facial
  Bones 0N8
see Division, Lower Bones 0Q8
see Division, Upper Bones 0P8
see Drainage, Head and Facial
  Bones 0N9
see Drainage, Lower Bones 0Q9
see Drainage, Upper Bones 0P9

Condylysis
see Release, Head and Facial
  Bones 0NN
see Release, Lower Bones 0QN
see Release, Upper Bones 0PN

Conization, cervix
see Excision, Cervix 0UBC

Conjunctivoplasty
see Repair, Eye 08Q
see Replacement, Eye 08R

CONSERVE® PLUS Total
  Resurfacing Hip System
use Resurfacing Device in Lower
  Joints

Construction
Auricle, ear
  see Bypass, Urinary System 0T1

Construction *(continued)*
Ileal conduit
  see Replacement, Ear, Nose,
  Sinus 09R

Consulta CRT-D
use Cardiac Resynchronization
  Defibrillator Pulse Generator in
  0JH

Consulta CRT-P
use Cardiac Resynchronization
  Pacemaker Pulse Generator
  in 0JH

Contact Radiation
Abdomen DWY37ZZ
Adrenal Gland DGY27ZZ
Bile Ducts DFY27ZZ
Bladder DTY27ZZ
Bone, Other DPYC7ZZ
Brain D0Y07ZZ
Brain Stem D0Y17ZZ
Breast
  Left DMY07ZZ
  Right DMY17ZZ
Bronchus DBY17ZZ
Cervix DUY17ZZ
Chest DWY27ZZ
Chest Wall DBY77ZZ
Colon DDY57ZZ
Diaphragm DBY87ZZ
Duodenum DDY27ZZ
Ear D9Y07ZZ
Esophagus DDY07ZZ
Eye D8Y07ZZ
Femur DPY97ZZ
Fibula DPYB7ZZ
Gallbladder DFY17ZZ
Gland
  Adrenal DGY27ZZ
  Parathyroid DGY47ZZ
  Pituitary DGY07ZZ
  Thyroid DGY57ZZ
Glands, Salivary D9Y67ZZ
Head and Neck DWY17ZZ
Hemibody DWY47ZZ
Humerus DPY67ZZ
Hypopharynx D9Y37ZZ
Ileum DDY47ZZ
Jejunum DDY37ZZ
Kidney DTY07ZZ
Larynx D9YB7ZZ
Liver DFY07ZZ
Lung DBY27ZZ
Mandible DPY37ZZ
Maxilla DPY27ZZ
Mediastinum DBY67ZZ
Mouth D9Y47ZZ
Nasopharynx D9YD7ZZ
Neck and Head DWY17ZZ
Nerve, Peripheral D0Y77ZZ
Nose D9Y17ZZ
Oropharynx D9YF7ZZ
Ovary DUY07ZZ
Palate
  Hard D9Y87ZZ
  Soft D9Y97ZZ
Pancreas DFY37ZZ
Parathyroid Gland
  DGY47ZZ
Pelvic Bones DPY87ZZ
Pelvic Region DWY67ZZ
Pineal Body DGY17ZZ
Pituitary Gland DGY07ZZ
Pleura DBY57ZZ
Prostate DVY07ZZ
Radius DPY77ZZ
Rectum DDY77ZZ
Rib DPY57ZZ
Sinuses D9Y77ZZ
Skin
  Abdomen DHY87ZZ
  Arm DHY47ZZ
  Back DHY77ZZ

Contact Radiation *(continued)*
Skin *(continued)*
  Buttock DHY97ZZ
  Chest DHY67ZZ
  Face DHY27ZZ
  Leg DHYB7ZZ
  Neck DHY37ZZ
Skull DPY07ZZ
Spinal Cord D0Y67ZZ
Sternum DPY47ZZ
Stomach DDY17ZZ
Testis DVY17ZZ
Thyroid Gland DGY57ZZ
Tibia DPYB7ZZ
Tongue D9Y57ZZ
Trachea DBY07ZZ
Ulna DPY77ZZ
Ureter DTY17ZZ
Urethra DTY37ZZ
Uterus DUY27ZZ
Whole Body DWY57ZZ

ContaCT software (Measurement
  of intracranial arterial flow)
  4A03X5D

CONTAK RENEWAL® 3 RF (HE)
  CRT-D
use Cardiac Resynchronization
  Defibrillator Pulse Generator
  in 0JH

Contegra Pulmonary Valved Conduit
use Zooplastic Tissue in Heart and
  Great Vessels

CONTEPO™
use Fosfomycin Anti-infective

Continent ileostomy *see* Bypass,
  Ileum 0D1B

Continuous Glucose Monitoring
  (CGM) device
use Monitoring Device

Continuous Negative Airway Pressure
24-96 Consecutive Hours,
  Ventilation 5A09459
Greater than 96 Consecutive Hours,
  Ventilation 5A09559
Less than 24 Consecutive Hours,
  Ventilation 5A09359

Continuous Positive Airway Pressure
24-96 Consecutive Hours,
  Ventilation 5A09457
Greater than 96 Consecutive Hours,
  Ventilation 5A09557
Less than 24 Consecutive Hours,
  Ventilation 5A09357

Continuous renal replacement
  therapy (CRRT) 5A1D90Z

Contraceptive Device
Change device in, Uterus and
  Cervix 0U2DXHZ
Insertion of device in
  Cervix 0UHC
  Subcutaneous Tissue and Fascia
    Abdomen 0JH8
    Chest 0JH6
    Lower Arm
      Left 0JHH
      Right 0JHG
    Lower Leg
      Left 0JHP
      Right 0JHN
    Upper Arm
      Left 0JHF
      Right 0JHD
    Upper Leg
      Left 0JHM
      Right 0JHL
  Uterus 0UH9
Removal of device from
  Subcutaneous Tissue and Fascia
    Lower Extremity 0JPW
    Trunk 0JPT
    Upper Extremity 0JPV
  Uterus and Cervix 0UPD

Contraceptive Device *(continued)*
Revision of device in
  Subcutaneous Tissue and Fascia
    Lower Extremity 0JWW
    Trunk 0JWT
    Upper Extremity 0JWV
  Uterus and Cervix 0UWD

Contractility Modulation Device
Abdomen 0JH8
Chest 0JH6

Control, Epistaxis
see Control bleeding in, Nasal
  Mucosa and Soft Tissue 093K

Control bleeding in
Abdominal Wall 0W3F
Ankle Region
  Left 0Y3L
  Right 0Y3K
Arm
  Lower
    Left 0X3F
    Right 0X3D
  Upper
    Left 0X39
    Right 0X38
Axilla
  Left 0X35
  Right 0X34
Back
  Lower 0W3L
  Upper 0W3K
Buttock
  Left 0Y31
  Right 0Y30
Cavity, Cranial 0W31
Chest Wall 0W38
Elbow Region
  Left 0X3C
  Right 0X3B
Extremity
  Lower
    Left 0Y3B
    Right 0Y39
  Upper
    Left 0X37
    Right 0X36
Face 0W32
Femoral Region
  Left 0Y38
  Right 0Y37
Foot
  Left 0Y3N
  Right 0Y3M
Gastrointestinal Tract 0W3P
Genitourinary Tract 0W3R
Hand
  Left 0X3K
  Right 0X3J
Head 0W30
Inguinal Region
  Left 0Y36
  Right 0Y35
Jaw
  Lower 0W35
  Upper 0W34
Knee Region
  Left 0Y3G
  Right 0Y3F
Leg
  Lower
    Left 0Y3J
    Right 0Y3H
  Upper
    Left 0Y3D
    Right 0Y3C
Mediastinum 0W3C
Nasal Mucosa and Soft Tissue
  093K
Neck 0W36
Oral Cavity and Throat 0W33
Pelvic Cavity 0W3J
Pericardial Cavity 0W3D

Control bleeding in *(continued)*
  Perineum
    Female 0W3N
    Male 0W3M
  Peritoneal Cavity 0W3G
  Pleural Cavity
    Left 0W3B
    Right 0W39
  Respiratory Tract 0W3Q
  Retroperitoneum 0W3H
  Shoulder Region
    Left 0X33
    Right 0X32
  Wrist Region
    Left 0X3H
    Right 0X3G
Control bleeding using Tourniquet, External *see* Compression, Anatomical Regions 2W1
Conus arteriosus
  use Ventricle, Right
Conus medullaris
  use Spinal Cord, Lumbar
Convalescent Plasma (Nonautologous)
  see New Technology, Anatomical Regions XW1
Conversion
  Cardiac rhythm 5A2204Z
  Gastrostomy to jejunostomy feeding device
    see Insertion of device in, Jejunum 0DHA
Cook Biodesign® Fistula Plug(s)
  use Nonautologous Tissue Substitute
Cook Biodesign® Hernia Graft(s)
  use Nonautologous Tissue Substitute
Cook Biodesign® Layered Graft(s)
  use Nonautologous Tissue Substitute
Cook Zenapro™ Layered Graft(s)
  use Nonautologous Tissue Substitute
Cook Zenith AAA Endovascular Graft
  use Intraluminal Device
Cook Zenith® Fenestrated AAA Endovascular Graft
  use Intraluminal Device, Branched or Fenestrated, One or Two Arteries in 04V
  use Intraluminal Device, Branched or Fenestrated, Three or More Arteries in 04V
Coracoacromial ligament
  use Bursa and Ligament, Shoulder, Left
  use Bursa and Ligament, Shoulder, Right
Coracobrachialis muscle
  use Muscle, Upper Arm, Left
  use Muscle, Upper Arm, Right
Coracoclavicular ligament
  use Bursa and Ligament, Shoulder, Left
  use Bursa and Ligament, Shoulder, Right
Coracohumeral ligament
  use Bursa and Ligament, Shoulder, Left
  use Bursa and Ligament, Shoulder, Right
Coracoid process
  use Scapula, Left
  use Scapula, Right
Cordotomy
  see Division, Central Nervous System and Cranial Nerves 008
Core needle biopsy
  see Biopsy

CoreValve transcatheter aortic valve
  use Zooplastic Tissue in Heart and Great Vessels
Cormet Hip Resurfacing System
  use Resurfacing Device in Lower Joints
Corniculate cartilage
  use Larynx
CoRoent® XL
  use Interbody Fusion Device in Lower Joints
Coronary arteriography
  see Fluoroscopy, Heart B21
  see Plain Radiography, Heart B20
Corox (OTW) Bipolar Lead
  use Cardiac Lead, Defibrillator in 02H
  use Cardiac Lead, Pacemaker in 02H
Corpus callosum
  use Brain
Corpus cavernosum
  use Penis
Corpus spongiosum
  use Penis
Corpus striatum
  use Basal Ganglia
Corrugator supercilii muscle
  use Muscle, Facial
Cortical strip neurostimulator lead
  use Neurostimulator Lead in Central Nervous System and Cranial Nerves
Corvia IASD®
  use Synthetic Substitute
COSELA™ *use* Trilaciclib
Costatectomy
  see Excision, Upper Bones 0PB
  see Resection, Upper Bones 0PT
Costectomy
  see Excision, Upper Bones 0PB
  see Resection, Upper Bones 0PT
Costocervical trunk
  use Artery, Subclavian, Left
  use Artery, Subclavian, Right
Costochondrectomy
  see Excision, Upper Bones 0PB
  see Resection, Upper Bones 0PT
Costoclavicular ligament
  use Bursa and Ligament, Shoulder, Left
  use Bursa and Ligament, Shoulder, Right
Costosternoplasty
  see Repair, Upper Bones 0PQ
  see Replacement, Upper Bones 0PR
  see Supplement, Upper Bones 0PU
Costotomy
  see Division, Upper Bones 0P8
  see Drainage, Upper Bones 0P9
Costotransverse joint
  use Joint, Thoracic Vertebral
Costotransverse ligament
  use Rib(s) Bursa and Ligament
Costovertebral joint
  use Joint, Thoracic Vertebral
Costoxiphoid ligament
  use Sternum Bursa and Ligament
Counseling
  Family, for substance abuse; Other Family Counseling HZ63ZZZ
  Group
    12-Step HZ43ZZZ
    Behavioral HZ41ZZZ
    Cognitive HZ40ZZZ
    Cognitive-Behavioral HZ42ZZZ
    Confrontational HZ48ZZZ
    Continuing Care HZ49ZZZ
    Infectious Disease
      Post-Test HZ4CZZZ
      Pre-Test HZ4CZZZ
    Interpersonal HZ44ZZZ
    Motivational Enhancement HZ47ZZZ

Counseling *(continued)*
  Group *(continued)*
    Psychoeducation HZ46ZZZ
    Spiritual HZ4BZZZ
    Vocational HZ45ZZZ
  Individual
    12-Step HZ33ZZZ
    Behavioral HZ31ZZZ
    Cognitive HZ30ZZZ
    Cognitive-Behavioral HZ32ZZZ
    Confrontational HZ38ZZZ
    Continuing Care HZ39ZZZ
    Infectious Disease
      Post-Test HZ3CZZZ
      Pre-Test HZ3CZZZ
    Interpersonal HZ34ZZZ
    Motivational Enhancement HZ37ZZZ
    Psychoeducation HZ36ZZZ
    Spiritual HZ3BZZZ
    Vocational HZ35ZZZ
  Mental Health Services
    Educational GZ60ZZZ
    Other Counseling GZ63ZZZ
    Vocational GZ61ZZZ
Countershock, cardiac 5A2204Z
COVID-19 Vaccine XW0
COVID-19 Vaccine Booster XW0
COVID-19 Vaccine Dose 1 XW0
COVID-19 Vaccine Dose 2 XW0
COVID-19 Vaccine Dose 3 XW0
Cowper's (bulbourethral) gland
  use Urethra
CPAP (continuous positive airway pressure)
  see Assistance, Respiratory 5A09
Craniectomy
  see Excision, Head and Facial Bones 0NB
  see Resection, Head and Facial Bones 0NT
Cranioplasty
  see Repair, Head and Facial Bones 0NQ
  see Replacement, Head and Facial Bones 0NR
  see Supplement, Head and Facial Bones 0NU
Craniotomy
  see Drainage, Central Nervous System and Cranial Nerves 009
  see Division, Head and Facial Bones 0N8
  see Drainage, Head and Facial Bones 0N9
Creation
  Perineum
    Female 0W4N0
    Male 0W4M0
  Valve
    Aortic 024F0
    Mitral 024G0
    Tricuspid 024J0
Cremaster muscle
  use Muscle, Perineum
CRESEMBA® (isavuconazonium sulfate)
  use Other Anti-infective
Cribriform plate
  use Bone, Ethmoid, Left
  use Bone, Ethmoid, Right
Cricoid cartilage
  use Trachea
Cricoidectomy
  see Excision, Larynx 0CBS
Cricothyroid artery
  use Artery, Thyroid, Left
  use Artery, Thyroid, Right
Cricothyroid muscle
  use Muscle, Neck, Left
  use Muscle, Neck, Right

Crisis Intervention GZ2ZZZZ
CRRT (Continuous renal replacement therapy) 5A1D90Z
Crural fascia
  use Subcutaneous Tissue and Fascia, Upper Leg, Left
  use Subcutaneous Tissue and Fascia, Upper Leg, Right
Crushing, nerve
  Cranial
    see Destruction, Central Nervous System and Cranial Nerves 005
  Peripheral
    see Destruction, Peripheral Nervous System 015
Cryoablation
  see Destruction
Cryotherapy
  see Destruction
Cryptorchidectomy
  see Excision, Male Reproductive System 0VB
  see Resection, Male Reproductive System 0VT
Cryptorchiectomy
  see Excision, Male Reproductive System 0VB
  see Resection, Male Reproductive System 0VT
Cryptotomy
  see Division, Gastrointestinal System 0D8
  see Drainage, Gastrointestinal System 0D9
CT scan
  see Computerized Tomography (CT Scan)
CT sialogram
  see Computerized Tomography (CT Scan), Ear, Nose, Mouth and Throat B92
CTX001™
  use Exagamglogene Autotemcel
Cubital lymph node
  use Lymphatic, Upper Extremity, Left
  use Lymphatic, Upper Extremity, Right
Cubital nerve
  use Nerve, Ulnar
Cuboid bone
  use Tarsal, Left
  use Tarsal, Right
Cuboideonavicular joint
  use Joint, Tarsal, Left
  use Joint, Tarsal, Right
Culdocentesis
  see Drainage, Cul-de-sac 0U9F
Culdoplasty
  see Repair, Cul-de-sac 0UQF
  see Supplement, Cul-de-sac 0UUF
Culdoscopy 0UJH8ZZ
Culdotomy
  see Drainage, Cul-de-sac 0U9F
Culmen
  use Cerebellum
Cultured epidermal cell autograft
  use Autologous Tissue Substitute
Cuneiform cartilage
  use Larynx
Cuneonavicular joint
  use Joint, Tarsal, Left
  use Joint, Tarsal, Right
Cuneonavicular ligament
  use Bursa and Ligament, Foot, Left
  use Bursa and Ligament, Foot, Right
Curettage
  see Excision
  see Extraction
Cutaneous (transverse) cervical nerve
  use Nerve, Cervical Plexus
CVP (central venous pressure)
  see Measurement, Venous 4A04

Cyclodiathermy
see Destruction, Eye 085
Cyclophotocoagulation
see Destruction, Eye 085
CYPHER® Stent
use Intraluminal Device, Drug-eluting in Heart and Great Vessels
Cystectomy
see Excision, Bladder 0TBB
see Resection, Bladder 0TTB
Cystocele repair
see Repair, Subcutaneous Tissue and Fascia, Pelvic Region 0JQC
Cystography
see Fluoroscopy, Urinary System BT1
see Plain Radiography, Urinary System BT0
Cystolithotomy
see Extirpation, Bladder 0TCB
Cystopexy
see Repair, Bladder 0TQB
see Reposition, Bladder 0TSB
Cystoplasty
see Repair, Bladder 0TQB
see Replacement, Bladder 0TRB
see Supplement, Bladder 0TUB
Cystorrhaphy
see Repair, Bladder 0TQB
Cystoscopy 0TJB8ZZ
Cystostomy
see Bypass, Bladder 0T1B
Cystostomy tube
use Drainage Device
Cystotomy
see Drainage, Bladder 0T9B
Cystourethrography
see Fluoroscopy, Urinary System BT1
see Plain Radiography, Urinary System BT0
Cystourethroplasty
see Repair, Urinary System 0TQ
see Replacement, Urinary System 0TR
see Supplement, Urinary System 0TU
CYTALUX® (Pafolacianine), in Fluorescence Guided Procedure
see Fluorescence Guided Procedure
Cytarabine and Daunorubicin Liposome Antineoplastic XW0

D

Daratumumab and Hyaluronidase-fihj XW01318
Darzalex Faspro® *use* Daratumumab and Hyaluronidase-fihj
DBS lead
use Neurostimulator Lead in Central Nervous System and Cranial Nerves
DeBakey Left Ventricular Assist Device
use Implantable Heart Assist System in Heart and Great Vessels
Debridement
Excisional
see Excision
Non-excisional
see Extraction
Decompression, Circulatory 6A15
Decortication, lung
see Extirpation, Respiratory System 0BC
see Release, Respiratory System 0BN
Deep brain neurostimulator lead
use Neurostimulator Lead in Central Nervous System and Cranial Nerves
Deep cervical fascia
use Subcutaneous Tissue and Fascia, Neck, Left
use Subcutaneous Tissue and Fascia, Neck, Right

Deep cervical vein
use Vein, Vertebral, Left
use Vein, Vertebral, Right
Deep circumflex iliac artery
use Artery, External Iliac, Left
use Artery, External Iliac, Right
Deep facial vein
use Vein, Face, Left
use Vein, Face, Right
Deep femoral (profunda femoris) vein
use Vein, Femoral, Left
use Vein, Femoral, Right
Deep femoral artery
use Artery, Femoral, Left
use Artery, Femoral, Right
Deep Inferior Epigastric Artery Perforator Flap
Replacement
Bilateral 0HRV077
Left 0HRU077
Right 0HRT077
Transfer
Left 0KXG
Right 0KXF
Deep palmar arch
use Artery, Hand, Left
use Artery, Hand, Right
Deep transverse perineal muscle
use Muscle, Perineum
DefenCath™ *use* Taurolidine Anti-infective and Heparin Anticoagulant
Deferential artery
use Artery, Internal Iliac, Left
use Artery, Internal Iliac, Right
Defibrillator Generator
Abdomen 0JH8
Chest 0JH6
Defibrillator Lead
Insertion of device in, Mediastinum 0WHC
Removal of device from, Mediastinum 0WPC
Revision of device in, Mediastinum 0WWC
Defibtech Automated Chest Compression (ACC) device 5A1221J
Defitelio
use Other Substance
Defitelio® infusion *see* Introduction of substance in or on, Physiological Systems and Anatomical Regions 3E0
Delivery
Cesarean
see Extraction, Products of Conception 10D0
Forceps
see Extraction, Products of Conception 10D0
Manually assisted 10E0XZZ
Products of Conception 10E0XZZ
Vacuum assisted
see Extraction, Products of Conception 10D0
Delta frame external fixator
use External Fixation Device, Hybrid in 0PH
use External Fixation Device, Hybrid in 0PS
use External Fixation Device, Hybrid in 0QH
use External Fixation Device, Hybrid in 0QS
Delta III Reverse shoulder prosthesis
use Synthetic Substitute, Reverse Ball and Socket in 0RR
Deltoid fascia
use Subcutaneous Tissue and Fascia, Upper Arm, Left

Deltoid fascia (*continued*)
use Subcutaneous Tissue and Fascia, Upper Arm, Right
Deltoid ligament
use Bursa and Ligament, Ankle, Left
use Bursa and Ligament, Ankle, Right
Deltoid muscle
use Muscle, Shoulder, Left
use Muscle, Shoulder, Right
Deltopectoral (infraclavicular) lymph node
use Lymphatic, Upper Extremity, Left
use Lymphatic, Upper Extremity, Right
Denervation
Cranial nerve
see Destruction, Central Nervous System and Cranial Nerves 005
Peripheral nerve
see Destruction, Peripheral Nervous System 015
Dens
use Cervical Vertebra
Densitometry
Plain Radiography
Femur
Left BQ04ZZ1
Right BQ03ZZ1
Hip
Left BQ01ZZ1
Right BQ00ZZ1
Spine
Cervical BR00ZZ1
Lumbar BR09ZZ1
Thoracic BR07ZZ1
Whole BR0GZZ1
Ultrasonography
Elbow
Left BP4HZZ1
Right BP4GZZ1
Hand
Left BP4PZZ1
Right BP4NZZ1
Shoulder
Left BP49ZZ1
Right BP48ZZ1
Wrist
Left BP4MZZ1
Right BP4LZZ1
Denticulate (dentate) ligament
use Spinal Meninges
Depressor anguli oris muscle
use Muscle, Facial
Depressor labii inferioris muscle
use Muscle, Facial
Depressor septi nasi muscle
use Muscle, Facial
Depressor supercilii muscle
use Muscle, Facial
Dermabrasion
see Extraction, Skin and Breast 0HD
Dermis
use Skin
Descending genicular artery
use Artery, Femoral, Left
use Artery, Femoral, Right
Destruction
Acetabulum
Left 0Q55
Right 0Q54
Adenoids 0C5Q
Ampulla of Vater 0F5C
Anal Sphincter 0D5R
Anterior Chamber
Left 08533ZZ
Right 08523ZZ
Anus 0D5Q

Destruction (*continued*)
Aorta
Abdominal 0450
Thoracic
Ascending/Arch 025X
Descending 025W
Aortic Body 0G5D
Appendix 0D5J
Artery
Anterior Tibial
Left 045Q
Right 045P
Axillary
Left 0356
Right 0355
Brachial
Left 0358
Right 0357
Celiac 0451
Colic
Left 0457
Middle 0458
Right 0456
Common Carotid
Left 035J
Right 035H
Common Iliac
Left 045D
Right 045C
External Carotid
Left 035N
Right 035M
External Iliac
Left 045J
Right 045H
Face 035R
Femoral
Left 045L
Right 045K
Foot
Left 045W
Right 045V
Gastric 0452
Hand
Left 035F
Right 035D
Hepatic 0453
Inferior Mesenteric 045B
Innominate 0352
Internal Carotid
Left 035L
Right 035K
Internal Iliac
Left 045F
Right 045E
Internal Mammary
Left 0351
Right 0350
Intracranial 035G
Lower 045Y
Peroneal
Left 045U
Right 045T
Popliteal
Left 045N
Right 045M
Posterior Tibial
Left 045S
Right 045R
Pulmonary
Left 025R
Right 025Q
Pulmonary Trunk 025P
Radial
Left 035C
Right 035B
Renal
Left 045A
Right 0459
Splenic 0454
Subclavian
Left 0354
Right 0353

Destruction *(continued)*

Artery *(continued)*
Superior Mesenteric 0455
Temporal
Left 035T
Right 035S
Thyroid
Left 035V
Right 035U
Ulnar
Left 035A
Right 0359
Upper 035Y
Vertebral
Left 035Q
Right 035P
Atrium
Left 0257
Right 0256
Auditory Ossicle
Left 095A
Right 0959
Basal Ganglia 0058
Bladder 0T5B
Bladder Neck 0T5C
Bone
Ethmoid
Left 0N5G
Right 0N5F
Frontal 0N51
Hyoid 0N5X
Lacrimal
Left 0N5J
Right 0N5H
Nasal 0N5B
Occipital 0N57
Palatine
Left 0N5L
Right 0N5K
Parietal
Left 0N54
Right 0N53
Pelvic
Left 0Q53
Right 0Q52
Sphenoid 0N5C
Temporal
Left 0N56
Right 0N55
Zygomatic
Left 0N5N
Right 0N5M
Brain 0050
Breast
Bilateral 0H5V
Left 0H5U
Right 0H5T
Bronchus
Lingula 0B59
Lower Lobe
Left 0B5B
Right 0B56
Main
Left 0B57
Right 0B53
Middle Lobe, Right 0B55
Upper Lobe
Left 0B58
Right 0B54
Buccal Mucosa 0C54
Bursa and Ligament
Abdomen
Left 0M5J
Right 0M5H
Ankle
Left 0M5R
Right 0M5Q
Elbow
Left 0M54
Right 0M53
Foot
Left 0M5T

Destruction *(continued)*

Bursa and Ligament *(continued)*
Foot *(continued)*
Right 0M5S
Hand
Left 0M58
Right 0M57
Head and Neck 0M50
Hip
Left 0M5M
Right 0M5L
Knee
Left 0M5P
Right 0M5N
Lower Extremity
Left 0M5W
Right 0M5V
Rib(s) 0M5G
Shoulder
Left 0M52
Right 0M51
Spine
Lower 0M5D
Upper 0M5C
Sternum 0M5F
Upper Extremity
Left 0M5B
Right 0M59
Wrist
Left 0M56
Right 0M55
Carina 0B52
Carotid Bodies, Bilateral 0G58
Carotid Body
Left 0G56
Right 0G57
Carpal
Left 0P5N
Right 0P5M
Cecum 0D5H
Cerebellum 005C
Cerebral Hemisphere 0057
Cerebral Meninges 0051
Cerebral Ventricle 0056
Cervix 0U5C
Chordae Tendineae 0259
Choroid
Left 085B
Right 085A
Cisterna Chyli 075L
Clavicle
Left 0P5B
Right 0P59
Clitoris 0U5J
Coccygeal Glomus 0G5B
Coccyx 0Q5S
Colon
Ascending 0D5K
Descending 0D5M
Sigmoid 0D5N
Transverse 0D5L
Conduction Mechanism 0258
Conjunctiva
Left 085TXZZ
Right 085SXZZ
Cord
Bilateral 0V5H
Left 0V5G
Right 0V5F
Cornea
Left 0859XZZ
Right 0858XZZ
Cul-de-sac 0U5F
Diaphragm 0B5T
Disc
Cervical Vertebral 0R53
Cervicothoracic Vertebral 0R55
Lumbar Vertebral 0S52
Lumbosacral 0S54
Thoracic Vertebral 0R59
Thoracolumbar Vertebral
0R5B

Destruction *(continued)*

Duct
Common Bile 0F59
Cystic 0F58
Hepatic
Common 0F57
Left 0F56
Right 0F55
Lacrimal
Left 085Y
Right 085X
Pancreatic 0F5D
Accessory 0F5F
Parotid
Left 0C5C
Right 0C5B
Duodenum 0D59
Dura Mater 0052
Ear
External
Left 0951
Right 0950
External Auditory Canal
Left 0954
Right 0953
Inner
Left 095E
Right 095D
Middle
Left 0956
Right 0955
Endometrium 0U5B
Epididymis
Bilateral 0V5L
Left 0V5K
Right 0V5J
Epiglottis 0C5R
Esophagogastric Junction 0D54
Esophagus 0D55
Lower 0D53
Middle 0D52
Upper 0D51
Eustachian Tube
Left 095G
Right 095F
Eye
Left 0851XZZ
Right 0850XZZ
Eyelid
Lower
Left 085R
Right 085Q
Upper
Left 085P
Right 085N
Fallopian Tube
Left 0U56
Right 0U55
Fallopian Tubes, Bilateral 0U57
Femoral Shaft
Left 0Q59
Right 0Q58
Femur
Lower
Left 0Q5C
Right 0Q5B
Upper
Left 0Q57
Right 0Q56
Fibula
Left 0Q5K
Right 0Q5J
Finger Nail 0H5QXZZ
Gallbladder 0F54
Gingiva
Lower 0C56
Upper 0C55
Gland
Adrenal
Bilateral 0G54
Left 0G52
Right 0G53

Destruction *(continued)*

Gland *(continued)*
Lacrimal
Left 085W
Right 085V
Minor Salivary 0C5J
Parotid
Left 0C59
Right 0C58
Pituitary 0G50
Sublingual
Left 0C5F
Right 0C5D
Submaxillary
Left 0C5H
Right 0C5G
Vestibular 0U5L
Glenoid Cavity
Left 0P58
Right 0P57
Glomus Jugulare 0G5C
Humeral Head
Left 0P5D
Right 0P5C
Humeral Shaft
Left 0P5G
Right 0P5F
Hymen 0U5K
Hypothalamus 005A
Ileocecal Valve 0D5C
Ileum 0D5B
Intestine
Large 0D5E
Left 0D5G
Right 0D5F
Small 0D58
Iris
Left 085D3ZZ
Right 085C3ZZ
Jejunum 0D5A
Joint
Acromioclavicular
Left 0R5H
Right 0R5G
Ankle
Left 0S5G
Right 0S5F
Carpal
Left 0R5R
Right 0R5Q
Carpometacarpal
Left 0R5T
Right 0R5S
Cervical Vertebral 0R51
Cervicothoracic Vertebral
0R54
Coccygeal 0S56
Elbow
Left 0R5M
Right 0R5L
Finger Phalangeal
Left 0R5X
Right 0R5W
Hip
Left 0S5B
Right 0S59
Knee
Left 0S5D
Right 0S5C
Lumbar Vertebral 0S50
Lumbosacral 0S53
Metacarpophalangeal
Left 0R5V
Right 0R5U
Metatarsal-Phalangeal
Left 0S5N
Right 0S5M
Occipital-cervical 0R50
Sacrococcygeal 0S55
Sacroiliac
Left 0S58
Right 0S57

Destruction–Destruction

13

Destruction (*continued*)
Joint (*continued*)
Shoulder
Left 0R5K
Right 0R5J
Sternoclavicular
Left 0R5F
Right 0R5E
Tarsal
Left 0S5J
Right 0S5H
Tarsometatarsal
Left 0S5L
Right 0S5K
Temporomandibular
Left 0R5D
Right 0R5C
Thoracic Vertebral 0R56
Thoracolumbar Vertebral
0R5A
Toe Phalangeal
Left 0S5Q
Right 0S5P
Wrist
Left 0R5P
Right 0R5N
Kidney
Left 0T51
Right 0T50
Kidney Pelvis
Left 0T54
Right 0T53
Larynx 0C5S
Lens
Left 085K3ZZ
Right 085J3ZZ
Lip
Lower 0C51
Upper 0C50
Liver 0F50
Left Lobe 0F52
Right Lobe 0F51
Ultrasound-guided Cavitation
XF5
Lung
Bilateral 0B5M
Left 0B5L
Lower Lobe
Left 0B5J
Right 0B5F
Middle Lobe, Right 0B5D
Right 0B5K
Upper Lobe
Left 0B5G
Right 0B5C
Lung Lingula 0B5H
Lymphatic
Aortic 075D
Axillary
Left 0756
Right 0755
Head 0750
Inguinal
Left 075J
Right 075H
Internal Mammary
Left 0759
Right 0758
Lower Extremity
Left 075G
Right 075F
Mesenteric 075B
Neck
Left 0752
Right 0751
Pelvis 075C
Thoracic Duct 075K
Thorax 0757
Upper Extremity
Left 0754
Right 0753

Destruction (*continued*)
Mandible
Left 0N5V
Right 0N5T
Maxilla 0N5R
Medulla Oblongata 005D
Mesentery 0D5V
Metacarpal
Left 0P5Q
Right 0P5P
Metatarsal
Left 0Q5P
Right 0Q5N
Muscle
Abdomen
Left 0K5L
Right 0K5K
Extraocular
Left 085M
Right 085L
Facial 0K51
Foot
Left 0K5W
Right 0K5V
Hand
Left 0K5D
Right 0K5C
Head 0K50
Hip
Left 0K5P
Right 0K5N
Lower Arm and Wrist
Left 0K5B
Right 0K59
Lower Leg
Left 0K5T
Right 0K5S
Neck
Left 0K53
Right 0K52
Papillary 025D
Perineum 0K5M
Shoulder
Left 0K56
Right 0K55
Thorax
Left 0K5J
Right 0K5H
Nasal Mucosa and Soft Tissue 095K
Tongue, Palate, Pharynx 0K54
Trunk
Left 0K5G
Right 0K5F
Upper Arm
Left 0K58
Right 0K57
Upper Leg
Left 0K5R
Right 0K5Q
Nasal Mucosa and Soft Tissue 095K
Nasopharynx 095N
Nerve
Abdominal Sympathetic 015M
Abducens 005L
Accessory 005R
Acoustic 005N
Brachial Plexus 0153
Cervical 0151
Cervical Plexus 0150
Facial 005M
Femoral 015D
Glossopharyngeal 005P
Head and Neck Sympathetic
015K
Hypoglossal 005S
Lumbar 015B
Lumbar Plexus 0159
Lumbar Sympathetic 015N
Lumbosacral Plexus 015A
Median 0155
Oculomotor 005H

Destruction (*continued*)
Nerve (*continued*)
Olfactory 005F
Optic 005G
Peroneal 015H
Phrenic 0152
Pudendal 015C
Radial 0156
Sacral 015R
Sacral Plexus 015Q
Sacral Sympathetic 015P
Sciatic 015F
Thoracic 0158
Thoracic Sympathetic 015L
Tibial 015G
Trigeminal 005K
Trochlear 005J
Ulnar 0154
Vagus 005Q
Nipple
Left 0H5X
Right 0H5W
Omentum 0D5U
Orbit
Left 0N5Q
Right 0N5P
Ovary
Bilateral 0U52
Left 0U51
Right 0U50
Palate
Hard 0C52
Soft 0C53
Pancreas 0F5G
Para-aortic Body 0G59
Paraganglion Extremity
0G5F
Parathyroid Gland 0G5R
Inferior
Left 0G5P
Right 0G5N
Multiple 0G5Q
Superior
Left 0G5M
Right 0G5L
Patella
Left 0Q5F
Right 0Q5D
Penis 0V5S
Pericardium 025N
Peritoneum 0D5W
Phalanx
Finger
Left 0P5V
Right 0P5T
Thumb
Left 0P5S
Right 0P5R
Toe
Left 0Q5R
Right 0Q5Q
Pharynx 0C5M
Pineal Body 0G51
Pleura
Left 0B5P
Right 0B5N
Pons 005B
Prepuce 0V5T
Prostate 0V50
Radius
Left 0P5J
Right 0P5H
Rectum 0D5P
Renal Sympathetic Nerve(s),
Ultrasound Ablation X051329
Retina
Left 085F3ZZ
Right 085E3ZZ
Retinal Vessel
Left 085H3ZZ
Right 085G3ZZ

Destruction (*continued*)
Rib (s)
1 to 2 0P51
3 or More 0P52
Sacrum 0Q51
Scapula
Left 0P56
Right 0P55
Sclera
Left 0857XZZ
Right 0856XZZ
Scrotum 0V55
Septum
Atrial 0255
Nasal 095M
Ventricular 025M
Sinus
Accessory 095P
Ethmoid
Left 095V
Right 095U
Frontal
Left 095T
Right 095S
Mastoid
Left 095C
Right 095B
Maxillary
Left 095R
Right 095Q
Sphenoid
Left 095X
Right 095W
Skin
Abdomen 0H57XZ
Back 0H56XZ
Buttock 0H58XZ
Chest 0H55XZ
Ear
Left 0H53XZ
Right 0H52XZ
Face 0H51XZ
Foot
Left 0H5NXZ
Right 0H5MXZ
Hand
Left 0H5GXZ
Right 0H5FXZ
Inguinal 0H5AXZ
Lower Arm
Left 0H5EXZ
Right 0H5DXZ
Lower Leg
Left 0H5LXZ
Right 0H5KXZ
Neck 0H54XZ
Perineum 0H59XZ
Scalp 0H50XZ
Upper Arm
Left 0H5CXZ
Right 0H5BXZ
Upper Leg
Left 0H5JXZ
Right 0H5HXZ
Skull 0N50
Spinal Cord
Cervical 005W
Lumbar 005Y
Thoracic 005X
Spinal Meninges 005T
Spleen 075P
Sternum 0P50
Stomach 0D56
Pylorus 0D57
Subcutaneous Tissue and Fascia
Abdomen 0J58
Back 0J57
Buttock 0J59
Chest 0J56
Face 0J51

Destruction *(continued)*
Subcutaneous Tissue and
  Fascia *(continued)*
    Foot
      Left 0J5R
      Right 0J5Q
    Hand
      Left 0J5K
      Right 0J5J
    Lower Arm
      Left 0J5H
      Right 0J5G
    Lower Leg
      Left 0J5P
      Right 0J5N
    Neck
      Left 0J55
      Right 0J54
    Pelvic Region 0J5C
    Perineum 0J5B
    Scalp 0J50
    Upper Arm
      Left 0J5F
      Right 0J5D
    Upper Leg
      Left 0J5M
      Right 0J5L
Tarsal
  Left 0Q5M
  Right 0Q5L
Tendon
  Abdomen
    Left 0L5G
    Right 0L5F
  Ankle
    Left 0L5T
    Right 0L5S
  Foot
    Left 0L5W
    Right 0L5V
  Hand
    Left 0L58
    Right 0L57
  Head and Neck 0L50
  Hip
    Left 0L5K
    Right 0L5J
  Knee
    Left 0L5R
    Right 0L5Q
  Lower Arm and Wrist
    Left 0L56
    Right 0L55
  Lower Leg
    Left 0L5P
    Right 0L5N
  Perineum 0L5H
  Shoulder
    Left 0L52
    Right 0L51
  Thorax
    Left 0L5D
    Right 0L5C
  Trunk
    Left 0L5B
    Right 0L59
  Upper Arm
    Left 0L54
    Right 0L53
  Upper Leg
    Left 0L5M
    Right 0L5L
Testis
  Bilateral 0V5C
  Left 0V5B
  Right 0V59
Thalamus 0059
Thymus 075M
Thyroid Gland 0G5K
  Left Lobe 0G5G
  Right Lobe 0G5H

Destruction *(continued)*
Tibia
  Left 0Q5H
  Right 0Q5G
Toe Nail 0H5RXZZ
Tongue 0C57
Tonsils 0C5P
Tooth
  Lower 0C5X
  Upper 0C5W
Trachea 0B51
Tunica Vaginalis
  Left 0V57
  Right 0V56
Turbinate, Nasal 095L
Tympanic Membrane
  Left 0958
  Right 0957
Ulna
  Left 0P5L
  Right 0P5K
Ureter
  Left 0T57
  Right 0T56
Urethra 0T5D
Uterine Supporting Structure 0U54
Uterus 0U59
Uvula 0C5N
Vagina 0U5G
Valve
  Aortic 025F
  Mitral 025G
  Pulmonary 025H
  Tricuspid 025J
Vas Deferens
  Bilateral 0V5Q
  Left 0V5P
  Right 0V5N
Vein
  Axillary
    Left 0558
    Right 0557
  Azygos 0550
  Basilic
    Left 055C
    Right 055B
  Brachial
    Left 055A
    Right 0559
  Cephalic
    Left 055F
    Right 055D
  Colic 0657
  Common Iliac
    Left 065D
    Right 065C
  Coronary 0254
  Esophageal 0653
  External Iliac
    Left 065G
    Right 065F
  External Jugular
    Left 055Q
    Right 055P
  Face
    Left 055V
    Right 055T
  Femoral
    Left 065N
    Right 065M
  Foot
    Left 065V
    Right 065T
  Gastric 0652
  Hand
    Left 055H
    Right 055G
  Hemiazygos 0551
  Hepatic 0654
  Hypogastric
    Left 065J
    Right 065H

Destruction *(continued)*
Vein *(continued)*
  Inferior Mesenteric 0656
  Innominate
    Left 0554
    Right 0553
  Internal Jugular
    Left 055N
    Right 055M
  Intracranial 055L
  Lower 065Y
  Portal 0658
  Pulmonary
    Left 025T
    Right 025S
  Renal
    Left 065B
    Right 0659
  Saphenous
    Left 065Q
    Right 065P
  Splenic 0651
  Subclavian
    Left 0556
    Right 0555
  Superior Mesenteric 0655
  Upper 055Y
  Vertebral
    Left 055S
    Right 055R
Vena Cava
  Inferior 0650
  Superior 025V
Ventricle
  Left 025L
  Right 025K
Vertebra
  Cervical 0P53
  Lumbar 0Q50
  Thoracic 0P54
Vesicle
  Bilateral 0V53
  Left 0V52
  Right 0V51
Vitreous
  Left 08553ZZ
  Right 08543ZZ
Vocal Cord
  Left 0C5V
  Right 0C5T
Vulva 0U5M
Detachment
Arm
  Lower
    Left 0X6F0Z
    Right 0X6D0Z
  Upper
    Left 0X690Z
    Right 0X680Z
Elbow Region
  Left 0X6C0ZZ
  Right 0X6B0ZZ
Femoral Region
  Left 0Y680ZZ
  Right 0Y670ZZ
Finger
  Index
    Left 0X6P0Z
    Right 0X6N0Z
  Little
    Left 0X6W0Z
    Right 0X6V0Z
  Middle
    Left 0X6R0Z
    Right 0X6Q0Z
  Ring
    Left 0X6T0Z
    Right 0X6S0Z
Foot
  Left 0Y6N0Z
  Right 0Y6M0Z

Detachment *(continued)*
Forequarter
  Left 0X610ZZ
  Right 0X600ZZ
Hand
  Left 0X6K0Z
  Right 0X6J0Z
Hindquarter
  Bilateral 0Y640ZZ
  Left 0Y630ZZ
  Right 0Y620ZZ
Knee Region
  Left 0Y6G0ZZ
  Right 0Y6F0ZZ
Leg
  Lower
    Left 0Y6J0Z
    Right 0Y6H0Z
  Upper
    Left 0Y6D0Z
    Right 0Y6C0Z
Shoulder Region
  Left 0X630ZZ
  Right 0X620ZZ
Thumb
  Left 0X6M0Z
  Right 0X6L0Z
Toe
  1st
    Left 0Y6Q0Z
    Right 0Y6P0Z
  2nd
    Left 0Y6S0Z
    Right 0Y6R0Z
  3rd
    Left 0Y6U0Z
    Right 0Y6T0Z
  4th
    Left 0Y6W0Z
    Right 0Y6V0Z
  5th
    Left 0Y6Y0Z
    Right 0Y6X0Z
Determination, Mental status
  GZ14ZZZ
Detorsion
  see Release
  see Reposition
DETOUR® System
  use Conduit through Femoral Vein to
    Popliteal Artery in New Technology
  use Conduit through Femoral Vein
    to Superficial Femoral Artery in
    New Technology
Detoxification Services, for
  substance abuse HZ2ZZZZ
Device Fitting F0DZ
Diagnostic Audiology
  see Audiology, Diagnostic
Diagnostic imaging
  see Imaging, Diagnostic
Diagnostic radiology
  see Imaging, Diagnostic
Dialysis
  Hemodialysis *see* Performance,
    Urinary 5A1D
  Peritoneal 3E1M39Z
Diaphragma sellae
  use Dura Mater
Diaphragmatic pacemaker
  generator
  use Stimulator Generator in
    Subcutaneous Tissue and Fascia
Diaphragmatic Pacemaker Lead
  Insertion of device in, Diaphragm
    0BHT
  Removal of device from, Diaphragm
    0BPT
  Revision of device in, Diaphragm
    0BWT
Digital radiography, plain
  see Plain Radiography

Dilation

Ampulla of Vater 0F7C
Anus 0D7Q
Aorta
  Abdominal 0470
  Thoracic
    Ascending/Arch 027X
    Descending 027W
Artery
  Anterior Tibial
    Left 047Q
      Sustained Release Drug-eluting Intraluminal Device X27Q385
        Four or More X27Q3C5
        Three X27Q3B5
        Two X27Q395
    Right 047P
      Sustained Release Drug-eluting Intraluminal Device X27P385
        Four or More X27P3C5
        Three X27P3B5
        Two X27P395
  Axillary
    Left 0376
    Right 0375
  Brachial
    Left 0378
    Right 0377
  Celiac 0471
  Colic
    Left 0477
    Middle 0478
    Right 0476
  Common Carotid
    Left 037J
    Right 037H
  Common Iliac
    Left 047D
    Right 047C
  Coronary
    Four or More Arteries 0273
    One Artery 0270
    Three Arteries 0272
    Two Arteries 0271
  External Carotid
    Left 037N
    Right 037M
  External Iliac
    Left 047J
    Right 047H
  Face 037R
  Femoral
    Left 047L
      Sustained Release Drug-eluting Intraluminal Device X27J385
        Four or More X27J3C5
        Three X27J3B5
        Two X27J395
    Right 047K
      Sustained Release Drug-eluting Intraluminal Device X27H385
        Four or More X27H3C5
        Three X27H3B5
        Two X27H395
  Foot
    Left 047W
    Right 047V
  Gastric 0472
  Hand
    Left 037F
    Right 037D
  Hepatic 0473
  Inferior Mesenteric 047B
  Innominate 0372
  Internal Carotid
    Left 037L
    Right 037K

Dilation *(continued)*

Artery *(continued)*
  Internal Iliac
    Left 047F
    Right 047E
  Internal Mammary
    Left 0371
    Right 0370
  Intracranial 037G
  Lower 047Y
  Peroneal
    Left 047U
      Sustained Release Drug-eluting Intraluminal Device X27U385
        Four or More X27U3C5
        Three X27U3B5
        Two X27U395
    Right 047T
      Sustained Release Drug-eluting Intraluminal Device X27T385
        Four or More X27T3C5
        Three X27T3B5
        Two X27T395
  Popliteal
    Left 047N
    Left Distal
      Sustained Release Drug-eluting Intraluminal Device X27N385
        Four or More X27N3C5
        Three X27N3B5
        Two X27N395
    Left Proximal
      Sustained Release Drug-eluting Intraluminal Device X27L385
        Four or More X27L3C5
        Three X27L3B5
        Two X27L395
    Right 047M
    Right Distal
      Sustained Release Drug-eluting Intraluminal Device X27M385
        Four or More X27M3C5
        Three X27M3B5
        Two X27M395
    Right Proximal
      Sustained Release Drug-eluting Intraluminal Device X27K385
        Four or More X27K3C5
        Three X27K3B5
        Two X27K395
  Posterior Tibial
    Left 047S
      Sustained Release Drug-eluting Intraluminal Device X27S385
        Four or More X27S3C5
        Three X27S3B5
        Two X27S395
    Right 047R
      Sustained Release Drug-eluting Intraluminal Device X27R385
        Four or More X27R3C5
        Three X27R3B5
        Two X27R395
  Pulmonary
    Left 027R
    Right 027Q
  Pulmonary Trunk 027P
  Radial
    Left 037C
    Right 037B
  Renal
    Left 047A
    Right 0479
  Splenic 0474

Dilation *(continued)*

Artery *(continued)*
  Subclavian
    Left 0374
    Right 0373
  Superior Mesenteric 0475
  Temporal
    Left 037T
    Right 037S
  Thyroid
    Left 037V
    Right 037U
  Ulnar
    Left 037A
    Right 0379
  Upper 037Y
  Vertebral
    Left 037Q
    Right 037P
Bladder 0T7B
Bladder Neck 0T7C
Bronchus
  Lingula 0B79
  Lower Lobe
    Left 0B7B
    Right 0B76
  Main
    Left 0B77
    Right 0B73
  Middle Lobe, Right 0B75
  Upper Lobe
    Left 0B78
    Right 0B74
Carina 0B72
Cerebral Ventricle 0076
Cecum 0D7H
Cervix 0U7C
Colon
  Ascending 0D7K
  Descending 0D7M
  Sigmoid 0D7N
  Transverse 0D7L
Duct
  Common Bile 0F79
  Cystic 0F78
  Hepatic
    Common 0F77
    Left 0F76
    Right 0F75
  Lacrimal
    Left 087Y
    Right 087X
  Pancreatic 0F7D
    Accessory 0F7F
  Parotid
    Left 0C7C
    Right 0C7B
Duodenum 0D79
Esophagogastric Junction 0D74
Esophagus 0D75
  Lower 0D73
  Middle 0D72
  Upper 0D71
Eustachian Tube
  Left 097G
  Right 097F
Fallopian Tube
  Left 0U76
  Right 0U75
Fallopian Tubes, Bilateral 0U77
Hymen 0U7K
Ileocecal Valve 0D7C
Ileum 0D7B
Intestine
  Large 0D7E
    Left 0D7G
    Right 0D7F
  Small 0D78
Jejunum 0D7A
Kidney Pelvis
  Left 0T74

Dilation *(continued)*

Kidney Pelvis *(continued)*
  Right 0T73
Larynx 0C7S
Pharynx 0C7M
Rectum 0D7P
Stomach 0D76
  Pylorus 0D77
Trachea 0B71
Ureter
  Left 0T77
  Right 0T76
Ureters, Bilateral 0T78
Urethra 0T7D
Uterus 0U79
Vagina 0U7G
Valve
  Aortic 027F
  Mitral 027G
  Pulmonary 027H
  Tricuspid 027J
Vas Deferens
  Bilateral 0V7Q
  Left 0V7P
  Right 0V7N
Vein
  Axillary
    Left 0578
    Right 0577
  Azygos 0570
  Basilic
    Left 057C
    Right 057B
  Brachial
    Left 057A
    Right 0579
  Cephalic
    Left 057F
    Right 057D
  Colic 0677
  Common Iliac
    Left 067D
    Right 067C
  Esophageal 0673
  External Iliac
    Left 067G
    Right 067F
  External Jugular
    Left 057Q
    Right 057P
  Face
    Left 057V
    Right 057T
  Femoral
    Left 067N
    Right 067M
  Foot
    Left 067V
    Right 067T
  Gastric 0672
  Hand
    Left 057H
    Right 057G
  Hemiazygos 0571
  Hepatic 0674
  Hypogastric
    Left 067J
    Right 067H
  Inferior Mesenteric 0676
  Innominate
    Left 0574
    Right 0573
  Internal Jugular
    Left 057N
    Right 057M
  Intracranial 057L
  Lower 067Y
  Portal 0678
  Pulmonary
    Left 027T
    Right 027S

Dilation *(continued)*
Vein *(continued)*
Renal
Left 067B
Right 0679
Saphenous
Left 067Q
Right 067P
Splenic 0671
Subclavian
Left 0576
Right 0575
Superior Mesenteric 0675
Upper 057Y
Vertebral
Left 057S
Right 057R
Vena Cava
Inferior 0670
Superior 027V
Ventricle
Left 027L
Right 027K
Direct Lateral Interbody Fusion (DLIF) device
use Interbody Fusion Device in Lower Joints
Disarticulation
see Detachment
Discectomy, diskectomy
see Excision, Lower Joints 0SB
see Excision, Upper Joints 0RB
see Resection, Lower Joints 0ST
see Resection, Upper Joints 0RT
Discography
see Fluoroscopy, Axial Skeleton, Except Skull and Facial Bones BR1
see Plain Radiography, Axial Skeleton, Except Skull and Facial Bones BR0
Dismembered pyeloplasty
see Repair, Kidney Pelvis
Distal humerus
use Humeral Shaft, Left
use Humeral Shaft, Right
Distal humerus, involving joint
use Joint, Elbow, Left
use Joint, Elbow, Right
Distal radioulnar joint
use Joint, Wrist, Left
use Joint, Wrist, Right
Diversion
see Bypass
Diverticulectomy
see Excision, Gastrointestinal System 0DB
Division
Acetabulum
Left 0Q85
Right 0Q84
Anal Sphincter 0D8R
Basal Ganglia 0088
Bladder Neck 0T8C
Bone
Ethmoid
Left 0N8G
Right 0N8F
Frontal 0N81
Hyoid 0N8X
Lacrimal
Left 0N8J
Right 0N8H
Nasal 0N8B
Occipital 0N87
Palatine
Left 0N8L
Right 0N8K
Parietal
Left 0N84
Right 0N83

Division *(continued)*
Bone *(continued)*
Pelvic
Left 0Q83
Right 0Q82
Sphenoid 0N8C
Temporal
Left 0N86
Right 0N85
Zygomatic
Left 0N8N
Right 0N8M
Brain 0080
Bursa and Ligament
Abdomen
Left 0M8J
Right 0M8H
Ankle
Left 0M8R
Right 0M8Q
Elbow
Left 0M84
Right 0M83
Foot
Left 0M8T
Right 0M8S
Hand
Left 0M88
Right 0M87
Head and Neck 0M80
Hip
Left 0M8M
Right 0M8L
Knee
Left 0M8P
Right 0M8N
Lower Extremity
Left 0M8W
Right 0M8V
Perineum 0M8K
Rib(s) 0M8G
Shoulder
Left 0M82
Right 0M81
Spine
Lower 0M8D
Upper 0M8C
Sternum 0M8F
Upper Extremity
Left 0M8B
Right 0M89
Wrist
Left 0M86
Right 0M85
Carpal
Left 0P8N
Right 0P8M
Cerebral Hemisphere 0087
Chordae Tendineae 0289
Clavicle
Left 0P8B
Right 0P89
Coccyx 0Q8S
Conduction Mechanism 0288
Esophagogastric Junction 0D84
Femoral Shaft
Left 0Q89
Right 0Q88
Femur
Lower
Left 0Q8C
Right 0Q8B
Upper
Left 0Q87
Right 0Q86
Fibula
Left 0Q8K
Right 0Q8J
Gland, Pituitary 0G80
Glenoid Cavity
Left 0P88

Division *(continued)*
Glenoid Cavity *(continued)*
Right 0P87
Humeral Head
Left 0P8D
Right 0P8C
Humeral Shaft
Left 0P8G
Right 0P8F
Hymen 0U8K
Kidneys, Bilateral 0T82
Liver 0F80
Left Lobe 0F82
Right Lobe 0F81
Mandible
Left 0N8V
Right 0N8T
Maxilla 0N8R
Metacarpal
Left 0P8Q
Right 0P8P
Metatarsal
Left 0Q8P
Right 0Q8N
Muscle
Abdomen
Left 0K8L
Right 0K8K
Facial 0K81
Foot
Left 0K8W
Right 0K8V
Hand
Left 0K8D
Right 0K8C
Head 0K80
Hip
Left 0K8P
Right 0K8N
Lower Arm and Wrist
Left 0K8B
Right 0K89
Lower Leg
Left 0K8T
Right 0K8S
Neck
Left 0K83
Right 0K82
Papillary 028D
Perineum 0K8M
Shoulder
Left 0K86
Right 0K85
Thorax
Left 0K8J
Right 0K8H
Tongue, Palate, Pharynx 0K84
Trunk
Left 0K8G
Right 0K8F
Upper Arm
Left 0K88
Right 0K87
Upper Leg
Left 0K8R
Right 0K8Q
Nerve
Abdominal Sympathetic 018M
Abducens 008L
Accessory 008R
Acoustic 008N
Brachial Plexus 0183
Cervical 0181
Cervical Plexus 0180
Facial 008M
Femoral 018D
Glossopharyngeal 008P
Head and Neck Sympathetic 018K
Hypoglossal 008S
Lumbar 018B
Lumbar Plexus 0189

Division *(continued)*
Nerve *(continued)*
Lumbar Sympathetic 018N
Lumbosacral Plexus 018A
Median 0185
Oculomotor 008H
Olfactory 008F
Optic 008G
Peroneal 018H
Phrenic 0182
Pudendal 018C
Radial 0186
Sacral 018R
Sacral Plexus 018Q
Sacral Sympathetic 018P
Sciatic 018F
Thoracic 0188
Thoracic Sympathetic 018L
Tibial 018G
Trigeminal 008K
Trochlear 008J
Ulnar 0184
Vagus 008Q
Orbit
Left 0N8Q
Right 0N8P
Ovary
Bilateral 0U82
Left 0U81
Right 0U80
Pancreas 0F8G
Patella
Left 0Q8F
Right 0Q8D
Perineum, Female 0W8NXZZ
Phalanx
Finger
Left 0P8V
Right 0P8T
Thumb
Left 0P8S
Right 0P8R
Toe
Left 0Q8R
Right 0Q8Q
Radius
Left 0P8J
Right 0P8H
Ribs
1 to 2 0P81
3 or More 0P82
Sacrum 0Q81
Scapula
Left 0P86
Right 0P85
Skin
Abdomen 0H87XZZ
Back 0H86XZZ
Buttock 0H88XZZ
Chest 0H85XZZ
Ear
Left 0H83XZZ
Right 0H82XZZ
Face 0H81XZZ
Foot
Left 0H8NXZZ
Right 0H8MXZZ
Hand
Left 0H8GXZZ
Right 0H8FXZZ
Inguinal 0H8AXZZ
Lower Arm
Left 0H8EXZZ
Right 0H8DXZZ
Lower Leg
Left 0H8LXZZ
Right 0H8KXZZ
Neck 0H84XZZ
Perineum 0H89XZZ
Scalp 0H80XZZ

Division *(continued)*

Skin *(continued)*
Upper Arm
Left 0H8CXZZ
Right 0H8BXZZ
Upper Leg
Left 0H8JXZZ
Right 0H8HXZZ
Skull 0N80
Spinal Cord
Cervical 008W
Lumbar 008Y
Thoracic 008X
Sternum 0P80
Stomach, Pylorus 0D87
Subcutaneous Tissue and Fascia
Abdomen 0J88
Back 0J87
Buttock 0J89
Chest 0J86
Face 0J81
Foot
Left 0J8R
Right 0J8Q
Hand
Left 0J8K
Right 0J8J
Head and Neck 0J8S
Lower Arm
Left 0J8H
Right 0J8G
Lower Extremity 0J8W
Lower Leg
Left 0J8P
Right 0J8N
Neck
Left 0J85
Right 0J84
Pelvic Region 0J8C
Perineum 0J8B
Scalp 0J80
Trunk 0J8T
Upper Arm
Left 0J8F
Right 0J8D
Upper Extremity 0J8V
Upper Leg
Left 0J8M
Right 0J8L
Tarsal
Left 0Q8M
Right 0Q8L
Tendon
Abdomen
Left 0L8G
Right 0L8F
Ankle
Left 0L8T
Right 0L8S
Foot
Left 0L8W
Right 0L8V
Hand
Left 0L88
Right 0L87
Head and Neck 0L80
Hip
Left 0L8K
Right 0L8J
Knee
Left 0L8R
Right 0L8Q
Lower Arm and Wrist
Left 0L86
Right 0L85
Lower Leg
Left 0L8P
Right 0L8N
Perineum 0L8H
Shoulder
Left 0L82

Division *(continued)*

Tendon *(continued)*
Shoulder *(continued)*
Right 0L81
Thorax
Left 0L8D
Right 0L8C
Trunk
Left 0L8B
Right 0L89
Upper Arm
Left 0L84
Right 0L83
Upper Leg
Left 0L8M
Right 0L8L
Thyroid Gland Isthmus 0G8J
Tibia
Left 0Q8H
Right 0Q8G
Turbinate, Nasal 098L
Ulna
Left 0P8L
Right 0P8K
Uterine Supporting Structure
0U84
Vertebra
Cervical 0P83
Lumbar 0Q80
Thoracic 0P84
Doppler study
see Ultrasonography
Dorsal digital nerve
use Nerve, Radial
Dorsal metacarpal vein
use Vein, Hand, Left
use Vein, Hand, Right
Dorsal metatarsal artery
use Artery, Foot, Left
use Artery, Foot, Right
Dorsal metatarsal vein
use Vein, Foot, Left
use Vein, Foot, Right
Dorsal root ganglion
use Cervical Spinal Cord
use Lumbar Spinal Cord
use Spinal Cord
use Thoracic Spinal Cord
Dorsal scapular artery
use Artery, Subclavian, Left
use Artery, Subclavian, Right
Dorsal scapular nerve
use Nerve, Brachial Plexus
Dorsal venous arch
use Vein, Foot, Left
use Vein, Foot, Right
Dorsalis pedis artery
use Artery, Anterior Tibial, Left
use Artery, Anterior Tibial,
Right
DownStream® System
5A0512C
5A0522C
Drainage
Abdominal Wall 0W9F
Acetabulum
Left 0Q95
Right 0Q94
Adenoids 0C9Q
Ampulla of Vater 0F9C
Anal Sphincter 0D9R
Ankle Region
Left 0Y9L
Right 0Y9K
Anterior Chamber
Left 0893
Right 0892
Anus 0D9Q
Aorta, Abdominal 0490
Aortic Body 0G9D
Appendix 0D9J

Drainage *(continued)*

Arm
Lower
Left 0X9F
Right 0X9D
Upper
Left 0X99
Right 0X98
Artery
Anterior Tibial
Left 049Q
Right 049P
Axillary
Left 0396
Right 0395
Brachial
Left 0398
Right 0397
Celiac 0491
Colic
Left 0497
Middle 0498
Right 0496
Common Carotid
Left 039J
Right 039H
Common Iliac
Left 049D
Right 049C
External Carotid
Left 039N
Right 039M
External Iliac
Left 049J
Right 049H
Face 039R
Femoral
Left 049L
Right 049K
Foot
Left 049W
Right 049V
Gastric 0492
Hand
Left 039F
Right 039D
Hepatic 0493
Inferior Mesenteric 049B
Innominate 0392
Internal Carotid
Left 039L
Right 039K
Internal Iliac
Left 049F
Right 049E
Internal Mammary
Left 0391
Right 0390
Intracranial 039G
Lower 049Y
Peroneal
Left 049U
Right 049T
Popliteal
Left 049N
Right 049M
Posterior Tibial
Left 049S
Right 049R
Radial
Left 039C
Right 039B
Renal
Left 049A
Right 0499
Splenic 0494
Subclavian
Left 0394
Right 0393
Superior Mesenteric
0495

Drainage *(continued)*

Artery *(continued)*
Temporal
Left 039T
Right 039S
Thyroid
Left 039V
Right 039U
Ulnar
Left 039A
Right 0399
Upper 039Y
Vertebral
Left 039Q
Right 039P
Auditory Ossicle
Left 099A
Right 0999
Axilla
Left 0X95
Right 0X94
Back
Lower 0W9L
Upper 0W9K
Basal Ganglia 0098
Bladder 0T9B
Bladder Neck 0T9C
Bone
Ethmoid
Left 0N9G
Right 0N9F
Frontal 0N91
Hyoid 0N9X
Lacrimal
Left 0N9J
Right 0N9H
Nasal 0N9B
Occipital 0N97
Palatine
Left 0N9L
Right 0N9K
Parietal
Left 0N94
Right 0N93
Pelvic
Left 0Q93
Right 0Q92
Sphenoid 0N9C
Temporal
Left 0N96
Right 0N95
Zygomatic
Left 0N9N
Right 0N9M
Bone Marrow 079T
Brain 0090
Breast
Bilateral 0H9V
Left 0H9U
Right 0H9T
Bronchus
Lingula 0B99
Lower Lobe
Left 0B9B
Right 0B96
Main
Left 0B97
Right 0B93
Middle Lobe, Right
0B95
Upper Lobe
Left 0B98
Right 0B94
Buccal Mucosa 0C94
Bursa and Ligament
Abdomen
Left 0M9J
Right 0M9H
Ankle
Left 0M9R
Right 0M9Q

Drainage *(continued)*

Bursa and Ligament *(continued)*
Elbow
Left 0M94
Right 0M93
Foot
Left 0M9T
Right 0M9S
Hand
Left 0M98
Right 0M97
Head and Neck 200M90
Hip
Left 0M9M
Right 0M9L
Knee
Left 0M9P
Right 0M9N
Lower Extremity
Left 0M9W
Right 0M9V
Perineum 0M9K
Rib(s) 0M9G
Shoulder
Left 0M92
Right 0M91
Spine
Lower 0M9D
Upper 0M9C
Sternum 0M9F
Upper Extremity
Left 0M9B
Right 0M99
Wrist
Left 0M96
Right 0M95
Buttock
Left 0Y91
Right 0Y90
Carina 0B92
Carotid Bodies, Bilateral 0G98
Carotid Body
Left 0G96
Right 0G97
Carpal
Left 0P9N
Right 0P9M
Cavity, Cranial 0W91
Cecum 0D9H
Cerebellum 009C
Cerebral Hemisphere 0097
Cerebral Meninges 0091
Cerebral Ventricle 0096
Cervix 0U9C
Chest Wall 0W98
Choroid
Left 089B
Right 089A
Cisterna Chyli 079L
Clavicle
Left 0P9B
Right 0P99
Clitoris 0U9J
Coccygeal Glomus 0G9B
Coccyx 0Q9S
Colon
Ascending 0D9K
Descending 0D9M
Sigmoid 0D9N
Transverse 0D9L
Conjunctiva
Left 089T
Right 089S
Cord
Bilateral 0V9H
Left 0V9G
Right 0V9F
Cornea
Left 0899
Right 0898
Cul-de-sac 0U9F

Drainage *(continued)*

Diaphragm 0B9T
Disc
Cervical Vertebral 0R93
Cervicothoracic Vertebral 0R95
Lumbar Vertebral 0S92
Lumbosacral 0S94
Thoracic Vertebral 0R99
Thoracolumbar Vertebral 0R9B
Duct
Common Bile 0F99
Cystic 0F98
Hepatic
Common 0F97
Left 0F96
Right 0F95
Lacrimal
Left 089Y
Right 089X
Pancreatic 0F9D
Accessory 0F9F
Parotid
Left 0C9C
Right 0C9B
Duodenum 0D99
Dura Mater 0092
Ear
External
Left 0991
Right 0990
External Auditory Canal
Left 0994
Right 0993
Inner
Left 099E
Right 099D
Middle
Left 0996
Right 0995
Elbow Region
Left 0X9C
Right 0X9B
Epididymis
Bilateral 0V9L
Left 0V9K
Right 0V9J
Epidural Space, Intracranial 0093
Epiglottis 0C9R
Esophagogastric Junction 0D94
Esophagus 0D95
Lower 0D93
Middle 0D92
Upper 0D91
Eustachian Tube
Left 099G
Right 099F
Extremity
Lower
Left 0Y9B
Right 0Y99
Upper
Left 0X97
Right 0X96
Eye
Left 0891
Right 0890
Eyelid
Lower
Left 089R
Right 089Q
Upper
Left 089P
Right 089N
Face 0W92
Fallopian Tube
Left 0U96
Right 0U95
Fallopian Tubes, Bilateral 0U97
Femoral Region
Left 0Y98
Right 0Y97

Drainage *(continued)*

Femoral Shaft
Left 0Q99
Right 0Q98
Femur
Lower
Left 0Q9C
Right 0Q9B
Upper
Left 0Q97
Right 0Q96
Fibula
Left 0Q9K
Right 0Q9J
Finger Nail 0H9Q
Foot
Left 0Y9N
Right 0Y9M
Gallbladder 0F94
Gingiva
Lower 0C96
Upper 0C95
Gland
Adrenal
Bilateral 0G94
Left 0G92
Right 0G93
Lacrimal
Left 089W
Right 089V
Minor Salivary
0C9J
Parotid
Left 0C99
Right 0C98
Pituitary 0G90
Sublingual
Left 0C9F
Right 0C9D
Submaxillary
Left 0C9H
Right 0C9G
Vestibular 0U9L
Glenoid Cavity
Left 0P98
Right 0P97
Glomus Jugulare
0G9C
Hand
Left 0X9K
Right 0X9J
Head 0W90
Humeral Head
Left 0P9D
Right 0P9C
Humeral Shaft
Left 0P9G
Right 0P9F
Hymen 0U9K
Hypothalamus 009A
Ileocecal Valve 0D9C
Ileum 0D9B
Inguinal Region
Left 0Y96
Right 0Y95
Intestine
Large 0D9E
Left 0D9G
Right 0D9F
Small 0D98
Iris
Left 089D
Right 089C
Jaw
Lower 0W95
Upper 0W94
Jejunum 0D9A
Joint
Acromioclavicular
Left 0R9H
Right 0R9G

Drainage *(continued)*

Joint *(continued)*
Ankle
Left 0S9G
Right 0S9F
Carpal
Left 0R9R
Right 0R9Q
Carpometacarpal
Left 0R9T
Right 0R9S
Cervical Vertebral 0R91
Cervicothoracic Vertebral
0R94
Coccygeal 0S96
Elbow
Left 0R9M
Right 0R9L
Finger Phalangeal
Left 0R9X
Right 0R9W
Hip
Left 0S9B
Right 0S99
Knee
Left 0S9D
Right 0S9C
Lumbar Vertebral 0S90
Lumbosacral 0S93
Metacarpophalangeal
Left 0R9V
Right 0R9U
Metatarsal-Phalangeal
Left 0S9N
Right 0S9M
Occipital-cervical 0R90
Sacrococcygeal 0S95
Sacroiliac
Left 0S98
Right 0S97
Shoulder
Left 0R9K
Right 0R9J
Sternoclavicular
Left 0R9F
Right 0R9E
Tarsal
Left 0S9J
Right 0S9H
Tarsometatarsal
Left 0S9L
Right 0S9K
Temporomandibular
Left 0R9D
Right 0R9C
Thoracic Vertebral 0R96
Thoracolumbar Vertebral
0R9A
Toe Phalangeal
Left 0S9Q
Right 0S9P
Wrist
Left 0R9P
Right 0R9N
Kidney
Left 0T91
Right 0T90
Kidney Pelvis
Left 0T94
Right 0T93
Knee Region
Left 0Y9G
Right 0Y9F
Larynx 0C9S
Leg
Lower
Left 0Y9J
Right 0Y9H
Upper
Left 0Y9D
Right 0Y9C

Drainage (continued)

Lens
Left 089K
Right 089J
Lip
Lower 0C91
Upper 0C90
Liver 0F90
Left Lobe 0F92
Right Lobe 0F91
Lung
Bilateral 0B9M
Left 0B9L
Lower Lobe
Left 0B9J
Right 0B9F
Middle Lobe, Right 0B9D
Right 0B9K
Upper Lobe
Left 0B9G
Right 0B9C
Lung Lingula 0B9H
Lymphatic
Aortic 079D
Axillary
Left 0796
Right 0795
Head 0790
Inguinal
Left 079J
Right 079H
Internal Mammary
Left 0799
Right 0798
Lower Extremity
Left 079G
Right 079F
Mesenteric 079B
Neck
Left 0792
Right 0791
Pelvis 079C
Thoracic Duct 079K
Thorax 0797
Upper Extremity
Left 0794
Right 0793
Mandible
Left 0N9V
Right 0N9T
Maxilla 0N9R
Mediastinum 0W9C
Medulla Oblongata 009D
Mesentery 0D9V
Metacarpal
Left 0P9Q
Right 0P9P
Metatarsal
Left 0Q9P
Right 0Q9N
Muscle
Abdomen
Left 0K9L
Right 0K9K
Extraocular
Left 089M
Right 089L
Facial 0K91
Foot
Left 0K9W
Right 0K9V
Hand
Left 0K9D
Right 0K9C
Head 0K90
Hip
Left 0K9P
Right 0K9N
Lower Arm and Wrist
Left 0K9B
Right 0K99

Drainage (continued)

Muscle (continued)
Lower Leg
Left 0K9T
Right 0K9S
Neck
Left 0K93
Right 0K92
Perineum 0K9M
Shoulder
Left 0K96
Right 0K95
Thorax
Left 0K9J
Right 0K9H
Tongue, Palate, Pharynx 0K94
Trunk
Left 0K9G
Right 0K9F
Upper Arm
Left 0K98
Right 0K97
Upper Leg
Left 0K9R
Right 0K9Q
Nasal Mucosa and Soft Tissue 099K
Nasopharynx 099N
Neck 0W96
Nerve
Abdominal Sympathetic 019M
Abducens 009L
Accessory 009R
Acoustic 009N
Brachial Plexus 0193
Cervical 0191
Cervical Plexus 0190
Facial 009M
Femoral 019D
Glossopharyngeal 009P
Head and Neck Sympathetic 019K
Hypoglossal 009S
Lumbar 019B
Lumbar Plexus 0199
Lumbar Sympathetic 019N
Lumbosacral Plexus 019A
Median 0195
Oculomotor 009H
Olfactory 009F
Optic 009G
Peroneal 019H
Phrenic 0192
Pudendal 019C
Radial 0196
Sacral 019R
Sacral Plexus 019Q
Sacral Sympathetic 019P
Sciatic 019F
Thoracic 0198
Thoracic Sympathetic 019L
Tibial 019G
Trigeminal 009K
Trochlear 009J
Ulnar 0194
Vagus 009Q
Nipple
Left 0H9X
Right 0H9W
Omentum 0D9U
Oral Cavity and Throat 0W93
Orbit
Left 0N9Q
Right 0N9P
Ovary
Bilateral 0U92
Left 0U91
Right 0U90
Palate
Hard 0C92
Soft 0C93
Pancreas 0F9G

Drainage (continued)

Para-aortic Body 0G99
Paraganglion Extremity 0G9F
Parathyroid Gland 0G9R
Inferior
Left 0G9P
Right 0G9N
Multiple 0G9Q
Superior
Left 0G9M
Right 0G9L
Patella
Left 0Q9F
Right 0Q9D
Pelvic Cavity 0W9J
Penis 0V9S
Pericardial Cavity 0W9D
Perineum
Female 0W9N
Male 0W9M
Peritoneal Cavity 0W9G
Peritoneum 0D9W
Phalanx
Finger
Left 0P9V
Right 0P9T
Thumb
Left 0P9S
Right 0P9R
Toe
Left 0Q9R
Right 0Q9Q
Pharynx 0C9M
Pineal Body 0G91
Pleura
Left 0B9P
Right 0B9N
Pleural Cavity
Left 0W9B
Right 0W99
Pons 009B
Prepuce 0V9T
Products of Conception
Amniotic Fluid
Diagnostic 1090
Therapeutic 1090
Fetal Blood 1090
Fetal Cerebrospinal Fluid 1090
Fetal Fluid, Other 1090
Fluid, Other 1090
Prostate 0V90
Radius
Left 0P9J
Right 0P9H
Rectum 0D9P
Retina
Left 089F
Right 089E
Retinal Vessel
Left 089H
Right 089G
Retroperitoneum 0W9H
Ribs
1 to 2 0P91
3 or More 0P92
Sacrum 0Q91
Scapula
Left 0P96
Right 0P95
Sclera
Left 0897
Right 0896
Scrotum 0V95
Septum, Nasal 099M
Shoulder Region
Left 0X93
Right 0X92
Sinus
Accessory 099P

Drainage (continued)

Sinus (continued)
Ethmoid
Left 099V
Right 099U
Frontal
Left 099T
Right 099S
Mastoid
Left 099C
Right 099B
Maxillary
Left 099R
Right 099Q
Sphenoid
Left 099X
Right 099W
Skin
Abdomen 0H97
Back 0H96
Buttock 0H98
Chest 0H95
Ear
Left 0H93
Right 0H92
Face 0H91
Foot
Left 0H9N
Right 0H9M
Hand
Left 0H9G
Right 0H9F
Inguinal 0H9A
Lower Arm
Left 0H9E
Right 0H9D
Lower Leg
Left 0H9L
Right 0H9K
Neck 0H94
Perineum 0H99
Scalp 0H90
Upper Arm
Left 0H9C
Right 0H9B
Upper Leg
Left 0H9J
Right 0H9H
Skull 0N90
Spinal Canal 009U
Spinal Cord
Cervical 009W
Lumbar 009Y
Thoracic 009X
Spinal Meninges 009T
Spleen 079P
Sternum 0P90
Stomach 0D96
Pylorus 0D97
Subarachnoid Space, Intracranial 0095
Subcutaneous Tissue and Fascia
Abdomen 0J98
Back 0J97
Buttock 0J99
Chest 0J96
Face 0J91
Foot
Left 0J9R
Right 0J9Q
Hand
Left 0J9K
Right 0J9J
Lower Arm
Left 0J9H
Right 0J9G
Lower Leg
Left 0J9P
Right 0J9N
Neck
Left 0J95

Drainage *(continued)*
Subcutaneous Tissue and
Fascia *(continued)*
Neck *(continued)*
Right 0J94
Pelvic Region 0J9C
Perineum 0J9B
Scalp 0J90
Upper Arm
Left 0J9F
Right 0J9D
Upper Leg
Left 0J9M
Right 0J9L
Subdural Space, Intracranial 0094
Tarsal
Left 0Q9M
Right 0Q9L
Tendon
Abdomen
Left 0L9G
Right 0L9F
Ankle
Left 0L9T
Right 0L9S
Foot
Left 0L9W
Right 0L9V
Hand
Left 0L98
Right 0L97
Head and Neck 0L90
Hip
Left 0L9K
Right 0L9J
Knee
Left 0L9R
Right 0L9Q
Lower Arm and Wrist
Left 0L96
Right 0L95
Lower Leg
Left 0L9P
Right 0L9N
Perineum 0L9H
Shoulder
Left 0L92
Right 0L91
Thorax
Left 0L9D
Right 0L9C
Electrocautery
Right 0L99
Upper Arm
Left 0L94
Right 0L93
Upper Leg
Left 0L9M
Right 0L9L
Testis
Bilateral 0V9C
Left 0V9B
Right 0V99
Thalamus 0099
Thymus 079M
Thyroid Gland 0G9K
Left Lobe 0G9G
Right Lobe 0G9H
Tibia
Left 0Q9H
Right 0Q9G
Toe Nail 0H9R
Tongue 0C97
Tonsils 0C9P
Tooth
Lower 0C9X
Upper 0C9W
Trachea 0B91
Tunica Vaginalis
Left 0V97
Right 0V96

Drainage *(continued)*
Turbinate, Nasal 099L
Tympanic Membrane
Left 0998
Right 0997
Ulna
Left 0P9L
Right 0P9K
Ureter
Left 0T97
Right 0T96
Ureters, Bilateral 0T98
Urethra 0T9D
Uterine Supporting Structure 0U94
Uterus 0U99
Uvula 0C9N
Vagina 0U9G
Vas Deferens
Bilateral 0V9Q
Left 0V9P
Right 0V9N
Vein
Axillary
Left 0598
Right 0597
Azygos 0590
Basilic
Left 059C
Right 059B
Brachial
Left 059A
Right 0599
Cephalic
Left 059F
Right 059D
Colic 0697
Common Iliac
Left 069D
Right 069C
Esophageal 0693
External Iliac
Left 069G
Right 069F
External Jugular
Left 059Q
Right 059P
Face
Left 059V
Right 059T
Femoral
Left 069N
Right 069M
Foot
Left 069V
Right 069T
Gastric 0692
Hand
Left 059H
Right 059G
Hemiazygos 0591
Hepatic 0694
Hypogastric
Left 069J
Right 069H
Inferior Mesenteric 0696
Innominate
Left 0594
Right 0593
Internal Jugular
Left 059N
Right 059M
Intracranial 059L
Lower 069Y
Portal 0698
Renal
Left 069B
Right 0699
Saphenous
Left 069Q
Right 069P
Splenic 0691

Drainage *(continued)*
Vein *(continued)*
Subclavian
Left 0596
Right 0595
Superior Mesenteric 0695
Upper 059Y
Vertebral
Left 059S
Right 059R
Vena Cava, Inferior 0690
Vertebra
Cervical 0P93
Lumbar 0Q90
Thoracic 0P94
Vesicle
Bilateral 0V93
Left 0V92
Right 0V91
Vitreous
Left 0895
Right 0894
Vocal Cord
Left 0C9V
Right 0C9T
Vulva 0U9M
Wrist Region
Left 0X9H
Right 0X9G
Dressing
Abdominal Wall 2W23X4Z
Arm
Lower
Left 2W2DX4Z
Right 2W2CX4Z
Upper
Left 2W2BX4Z
Right 2W2AX4Z
Back 2W25X4Z
Chest Wall 2W24X4Z
Extremity
Lower
Left 2W2MX4Z
Right 2W2LX4Z
Upper
Left 2W29X4Z
Right 2W28X4Z
Face 2W21X4Z
Finger
Left 2W2KX4Z
Right 2W2JX4Z
Foot
Left 2W2TX4Z
Right 2W2SX4Z
Hand
Left 2W2FX4Z
Right 2W2EX4Z
Head 2W20X4Z
Inguinal Region
Left 2W27X4Z
Right 2W26X4Z
Leg
Lower
Left 2W2RX4Z
Right 2W2QX4Z
Upper
Left 2W2PX4Z
Right 2W2NX4Z
Neck 2W22X4Z
Thumb
Left 2W2HX4Z
Right 2W2GX4Z
Toe
Left 2W2VX4Z
Right 2W2UX4Z
Driver stent (RX) (OTW)
use Intraluminal Device
Drotrecogin alfa, infusion
see Introduction of Recombinant
Human-activated
Protein C

Duct of Santorini
use Duct, Pancreatic, Accessory
Duct of Wirsung
use Duct, Pancreatic
Ductogram, mammary
see Plain Radiography, Skin,
Subcutaneous Tissue and Breast
BH0
Ductography, mammary
see Plain Radiography, Skin,
Subcutaneous Tissue and Breast
BH0
Ductus deferens
use Vas Deferens
use Vas Deferens, Bilateral
use Vas Deferens, Left
use Vas Deferens, Right
Duodenal ampulla
use Ampulla of Vater
Duodenectomy
see Excision, Duodenum 0DB9
see Resection, Duodenum 0DT9
Duodenocholedochotomy
see Drainage, Gallbladder 0F94
Duodenocystostomy
see Bypass, Gallbladder 0F14
see Drainage, Gallbladder 0F94
Duodenoenterostomy
see Bypass, Gastrointestinal System
0D1
see Drainage, Gastrointestinal
System 0D9
Duodenojejunal flexure
use Jejunum
Duodenolysis
see Release, Duodenum 0DN9
Duodenorrhaphy
see Repair, Duodenum 0DQ9
Duodenoscopy, single-use (aScope™
Duodeno) (EXALT™) Model
D) *see* New Technology,
Hepatobiliary System and
Pancreas XFJ
Duodenostomy
see Bypass, Duodenum 0D19
see Drainage, Duodenum 0D99
Duodenotomy
see Drainage, Duodenum 0D99
**DuraGraft® Endothelial Damage
Inhibitor**
use Endothelial Damage Inhibitor
**DuraHeart Left Ventricular Assist
System**
use Implantable Heart Assist System
in Heart and Great Vessels
Dural venous sinus
use Vein, Intracranial
Dura mater, intracranial
use Dura Mater
Dura mater, spinal
use Spinal Meninges
Durata® Defibrillation Lead
use Cardiac Lead, Defibrillator in
02H
Durvalumab Antineoplastic XW0
DynaClip® (Forte)
use Internal Fixation Device,
Sustained Compression in 0RG
use Internal Fixation Device,
Sustained Compression in 0SG
DynaNail® (Helix) (Hybrid)(Mini)
use Internal Fixation Device,
Sustained Compression in 0RG
use Internal Fixation Device,
Sustained Compression in 0SG
**Dynesys® Dynamic Stabilization
System**
use Spinal Stabilization Device,
Pedicle-Based in 0RH
use Spinal Stabilization Device,
Pedicle-Based in 0SH

E

E-Luminexx™ (Biliary)(Vascular) Stent
use Intraluminal Device

Earlobe
use Ear, External, Bilateral
use Ear, External, Left
use Ear, External, Right

ECC02R (Extracorporeal Carbon Dioxide Removal) 5A0920Z

Echocardiogram
see Ultrasonography, Heart B24

EchoGo Heart Failure 1.0 software XXE2X19

Echography
see Ultrasonography

EchoTip® Insight™ Portosystemic Pressure Gradient Measurement System 4A044B2

ECMO
see Performance, Circulatory 5A15

ECMO, intraoperative
see Performance, Circulatory 5A15A

Eculizumab XW0

EDWARDS INTUITY Elite valve system (rapid deployment technique) *see* Replacement, Valve, Aortic 02RF

EEG (electroencephalogram)
see Measurement, Central Nervous 4A00

EGD (esophagogastroduodenoscopy) 0DJ08ZZ

Eighth cranial nerve
use Nerve, Acoustic

Ejaculatory duct
use Vas Deferens
use Vas Deferens, Bilateral
use Vas Deferens, Left
use Vas Deferens, Right

EKG (electrocardiogram)
see Measurement, Cardiac 4A02

EKOS™ EkoSonic® Endovascular System
see Fragmentation, Artery

Eladocagene exuparvovec XW0Q316

Electrical bone growth stimulator (EBGS)
use Bone Growth Stimulator in Head and Facial Bones
use Bone Growth Stimulator in Lower Bones
use Bone Growth Stimulator in Upper Bones

Electrical muscle stimulation (EMS) lead
use Stimulator Lead in Muscles

Electrocautery
Destruction
see Destruction
Repair
see Repair

Electroconvulsive Therapy
Bilateral-Multiple Seizure GZB3ZZZ
Bilateral-Single Seizure GZB2ZZZ
Electroconvulsive Therapy, Other GZB4ZZZ
Unilateral-Multiple Seizure GZB1ZZZ
Unilateral-Single Seizure GZB0ZZZ

Electroencephalogram (EEG)
see Measurement, Central Nervous 4A00

Electromagnetic Therapy
Central Nervous 6A22
Urinary 6A21

Electronic muscle stimulator lead
use Stimulator Lead in Muscles

Electrophysiologic stimulation (EPS)
see Measurement, Cardiac 4A02

Electroshock therapy
see Electroconvulsive Therapy

Elevation, bone fragments, skull
see Reposition, Head and Facial Bones 0NS

Eleventh cranial nerve
use Nerve, Accessory

Ellipsys® vascular access system
see New Technology, Cardiovascular System X2K

Elranatamab Antineoplastic XW013L9

Eluvia™ Drug-Eluting Vascular Stent System
use Intraluminal Device, Sustained Release Drug-eluting in New Technology
use Intraluminal Device, Sustained Release Drug-eluting, Two in New Technology
use Intraluminal Device, Sustained Release Drug-eluting, Three in New Technology
use Intraluminal Device, Sustained Release Drug-eluting, Four or More in New Technology

ELZONRIS™
use Tagraxofusp-erzs Antineoplastic

Embolectomy
see Extirpation

Embolization
see Occlusion
see Restriction

Embolization coil(s)
use Intraluminal Device

EMG (electromyogram)
see Measurement, Musculoskeletal 4A0F

Encephalon
use Brain

Endarterectomy
see Extirpation, Lower Arteries 04C
see Extirpation, Upper Arteries 03C

Endeavor® (III)(IV) (Sprint) Zotarolimus-eluting Coronary Stent System
use Intraluminal Device, Drug-eluting in Heart and Great Vessels

EndoAVF procedure, using magnetic-guided radiofrequency
see Bypass, Upper Arteries 031

EndoAVF procedure, using thermal resistance energy
see New Technology, Cardiovascular System X2K

Endologix AFX® Endovascular AAA System
use Intraluminal Device

EndoSure® sensor
use Monitoring Device, Pressure Sensor in 02H

ENDOTAK RELIANCE® (G) Defibrillation Lead
use Cardiac Lead, Defibrillator in 02H

Endothelial damage inhibitor, applied to vein graft XY0VX83

Endotracheal tube (cuffed)(double-lumen)
use Intraluminal Device, Endotracheal Airway in Respiratory System

Endovascular fistula creation, using magnetic-guided radiofrequency
see Bypass, Upper Arteries 031

Endovascular fistula creation, using thermal resistance energy
see New Technology, Cardiovascular System X2K

Endurant® II AAA stent graft system
use Intraluminal Device

Endurant® Endovascular Stent Graft
use Intraluminal Device

Engineered Allogeneic Thymus Tissue XW020D8

Engineered Chimeric Antigen Receptor T-cell Immunotherapy
Allogeneic XW0
Autologous XW0

Enlargement
see Dilation
see Repair

EnRhythm
use Pacemaker, Dual Chamber in 0JH

ENROUTE® Transcarotid Neuroprotection System
see New Technology, Cardiovascular System X2A

ENSPRYNG™
use Satralizumab-mwge

Enterorrhaphy
see Repair, Gastrointestinal System 0DQ

Enterra gastric neurostimulator
use Stimulator Generator, Multiple Array in 0JH

Enucleation
Eyeball
see Resection, Eye 08T
Eyeball with prosthetic implant
see Replacement, Eye 08R

Epcoritamab Monoclonal Antibody XW013S9

Ependyma
use Cerebral Ventricle

Epicel® cultured epidermal autograft
use Autologous Tissue Substitute

Epic™ Stented Tissue Valve (aortic)
use Zooplastic Tissue in Heart and Great Vessels

Epidermis
use Skin

Epididymectomy
see Excision, Male Reproductive System 0VB
see Resection, Male Reproductive System 0VT

Epididymoplasty
see Repair, Male Reproductive System 0VQ
see Supplement, Male Reproductive System 0VU

Epididymorrhaphy
see Repair, Male Reproductive System 0VQ

Epididymotomy
see Drainage, Male Reproductive System 0V9

Epidural space, spinal
use Spinal Canal

Epiphysiodesis
see Insertion of device in Lower Bones 0QH
see Insertion of device in Upper Bones 0PH
see Repair, Lower Bones 0QQ
see Repair, Upper Bones 0PQ

Epiploic foramen
use Peritoneum

Epiretinal Visual Prosthesis
Left 08H105Z
Right 08H005Z

Episiorrhaphy
see Repair, Perineum, Female 0WQN

Episiotomy
see Division, Perineum, Female 0W8N

Epithalamus
use Thalamus

Epitrochlear lymph node
use Lymphatic, Upper Extremity, Left
use Lymphatic, Upper Extremity, Right

EPS (electrophysiologic stimulation)
see Measurement, Cardiac 4A02

Eptifibatide, infusion
see Introduction of Platelet Inhibitor

ERCP (endoscopic retrograde cholangiopancreatography)
see Fluoroscopy, Hepatobiliary System and Pancreas BF1

Erdafitinib Antineoplastic XW0DXL5

Erector spinae muscle
use Muscle, Trunk, Left
use Muscle, Trunk, Right

ERLEADA™
use Apalutamide Antineoplastic

Esketamine Hydrochloride XW097M5

Esophageal artery
use Upper Artery

Esophageal obturator airway (EOA)
use Intraluminal Device, Airway in Gastrointestinal System

Esophageal plexus
use Nerve, Thoracic Sympathetic

Esophagectomy
see Excision, Gastrointestinal System 0DB
see Resection, Gastrointestinal System 0DT

Esophagocoloplasty
see Repair, Gastrointestinal System 0DQ
see Supplement, Gastrointestinal System 0DU

Esophagoenterostomy
see Bypass, Gastrointestinal System 0D1
see Drainage, Gastrointestinal System 0D9

Esophagoesophagostomy
see Bypass, Gastrointestinal System 0D1
see Drainage, Gastrointestinal System 0D9

Esophagogastrectomy
see Excision, Gastrointestinal System 0DB
see Resection, Gastrointestinal System 0DT

Esophagogastroduodenoscopy (EGD) 0DJ08ZZ

Esophagogastroplasty
see Repair, Gastrointestinal System 0DQ
see Supplement, Gastrointestinal System 0DU

Esophagogastroscopy 0DJ68ZZ

Esophagogastrostomy
see Bypass, Gastrointestinal System 0D1
see Drainage, Gastrointestinal System 0D9

Esophagojejunoplasty
see Supplement, Gastrointestinal System 0DU

Esophagojejunostomy
see Bypass, Gastrointestinal System 0D1
see Drainage, Gastrointestinal System 0D9

Esophagomyotomy
see Division, Esophagogastric Junction 0D84

Esophagoplasty
see Repair, Gastrointestinal System 0DQ
see Replacement, Esophagus 0DR5
see Supplement, Gastrointestinal System 0DU
Esophagoplication
see Restriction, Gastrointestinal System 0DV
Esophagorrhaphy
see Repair, Gastrointestinal System 0DQ
Esophagoscopy 0DJ08ZZ
Esophagotomy
see Drainage, Gastrointestinal System 0D9
Esteem® implantable hearing system
use Hearing Device in Ear, Nose, Sinus
ESWL (extracorporeal shock wave lithotripsy)
see Fragmentation
Ethmoidal air cell
use Sinus, Ethmoid, Left
use Sinus, Ethmoid, Right
Ethmoidectomy
see Excision, Ear, Nose, Sinus 09B
see Excision, Head and Facial Bones 0NB
see Resection, Ear, Nose, Sinus 09T
see Resection, Head and Facial Bones 0NT
Ethmoidotomy
see Drainage, Ear, Nose, Sinus 099
Evacuation
Hematoma
see Extirpation
Other Fluid
see Drainage
Evera (XT)(S)(DR/VR)
use Defibrillator Generator in 0JH
Everolimus-eluting coronary stent
use Intraluminal Device, Drug-eluting in Heart and Great Vessels
EV ICD System (Extravascular implantable defibrillator lead) use Defibrillator Lead in Anatomical Regions, General
Evisceration
Eyeball
see Resection, Eye 08T
Eyeball with prosthetic implant
see Replacement, Eye 08R
EVUSHELD™ use Tixagevimab and Cilgavimab Monoclonal Antibody
Ex-PRESS™ mini glaucoma shunt
use Synthetic Substitute
Exagamglogene Autotemcel XW1
EXALT™ Model D Single-Use Duodenoscope
see New Technology, Hepatobiliary System and Pancreas XFJ
Examination
see Inspection
Exchange
see Change device in
Excision
Abdominal Wall 0WBF
Acetabulum
Left 0QB5
Right 0QB4
Adenoids 0CBQ
Ampulla of Vater 0FBC
Anal Sphincter 0DBR
Ankle Region
Left 0YBL
Right 0YBK
Anus 0DBQ
Aorta
Abdominal 04B0

Excision (continued)
Aorta (continued)
Thoracic
Ascending/Arch 02BX
Descending 02BW
Aortic Body 0GBD
Appendix 0DBJ
Arm
Lower
Left 0XBF
Right 0XBD
Upper
Left 0XB9
Right 0XB8
Artery
Anterior Tibial
Left 04BQ
Right 04BP
Axillary
Left 03B6
Right 03B5
Brachial
Left 03B8
Right 03B7
Celiac 04B1
Colic
Left 04B7
Middle 04B8
Right 04B6
Common Carotid
Left 03BJ
Right 03BH
Common Iliac
Left 04BD
Right 04BC
External Carotid
Left 03BN
Right 03BM
External Iliac
Left 04BJ
Right 04BH
Face 03BR
Femoral
Left 04BL
Right 04BK
Foot
Left 04BW
Right 04BV
Gastric 04B2
Hand
Left 03BF
Right 03BD
Hepatic 04B3
Inferior Mesenteric 04BB
Innominate 03B2
Internal Carotid
Left 03BL
Right 03BK
Internal Iliac
Left 04BF
Right 04BE
Internal Mammary
Left 03B1
Right 03B0
Intracranial 03BG
Lower 04BY
Peroneal
Left 04BU
Right 04BT
Popliteal
Left 04BN
Right 04BM
Posterior Tibial
Left 04BS
Right 04BR
Pulmonary
Left 02BR
Right 02BQ
Pulmonary Trunk 02BP
Radial
Left 03BC
Right 03BB

Excision (continued)
Artery (continued)
Renal
Left 04BA
Right 04B9
Splenic 04B4
Subclavian
Left 03B4
Right 03B3
Superior Mesenteric 04B5
Temporal
Left 03BT
Right 03BS
Thyroid
Left 03BV
Right 03BU
Ulnar
Left 03BA
Right 03B9
Upper 03BY
Vertebral
Left 03BQ
Right 03BP
Atrium
Left 02B7
Right 02B6
Auditory Ossicle
Left 09BA
Right 09B9
Axilla
Left 0XB5
Right 0XB4
Back
Lower 0WBL
Upper 0WBK
Basal Ganglia 00B8
Bladder 0TBB
Bladder Neck 0TBC
Bone
Ethmoid
Left 0NBG
Right 0NBF
Frontal 0NB1
Hyoid 0NBX
Lacrimal
Left 0NBJ
Right 0NBH
Nasal 0NBB
Occipital 0NB7
Palatine
Left 0NBL
Right 0NBK
Parietal
Left 0NB4
Right 0NB3
Pelvic
Left 0QB3
Right 0QB2
Sphenoid 0NBC
Temporal
Left 0NB6
Right 0NB5
Zygomatic
Left 0NBN
Right 0NBM
Brain 00B0
Breast
Bilateral 0HBV
Left 0HBU
Right 0HBT
Supernumerary 0HBY
Bronchus
Lingula 0BB9
Lower Lobe
Left 0BBB
Right 0BB6
Main
Left 0BB7
Right 0BB3
Middle Lobe, Right 0BB5
Upper Lobe
Left 0BB8
Right 0BB4

Excision (continued)
Buccal Mucosa 0CB4
Bursa and Ligament
Abdomen
Left 0MBJ
Right 0MBH
Ankle
Left 0MBR
Right 0MBQ
Elbow
Left 0MB4
Right 0MB3
Foot
Left 0MBT
Right 0MBS
Hand
Left 0MB8
Right 0MB7
Head and Neck 0MB0
Hip
Left 0MBM
Right 0MBL
Knee
Left 0MBP
Right 0MBN
Lower Extremity
Left 0MBW
Right 0MBV
Rib(s) 0MBG
Perineum 0MBK
Shoulder
Left 0MB2
Right 0MB1
Spine
Lower 0MBD
Upper 0MBC
Sternum 0MBF
Upper Extremity
Left 0MB8
Right 0MB9
Wrist
Left 0MB6
Right 0MB5
Buttock
Left 0YB1
Right 0YB0
Carina 0BB2
Carotid Bodies, Bilateral 0GB8
Carotid Body
Left 0GB6
Right 0GB7
Carpal
Left 0PBN
Right 0PBM
Cecum 0DBH
Cerebellum 00BC
Cerebral Hemisphere 00B7
Cerebral Meninges 00B1
Cerebral Ventricle 00B6
Cervix 0UBC
Chest Wall 0WB8
Chordae Tendineae 02B9
Choroid
Left 08BB
Right 08BA
Cisterna Chyli 07BL
Clavicle
Left 0PBB
Right 0PB9
Clitoris 0UBJ
Coccygeal Glomus 0GBB
Coccyx 0QBS
Colon
Ascending 0DBK
Descending 0DBM
Sigmoid 0DBN
Transverse 0DBL
Conduction Mechanism 02B8
Conjunctiva
Left 08BTXZ
Right 08BSXZ

Excision (continued)

Cord
  Bilateral 0VBH
  Left 0VBG
  Right 0VBF
Cornea
  Left 08B9XZ
  Right 08B8XZ
Cul-de-sac 0UBF
Diaphragm 0BBT
Disc
  Cervical Vertebral 0RB3
  Cervicothoracic Vertebral 0RB5
  Lumbar Vertebral 0SB2
  Lumbosacral 0SB4
  Thoracic Vertebral 0RB9
  Thoracolumbar Vertebral 0RBB
Duct
  Common Bile 0FB9
  Cystic 0FB8
  Hepatic
    Common 0FB7
    Left 0FB6
    Right 0FB5
  Lacrimal
    Left 08BY
    Right 08BX
  Pancreatic 0FBD
    Accessory 0FBF
  Parotid
    Left 0CBC
    Right 0CBB
Duodenum 0DB9
Dura Mater 00B2
Ear
  External
    Left 09B1
    Right 09B0
  External Auditory Canal
    Left 09B4
    Right 09B3
  Inner
    Left 09BE
    Right 09BD
  Middle
    Left 09B6
    Right 09B5
Elbow Region
  Left 0XBC
  Right 0XBB
Epididymis
  Bilateral 0VBL
  Left 0VBK
  Right 0VBJ
Epiglottis 0CBR
Esophagogastric Junction 0DB4
Esophagus 0DB5
  Lower 0DB3
  Middle 0DB2
  Upper 0DB1
Eustachian Tube
  Left 09BG
  Right 09BF
Extremity
  Lower
    Left 0YBB
    Right 0YB9
  Upper
    Left 0XB7
    Right 0XB6
Eye
  Left 08B1
  Right 08B0
Eyelid
  Lower
    Left 08BR
    Right 08BQ
  Upper
    Left 08BP
    Right 08BN
Face 0WB2

Excision (continued)

Fallopian Tube
  Left 0UB6
  Right 0UB5
Fallopian Tubes, Bilateral 0UB7
Femoral Region
  Left 0YB8
  Right 0YB7
Femoral Shaft
  Left 0QB9
  Right 0QB8
Femur
  Lower
    Left 0QBC
    Right 0QBB
  Upper
    Left 0QB7
    Right 0QB6
Fibula
  Left 0QBK
  Right 0QBJ
Finger Nail 0HBQXZ
Floor of mouth
  see Excision, Oral Cavity and
    Throat 0WB3
Foot
  Left 0YBN
  Right 0YBM
Gallbladder 0FB4
Gingiva
  Lower 0CB6
  Upper 0CB5
Gland
  Adrenal
    Bilateral 0GB4
    Left 0GB2
    Right 0GB3
  Lacrimal
    Left 08BW
    Right 08BV
  Minor Salivary 0CBJ
  Parotid
    Left 0CB9
    Right 0CB8
  Pituitary 0GB0
  Sublingual
    Left 0CBF
    Right 0CBD
  Submaxillary
    Left 0CBH
    Right 0CBG
  Vestibular 0UBL
Glenoid Cavity
  Left 0PB8
  Right 0PB7
Glomus Jugulare 0GBC
Hand
  Left 0XBK
  Right 0XBJ
Head 0WB0
Humeral Head
  Left 0PBD
  Right 0PBC
Humeral Shaft
  Left 0PBG
  Right 0PBF
Hymen 0UBK
Hypothalamus 00BA
Ileocecal Valve 0DBC
Ileum 0DBB
Inguinal Region
  Left 0YB6
  Right 0YB5
Intestine
  Large 0DBE
    Left 0DBG
    Right 0DBF
  Small 0DB8
Iris
  Left 08BD3Z
  Right 08BC3Z

Excision (continued)

Jaw
  Lower 0WB5
  Upper 0WB4
Jejunum 0DBA
Joint
  Acromioclavicular
    Left 0RBH
    Right 0RBG
  Ankle
    Left 0SBG
    Right 0SBF
  Carpal
    Left 0RBR
    Right 0RBQ
  Carpometacarpal
    Left 0RBT
    Right 0RBS
  Cervical Vertebral 0RB1
  Cervicothoracic Vertebral 0RB4
  Coccygeal 0SB6
  Elbow
    Left 0RBM
    Right 0RBL
  Finger Phalangeal
    Left 0RBX
    Right 0RBW
  Hip
    Left 0SBB
    Right 0SB9
  Knee
    Left 0SBD
    Right 0SBC
  Lumbar Vertebral
    0SB0
  Lumbosacral 0SB3
  Metacarpophalangeal
    Left 0RBV
    Right 0RBU
  Metatarsal-Phalangeal
    Left 0SBN
    Right 0SBM
  Occipital-cervical
    0RB0
  Sacrococcygeal 0SB5
  Sacroiliac
    Left 0SB8
    Right 0SB7
  Shoulder
    Left 0RBK
    Right 0RBJ
  Sternoclavicular
    Left 0RBF
    Right 0RBE
  Tarsal
    Left 0SBJ
    Right 0SBH
  Tarsometatarsal
    Left 0SBL
    Right 0SBK
  Temporomandibular
    Left 0RBD
    Right 0RBC
  Thoracic Vertebral 0RB6
  Thoracolumbar Vertebral 0RBA
  Toe Phalangeal
    Left 0SBQ
    Right 0SBP
  Wrist
    Left 0RBP
    Right 0RBN
Kidney
  Left 0TB1
  Right 0TB0
Kidney Pelvis
  Left 0TB4
  Right 0TB3
Knee Region
  Left 0YBG
  Right 0YBF
Larynx 0CBS

Excision (continued)

Leg
  Lower
    Left 0YBJ
    Right 0YBH
  Upper
    Left 0YBD
    Right 0YBC
Lens
  Left 08BK3Z
  Right 08BJ3Z
Lip
  Lower 0CB1
  Upper 0CB0
Liver 0FB0
  Left Lobe 0FB2
  Right Lobe 0FB1
Lung
  Bilateral 0BBM
  Left 0BBL
  Lower Lobe
    Left 0BBJ
    Right 0BBF
  Middle Lobe, Right 0BBD
  Right 0BBK
  Upper Lobe
    Left 0BBG
    Right 0BBC
Lung Lingula 0BBH
Lymphatic
  Aortic 07BD
  Axillary
    Left 07B6
    Right 07B5
  Head 07B0
  Inguinal
    Left 07BJ
    Right 07BH
  Internal Mammary
    Left 07B9
    Right 07B8
  Lower Extremity
    Left 07BG
    Right 07BF
  Mesenteric 07BB
  Neck
    Left 07B2
    Right 07B1
  Pelvis 07BC
  Thoracic Duct 07BK
  Thorax 07B7
  Upper Extremity
    Left 07B4
    Right 07B3
Mandible
  Left 0NBV
  Right 0NBT
Maxilla 0NBR
Mediastinum 0WBC
Medulla Oblongata 00BD
Mesentery 0DBV
Metacarpal
  Left 0PBQ
  Right 0PBP
Metatarsal
  Left 0QBP
  Right 0QBN
Muscle
  Abdomen
    Left 0KBL
    Right 0KBK
  Extraocular
    Left 08BM
    Right 08BL
  Facial 0KB1
  Foot
    Left 0KBW
    Right 0KBV
  Hand
    Left 0KBD
    Right 0KBC

Excision (*continued*)

Head 0KB0
Hip
  Left 0KBP
  Right 0KBN
Lower Arm and Wrist
  Left 0KBB
  Right 0KB9
Lower Leg
  Left 0KBT
  Right 0KBS
Neck
  Left 0KB3
  Right 0KB2
Papillary 02BD
Perineum 0KBM
Shoulder
  Left 0KB6
  Right 0KB5
Thorax
  Left 0KBJ
  Right 0KBH
Tongue, Palate, Pharynx 0KB4
Trunk
  Left 0KBG
  Right 0KBF
Upper Arm
  Left 0KB8
  Right 0KB7
Upper Leg
  Left 0KBR
  Right 0KBQ
Nasal Mucosa and Soft Tissue 09BK
Nasopharynx 09BN
Neck 0WB6
Nerve
  Abdominal Sympathetic 01BM
  Abducens 00BL
  Accessory 00BR
  Acoustic 00BN
  Brachial Plexus 01B3
  Cervical 01B1
  Cervical Plexus 01B0
  Facial 00BM
  Femoral 01BD
  Glossopharyngeal 00BP
  Head and Neck Sympathetic 01BK
  Hypoglossal 00BS
  Lumbar 01BB
  Lumbar Plexus 01B9
  Lumbar Sympathetic 01BN
  Lumbosacral Plexus 01BA
  Median 01B5
  Oculomotor 00BH
  Olfactory 00BF
  Optic 00BG
  Peroneal 01BH
  Phrenic 01B2
  Pudendal 01BC
  Radial 01B6
  Sacral 01BR
  Sacral Plexus 01BQ
  Sacral Sympathetic 01BP
  Sciatic 01BF
  Thoracic 01B8
  Thoracic Sympathetic 01BL
  Tibial 01BG
  Trigeminal 00BK
  Trochlear 00BJ
  Ulnar 01B4
  Vagus 00BQ
Nipple
  Left 0HBX
  Right 0HBW
Omentum 0DBU
Oral Cavity and Throat 0WB3
Orbit
  Left 0NBQ
  Right 0NBP

Excision (*continued*)

Ovary
  Bilateral 0UB2
  Left 0UB1
  Right 0UB0
Palate
  Hard 0CB2
  Soft 0CB3
Pancreas 0FBG
Para-aortic Body 0GB9
Paraganglion Extremity 0GBF
Parathyroid Gland 0GBR
  Inferior
    Left 0GBP
    Right 0GBN
  Multiple 0GBQ
  Superior
    Left 0GBM
    Right 0GBL
Patella
  Left 0QBF
  Right 0QBD
Penis 0VBS
Pericardium 02BN
Perineum
  Female 0WBN
  Male 0WBM
Peritoneum 0DBW
Phalanx
  Finger
    Left 0PBV
    Right 0PBT
  Thumb
    Left 0PBS
    Right 0PBR
  Toe
    Left 0QBR
    Right 0QBQ
Pharynx 0CBM
Pineal Body 0GB1
Pleura
  Left 0BBP
  Right 0BBN
Pons 00BB
Prepuce 0VBT
Prostate 0VB0
Radius
  Left 0PBJ
  Right 0PBH
Rectum 0DBP
Retina
  Left 08BF3Z
  Right 08BE3Z
Retroperitoneum 0WBH
Ribs
  1 to 2 0PB1
  3 or More 0PB2
Sacrum 0QB1
Scapula
  Left 0PB6
  Right 0PB5
Sclera
  Left 08B7XZ
  Right 08B6XZ
Scrotum 0VB5
Septum
  Atrial 02B5
  Nasal 09BM
  Ventricular 02BM
Shoulder Region
  Left 0XB3
  Right 0XB2
Sinus
  Accessory 09BP
  Ethmoid
    Left 09BV
    Right 09BU
  Frontal
    Left 09BT
    Right 09BS

Excision (*continued*)

Sinus (*continued*)
  Mastoid
    Left 09BC
    Right 09BB
  Maxillary
    Left 09BR
    Right 09BQ
  Sphenoid
    Left 09BX
    Right 09BW
Skin
  Abdomen 0HB7XZ
  Back 0HB6XZ
  Buttock 0HB8XZ
  Chest 0HB5XZ
  Ear
    Left 0HB3XZ
    Right 0HB2XZ
  Face 0HB1XZ
  Foot
    Left 0HBNXZ
    Right 0HBMXZ
  Hand
    Left 0HBGXZ
    Right 0HBFXZ
  Inguinal 0HBAXZ
  Lower Arm
    Left 0HBEXZ
    Right 0HBDXZ
  Lower Leg
    Left 0HBLXZ
    Right 0HBKXZ
  Neck 0HB4XZ
  Perineum 0HB9XZ
  Scalp 0HB0XZ
  Upper Arm
    Left 0HBCXZ
    Right 0HBBXZ
  Upper Leg
    Left 0HBJXZ
    Right 0HBHXZ
Skull 0NB0
Spinal Cord
  Cervical 00BW
  Lumbar 00BY
  Thoracic 00BX
Spinal Meninges 00BT
Spleen 07BP
Sternum 0PB0
Stomach 0DB6
  Pylorus 0DB7
Subcutaneous Tissue and Fascia
  Abdomen 0JB8
  Back 0JB7
  Buttock 0JB9
  Chest 0JB6
  Face 0JB1
  Foot
    Left 0JBR
    Right 0JBQ
  Hand
    Left 0JBK
    Right 0JBJ
  Lower Arm
    Left 0JBH
    Right 0JBG
  Lower Leg
    Left 0JBP
    Right 0JBN
  Neck
    Left 0JB5
    Right 0JB4
  Pelvic Region 0JBC
  Perineum 0JBB
  Scalp 0JB0
  Upper Arm
    Left 0JBF
    Right 0JBD
  Upper Leg
    Left 0JBM

Excision (*continued*)

Subcutaneous Tissue and Fascia (*continued*)
  Upper Leg (*continued*)
    Right 0JBL
Tarsal
  Left 0QBM
  Right 0QBL
Tendon
  Abdomen
    Left 0LBG
    Right 0LBF
  Ankle
    Left 0LBT
    Right 0LBS
  Foot
    Left 0LBW
    Right 0LBV
  Hand
    Left 0LB8
    Right 0LB7
  Head and Neck 0LB0
  Hip
    Left 0LBK
    Right 0LBJ
  Knee
    Left 0LBR
    Right 0LBQ
  Lower Arm and Wrist
    Left 0LB6
    Right 0LB5
  Lower Leg
    Left 0LBP
    Right 0LBN
  Perineum 0LBH
  Shoulder
    Left 0LB2
    Right 0LB1
  Thorax
    Left 0LBD
    Right 0LBC
  Trunk
    Left 0LBB
    Right 0LB9
  Upper Arm
    Left 0LB4
    Right 0LB3
  Upper Leg
    Left 0LBM
    Right 0LBL
Testis
  Bilateral 0VBC
  Left 0VBB
  Right 0VB9
Thalamus 00B9
Thymus 07BM
Thyroid Gland
  Left Lobe 0GBG
  Right Lobe 0GBH
Thyroid Gland Isthmus 0GBJ
Tibia
  Left 0QBH
  Right 0QBG
Toe Nail 0HBRXZ
Tongue 0CB7
Tonsils 0CBP
Tooth
  Lower 0CBX
  Upper 0CBW
Trachea 0BB1
Tunica Vaginalis
  Left 0VB7
  Right 0VB6
Turbinate, Nasal 09BL
Tympanic Membrane
  Left 09B8
  Right 09B7
Ulna
  Left 0PBL
  Right 0PBK

Excision (continued)

Ureter
  Left 0TB7
  Right 0TB6
Urethra 0TBD
Uterine Supporting Structure
  0UB4
Uterus 0UB9
Uvula 0CBN
Vagina 0UBG
Valve
  Aortic 02BF
  Mitral 02BG
  Pulmonary 02BH
  Tricuspid 02BJ
Vas Deferens
  Bilateral 0VBQ
  Left 0VBP
  Right 0VBN
Vein
  Axillary
    Left 05B8
    Right 05B7
  Azygos 05B0
  Basilic
    Left 05BC
    Right 05BB
  Brachial
    Left 05BA
    Right 05B9
  Cephalic
    Left 05BF
    Right 05BD
  Colic 06B7
  Common Iliac
    Left 06BD
    Right 06BC
  Coronary 02B4
  Esophageal 06B3
  External Iliac
    Left 06BG
    Right 06BF
  External Jugular
    Left 05BQ
    Right 05BP
  Face
    Left 05BV
    Right 05BT
  Femoral
    Left 06BN
    Right 06BM
  Foot
    Left 06BV
    Right 06BT
  Gastric 06B2
  Hand
    Left 05BH
    Right 05BG
  Hemiazygos
    05B1
  Hepatic 06B4
  Hypogastric
    Left 06BJ
    Right 06BH
  Inferior Mesenteric
    06B6
  Innominate
    Left 05B4
    Right 05B3
  Internal Jugular
    Left 05BN
    Right 05BM
  Intracranial 05BL
  Lower 06BY
  Portal 06B8
  Pulmonary
    Left 02BT
    Right 02BS
  Renal
    Left 06BB
    Right 06B9

Excision (continued)

Vein (continued)
  Saphenous
    Left 06BQ
    Right 06BP
  Splenic 06B1
  Subclavian
    Left 05B6
    Right 05B5
  Superior Mesenteric 06B5
  Upper 05BY
  Vertebral
    Left 05BS
    Right 05BR
Vena Cava
  Inferior 06B0
  Superior 02BV
Ventricle
  Left 02BL
  Right 02BK
Vertebra
  Cervical 0PB3
  Lumbar 0QB0
  Thoracic 0PB4
Vesicle
  Bilateral 0VB3
  Left 0VB2
  Right 0VB1
Vitreous
  Left 08B53Z
  Right 08B43Z
Vocal Cord
  Left 0CBV
  Right 0CBT
Vulva 0UBM
Wrist Region
  Left 0XBH
  Right 0XBG

EXCLUDER® AAA Endoprosthesis
  use Intraluminal Device
  use Intraluminal Device, Branched
    or Fenestrated, One or Two
    Arteries in 04V
  use Intraluminal Device, Branched
    or Fenestrated, Three or More
    Arteries in 04V

EXCLUDER® IBE Endoprosthesis
  use Intraluminal Device, Branched
    or Fenestrated, One or Two
    Arteries in 04V

Exclusion, Left atrial appendage (LAA)
  see Occlusion, Atrium, Left 02L7

Exercise, rehabilitation
  see Motor Treatment, Rehabilitation
    F07

Exploration
  see Inspection

Express® (LD) Premounted Stent System
  use Intraluminal Device

Express® Biliary SD Monorail® Premounted Stent System
  use Intraluminal Device

Express® SD Renal Monorail® Premounted Stent System
  use Intraluminal Device

Extensor carpi radialis muscle
  use Muscle, Lower Arm and Wrist,
    Left

Extensor carpi radialis muscle
  use Muscle, Lower Arm and Wrist,
    Right

Extensor carpi ulnaris muscle
  use Muscle, Lower Arm and Wrist,
    Left
  use Muscle, Lower Arm and Wrist,
    Right

Extensor digitorum brevis muscle
  use Muscle, Foot, Left
  use Muscle, Foot, Right

Extensor digitorum longus muscle
  use Muscle, Lower Leg, Left
  use Muscle, Lower Leg, Right

Extensor hallucis brevis muscle
  use Muscle, Foot, Left
  use Muscle, Foot, Right

Extensor hallucis longus muscle
  use Muscle, Lower Leg, Left
  use Muscle, Lower Leg, Right

External anal sphincter
  use Anal Sphincter

External auditory meatus
  use Ear, External Auditory Canal,
    Left
  use Ear, External Auditory Canal,
    Right

External fixator
  use External Fixation Device in
    Head and Facial Bones
  use External Fixation Device in
    Lower Bones
  use External Fixation Device in
    Lower Joints
  use External Fixation Device in
    Upper Bones
  use External Fixation Device in
    Upper Joints

External maxillary artery
  use Artery, Face

External naris
  use Nasal Mucosa and Soft
    Tissue

External oblique aponeurosis
  use Subcutaneous Tissue and Fascia,
    Trunk

External oblique muscle
  use Muscle, Abdomen, Left
  use Muscle, Abdomen, Right

External popliteal nerve
  use Nerve, Peroneal

External pudendal artery
  use Artery, Femoral, Left
  use Artery, Femoral, Right

External pudendal vein
  use Vein, Saphenous, Left
  use Vein, Saphenous, Right

External urethral sphincter
  use Urethra

Extirpation

Acetabulum
  Left 0QC5
  Right 0QC4
Adenoids 0CCQ
Ampulla of Vater 0FCC
Anal Sphincter 0DCR
Anterior Chamber
  Left 08C3
  Right 08C2
Anus 0DCQ
Aorta
  Abdominal 04C0
  Thoracic
    Ascending/Arch 02CX
    Descending 02CW
Aortic Body 0GCD
Appendix 0DCJ
Artery
  Anterior Tibial
    Left 04CQ
    Right 04CP
  Axillary
    Left 03C6
    Right 03C5
  Brachial
    Left 03C8
    Right 03C7
  Celiac 04C1
  Colic
    Left 04C7
    Middle 04C8
    Right 04C6

Extirpation (continued)

Artery (continued)
  Common Carotid
    Left 03CJ
    Right 03CH
  Common Iliac
    Left 04CD
    Right 04CC
  Coronary
    Four or More Arteries 02C3
    One Artery 02C0
    Three Arteries 02C2
    Two Arteries 02C1
  External Carotid
    Left 03CN
    Right 03CM
  External Iliac
    Left 04CJ
    Right 04CH
  Face 03CR
  Femoral
    Left 04CL
    Right 04CK
  Foot
    Left 04CW
    Right 04CV
  Gastric 04C2
  Hand
    Left 03CF
    Right 03CD
  Hepatic 04C3
  Inferior Mesenteric 04CB
  Innominate 03C2
  Internal Carotid
    Left 03CL
    Right 03CK
  Internal Iliac
    Left 04CF
    Right 04CE
  Internal Mammary
    Left 03C1
    Right 03C0
  Intracranial 03CG
  Lower 04CY
  Peroneal
    Left 04CU
    Right 04CT
  Popliteal
    Left 04CN
    Right 04CM
  Posterior Tibial
    Left 04CS
    Right 04CR
  Pulmonary
    Left 02CR
    Right 02CQ
  Pulmonary Trunk 02CP
  Radial
    Left 03CC
    Right 03CB
  Renal
    Left 04CA
    Right 04C9
  Splenic 04C4
  Subclavian
    Left 03C4
    Right 03C3
  Superior Mesenteric 04C5
  Temporal
    Left 03CT
    Right 03CS
  Thyroid
    Left 03CV
    Right 03CU
  Ulnar
    Left 03CA
    Right 03C9
  Upper 03CY
  Vertebral
    Left 03CQ
    Right 03CP

Extirpation *(continued)*

Atrium
  Left 02C7
  Right 02C6
Auditory Ossicle
  Left 09CA
  Right 09C9
Basal Ganglia 00C8
Bladder 0TCB
Bladder Neck
  0TCC
Bone
  Ethmoid
    Left 0NCG
    Right 0NCF
  Frontal 0NC1
  Hyoid 0NCX
  Lacrimal
    Left 0NCJ
    Right 0NCH
  Nasal 0NCB
  Occipital 0NC7
  Palatine
    Left 0NCL
    Right 0NCK
  Parietal
    Left 0NC4
    Right 0NC3
  Pelvic
    Left 0QC3
    Right 0QC2
  Sphenoid 0NCC
  Temporal
    Left 0NC6
    Right 0NC5
  Zygomatic
    Left 0NCN
    Right 0NCM
Brain 00C0
Breast
  Bilateral 0HCV
  Left 0HCU
  Right 0HCT
Bronchus
  Lingula 0BC9
  Lower Lobe
    Left 0BCB
    Right 0BC6
  Main
    Left 0BC7
    Right 0BC3
  Middle Lobe, Right
    0BC5
  Upper Lobe
    Left 0BC8
    Right 0BC4
Buccal Mucosa 0CC4
Bursa and Ligament
  Abdomen
    Left 0MCJ
    Right 0MCH
  Ankle
    Left 0MCR
    Right 0MCQ
  Elbow
    Left 0MC4
    Right 0MC3
  Foot
    Left 0MCT
    Right 0MCS
  Hand
    Left 0MC8
    Right 0MC7
  Head and Neck
    0MC0
  Hip
    Left 0MCM
    Right 0MCL
  Knee
    Left 0MCP
    Right 0MCN

Extirpation *(continued)*

Bursa and Ligament *(continued)*
  Lower Extremity
    Left 0MCW
    Right 0MCV
  Perineum 0MCK
  Rib(s) 0MCG
  Shoulder
    Left 0MC2
    Right 0MC1
  Spine
    Lower 0MCD
    Upper 0MCC
  Sternum 0MCF
  Upper Extremity
    Left 0MCB
    Right 0MC9
  Wrist
    Left 0MC6
    Right 0MC5
Carina 0BC2
Carotid Bodies, Bilateral
  0GC8
Carotid Body
  Left 0GC6
  Right 0GC7
Carpal
  Left 0PCN
  Right 0PCM
Cavity, Cranial 0WC1
Cecum 0DCH
Cerebellum 00CC
Cerebral Hemisphere 00C7
Cerebral Meninges 00C1
Cerebral Ventricle 00C6
Cervix 0UCC
Chordae Tendineae 02C9
Choroid
  Left 08CB
  Right 08CA
Cisterna Chyli 07CL
Clavicle
  Left 0PCB
  Right 0PC9
Clitoris 0UCJ
Coccygeal Glomus 0GCB
Coccyx 0QCS
Colon
  Ascending 0DCK
  Descending 0DCM
  Sigmoid 0DCN
  Transverse 0DCL
Computer-aided Mechanical
  Aspiration X2C
Conduction Mechanism 02C8
Conjunctiva
  Left 08CTXZZ
  Right 08CSXZZ
Cord
  Bilateral 0VCH
  Left 0VCG
  Right 0VCF
Cornea
  Left 08C9XZZ
  Right 08C8XZZ
Cul-de-sac 0UCF
Diaphragm 0BCT
Disc
  Cervical Vertebral 0RC3
  Cervicothoracic Vertebral 0RC5
  Lumbar Vertebral 0SC2
  Lumbosacral 0SC4
  Thoracic Vertebral 0RC9
  Thoracolumbar Vertebral 0RCB
Duct
  Common Bile 0FC9
  Cystic 0FC8
  Hepatic
    Common 0FC7
    Left 0FC6
    Right 0FC5

Extirpation *(continued)*

Duct *(continued)*
  Lacrimal
    Left 08CY
    Right 08CX
  Pancreatic 0FCD
    Accessory 0FCF
  Parotid
    Left 0CCC
    Right 0CCB
Duodenum 0DC9
Dura Mater 00C2
Ear
  External
    Left 09C1
    Right 09C0
  External Auditory Canal
    Left 09C4
    Right 09C3
  Inner
    Left 09CE
    Right 09CD
  Middle
    Left 09C6
    Right 09C5
Endometrium 0UCB
Epididymis
  Bilateral 0VCL
  Left 0VCK
  Right 0VCJ
Epidural Space, Intracranial 00C3
Epiglottis 0CCR
Esophagogastric Junction 0DC4
Esophagus 0DC5
  Lower 0DC3
  Middle 0DC2
  Upper 0DC1
Eustachian Tube
  Left 09CG
  Right 09CF
Eye
  Left 08C1XZZ
  Right 08C0XZZ
Eyelid
  Lower
    Left 08CR
    Right 08CQ
  Upper
    Left 08CP
    Right 08CN
Fallopian Tube
  Left 0UC6
  Right 0UC5
Fallopian Tubes, Bilateral 0UC7
Femoral Shaft
  Left 0QC9
  Right 0QC8
Femur
  Lower
    Left 0QCC
    Right 0QCB
  Upper
    Left 0QC7
    Right 0QC6
Fibula
  Left 0QCK
  Right 0QCJ
Finger Nail 0HCQXZZ
Gallbladder 0FC4
Gastrointestinal Tract
  0WCP
Genitourinary Tract
  0WCR
Gingiva
  Lower 0CC6
  Upper 0CC5
Gland
  Adrenal
    Bilateral 0GC4
    Left 0GC2
    Right 0GC3

Extirpation *(continued)*

Gland *(continued)*
  Lacrimal
    Left 08CW
    Right 08CV
  Minor Salivary 0CCJ
  Parotid
    Left 0CC9
    Right 0CC8
  Pituitary 0GC0
  Sublingual
    Left 0CCF
    Right 0CCD
  Submaxillary
    Left 0CCH
    Right 0CCG
  Vestibular 0UCL
Glenoid Cavity
  Left 0PC8
  Right 0PC7
Glomus Jugulare 0GCC
Humeral Head
  Left 0PCD
  Right 0PCC
Humeral Shaft
  Left 0PCG
  Right 0PCF
Hymen 0UCK
Hypothalamus 00CA
Ileocecal Valve 0DCC
Ileum 0DCB
Intestine
  Large 0DCE
    Left 0DCG
    Right 0DCF
  Small 0DC8
Iris
  Left 08CD
  Right 08CC
Jaw
  Lower 0WC5
  Upper 0WC4
Jejunum 0DCA
Joint
  Acromioclavicular
    Left 0RCH
    Right 0RCG
  Ankle
    Left 0SCG
    Right 0SCF
  Carpal
    Left 0RCR
    Right 0RCQ
  Carpometacarpal
    Left 0RCT
    Right 0RCS
  Cervical Vertebral 0RC1
  Cervicothoracic Vertebral 0RC4
  Coccygeal 0SC6
  Elbow
    Left 0RCM
    Right 0RCL
  Finger Phalangeal
    Left 0RCX
    Right 0RCW
  Hip
    Left 0SCB
    Right 0SC9
  Knee
    Left 0SCD
    Right 0SCC
  Lumbar Vertebral 0SC0
  Lumbosacral 0SC3
  Metacarpophalangeal
    Left 0RCV
    Right 0RCU
  Metatarsal-Phalangeal
    Left 0SCN
    Right 0SCM
  Occipital-cervical 0RC0
  Sacrococcygeal 0SC5

Extirpation *(continued)*
Joint *(continued)*
Sacroiliac
Left 0SC8
Right 0SC7
Shoulder
Left 0RCK
Right 0RCJ
Sternoclavicular
Left 0RCF
Right 0RCE
Tarsal
Left 0SCJ
Right 0SCH
Tarsometatarsal
Left 0SCL
Right 0SCK
Temporomandibular
Left 0RCD
Right 0RCC
Thoracic Vertebral 0RC6
Thoracolumbar Vertebral 0RCA
Toe Phalangeal
Left 0SCQ
Right 0SCP
Wrist
Left 0RCP
Right 0RCN
Kidney
Left 0TC1
Right 0TC0
Kidney Pelvis
Left 0TC4
Right 0TC3
Larynx 0CCS
Lens
Left 08CK
Right 08CJ
Lip
Lower 0CC1
Upper 0CC0
Liver 0FC0
Left Lobe 0FC2
Right Lobe 0FC1
Lung
Bilateral 0BCM
Left 0BCL
Lower Lobe
Left 0BCJ
Right 0BCF
Middle Lobe, Right 0BCD
Right 0BCK
Upper Lobe
Left 0BCG
Right 0BCC
Lung Lingula 0BCH
Lymphatic
Aortic 07CD
Axillary
Left 07C6
Right 07C5
Head 07C0
Inguinal
Left 07CJ
Right 07CH
Internal Mammary
Left 07C9
Right 07C8
Lower Extremity
Left 07CG
Right 07CF
Mesenteric 07CB
Neck
Left 07C2
Right 07C1
Pelvis 07CC
Thoracic Duct 07CK
Thorax 07C7
Upper Extremity
Left 07C4
Right 07C3

Extirpation *(continued)*
Mandible
Left 0NCV
Right 0NCT
Maxilla 0NCR
Mediastinum 0WCC
Medulla Oblongata 00CD
Mesentery 0DCV
Metacarpal
Left 0PCQ
Right 0PCP
Metatarsal
Left 0QCP
Right 0QCN
Muscle
Abdomen
Left 0KCL
Right 0KCK
Extraocular
Left 08CM
Right 08CL
Facial 0KC1
Foot
Left 0KCW
Right 0KCV
Hand
Left 0KCD
Right 0KCC
Head 0KC0
Hip
Left 0KCP
Right 0KCN
Lower Arm and Wrist
Left 0KCB
Right 0KC9
Lower Leg
Left 0KCT
Right 0KCS
Neck
Left 0KC3
Right 0KC2
Papillary 02CD
Perineum 0KCM
Shoulder
Left 0KC6
Right 0KC5
Thorax
Left 0KCJ
Right 0KCH
Tongue, Palate, Pharynx 0KC4
Trunk
Left 0KCG
Right 0KCF
Upper Arm
Left 0KC8
Right 0KC7
Upper Leg
Left 0KCR
Right 0KCQ
Nasal Mucosa and Soft Tissue
09CK
Nasopharynx 09CN
Nerve
Abdominal Sympathetic
01CM
Abducens 00CL
Accessory 00CR
Acoustic 00CN
Brachial Plexus 01C3
Cervical 01C1
Cervical Plexus 01C0
Facial 00CM
Femoral 01CD
Glossopharyngeal 00CP
Head and Neck Sympathetic
01CK
Hypoglossal 00CS
Lumbar 01CB
Lumbar Plexus 01C9
Lumbar Sympathetic 01CN
Lumbosacral Plexus 01CA

Extirpation *(continued)*
Nerve *(continued)*
Median 01C5
Oculomotor 00CH
Olfactory 00CF
Optic 00CG
Peroneal 01CH
Phrenic 01C2
Pudendal 01CC
Radial 01C6
Sacral 01CR
Sacral Plexus 01CQ
Sacral Sympathetic 01CP
Sciatic 01CF
Thoracic 01C8
Thoracic Sympathetic 01CL
Tibial 01CG
Trigeminal 00CK
Trochlear 00CJ
Ulnar 01C4
Vagus 00CQ
Nipple
Left 0HCX
Right 0HCW
Omentum 0DCU
Oral Cavity and Throat
0WC3
Orbit
Left 0NCQ
Right 0NCP
Orbital Atherectomy *see* Extirpation,
Heart and Great Vessels 02C
Ovary
Bilateral 0UC2
Left 0UC1
Right 0UC0
Palate
Hard 0CC2
Soft 0CC3
Pancreas 0FCG
Para-aortic Body 0GC9
Paraganglion Extremity 0GCF
Parathyroid Gland 0GCR
Inferior
Left 0GCP
Right 0GCN
Multiple 0GCQ
Superior
Left 0GCM
Right 0GCL
Patella
Left 0QCF
Right 0QCD
Pelvic Cavity 0WCJ
Penis 0VCS
Pericardial Cavity 0WCD
Pericardium 02CN
Peritoneal Cavity
0WCG
Peritoneum 0DCW
Phalanx
Finger
Left 0PCV
Right 0PCT
Thumb
Left 0PCS
Right 0PCR
Toe
Left 0QCR
Right 0QCQ
Pharynx 0CCM
Pineal Body 0GC1
Pleura
Left 0BCP
Right 0BCN
Pleural Cavity
Left 0WCB
Right 0WC9
Pons 00CB
Prepuce 0VCT
Prostate 0VC0

Extirpation *(continued)*
Radius
Left 0PCJ
Right 0PCH
Rectum 0DCP
Respiratory Tract 0WCQ
Retina
Left 08CF
Right 08CE
Retinal Vessel
Left 08CH
Right 08CG
Retroperitoneum 0WCH
Ribs
1 to 2 0PC1
3 or More 0PC2
Sacrum 0QC1
Scapula
Left 0PC6
Right 0PC5
Sclera
Left 08C7XZZ
Right 08C6XZZ
Scrotum 0VC5
Septum
Atrial 02C5
Nasal 09CM
Ventricular 02CM
Sinus
Accessory 09CP
Ethmoid
Left 09CV
Right 09CU
Frontal
Left 09CT
Right 09CS
Mastoid
Left 09CC
Right 09CB
Maxillary
Left 09CR
Right 09CQ
Sphenoid
Left 09CX
Right 09CW
Skin
Abdomen 0HC7XZZ
Back 0HC6XZZ
Buttock 0HC8XZZ
Chest 0HC5XZZ
Ear
Left 0HC3XZZ
Right 0HC2XZZ
Face 0HC1XZZ
Foot
Left 0HCNXZZ
Right 0HCMXZZ
Hand
Left 0HCGXZZ
Right 0HCFXZZ
Inguinal 0HCAXZZ
Lower Arm
Left 0HCEXZZ
Right 0HCDXZZ
Lower Leg
Left 0HCLXZZ
Right 0HCKXZZ
Neck 0HC4XZZ
Perineum 0HC9XZZ
Scalp 0HC0XZZ
Upper Arm
Left 0HCCXZZ
Right 0HCBXZZ
Upper Leg
Left 0HCJXZZ
Right 0HCHXZZ
Spinal Canal 00CU
Spinal Cord
Cervical 00CW
Lumbar 00CY
Thoracic 00CX

Extirpation *(continued)*
Spinal Meninges 00CT
Spleen 07CP
Sternum 0PC0
Stomach 0DC6
  Pylorus 0DC7
Subarachnoid Space, Intracranial
  00C5
Subcutaneous Tissue and Fascia
  Abdomen 0JC8
  Back 0JC7
  Buttock 0JC9
  Chest 0JC6
  Face 0JC1
  Foot
    Left 0JCR
    Right 0JCQ
  Hand
    Left 0JCK
    Right 0JCJ
  Lower Arm
    Left 0JCH
    Right 0JCG
  Lower Leg
    Left 0JCP
    Right 0JCN
  Neck
    Left 0JC5
    Right 0JC4
  Pelvic Region 0JCC
  Perineum 0JCB
  Scalp 0JC0
  Upper Arm
    Left 0JCF
    Right 0JCD
  Upper Leg
    Left 0JCM
    Right 0JCL
Subdural Space, Intracranial 00C4
Tarsal
  Left 0QCM
  Right 0QCL
Tendon
  Abdomen
    Left 0LCG
    Right 0LCF
  Ankle
    Left 0LCT
    Right 0LCS
  Foot
    Left 0LCW
    Right 0LCV
  Hand
    Left 0LC8
    Right 0LC7
  Head and Neck 0LC0
  Hip
    Left 0LCK
    Right 0LCJ
  Knee
    Left 0LCR
    Right 0LCQ
  Lower Arm and Wrist
    Left 0LC6
    Right 0LC5
  Lower Leg
    Left 0LCP
    Right 0LCN
  Perineum 0LCH
  Shoulder
    Left 0LC2
    Right 0LC1
  Thorax
    Left 0LCD
    Right 0LCC
  Trunk
    Left 0LCB
    Right 0LC9
  Upper Arm
    Left 0LC4
    Right 0LC3

Extirpation *(continued)*
Tendon *(continued)*
  Upper Leg
    Left 0LCM
    Right 0LCL
Testis
  Bilateral 0VCC
  Left 0VCB
  Right 0VC9
Thalamus 00C9
Thymus 07CM
Thyroid Gland 0GCK
  Left Lobe 0GCG
  Right Lobe 0GCH
Tibia
  Left 0QCH
  Right 0QCG
Toe Nail 0HCRXZZ
Tongue 0CC7
Tonsils 0CCP
Tooth
  Lower 0CCX
  Upper 0CCW
Trachea 0BC1
Tunica Vaginalis
  Left 0VC7
  Right 0VC6
Turbinate, Nasal 09CL
Tympanic Membrane
  Left 09C8
  Right 09C7
Ulna
  Left 0PCL
  Right 0PCK
Ureter
  Left 0TC7
  Right 0TC6
Urethra 0TCD
Uterine Supporting Structure
  0UC4
Uterus 0UC9
Uvula 0CCN
Vagina 0UCG
Valve
  Aortic 02CF
  Mitral 02CG
  Pulmonary 02CH
  Tricuspid 02CJ
Vas Deferens
  Bilateral 0VCQ
  Left 0VCP
  Right 0VCN
Vein
  Axillary
    Left 05C8
    Right 05C7
  Azygos 05C0
  Basilic
    Left 05CC
    Right 05CB
  Brachial
    Left 05CA
    Right 05C9
  Cephalic
    Left 05CF
    Right 05CD
  Colic 06C7
  Common Iliac
    Left 06CD
    Right 06CC
  Coronary 02C4
  Esophageal 06C3
  External Iliac
    Left 06CG
    Right 06CF
  External Jugular
    Left 05CQ
    Right 05CP
  Face
    Left 05CV
    Right 05CT

Extirpation *(continued)*
Vein *(continued)*
  Femoral
    Left 06CN
    Right 06CM
  Foot
    Left 06CV
    Right 06CT
  Gastric 06C2
  Hand
    Left 05CH
    Right 05CG
  Hemiazygos 05C1
  Hepatic 06C4
  Hypogastric
    Left 06CJ
    Right 06CH
  Inferior Mesenteric
    06C6
  Innominate
    Left 05C4
    Right 05C3
  Internal Jugular
    Left 05CN
    Right 05CM
  Intracranial 05CL
  Lower 06CY
  Portal 06C8
  Pulmonary
    Left 02CT
    Right 02CS
  Renal
    Left 06CB
    Right 06C9
  Saphenous
    Left 06CQ
    Right 06CP
  Splenic 06C1
  Subclavian
    Left 05C6
    Right 05C5
  Superior Mesenteric
    06C5
  Upper 05CY
  Vertebral
    Left 05CS
    Right 05CR
Vena Cava
  Inferior 06C0
  Superior 02CV
Ventricle
  Left 02CL
  Right 02CK
Vertebra
  Cervical 0PC3
  Lumbar 0QC0
  Thoracic 0PC4
Vesicle
  Bilateral 0VC3
  Left 0VC2
  Right 0VC1
Vitreous
  Left 08C5
  Right 08C4
Vocal Cord
  Left 0CCV
  Right 0CCT
Vulva 0UCM
Extracorporeal shock wave lithotripsy
see Fragmentation
Extracranial-intracranial bypass
  (EC-IC)
see Bypass, Upper Arteries 031
Extracorporeal Carbon Dioxide
  Removal (ECC02R) 5A0920Z
Extraction
Acetabulum
  Left 0QD50ZZ
  Right 0QD40ZZ
Ampulla of Vater 0FDC
Anus 0DDQ

Extraction *(continued)*
Appendix 0DDJ
Auditory Ossicle
  Left 09DA0ZZ
  Right 09D90ZZ
Bone
  Ethmoid
    Left 0NDG0ZZ
    Right 0NDF0ZZ
  Frontal 0ND10ZZ
  Hyoid 0NDX0ZZ
  Lacrimal
    Left 0NDJ0ZZ
    Right 0NDH0ZZ
  Nasal 0NDB0ZZ
  Occipital 0ND70ZZ
  Palatine
    Left 0NDL0ZZ
    Right 0NDK0ZZ
  Parietal
    Left 0ND40ZZ
    Right 0ND30ZZ
  Pelvic
    Left 0QD30ZZ
    Right 0QD20ZZ
  Sphenoid 0NDC0ZZ
  Temporal
    Left 0ND60ZZ
    Right 0ND50ZZ
  Zygomatic
    Left 0NDN0ZZ
    Right 0NDM0ZZ
Bone Marrow 07DT
  Iliac 07DR
  Sternum 07DQ
  Vertebral 07DS
Brain 00D0
Breast
  Bilateral 0HDV
  Left 0HDU
  Right 0HDT
  Supernumerary 0HDY
Bronchus
  Lingula 0BD9
  Lower Lobe
    Left 0BDB
    Right 0BD6
  Main
    Left 0BD7
    Right 0BD3
  Middle Lobe, Right 0BD5
  Upper Lobe
    Left 0BD8
    Right 0BD4
Bursa and Ligament
  Abdomen
    Left 0MDJ
    Right 0MDH
  Ankle
    Left 0MDR
    Right 0MDQ
  Elbow
    Left 0MD4
    Right 0MD3
  Foot
    Left 0MDT
    Right 0MDS
  Hand
    Left 0MD8
    Right 0MD7
  Head and Neck 0MD0
  Hip
    Left 0MDM
    Right 0MDL
  Knee
    Left 0MDP
    Right 0MDN
  Lower Extremity
    Left 0MDW
    Right 0MDV
  Perineum 0MDK

Extraction *(continued)*

Bursa and Ligament *(continued)*
Rib(s) 0MDG
Shoulder
Left 0MD2
Right 0MD1
Spine
Lower 0MDD
Upper 0MDC
Sternum 0MDF
Upper Extremity
Left 0MDB
Right 0MD9
Wrist
Left 0MD6
Right 0MD5
Carina 0BD2
Carpal
Left 0PDN0ZZ
Right 0PDM0ZZ
Cecum 0DDH
Cerebellum 00DC
Cerebral Hemisphere 00D7
Cerebral Meninges 00D1
Cisterna Chyli 07DL
Clavicle
Left 0PDB0ZZ
Right 0PD90ZZ
Coccyx 0QDS0ZZ
Colon
Ascending 0DDK
Descending 0DDM
Sigmoid 0DDN
Transverse 0DDL
Cornea
Left 08D9XZ
Right 08D8XZ
Duct
Common Bile 0FD9
Cystic 0FD8
Hepatic
Common 0FD7
Left 0FD6
Right 0FD5
Pancreatic 0FDD
Accessory 0FDF
Duodenum 0DD9
Dura Mater 00D2
Endometrium 0UDB
Esophagogastric Junction 0DD4
Esophagus 0DD5
Lower 0DD3
Middle 0DD2
Upper 0DD1
Femoral Shaft
Left 0QD90ZZ
Right 0QD80ZZ
Femur
Lower
Left 0QDC0ZZ
Right 0QDB0ZZ
Upper
Left 0QD70ZZ
Right 0QD60ZZ
Fibula
Left 0QDK0ZZ
Right 0QDJ0ZZ
Finger Nail 0HDQXZZ
Gallbladder 0FD4
Glenoid Cavity
Left 0PD80ZZ
Right 0PD70ZZ
Hair 0HDSXZZ
Humeral Head
Left 0PDD0ZZ
Right 0PDC0ZZ
Humeral Shaft
Left 0PDG0ZZ
Right 0PDF0ZZ
Ileocecal Valve 0DDC
Ileum 0DDB

Intestine
Large 0DDE
Left 0DDG
Right 0DDF
Small 0DD8
Jejunum 0DDA
Kidney
Left 0TD1
Right 0TD0
Lens
Left 08DK3ZZ
Right 08DJ3ZZ
Liver 0FD0
Left Lobe 0FD2
Right Lobe 0FD1
Lung
Bilateral 0BDM
Left 0BDL
Lower Lobe
Left 0BDJ
Right 0BDF
Middle Lobe, Right 0BDD
Right 0BDK
Upper Lobe
Left 0BDG
Right 0BDC
Lung Lingula 0BDH
Lymphatic
Aortic 07DD
Axillary
Left 07D6
Right 07D5
Head 07D0
Inguinal
Left 07DJ
Right 07DH
Internal Mammary
Left 07D9
Right 07D8
Lower Extremity
Left 07DG
Right 07DF
Mesenteric 07DB
Neck
Left 07D2
Right 07D1
Pelvis 07DC
Thoracic Duct 07DK
Thorax 07D7
Upper Extermity
Left 07D4
Right 07D3
Mandible
Left 0NDV0ZZ
Right 0NDT0ZZ
Maxilla 0NDR0ZZ
Metacarpal
Left 0PDQ0ZZ
Right 0PDP0ZZ
Metatarsal
Left 0QDP0ZZ
Right 0QDN0ZZ
Muscle
Abdomen
Left 0KDL0ZZ
Right 0KDK0ZZ
Facial 0KD10ZZ
Foot
Left 0KDW0ZZ
Right 0KDV0ZZ
Hand
Left 0KDD0ZZ
Right 0KDC0ZZ
Head 0KD00ZZ
Hip
Left 0KDP0ZZ
Right 0KD90ZZ
Lower Arm and Wrist
Left 0KDB0ZZ
Right 0KD90ZZ

Muscle *(continued)*
Lower Leg
Left 0KDT0ZZ
Right 0KDS0ZZ
Neck
Left 0KD30ZZ
Right 0KD20ZZ
Perineum 0KDM0ZZ
Shoulder
Left 0KD60ZZ
Right 0KD50ZZ
Thorax
Left 0KDJ0ZZ
Right 0KDH0ZZ
Tongue, Palate, Pharynx
0KD40ZZ
Trunk
Left 0KDG0ZZ
Right 0KDF0ZZ
Upper Arm
Left 0KD80ZZ
Right 0KD70ZZ
Upper Leg
Left 0KDR0ZZ
Right 0KDQ0ZZ
Nerve
Abdominal Sympathetic 01DM
Abducens 00DL
Accessory 00DR
Acoustic 00DN
Brachial Plexus 01D3
Cervical 01D1
Cervical Plexus 01D0
Facial 00DM
Femoral 01DD
Glossopharyngeal 00DP
Head and Neck Sympathetic
01DK
Hypoglossal 00DS
Lumbar 01DB
Lumbar Plexus 01D9
Lumbar Sympathetic 01DN
Lumbosacral Plexus 01DA
Median 01D5
Oculomotor 00DH
Olfactory 00DF
Optic 00DG
Peroneal 01DH
Phrenic 01D2
Pudendal 01DC
Radial 01D6
Sacral 01DR
Sacral Plexus 01DQ
Sacral Sympathetic 01DP
Sciatic 01DF
Thoracic 01D8
Thoracic Sympathetic 01DL
Tibial 01DG
Trigeminal 00DK
Trochlear 00DJ
Ulnar 01D4
Vagus 00DQ
Orbit
Left 0NDQ0ZZ
Right 0NDP0ZZ
Ova 0UDN
Pancreas 0FDG
Patella
Left 0QDF0ZZ
Right 0QDD0ZZ
Phalanx
Finger
Left 0PDV0ZZ
Right 0PDT0ZZ
Thumb
Left 0PDS0ZZ
Right 0PDR0ZZ
Toe
Left 0QDR0ZZ
Right 0QDQ0ZZ

Pleura
Left 0BDP
Right 0BDN
Products of Conception
Ectopic 10D2
Extraperitoneal 10D00Z2
High 10D00Z0
High Forceps 10D07Z5
Internal Version 10D07Z7
Low 10D00Z1
Low Forceps
10D07Z3
Mid Forceps 10D07Z4
Other 10D07Z8
Retained 10D1
Vacuum 10D07Z6
Radius
Left 0PDJ0ZZ
Right 0PDH0ZZ
Rectum 0DDP
Ribs
1 to 2 0PD10ZZ
3 or More 0PD20ZZ
Sacrum 0QD10ZZ
Scapula
Left 0PD60ZZ
Right 0PD50ZZ
Septum, Nasal 09DM
Sinus
Accessory 09DP
Ethmoid
Left 09DV
Right 09DU
Frontal
Left 09DT
Right 09DS
Mastoid
Left 09DC
Right 09DB
Maxillary
Left 09DR
Right 09DQ
Sphenoid
Left 09DX
Right 09DW
Skin
Abdomen 0HD7XZZ
Back 0HD6XZZ
Buttock 0HD8XZZ
Chest 0HD5XZZ
Ear
Left 0HD3XZZ
Right 0HD2XZZ
Face 0HD1XZZ
Foot
Left 0HDNXZZ
Right 0HDMXZZ
Hand
Left 0HDGXZZ
Right 0HDFXZZ
Inguinal 0HDAXZZ
Lower Arm
Left 0HDEXZZ
Right 0HDDXZZ
Lower Leg
Left 0HDLXZZ
Right 0HDKXZZ
Neck 0HD4XZZ
Perineum 0HD9XZZ
Scalp 0HD0XZZ
Upper Arm
Left 0HDCXZZ
Right 0HDBXZZ
Upper Leg
Left 0HDJXZZ
Right 0HDHXZZ
Skull 0ND00ZZ
Spinal Meninges 00DT
Spleen 07DP
Sternum 0PD00ZZ

Extraction (continued)
Stomach 0DD6
  Pylorus 0DD7
Subcutaneous Tissue and Fascia
  Abdomen 0JD8
  Back 0JD7
  Buttock 0JD9
  Chest 0JD6
  Face 0JD1
  Foot
    Left 0JDR
    Right 0JDQ
  Hand
    Left 0JDK
    Right 0JDJ
  Lower Arm
    Left 0JDH
    Right 0JDG
  Lower Leg
    Left 0JDP
    Right 0JDN
  Neck
    Left 0JD5
    Right 0JD4
  Pelvic Region 0JDC
  Perineum 0JDB
  Scalp 0JD0
  Upper Arm
    Left 0JDF
    Right 0JDD
  Upper Leg
    Left 0JDM
    Right 0JDL
Tarsal
  Left 0QDM0ZZ
  Right 0QDL0ZZ
Tendon
  Abdomen
    Left 0LDG0ZZ
    Right 0LDF0ZZ
  Ankle
    Left 0LDT0ZZ
    Right 0LDS0ZZ
  Foot
    Left 0LDW0ZZ
    Right 0LDV0ZZ
  Hand
    Left 0LD80ZZ
    Right 0LD70ZZ
  Head and Neck
    0LD00ZZ
  Hip
    Left 0LDK0ZZ
    Right 0LDJ0ZZ
  Knee
    Left 0LDR0ZZ
    Right 0LDQ0ZZ
  Lower Arm and
    Wrist
    Left 0LD60ZZ
    Right 0LD50ZZ
  Lower Leg
    Left 0LDP0ZZ
    Right 0LDN0ZZ
  Perineum 0LDH0ZZ
  Shoulder
    Left 0LD20ZZ
    Right 0LD10ZZ
  Thorax
    Left 0LDD0ZZ
    Right 0LDC0ZZ
  Trunk
    Left 0LDB0ZZ
    Right 0LD90ZZ
  Upper Arm
    Left 0LD40ZZ
    Right 0LD30ZZ
  Upper Leg
    Left 0LDM0ZZ
    Right 0LDL0ZZ
Thymus 07DM

Extraction (continued)
Tibia
  Left 0QDH0ZZ
  Right 0QDG0ZZ
Toe Nail 0HDRXZZ
Tooth
  Lower 0CDXXZ
  Upper 0CDWXZ
Trachea 0BD1
Turbinate, Nasal 09DL
Tympanic Membrane
  Left 09D8
  Right 09D7
Ulna
  Left 0PDL0ZZ
  Right 0PDK0ZZ
Vein
  Basilic
    Left 05DC
    Right 05DB
  Brachial
    Left 05DA
    Right 05D9
  Cephalic
    Left 05DF
    Right 05DD
  Femoral
    Left 06DN
    Right 06DM
  Foot
    Left 06DV
    Right 06DT
  Hand
    Left 05DH
    Right 05DG
  Lower 06DY
  Saphenous
    Left 06DQ
    Right 06DP
  Upper 05DY
Vertebra
  Cervical 0PD30ZZ
  Lumbar 0QD00ZZ
  Thoracic 0PD40ZZ
Vocal Cord
  Left 0CDV
  Right 0CDT

Extradural space, intracranial
  use Epidural Space, Intracranial
Extradural space, spinal
  use Spinal Canal
EXtreme Lateral Interbody Fusion
  (XLIF) device
  use Interbody Fusion Device in
    Lower Joints

F

Face lift
  see Alteration, Face 0W02
Facet replacement spinal stabilization
  device
  use Spinal Stabilization Device,
    Facet Replacement in 0RH
  use Spinal Stabilization Device, Facet
    Replacement in 0SH
Facial artery
  use Artery, Face
Factor Xa Inhibitor Reversal Agent,
  Andexanet Alfa
  use Coagulation Factor Xa,
    Inactivated
False vocal cord
  use Larynx
Falx cerebri
  use Dura Mater
Fascia lata
  use Subcutaneous Tissue and Fascia,
    Upper Leg, Left
  use Subcutaneous Tissue and Fascia,
    Upper Leg, Right

Fasciaplasty, fascioplasty
  see Repair, Subcutaneous Tissue
    and Fascia 0JQ
  see Replacement,
    Subcutaneous Tissue and
    Fascia 0JR
Fasciectomy
  see Excision, Subcutaneous Tissue
    and Fascia 0JB
  see Release
Fasciorrhaphy
  see Repair, Subcutaneous Tissue
    and Fascia 0JQ
Fasciotomy
  see Division, Subcutaneous Tissue
    and Fascia 0J8
  see Drainage, Subcutaneous Tissue
    and Fascia 0J9
  see Release
Feeding Device
  Change device in
    Lower Intestinal Tract 0D2DXUZ
    Upper Intestinal Tract 0D20XUZ
  Insertion of device in
    Duodenum 0DH9
    Esophagus 0DH5
    Ileum 0DHB
    Intestine, Small 0DH8
    Jejunum 0DHA
    Stomach 0DH6
  Removal of device from
    Esophagus 0DP5
    Intestinal Tract
      Lower Intestinal Tract 0DPD
      Upper Intestinal Tract 0DP0
    Stomach 0DP6
  Revision of device in
    Intestinal Tract
      Lower Intestinal Tract 0DWD
      Upper Intestinal Tract 0DW0
    Stomach 0DW6
Femoral head
  use Femur, Upper, Left
  use Femur, Upper, Right
Femoral lymph node
  use Lymphatic, Lower Extremity,
    Left
  use Lymphatic, Lower Extremity,
    Right
Femoropatellar joint
  use Joint, Knee, Left
  use Joint, Knee, Left, Femoral
    Surface
  use Joint, Knee, Right
  use Joint, Knee, Right, Femoral
    Surface
Femorotibial joint
  use Joint, Knee, Left
  use Joint, Knee, Left, Tibial Surface
  use Joint, Knee, Right
  use Joint, Knee, Right, Tibial Surface
FETROJA®
  use Cefiderocol Anti-infective
FGS (fluorescence-guided surgery)
  see Fluorescence Guided Procedure
Fibular artery
  use Artery, Peroneal, Left
  use Artery, Peroneal, Right
Fibular sesamoid
  use Metatarsal, Left
  use Metatarsal, Right
Fibularis brevis muscle
  use Muscle, Lower Leg, Left
  use Muscle, Lower Leg, Right
Fibularis longus muscle
  use Muscle, Lower Leg, Left
  use Muscle, Lower Leg, Right
Fifth cranial nerve
  use Nerve, Trigeminal
Filum terminale
  use Spinal Meninges

Fimbriectomy
  see Excision, Female Reproductive
    System 0UB
  see Resection, Female Reproductive
    System 0UT
Fine needle aspiration
  Fluid or gas
    see Drainage
  Tissue biopsy
    see Excision
    see Extraction
First cranial nerve
  use Nerve, Olfactory
First intercostal nerve
  use Nerve, Brachial Plexus
Fistulization
  see Bypass
  see Drainage
  see Repair
Fitting
  Arch bars, for fracture reduction
    see Reposition, Mouth and Throat
    0CS
  Arch bars, for immobilization
    see Immobilization, Face 2W31
  Artificial limb
    see Device Fitting, Rehabilitation
    F0D
  Hearing aid
    see Device Fitting, Rehabilitation
    F0D
  Ocular prosthesis F0DZ8UZ
  Prosthesis, limb
    see Device Fitting, Rehabilitation
    F0D
  Prosthesis, ocular F0DZ8UZ
Fixation, bone
  External, with fracture reduction
    see Reposition
  External, without fracture reduction
    see Insertion
  Internal, with fracture reduction
    see Reposition
  Internal, without fracture
    reduction
    see Insertion
FLAIR® Endovascular Stent Graft
  use Intraluminal Device
Flexible Composite Mesh
  use Synthetic Substitute
Flexor carpi radialis muscle
  use Muscle, Lower Arm and Wrist,
    Left
  use Muscle, Lower Arm and Wrist,
    Right
Flexor carpi ulnaris muscle
  use Muscle, Lower Arm and Wrist,
    Left
  use Muscle, Lower Arm and Wrist,
    Right
Flexor digitorum brevis muscle
  use Muscle, Foot, Left
  use Muscle, Foot, Right
Flexor digitorum longus muscle
  use Muscle, Lower Leg, Left
  use Muscle, Lower Leg, Right
Flexor hallucis brevis muscle
  use Muscle, Foot, Left
  use Muscle, Foot, Right
Flexor hallucis longus muscle
  use Muscle, Lower Leg, Left
  use Muscle, Lower Leg, Right
Flexor pollicis longus muscle
  use Muscle, Lower Arm and Wrist,
    Left
  use Muscle, Lower Arm and Wrist,
    Right
Flourish® Pediatric Esophageal
  Atresia Device *use* Magnetic
    Lengthening Device in
    Gastrointestinal System

Extraction–Flourish® Pediatric Esophageal Altresia Device

31

Flow Diverter embolization device
use Intraluminal Device, Flow
 Diverter in 03V
FlowSense Noninvasive Thermal
 Sensor 4B00XW0
Fluorescence Guided Procedure
 Extremity
 Lower 8E0Y
 Upper 8E0X
 Head and Neck Region 8E09
 Aminolevulinic Acid 8E09
 No Qualifier 8E09
 Reproductive System, Female,
 Pafolacianine (CYTALUX®) 8E0U
 Trunk Region
 No Qualifier 8E0W
 Pafolacianine (CYTALUX®)
 8E0W
Fluorescent Pyrazine, Kidney
 XT25XE5
Fluoroscopy
 Abdomen and Pelvis BW11
 Airway, Upper BB1DZZZ
 Ankle
 Left BQ1
 Right BQ1G
 Aorta
 Abdominal B410
 Laser, Intraoperative B410
 Thoracic B310
 Laser, Intraoperative B310
 Thoraco-Abdominal B31P
 Laser, Intraoperative B31P
 Aorta and Bilateral Lower
 Extremity Arteries B41D
 Laser, Intraoperative B41D
 Arm
 Left BP1FZZZ
 Right BP1EZZZ
 Artery
 Brachiocephalic-Subclavian
 Right B311
 Laser, Intraoperative B311
 Bronchial B31L
 Laser, Intraoperative B31L
 Bypass Graft, Other B21F
 Cervico-Cerebral Arch B31Q
 Laser, Intraoperative B31Q
 Common Carotid
 Bilateral B315
 Laser, Intraoperative B315
 Left B314
 Laser, Intraoperative B314
 Right B313
 Laser, Intraoperative B313
 Coronary
 Bypass Graft
 Multiple B213
 Laser, Intraoperative B213
 Single B212
 Laser, Intraoperative B212
 Multiple B211
 Laser, Intraoperative B211
 Single B210
 Laser, Intraoperative B210
 External Carotid
 Bilateral B31C
 Laser, Intraoperative B31C
 Left B31B
 Laser, Intraoperative B31B
 Right B319
 Laser, Intraoperative B319
 Hepatic B412
 Laser, Intraoperative B412
 Inferior Mesenteric B415
 Laser, Intraoperative B415
 Intercostal B31L
 Laser, Intraoperative B31L
 Internal Carotid
 Bilateral B318
 Laser, Intraoperative B318

Fluoroscopy *(continued)*
 Artery *(continued)*
 Internal Carotid *(continued)*
 Left B317
 Laser, Intraoperative B317
 Right B316
 Laser, Intraoperative B316
 Internal Mammary Bypass Graft
 Left B218
 Right B217
 Intra-Abdominal
 Laser, Intraoperative B41B
 Other B41B
 Intracranial B31R
 Laser, Intraoperative B31R
 Lower
 Laser, Intraoperative B41J
 Other B41J
 Lower Extremity
 Bilateral and Aorta B41D
 Laser, Intraoperative B41D
 Left B41G
 Laser, Intraoperative B41G
 Right B41F
 Laser, Intraoperative B41F
 Lumbar B419
 Laser, Intraoperative B419
 Pelvic B41C
 Laser, Intraoperative B41C
 Pulmonary
 Left B31T
 Laser, Intraoperative B31T
 Right B31S
 Laser, Intraoperative B31S
 Pulmonary Trunk B31U
 Laser, Intraoperative B31U
 Renal
 Bilateral B418
 Laser, Intraoperative B418
 Left B417
 Laser, Intraoperative B417
 Right B416
 Laser, Intraoperative B416
 Spinal B31M
 Laser, Intraoperative B31M
 Splenic B413
 Laser, Intraoperative B413
 Subclavian
 Laser, Intraoperative B312
 Left B312
 Superior Mesenteric B414
 Laser, Intraoperative B414
 Upper
 Laser, Intraoperative B31N
 Other B31N
 Upper Extremity
 Bilateral B31K
 Laser, Intraoperative B31K
 Left B31J
 Laser, Intraoperative B31J
 Right B31H
 Laser, Intraoperative B31H
 Vertebral
 Bilateral B31G
 Laser, Intraoperative B31G
 Left B31F
 Laser, Intraoperative B31F
 Right B31D
 Laser, Intraoperative
 B31D
 Bile Duct BF10
 Pancreatic Duct and Gallbladder
 BF14
 Bile Duct and Gallbladder BF13
 Biliary Duct BF11
 Bladder BT10
 Kidney and Ureter BT14
 Left BT1F
 Right BT1D
 Bladder and Urethra BT1B
 Bowel, Small BD1

Fluoroscopy *(continued)*
 Calcaneus
 Left BQ1KZZZ
 Right BQ1JZZZ
 Clavicle
 Left BP15ZZZ
 Right BP14ZZZ
 Coccyx BR1F
 Colon BD14
 Corpora Cavernosa BV10
 Dialysis Fistula B51W
 Dialysis Shunt B51W
 Diaphragm BB16ZZZ
 Disc
 Cervical BR11
 Lumbar BR13
 Thoracic BR12
 Duodenum BD19
 Elbow
 Left BP1H
 Right BP1G
 Epiglottis B91G
 Esophagus BD11
 Extremity
 Lower BW1C
 Upper BW1J
 Facet Joint
 Cervical BR14
 Lumbar BR16
 Thoracic BR15
 Fallopian Tube
 Bilateral BU12
 Left BU11
 Right BU10
 Fallopian Tube and Uterus BU18
 Femur
 Left BQ14ZZZ
 Right BQ13ZZZ
 Finger
 Left BP1SZZZ
 Right BP1RZZZ
 Foot
 Left BQ1MZZZ
 Right BQ1LZZZ
 Forearm
 Left BP1KZZZ
 Right BP1JZZZ
 Gallbladder BF12
 Bile Duct and Pancreatic Duct
 BF14
 Gallbladder and Bile Duct BF13
 Gastrointestinal, Upper BD1
 Hand
 Left BP1PZZZ
 Right BP1NZZZ
 Head and Neck BW19
 Heart
 Left B215
 Right B214
 Right and Left B216
 Hip
 Left BQ11
 Right BQ10
 Humerus
 Left BP1BZZZ
 Right BP1AZZZ
 Ileal Diversion Loop BT1C
 Ileal Loop, Ureters and Kidney BT1G
 Intracranial Sinus B512
 Joint
 Acromioclavicular, Bilateral
 BP13ZZZ
 Finger
 Left BP1D
 Right BP1C
 Foot
 Left BQ1Y
 Right BQ1X
 Hand
 Left BP1D
 Right BP1C

Fluoroscopy *(continued)*
 Joint *(continued)*
 Lumbosacral BR1B
 Sacroiliac BR1D
 Sternoclavicular
 Bilateral BP12ZZZ
 Left BP11ZZZ
 Right BP10ZZZ
 Temporomandibular
 Bilateral BN19
 Left BN18
 Right BN17
 Thoracolumbar BR18
 Toe
 Left BQ1Y
 Right BQ1X
 Kidney
 Bilateral BT13
 Ileal Loop and Ureter BT1G
 Left BT12
 Right BT11
 Ureter and Bladder BT14
 Left BT1F
 Right BT1D
 Knee
 Left BQ18
 Right BQ17
 Larynx B91J
 Leg
 Left BQ1FZZZ
 Right BQ1DZZZ
 Liver BF15
 Lung
 Bilateral BB14ZZZ
 Left BB13ZZZ
 Right BB12ZZZ
 Mediastinum BB1CZZZ
 Mouth BD1B
 Neck and Head BW19
 Oropharynx BD1B
 Pancreatic Duct BF1
 Gallbladder and Bile Buct BF14
 Patella
 Left BQ1WZZZ
 Right BQ1VZZZ
 Pelvis BR1C
 Pelvis and Abdomen BW11
 Pharynix B91G
 Ribs
 Left BP1YZZZ
 Right BP1XZZZ
 Sacrum BR1F
 Scapula
 Left BP17ZZZ
 Right BP16ZZZ
 Shoulder
 Left BP19
 Right BP18
 Sinus, Intracranial B512
 Spinal Cord B01B
 Spine
 Cervical BR10
 Lumbar BR19
 Thoracic BR17
 Whole BR1G
 Sternum BR1H
 Stomach BD12
 Toe
 Left BQ1QZZZ
 Right BQ1PZZZ
 Tracheobronchial Tree
 Bilateral BB19YZZ
 Left BB18YZZ
 Right BB17YZZ
 Ureter
 Ileal Loop and Kidney BT1G
 Kidney and Bladder BT14
 Left BT1F
 Right BT1D
 Left BT17
 Right BT16

Flow Diverter embolization device–Fluoroscopy

32

Fluoroscopy (*continued*)
    Urethra BT15
    Urethra and Bladder BT1B
    Uterus BU16
    Uterus and Fallopian Tube BU18
    Vagina BU19
    Vasa Vasorum BV18
    Vein
        Cerebellar B511
        Cerebral B511
        Epidural B510
        Jugular
            Bilateral B515
            Left B514
            Right B513
        Lower Extremity
            Bilateral B51D
            Left B51C
            Right B51B
        Other B51V
        Pelvic (Iliac)
            Left B51G
            Right B51F
        Pelvic (Iliac) Bilateral B51H
        Portal B51T
        Pulmonary
            Bilateral B51S
            Left B51R
            Right B51Q
        Renal
            Bilateral B51L
            Left B51K
            Right B51J
        Spanchnic B51T
        Subclavian
            Left B517
            Right B516
        Upper Extremity
            Bilateral B51P
            Left B51N
            Right B51M
    Vena Cava
        Inferior B519
        Superior B518
    Wrist
        Left BP1M
        Right BP1L
Fluoroscopy, laser intraoperative
    Fluoroscopy, Heart B21
    Fluoroscopy, Lower Arteries B41
    Fluoroscopy, Upper Arteries B31
Flushing
    see Irrigation
Foley catheter
    use Drainage Device
Fontan completion procedure
    Stage II
    see Bypass, Vena Cava, Inferior 0610
Foramen magnum
    use Occipital Bone
Foramen of Monro (intraventricular)
    use Cerebral Ventricle
Foreskin
    use Prepuce
Formula™ Balloon-Expandable Renal Stent System
    use Intraluminal Device
Fosfomycin Anti-infective XW0
Fosfomycin injection
    use Fosfomycin Anti-infective
Fossa of Rosenmuller
    use Nasopharynx
Fostamatinib XW0
Fourth cranial nerve
    use Nerve, Trochlear
Fourth ventricle
    use Cerebral Ventricle
Fovea
    use Retina, Left
    use Retina, Right

Fragmentation
    Ampulla of Vater 0FFC
    Anus 0DFQ
    Appendix 0DFJ
    Artery
        Anterior Tibial
            Left 04FQ3Z
            Right 04FP3Z
        Axillary
            Left 03F63Z
            Right 03F53Z
        Brachial
            Left 03F83Z
            Right 03F73Z
        Common Illiac
            Left 04FD3Z
            Right 04FC3Z
        Coronary
            Four or More Arteries 02F33ZZ
            One Artery 02F03ZZ
            Three Arteries 02F23ZZ
            Two Arteries 02F13ZZ
        External Illiac
            Left 04FJ3Z
            Right 04FH3Z
        Femoral
            Left 04FL3Z
            Right 04FK3Z
        Innominate 03F23Z
        Internal Illiac
            Left 04FF3Z
            Right 04FE3Z
        Intracranial 03FG3Z
        Lower 04FY3Z
        Peroneal
            Left 04FU3Z
            Right 04FT3Z
        Popliteal
            Left 04FN3Z
            Right 04FM3Z
        Posterior Tibial
            Left 04FS3Z
            Right 04FR3Z
        Pulmonary
            Left 02FR3Z
            Right 02FQ3Z
        Pulmonary Trunk 02FP3Z
        Radial
            Left 03FC3Z
            Right 03FB3Z
        Subclavian
            Left 03F43Z
            Right 03F33Z
        Ulnar
            Left 03FA3Z
            Right 03F93Z
        Upper 03FY3Z
    Bladder 0TFB
    Bladder Neck 0TFC
    Bronchus
        Lingula 0BF9
        Lower Lobe
            Left 0BFB
            Right 0BF6
        Main
            Left 0BF7
            Right 0BF3
        Middle Lobe, Right 0BF5
        Upper Lobe
            Left 0BF8
            Right 0BF4
    Carina 0BF2
    Cavity, Cranial 0WF1
    Cecum 0DFH
    Cerebral Ventricle 00F6
    Colon
        Ascending 0DFK
        Descending 0DFM
        Sigmoid 0DFN
        Transverse 0DFL

Fragmentation (*continued*)
    Duct
        Common Bile 0FF9
        Cystic 0FF8
        Hepatic
            Common 0FF7
            Left 0FF6
            Right 0FF5
        Pancreatic 0FFD
            Accessory 0FFF
        Parotid
            Left 0CFC
            Right 0CFB
    Duodenum 0DF9
    Epidural Space, Intracranial 00F3
    Esophagus 0DF5
    Fallopian Tube
        Left 0UF6
        Right 0UF5
    Fallopian Tubes, Bilateral 0UF7
    Gallbladder 0FF4
    Gastrointestinal Tract 0WFP
    Genitourinary Tract 0WFR
    Ileum 0DFB
    Intestine
        Large 0DFE
            Left 0DFG
            Right 0DFF
        Small 0DF8
    Jejunum 0DFA
    Kidney Pelvis
        Left 0TF4
        Right 0TF3
    Mediastinum 0WFC
    Oral Cavity and Throat 0WF3
    Pelvic Cavity 0WFJ
    Pericardial Cavity 0WFD
    Pericardium 02FN
    Peritoneal Cavity 0WFG
    Pleural Cavity
        Left 0WFB
        Right 0WF9
    Rectum 0DFP
    Respiratory Tract 0WFQ
    Spinal Canal 00FU
    Stomach 0DF6
    Subarachnoid Space, Intracranial 00F5
    Subdural Space, Intracranial 00F4
    Trachea 0BF1
    Ureter
        Left 0TF7
        Right 0TF6
    Urethra 0TFD
    Uterus 0UF9
    Vein
        Axillary
            Left 05F83Z
            Right 05F73Z
        Basilic
            Left 05FC3Z
            Right 05FB3Z
        Brachial
            Left 05FA3Z
            Right 05F93Z
        Cephalic
            Left 05FF3Z
            Right 05FD3Z
        Common Iliac
            Left 06FD3Z
            Right 06FC3Z
        External Iliac
            Left 06FG3Z
            Right 06FF3Z
        Femoral
            Left 06FN3Z
            Right 06FM3Z
        Hypogastric
            Left 06FJ3Z
            Right 06FH3Z

Fragmentation (*continued*)
    Vein (*continued*)
        Innominate
            Left 05F43Z
            Right 05F33Z
        Lower 06FY3Z
        Pulmonary
            Left 02FT3Z
            Right 02FS3Z
        Saphenous
            Left 06FQ3Z
            Right 06FP3Z
        Subclavian
            Left 05F63Z
            Right 05F53Z
        Upper 05FY3Z
        Vitreous
            Left 08F5
            Right 08F4
Fragmentation, Ultrasonic
    see Fragmentation, Artery
Freestyle (Stentless) Aortic Root Bioprosthesis
    use Zooplastic Tissue in Heart and Great Vessels
Frenectomy
    see Excision, Mouth and Throat 0CB
    see Resection, Mouth and Throat 0CT
Frenoplasty, frenuloplasty
    see Repair, Mouth and Throat 0CQ
    see Replacement, Mouth and Throat 0CR
    see Supplement, Mouth and Throat 0CU
Frenotomy
    see Drainage, Mouth and Throat 0C9
    see Release, Mouth and Throat 0CN
Frenulotomy
    see Drainage, Mouth and Throat 0C9
    see Release, Mouth and Throat 0CN
Frenulum labii inferioris
    use Lip, Lower
Frenulum labii superioris
    use Lip, Upper
Frenulum linguae
    use Tongue
Frenulumectomy
    see Excision, Mouth and Throat 0CB
    see Resection, Mouth and Throat 0CT
Frontal lobe
    use Cerebral Hemisphere
Frontal vein
    use Vein, Face, Left
    use Vein, Face, Right
Frozen elephant trunk (FET) technique, aortic arch replacement
    see New Technology, Cardiovascular System X2R
    see Replacement, Heart and Great Vessels 02R
Frozen elephant trunk (FET) technique, thoracic aorta restriction
    see New Technology, Cardiovascular System X2V
    see Restriction, Heart and Great Vessels 02V
FUJIFILM EP-7000X System for Oxygen Saturation Endoscopic Imaging (OXEI)
    see New Technology, Gastrointestinal System XD2
Fulguration
    see Destruction
Fundoplication, gastroesophageal
    see Restriction, Esophagogastric Junction 0DV4

Fundus uteri
use Uterus
Fusion
Acromioclavicular
Left 0RGH
Right 0RGG
Ankle
Left 0SGG
Open-truss Design Internal
Fixation Device XRGK0B9
Right 0SGF
Open-truss Design Internal
Fixation Device XRGJ0B9
Carpal
Left 0RGR
Right 0RGQ
Carpometacarpal
Left 0RGT
Right 0RGS
Cervical Vertebral 0RG1
2 or more 0RG2
Cervicothoracic Vertebral 0RG4
Coccygeal 0SG6
Elbow
Left 0RGM
Right 0RGL
Finger Phalangeal
Left 0RGX
Right 0RGW
Hip
Left 0SGB
Right 0SG9
Knee
Left 0SGD
Right 0SGC
Lumbar Vertebral 0SG0
2 or more 0SG1
Interbody Fusion
Device, Custom-Made
Anatomically Designed
XRGC
Interbody Fusion
Device, Custom-Made
Anatomically Designed XRGB
Lumbosacral 0SG3
Interbody Fusion
Device, Custom-Made
Anatomically Designed
XRGD
Metacarpophalangeal
Left 0RGV
Right 0RGU
Metatarsal-Phalangeal
Left 0SGN
Right 0SGM
Occipital-cervical 0RG0
Sacrococcygeal 0SG5
Sacroiliac
Internal Fixation Device
with Tulip Connector XRG
Left 0SG8
Right 0SG7
Shoulder
Left 0RGK
Right 0RGJ
Sternoclavicular
Left 0RGF
Right 0RGE
Tarsal
Left 0SGJ
Open-truss Design Internal
Fixation Device XRGM0B9
Right 0SGH
Open-truss Design Internal
Fixation Device XRGL0B9
Tarsometatarsal
Left 0SGL
Right 0SGK
Temporomandibular
Left 0RGD
Right 0RGC

Fusion *(continued)*
Thoracic Vertebral 0RG6
2 to 7 0RG7
8 or more 0RG8
Thoracolumbar Vertebral
0RGA
Interbody Fusion Device,
Custom-Made Anatomically
Designed XRGA
Toe Phalangeal
Left 0SGQ
Right 0SGP
Wrist
Left 0RGP
Right 0RGN
**Fusion screw (compression)(lag)
(locking)**
use Internal Fixation Device in
Lower Joints
use Internal Fixation Device in
Upper Joints

G

Gait training
see Motor Treatment, Rehabilitation
F07
Galea aponeurotica
use Subcutaneous Tissue and Fascia,
Scalp
Gammaglobulin
use Globulin
GammaTile™
use Radioactive Element,
Cesium-131 Collagen Implant
in 00H
**GAMUNEX-C, for COVID-19
treatment**
use High-Dose Intravenous Immune
Globulin
**Ganglion impar (ganglion of
Walther)**
use Nerve, Sacral Sympathetic
Ganglionectomy
Destruction of lesion
see Destruction
Excision of lesion
see Excision
Gasserian ganglion
use Nerve, Trigeminal
Gastrectomy
Partial
see Excision, Stomach 0DB6
Total
see Resection, Stomach 0DT6
Vertical (sleeve)
see Excision, Stomach 0DB6
**Gastric electrical stimulation (GES)
lead**
use Stimulator Lead in
Gastrointestinal System
Gastric lymph node
use Lymphatic, Aortic
Gastric pacemaker lead
use Stimulator Lead in
Gastrointestinal System
Gastric plexus
use Nerve, Abdominal
Sympathetic
Gastrocnemius muscle
use Muscle, Lower Leg, Left
use Muscle, Lower Leg, Right
Gastrocolic ligament
use Omentum
Gastrocolic omentum
use Omentum
Gastrocolostomy
see Bypass, Gastrointestinal System
0D1
see Drainage, Gastrointestinal
System 0D9

Gastroduodenal artery
use Artery, Hepatic
Gastroduodenectomy
see Excision, Gastrointestinal
System 0DB
see Resection, Gastrointestinal
System 0DT
Gastroduodenoscopy 0DJ08ZZ
Gastroenteroplasty
see Repair, Gastrointestinal System
0DQ
see Supplement, Gastrointestinal
System 0DU
Gastroenterostomy
see Bypass, Gastrointestinal System
0D1
see Drainage, Gastrointestinal
System 0D9
Gastroesophageal (GE) junction
use Esophagogastric Junction
Gastrogastrostomy
see Bypass, Stomach 0D16
see Drainage, Stomach 0D96
Gastrohepatic omentum
use Omentum
Gastrojejunostomy
see Bypass, Stomach 0D16
see Drainage, Stomach 0D96
Gastrolysis
see Release, Stomach 0DN6
Gastropexy
see Repair, Stomach 0DQ6
see Reposition, Stomach
0DS6
Gastrophrenic ligament
use Omentum
Gastroplasty
see Repair, Stomach 0DQ6
see Supplement, Stomach 0DU6
Gastroplication
see Restriction, Stomach 0DV6
Gastropylorectomy
see Excision, Gastrointestinal
System 0DB
Gastrorrhaphy
see Repair, Stomach 0DQ6
Gastroscopy 0DJ68ZZ
Gastrosplenic ligament
use Omentum
Gastrostomy
see Bypass, Stomach 0D16
see Drainage, Stomach 0D96
Gastrotomy
see Drainage, Stomach 0D96
Gemellus muscle
use Muscle, Hip, Left
use Muscle, Hip, Right
Geniculate ganglion
use Nerve, Facial
Geniculate nucleus
use Thalamus
Genioglossus muscle
use Muscle, Tongue, Palate,
Pharynx
Genioplasty
see Alteration, Jaw, Lower 0W05
Genitofemoral nerve
use Nerve, Lumbar Plexus
GIAPREZA™
use Vasopressor
Gilteritinib Antineoplastic
XW0DXV5
Gingivectomy
see Excision, Mouth and Throat
0CB
Gingivoplasty
see Repair, Mouth and Throat 0CQ
see Replacement, Mouth and Throat
0CR
see Supplement, Mouth and Throat
0CU

Glans penis
use Prepuce
Glenohumeral joint
use Joint, Shoulder, Left
use Joint, Shoulder, Right
Glenohumeral ligament
use Bursa and Ligament, Shoulder,
Left
use Bursa and Ligament, Shoulder,
Right
Glenoid fossa (of scapula)
use Glenoid Cavity, Left
use Glenoid Cavity, Right
Glenoid ligament (labrum)
use Shoulder Joint, Left
use Shoulder Joint, Right
Globus pallidus
use Basal Ganglia
Glofitamab Antineoplastic XW0
Glomectomy
see Excision, Endocrine System
0GB
see Resection, Endocrine System
0GT
Glossectomy
see Excision, Tongue 0CB7
see Resection, Tongue 0CT7
Glossoepiglottic fold
use Epiglottis
Glossopexy
see Repair, Tongue 0CQ7
see Reposition, Tongue
0CS7
Glossoplasty
see Repair, Tongue 0CQ7
see Replacement, Tongue
0CR7
see Supplement, Tongue
0CU7
Glossorrhaphy
see Repair, Tongue 0CQ7
Glossotomy
see Drainage, Tongue 0C97
Glottis
use Larynx
**Gluteal Artery Perforator
Flap**
Replacement
Bilateral 0HRV079
Left 0HRU079
Right 0HRT079
Transfer
Left 0KXG
Right 0KXF
Gluteal lymph node
use Lymphatic, Pelvis
Gluteal vein
use Vein, Hypogastric,
Left
use Vein, Hypogastric,
Right
Gluteus maximus muscle
use Muscle, Hip, Left
use Muscle, Hip, Right
Gluteus medius muscle
use Muscle, Hip, Left
use Muscle, Hip, Right
Gluteus minimus muscle
use Muscle, Hip, Left
use Muscle, Hip, Right
GORE® DUALMESH®
use Synthetic Substitute
**GORE EXCLUDER® AAA
Endoprosthesis**
use Intraluminal Device
use Intraluminal Device, Branched
or Fenestrated, One or Two
Arteries in 04V
use Intraluminal Device, Branched
or Fenestrated, Three or More
Arteries in 04V

GORE EXCLUDER® IBE Endoprosthesis
use Intraluminal Device, Branched or Fenestrated, One or Two Arteries in 04V

GORE TAG® Thoracic Endoprosthesis
use Intraluminal Device

Gracilis muscle
use Muscle, Upper Leg, Left
use Muscle, Upper Leg, Right

Graft
see Replacement
see Supplement

Great auricular nerve
use Nerve, Cervical Plexus

Great cerebral vein
use Vein, Intracranial

Great(er) saphenous vein
use Vein, Saphenous, Left
use Vein, Saphenous, Right

Greater alar cartilage
use Nasal Mucosa and Soft Tissue

Greater occipital nerve
use Nerve, Cervical

Greater Omentum
use Omentum

Greater splanchnic nerve
use Nerve, Thoracic Sympathetic

Greater superficial petrosal nerve
use Nerve, Facial

Greater trochanter
use Femur, Upper, Left
use Femur, Upper, Right

Greater tuberosity
use Humeral Head, Left
use Humeral Head, Right

Greater vestibular (Bartholin's) gland
use Gland, Vestibular

Greater wing
use Bone, Sphenoid

GS-5734 *use* Remdesivir Anti-infective

Guedel airway
use Intraluminal Device, Airway in Mouth and Throat

Guidance, catheter placement
EKG
see Measurement, Physiological Systems 4A0
Fluoroscopy
see Fluoroscopy, Veins B51
Ultrasound
see Ultrasonography, Veins B54

H

Hallux
use Toe, 1st, Left
use Toe, 1st, Right

Hamate bone
use Carpal, Left
use Carpal, Right

Hancock Bioprosthesis (aortic) (mitral) valve
use Zooplastic Tissue in Heart and Great Vessels

Hancock Bioprosthetic Valved Conduit
use Zooplastic Tissue in Heart and Great Vessels

Harmony™ transcatheter pulmonary valve (TPV) placement 02RH38M

Harvesting, stem cells
see Pheresis, Circulatory 6A55

hdIVIG (high-dose intravenous immunogloblin), for COVID-19 treatment
use High-Dose Intravenous Immune Globulin

Head of fibula
use Fibula, Left
use Fibula, Right

Hearing Aid Assessment F14Z

Hearing Assessment F13Z

Hearing Device
Bone Conduction
Left 09HE
Right 09HD
Insertion of device in
Left 0NH6
Right 0NH5
Multiple Channel Cochlear Prosthesis
Left 09HE
Right 09HD
Removal of device from, Skull 0NP0
Revision of device in, Skull 0NW0
Single Channel Cochlear Prosthesis
Left 09HE
Right 09HD

Hearing Treatment F09Z

Heart Assist System
Implantable
Insertion of device in, Heart 02HA
Removal of device from, Heart 02PA
Revision of device in, Heart 02WA
Short-term External
Insertion of device in
Aorta, Thoracic, Descending 02HW3RZ
Heart 02HA
Removal of device from
Aorta, Thoracic, Descending 02PW3RZ
Heart 02PA
Revision of device in
Aorta, Thoracic, Descending 02WW3RZ
Heart 02WA

HeartMate II® Left Ventricular Assist Device (LVAD)
use Implantable Heart Assist System in Heart and Great Vessels

HeartMate 3™ LVAS
use Implantable Heart Assist System in Heart and Great Vessels

HeartMate XVE® Left Ventricular Assist Device (LVAD)
use Implantable Heart Assist System in Heart and Great Vessels

HeartMate® implantable heart assist system
see Insertion of device in, Heart 02HA

Helix
use Ear, External, Bilateral
use Ear, External, Left
use Ear, External, Right

Hematopoietic cell transplant (HCT)
see Transfusion, Circulatory 302

Hemicolectomy
see Resection, Gastrointestinal System 0DT

Hemicystectomy
see Excision, Urinary System 0TB

Hemigastrectomy
see Excision, Gastrointestinal System 0DB

Hemiglossectomy
see Excision, Mouth and Throat 0CB

Hemilaminectomy
see Excision, Lower Bones 0QB
see Excision, Upper Bones 0PB

Hemilaminotomy
see Drainage, Lower Bones 0Q9
see Drainage, Upper Bones 0P9
see Excision, Lower Bones 0QB
see Excision, Upper Bones 0PB
see Release, Central Nervous System and Cranial Nerves 00N
see Release, Lower Bones 0QN
see Release, Peripheral Nervous System 01N
see Release, Upper Bones 0PN

Hemilaryngectomy
see Excision, Larynx 0CBS

Hemimandibulectomy
see Excision, Head and Facial Bones 0NB

Hemimaxillectomy
see Excision, Head and Facial Bones 0NB

Hemipylorectomy
see Excision, Gastrointestinal System 0DB

Hemispherectomy
see Excision, Central Nervous System and Cranial Nerves 00B
see Resection, Central Nervous System and Cranial Nerves 00T

Hemithyroidectomy
see Resection, Endocrine System 0GT
see Excision, Endocrine System 0GB

Hemodialysis
see Performance, Urinary 5A1D

Hemolung® Respiratory Assist System (RAS) 5A0920Z

Hemospray® Endoscopic Hemostat
use Mineral-based Topical Hemostatic Agent

Hepatectomy
see Excision, Hepatobiliary System and Pancreas 0FB
see Resection, Hepatobiliary System and Pancreas 0FT

Hepatic artery proper
use Artery, Hepatic

Hepatic flexure
use Colon, Transverse

Hepatic lymph node
use Lymphatic, Aortic

Hepatic plexus
use Nerve, Abdominal Sympathetic

Hepatic portal vein
use Vein, Portal

Hepaticoduodenostomy
see Bypass, Hepatobiliary System and Pancreas 0F1
see Drainage, Hepatobiliary System and Pancreas 0F9

Hepaticotomy
see Drainage, Hepatobiliary System and Pancreas 0F9

Hepatocholedochostomy
see Drainage, Duct, Common Bile 0F99

Hepatogastric ligament
use Omentum

Hepatopancreatic ampulla
use Ampulla of Vater

Hepatopexy
see Repair, Hepatobiliary System and Pancreas 0FQ
see Reposition, Hepatobiliary System and Pancreas 0FS

Hepatorrhaphy
see Repair, Hepatobiliary System and Pancreas 0FQ

Hepatotomy
see Drainage, Hepatobiliary System and Pancreas 0F9

HEPZATO™ KIT (melphalan hydrochloride Hepatic Delivery System) *use* Melphalan Hydrochloride Antineoplastic

Herculink (RX) Elite Renal Stent System
use Intraluminal Device

Herniorrhaphy
see Repair, Anatomical Regions, General 0WQ
see Repair, Anatomical Regions, Lower Extremities 0YQ
With synthetic substitute
see Supplement, Anatomical Regions, General 0WU
see Supplement, Anatomical Regions, Lower Extremities 0YU

HIG (hyperimmune globulin), for COVID-19 treatment
use Hyperimmune Globulin

High-Dose intravenous Immune Globulin, for COVID-19 treatment XW1

High-dose intravenous immunoglobulin (hdIVIG), for COVID-19 treatment
use High-Dose Intravenous Immune Globulin

Hip (joint) liner
use Liner in Lower Joints

HIPEC (hyperthermic intraperitoneal chemotherapy) 3E0M30Y

HistoSonics® System *see* New Technology, Hepatobiliary System and Pancreas XF5

Histotripsy, liver *see* New Technology, Hepatobiliary System and Pancreas XF5

hIVIG (hyperimmune intravenous immunoglobulin), for COVID-19 treatment,
use Hyperimmune Globulin

Holter monitoring 4A12X45

Holter valve ventricular shunt
use Synthetic Substitute

Human angiotensin II, synthetic
use Vasopressor

Humeroradial joint
use Joint, Elbow, Left
use Joint, Elbow, Right

Humeroulnar joint
use Joint, Elbow, Left
use Joint, Elbow, Right

Humerus, distal
use Humeral Shaft, Left
use Humeral Shaft, Right

Hydrocelectomy
see Excision, Male Reproductive System 0VB

Hydrotherapy
Assisted exercise in pool
see Motor Treatment, Rehabilitation F07
Whirlpool
see Activities of Daily Living Treatment, Rehabilitation F08

Hymenectomy
see Excision, Hymen 0UBK
see Resection, Hymen 0UTK

Hymenoplasty
see Repair, Hymen 0UQK
see Supplement, Hymen 0UUK
Hymenorrhaphy
see Repair, Hymen 0UQK
Hymenotomy
see Division, Hymen 0U8K
see Drainage, Hymen 0U9K
Hyoglossus muscle
use Muscle, Tongue, Palate,
Pharynx
Hyoid artery
use Artery, Thyroid, Left
use Artery, Thyroid, Right
Hyperalimentation
see Introduction of substance in or on
Hyperbaric oxygenation
Decompression sickness treatment
see Decompression, Circulatory
6A15
Other treatment
see Assistance, Circulatory 5A05
Hyperimmune globulin
use Globulin
Hyperimmune globulin, for
COVID-19 treatment XW1
Hyperimmune intravenous
immunoglobulin (hIVIG), for
COVID-19 treatment
use Hyperimmune Globulin
Hyperthermia
Radiation Therapy
Abdomen DWY38ZZ
Adrenal Gland DGY28ZZ
Bile Ducts DFY28ZZ
Bladder DTY28ZZ
Bone, Other DPYC8ZZ
Bone Marrow D7Y08ZZ
Brain D0Y08ZZ
Brain Stem D0Y18ZZ
Breast
Left DMY08ZZ
Right DMY18ZZ
Bronchus DBY18ZZ
Cervix DUY18ZZ
Chest DWY28ZZ
Chest Wall DBY78ZZ
Colon DDY58ZZ
Diaphragm DBY88ZZ
Duodenum DDY28ZZ
Ear D9Y08ZZ
Esophagus DDY08ZZ
Eye D8Y08ZZ
Femur DPY98ZZ
Fibula DPYB8ZZ
Gallbladder DFY18ZZ
Gland
Adrenal DGY28ZZ
Parathyroid DGY48ZZ
Pituitary DGY08ZZ
Thyroid DGY58ZZ
Glands, Salivary D9Y68ZZ
Head and Neck DWY18ZZ
Hemibody DWY48ZZ
Humerus DPY68ZZ
Hypopharynx D9Y38ZZ
Ileum DDY48ZZ
Jejunum DDY38ZZ
Kidney DTY08ZZ
Larynx D9YB8ZZ
Liver DFY08ZZ
Lung DBY28ZZ
Lymphatics
Abdomen D7Y68ZZ
Axillary D7Y48ZZ
Inguinal D7Y88ZZ
Neck D7Y38ZZ
Pelvis D7Y78ZZ
Thorax D7Y58ZZ
Mandible DPY38ZZ
Maxilla DPY28ZZ
Mediastinum DBY68ZZ

Hyperthermia *(continued)*
Radiation Therapy *(continued)*
Mouth D9Y48ZZ
Nasopharynx D9YD8ZZ
Neck and Head DWY18ZZ
Nerve, Peripheral D0Y78ZZ
Nose D9Y18ZZ
Oropharynx D9YF8ZZ
Ovary DUY08ZZ
Palate
Hard D9Y88ZZ
Soft D9Y98ZZ
Pancreas DFY38ZZ
Parathyroid Gland DGY48ZZ
Pelvic Bones DPY88ZZ
Pelvic Region DWY68ZZ
Pineal Body DGY18ZZ
Pituitary Gland DGY08ZZ
Pleura DBY58ZZ
Prostate DVY08ZZ
Radius DPY78ZZ
Rectum DDY78ZZ
Rib DPY58ZZ
Sinuses D9Y78ZZ
Skin
Abdomen DHY88ZZ
Arm DHY48ZZ
Back DHY78ZZ
Buttock DHY98ZZ
Chest DHY68ZZ
Face DHY28ZZ
Leg DHYB8ZZ
Neck DHY38ZZ
Skull DPY08ZZ
Spinal Cord D0Y68ZZ
Spleen D7Y28ZZ
Sternum DPY48ZZ
Stomach DDY18ZZ
Testis DVY18ZZ
Thymus D7Y18ZZ
Thyroid Gland DGY58ZZ
Tibia DPYB8ZZ
Tongue D9Y58ZZ
Trachea DBY08ZZ
Ulna DPY78ZZ
Ureter DTY18ZZ
Urethra DTY38ZZ
Uterus DUY28ZZ
Whole Body DWY58ZZ
Whole Body 6A3Z
Hyperthermic intraperitoneal
chemotherapy (HIPEC)
3E0M30Y
Hypnosis GZFZZZZZ
Hypogastric artery
use Artery, Internal Iliac, Left
use Artery, Internal Iliac, Right
Hypopharynx
use Pharynx
Hypophysectomy
see Excision, Gland, Pituitary 0GB0
see Resection, Gland, Pituitary 0GT0
Hypophysis
use Gland, Pituitary
Hypothalamotomy
see Destruction, Thalamus 0059
Hypothenar muscle
use Muscle, Hand, Left
use Muscle, Hand, Right
Hypothermia, Whole Body 6A4Z
Hysterectomy
Supracervical
see Resection, Uterus 0UT9
Total
see Resection, Uterus 0UT9
Hysterolysis
see Release, Uterus 0UN9
Hysteropexy
see Repair, Uterus 0UQ9
see Reposition, Uterus 0US9
Hysteroplasty
see Repair, Uterus 0UQ9

Hysterorrhaphy
see Repair, Uterus 0UQ9
Hysteroscopy 0UJD8ZZ
Hysterotomy
see Drainage, Uterus 0U99
Hysterotrachelectomy
see Resection, Cervix 0UTC
see Resection, Uterus 0UT9
Hysterotracheloplasty
see Repair, Uterus 0UQ9
Hysterotrachelorrhaphy
see Repair, Uterus 0UQ9

I

IABP (Intra-aortic balloon pump)
see Assistance, Cardiac 5A02
IAEMT (Intraoperative anesthetic
effect monitoring and titration)
see Monitoring, Central Nervous
4A10
IASD® (InterAtrial Shunt Device),
Corvia
use Synthetic Substitute
Idarucizumab, Pradaxa®
(dabigatran) reversal agent
use Other Therapeutic Substance
Ide-cel
use Idecabtagene Vicleucel
Immunotherapy
Idecabtagene Vicleucel
use Idecabtagene Vicleucel
Immunotherapy
Idecabtagene Vicleucel
Immunotherapy XW0
iFuse Bedrock™ Granite Implant
System *use* Internal Fixation
Device with Tulip Connector in
New Technology
IGIV-C, for COVID-19 treatment
use Hyperimmune Globulin
IHD (Intermittent hemodialysis)
5A1D70Z
Ileal artery
use Artery, Superior Mesenteric
Ileectomy
see Excision, Ileum 0DBB
see Resection, Ileum 0DTB
Ileocolic artery
use Artery, Superior Mesenteric
Ileocolic vein
use Vein, Colic
Ileopexy
see Repair, Ileum 0DQB
see Reposition, Ileum 0DSB
Ileorrhaphy
see Repair, Ileum 0DQB
Ileoscopy 0DJD8ZZ
Ileostomy
see Bypass, Ileum 0D1B
see Drainage, Ileum 0D9B
Ileotomy
see Drainage, Ileum 0D9B
Ileoureterostomy
see Bypass, Urinary System
0T1
Iliac crest
use Bone, Pelvic, Left
use Bone, Pelvic, Right
Iliac fascia
use Subcutaneous Tissue and Fascia,
Upper Leg, Left
use Subcutaneous Tissue and Fascia,
Upper Leg, Right
Iliac lymph node
use Lymphatic, Pelvis
Iliacus muscle
use Muscle, Hip, Left
use Muscle, Hip, Right
Iliofemoral ligament
use Bursa and Ligament, Hip, Left
use Bursa and Ligament, Hip, Right

Iliohypogastric nerve
use Nerve, Lumbar Plexus
Ilioinguinal nerve
use Nerve, Lumbar Plexus
Iliolumbar artery
use Artery, Internal Iliac, Left
use Artery, Internal Iliac, Right
Iliolumbar ligament
use Bursa and Ligament, Lower Spine
Iliotibial tract (band)
use Subcutaneous Tissue and Fascia,
Upper Leg, Left
use Subcutaneous Tissue and Fascia,
Upper Leg, Right
Ilium
use Bone, Pelvic, Left
use Bone, Pelvic, Right
Ilizarov external fixator
use External Fixation Device, Ring
in 0PH
use External Fixation Device, Ring
in 0PS
use External Fixation Device, Ring
in 0QH
use External Fixation Device, Ring
in 0QS
Ilizarov-Vecklich device
use External Fixation Device, Limb
Lengthening in 0QH
use External Fixation Device, Limb
Lengthening in 0PH
Imaging, diagnostic
see Computerized Tomography
(CT Scan)
see Fluoroscopy
see Magnetic Resonance Imaging
(MRI)
see Plain Radiography
see Ultrasonography
Imdevimab (REGN10987) and
Casirivimab (REGN10933)
use REGN-COV2 Monoclonal
Antibody
IMFINZI®
use Durvalumab Antineoplastic
IMI/REL
use Imipenem-cilastatin-relebactam
Anti-infective
Imipenem-cilastatin-relebactam
Anti-infective XW0
Immobilization
Abdominal Wall 2W33X
Arm
Lower
Left 2W3DX
Right 2W3CX
Upper
Left 2W3BX
Right 2W3AX
Back 2W35X
Chest Wall 2W34X
Extremity
Lower
Left 2W3MX
Right 2W3LX
Upper
Left 2W39X
Right 2W38X
Face 2W31X
Finger
Left 2W3KX
Right 2W3JX
Foot
Left 2W3TX
Right 2W3SX
Hand
Left 2W3FX
Right 2W3EX
Head 2W30X
Inguinal Region
Left 2W37X
Right 2W36X

Immobilization *(continued)*
Leg
  Lower
    Left 2W3RX
    Right 2W3QX
  Upper
    Left 2W3PX
    Right 2W3NX
Neck 2W32X
Thumb
  Left 2W3H
  Right 2W3GX
Toe
  Left 2W3VX
  Right 2W3UX
Immunization
  see Introduction of Serum, Toxoid, and Vaccine
Immunoglobulin
  use Globulin
Immunotherapy
  see Introduction of Immunotherapeutic Substance
Immunotherapy, antineoplastic
Interferon
  see Introduction of Low-dose Interleukin-2
Interleukin-2, high-dose
  see Introduction of High-dose Interleukin-2
Interleukin-2, low-dose
  see Introduction of Low-dose Interleukin-2
Monoclonal antibody
  see Introduction of Monoclonal Antibody
Proleukin, high-dose
  see Introduction of High-dose Interleukin-2
Proleukin, low-dose
  see Introduction of Low-dose Interleukin-2
Impella® 5.5 with SmartAssist® System *use* Conduit to Short-term External Heart Assist System in New Technology
Impella® heart pump
  use Short-term External Heart Assist System in Heart and Great Vessels
Impeller Pump
Continuous, Output 5A0221D
Intermittent, Output 5A0211D
Implantable cardioverter-defibrillator (ICD)
  use Defibrillator Generator in 0JH
Implantable drug infusion pump (anti-spasmodic) (chemotherapy)(pain)
  use Infusion Device, Pump in Subcutaneous Tissue and Fascia
Implantable glucose monitoring device
  use Monitoring Device
Implantable hemodynamic monitor (IHM)
  use Monitoring Device, Hemodynamic in 0JH
Implantable hemodynamic monitoring system (IHMS)
  use Monitoring Device, Hemodynamic in 0JH
Implantable Miniature Telescope™ (IMT)
  use Synthetic Substitute, Intraocular Telescope in 08R
Implantation
  see Insertion
  see Replacement
Implanted (venous)(access) port
  use Vascular Access Device, Totally Implantable in Subcutaneous Tissue and Fascia

IMV (intermittent mandatory ventilation)
  see Assistance, Respiratory 5A09
In Vitro Fertilization 8E0ZXY1
Incision, abscess
  see Drainage
Incudectomy
  see Excision, Ear, Nose, Sinus 09B
  see Resection, Ear, Nose, Sinus 09T
Incudopexy
  see Reposition, Ear, Nose, Sinus 09S
  see Repair, Ear, Nose, Sinus 09Q
Incus
  use Auditory Ossicle, Left
  use Auditory Ossicle, Right
Induction of labor
Artificial rupture of membranes
  see Drainage, Pregnancy 109
Oxytocin
  see Introduction of Hormone
InDura, intrathecal catheter (1P) (spinal)
  use Infusion Device
Inebilizumab-cdon XW0
Inferior cardiac nerve
  use Nerve, Thoracic Sympathetic
Inferior cerebellar vein
  use Vein, Intracranial
Inferior cerebral vein
  use Vein, Intracranial
Inferior epigastric artery
  use Artery, External Iliac, Left
  use Artery, External Iliac, Right
Inferior epigastric lymph node
  use Lymphatic, Pelvis
Inferior genicular artery
  use Artery, Popliteal, Left
  use Artery, Popliteal, Right
Inferior gluteal artery
  use Artery, Internal Iliac, Left
  use Artery, Internal Iliac, Right
Inferior gluteal nerve
  use Nerve, Sacral Plexus
Inferior hypogastric plexus
  use Nerve, Abdominal Sympathetic
Inferior labial artery
  use Artery, Face
Inferior longitudinal muscle
  use Muscle, Tongue, Palate, Pharynx
Inferior mesenteric ganglion
  use Nerve, Abdominal Sympathetic
Inferior mesenteric lymph node
  use Lymphatic, Mesenteric
Inferior mesenteric plexus
  use Nerve, Abdominal Sympathetic
Inferior oblique muscle
  use Muscle, Extraocular, Left
  use Muscle, Extraocular, Right
Inferior pancreaticoduodenal artery
  use Artery, Superior Mesenteric
Inferior phrenic artery
  use Aorta, Abdominal
Inferior rectus muscle
  use Muscle, Extraocular, Left
  use Muscle, Extraocular, Right
Inferior suprarenal artery
  use Artery, Renal, Left
  use Artery, Renal, Right
Inferior tarsal plate
  use Eyelid, Lower, Left
  use Eyelid, Lower, Right
Inferior thyroid vein
  use Vein, Innominate, Left
  use Vein, Innominate, Right
Inferior tibiofibular joint
  use Joint, Ankle, Left
  use Joint, Ankle, Right
Inferior turbinate
  use Turbinate, Nasal
Inferior ulnar collateral artery
  use Artery, Brachial, Left
  use Artery, Brachial, Right

Inferior vesical artery
  use Artery, Internal Iliac, Left
  use Artery, Internal Iliac, Right
Infraauricular lymph node
  use Lymphatic, Head
Infraclavicular (deltopectoral) lymph node
  use Lymphatic, Upper Extremity, Left
  use Lymphatic, Upper Extremity, Right
Infrahyoid muscle
  use Muscle, Neck, Left
  use Muscle, Neck, Right
Infraparotid lymph node
  use Lymphatic, Head
Infraspinatus fascia
  use Subcutaneous Tissue and Fascia, Upper Arm, Left
  use Subcutaneous Tissue and Fascia, Upper Arm, Right
Infraspinatus muscle
  use Muscle, Shoulder, Left
  use Muscle, Shoulder, Right
Infundibulopelvic ligament
  use Uterine Supporting Structure
Infusion
  see Introduction of substance in or on
Infusion Device, Pump
Insertion of device in
  Abdomen 0JH8
  Back 0JH7
  Chest 0JH6
  Lower Arm
    Left 0JHH
    Right 0JHG
  Lower Leg
    Left 0JHP
    Right 0JHN
  Trunk 0JHT
  Upper Arm
    Left 0JHF
    Right 0JHD
  Upper Leg
    Left 0JHM
    Right 0JHL
Removal of device from
  Lower Extremity 0JPW
  Trunk 0JPT
  Upper Extremity 0JPV
Revision of device in
  Lower Extremity 0JWW
  Trunk 0JWT
  Upper Extremity 0JWV
Infusion, glucarpidase
Central vein 3E043GQ
Peripheral vein 3E033GQ
Inguinal canal
  use Inguinal Region, Bilateral
  use Inguinal Region, Left
  use Inguinal Region, Right
Inguinal triangle
  use Inguinal Region, Bilateral
  use Inguinal Region, Left
  use Inguinal Region, Right
Injection
  see Introduction of substance in or on
Injection reservoir, port
  use Vascular Access Device, Totally Implantable in Subcutaneous Tissue and Fascia
Injection reservoir, pump
  use Infusion Device, Pump in Subcutaneous Tissue and Fascia
Insemination, artificial 3E0P7LZ
Insertion
Antimicrobial envelope
  see Introduction of Anti-infective
Aqueous drainage shunt
  see Bypass, Eye 081
  see Drainage, Eye 089
Bone, Pelvic, Internal Fixation Device with Tulip Connector XNH

Insertion *(continued)*
Conduit to Short-term External Heart Assist System X2H
Intracardiac Pacemaker, Dual-Chamber X2H
Intraluminal Device, Bioprosthetic Valve X2H
Joint
  Lumbar Vertebral, Posterior Spinal Motion Preservation Device XRHB018
  Lumbosacral, Posterior Spinal Motion Preservation Device XRHD018
Neurostimulator Lead, Sphenopalatine Ganglion X0HK3Q8
Neurostimulator Lead with Paired Stimulation System X0HQ3R8
Products of Conception 10H0
Spinal Stabilization Device
  see Insertion of device in, Upper Joints 0RH
  see Insertion of device in, Lower Joints 0SH
Tibial Extension with Motion Sensors XNH
Insertion of device in
Abdominal Wall 0WHF
Acetabulum
  Left 0QH5
  Right 0QH4
Anal Sphincter 0DHR
Ankle Region
  Left 0YHL
  Right 0YHK
Anus 0DHQ
Aorta
  Abdominal 04H0
  Thoracic
    Ascending/Arch 02HX
    Descending 02HW
Arm
  Lower
    Left 0XHF
    Right 0XHD
  Upper
    Left 0XH9
    Right 0XH8
Artery
  Anterior Tibial
    Left 04HQ
    Right 04HP
  Axillary
    Left 03H6
    Right 03H5
  Brachial
    Left 03H8
    Right 03H7
  Celiac 04H1
  Colic
    Left 04H7
    Middle 04H8
    Right 04H6
  Common Carotid
    Left 03HJ
    Right 03HH
  Common Iliac
    Left 04HD
    Right 04HC
  Coronary
    Four or More Arteries 02H3
    One Artery 02H0
    Three Arteries 02H2
    Two Arteries 02H1
  External Carotid
    Left 03HN
    Right 03HM
  External Iliac
    Left 04HJ
    Right 04HH

Insertion of device in (continued)
  Artery (continued)
    Face 03HR
    Femoral
      Left 04HL
      Right 04HK
    Foot
      Left 04HW
      Right 04HV
    Gastric 04H2
    Hand
      Left 03HF
      Right 03HD
    Hepatic 04H3
    Inferior Mesenteric 04HB
    Innominate 03H2
    Internal Carotid
      Left 03HL
      Right 03HK
    Internal Iliac
      Left 04HF
      Right 04HE
    Internal Mammary
      Left 03H1
      Right 03H0
    Intracranial 03HG
    Lower 04HY
    Peroneal
      Left 04HU
      Right 04HT
    Popliteal
      Left 04HN
      Right 04HM
    Posterior Tibial
      Left 04HS
      Right 04HR
    Pulmonary
      Left 02HR
      Right 02HQ
    Pulmonary Trunk 02HP
    Radial
      Left 03HC
      Right 03HB
    Renal
      Left 04HA
      Right 04H9
    Splenic 04H4
    Subclavian
      Left 03H4
      Right 03H3
    Superior Mesenteric 04H5
    Temporal
      Left 03HT
      Right 03HS
    Thyroid
      Left 03HV
      Right 03HU
    Ulnar
      Left 03HA
      Right 03H9
    Upper 03HY
    Vertebral
      Left 03HQ
      Right 03HP
  Atrium
    Left 02H7
    Right 02H6
  Axilla
    Left 0XH5
    Right 0XH4
  Back
    Lower 0WHL
    Upper 0WHK
  Bladder 0THB
  Bladder Neck 0THC
  Bone
    Ethmoid
      Left 0NHG
      Right 0NHF
    Facial 0NHW
    Frontal 0NH1
    Hyoid 0NHX

  Bone (continued)
    Lacrimal
      Left 0NHJ
      Right 0NHH
    Lower 0QHY
    Nasal 0NHB
    Occipital 0NH7
    Palatine
      Left 0NHL
      Right 0NHK
    Parietal
      Left 0NH4
      Right 0NH3
    Pelvic
      Left 0QH3
      Right 0QH2
    Sphenoid 0NHC
    Temporal
      Left 0NH6
      Right 0NH5
    Upper 0PHY
    Zygomatic
      Left 0NHN
      Right 0NHM
  Bone Marrow 07HT
  Brain 00H0
  Breast
    Bilateral 0HHV
    Left 0HHU
    Right 0HHT
  Bronchus
    Lingula 0BH9
    Lower Lobe
      Left 0BHB
      Right 0BH6
    Main
      Left 0BH7
      Right 0BH3
    Middle Lobe, Right 0BH5
    Upper Lobe
      Left 0BH8
      Right 0BH4
  Bursa and Ligament
    Lower 0MHY
    Upper 0MHX
  Buttock
    Left 0YH1
    Right 0YH0
  Carpal
    Left 0PHN
    Right 0PHM
  Cavity, Cranial 0WH1
  Cerebral Ventricle 00H6
  Cervix 0UHC
  Chest Wall 0WH8
  Cisterna Chyli 07HL
  Clavicle
    Left 0PHB
    Right 0PH9
  Coccyx 0QHS
  Cul-de-sac 0UHF
  Diaphragm 0BHT
  Disc
    Cervical Vertebral 0RH3
    Cervicothoracic Vertebral
      0RH5
    Lumbar Vertebral 0SH2
    Lumbosacral 0SH4
    Thoracic Vertebral 0RH9
    Thoracolumbar Vertebral
      0RHB
  Duct
    Hepatobiliary 0FHB
    Pancreatic 0FHD
  Duodenum 0DH9
  Ear
    Inner
      Left 09HE
      Right 09HD
    Left 09HJ
    Right 09HH

  Elbow Region
    Left 0XHC
    Right 0XHB
  Epididymis and Spermatic Cord
    0VHM
  Esophagus 0DH5
    Lower, Magnetic Lengthening
      Device 0DH37JZ
    Middle, Magnetic Lengthening
      Device 0DH27JZ
    Upper, Magnetic Lengthening
      Device 0DH17JZ
  Extremity
    Lower
      Left 0YHB
      Right 0YH9
    Upper
      Left 0XH7
      Right 0XH6
  Eye
    Left 08H1
    Right 08H0
  Face 0WH2
  Fallopian Tube 0UH8
  Femoral Region
    Left 0YH8
    Right 0YH7
  Femoral Shaft
    Left 0QH9
    Right 0QH8
  Femur
    Lower
      Left 0QHC
      Right 0QHB
    Upper
      Left 0QH7
      Right 0QH6
  Fibula
    Left 0QHK
    Right 0QHJ
  Foot
    Left 0YHN
    Right 0YHM
  Gallbladder 0FH4
  Gastrointestinal Tract 0WHP
  Genitourinary Tract 0WHR
  Gland
    Endocrine 0GHS
    Salivary 0CHA
  Glenoid Cavity
    Left 0PH8
    Right 0PH7
  Hand
    Left 0XHK
    Right 0XHJ
  Head 0WH0
  Heart 02HA
  Humeral Head
    Left 0PHD
    Right 0PHC
  Humeral Shaft
    Left 0PHG
    Right 0PHF
  Ileum 0DHB
  Inguinal Region
    Left 0YH6
    Right 0YH5
  Intestinal Tract
    Lower Intestinal Tract 0DHD
    Upper Intestinal Tract 0DH0
  Intestine
    Large 0DHE
    Small 0DH8
  Jaw
    Lower 0WH5
    Upper 0WH4
  Jejunum 0DHA
  Joint
    Acromioclavicular
      Left 0RHH
      Right 0RHG

  Joint (continued)
    Ankle
      Left 0SHG
      Right 0SHF
    Carpal
      Left 0RHR
      Right 0RHQ
    Carpometacarpal
      Left 0RHT
      Right 0RHS
    Cervical Vertebral 0RH1
    Cervicothoracic Vertebral 0RH4
    Coccygeal 0SH6
    Elbow
      Left 0RHM
      Right 0RHL
    Finger Phalangeal
      Left 0RHX
      Right 0RHW
    Hip
      Left 0SHB
      Right 0SH9
    Knee
      Left 0SHD
      Right 0SHC
    Lumbar Vertebral 0SH0
    Lumbosacral 0SH3
    Metacarpophalangeal
      Left 0RHV
      Right 0RHU
    Metatarsal-Phalangeal
      Left 0SHN
      Right 0SHM
    Occipital-cervical 0RH0
    Sacrococcygeal 0SH5
    Sacroiliac
      Left 0SH8
      Right 0SH7
    Shoulder
      Left 0RHK
      Right 0RHJ
    Sternoclavicular
      Left 0RHF
      Right 0RHE
    Tarsal
      Left 0SHJ
      Right 0SHH
    Tarsometatarsal
      Left 0SHL
      Right 0SHK
    Temporomandibular
      Left 0RHD
      Right 0RHC
    Thoracic Vertebral 0RH6
    Thoracolumbar Vertebral
    Toe Phalangeal
      Left 0SHQ
      Right 0SHP
    Wrist
      Left 0RHP
      Right 0RHN
  Kidney 0TH5
  Knee Region
    Left 0YHG
    Right 0YHF
  Larynx 0CHS
  Leg
    Lower
      Left 0YHJ
      Right 0YHH
    Upper
      Left 0YHD
      Right 0YHC
  Liver 0FH0
    Left Lobe 0FH2
    Right Lobe 0FH1
  Lung
    Left 0BHL
    Right 0BHK
  Lymphatic 07HN3
    Thoracic Duct 07HK

Insertion of device in (continued)

Mandible
  Left 0NHV
  Right 0NHT
Maxilla 0NHR
Mediastinum 0WHC
Metacarpal
  Left 0PHQ
  Right 0PHP
Metatarsal
  Left 0QHP
  Right 0QHN
Mouth and Throat 0CHY
Muscle
  Lower 0KHY
  Upper 0KHX
Nasal Mucosa and Soft Tissue 09HK
Nasopharynx 09HN
Neck 0WH6
Nerve
  Cranial 00HE
  Peripheral 01HY
Nipple
  Left 0HHX
  Right 0HHW
Oral Cavity and Throat 0WH3
Orbit
  Left 0NHQ
  Right 0NHP
Ovary 0UH3
Pancreas 0FHG
Patella
  Left 0QHF
  Right 0QHD
Pelvic Cavity 0WHJ
Penis 0VHS
Pericardial Cavity 0WHD
Pericardium 02HN
Perineum
  Female 0WHN
  Male 0WHM
Peritoneal Cavity 0WHG
Phalanx
  Finger
    Left 0PHV
    Right 0PHT
  Thumb
    Left 0PHS
    Right 0PHR
  Toe
    Left 0QHR
    Right 0QHQ
Pleura 0BHQ
Pleural Cavity
  Left 0WHB
  Right 0WH9
Prostate 0VH0
Prostate and Seminal Vesicles 0VH4
Radius
  Left 0PHJ
  Right 0PHH
Rectum 0DHP
Respiratory Tract 0WHQ
Retroperitoneum 0WHH
Ribs
  1 to 2 0PH1
  3 or More 0PH2
Sacrum 0QH1
Scapula
  Left 0PH6
  Right 0PH5
Scrotum and Tunica Vaginalis 0VH8
Shoulder Region
  Left 0XH3
  Right 0XH2
Sinus 09HY
Skin 0HHPXYZ
Skull 0NH0
Spinal Canal 00HU
Spinal Cord 00HV
Spleen 07HP
Sternum 0PH0

Insertion of device in (continued)

Stomach 0DH6
Subcutaneous Tissue and Fascia
  Abdomen 0JH8
  Back 0JH7
  Buttock 0JH9
  Chest 0JH6
  Face 0JH1
  Foot
    Left 0JHR
    Right 0JHQ
  Hand
    Left 0JHK
    Right 0JHJ
  Head and Neck 0JHS
  Lower Arm
    Left 0JHH
    Right 0JHG
  Lower Extremity 0JHW
  Lower Leg
    Left 0JHP
    Right 0JHN
  Neck
    Left 0JH5
    Right 0JH4
  Pelvic Region 0JHC
  Perineum 0JHB
  Scalp 0JH0
  Trunk 0JHT
  Upper Arm
    Left 0JHF
    Right 0JHD
  Upper Extremity 0JHV
  Upper Leg
    Left 0JHM
    Right 0JHL
Tarsal
  Left 0QHM
  Right 0QHL
Tendon
  Lower 0LHY
  Upper 0LHX
Testis 0VHD
Thymus 07HM
Tibia
  Left 0QHH
  Right 0QHG
Tongue 0CH7
Trachea 0BH1
Tracheobronchial Tree 0BH0
Ulna
  Left 0PHL
  Right 0PHK
Ureter 0TH9
Urethra 0THD
Uterus 0UH9
Uterus and Cervix 0UHD
Vagina 0UHG
Vagina and Cul-de-sac 0UHH
Vas Deferens 0VHR
Vein
  Axillary
    Left 05H8
    Right 05H7
  Azygos 05H0
  Basilic
    Left 05HC
    Right 05HB
  Brachial
    Left 05HA
    Right 05H9
  Cephalic
    Left 05HF
    Right 05HD
  Colic 06H7
  Common Iliac
    Left 06HD
    Right 06HC
  Coronary 02H4
  Esophageal 06H3
  External Iliac
    Left 06HG
    Right 06HF

Insertion of device in (continued)

Vein (continued)
  External Jugular
    Left 05HQ
    Right 05HP
  Face
    Left 05HV
    Right 05HT
  Femoral
    Left 06HN
    Right 06HM
  Foot
    Left 06HV
    Right 06HT
  Gastric 06H2
  Hand
    Left 05HH
    Right 05HG
  Hemiazygos 05H1
  Hepatic 06H4
  Hypogastric
    Left 06HJ
    Right 06HH
  Inferior Mesenteric 06H6
  Innominate
    Left 05H4
    Right 05H3
  Internal Jugular
    Left 05HN
    Right 05HM
  Intracranial 05HL
  Lower 06HY
  Portal 06H8
  Pulmonary
    Left 02HT
    Right 02HS
  Renal
    Left 06HB
    Right 06H9
  Saphenous
    Left 06HQ
    Right 06HP
  Splenic 06H1
  Subclavian
    Left 05H6
    Right 05H5
  Superior Mesenteric 06H5
  Upper 05HY
  Vertebral
    Left 05HS
    Right 05HR
Vena Cava
  Inferior 06H0
  Superior 02HV
Ventricle
  Left 02HL
  Right 02HK
Vertebra
  Cervical 0PH3
  Lumbar 0QH0
  Thoracic 0PH4
Wrist Region
  Left 0XHH
  Right 0XHG

Inspection

Abdominal Wall 0WJF
Ankle Region
  Left 0YJL
  Right 0YJK
Arm
  Lower
    Left 0XJF
    Right 0XJD
  Upper
    Left 0XJ9
    Right 0XJ8
Artery
  Lower 04JY
  Upper 03JY
Axilla
  Left 0XJ5
  Right 0XJ4

Inspection (continued)

Back
  Lower 0WJL
  Upper 0WJK
Bladder 0TJB
Bone
  Facial 0NJW
  Lower 0QJY
  Nasal 0NJB
  Upper 0PJY
Bone Marrow 07JT
Brain 00J0
Breast
  Left 0HJU
  Right 0HJT
Bursa and Ligament
  Lower 0MJY
  Upper 0MJX
Buttock
  Left 0YJ1
  Right 0YJ0
Cavity, Cranial 0WJ1
Chest Wall 0WJ8
Cisterna Chyli 07JL
Diaphragm 0BJT
Disc
  Cervical Vertebral 0RJ3
  Cervicothoracic Vertebral
    0RJ5
  Lumbar Vertebral 0SJ2
  Lumbosacral 0SJ4
  Thoracic Vertebral 0RJ9
  Thoracolumbar Vertebral
    0RJB
Duct
  Hepatobiliary 0FJB
  Pancreatic 0FJD
Ear
  Inner
    Left 09JE
    Right 09JD
  Left 09JJ
  Right 09JH
Elbow Region
  Left 0XJC
  Right 0XJB
Epididymis and Spermatic Cord
  0VJM
Extremity
  Lower
    Left 0YJB
    Right 0YJ9
  Upper
    Left 0XJ7
    Right 0XJ6
Eye
  Left 08J1XZZ
  Right 08J0XZZ
Face 0WJ2
Fallopian Tube 0UJ8
Femoral Region
  Bilateral 0YJE
  Left 0YJ8
  Right 0YJ7
Finger Nail 0HJQXZZ
Foot
  Left 0YJN
  Right 0YJM
Gallbladder 0FJ4
Gastrointestinal Tract 0WJP
Genitourinary Tract 0WJR
Gland
  Adrenal 0GJ5
  Endocrine 0GJS
  Pituitary 0GJ0
  Salivary 0CJA
Great Vessel 02JY
Hand
  Left 0XJK
  Right 0XJJ
Head 0WJ0
Heart 02JA

Inspection (continued)

Inguinal Region
  Bilateral 0YJA
  Left 0YJ6
  Right 0YJ5
Intestinal Tract
  Lower Intestinal Tract 0DJD
  Upper Intestinal Tract 0DJ0
Jaw
  Lower 0WJ5
  Upper 0WJ4
Joint
  Acromioclavicular
    Left 0RJH
    Right 0RJG
  Ankle
    Left 0SJG
    Right 0SJF
  Carpal
    Left 0RJR
    Right 0RJQ
  Carpometacarpal
    Left 0RJT
    Right 0RJS
  Cervical Vertebral 0RJ1
  Cervicothoracic Vertebral 0RJ4
  Coccygeal 0SJ6
  Elbow
    Left 0RJM
    Right 0RJL
  Finger Phalangeal
    Left 0RJX
    Right 0RJW
  Hip
    Left 0SJB
    Right 0SJ9
  Knee
    Left 0SJD
    Right 0SJC
  Lumbar Vertebral 0SJ0
  Lumbosacral 0SJ3
  Metacarpophalangeal
    Left 0RJV
    Right 0RJU
  Metatarsal-Phalangeal
    Left 0SJN
    Right 0SJM
  Occipital-cervical 0RJ0
  Sacrococcygeal 0SJ5
  Sacroiliac
    Left 0SJ8
    Right 0SJ7
  Shoulder
    Left 0RJK
    Right 0RJJ
  Sternoclavicular
    Left 0RJF
    Right 0RJE
  Tarsal
    Left 0SJJ
    Right 0SJH
  Tarsometatarsal
    Left 0SJL
    Right 0SJK
  Temporomandibular
    Left 0RJD
    Right 0RJC
  Thoracic Vertebral 0RJ6
  Thoracolumbar Vertebral
    0RJA
  Toe Phalangeal
    Left 0SJQ
    Right 0SJP
  Wrist
    Left 0RJP
    Right 0RJN
Kidney 0TJ5
Knee Region
  Left 0YJG
  Right 0YJF
Larynx 0CJS

Inspection (continued)

Leg
  Lower
    Left 0YJJ
    Right 0YJH
  Upper
    Left 0YJD
    Right 0YJC
Lens
  Left 08JKXZZ
  Right 08JJXZZ
Liver 0FJ0
Lung
  Left 0BJL
  Right 0BJK
Lymphatic 07JN
  Thoracic Duct 07JK
Mediastinum 0WJC
Mesentery 0DJV
Mouth and Throat 0CJY
Muscle
  Extraocular
    Left 08JM
    Right 08JL
  Lower 0KJY
  Upper 0KJX
Nasal Mucosa and Soft Tissue
  09JK
Neck 0WJ6
Nerve
  Cranial 00JE
  Peripheral 01JY
Omentum 0DJU
Oral Cavity and Throat 0WJ3
Ovary 0UJ3
Pancreas 0FJG
Parathyroid Gland 0GJR
Pelvic Cavity 0WJJ
Penis 0VJS
Pericardial Cavity 0WJD
Perineum
  Female 0WJN
  Male 0WJM
Peritoneal Cavity 0WJG
Peritoneum 0DJW
Pineal Body 0GJ1
Pleura 0BJQ
Pleural Cavity
  Left 0WJB
  Right 0WJ9
Products of Conception 10J0
  Ectopic 10J2
  Retained 10J1
Prostate and Seminal Vesicles 0VJ4
Respiratory Tract 0WJQ
Retroperitoneum 0WJH
Scrotum and Tunica Vaginalis
  0VJ8
Shoulder Region
  Left 0XJ3
  Right 0XJ2
Sinus 09JY
Skin 0HJPXZZ
Skull 0NJ0
Spinal Canal 00JU
Spinal Cord 00JV
Spleen 07JP
Stomach 0DJ6
Subcutaneous Tissue and Fascia
  Head and Neck 0JJS
  Lower Extremity 0JJW
  Trunk 0JJT
  Upper Extremity 0JJV
Tendon
  Lower 0LJY
  Upper 0LJX
Testis 0VJD
Thymus 07JM
Thyroid Gland 0GJK
Toe Nail 0HJRX
Trachea 0BJ1

Inspection (continued)

Tracheobronchial Tree
  0BJ0
Tympanic Membrane
  Left 09J8
  Right 09J7
Ureter 0TJ9
Urethra 0TJD
Uterus and Cervix 0UJD
Vagina and Cul-de-sac
  0UJH
Vas Deferens 0VJR
Vein
  Lower 06JY
  Upper 05JY
Vulva 0UJM
Wrist Region
  Left 0XJH
  Right 0XJG
Instillation
  see Introduction of substance in
  or on
Insufflation
  see Introduction of substance in
  or on
Intellis™ neurostimulator *use*
  Stimulator Generator, Multiple
  Array Rechargeable in 0JH
Interatrial septum
  use Septum, Atrial
InterAtrial Shunt Device IASD®,
  Corvia
  use Synthetic Substitute
Interbody fusion (spine)
  cage
  use Interbody Fusion Device in
  Lower Joints
  use Interbody Fusion Device in
  Upper Joints
Interbody Fusion Device, Custom-
  Made Anatomically Designed
  Lumbar Vertebral
    XRGB
    2 or more XRGC
  Lumbosacral XRGD
  Thoracolumbar Vertebral
    XRGA
Intercarpal joint
  use Joint, Carpal, Left
  use Joint, Carpal, Right
Intercarpal ligament
  use Bursa and Ligament, Hand,
  Left
  use Bursa and Ligament, Hand,
  Right
INTERCEPT Blood System for
  Plasma Pathogen Reduced
  Cryoprecipitated Fibrinogen
  Complex
  use Pathogen Reduced
  Cryoprecipitated Fibrinogen
  Complex
INTERCEPT Fibrinogen
  Complex
  use Pathogen Reduced
  Cryoprecipitated Fibrinogen
  Complex
Interclavicular ligament
  use Bursa and Ligament, Shoulder,
  Left
  use Bursa and Ligament, Shoulder,
  Right
Intercostal lymph node
  use Lymphatic, Thorax
Intercostal muscle
  use Muscle, Thorax, Left
  use Muscle, Thorax, Right
Intercostal nerve
  use Nerve, Thoracic
Intercostobrachial nerve
  use Nerve, Thoracic

Intercuneiform joint
  use Joint, Tarsal, Left
  use Joint, Tarsal, Right
Intercuneiform ligament
  use Bursa and Ligament, Foot,
  Left
  use Bursa and Ligament, Foot,
  Right
Intermediate bronchus
  use Main Bronchus, Right
Intermediate cuneiform bone
  use Tarsal, Left
  use Tarsal, Right
Intermittent Coronary Sinus
  Occlusion X2A7358
Intermittent hemodialysis (IHD)
  5A1D70Z
Intermittent mandatory
  ventilation
  see Assistance, Respiratory
  5A09
Intermittent Negative Airway
  Pressure
  24-96 Consecutive Hours,
  Ventilation 5A0945B
  Greater than 96 Consecutive Hours,
  Ventilation 5A0955B
  Less than 24 Consecutive Hours,
  Ventilation 5A0935B
Intermittent Positive Airway
  Pressure
  24-96 Consecutive Hours,
  Ventilation 5A09458
  Greater than 96 Consecutive Hours,
  Ventilation 5A09558
  Less than 24 Consecutive Hours,
  Ventilation 5A09358
Intermittent positive pressure
  breathing
  see Assistance, Respiratory
  5A09
Internal anal sphincter
  use Anal Sphincter
Internal (basal) cerebral vein
  use Vein, Intracranial
Internal carotid artery, intracranial
  portion
  use Intracranial Artery
Internal carotid plexus
  use Nerve, Head and Neck
  Sympathetic
Internal Fixation Device with Tulip
  Connector
  Fusion, Joint, Sacroiliac XRG
  Insertion, Bone, Pelvic XNH
Internal iliac vein
  use Vein, Hypogastric, Left
  use Vein, Hypogastric, Right
Internal maxillary artery
  use Artery, External Carotid,
  Left
  use Artery, External Carotid,
  Right
Internal naris
  use Nasal Mucosa and Soft
  Tissue
Internal oblique muscle
  use Muscle, Abdomen, Left
  use Muscle, Abdomen, Right
Internal pudendal artery
  use Artery, Internal Iliac,
  Left
  use Artery, Internal Iliac,
  Right
Internal pudendal vein
  use Vein, Hypogastric, Left
  use Vein, Hypogastric, Right
Internal thoracic artery
  use Artery, Internal Mammary, Left
  use Artery, Internal Mammary,
  Right

Internal thoracic artery *(continued)*
  use Artery, Subclavian, Left
  use Artery, Subclavian, Right
Internal urethral sphincter
  use Urethra
Interphalangeal (IP) joint
  use Joint, Finger Phalangeal, Left
  use Joint, Finger Phalangeal, Right
  use Joint, Toe Phalangeal, Left
  use Joint, Toe Phalangeal, Right
Interphalangeal ligament
  use Bursa and Ligament, Foot, Left
  use Bursa and Ligament, Foot, Right
  use Bursa and Ligament, Hand, Left
  use Bursa and Ligament, Hand, Right
Interrogation, cardiac rhythm related device
  Interrogation only
    see Measurement, Cardiac 4B02
  With cardiac function testing
    see Measurement, Cardiac 4A02
Interruption
  see Occlusion
Interspinalis muscle
  use Muscle, Trunk, Left
  use Muscle, Trunk, Right
Interspinous ligament, cervical
  use Head and Neck Bursa and Ligament
Interspinous ligament, lumbar
  use Lower Spine Bursa and Ligament
Interspinous ligament, thoracic
  use Upper Spine Bursa and Ligament
Interspinous process spinal stabilization device
  use Spinal Stabilization Device, Interspinous Process in 0RH
  use Spinal Stabilization Device, Interspinous Process in 0SH
InterStim® Therapy lead
  use Neurostimulator Lead in Peripheral Nervous System
InterStim® II Therapy neurostimulator
  use Stimulator Generator, Single Array in 0JH
InterStim™ Micro Therapy neurostimulator
  use Stimulator Generator, Single Array Rechargeable in 0JH
Intertransversarius muscle
  use Muscle, Trunk, Left
  use Muscle, Trunk, Right
Intertransverse ligament, cervical
  use Head and Neck Bursa and Ligament
Intertransverse ligament, lumbar
  use Lower Spine Bursa and Ligament
Intertransverse ligament, thoracic
  use Upper Spine Bursa and Ligament
Interventricular foramen (Monro)
  use Cerebral Ventricle
Interventricular septum
  use Septum, Ventricular
Intestinal lymphatic trunk
  use Cisterna Chyli
Intracardiac Pacemaker, Dual-Chamber, Insertion X2H
Intracranial Arterial Flow, Whole Blood mRNA XXE5XT7
Intraluminal Device
  Airway
    Esophagus 0DH5
    Mouth and Throat 0CHY

Intraluminal Device *(continued)*
  Airway *(continued)*
    Nasopharynx 09HN
  Bioactive
    Occlusion
      Common Carotid
        Left 03LJ
        Right 03LH
      External Carotid
        Left 03LN
        Right 03LM
      Internal Carotid
        Left 03LL
        Right 03LK
      Intracranial 03LG
      Vertebral
        Left 03LQ
        Right 03LP
    Restriction
      Common Carotid
        Left 03VJ
        Right 03VH
      External Carotid
        Left 03VN
        Right 03VM
      Internal Carotid
        Left 03VL
        Right 03VK
      Intracranial 03VG
      Vertebral
        Left 03VQ
        Right 03VP
  Bioprosthetic Valve, Insertion X2H
  Endobronchial Valve
    Lingula 0BH9
    Lower Lobe
      Left 0BHB
      Right 0BH6
    Main
      Left 0BH7
      Right 0BH3
    Middle Lobe, Right 0BH5
    Upper Lobe
      Left 0BH8
      Right 0BH4
  Endotracheal Airway
    Change device in, Trachea 0B21XEZ
    Insertion of device in, Trachea 0BH1
  Pessary
    Change device in, Vagina and Cul-de-sac 0U2HXGZ
    Insertion of device in Cul-de-sac 0UHF
    Vagina 0UHG
Intramedullary (IM) rod (nail)
  use Internal Fixation Device, Intramedullary in Lower Bones
  use Internal Fixation Device, Intramedullary in Upper Bones
Intramedullary skeletal kinetic distractor (ISKD)
  use Internal Fixation Device, Intramedullary in Lower Bones
  use Internal Fixation Device, Intramedullary in Upper Bones
Intraocular Telescope
  Left 08RK30Z
  Right 08RJ30Z
Intra.OX 8E02XDZ
Intraoperative Radiation Therapy (IORT)
  Anus DDY8CZZ
  Bile Ducts DFY2CZZ
  Bladder DTY2CZZ
  Brain D0Y0CZZ
  Brain Stem D0Y1CZZ
  Cervix DUY1CZZ
  Colon DDY5CZZ
  Duodenum DDY2CZZ

Intraoperative Radiation Therapy (IORT) *(continued)*
  Gallbladder DFY1CZZ
  Ileum DDY4CZZ
  Jejunum DDY3CZZ
  Kidney DTY0CZZ
  Larynx D9YBCZZ
  Liver DFY0CZZ
  Mouth D9Y4CZZ
  Nasopharynx D9YDCZZ
  Nerve, Peripheral D0Y7CZZ
  Ovary DUY0CZZ
  Pancreas DFY3CZZ
  Pharynx D9YCCZZ
  Prostate DVY0CZZ
  Rectum DDY7CZZ
  Spinal Cord D0Y6CZZ
  Stomach DDY1CZZ
  Ureter DTY1CZZ
  Urethra DTY3CZZ
  Uterus DUY2CZZ
Intrauterine device (IUD)
  use Contraceptive Device in Female Reproductive System
Intravascular fluorescence angiography (IFA)
  see Monitoring, Physiological Systems 4A1
Intravascular Lithotripsy (IVL)
  see Fragmentation
Intravascular ultrasound assisted thrombolysis
  see Fragmentation, Artery
Introduction of substance in or on
  Artery
    Central 3E06
      Analgesics 3E06
      Anesthetic, Intracirculatory 3E06
      Anti-infective 3E06
      Anti-inflammatory 3E06
      Antiarrhythmic 3E06
      Antineoplastic 3E06
      Destructive Agent 3E06
      Diagnostic Substance, Other 3E06
      Electrolytic Substance 3E06
      Hormone 3E06
      Hypnotics 3E06
      Immunotherapeutic 3E06
      Nutritional Substance 3E06
      Platelet Inhibitor 3E06
      Radioactive Substance 3E06
      Sedatives 3E06
      Serum 3E06
      Thrombolytic 3E06
      Toxoid 3E06
      Vaccine 3E06
      Vasopressor 3E06
      Water Balance Substance 3E06
    Coronary 3E07
      Diagnostic Substance, Other 3E07
      Platelet Inhibitor 3E07
      Thrombolytic 3E07
    Peripheral 3E05
      Analgesics 3E05
      Anesthetic, Intracirculatory 3E05
      Anti-infective 3E052
      Anti-inflammatory 3E05
      Antiarrhythmic 3E05
      Antineoplastic 3E05
      Destructive Agent 3E05
      Diagnostic Substance, Other 3E05

Introduction of substance in or on *(continued)*
  Artery *(continued)*
    Peripheral 3E05 *(continued)*
      Electrolytic Substance 3E05
      Hormone 3E05
      Hypnotics 3E05
      Immunotherapeutic 3E05
      Nutritional Substance 3E05
      Platelet Inhibitor 3E05
      Radioactive Substance 3E05
      Sedatives 3E05
      Serum 3E05
      Thrombolytic 3E05
      Toxoid 3E05
      Vaccine 3E05
      Vasopressor 3E05
      Water Balance Substance 3E05
  Biliary Tract 3E0J
    Analgesics 3E0J
    Anesthetic, Agent 3E0J
    Anti-infective 3E0J
    Anti-inflammatory 3E0J
    Antineoplastic 3E0J
    Destructive Agent 3E0J
    Diagnostic Substance, Other 3E0J
    Electrolytic Substance 3E0J
    Gas 3E0J
    Hypnotics 3E0J
    Islet Cells, Pancreatic 3E0J
    Nutritional Substance 3E0J
    Radioactive Substance 3E0J
    Sedatives 3E0J
    Water Balance Substance 3E0J
  Bone 3E0V
    Analgesics 3E0V3NZ
    Anesthetic, Agent 3E0V3BZ
    Anti-infective 3E0V32
    Anti-inflammatory 3E0V33Z
    Antineoplastic 3E0V30
    Destructive Agent 3E0V3TZ
    Diagnostic Substance, Other 3E0V3KZ
    Electrolytic Substance 3E0V37Z
    Hypnotics 3E0V3NZ
    Nutritional Substance 3E0V36Z
    Radioactive Substance 3E0V3HZ
    Sedatives 3E0V3NZ
    Water Balance Substance 3E0V37Z
  Bone Marrow 3E0A3GC
    Antineoplastic 3E0A30
  Brain 3E0Q
    Analgesics 3E0Q
    Anesthetic, Agent 3E0Q
    Anti-infective 3E0Q
    Anti-inflammatory 3E0Q
    Antineoplastic 3E0Q
    Destructive Agent 3E0Q
    Diagnostic Substance, Other 3E0Q
    Electrolytic Substance 3E0Q
    Gas 3E0Q
    Hypnotics 3E0Q
    Nutritional Substance 3E0Q
    Radioactive Substance 3E0Q
    Sedatives 3E0Q
    Stem Cells
      Embryonic 3E0Q
      Somatic 3E0Q
    Water Balance Substance 3E0Q
  Cranial Cavity 3E0Q
    Analgesics 3E0Q
    Anesthetic Agent 3E0Q
    Anti-infective 3E0Q

Introduction of substance in or on (continued)

Cranial Cavity 3E0Q (continued)
Anti-inflammatory 3E0Q
Antineoplastic 3E0Q
Destructive Agent 3E0Q
Diagnostic Substance, Other
   3E0Q
Electrolytic Substance 3E0Q
Gas 3E0Q
Hypnotics 3E0Q
Nutritional Substance
   3E0Q
Radioactive Substance 3E0Q
Sedatives 3E0Q
Stem Cells
   Embryonic 3E0Q
   Somatic 3E0Q
Water Balance Substance 3E0Q

Ear 3E0B
Analgesics 3E0B
Anesthetic Agentl 3E0B
Anti-infective 3E0B
Anti-inflammatory 3E0B
Antineoplastic 3E0B
Destructive Agent 3E0B
Diagnostic Substance, Other
   3E0B
Hypnotics 3E0B
Radioactive Substance 3E0B
Sedatives 3E0B

Epidural Space 3E0S3GC
Analgesics 3E0S3NZ
Anesthetic Agent 3E0S3BZ
Anti-infective 3E0S32
Anti-inflammatory 3E0S33Z
Antineoplastic 3E0S30
Destructive Agent 3E0S3TZ
Diagnostic Substance, Other
   3E0S3KZ
Electrolytic Substance 3E0S37Z
Gas 3E0S
Hypnotics 3E0S3NZ
Nutritional Substance 3E0S36Z
Radioactive Substance 3E0S3HZ
Sedatives 3E0S3NZ
Water Balance Substance
   3E0S37Z

Eye 3E0C
Analgesics 3E0C
Anesthetic Agent 3E0C
Anti-infective 3E0C
Anti-inflammatory 3E0C
Antineoplastic 3E0C
Destructive Agent 3E0C
Diagnostic Substance, Other
   3E0C
Gas 3E0C
Hypnotics 3E0C
Pigment 3E0C
Radioactive Substance
   3E0C
Sedatives 3E0C

Gastrointestinal Tract
Lower 3E0H
   Analgesics 3E0H
   Anesthetic Agent 3E0H
   Anti-infective 3E0H
   Anti-inflammatory 3E0H
   Antineoplastic 3E0H
   Destructive Agent 3E0H
   Diagnostic Substance, Other
      3E0H
   Electrolytic Substance 3E0H
   Gas 3E0H
   Hypnotics 3E0H
   Nutritional Substance 3E0H
   Radioactive Substance 3E0H
   Sedatives 3E0H
   Water Balance Substance
      3E0H

Gastrointestinal Tract (continued)
Upper 3E0G
   Analgesics 3E0G
   Anesthetic Agent 3E0G
   Anti-infective 3E0G
   Anti-inflammatory 3E0G
   Antineoplastic 3E0G
   Destructive Agent 3E0G
   Diagnostic Substance, Other
      3E0G
   Electrolytic Substance 3E0G
   Gas 3E0G
   Hypnotics 3E0G
   Nutritional Substance 3E0G
   Radioactive Substance 3E0G
   Sedatives 3E0G
   Water Balance Substance
      3E0G

Genitourinary Tract 3E0K
Analgesics 3E0K
Anesthetic Agent 3E0K
Anti-infective 3E0K
Anti-inflammatory 3E0K
Antineoplastic 3E0K
Destructive Agent 3E0K
Diagnostic Substance, Other
   3E0K
Electrolytic Substance 3E0K
Gas 3E0K
Hypnotics 3E0K
Nutritional Substance 3E0K
Radioactive Substance 3E0K
Sedatives 3E0K
Water Balance Substance 3E0K

Heart 3E08
Diagnostic Substance, Other
   3E08
Platelet Inhibitor 3E08
Thrombolytic 3E08

Joint 3E0U
Analgesics 3E0U3NZ
Anesthetic Agent 3E0U3BZ
Anti-infective 3E0U
Anti-inflammatory 3E0U33Z
Antineoplastic 3E0U30
Destructive Agent 3E0U3TZ
Diagnostic Substance, Other
   3E0U3KZ
Electrolytic Substance 3E0U37Z
Gas 3E0U3SF
Hypnotics 3E0U3NZ
Nutritional Substance 3E0U36Z
Radioactive Substance 3E0U3HZ
Sedatives 3E0U3NZ
Water Balance Substance
   3E0U37Z

Lymphatic 3E0W3GC
Analgesics 3E0W3NZ
Anesthetic Agent 3E0W3BZ
Anti-infective 3E0W32
Anti-inflammatory 3E0W33Z
Antineoplastic 3E0W30
Destructive Agent 3E0W3TZ
Diagnostic Substance, Other
   3E0W3KZ
Electrolytic Substance 3E0W37Z
Hypnotics 3E0W3NZ
Nutritional Substance 3E0W36Z
Radioactive Substance
   3E0W3HZ
Sedatives 3E0W3NZ
Water Balance Substance
   3E0W37Z

Mouth 3E0D
Analgesics 3E0D
Anesthetic Agent 3E0D
Anti-infective 3E0D
Anti-inflammatory 3E0D
Antiarrhythmic 3E0D

Mouth 3E0D (continued)
Antineoplastic 3E0D
Destructive Agent 3E0D
Diagnostic Substance, Other
   3E0D
Electrolytic Substance 3E0D
Hypnotics 3E0D
Nutritional Substance 3E0D
Radioactive Substance 3E0D
Sedatives 3E0D
Serum 3E0D
Toxoid 3E0D
Vaccine 3E0D
Water Balance Substance 3E0D

Mucous Membrane 3E00XGC
Analgesics 3E00XNZ
Anesthetic Agent 3E00XBZ
Anti-infective 3E00X2
Anti-inflammatory 3E00X3Z
Antineoplastic 3E00X0
Destructive Agent 3E00XTZ
Diagnostic Substance, Other
   3E00XKZ
Hypnotics 3E00XNZ
Pigment 3E00XMZ
Sedatives 3E00XNZ
Serum 3E00X4Z
Toxoid 3E00X4Z
Vaccine 3E00X4Z

Muscle 3E023GC
Analgesics 3E023NZ
Anesthetic Agent 3E023BZ
Anti-infective 3E0232
Anti-inflammatory 3E0233Z
Antineoplastic 3E0230
Destructive Agent 3E023TZ
Diagnostic Substance, Other
   3E023KZ
Electrolytic Substance 3E0237Z
Hypnotics 3E023NZ
Nutritional Substance 3E0236Z
Radioactive Substance 3E023HZ
Sedatives 3E023NZ
Serum 3E0234Z
Toxoid 3E0234Z
Vaccine 3E0234Z
Water Balance Substance
   3E0237Z

Nerve
Cranial 3E0X3GC
   Anesthetic Agent 3E0X3BZ
   Anti-inflammatory 3E0X33Z
   Destructive Agent 3E0X3TZ
Peripheral 3E0T3GC
   Anesthetic Agent 3E0T3BZ
   Anti-inflammatory 3E0T33Z
   Destructive Agent 3E0T3TZ
Plexus 3E0T3GC Agent
   3E0T3BZ
   Anti-inflammatory 3E0T33Z
   Destructive Agent 3E0T3TZ

Nose 3E09
Analgesics 3E09
Anesthetic Agent 3E09
Anti-infective 3E09
Anti-inflammatory 3E09
Antineoplastic 3E09
Destructive Agent 3E09
Diagnostic Substance, Other
   3E09
Hypnotics 3E09
Radioactive Substance 3E09
Sedatives 3E09
Serum 3E09
Toxoid 3E09
Vaccine 3E09

Pancreatic Tract 3E0J
Analgesics 3E0J
Anesthetic Agent 3E0J

Pancreatic Tract 3E0J (continued)
Anti-infective 3E0J
Anti-inflammatory 3E0J
Antineoplastic 3E0J0
Destructive Agent 3E0J
Diagnostic Substance, Other
   3E0J
Electrolytic Substance 3E0J
Gas 3E0J
Hypnotics 3E0J
Islet Cells, Pancreatic 3E0JU
Nutritional Substance 3E0J
Radioactive Substance 3E0J
Sedatives 3E0J
Water Balance Substance 3E0J

Pericardial Cavity 3E0Y
Analgesics 3E0Y3NZ
Anesthetic Agent 3E0Y3BZ
Anti-infective 3E0Y32
Anti-inflammatory 3E0Y33Z
Antineoplastic 3E0Y
Destructive Agent 3E0Y3TZ
Diagnostic Substance, Other
   3E0Y3KZ
Electrolytic Substance 3E0Y37Z
Gas 3E0Y
Hypnotics 3E0Y3NZ
Nutritional Substance 3E0Y36Z
Radioactive Substance 3E0Y3HZ
Sedatives 3E0Y3NZ
Water Balance Substance
   3E0Y37Z

Peritoneal Cavity 3E0M
Adhesion Barrier 3E0M
Analgesics 3E0M3NZ
Anesthetic Agent 3E0M3BZ
Anti-infective 3E0M32
Anti-inflammatory 3E0M33Z
Antineoplastic 3E0M
Destructive Agent 3E0M3TZ
Diagnostic Substance, Other
   3E0M3KZ
Electrolytic Substance 3E0M37Z
Gas 3E0M
Hypnotics 3E0M3NZ
Nutritional Substance 3E0M36Z
Radioactive Substance 3E0M3HZ
Sedatives 3E0M3NZ
Water Balance Substance
   3E0M37Z

Pharynx 3E0D
Analgesics 3E0D
Anesthetic Agent 3E0D
Anti-infective 3E0D
Anti-inflammatory 3E0D
Antiarrhythmic 3E0D
Antineoplastic 3E0D
Destructive Agent 3E0D
Diagnostic Substance, Other
   3E0D
Electrolytic Substance 3E0D
Hypnotics 3E0D
Nutritional Substance 3E0D
Radioactive Substance 3E0D
Sedatives 3E0D
Serum 3E0D
Toxoid 3E0D
Vaccine 3E0D
Water Balance Substance 3E0D

Pleural Cavity 3E0L
Adhesion Barrier 3E0L
Analgesics 3E0L3NZ
Anesthetic Agent 3E0L3BZ
Anti-infective 3E0L32
Anti-inflammatory 3E0L33Z
Antineoplastic 3E0L
Destructive Agent 3E0L3TZ
Diagnostic Substance, Other
   3E0L3KZ

Introduction of substance in or on (continued)

Pleural Cavity 3E0L (continued)
- Electrolytic Substance 3E0L37Z
- Gas 3E0L
- Hypnotics 3E0L3NZ
- Nutritional Substance 3E0L36Z
- Radioactive Substance 3E0L3HZ
- Sedatives 3E0L3NZ
- Water Balance Substance 3E0L37Z

Products of Conception 3E0E
- Analgesics 3E0E
- Anesthetic Agent 3E0E
- Anti-infective 3E0E2
- Anti-inflammatory 3E0E
- Antineoplastic 3E0E0
- Destructive Agent 3E0E
- Diagnostic Substance, Other 3E0E
- Electrolytic Substance 3E0E
- Gas 3E0E
- Hypnotics 3E0E
- Nutritional Substance 3E0E
- Radioactive Substance 3E0E
- Sedatives 3E0E
- Water Balance Substance 3E0E

Reproductive
- Female 3E0P
  - Adhesion Barrier 3E0P0
  - Analgesics 3E0P
  - Anesthetic Agent 3E0P
  - Anti-infective 3E0P
  - Anti-inflammatory 3E0P
  - Antineoplastic 3E0P
  - Destructive Agent 3E0P
  - Diagnostic Substance, Other 3E0P
  - Electrolytic Substance 3E0P
  - Gas 3E0P
  - Hormone 3E0P
  - Hypnotics 3E0P
  - Nutritional Substance 3E0P
  - Ovum, Fertilized 3E0P
  - Radioactive Substance 3E0P
  - Sedatives 3E0P
  - Sperm 3E0P
  - Water Balance Substance 3E0P
- Male 3E0N
  - Analgesics 3E0N
  - Anesthetic Agent 3E0N
  - Anti-infective 3E0N
  - Anti-inflammatory 3E0N
  - Antineoplastic 3E0N0
  - Destructive Agent 3E0N
  - Diagnostic Substance, Other 3E0N
  - Electrolytic Substance 3E0N
  - Gas 3E0N
  - Hypnotics 3E0N
  - Nutritional Substance 3E0N
  - Radioactive Substance 3E0N
  - Sedatives 3E0N
  - Water Balance Substance 3E0N

Respiratory Tract 3E0F
- Analgesics 3E0F
- Anesthetic Agent 3E0F
- Anti-infective 3E0F
- Anti-inflammatory 3E0F
- Antineoplastic 3E0F
- Destructive Agent 3E0F
- Diagnostic Substance, Other 3E0F
- Electrolytic Substance 3E0F
- Gas 3E0F
- Hypnotics 3E0F
- Nutritional Substance 3E0F
- Radioactive Substance 3E0F
- Sedatives 3E0F
- Water Balance Substance 3E0F

Introduction of substance in or on (continued)

Skin 3E00XGC
- Analgesics 3E00XNZ
- Anesthetic Agent 3E00XBZ
- Anti-infective 3E00X2
- Anti-inflammatory 3E00X3Z
- Antineoplastic 3E00X0
- Destructive Agent 3E00XTZ
- Diagnostic Substance, Other 3E00XKZ
- Hypnotics 3E00XNZ
- Pigment 3E00XMZ
- Sedatives 3E00XNZ
- Serum 3E00X4Z
- Toxoid 3E00X4Z
- Vaccine 3E00X4Z

Spinal Canal 3E0R3GC
- Analgesics 3E0R3NZ
- Anesthetic Agent 3E0R3BZ
- Anti-infective 3E0R32
- Anti-inflammatory 3E0R33Z
- Antineoplastic 3E0R30
- Destructive Agent 3E0R3TZ
- Diagnostic Substance, Other 3E0R3KZ
- Electrolytic Substance 3E0R37Z
- Gas 3E0R
- Hypnotics 3E0R3NZ
- Nutritional Substance 3E0R36Z
- Radioactive Substance 3E0R3HZ
- Sedatives 3E0R3NZ
- Stem Cells
  - Embryonic 3E0R
  - Somatic 3E0R
- Water Balance Substance 3E0R37Z

Subcutaneous Tissue 3E013GC
- Analgesics 3E013NZ
- Anesthetic Agent 3E013BZ
- Anti-infective 3E01
- Anti-inflammatory 3E0133Z
- Antineoplastic 3E0130
- Destructive Agent 3E013TZ
- Diagnostic Substance, Other 3E013KZ
- Electrolytic Substance 3E0137Z
- Hormone 3E013V
- Hypnotics 3E013NZ
- Nutritional Substance 3E0136Z
- Radioactive Substance 3E013HZ
- Sedatives 3E013NZ
- Serum 3E0134Z
- Toxoid 3E0134Z
- Vaccine 3E0134Z
- Water Balance Substance 3E0137Z

Vein
- Central 3E04
  - Analgesics 3E04
  - Anesthetic, Intracirculatory 3E04
  - Anti-infective 3E04
  - Anti-inflammatory 3E04
  - Antiarrhythmic 3E04
  - Antineoplastic 3E04
  - Destructive Agent 3E04
  - Diagnostic Substance, Other 3E04
  - Electrolytic Substance 3E04
  - Hormone 3E04
  - Hypnotics 3E04
  - Immunotherapeutic 3E04
  - Nutritional Substance 3E04
  - Platelet Inhibitor 3E04
  - Radioactive Substance 3E04
  - Sedatives 3E04
  - Serum 3E04
  - Thrombolytic 3E04
  - Toxoid 3E04
  - Vaccine 3E04
  - Vasopressor 3E04

Introduction of substance in or on (continued)

Vein (continued)
- Central 3E04 (continued)
  - Water Balance Substance 3E04
- Peripheral 3E03
  - Analgesics 3E03
  - Anesthetic, Intracirculatory 3E03
  - Anti-infective 3E03
  - Anti-inflammatory 3E03
  - Antiarrhythmic 3E03
  - Antineoplastic 3E03
  - Destructive Agent 3E03
  - Diagnostic Substance, Other 3E03
  - Electrolytic Substance 3E03
  - Hormone 3E03
  - Hypnotics 3E03
  - Immunotherapeutic 3E03
  - Islet Cells, Pancreatic 3E03
  - Nutritional Substance 3E03
  - Platelet Inhibitor 3E03
  - Radioactive Substance 3E03
  - Sedatives 3E03
  - Serum 3E03
  - Thrombolytic 3E03
  - Toxoid 3E03
  - Vaccine 3E03
  - Vasopressor 3E03
  - Water Balance Substance 3E03

Intubated prone positioning *see* Assistance, Respiratory 5A09

Intubation
- Airway
  - *see* Insertion of device in, Esophagus 0DH5
  - *see* Insertion of device in, Mouth and Throat 0CHY
  - *see* Insertion of device in, Trachea 0BH1
- Drainage device
  - *see* Drainage
- Feeding Device
  - *see* Insertion of device in, Gastrointestinal System 0DH

INTUITY Elite valve system, EDWARDS (rapid deployment technique) *see* Replacement, Valve, Aortic 02RF

Iobenguane I-131 Antineoplastic XW0

Iobenguane I-131, High Specific Activity (HSA) *use* Iobenguane I-131 Antineoplastic

IPPB (intermittent positive pressure breathing) *see* Assistance, Respiratory 5A09

IRE (Irreversible Electroporation) *see* Destruction, Hepatobiliary System and Pancreas 0F5

Iridectomy
- *see* Excision, Eye 08B
- *see* Resection, Eye 08T

Iridoplasty
- *see* Repair, Eye 08Q
- *see* Replacement, Eye 08R
- *see* Supplement, Eye 08U

Iridotomy
- *see* Drainage, Eye 089

Irreversible Electroporation (IRE) *see* Destruction, Hepatobiliary System and Pancreas 0F5

Irrigation
- Biliary Tract, Irrigating Substance 3E1J
- Brain, Irrigating Substance 3E1Q38Z
- Cranial Cavity, Irrigating Substance 3E1Q38Z
- Ear, Irrigating Substance 3E1B
- Epidural Space, Irrigating Substance 3E1S38Z
- Eye, Irrigating Substance 3E1C

Irrigation (continued)

- Gastrointestinal Tract
  - Lower, Irrigating Substance 3E1H
  - Upper, Irrigating Substance 3E1G
- Genitourinary Tract, Irrigating Substance 3E1K
- Irrigating Substance 3C1ZX8Z
- Joint, Irrigating Substance 3E1U
- Mucous Membrane, Irrigating Substance 3E10
- Nose, Irrigating Substance 3E19
- Pancreatic Tract, Irrigating Substance 3E1J
- Pericardial Cavity, Irrigating Substance 3E1Y38Z
- Peritoneal Cavity
  - Dialysate 3E1M39Z
  - Irrigating Substance 3E1M
- Pleural Cavity, Irrigating Substance 3E1L38Z
- Reproductive
  - Female, Irrigating Substance 3E1P
  - Male, Irrigating Substance 3E1N
- Respiratory Tract, Irrigating Substance 3E1F
- Skin, Irrigating Substance 3E10
- Spinal Canal, Irrigating Substance 3E1R38Z

Isavuconazole (isavuconazonium sulfate) *use* Other Anti-Infective

ISC-REST kit
- ISCDx XXE5XT7
- QIAGEN Access Anti-SARS-CoV-2 Total Test XXE5XV7
- QIAstat-Dx Respiratory SARS-CoV-2 Panel XXE97U7

Ischemic Stroke System (ISS500) *use* Neurostimulator Lead in New Technology

Ischiatic nerve *use* Nerve, Sciatic

Ischiocavernosus muscle *use* Muscle, Perineum

Ischiofemoral ligament *use* Bursa and Ligament, Hip, Left *use* Bursa and Ligament, Hip, Right

Ischium *use* Bone, Pelvic, Left *use* Bone, Pelvic, Right

Isolation 8E0ZXY6

Isotope Administration, Other Radiation, Whole Body DWY5G

ISS500 (Ischemic Stroke System) *use* Neurostimulator Lead in New Technology

Itrel (3)(4) neurostimulator *use* Stimulator Generator, Single Array in 0JH

J

Jakafi® *use* Ruxolitinib

Jejunal artery *use* Artery, Superior Mesenteric

Jejunectomy
- *see* Excision, Jejunum 0DBA
- *see* Resection, Jejunum 0DTA

Jejunocolostomy
- *see* Bypass, Gastrointestinal System 0D1
- *see* Drainage, Gastrointestinal System 0D9

Jejunopexy
- *see* Repair, Jejunum 0DQA
- *see* Reposition, Jejunum 0DSA

Jejunostomy
- *see* Bypass, Jejunum 0D1A
- *see* Drainage, Jejunum 0D9A

Jejunotomy
- *see* Drainage, Jejunum 0D9A

Joint fixation plate
use Internal Fixation Device in Lower Joints
use Internal Fixation Device in Upper Joints
Joint liner (insert)
use Liner in Lower Joints
Joint spacer (antibiotic)
use Spacer in Lower Joints
use Spacer in Upper Joints
Jugular body
use Glomus Jugulare
Jugular lymph node
use Lymphatic, Neck, Left
use Lymphatic, Neck, Right

K

Kappa
use Pacemaker, Dual Chamber in 0JH
Kcentra
use 4-Factor Prothrombin Complex Concentrate
Keratectomy, kerectomy
see Excision, Eye 08B
see Resection, Eye 08T
Keratocentesis
see Drainage, Eye 089
Keratoplasty
see Repair, Eye 08Q
see Replacement, Eye 08R
see Supplement, Eye 08U
Keratotomy
see Drainage, Eye 089
see Repair, Eye 08Q
KEVZARA® use Sarilumab
Keystone Heart TriGuard 3™ CEPD (cerebral embolic protection device) X2A6325
Kirschner wire (K-wire)
use Internal Fixation Device in Head and Facial Bones
use Internal Fixation Device in Lower Bones
use Internal Fixation Device in Lower Joints
use Internal Fixation Device in Upper Bones
use Internal Fixation Device in Upper Joints
Knee (implant) insert
use Liner in Lower Joints
KUB x-ray
see Plain Radiography, Kidney, Ureter and Bladder BT04
Kuntscher nail
use Internal Fixation Device, Intramedullary in Lower Bones
use Internal Fixation Device, Intramedullary in Upper Bones
KYMRIAH®
use Tisagenlecleucel Immunotherapy

L

Labia majora
use Vulva
Labia minora
use Vulva
Labial gland
use Lip, Lower
use Lip, Upper
Labiectomy
see Excision, Female Reproductive System 0UB
see Resection, Female Reproductive System 0UT
see Release, Central Nervous System 00N
see Release, Peripheral Nervous System 01N

Lacrimal canaliculus
use Duct, Lacrimal, Left
use Duct, Lacrimal, Right
Lacrimal punctum
use Duct, Lacrimal, Left
use Duct, Lacrimal, Right
Lacrimal sac
use Duct, Lacrimal, Left
use Duct, Lacrimal, Right
LAGB (laparoscopic adjustable gastric banding)
Initial procedure 0DV64CZ
Surgical correction
see Revision of device in, Stomach 0DW6
Laminectomy
see Excision, Lower Bones 0QB
see Excision, Upper Bones 0PB
see Release, Central Nervous System and Cranial Nerves 00N
see Release, Peripheral Nervous System 01N
Laminotomy
see Drainage, Lower Bones 0Q9
see Drainage, Upper Bones 0P9
see Excision, Lower Bones 0QB
see Excision, Upper Bones 0PB
see Release, Central Nervous System and Cranial Nerves 00N
see Release, Lower Bones 0QN
see Release, Peripheral Nervous System 01N
see Release, Upper Bones 0PN
LAP-BAND® adjustable gastric banding system
use Extraluminal Device
Laparoscopic-assisted transanal pull-through
see Excision, Gastrointestinal System 0DB
see Resection, Gastrointestinal System 0DT
Laparoscopy
see Inspection
Laparotomy
Drainage
see Drainage, Peritoneal Cavity 0W9G
Exploratory
see Inspection, Peritoneal Cavity 0WJG
Laryngectomy
see Excision, Larynx 0CBS
see Resection, Larynx 0CTS
Laryngocentesis
see Drainage, Larynx 0C9S
Laryngogram
see Fluoroscopy, Larynx B91J
Laryngopexy
see Repair, Larynx 0CQS
Laryngopharynx
use Pharynx
Laryngoplasty
see Repair, Larynx 0CQS
see Replacement, Larynx 0CRS
see Supplement, Larynx 0CUS
Laryngorrhaphy
see Repair, Larynx 0CQS
Laryngoscopy 0CJS8ZZ
Laryngotomy
see Drainage, Larynx 0C9S
Laser Interstitial Thermal Therapy
Ampulla of Vater 0F5C
Anus 0D5Q
Aortic Body 0G5D
Appendix 0D5J
Brain 0050
Breast
Bilateral 0H5V
Left 0H5U
Right 0H5T
Carotid Bodies, Bilateral 0G58

Laser Interstitial Thermal Therapy
(continued)
Carotid Body
Left 0G56
Right 0G57
Cecum 0D5H
Coccygeal Glomus 0G5B
Colon
Ascending 0D5K
Descending 0D5M
Sigmoid 0D5N
Transverse 0D5L
Duct
Common Bile 0F59
Cystic 0F58
Hepatic
Common 0F57
Left 0F56
Right 0F55
Pancreatic 0F5D
Accessory 0F5F
Duodenum 0D59
Esophagogastric Junction 0D54
Esophagus 0D55
Lower 0D53
Middle 0D52
Upper 0D51
Gallbladder 0F54
Gland
Adrenal
Bilateral 0G54
Left 0G52
Right 0G53
Pituitary 0G50
Glomus Jugulare 0G5C
Ileocecal Valve 0D5C
Ileum 0D5B
Intestine
Large 0D5E
Left 0D5G
Right 0D5F
Small 0D58
Jejunum 0D5A
Liver 0F50
Left Lobe 0F52
Right Lobe 0F51
Lung
Bilateral 0B5M
Left 0B5L
Lower Lobe
Left 0B5J
Right 0B5F
Middle Lobe, Right 0B5D
Right 0B5K
Upper Lobe
Left 0B5G
Right 0B5C
Lung Lingula 0B5H
Pancreas 0F5G
Para-aortic Body 0G59
Paraganglion Extremity 0G5F
Parathyroid Gland 0G5R
Inferior
Left 0G5P
Right 0G5N
Multiple 0G5Q
Superior
Left 0G5M
Right 0G5L
Pineal Body 0G51
Prostate 0V50
Rectum 0D5P
Sacrum 0Q51
Spinal Cord
Cervical 005W
Lumbar 005Y
Thoracic 005X
Stomach 0D56
Pylorus 0D57
Thyroid Gland 0G5K
Left Lobe 0G5G
Right Lobe 0G5H

Laser Interstitial Thermal Therapy
(continued)
Vertebra
Cervical 0P53
Lumbar 0Q50
Thoracic 0P54
Lateral (brachial) lymph node
use Lymphatic, Axillary, Left
use Lymphatic, Axillary, Right
Lateral canthus
use Eyelid, Upper, Left
use Eyelid, Upper, Right
Lateral collateral ligament (LCL)
use Bursa and Ligament, Knee, Left
use Bursa and Ligament, Knee, Right
Lateral condyle of femur
use Femur, Lower, Left
use Femur, Lower, Right
Lateral condyle of tibia
use Tibia, Left
use Tibia, Right
Lateral cuneiform bone
use Tarsal, Left
use Tarsal, Right
Lateral epicondyle of femur
use Femur, Lower, Left
use Femur, Lower, Right
Lateral epicondyle of humerus
use Humeral Shaft, Left
use Humeral Shaft, Right
Lateral femoral cutaneous nerve
use Nerve, Lumbar Plexus
Lateral malleolus
use Fibula, Left
use Fibula, Right
Lateral meniscus
use Joint, Knee, Left
use Joint, Knee, Right
Lateral nasal cartilage
use Nasal Mucosa and Soft Tissue
Lateral plantar artery
use Artery, Foot, Left
use Artery, Foot, Right
Lateral plantar nerve
use Nerve, Tibial
Lateral rectus muscle
use Muscle, Extraocular, Left
use Muscle, Extraocular, Right
Lateral sacral artery
use Artery, Internal Iliac, Left
use Artery, Internal Iliac, Right
Lateral sacral vein
use Vein, Hypogastric, Left
use Vein, Hypogastric, Right
Lateral sural cutaneous nerve
use Nerve, Peroneal
Lateral tarsal artery
use Artery, Foot, Left
use Artery, Foot, Right
Lateral temporomandibular ligament
use Bursa and Ligament, Head and Neck
Lateral thoracic artery
use Artery, Axillary, Left
use Artery, Axillary, Right
Latissimus dorsi muscle
use Muscle, Trunk, Left
use Muscle, Trunk, Right
Latissimus Dorsi Myocutaneous Flap
Replacement
Bilateral 0HRV075
Left 0HRU075
Right 0HRT075
Transfer
Left 0KXG
Right 0KXF
Lavage
see Irrigation
Bronchial alveolar, diagnostic
see Drainage, Respiratory System 0B9

Least splanchnic nerve
use Nerve, Thoracic Sympathetic
Lefamulin Anti-infective XW0
Left ascending lumbar vein
use Vein, Hemiazygos
Left atrioventricular valve
use Valve, Mitral
Left auricular appendix
use Atrium, Left
Left colic vein
use Vein, Colic
Left coronary sulcus
use Heart, Left
Left gastric artery
use Artery, Gastric
Left gastroepiploic artery
use Artery, Splenic
Left gastroepiploic vein
use Vein, Splenic
Left inferior phrenic vein
use Vein, Renal, Left
Left inferior pulmonary vein
use Vein, Pulmonary, Left
Left jugular trunk
use Lymphatic, Thoracic Duct
Left lateral ventricle
use Cerebral Ventricle
Left ovarian vein
use Vein, Renal, Left
Left second lumbar vein
use Vein, Renal, Left
Left subclavian trunk
use Lymphatic, Thoracic Duct
Left subcostal vein
use Vein, Hemiazygos
Left superior pulmonary vein
use Vein, Pulmonary, Left
Left suprarenal vein
use Vein, Renal, Left
Left testicular vein
use Vein, Renal, Left
Lengthening
Bone, with device
see Insertion of Limb
Lengthening Device
Muscle, by incision
see Division, Muscles 0K8
Tendon, by incision
see Division, Tendons 0L8
Leptomeninges, intracranial
use Cerebral Meninges
Leptomeninges, spinal
use Spinal Meninges
Lesser alar cartilage
use Nasal Mucosa and Soft Tissue
Lesser occipital nerve
use Nerve, Cervical Plexus
Lesser Omentum
use Omentum
Lesser saphenous vein
use Saphenous Vein, Left
use Saphenous Vein, Right
Lesser splanchnic nerve
use Nerve, Thoracic Sympathetic
Lesser trochanter
use Femur, Upper, Left
use Femur, Upper, Right
Lesser tuberosity
use Humeral Head, Left
use Humeral Head, Right
Lesser wing
use Bone, Sphenoid
Leukopheresis, therapeutic
see Pheresis, Circulatory 6A55
Levator anguli oris muscle
use Muscle, Facial
Levator ani muscle
use Perineum Muscle
Levator labii superioris alaeque nasi muscle
use Muscle, Facial

Levator labii superioris muscle
use Muscle, Facial
Levator palpebrae superioris muscle
use Eyelid, Upper, Left
use Eyelid, Upper, Right
Levator scapulae muscle
use Muscle, Neck, Left
use Muscle, Neck, Right
Levator veli palatini muscle
use Muscle, Tongue, Palate, Pharynx
Levatores costarum muscle
use Muscle, Thorax, Left
use Muscle, Thorax, Right
Lifeline ARM Automated Chest Compression (ACC) device 5A1221J
LifeStent® (Flexstar)(XL) Vascular Stent System
use Intraluminal Device
Lifileucel *use* Lifileucel Immunotherapy
Lifileucel Immunotherapy XW0
Ligament of head of fibula
use Bursa and Ligament, Knee, Left
use Bursa and Ligament, Knee, Right
Ligament of the lateral malleolus
use Bursa and Ligament, Ankle, Left
use Bursa and Ligament, Ankle, Right
Ligamentum flavum, cervical
use Head and Neck Bursa and Ligament
Ligamentum flavum, lumbar
use Lower Spine Bursa and Ligament
Ligamentum flavum, thoracic
use Upper Spine Bursa and Ligament
LigaPASS 2.0™ PJK Prevention System *use* Posterior Vertebral Tether in New Technology
Ligation
see Occlusion
Ligation, hemorrhoid
see Occlusion, Lower Veins, Hemorrhoidal Plexus
Light Therapy GZJZZZZ
Liner
Removal of device from
Hip
Left 0SPB09Z
Right 0SP909Z
Knee
Left 0SPD09Z
Right 0SPC09Z
Revision of device in
Hip
Left 0SWB09Z
Right 0SW909Z
Knee
Left 0SWD09Z
Right 0SWC09Z
Supplement
Hip
Left 0SUB09Z
Acetabular Surface 0SUE09Z
Femoral Surface 0SUS09Z
Right 0SU909Z
Acetabular Surface 0SUA09Z
Femoral Surface 0SUR09Z
Knee
Left 0SUD09
Femoral Surface 0SUU09Z
Tibial Surface 0SUW09Z
Right 0SUC09
Femoral Surface 0SUT09Z
Tibial Surface 0SUV09Z
Lingual artery
use Artery, External Carotid, Left
use Artery, External Carotid, Right

Lingual tonsil
use Pharynx
Lingulectomy, lung
see Excision, Lung Lingula 0BBH
see Resection, Lung Lingula 0BTH
Lisocabtagene Maraleucel
use Lisocabtagene Maraleucel Immunotherapy
Lisocabtagene Maraleucel Immunotherapy XW0
Lithoplasty
see Fragmentation
Lithotripsy
see Fragmentation
With removal of fragments
see Extirpation
LITT (laser interstitial thermal therapy)
see Destruction
see Laser Interstitial Thermal Therapy
LIVIAN™ CRT-D
use Cardiac Resynchronization Defibrillator Pulse Generator in 0JH
LIVTENCITY™ *use* Maribavir Anti-infective
Lobectomy
see Excision, Central Nervous System and Cranial Nerves 00B
see Excision, Endocrine System 0GB
see Excision, Hepatobiliary System and Pancreas 0FB
see Excision, Respiratory System 0BB
see Resection, Endocrine System 0GT
see Resection, Hepatobiliary System and Pancreas 0FT
see Resection, Respiratory System 0BT
Lobotomy
see Division, Brain 0080
Localization
see Map
see Imaging
Locus ceruleus
use Pons
Long thoracic nerve
use Nerve, Brachial Plexus
Longeviti ClearFit® Cranial Implant
use Synthetic Substitute, Ultrasound Penetrable in New Technology
Longeviti ClearFit® OTS Cranial Implant *use* Synthetic Substitute, Ultrasound Penetrable in New Technology
Loop ileostomy
see Bypass, Ileum 0D1B
Loop recorder, implantable
use Monitoring Device
Lovotibeglogene Autotemcel XW1
Lower GI series
see Fluoroscopy, Colon BD14
Lower Respiratory Fluid Nucleic Acid-base Microbial Detection XXEBXQ6
LTX Regional Anticoagulant
use Nafamostat Anticoagulant
LUCAS® Chest Compression System 5A1221J
Lumbar artery
use Aorta, Abdominal
Lumbar facet joint
use Joint, Lumbar Vertebral
Lumbar ganglion
use Nerve, Lumbar Sympathetic
Lumbar lymph node
use Lymphatic, Aortic
Lumbar lymphatic trunk
use Cisterna Chyli
Lumbar splanchnic nerve
use Nerve, Lumbar Sympathetic

Lumbosacral facet joint
use Joint, Lumbosacral
Lumbosacral trunk
use Nerve, Lumbar
Lumpectomy
see Excision
Lunate bone
use Carpal, Left
use Carpal, Right
Lunotriquetral ligament
use Bursa and Ligament, Hand, Left
use Bursa and Ligament, Hand, Right
LUNSUMIO™ *use* Mosunetuzumab Antineoplastic
Lurbinectedin XW0
Lymphadenectomy
see Excision, Lymphatic and Hemic Systems 07B
see Resection, Lymphatic and Hemic Systems 07T
Lymphadenotomy
see Drainage, Lymphatic and Hemic Systems 079
Lymphangiectomy
see Excision, Lymphatic and Hemic Systems 07B
see Resection, Lymphatic and Hemic Systems 07T
Lymphangiogram
see Plain Radiography, Lymphatic System B70
Lymphangioplasty
see Repair, Lymphatic and Hemic Systems 07Q
see Supplement, Lymphatic and Hemic Systems 07U
Lymphangiorrhaphy
see Repair, Lymphatic and Hemic Systems 07Q
Lymphangiotomy
see Drainage, Lymphatic and Hemic Systems 079
Lysis
see Release

M

Macula
use Retina, Left
use Retina, Right
MAGEC® Spinal Bracing and Distraction System
use Magnetically Controlled Growth Rod(s) in New Technology
Magnet extraction, ocular foreign body
see Extirpation, Eye 08C
Magnetic-guided radiofrequency endovascular fistula
Radial Artery, Left 031C
Radial Artery, Right 031B
Ulnar Artery, Left 031A
Ulnar Artery, Right 0319
Magnetic Resonance Imaging (MRI)
Abdomen BW30
Ankle
Left BQ3H
Right BQ3G
Aorta
Abdominal B430
Thoracic B330
Arm
Left BP3F
Right BP3E
Artery
Celiac B431
Cervico-Cerebral Arch B33Q
Common Carotid, Bilateral B335
Coronary
Bypass Graft, Multiple B233
Multiple B231

45

Magnetic Resonance Imaging (MRI) (continued)

Artery (continued)
  Internal Carotid, Bilateral B338
  Intracranial B33R
  Lower Extremity
    Bilateral B43H
    Left B43G
    Right B43F
  Pelvic B43C
  Renal, Bilateral B438
  Spinal B33M
  Superior Mesenteric B434
  Upper Extremity
    Bilateral B33K
    Left B33J
    Right B33H
  Vertebral, Bilateral B33G
Bladder BT30
Brachial Plexus BW3P
Brain B030
Breast
  Bilateral BH32
  Left BH31
  Right BH30
Calcaneus
  Left BQ3K
  Right BQ3J
Chest BW33Y
Coccyx BR3F
Connective Tissue
  Lower Extremity BL31
  Upper Extremity BL30
Corpora Cavernosa BV30
Disc
  Cervical BR31
  Lumbar BR33
  Thoracic BR32
Ear B930
Elbow
  Left BP3H
  Right BP3G
Eye
  Bilateral B837
  Left B836
  Right B835
Femur
  Left BQ34
  Right BQ33
Fetal Abdomen BY33
Fetal Extremity BY35
Fetal Head BY30
Fetal Heart BY31
Fetal Spine BY34
Fetal Thorax BY32
Fetus, Whole BY36
Foot
  Left BQ3M
  Right BQ3L
Forearm
  Left BP3K
  Right BP3J
Gland
  Adrenal, Bilateral BG32
  Parathyroid BG33
  Parotid, Bilateral B936
  Salivary, Bilateral B93D
  Submandibular, Bilateral B939
  Thyroid BG34
Head BW38
Heart, Right and Left B236
Hip
  Left BQ31
  Right BQ30
Intracranial Sinus B532
Joint
  Finger
    Left BP3D
    Right BP3C
  Hand
    Left BP3D
    Right BP3C

Magnetic Resonance Imaging (MRI) (continued)

Joint (continued)
  Temporomandibular, Bilateral BN39
Kidney
  Bilateral BT33
  Left BT32
  Right BT31
  Transplant BT39
Knee
  Left BQ38
  Right BQ37
Larynx B93J
Leg
  Left BQ3F
  Right BQ3D
Liver BF35
Liver and Spleen BF36
Lung Apices BB3G
Lung, Bilateral, Hyperpolarized Xenon 129 (Xe-129) BB34Z3Z
Nasopharynx B93F
Neck BW3F
Nerve
  Acoustic B03C
  Brachial Plexus BW3P
Oropharynx B93F
Ovary
  Bilateral BU35
  Left BU34
  Right BU33
Ovary and Uterus BU3C
Pancreas BF37
Patella
  Left BQ3W
  Right BQ3V
Pelvic Region BW3G
Pelvis BR3C
Pituitary Gland B039
Plexus, Brachial BW3P
Prostate BV33
Retroperitoneum BW3H
Sacrum BR3F
Scrotum BV34
Sella Turcica B039
Shoulder
  Left BP39
  Right BP38
Sinus
  Intracranial B532
  Paranasal B932
Spinal Cord B03B
Spine
  Cervical BR30
  Lumbar BR39
  Thoracic BR37
Spleen and Liver BF36
Subcutaneous Tissue
  Abdomen BH3H
  Extremity
    Lower BH3J
    Upper BH3F
  Head BH3D
  Neck BH3D
  Pelvis BH3H
  Thorax BH3G
Tendon
  Lower Extremity BL33
  Upper Extremity BL32
Testicle
  Bilateral BV37
  Left BV36
  Right BV35
Toe
  Left BQ3Q
  Right BQ3P
Uterus BU36
  Pregnant BU3B
Uterus and Ovary BU3C
Vagina BU39

Magnetic Resonance Imaging (MRI) (continued)

Vein
  Cerebellar B531
  Cerebral B531
  Jugular, Bilateral B535
  Lower Extremity
    Bilateral B53D
    Left B53C
    Right B53B
  Other B53V
  Pelvic (Iliac) Bilateral B53H
  Portal B53T
  Pulmonary, Bilateral B53S
  Renal, Bilateral B53L
  Spanchnic B53T
  Upper Extremity
    Bilateral B53P
    Left B53N
    Right B53M
Vena Cava
  Inferior B539
  Superior B538
Wrist
  Left BP3M
  Right BP3L

Magnetically Controlled Growth Rod(s)
  Cervical XNS3
  Lumbar XNS0
  Thoracic XNS4

Magnus Neuromodulation System (MNS) X0Z0X18

Malleotomy
  see Drainage, Ear, Nose, Sinus 099

Malleus
  use Auditory Ossicle, Left
  use Auditory Ossicle, Right

Mammaplasty, mammoplasty
  see Alteration, Skin and Breast 0H0
  see Repair, Skin and Breast 0HQ
  see Replacement, Skin and Breast 0HR
  see Supplement, Skin and Breast 0HU

Mammary duct
  use Breast, Bilateral
  use Breast, Left
  use Breast, Right

Mammary gland
  use Breast, Bilateral
  use Breast, Left
  use Breast, Right

Mammectomy
  see Excision, Skin and Breast 0HB
  see Resection, Skin and Breast 0HT

Mammillary body
  use Hypothalamus

Mammography
  see Plain Radiography, Skin, Subcutaneous Tissue and Breast BH0

Mammotomy
  see Drainage, Skin and Breast 0H9

Mandibular nerve
  use Nerve, Trigeminal

Mandibular notch
  use Mandible, Left
  use Mandible, Right

Mandibulectomy
  see Excision, Head and Facial Bones 0NB
  see Resection, Head and Facial Bones 0NT

Manipulation
  Adhesions
    see Release
  Chiropractic
    see Chiropractic Manipulation

Manual removal, retained placenta
  see Extraction, Products of Conception, Retained 10D1

Manubrium
  use Sternum

Map
  Basal Ganglia 00K8
  Brain 00K0
  Cerebellum 00KC
  Cerebral Hemisphere 00K7
  Conduction Mechanism 02K8
  Hypothalamus 00KA
  Medulla Oblongata 00KD
  Pons 00KB
  Thalamus 00K9

Mapping
  Doppler ultrasound
    see Ultrasonography
  Electrocardiogram only
    see Measurement, Cardiac 4A02

Maribavir Anti-infective XW0

Mark IV Breathing Pacemaker System
  use Stimulator Generator in Subcutaneous Tissue and Fascia

MarrowStim™ PAD Kit for CBMA (Concentrated Bone Marrow Aspirate) *use* Other Substance

MarrowStim™ PAD Kit, for injection of concentration bone marrow aspirate *see* Introduction of substance in or on, Muscle 3E02

Marsupialization
  see Drainage
  see Excision

Massage, cardiac
  External 5A12012
  Open 02QA0ZZ

Masseter muscle
  use Muscle, Head

Masseteric fascia
  use Subcutaneous Tissue and Fascia, Face

Mastectomy
  see Excision, Skin and Breast 0HB
  see Resection, Skin and Breast 0HT

Mastoid (postauricular) lymph node
  use Lymphatic, Neck, Left
  use Lymphatic, Neck, Right

Mastoid air cells
  use Sinus, Mastoid, Left
  use Sinus, Mastoid, Right

Mastoid process
  use Bone, Temporal, Left
  use Bone, Temporal, Right

Mastoidectomy
  see Excision, Ear, Nose, Sinus 09B
  see Resection, Ear, Nose, Sinus 09T

Mastoidotomy
  see Drainage, Ear, Nose, Sinus 099

Mastopexy
  see Repair, Skin and Breast 0HQ
  see Reposition, Skin and Breast 0HS

Mastorrhaphy
  see Repair, Skin and Breast 0HQ

Mastotomy
  see Drainage, Skin and Breast 0H9

Maxillary artery
  use Artery, External Carotid, Left
  use Artery, External Carotid, Right

Maxillary nerve
  use Nerve, Trigeminal

Maximo II DR (VR)
  use Defibrillator Generator in 0JH

Maximo II DR CRT-D
  use Cardiac Resynchronization Defibrillator Pulse Generator in 0JH

Measurement
  Arterial
    Flow
      Coronary 4A03
      Intracranial 4A03X5D
      Peripheral 4A03
      Pulmonary 4A03

Measurement *(continued)*
  Arterial *(continued)*
    Pressure
      Coronary 4A03
      Peripheral 4A03
      Pulmonary 4A03
      Thoracic, Other 4A03
    Pulse
      Coronary 4A03
      Peripheral 4A03
      Pulmonary 4A03
    Saturation, Peripheral 4A03
    Sound, Peripheral 4A03
  Biliary
    Flow 4A0C
    Pressure 4A0C
  Cardiac
    Action Currents 4A02
    Defibrillator 4B02XTZ
    Electrical Activity 4A02
      Guidance 4A02X4A
      No Qualifier 4A02X4Z
    Output 4A02
    Pacemaker 4B02XSZ
    Rate 4A02
    Rhythm 4A02
    Sampling and Pressure
      Bilateral 4A02
      Left Heart 4A02
      Right Heart 4A02
    Sound 4A02
    Total Activity, Stress 4A02XM4
  Central Nervous
    Cerebrospinal Fluid Shunt,
      Wireless Sensor 4B00XW0
    Conductivity 4A00
    Electrical Activity 4A00
    Pressure 4A000BZ
      Intracranial 4A00
    Saturation, Intracranial 4A00
    Stimulator 4B00XVZ
    Temperature, Intracranial 4A00
  Circulatory, Volume 4A05XLZ
  Gastrointestinal
    Motility 4A0B
    Pressure 4A0B
    Secretion 4A0B
  Lower Respiratory Fluid Nucleic
    Acid-base Microbial Detection
    XXEBXQ6
  Lymphatic
    Flow 4A06
    Pressure 4A06
  Metabolism 4A0Z
  Musculoskeletal
    Contractility 4A0F
    Pressure 4A0F3BE
    Stimulator 4B0FXVZ
  Olfactory, Acuity 4A08X0Z
  Peripheral Nervous
    Conductivity
      Motor 4A01
      Sensory 4A01
    Electrical Activity 4A01
    Stimulator 4B01XVZ
  Positive Blood Culture Fluorescence
    Hybridization for Organism
    Identification, Concentration and
    Susceptibility XXE5XN6
  Products of Conception
    Cardiac
      Electrical Activity 4A0H
      Rate 4A0H
      Rhythm 4A0H
      Sound 4A0HH
    Nervous
      Conductivity 4A0J
      Electrical Activity 4A0J
      Pressure 4A0J
  Respiratory
    Capacity 4A09
    Flow 4A09

Measurement *(continued)*
  Respiratory *(continued)*
    Pacemaker 4B09X
    Rate 4A09
    Resistance 4A09
    Total Activity 4A09
    Volume 4A09
    Sleep 4A0ZXQZ
    Temperature 4A0Z
  Urinary
    Contractility 4A0D
    Flow 4A0D
    Pressure 4A0D
    Resistance 4A0D
    Volume 4A0D
  Venous
    Flow
      Central 4A04
      Peripheral 4A04
      Portal 4A04
      Pulmonary 4A04
    Pressure
      Central 4A04
      Peripheral 4A04
      Portal 4A04
      Pulmonary 4A04
    Pulse
      Central 4A04
      Peripheral 4A04
      Portal 4A04
      Pulmonary 4A04
    Saturation, Peripheral 4A04
  Visual
    Acuity 4A07X0Z
    Mobility 4A07X7Z
    Pressure 4A07XBZ
  Whole Blood Nucleic Acid-base
    Microbial Detection XXE5XM5
Meatoplasty, urethra
  see Repair, Urethra 0TQD
Meatotomy
  see Drainage, Urinary System 0T9
Mechanical chest compression
  (mCPR) 5A1221J
Mechanical Initial Specimen
  Diversion Technique Using
  Active Negative Pressure (blood
  collection) XXE5XR7
Mechanical ventilation
  see Performance, Respiratory 5A19
Medial canthus
  use Eyelid, Lower, Left
  use Eyelid, Lower, Right
Medial collateral ligament (MCL)
  use Bursa and Ligament, Knee, Left
  use Bursa and Ligament, Knee, Right
Medial condyle of femur
  use Femur, Lower, Left
  use Femur, Lower, Right
Medial condyle of tibia
  use Tibia, Left
  use Tibia, Right
Medial cuneiform bone
  use Tarsal, Left
  use Tarsal, Right
Medial epicondyle of femur
  use Femur, Lower, Left
  use Femur, Lower, Right
Medial epicondyle of humerus
  use Humeral Shaft, Left
  use Humeral Shaft, Right
Medial malleolus
  use Tibia, Left
  use Tibia, Right
Medial meniscus
  use Joint, Knee, Left
  use Joint, Knee, Right
Medial plantar artery
  use Artery, Foot, Left
  use Artery, Foot, Right
Medial plantar nerve
  use Nerve, Tibial

Medial popliteal nerve
  use Nerve, Tibial
Medial rectus muscle
  use Muscle, Extraocular, Left
  use Muscle, Extraocular, Right
Medial sural cutaneous nerve
  use Nerve, Tibial
Median antebrachial vein
  use Vein, Basilic, Left
  use Vein, Basilic, Right
Median cubital vein
  use Vein, Basilic, Left
  use Vein, Basilic, Right
Median sacral artery
  use Aorta, Abdominal
Mediastinal cavity
  use Mediastinum
Mediastinal lymph node
  use Lymphatic, Thorax
Mediastinal space
  use Mediastinum
Mediastinoscopy 0WJC4ZZ
Medication Management GZ3ZZZZ
  for substance abuse
    Antabuse HZ83ZZZ
    Bupropion HZ87ZZZ
    Clonidine HZ86ZZZ
    Levo-alpha-acetyl-methadol
      (LAAM) HZ82ZZZ
    Methadone Maintenance
      HZ81ZZZ
    Naloxone HZ85ZZZ
    Naltrexone HZ84ZZZ
    Nicotine Replacement HZ80ZZZ
    Other Replacement Medication
      HZ89ZZZ
    Psychiatric Medication
      HZ88ZZZ
Meditation 8E0ZXY5
Medtronic Endurant® II AAA stent
  graft system
  use Intraluminal Device
Meissner's (submucous) plexus
  use Nerve, Abdominal Sympathetic
Melody® transcatheter pulmonary
  valve
  use Zooplastic Tissue in Heart and
    Great Vessels
Melphalan Hydrochloride
  Antineoplastic XW053T9
Membranous urethra
  use Urethra
Meningeorrhaphy
  see Repair, Cerebral Meninges 00Q1
  see Repair, Spinal Meninges 00QT
Meniscectomy, knee
  see Excision, Joint, Knee, Left 0SBD
  see Excision, Joint, Knee, Right
    0SBC
Mental foramen
  use Mandible, Left
  use Mandible, Right
Mentalis muscle
  use Muscle, Facial
Mentoplasty
  see Alteration, Jaw, Lower 0W05
Meropenem-vaborbactam Anti-
  infective XW0
Mesenterectomy
  see Excision, Mesentery 0DBV
Mesenteriorrhaphy,
  mesenterorrhaphy
  see Repair, Mesentery 0DQV
Mesenteriplication
  see Repair, Mesentery 0DQV
Mesoappendix
  use Mesentery
Mesocolon
  use Mesentery
Metacarpal ligament
  use Bursa and Ligament, Hand, Left
  use Bursa and Ligament, Hand, Right

Metacarpophalangeal ligament
  use Bursa and Ligament, Hand, Left
  use Bursa and Ligament, Hand,
    Right
Metal on metal bearing surface
  use Synthetic Substitute, Metal in
    0SR
Metatarsal ligament
  use Bursa and Ligament, Foot, Left
  use Bursa and Ligament, Foot, Right
Metatarsectomy
  see Excision, Lower Bones 0QB
  see Resection, Lower Bones 0QT
Metatarsophalangeal (MTP) joint
  use Joint, Metatarsal-Phalangeal, Left
  use Joint, Metatarsal-Phalangeal,
    Right
Metatarsophalangeal ligament
  use Bursa and Ligament, Foot, Left
  use Bursa and Ligament, Foot, Right
Metathalamus
  use Thalamus
Micro-Driver stent (RX) (OTW)
  use Intraluminal Device
MicroMed HeartAssist
  use Implantable Heart Assist System
    in Heart and Great Vessels
Micrus CERECYTE microcoil
  use Intraluminal Device, Bioactive
    in Upper Arteries
Midcarpal joint
  use Joint, Carpal, Left
  use Joint, Carpal, Right
Middle cardiac nerve
  use Nerve, Thoracic Sympathetic
Middle cerebral artery
  use Artery, Intracranial
Middle cerebral vein
  use Vein, Intracranial
Middle colic vein
  use Vein, Colic
Middle genicular artery
  use Artery, Popliteal, Left
  use Artery, Popliteal, Right
Middle hemorrhoidal vein
  use Vein, Hypogastric, Left
  use Vein, Hypogastric, Right
Middle meningeal artery,
  intracranial portion *use*
  Intracranial Artery
Middle rectal artery
  use Artery, Internal Iliac, Left
  use Artery, Internal Iliac, Right
Middle suprarenal artery
  use Aorta, Abdominal
Middle temporal artery
  use Artery, Temporal, Left
  use Artery, Temporal, Right
Middle turbinate
  use Turbinate, Nasal
Mineral-based Topical Hemostatic
  Agent XW0
MIRODERM™ Biologic Wound
  Matrix
  use Nonautologous Tissue
    Substitute
MIRODERM™ skin graft *see*
  Replacement, Skin and Breast 0HR
MitraClip valve repair system
  use Synthetic Substitute
Mitral annulus
  use Valve, Mitral
Mitroflow® Aortic Pericardial Heart
  Valve
  use Zooplastic Tissue in Heart and
    Great Vessels
MNS (Magnus Neuromodulation
  System) X0Z0X18
Mobilization, adhesions
  see Release
Molar gland
  use Buccal Mucosa

MolecuLight i:X® wound imaging
see Other Imaging, Anatomical Regions BW5

Monitoring
Arterial
Flow
Coronary 4A13
Peripheral 4A13
Pulmonary 4A13
Pressure
Coronary 4A13
Peripheral 4A13
Pulmonary 4A13
Pulse
Coronary 4A13
Peripheral 4A13
Pulmonary 4A13
Saturation, Peripheral 4A13
Sound, Peripheral 4A13
Brain Electrical Activity, Computer-aided Detection and Notification XX20X89
Cardiac
Electrical Activity 4A12
Ambulatory 4A12X45
No Qualifier 4A12X4Z
Output 4A12
Rate 4A12
Rhythm 4A12
Sound 4A12
Total Activity, Stress 4A12XM4
Vascular Perfusion, Indocyanine Green Dye 4A12XSH
Central Nervous
Conductivity 4A10
Electrical Activity
Intraoperative 4A10
No Qualifier 4A10
Pressure 4A100BZ
Intracranial 4A10
Saturation, Intracranial 4A10
Temperature, Intracranial 4A10
Gastrointestinal
Motility 4A1B
Pressure 4A1B
Secretion 4A1B
Vascular Perfusion, Indocyanine Green Dye 4A1BXSH
Kidney, Fluorescent Pyrazine XT25XE5
Lymphatic
Flow
Indocyanine Green Dye 4A16
No Qualifier A416
Pressure 4A16
Muscle Compartment Pressure, Micro-Electro-Mechanical System XX2F3W9
Oxygen Saturation Endoscopic Imaging (OXEI) XD2
Peripheral Nervous
Conductivity
Motor 4A11
Sensory 4A11
Electrical Activity
Intraoperative 4A11
No Qualifier 4A11
Products of Conception
Cardiac
Electrical Activity 4A1H
Rate 4A1H
Rhythm 4A1H
Sound 4A1H
Nervous
Conductivity 4A1J
Electrical Activity 4A1J
Pressure 4A1J
Respiratory
Capacity 4A19
Flow 4A19
Rate 4A19

Monitoring (continued)
Respiratory (continued)
Resistance 4A19
Volume 4A19
Skin and Breast
Vascular Perfusion, Indocyanine Green Dye 4A1GXSH
Sleep 4A1ZXQZ
Temperature 4A1Z
Urinary
Contractility 4A1D
Flow 4A1D
Pressure 4A1D
Resistance 4A1D
Volume 4A1D
Venous
Flow
Central 4A14
Peripheral 4A14
Portal 4A14
Pulmonary 4A14
Pressure
Central 4A14
Peripheral 4A14
Portal 4A14
Pulmonary 4A14
Pulse
Central 4A14
Peripheral 4A14
Portal 4A14
Pulmonary 4A14
Saturation
Central 4A14
Portal 4A14
Pulmonary 4A14

Monitoring Device, Hemodynamic
Abdomen 0JH8
Chest 0JH6

Mosaic Bioprosthesis (aortic) (mitral) valve
use Zooplastic Tissue in Heart and Great Vessels

Mosunetuzumab Antineoplastic XW0

Motor Function Assessment F01
Motor Treatment F07
MR Angiography
see Magnetic Resonance Imaging (MRI), Heart B23
see Magnetic Resonance Imaging (MRI), Lower Arteries B43
see Magnetic Resonance Imaging (MRI), Upper Arteries B33

MULTI-LINK (VISION)(MINI-VISION)(ULTRA) Coronary Stent System
use Intraluminal Device

Multiple sleep latency test 4A0ZXQZ

Muscle Compartment Pressure, Micro-Electro-Mechanical System XX2F3W9

Musculocutaneous nerve
use Nerve, Brachial Plexus

Musculopexy
see Repair, Muscles 0KQ
see Reposition, Muscles 0KS

Musculophrenic artery
use Artery, Internal Mammary, Left
use Artery, Internal Mammary, Right

Musculoplasty
see Repair, Muscles 0KQ
see Supplement, Muscles 0KU

Musculorrhaphy
see Repair, Muscles 0KQ

Musculospiral nerve
use Nerve, Radial

MY01 Continuous Compartmental Pressure Monitor XX2F3W9

Myectomy
see Excision, Muscles 0KB
see Resection, Muscles 0KT

Myelencephalon
use Medulla Oblongata

Myelogram
CT
see Computerized Tomography (CT Scan), Central Nervous System B02
MRI
see Magnetic Resonance Imaging (MRI), Central Nervous System B03

Myenteric (Auerbach's) plexus
use Nerve, Abdominal Sympathetic

Myocardial Bridge Release
see Release, Artery, Coronary

Myomectomy
see Excision, Female Reproductive System 0UB

Myometrium
use Uterus

Myopexy
see Repair, Muscles 0KQ
see Reposition, Muscles 0KS

Myoplasty
see Repair, Muscles 0KQ
see Supplement, Muscles 0KU

Myorrhaphy
see Repair, Muscles 0KQ

Myoscopy
see Inspection, Muscles 0KJ

Myotomy
see Division, Muscles 0K8
see Drainage, Muscles 0K9

Myringectomy
see Excision, Ear, Nose, Sinus 09B
see Resection, Ear, Nose, Sinus 09T

Myringoplasty
see Repair, Ear, Nose, Sinus 09Q
see Replacement, Ear, Nose, Sinus 09R
see Supplement, Ear, Nose, Sinus 09U

Myringostomy
see Drainage, Ear, Nose, Sinus 099

Myringotomy
see Drainage, Ear, Nose, Sinus 099

N

NA-1 (Nerinitide)
use Nerinitide

Nafamostat Anticoagulant XY0YX37

Nail bed
use Finger Nail
use Toe Nail

Nail plate
use Finger Nail
use Toe Nail

nanoLOCK™ interbody fusion device
use Interbody Fusion Device in Lower Joints
use Interbody Fusion Device in Upper Joints

Narcosynthesis GZGZZZZ

Narsoplimab Monoclonal Antibody XW0

Nasal cavity
use Nasal Mucosa and Soft Tissue

Nasal concha
use Turbinate, Nasal

Nasalis muscle
use Muscle, Facial

Nasolacrimal duct
use Duct, Lacrimal, Left
use Duct, Lacrimal, Right

Nasopharyngeal airway (NPA)
use Intraluminal Device, Airway in Ear, Nose, Sinus

Navicular bone
use Tarsal, Left
use Tarsal, Right

Near Infrared Spectroscopy, Circulatory System 8E02

Neck of femur
use Femur, Upper, Left
use Femur, Upper, Right

Neck of humerus (anatomical) (surgical)
use Humeral Head, Left
use Humeral Head, Right

Nelli® Seizure Monitoring System XXE0X48

Neovasc Reducer™
use Reduction Device in New Technology

Nephrectomy
see Excision, Urinary System 0TB
see Resection, Urinary System 0TT

Nephrolithotomy
see Extirpation, Urinary System 0TC

Nephrolysis
see Release, Urinary System 0TN

Nephropexy
see Repair, Urinary System 0TQ
see Reposition, Urinary System 0TS

Nephroplasty
see Repair, Urinary System 0TQ
see Supplement, Urinary System 0TU

Nephropyeloureterostomy
see Bypass, Urinary System 0T1
see Drainage, Urinary System 0T9

Nephrorrhaphy
see Repair, Urinary System 0TQ

Nephroscopy, transurethral 0TJ58ZZ

Nephrostomy
see Bypass, Urinary System 0T1
see Drainage, Urinary System 0T9

Nephrotomography
see Fluoroscopy, Urinary System BT1
see Plain Radiography, Urinary System BT0

Nephrotomy
see Division, Urinary System 0T8
see Drainage, Urinary System 0T9

Nerinitide XW0

Nerve conduction study
see Measurement, Central Nervous 4A00
see Measurement, Peripheral Nervous 4A01

Nerve Function Assessment F01

Nerve to the stapedius
use Nerve, Facial

Nesiritide
use Human B-type Natriuretic Peptide

Neurectomy
see Excision, Central Nervous System and Cranial Nerves 00B
see Excision, Peripheral Nervous System 01B

Neurexeresis
see Extraction, Central Nervous System and Cranial Nerves 00D
see Extraction, Peripheral Nervous System 01D

NeuroBlate™ System see Destruction

Neurohypophysis
use Gland, Pituitary

Neurolysis
see Release, Central Nervous System and Cranial Nerves 00N
see Release, Peripheral Nervous System 01N

Neuromuscular electrical stimulation (NEMS) lead
use Stimulator Lead in Muscles

Neurophysiologic monitoring
see Monitoring, Central Nervous 4A10

Neuroplasty
see Repair, Central Nervous System and Cranial Nerves 00Q
see Repair, Peripheral Nervous System 01Q
see Supplement, Central Nervous System and Cranial Nerves 00U
see Supplement, Peripheral Nervous System 01U

Neurorrhaphy
see Repair, Central Nervous System and Cranial Nerves 00Q
see Repair, Peripheral Nervous System 01Q

Neurostimulator Generator
Insertion of device in, Skull 0NH00NZ
Removal of device from, Skull 0NP00NZ
Revision of device in, Skull 0NW00NZ

Neurostimulator generator, multiple channel
use Stimulator Generator, Multiple Array in 0JH

Neurostimulator generator, multiple channel rechargeable
use Stimulator Generator, Multiple Array Rechargeable in 0JH

Neurostimulator generator, single channel
use Stimulator Generator, Single Array in 0JH

Neurostimulator generator, single channel rechargeable
use Stimulator Generator, Single Array Rechargeable in 0JH

Neurostimulator Lead
Insertion of device in
Brain 00H0
Cerebral Ventricle 00H6
Nerve
Cranial 00HE
Peripheral 01HY
Spinal Canal 00HU
Spinal Cord 00HV
Vein
Azygos 05H0
Innominate
Left 05H4
Right 05H3
Removal of device from
Brain 00P0
Cerebral Ventricle 00P6
Nerve
Cranial 00PE
Peripheral 01PY
Spinal Canal 00PU
Spinal Cord 00PV
Vein
Azygos 05P0
Innominate
Left 05P4
Right 05HP3
Revision of device in
Brain 00W0
Cerebral Ventricle 00W6

Neurostimulator Lead *(continued)*
Revision of device in *(continued)*
Nerve
Cranial 00WE
Peripheral 01WY
Spinal Canal 00WU
Spinal Cord 00WV
Vein
Azygos 05W0
Innominate
Left 05W4
Right 05HW3
Sphenopalatine Ganglion, Insertion X0HK3Q8

Neurostimulator Lead in Oropharynx XWHD7Q7

Neurostimulator Lead with Paired Stimulation System, Insertion X0HQ3R8

Neurotomy
see Division, Central Nervous System and Cranial Nerves 008
see Division, Peripheral Nervous System and Cranial Nerves 018

Neurotripsy
see Destruction, Central Nervous System and Cranial Nerves 005
see Destruction, Peripheral Nervous System 015

Neutralization plate
use Internal Fixation Device in Head and Facial Bones
use Internal Fixation Device in Lower Bones
use Internal Fixation Device in Upper Bones

New Technology
Afamitresgene Autoleucel Immunotherapy XW0
Amivantamab Monoclonal Antibody XW0
Anacaulase-bcdb XW0
Antibiotic-eluting Bone Void Filler XW0V0P7
Aorta
Thoracic Arch using Branched Synthetic Substitute with Intraluminal Device X2RX0N7
Thoracic Descending using Branched Synthetic Substitute with Intraluminal Device X2VW0N7
Apalutamide Antineoplstic XW0DJX5
Atezolizumab Antineoplastic XW0
Axicabtagene Ciloleucel Immunotherapy XW0
Betibeglogene Autotemcel XW1
Bioengineered Allogeneic Construct, Skin XHRPXF7
Brain Electrical Activity
Computer-aided Detection and Notification XX20X89
Computer-aided Semiologic Analysis XXE0X48
Brexanolone XW0
Brexucabtagene Autoleucel Immunotherapy XW0
Broad Consortium Microbiota-based Live Biotherapeutic Suspension XW0H7X8
Bypass
Conduit through Femoral Vein to Popliteal Artery X2K
Conduit through Femoral Vein to Superficial Femoral Artery X2K
Caplacizumab XW0
Cefiderocol Anti-infective XW0
Ceftolozane/Tazobactam Anti-infective XW0

New Technology *(continued)*
Cerebral Embolic Filtration
Dual Filter X2A5312
Extracorporeal Flow Reversal Circuit X2A
Single Deflection Filter X2A6325
Ciltacabtagene Autoleucel XW0
Coagulation Factor Xa, Inactivated XW0
Computer-aided Assessment, Cardiac Output XXE2X19
Intracranial Vascular Activity XXE0X07
Computer-aided Guidance, Transthoracic Echocardiography X2JAX47
Computer-aided Mechanical Aspiration X2C
Computer-aided Triage and Notification, Pulmonary Artery Flow XXE3X27
Computer-aided Valve Modeling and Notification, Coronary Artery Flow XXE3X68
Computer-assisted Transcranial Magnetic Stimulation X0Z0X18
Coronary Sinus, Reduction Device X2V73Q7
COVID-19 Vaccine Booster XW0
COVID-19 Vaccine Dose 3 XW0
Cytarabine and Daunorubicin Liposome Antineoplastic XW0
Daratumumab and Hyaluronidase-fihj XW01318
Destruction
Liver, Ultrasound-guided Cavitation XF5
Renal Sympathetic Nerve(s), Ultrasound Ablation X051329
Dilation
Anterior Tibial
Left
Sustained Release Drug-eluting Intraluminal Device X27Q385
Four or More X27Q3C5
Three X27Q3B5
Two X27Q395
Right
Sustained Release Drug-eluting Intraluminal Device X27P385
Four or More X27P3C5
Three X27P3B5
Two X27P395
Femoral
Left
Sustained Release Drug-eluting Intraluminal Device X27J385
Four or More X27J3C5
Three X27J3B5
Two X27J395
Right
Sustained Release Drug-eluting Intraluminal Device X27H385
Four or More X27H3C5
Three X27H3B5
Two X27H395
Peroneal
Left
Sustained Release Drug-eluting Intraluminal Device X27U385
Four or More X27U3C5
Three X27U3B5
Two X27U395

New Technology *(continued)*
Dilation *(continued)*
Peroneal *(continued)*
Right
Sustained Release Drug-eluting Intraluminal Device X27T385
Four or More X27T3C5
Three X27T3B5
Two X27T395
Popliteal
Left Distal
Sustained Release Drug-eluting Intraluminal Device X27N385
Four or More X27N3C5
Three X27N3B5
Two X27N395
Left Proximal
Sustained Release Drug-eluting Intraluminal Device X27L385
Four or More X27L3C5
Three X27L3B5
Two X27L395
Right Distal
Sustained Release Drug-eluting Intraluminal Device X27M385
Four or More X27M3C5
Three X27M3B5
Two X27M395
Right Proximal
Sustained Release Drug-eluting Intraluminal Device X27K385
Four or More X27K3C5
Three X27QK3B5
Two X27K395
Posterior Tibial
Left
Sustained Release Drug-eluting Intraluminal Device X27S385
Four or More X27S3C5
Three X27S3B5
Two X27S395
Right
Sustained Release Drug-eluting Intraluminal Device X27R385
Four or More X27R3C5
Three X27R3B5
Two X27R395
Durvalumab Antineoplastic XW0
Eculizumab XW0
Eladocagene exuparvovec XW0Q316
Elranatamab Antineoplastic XW013L9
Endothelial Damage Inhibitor XY0VX83
Engineered Allogeneic Thymus Tissue XW020D8
Engineered Chimeric Antigen Receptor T-cell Immunotherapy Allogeneic XW0
Autologous XW0
Epcoritamab Monoclonal Antibody XW013S9
Erdafitinib Antineoplastic XW0DXL5
Esketamine Hydrochloride XW097M5
Exagamglogene Autotemcel XW1
Fosfomycin Anti-infective XW0
Fostamatinib XW0
Fusion
Ankle
Left, Open-truss Design Internal Fixation Device XRGK0B9
Right, Open-truss Design Internal Fixation Device XRGJ0B9

New Technology *(continued)*
Fusion *(continued)*
Lumbar Vertebral
2 or more, Interbody Fusion
Device, Custom-Made
Anatomically Designed
XRGC
Interbody Fusion Device
Custom-Made Anatomically
Designed XRGB
Lumbosacral, Interbody Fusion
Device, Custom-Made
Anatomically Designed
XRGD
Sacroiliac, Internal Fixation
Device with Tulip Connector
XRG
Tarsal
Left, Open-truss Design
Internal Fixation Device
XRGM0B9
Right, Open-truss Design
Internal Fixation Device
XRGL0B9
Thoracolumbar Vertebral,
Interbody Fusion Device,
Custom-Made Anatomically
Designed XRGA
Gilteritinib Antineoplastic
XW0DXV5
Glofitamab Antineoplastic XW0
High-Dose Intravenous Immune
Globulin, for COVID-19
treatment XW1
Hyperimmune Globulin, for
COVID-19 treatment XW1
Idecabtagene Vicleucel
Immunotherapy XW0
Imipenem-cilastatin-relebactam
Anti-infective XW0
Inebilizumab-cdon XW0
Insertion
Bone, Pelvic, Internal Fixation
Device with Tulip Connector
XNH
Conduit to Short-term External
Heart Assist System X2H
Intracardiac Pacemaker, Dual-
Chamber X2H
Intraluminal Device,
Bioprosthetic Valve X2H
Joint
Lumbar Vertebral, Posterior
Spinal Motion Preservation
Device XRHB018
Lumbosacral, Posterior Spinal
Motion Preservation Device
XRHD018
Neurostimulator Lead,
Sphenopalatine Ganglion
X0HK3Q8
Neurostimulator Lead with
Paired Stimulation System
X0HQ3R8
Tibial Extension with Motion
Sensors XNH
Intermittent Coronary Sinus
Occlusion X2A7358
Intracranial Arterial Flow, Whole
Blood mRNA XXE5XT7
Iobenguane I-131 Antineoplastic XW0
Kidney, Fluorescent Pyrazine
XT25XE5
Lefamulin Anti-infective XW0
Lifileucel Immunotherapy XW0
Lisocabtagene Maraleucel
Immunotherapy XW0
Lovotibeglogene Autotemcel XW1
Lower Respiratory Fluid Nucleic
Acid-base Microbial Detection
XXEBXQ6

New Technology *(continued)*
Lurbinectedin XW0
Maribavir Anti-infective XW0
Mechanical Initial Specimen
Diversion Technique Using
Active Negative Pressure (blood
collection) XXE5XR7
Melphalan Hydrochloride
Antineoplastic XW053T9
Meropenem-vaborbactam Anti-
infective XW0
Mineral-based Topical Hemostatic
Agent XW0
Mosunetuzumab Antineoplastic XW0
Muscle Compartment Pressure,
Micro-Electro-Mechanical System
XX2F3W9
Nafamostat Anticoagulant XY0YX37
Narsoplimab Monoclonal Antibody
XW0
Nerinitide XW0
Neurostimulator Lead in Oropharynx
XWHD7Q7
Omadacycline Anti-infective XW0
Omidubicel XW1
Other New Technology Therapeutic
Substance XW0
Other Positive Blood/Isolated
Colonies Bimodal Phenotypic
Susceptibility Technology
XXE5XY9
OTL-103 XW1
OTL-200 XW1
Oxygen Saturation Endoscopic
Imaging (OXEI) XD2
Plasma, Convalescent
(Nonautologous) XW1
Positive Blood Culture Fluorescence
Hybridization for Organism
Identification, Concentration and
Susceptibility XXE5XN6
Posoleucel XW0
Quantitative Flow Ratio Analysis,
Coronary Artery Flow XXE3X58
Quizartinib Antineoplastic
XW0DXJ9
Radial artery ateriovenous fistula,
using Thermal Resistance
Energy X2K
Remdesivir Anti-infective XW0
Replacement
Lateral Meniscus Synthetic
Substitute XRR
Medial Meniscus Synthetic
Substitute XRR
Reposition
Cervical, Magnetically Controlled
Growth Rod(s) XNS3
Lumbar
Magnetically Controlled
Growth Rod(s) XNS0
Posterior (Dynamic)
Distraction Device XNS0
Thoracic
Magnetically Controlled
Growth Rod(s) XNS4
Posterior (Dynamic)
Distraction Device XNS4
Rezafungin XW0
Ruxolitinib XW0DXT5
Sabizabulin XW0
Sarilumab XW0
SARS-CoV-2 Antibody Detection,
Serum/Plasma Nanoparticle
Fluorescence XXE5XV7
SARS-CoV-2 Polymerase Chain
Reaction, Nasopharyngeal Fluid
XXE97U7
Satralizumab-mwge XW01397
SER-109 XW0DXN9
Single-use Duodenoscope XFJ

New Technology *(continued)*
Single-use Oversleeve with
Intraoperative Colonic Irrigation
XDPH8K7
Spesolimab Monoclonal Antibody
XW0
Sulbactam-Durlobactam XW0
Supplement
Arteriovenous Fistula, Extraluminal
Support Device X2U
Bursa and Ligament, Spine,
Posterior Vertebral Tether XKU
Coronary Artery/Arteries, Vein
Graft Extraluminal Support
Device(s) X2U4079
Vertebra
Lumbar, Mechanically
Expandable (Paired)
Synthetic Substitute
XNU0356
Thoracic, Mechanically
Expandable (Paired)
Synthetic Substitute
XNU4356
Tabelecleucel Immunotherapy XW0
Tagraxofusp-erzs Antineoplastic XW0
Talar Prosthesis Synthetic
Substitute XNR
Taurolidine Anti-infective
and Heparin Anticoagulant
XY0YX28
Teclistamab Antineoplastic
XW01348
Terlipressin XW0
Tisagenlecleucel Immunotherapy
XW0
Tixagevimab and Cilgavimab
Monoclonal Antibody
XW023X7
Tocilizumab XW0
Treosulfan XW0
Trilaciclib XW0
Ultrasound Penetrable Synthetic
Substitute, Skull XNR80D9
Uridine Triacetate XW0DX82
Venetoclax Antineoplastic
XW0DXR5
Whole Blood Nucleic Acid-base
Microbial Detection XXE5XM5
Whole Blood Reverse Transcription
and Quantitative Real-time
Polymerase Chain Reaction
XXE5X38
NexoBrid™
use Anacaulase-bcdb
Ninth cranial nerve
use Nerve, Glossopharyngeal
NIRS (Near Infrared Spectroscopy)
see Physiological Systems and
Anatomical Regions 8E0
Nitinol framed polymer mesh
use Synthetic Substitute
Niyad™
use Nafamostat Anticoagulant
Non-tunneled central venous catheter
use Infusion Device
Nonimaging Nuclear Medicine Assay
Bladder, Kidneys and Ureters CT63
Blood C763
Kidneys, Ureters and Bladder CT63
Lymphatics and Hematologic
System C76YYZZ
Ureters, Kidneys and Bladder CT63
Urinary System CT6YYZZ
Nonimaging Nuclear Medicine Probe
Abdomen CW50
Abdomen and Chest CW54
Abdomen and Pelvis CW51
Brain C050
Central Nervous System C05YYZZ
Chest CW53ZZ

**Nonimaging Nuclear Medicine
Probe** *(continued)*
Chest and Abdomen CW54
Chest and Neck CW56
Extremity
Lower CP5PZZZ
Upper CP5NZZZ
Head and Neck CW5B
Heart C25YYZZ
Right and Left C256
Lymphatics
Head C75J
Head and Neck C755
Lower Extremity C75P
Neck C75K
Pelvic C75D
Trunk C75M
Upper Chest C75L
Upper Extremity C75N
Lymphatics and Hematologic
System C75YYZZ
Musculoskeletal System, Other
CP5YYZZ
Neck and Chest CW56
Neck and Head CW5B
Pelvic Region CW5J
Pelvis and Abdomen CW51
Spine CP55ZZZ
**Nonimaging Nuclear Medicine
Uptake**
Endocrine System CG4YYZZ
Gland, Thyroid CG42
Nostril
use Nasal Mucosa and Soft Tissue
**Novacor Left Ventricular Assist
Device**
use Implantable Heart Assist System
in Heart and Great Vessels
**Novation® Ceramic AHS®
(Articulation Hip System)**
use Synthetic Substitute, Ceramic
in 0SR
Nuclear medicine
see Nonimaging Nuclear Medicine
Assay
see Nonimaging Nuclear Medicine
Probe
see Nonimaging Nuclear Medicine
Uptake
see Planar Nuclear Medicine
Imaging
see Positron Emission Tomographic
(PET) Imaging
see Systemic Nuclear Medicine
Therapy
see Tomographic (Tomo) Nuclear
Medicine Imaging
Nuclear scintigraphy
see Nuclear Medicine
NUsurface® Meniscus Implant
use Synthetic Substitute, Lateral
Meniscus in New Technology
use Synthetic Substitute, Medical
Meniscus in New Technology
Nutrition, concentrated substances
Enteral infusion 3E0G36Z
Parenteral (peripheral) infusion
see Introduction of Nutritional
Substance
NUZYRA™
use Omadacycline Anti-infective

O

Obliteration
see Destruction
Obturator artery
use Artery, Internal Iliac, Left
use Artery, Internal Iliac, Right
Obturator lymph node
use Lymphatic, Pelvis

Obturator muscle
use Muscle, Hip, Left
use Muscle, Hip, Right
Obturator nerve
use Nerve, Lumbar Plexus
Obturator vein
use Vein, Hypogastric, Left
use Vein, Hypogastric, Right
Obtuse margin
use Heart, Left
Occipital artery
use Artery, External Carotid, Left
use Artery, External Carotid, Right
Occipital lobe
use Cerebral Hemisphere
Occipital lymph node
use Lymphatic, Neck, Left
use Lymphatic, Neck, Right
Occipitofrontalis muscle
use Muscle, Facial
Occlusion
Ampulla of Vater 0FLC
Anus 0DLQ
Aorta
  Abdominal 04L0
  Thoracic, Descending 02LW
Artery
  Anterior Tibial
    Left 04LQ
    Right 04LP
  Axillary
    Left 03L6
    Right 03L5
  Brachial
    Left 03L8
    Right 03L7
  Celiac 04L1
  Colic
    Left 04L7
    Middle 04L8
    Right 04L6
  Common Carotid
    Left 03LJ
    Right 03LH
  Common Iliac
    Left 04LD
    Right 04LC
  External Carotid
    Left 03LN
    Right 03LM
  External Iliac
    Left 04LJ
    Right 04LH
  Face 03LR
  Femoral
    Left 04LL
    Right 04LK
  Foot
    Left 04LW
    Right 04LV
  Gastric 04L2
  Hand
    Left 03LF
    Right 03LD
  Hepatic 04L3
  Inferior Mesenteric 04LB
  Innominate 03L2
  Internal Carotid
    Left 03LL
    Right 03LK
  Internal Iliac
    Left 04LF
    Right 04LE
  Internal Mammary
    Left 03L1
    Right 03L0
  Intracranial 03LG
  Lower 04LY
  Peroneal
    Left 04LU
    Right 04LT

Occlusion *(continued)*
Artery *(continued)*
  Popliteal
    Left 04LN
    Right 04LM
  Posterior Tibial
    Left 04LS
    Right 04LR
  Pulmonary
    Left 02LR
    Right 02LQ
  Pulmonary Trunk 02LP
  Radial
    Left 03LC
    Right 03LB
  Renal
    Left 04LA
    Right 04L9
  Splenic 04L4
  Subclavian
    Left 03L4
    Right 03L3
  Superior Mesenteric 04L5
  Temporal
    Left 03LT
    Right 03LS
  Thyroid
    Left 03LV
    Right 03LU
  Ulnar
    Left 03LA
    Right 03L9
  Upper 03LY
  Vertebral
    Left 03LQ
    Right 03LP
Atrium, Left 02L7
Bladder 0TLB
Bladder Neck 0TLC
Bronchus
  Lingula 0BL9
  Lower Lobe
    Left 0BLB
    Right 0BL6
  Main
    Left 0BL7
    Right 0BL3
  Middle Lobe, Right
    0BL5
  Upper Lobe
    Left 0BL8
    Right 0BL4
Carina 0BL2
Cecum 0DLH
Cisterna Chyli 07LL
Colon
  Ascending 0DLK
  Descending 0DLM
  Sigmoid 0DLN
  Transverse 0DLL
Cord
  Bilateral 0VLH
  Left 0VLG
  Right 0VLF
Cul-de-sac 0ULF
Duct
  Common Bile 0FL9
  Cystic 0FL8
  Hepatic
    Common 0FL7
    Left 0FL6
    Right 0FL5
  Lacrimal
    Left 08LY
    Right 08LX
  Pancreatic 0FLD
    Accessory 0FLF
  Parotid
    Left 0CLC
    Right 0CLB
Duodenum 0DL9

Occlusion *(continued)*
Esophagogastric Junction 0DL4
Esophagus 0DL5
  Lower 0DL3
  Middle 0DL2
  Upper 0DL1
Fallopian Tube
  Left 0UL6
  Right 0UL5
Fallopian Tubes, Bilateral 0UL7
Ileocecal Valve 0DLC
Ileum 0DLB
Intestine
  Large 0DLE
    Left 0DLG
    Right 0DLF
  Small 0DL8
Jejunum 0DLA
Kidney Pelvis
  Left 0TL4
  Right 0TL3
Left atrial appendage (LAA)
  see Occlusion, Atrium, Left 02L7
Lymphatic
  Aortic 07LD
  Axillary
    Left 07L6
    Right 07L5
  Head 07L0
  Inguinal
    Left 07LJ
    Right 07LH
  Internal Mammary
    Left 07L9
    Right 07L8
  Lower Extremity
    Left 07LG
    Right 07LF
  Mesenteric 07LB
  Neck
    Left 07L2
    Right 07L1
  Pelvis 07LC
  Thoracic Duct 07LK
  Thorax 07L7
  Upper Extremity
    Left 07L4
    Right 07L3
Rectum 0DLP
Stomach 0DL6
  Pylorus 0DL7
Trachea 0BL1
Ureter
  Left 0TL7
  Right 0TL6
Urethra 0TLD
Vagina 0ULG
Valve, Pulmonary 02LH
Vas Deferens
  Bilateral 0VLQ
  Left 0VLP
  Right 0VLN
Vein
  Axillary
    Left 05L8
    Right 05L7
  Azygos 05L0
  Basilic
    Left 05LC
    Right 05LB
  Brachial
    Left 05LA
    Right 05L9
  Cephalic
    Left 05LF
    Right 05LD
  Colic 06L7
  Common Iliac
    Left 06LD
    Right 06LC
  Esophageal 06L3

Occlusion *(continued)*
Vein *(continued)*
  External Iliac
    Left 06LG
    Right 06LF
  External Jugular
    Left 05LQ
    Right 05LP
  Face
    Left 05LV
    Right 05LT
  Femoral
    Left 06LN
    Right 06LM
  Foot
    Left 06LV
    Right 06LT
  Gastric 06L2
  Hand
    Left 05LH
    Right 05LG
  Hemiazygos 05L1
  Hepatic 06L4
  Hypogastric
    Left 06LJ
    Right 06LH
  Inferior Mesenteric 06L6
  Innominate
    Left 05L4
    Right 05L3
  Internal Jugular
    Left 05LN
    Right 05LM
  Intracranial 05LL
  Lower 06LY
  Portal 06L8
  Pulmonary
    Left 02LT
    Right 02LS
  Renal
    Left 06LB
    Right 06L9
  Saphenous
    Left 06LQ
    Right 06LP
  Splenic 06L1
  Subclavian
    Left 05L6
    Right 05L5
  Superior Mesenteric
    06L5
  Upper 05LY
  Vertebral
    Left 05LS
    Right 05LR
  Vena Cava
    Inferior 06L0
    Superior 02LV
Occlusion, REBOA (resuscitative endovascular balloon occlusion of the aorta)
02LW3DJ
04L03DJ
Occupational therapy
see Activities of Daily Living
  Treatment, Rehabilitation F08
Octagam 10%, for COVID-19 treatment
use High-Dose Intravenous Immune
  Globulin
Odentectomy
see Excision, Mouth and Throat 0CB
see Resection, Mouth and Throat 0CT
Odontoid process
use Cervical Vertebra
Olecranon bursa
use Bursa and Ligament, Elbow, Left
use Bursa and Ligament, Elbow, Right
Olecranon process
use Ulna, Left
use Ulna, Right

51

Olfactory bulb
use Nerve, Olfactory
Omadacycline Anti-infective XW0
Omentectomy, omentumectomy
see Excision, Gastrointestinal
System 0DB
see Resection, Gastrointestinal
System 0DT
Omentofixation
see Repair, Gastrointestinal System
0DQ
Omentoplasty
see Repair, Gastrointestinal System
0DQ
see Replacement, Gastrointestinal
System 0DR
see Supplement, Gastrointestinal
System 0DU
Omentorrhaphy
see Repair, Gastrointestinal System
0DQ
Omentotomy
see Drainage, Gastrointestinal
System 0D9
Omidubicel XW1
Omnilink Elite Vascular Balloon
Expandable Stent System
use Intraluminal Device
Onychectomy
see Excision, Skin and Breast 0HB
see Resection, Skin and Breast 0HT
Onychoplasty
see Repair, Skin and Breast 0HQ
see Replacement, Skin and Breast 0HR
Onychotomy
see Drainage, Skin and Breast 0H9
Oophorectomy
see Excision, Female Reproductive
System 0UB
see Resection, Female Reproductive
System 0UT
Oophoropexy
see Repair, Female Reproductive
System 0UQ
see Reposition, Female
Reproductive System 0US
Oophoroplasty
see Repair, Female Reproductive
System 0UQ
see Supplement, Female
Reproductive System 0UU
Oophororrhaphy
see Repair, Female Reproductive
System 0UQ
Oophorostomy
see Drainage, Female Reproductive
System 0U9
Oophorotomy
see Drainage, Female Reproductive
System 0U9
see Division, Female Reproductive
System 0U8
Oophorrhaphy
see Repair, Female Reproductive
System 0UQ
Open Pivot (mechanical) valve
use Synthetic Substitute
Open Pivot Aortic Valve Graft (AVG)
use Synthetic Substitute
Open-truss Design Internal Fixation
Device
Ankle
Left XRGK0B9
Right XRGJ0B9
Tarsal
Left XRGM0B9
Right XRGL0B9
Ophthalmic artery
use Intracranial Artery
Ophthalmic nerve
use Nerve, Trigeminal
Ophthalmic vein
use Vein, Intracranial

Opponensplasty
Tendon replacement
see Replacement, Tendons 0LR
Tendon transfer
see Transfer, Tendons 0LX
Optic chiasma
use Nerve, Optic
Optic disc
use Retina, Left
use Retina, Right
Optic foramen
use Bone, Sphenoid
Optical coherence tomography,
intravascular
see Computerized Tomography (CT
Scan)
Optimizer™ III implantable pulse
generator
use Contractility Modulation Device
in 0JH
Orbicularis oculi muscle
use Eyelid, Upper, Left
use Eyelid, Upper, Right
Orbicularis oris muscle
use Muscle, Facial
Orbital Atherectomy
see Extirpation, Heart and Great
Vessels 02C
Orbital fascia
use Subcutaneous Tissue and Fascia,
Face
Orbital portion of ethmoid bone
use Orbit, Left
use Orbit, Right
Orbital portion of frontal bone
use Orbit, Left
use Orbit, Right
Orbital portion of lacrimal bone
use Orbit, Left
use Orbit, Right
Orbital portion of maxilla
use Orbit, Left
use Orbit, Right
Orbital portion of palatine bone
use Orbit, Left
use Orbit, Right
Orbital portion of sphenoid bone
use Orbit, Left
use Orbit, Right
Orbital portion of zygomatic bone
use Orbit, Left
use Orbit, Right
Orchectomy, orchidectomy,
orchiectomy
see Excision, Male Reproductive
System 0VB
see Resection, Male Reproductive
System 0VT
Orchidoplasty, orchioplasty
see Repair, Male Reproductive
System 0VQ
see Replacement, Male
Reproductive System 0VR
see Supplement, Male Reproductive
System 0VU
Orchidorrhaphy, orchiorrhaphy
see Repair, Male Reproductive
System 0VQ
Orchidotomy, orchiotomy,
orchotomy
see Drainage, Male Reproductive
System 0V9
Orchiopexy
see Repair, Male Reproductive
System 0VQ
see Reposition, Male Reproductive
System 0VS
Oropharyngeal airway (OPA)
use Intraluminal Device, Airway in
Mouth and Throat
Oropharynx
use Pharynx

Ossiculectomy
see Excision, Ear, Nose, Sinus 09B
see Resection, Ear, Nose, Sinus 09T
Ossiculotomy
see Drainage, Ear, Nose, Sinus 099
Ostectomy
see Excision, Head and Facial
Bones 0NB
see Excision, Lower Bones 0QB
see Excision, Upper Bones 0PB
see Resection, Head and Facial
Bones 0NT
see Resection, Lower Bones 0QT
see Resection, Upper Bones 0PT
Osteoclasis
see Division, Head and Facial
Bones 0N8
see Division, Lower Bones 0Q8
see Division, Upper Bones 0P8
Osteolysis
see Release, Head and Facial Bones
0NN
see Release, Lower Bones 0QN
see Release, Upper Bones 0PN
Osteopathic Treatment
Abdomen 7W09X
Cervical 7W01X
Extremity
Lower 7W06X
Upper 7W07X
Head 7W00X
Lumbar 7W03X
Pelvis 7W05X
Rib Cage 7W08X
Sacrum 7W04X
Thoracic 7W02X
Osteopexy
see Repair, Head and Facial Bones
0NQ
see Repair, Lower Bones 0QQ
see Repair, Upper Bones 0PQ
see Reposition, Head and Facial
Bones 0NS
see Reposition, Lower Bones 0QS
see Reposition, Upper Bones 0PS
Osteoplasty
see Repair, Head and Facial Bones
0NQ
see Repair, Lower Bones 0QQ
see Repair, Upper Bones 0PQ
see Replacement, Head and Facial
Bones 0NR
see Replacement, Lower Bones
0QR
see Replacement, Upper Bones 0PR
see Supplement, Head and Facial
Bones 0NU
see Supplement, Lower Bones 0QU
see Supplement, Upper Bones 0PU
Osteorrhaphy
see Repair, Head and Facial Bones
0NQ
see Repair, Lower Bones 0QQ
see Repair, Upper Bones 0PQ
Osteotomy, ostotomy
see Division, Head and Facial
Bones 0N8
see Division, Lower Bones 0Q8
see Division, Upper Bones 0P8
see Drainage, Head and Facial
Bones 0N9
see Drainage, Lower Bones 0Q9
see Drainage, Upper Bones 0P9
Other Imaging
Bile Duct, Indocyanine Green Dye,
Intraoperative BF50200
Bile Duct and Gallbladder,
Indocyanine Green Dye,
Intraoperative BF53200
Extremity
Lower BW5CZ1Z
Upper BW5JZ1Z

Other Imaging *(continued)*
Gallbladder, Indocyanine Green
Dye, Intraoperative BF52200
Gallbladder and Bile Duct,
Indocyanine Green Dye,
Intraoperative BF53200
Head and Neck BW59Z1Z
Hepatobiliary System, All,
Indocyanine Green Dye,
Intraoperative BF5C200
Liver, Indocyanine Green Dye,
Intraoperative BF55200
Liver and Spleen, Indocyanine
Green Dye, Intraoperative
BF56200
Neck and Head BW59Z1Z
Pancreas, Indocyanine Green Dye,
Intraoperative BF57200
Spleen and Liver, Indocyanine
Green Dye, Intraoperative
BF56200
Trunk BW52Z1Z
Other New Technology Therapeutic
Substance XW0
Other Positive Blood/Isolated
Colonies Bimodal Phenotypic
Susceptibility Technology
XXE5XY9
Otic ganglion
use Nerve, Head and Neck
Sympathetic
OTL-101
use Hematopoietic Stem/Progenitor
Cells, Genetically Modified
OTL-103 XW1
OTL-200 XW1
Otoplasty
see Repair, Ear, Nose, Sinus 09Q
see Replacement, Ear, Nose, Sinus
09R
see Supplement, Ear, Nose, Sinus 09U
Otoscopy
see Inspection, Ear, Nose, Sinus 09J
Oval window
use Ear, Middle, Left
use Ear, Middle, Right
Ovarian artery
use Aorta, Abdominal
Ovarian ligament
use Uterine Supporting Structure
Ovariectomy
see Excision, Female Reproductive
System 0UB
see Resection, Female Reproductive
System 0UT
Ovariocentesis
see Drainage, Female Reproductive
System 0U9
Ovariopexy
see Repair, Female Reproductive
System 0UQ
see Reposition, Female
Reproductive System 0US
Ovariotomy
see Division, Female Reproductive
System 0U8
see Drainage, Female Reproductive
System 0U9
Ovatio™ CRT-D
use Cardiac Resynchronization
Defibrillator Pulse Generator in
0JH
Oversewing
Gastrointestinal ulcer
see Repair, Gastrointestinal
System 0DQ
Pleural bleb
see Repair, Respiratory System
0BQ
Oviduct
use Fallopian Tube, Left
use Fallopian Tube, Right

Oximetry, Fetal pulse 10H073Z
OXINIUM
  use Synthetic Substitute, Oxidized
    Zirconium on Polyethylene in 0SR
Oxygen Saturation Endoscopic
    Imaging (OXEI) XD2
Oxygenation
  Extracorporeal membrane (ECMO)
    see Performance, Circulatory 5A15
  Hyperbaric
    see Assistance, Circulatory 5A05
  Supersaturated
    see Assistance, Circulatory 5A02

P

Pacemaker
  Dual Chamber
    Abdomen 0JH8
    Chest 0JH6
  Intracardiac
    Insertion of device in
      Atrium
        Left 02H7
        Right 02H6
      Vein, Coronary 02H4
      Ventricle
        Left 02HL
        Right 02HK
    Removal of device from
      Heart 02PA
    Revision of device in
      Heart 02WA
  Single Chamber
    Abdomen 0JH8
    Chest 0JH6
  Single Chamber Rate Responsive
    Abdomen 0JH8
    Chest 0JH6
Packing
  Abdominal Wall 2W43X5Z
  Anorectal 2Y43X5Z
  Arm
    Lower
      Left 2W4DX5Z
      Right 2W4CX5Z
    Upper
      Left 2W4BX5Z
      Right 2W4AX5Z
  Back 2W45X5Z
  Chest Wall 2W44X5Z
  Ear 2Y42X5Z
  Extremity
    Lower
      Left 2W4MX5Z
      Right 2W4LX5Z
    Upper
      Left 2W49X5Z
      Right 2W48X5Z
  Face 2W41X5Z
  Finger
    Left 2W4KX5Z
    Right 2W4JX5Z
  Foot
    Left 2W4TX5Z
    Right 2W4SX5Z
  Genital Tract, Female 2Y44X5Z
  Hand
    Left 2W4FX5Z
    Right 2W4EX5Z
  Head 2W40X5Z
  Inguinal Region
    Left 2W47X5Z
    Right 2W46X5Z
  Leg
    Lower
      Left 2W4RX5Z
      Right 2W4QX5Z
    Upper
      Left 2W4PX5Z
      Right 2W4NX5Z
  Mouth and Pharynx 2Y40X5Z
  Nasal 2Y41X5Z

Packing *(continued)*
  Neck 2W42X5Z
  Thumb
    Left 2W4HX5Z
    Right 2W4GX5Z
  Toe
    Left 2W4VX5Z
    Right 2W4UX5Z
  Urethra 2Y45X5Z
Paclitaxel-eluting coronary stent
  use Intraluminal Device, Drug-eluting
    in Heart and Great Vessels
Paclitaxel-eluting peripheral
    stent
  use Intraluminal Device, Drug-
    eluting in Lower Arteries
  use Intraluminal Device, Drug-
    eluting in Upper Arteries
Palatine gland
  use Buccal Mucosa
Palatine tonsil
  use Tonsils
Palatine uvula
  use Uvula
Palatoglossal muscle
  use Muscle, Tongue, Palate, Pharynx
Palatopharyngeal muscle
  use Muscle, Tongue, Palate, Pharynx
Palatoplasty
  see Repair, Mouth and Throat 0CQ
  see Replacement, Mouth and Throat
    0CR
  see Supplement, Mouth and Throat
    0CU
Palatorrhaphy
  see Repair, Mouth and Throat 0CQ
Palmar (volar) digital vein
  use Vein, Hand, Left
  use Vein, Hand, Right
Palmar (volar) metacarpal vein
  use Vein, Hand, Left
  use Vein, Hand, Right
Palmar cutaneous nerve
  use Nerve, Median
  use Nerve, Radial
Palmar fascia (aponeurosis)
  use Subcutaneous Tissue and Fascia,
    Hand, Left
  use Subcutaneous Tissue and Fascia,
    Hand, Right
Palmar interosseous muscle
  use Muscle, Hand, Left
  use Muscle, Hand, Right
Palmar ulnocarpal ligament
  use Bursa and Ligament, Wrist, Left
  use Bursa and Ligament, Wrist,
    Right
Palmaris longus muscle
  use Muscle, Lower Arm and Wrist,
    Left
  use Muscle, Lower Arm and Wrist,
    Right
Pancreatectomy
  see Excision, Pancreas 0FBG
  see Resection, Pancreas 0FTG
Pancreatic artery
  use Artery, Splenic
Pancreatic plexus
  use Nerve, Abdominal Sympathetic
Pancreatic vein
  use Vein, Splenic
Pancreaticoduodenostomy
  see Bypass, Hepatobiliary
    System and Pancreas 0F1
Pancreaticosplenic lymph node
  use Lymphatic, Aortic
Pancreatogram, endoscopic
    retrograde
  see Fluoroscopy, Pancreatic Duct
    BF18
Pancreatolithotomy
  see Extirpation, Pancreas 0FCG

Pancreatotomy
  see Division, Pancreas 0F8G
  see Drainage, Pancreas 0F9G
Panniculectomy
  see Excision, Skin, Abdomen 0HB7
  see Excision, Subcutaneous Tissue
    and Fascia, Abdomen 0JB8
Paraaortic lymph node
  use Lymphatic, Aortic
Paracentesis
  Eye
    see Drainage, Eye 089
  Peritoneal Cavity
    see Drainage, Peritoneal Cavity
      0W9G
  Tympanum
    see Drainage, Ear, Nose, Sinus
      099
Paradise™ Ultrasound Renal
    Denervation System X051329
Parapharyngeal space
  use Neck
Pararectal lymph node
  use Lymphatic, Mesenteric
Parasternal lymph node
  use Lymphatic, Thorax
Parathyroidectomy
  see Excision, Endocrine System 0GB
  see Resection, Endocrine System 0GT
Paratracheal lymph node
  use Lymphatic, Thorax
Paraurethral (Skene's) gland
  use Gland, Vestibular
Parenteral nutrition, total
  see Introduction of Nutritional
    Substance
Parietal lobe
  use Cerebral Hemisphere
Parotid lymph node
  use Lymphatic, Head
Parotid plexus
  use Nerve, Facial
Parotidectomy
  see Excision, Mouth and Throat
    0CB
  see Resection, Mouth and Throat
    0CT
Pars flaccida
  use Tympanic Membrane, Left
  use Tympanic Membrane, Right
Partial joint replacement
  Hip
    see Replacement, Lower Joints
      0SR
  Knee
    see Replacement, Lower Joints
      0SR
  Shoulder
    see Replacement, Upper Joints
      0RR
Partially absorbable mesh
  use Synthetic Substitute
Patch, blood, spinal 3E0R3GC
Patellapexy
  see Repair, Lower Bones 0QQ
  see Reposition, Lower Bones 0QS
Patellaplasty
  see Repair, Lower Bones 0QQ
  see Replacement, Lower Bones
    0QR
  see Supplement, Lower Bones 0QU
Patellar ligament
  use Bursa and Ligament, Knee, Left
  use Bursa and Ligament, Knee,
    Right
Patellar tendon
  use Tendon, Knee, Left
  use Tendon, Knee, Right
Patellectomy
  see Excision, Lower Bones
    0QB
  see Resection, Lower Bones 0QT

Patellofemoral joint
  use Joint, Knee, Left
  use Joint, Knee, Left, Femoral
    Surface
  use Joint, Knee, Right
  use Joint, Knee, Right, Femoral
    Surface
pAVF (percutaneous arteriovenous
    fistula), using magnetic-guided
    radiofrequency
  see Bypass, Upper Arteries 031
pAVF (percutaneous arteriovenous
    fistula), using thermal
    resistance energy
  see New Technology,
    Cardiovascular System X2K
Pectineus muscle
  use Muscle, Upper Leg, Left
  use Muscle, Upper Leg, Right
Pectoral (anterior) lymph node
  use Lymphatic, Axillary, Left
  use Lymphatic, Axillary,
    Right
Pectoral fascia
  use Subcutaneous Tissue and Fascia,
    Chest
Pectoralis major muscle
  use Muscle, Thorax, Left
  use Muscle, Thorax, Right
Pectoralis minor muscle
  use Muscle, Thorax, Left
  use Muscle, Thorax, Right
Pedicle-based dynamic stabilization
    device
  use Spinal Stabilization Device,
    Pedicle-Based in 0RH
  use Spinal Stabilization Device,
    Pedicle-Based in 0SH
PEEP (positive end expiratory
    pressure)
  see Assistance, Respiratory
    5A09
PEG (percutaneous endoscopic
    gastrostomy) 0DH63UZ
PEJ (percutaneous endoscopic
    jejunostomy) 0DHA3UZ
Pelvic splanchnic nerve
  use Nerve, Abdominal Sympathetic
  use Nerve, Sacral Sympathetic
Penectomy
  see Excision, Male Reproductive
    System 0VB
  see Resection, Male Reproductive
    System 0VT
Penile urethra
  use Urethra
Penumbra Indigo® Aspiration
    System
  see New Technology,
    Cardiovascular System X2C
PERCEPT™ neurostimulator
  use Stimulator Generator, Multiple
    Array in 0JH
Perceval sutureless valve
  (rapid deployment technique) *see*
    Replacement, Valve, Aortic
    02RF
Percutaneous endoscopic
    gastrojejunostomy (PEG/J)
    tube
  use Feeding Device in
    Gastrointestinal System
Percutaneous endoscopic
    gastrostomy (PEG) tube
  use Feeding Device in
    Gastrointestinal System
Percutaneous nephrostomy catheter
  use Drainage Device
Percutaneous transluminal coronary
    angioplasty (PTCA)
  see Dilation, Heart and Great
    Vessels 027

Performance
  Biliary
    Multiple, Filtration 5A1C60Z
    Single, Filtration 5A1C00Z
  Cardiac
    Continuous
      Output 5A1221Z
      Pacing 5A1223Z
    Intermittent, Pacing 5A1213Z
    Single, Output, Manual 5A12012
  Circulatory
    Continuous
      Central Membrane 5A1522F
      Peripheral Veno-arterial
        Membrane 5A1522G
      Peripheral Veno-venous
        Membrane 5A1522H
    Intraoperative
      Central Membrane 5A15A2F
      Peripheral Veno-arterial
        Membrane 5A15A2G
      Peripheral Veno-venous
        Membrane 5A15A2H
  Respiratory
    24-96 Consecutive Hours,
      Ventilation 5A1945Z
    Greater than 96 Consecutive
      Hours, Ventilation 5A1955Z
    Less than 24 Consecutive Hours,
      Ventilation 5A1935Z
    Single, Ventilation,
      Nonmechanical5A19054
  Urinary
    Continuous, Greater than 18
      hours per day, Filtration
      5A1D90Z
    Intermittent, Less than 6 hours
      per day, Filtration 5A1D70Z
    Prolonged Intermittent, 6-18
      hours per day, Filtration
      5A1D80Z
Perfusion
  see Introduction of substance in or on
Perfusion, donor organ
  Heart 6AB50BZ
  Kidney(s) 6ABT0BZ
  Liver 6ABF0BZ
  Lung(s) 6ABB0BZ
Perianal skin *use* Skin, Perineum
Pericardiectomy
  see Excision, Pericardium 02BN
  see Resection, Pericardium 02TN
Pericardiocentesis
  see Drainage, Pericardial Cavity
    0W9D
Pericardiolysis
  see Release, Pericardium 02NN
Pericardiophrenic artery
  use Artery, Internal Mammary, Left
  use Artery, Internal Mammary, Right
Pericardioplasty
  see Repair, Pericardium 02QN
  see Replacement, Pericardium
    02RN
  see Supplement, Pericardium 02UN
Pericardiorrhaphy
  see Repair, Pericardium 02QN
Pericardiostomy
  see Drainage, Pericardial Cavity
    0W9D
Pericardiotomy
  see Drainage, Pericardial Cavity
    0W9D
Perimetrium
  use Uterus
Peripheral Intravascular Lithotripsy
  (Peripheral IVL)
  see Fragmentation
Peripheral parenteral nutrition
  see Introduction of Nutritional
    Substance

Peripherally inserted central
  catheter (PICC)
  use Infusion Device
Peritoneal dialysis 3E1M39Z
Peritoneocentesis
  see Drainage, Peritoneal Cavity
    0W9G
  see Drainage, Peritoneum
    0D9W
Peritoneoplasty
  see Repair, Peritoneum 0DQW
  see Replacement, Peritoneum
    0DRW
  see Supplement, Peritoneum
    0DUW
Peritoneoscopy 0DJW4ZZ
Peritoneotomy
  see Drainage, Peritoneum 0D9W
Peritoneumectomy
  see Excision, Peritoneum 0DBW
Peroneus brevis muscle
  use Muscle, Lower Leg, Left
  use Muscle, Lower Leg, Right
Peroneus longus muscle
  use Muscle, Lower Leg, Left
  use Muscle, Lower Leg, Right
Pessary ring
  use Intraluminal Device, Pessary in
    Female Reproductive System
PET scan
  see Positron Emission Tomographic
    (PET) Imaging
Petrous part of temporal bone
  use Bone, Temporal, Left
  use Bone, Temporal, Right
Phacoemulsification, lens
  With IOL implant
    see Replacement, Eye 08R
  Without IOL implant
    see Extraction, Eye 08D
Phagenyx® System XWHD7Q7
Phalangectomy
  see Excision, Lower Bones 0QB
  see Excision, Upper Bones 0PB
  see Resection, Lower Bones 0QT
  see Resection, Upper Bones 0PT
Phallectomy
  see Excision, Penis 0VBS
  see Resection, Penis 0VTS
Phalloplasty
  see Repair, Penis 0VQS
  see Supplement, Penis 0VUS
Phallotomy
  see Drainage, Penis 0V9S
Pharmacotherapy, for substance
  abuse
  Antabuse HZ93ZZZ
  Bupropion HZ97ZZZ
  Clonidine HZ96ZZZ
  Levo-alpha-acetyl-methadol
    (LAAM) HZ92ZZZ
  Methadone Maintenance
    HZ91ZZZ
  Naloxone HZ95ZZZ
  Naltrexone HZ94ZZZ
  Nicotine Replacement HZ90ZZZ
  Psychiatric Medication HZ98ZZZ
  Replacement Medication, Other
    HZ99ZZZ
Pharyngeal constrictor muscle
  use Muscle, Tongue, Palate,
    Pharynx
Pharyngeal plexus
  use Nerve, Vagus
Pharyngeal recess
  use Nasopharynx
Pharyngeal tonsil
  use Adenoids
Pharyngogram
  see Fluoroscopy, Pharynix
    B91G

Pharyngoplasty
  see Repair, Mouth and Throat 0CQ
  see Replacement, Mouth and Throat
    0CR
  see Supplement, Mouth and Throat
    0CU
Pharyngorrhaphy
  see Repair, Mouth and Throat 0CQ
Pharyngotomy
  see Drainage, Mouth and Throat 0C9
Pharyngotympanic tube
  use Eustachian Tube, Left
  use Eustachian Tube, Right
Pheresis
  Erythrocytes 6A55
  Leukocytes 6A55
  Plasma 6A55
  Platelets 6A55
  Stem Cells
    Cord Blood 6A55
    Hematopoietic 6A55
Phlebectomy
  see Excision, Lower Veins 06B
  see Excision, Upper Veins 05B
  see Extraction, Lower Veins 06D
  see Extraction, Upper Veins 05D
Phlebography
  see Plain Radiography, Veins B50
  Impedance 4A04X51
Phleborrhaphy
  see Repair, Lower Veins 06Q
  see Repair, Upper Veins 05Q
Phlebotomy
  see Drainage, Lower Veins 069
  see Drainage, Upper Veins 059
Photocoagulation
  For Destruction
    see Destruction
  For Repair
    see Repair
Photopheresis, therapeutic
  see Phototherapy, Circulatory
    6A65
Phototherapy
  Circulatory 6A65
  Skin 6A60
  Ultraviolet light
    see Ultraviolet Light Therapy,
      Physiological Systems 6A8
Phrenectomy, phrenoneurectomy
  see Excision, Nerve, Phrenic 01B2
Phrenemphraxis
  see Destruction, Nerve, Phrenic
    0152
Phrenic nerve stimulator generator
  use Stimulator Generator in
    Subcutaneous Tissue and Fascia
Phrenic nerve stimulator lead
  use Diaphragmatic Pacemaker Lead
    in Respiratory System
Phreniclasis
  see Destruction, Nerve, Phrenic
    0152
Phrenicoexeresis
  see Extraction, Nerve, Phrenic
    01D2
Phrenicotomy
  see Division, Nerve, Phrenic 0182
Phrenicotripsy
  see Destruction, Nerve, Phrenic 0152
Phrenoplasty
  see Repair, Respiratory System
    0BQ
  see Supplement, Respiratory System
    0BU
Phrenotomy
  see Drainage, Respiratory System
    0B9
Physiatry
  see Motor Treatment, Rehabilitation
    F07

Physical medicine
  see Motor Treatment, Rehabilitation
    F07
Physical therapy
  see Motor Treatment, Rehabilitation
    F07
PHYSIOMESH™ Flexible
  Composite Mesh
  use Synthetic Substitute
Pia mater, intracranial
  use Cerebral Meninges
Pia mater, spinal
  use Spinal Meninges
PiCSO® Impulse System X2A7358
Pinealectomy
  see Excision, Pineal Body 0GB1
  see Resection, Pineal Body 0GT1
Pinealoscopy 0GJ14ZZ
Pinealotomy
  see Drainage, Pineal Body 0G91
Pinna
  use Ear, External, Bilateral
  use Ear, External, Left
  use Ear, External, Right
Pipeline™ (Flex) embolization
  device
  use Intraluminal Device, Flow
    Diverter in 03V
Piriform recess (sinus)
  use Pharynx
Piriformis muscle
  use Muscle, Hip, Right
  use Muscle, Hip, Left
PIRRT (Prolonged intermittent
  renal replacement therapy)
  5A1D80Z
Pisiform bone
  use Carpal, Left
  use Carpal, Right
Pisohamate ligament
  use Bursa and Ligament, Hand,
    Left
  use Bursa and Ligament, Hand,
    Right
Pisometacarpal ligament
  use Bursa and Ligament, Hand, Left
  use Bursa and Ligament, Hand,
    Right
Pituitectomy
  see Excision, Gland, Pituitary 0GB0
  see Resection, Gland, Pituitary
    0GT0
Plain film radiology
  see Plain Radiography
Plain Radiography
  Abdomen BW00ZZZ
  Abdomen and Pelvis BW01ZZZ
  Abdominal Lymphatic
    Bilateral B701
    Unilateral B700
  Airway, Upper BB0DZZZ
  Ankle
    Left BQ0H
    Right BQ0G
  Aorta
    Abdominal B400
    Thoracic B300
    Thoraco-Abdominal B30P
  Aorta and Bilateral Lower
    Extremity Arteries B40D
  Arch
    Bilateral BN0DZZZ
    Left BN0CZZZ
    Right BN0BZZZ
  Arm
    Left BP0FZZZ
    Right BP0EZZZ
  Artery
    Brachiocephalic-Subclavian,
      Right B301
    Bronchial B30L

Plain Radiography *(continued)*

Artery *(continued)*
Bypass Graft, Other B20F
Cervico-Cerebral Arch B30Q
Common Carotid
Bilateral B305
Left B304
Right B303
Coronary
Bypass Graft
Multiple B203
Single B202
Multiple B201
Single B200
External Carotid
Bilateral B30C
Left B30B
Right B309
Hepatic B402
Inferior Mesenteric B405
Intercostal B30L
Internal Carotid
Bilateral B308
Left B307
Right B306
Internal Mammary Bypass Graft
Left B208
Right B207
Intra-Abdominal, Other B40B
Intracranial B30R
Lower, Other B40J
Lower Extremity
Bilateral and Aorta
B40D
Left B40G
Right B40F
Lumbar B409
Pelvic B40C
Pulmonary
Left B30T
Right B30S
Renal
Bilateral B408
Left B407
Right B406
Transplant B40M
Spinal B30M
Splenic B403
Subclavian, Left B302
Superior Mesenteric B404
Upper, Other B30N
Upper Extremity
Bilateral B30K
Left B30J
Right B30H
Vertebral
Bilateral B30G
Left B30F
Right B30D
Bile Duct BF00
Bile Duct and Gallbladder BF03
Bladder BT00
Kidney and Ureter BT04
Bladder and Urethra BT0B
Bone
Facial BN05ZZZ
Nasal BN04ZZZ
Bones, Long, All BW0BZZZ
Breast
Bilateral BH02ZZZ
Left BH01ZZZ
Right BH00ZZZ
Calcaneus
Left BQ0KZZZ
Right BQ0JZZZ
Chest BW03ZZZ
Clavicle
Left BP05ZZZ
Right BP04ZZZ
Coccyx BR0FZZZ
Corpora Cavernosa BV00

Plain Radiography *(continued)*

Dialysis Fistula B50W
Dialysis Shunt B50W
Disc
Cervical BR01
Lumbar BR03
Thoracic BR02
Duct
Lacrimal
Bilateral B802
Left B801
Right B800
Mammary
Multiple
Left BH06
Right BH05
Single
Left BH04
Right BH03
Elbow
Left BP0H
Right BP0G
Epididymis
Left BV02
Right BV01
Extremity
Lower BW0CZZZ
Upper BW0JZZZ
Eye
Bilateral B807ZZZ
Left B806ZZZ
Right B805ZZZ
Facet Joint
Cervical BR04
Lumbar BR06
Thoracic BR05
Fallopian Tube
Bilateral BU02
Left BU01
Right BU00
Fallopian Tube and Uterus BU08
Femur
Left, Densitometry BQ04ZZ1
Right, Densitometry BQ03ZZ1
Finger
Left BP0SZZZ
Right BP0RZZZ
Foot
Left BQ0MZZZ
Right BQ0LZZZ
Forearm
Left BP0KZZZ
Right BP0JZZZ
Gallbladder and Bile Duct BF03
Gland
Parotid
Bilateral B906
Left B905
Right B904
Salivary
Bilateral B90D
Left B90C
Right B90B
Submandibular
Bilateral B909
Left B908
Right B907
Hand
Left BP0PZZZ
Right BP0NZZZ
Heart
Left B205
Right B204
Right and Left B206
Hepatobiliary System, All
BF0C
Hip
Left BQ01
Densitometry BQ01ZZ1
Right BQ00
Densitometry BQ00ZZ1

Plain Radiography *(continued)*

Humerus
Left BP0BZZZ
Right BP0AZZZ
Ileal Diversion Loop BT0C
Intracranial Sinus B502
Joint
Acromioclavicular, Bilateral
BP03ZZZ
Finger
Left BP0D
Right BP0C
Foot
Left BQ0Y
Right BQ0X
Hand
Left BP0D
Right BP0C
Lumbosacral BR0BZZZ
Sacroiliac BR0D
Sternoclavicular
Bilateral BP02ZZZ
Left BP01ZZZ
Right BP00ZZZ
Temporomandibular
Bilateral BN09
Left BN08
Right BN07
Thoracolumbar BR08ZZZ
Toe
Left BQ0Y
Right BQ0X
Kidney
Bilateral BT03
Left BT02
Right BT01
Ureter and Bladder BT04
Knee
Left BQ08
Right BQ07
Leg
Left BQ0FZZZ
Right BQ0DZZZ
Lymphatic
Head B704
Lower Extremity
Bilateral B70B
Left B709
Right B708
Neck B704
Pelvic B70C
Upper Extremity
Bilateral B707
Left B706
Right B705
Mandible BN06ZZZ
Mastoid B90HZZZ
Nasopharynx B90FZZZ
Optic Foramina
Left B804ZZZ
Right B803ZZZ
Orbit
Bilateral BN03ZZZ
Left BN02ZZZ
Right BN01ZZZ
Oropharynx B90FZZZ
Patella
Left BQ0WZZZ
Right BQ0VZZZ
Pelvis BR0CZZZ
Pelvis and Abdomen BW01ZZZ
Prostate BV03
Retroperitoneal Lymphatic
Bilateral B701
Unilateral B700
Ribs
Left BP0YZZZ
Right BP0XZZZ
Sacrum BR0FZZZ
Scapula
Left BP07ZZZ
Right BP06ZZZ

Plain Radiography *(continued)*

Shoulder
Left BP09
Right BP08
Sinus
Intracranial B502
Paranasal B902ZZZ
Skull BN00ZZZ
Spinal Cord B00B
Spine
Cervical, Densitometry BR00ZZ1
Lumbar, Densitometry BR09ZZ1
Thoracic, Densitometry
BR07ZZ1
Whole, Densitometry BR0GZZ1
Sternum BR0HZZZ
Teeth
All BN0JZZZ
Multiple BN0HZZZ
Testicle
Left BV06
Right BV05
Toe
Left BQ0QZZZ
Right BQ0PZZZ
Tooth, Single BN0GZZZ
Tracheobronchial Tree
Bilateral BB09YZZ
Left BB08Y
Right BB07Y
Ureter
Bilateral BT08
Kidney and Bladder BT04
Left BT07
Right BT06
Urethra BT05
Urethra and Bladder BT0B
Uterus BU06
Uterus and Fallopian Tube BU08
Vagina BU09
Vasa Vasorum BV08
Vein
Cerebellar B501
Cerebral B501
Epidural B500
Jugular
Bilateral B505
Left B504
Right B503
Lower Extremity
Bilateral B50D
Left B50C
Right B50B
Other B50V
Pelvic (Iliac)
Left B50G
Right B50F
Pelvic (Iliac) Bilateral B50H
Portal B50T
Pulmonary
Bilateral B50S
Left B50R
Right B50Q
Renal
Bilateral B50L
Left B50K
Right B50J
Spanchnic B50T
Subclavian
Left B507
Right B506
Upper Extremity
Bilateral B50P
Left B50N
Right B50M
Vena Cava
Inferior B509
Superior B508
Whole Body BW0KZZZ
Infant BW0MZZZ
Whole Skeleton BW0LZZZ

Plain Radiography *(continued)*
 Wrist
  Left BP0M
  Right BP0L
Planar Nuclear Medicine Imaging
 Abdomen CW10
 Abdomen and Chest CW14
 Abdomen and Pelvis CW11
 Anatomical Regions, Multiple
  CW1YYZZ
 Anatomical Region, Other
  CW1ZZZZ
 Bladder, Kidneys and Ureters CT13
 Bladder and Ureters CT1H
 Blood C713
 Bone Marrow C710
 Brain C010
 Breast CH1YYZZ
  Bilateral CH12
  Left CH11
  Right CH10
 Bronchi and Lungs CB12
 Central Nervous System C01YYZZ
 Cerebrospinal Fluid C015
 Chest CW13
 Chest and Abdomen CW14
 Chest and Neck CW16
 Digestive System CD1YYZZ
 Ducts, Lacrimal, Bilateral C819
 Ear, Nose, Mouth and Throat
  C91YYZZ
 Endocrine System CG1YYZZ
 Extremity
  Lower CW1D
   Bilateral CP1F
   Left CP1D
   Right CP1C
  Upper CW1M
   Bilateral CP1B
   Left CP19
   Right CP18
 Eye C81YYZZ
 Gallbladder CF14
 Gastrointestinal Tract CD17
  Upper CD15
 Gland
  Adrenal, Bilateral CG14
  Parathyroid CG11
  Thyroid CG12
 Glands, Salivary, Bilateral C91B
 Head and Neck CW1B
 Heart C21YYZZ
  Right and Left C216
 Hepatobiliary System, All
  CF1C
 Hepatobiliary System and Pancreas
  CF1YYZZ
 Kidneys, Ureters and Bladder
  CT13
 Liver CF15
 Liver and Spleen CF16
 Lungs and Bronchi CB12
 Lymphatics
  Head C71J
  Head and Neck C715
  Lower Extremity C71P
  Neck C71K
  Pelvic C71D
  Trunk C71M
  Upper Chest C71L
  Upper Extremity C71N
 Lymphatics and Hematologic
  System C71YYZZ
 Musculoskeletal System
  All CP1Z
  Other CP1YYZZ
 Myocardium C21G
 Neck and Chest CW16
 Neck and Head CW1B
 Pancreas and Hepatobiliary System
  CF1YYZZ

Planar Nuclear Medicine Imaging *(continued)*
 Pelvic Region CW1J
 Pelvis CP16
 Pelvis and Abdomen CW11
 Pelvis and Spine CP17
 Reproductive System, Male
  CV1YYZZ
 Respiratory System CB1YYZZ
 Skin CH1YYZZ
 Skull CP11
 Spine CP15
 Spine and Pelvis CP17
 Spleen C712
 Spleen and Liver CF16
 Subcutaneous Tissue CH1YYZZ
 Testicles, Bilateral CV19
 Thorax CP14
 Ureters, Kidneys and Bladder CT13
 Ureters and Bladder CT1H
 Urinary System CT1YYZZ
 Veins C51YYZZ
  Central C51R
  Lower Extremity
   Bilateral C51D
   Left C51C
   Right C51B
  Upper Extremity
   Bilateral C51Q
   Left C51P
   Right C51N
 Whole Body CW1N
Plantar digital vein
 use Vein, Foot, Left
 use Vein, Foot, Right
Plantar fascia (aponeurosis)
 use Subcutaneous Tissue and Fascia,
  Foot, Left
 use Subcutaneous Tissue and Fascia,
  Foot, Right
Plantar metatarsal vein
 use Vein, Foot, Left
 use Vein, Foot, Right
Plantar venous arch
 use Vein, Foot, Left
 use Vein, Foot, Right
Plaque Radiation
 Abdomen DWY3FZZ
 Adrenal Gland DGY2FZZ
 Anus DDY8FZZ
 Bile Ducts DFY2FZZ
 Bladder DTY2FZZ
 Bone, Other DPYCFZZ
 Bone Marrow D7Y0FZZ
 Brain D0Y0FZZ
 Brain Stem D0Y1FZZ
 Breast
  Left DMY0FZZ
  Right DMY1FZZ
 Bronchus DBY1FZZ
 Cervix DUY1FZZ
 Chest DWY2FZZ
 Chest Wall DBY7FZZ
 Colon DDY5FZZ
 Diaphragm DBY8FZZ
 Duodenum DDY2FZZ
 Ear D9Y0FZZ
 Esophagus DDY0FZZ
 Eye D8Y0FZZ
 Femur DPY9FZZ
 Fibula DPYBFZZ
 Gallbladder DFY1FZZ
 Gland
  Adrenal DGY2FZZ
  Parathyroid DGY4FZZ
  Pituitary DGY0FZZ
  Thyroid DGY5FZZ
 Glands, Salivary D9Y6FZZ
 Head and Neck DWY1FZZ
 Hemibody DWY4FZZ
 Humerus DPY6FZZ

Plaque Radiation *(continued)*
 Ileum DDY4FZZ
 Jejunum DDY3FZZ
 Kidney DTY0FZZ
 Larynx D9YBFZZ
 Liver DFY0FZZ
 Lung DBY2FZZ
 Lymphatics
  Abdomen D7Y6FZZ
  Axillary D7Y4FZZ
  Inguinal D7Y8FZZ
  Neck D7Y3FZZ
  Pelvis D7Y7FZZ
  Thorax D7Y5FZZ
 Mandible DPY3FZZ
 Maxilla DPY2FZZ
 Mediastinum DBY6FZZ
 Mouth D9Y4FZZ
 Nasopharynx D9YDFZZ
 Neck and Head DWY1FZZ
 Nerve, Peripheral D0Y7FZZ
 Nose D9Y1FZZ
 Ovary DUY0FZZ
 Palate
  Hard D9Y8FZZ
  Soft D9Y9FZZ
 Pancreas DFY3FZZ
 Parathyroid Gland DGY4FZZ
 Pelvic Bones DPY8FZZ
 Pelvic Region DWY6FZZ
 Pharynx D9YCFZZ
 Pineal Body DGY1FZZ
 Pituitary Gland DGY0FZZ
 Pleura DBY5FZZ
 Prostate DVY0FZZ
 Radius DPY7FZZ
 Rectum DDY7FZZ
 Rib DPY5FZZ
 Sinuses D9Y7FZZ
 Skin
  Abdomen DHY8FZZ
  Arm DHY4FZZ
  Back DHY7FZZ
  Buttock DHY9FZZ
  Chest DHY6FZZ
  Face DHY2FZZ
  Foot DHYCFZZ
  Hand DHY5FZZ
  Leg DHYBFZZ
  Neck DHY3FZZ
 Skull DPY0FZZ
 Spinal Cord D0Y6FZZ
 Spleen D7Y2FZZ
 Sternum DPY4FZZ
 Stomach DDY1FZZ
 Testis DVY1FZZ
 Thymus D7Y1FZZ
 Thyroid Gland DGY5FZZ
 Tibia DPY5FZZ
 Tongue D9Y5FZZ
 Trachea DBY0FZZ
 Ulna DPY7FZZ
 Ureter DTY1FZZ
 Urethra DTY3FZZ
 Uterus DUY2FZZ
 Whole Body DWY5FZZ
**Plasma, Convalescent
 (Nonautologous)** XW1
Plasmapheresis, therapeutic
 see Pheresis, Physiological Systems
  6A5
Plateletpheresis, therapeutic
 see Pheresis, Physiological Systems
  6A5
Platysma muscle
 use Muscle, Neck, Left
 use Muscle, Neck, Right
Plazomicin *use* Other anti-infective
Pleurectomy
 see Excision, Respiratory System
  0BB

Pleurectomy *(continued)*
 see Resection, Respiratory System
  0BT
Pleurocentesis
 see Drainage, Anatomical Regions,
  General 0W9
Pleurodesis, pleurosclerosis
 Chemical injection
  see Introduction of substance in
   or on, Pleural Cavity 3E0L
 Surgical
  see Destruction, Respiratory
   System 0B5
Pleurolysis
 see Release, Respiratory System
  0BN
Pleuroscopy 0BJQ4ZZ
Pleurotomy
 see Drainage, Respiratory System
  0B9
Plica semilunaris
 use Conjunctiva, Left
 use Conjunctiva, Right
Plication
 see Restriction
Pneumectomy
 see Excision, Respiratory System
  0BB
 see Resection, Respiratory System
  0BT
Pneumocentesis
 see Drainage, Respiratory System
  0B9
Pneumogastric nerve
 use Nerve, Vagus
Pneumolysis
 see Release, Respiratory System 0BN
Pneumonectomy
 see Resection, Respiratory System
  0BT
Pneumonolysis
 see Release, Respiratory System
  0BN
Pneumonopexy
 see Repair, Respiratory System 0BQ
 see Reposition, Respiratory System
  0BS
Pneumonorrhaphy
 see Repair, Respiratory System
  0BQ
Pneumonotomy
 see Drainage, Respiratory System
  0B9
Pneumotaxic center
 use Pons
Pneumotomy
 see Drainage, Respiratory System
  0B9
Pollicization
 see Transfer, Anatomical Regions,
  Upper Extremities 0XX
Polyclonal hyperimmune globulin
 use Globulin
Polyethylene socket
 use Synthetic Substitute,
  Polyethylene in 0SR
**Polymethylmethacrylate
 (PMMA)**
 use Synthetic Substitute
Polypectomy, gastrointestinal
 see Excision, Gastrointestinal
  System 0DB
Polypropylene mesh
 use Synthetic Substitute
Polysomnogram 4A1ZXQZ
Pontine tegmentum
 use Pons
Popliteal ligament
 use Bursa and Ligament, Knee, Left
 use Bursa and Ligament, Knee,
  Right

Popliteal lymph node
  use Lymphatic, Lower Extremity, Left
  use Lymphatic, Lower Extremity, Right
Popliteal vein
  use Vein, Femoral, Left
  use Vein, Femoral, Right
Popliteus muscle
  use Muscle, Lower Leg, Left
  use Muscle, Lower Leg, Right
Porcine (bioprosthetic) valve
  use Zooplastic Tissue in Heart and Great Vessels
Positive Blood Culture Fluorescence Hybridization for Organism Identification, Concentration and Susceptibility XXE5XN6
Positive end expiratory pressure
  see Performance, Respiratory 5A19
Positron Emission Tomographic (PET) Imaging
  Brain C030
  Bronchi and Lungs CB32
  Central Nervous System C03YYZZ
  Heart C23YYZZ
  Lungs and Bronchi CB32
  Myocardium C23G
  Respiratory System CB3YYZZ
  Whole Body CW3NYZZ
Positron emission tomography
  see Positron Emission Tomographic (PET) Imaging
Posoleucel XW0
Postauricular (mastoid) lymph node
  use Lymphatic, Neck, Left
  use Lymphatic, Neck, Right
Postcava
  use Vena Cava, Inferior
Posterior (subscapular) lymph node
  use Lymphatic, Axillary, Left
  use Lymphatic, Axillary, Right
Posterior auricular artery
  use Artery, External Carotid, Left
  use Artery, External Carotid, Right
Posterior auricular nerve
  use Nerve, Facial
Posterior auricular vein
  use Vein, External Jugular, Left
  use Vein, External Jugular, Right
Posterior cerebral artery
  use Artery, Intracranial
Posterior chamber
  use Eye, Left
  use Eye, Right
Posterior circumflex humeral artery
  use Artery, Axillary, Left
  use Artery, Axillary, Right
Posterior communicating artery
  use Artery, Intracranial
Posterior cruciate ligament (PCL)
  use Bursa and Ligament, Knee, Left
  use Bursa and Ligament, Knee, Right
Posterior (Dynamic) Distraction Device
  Lumbar XNS0
  Thoracic XNS4
Posterior facial (retromandibular) vein
  use Vein, Face, Left
  use Vein, Face, Right
Posterior femoral cutaneous nerve
  use Nerve, Sacral Plexus
Posterior inferior cerebellar artery (PICA)
  use Artery, Intracranial
Posterior interosseous nerve
  use Nerve, Radial
Posterior labial nerve
  use Nerve, Pudendal

Posterior scrotal nerve
  use Nerve, Pudendal
Posterior spinal artery
  use Artery, Vertebral, Left
  use Artery, Vertebral, Right
Posterior tibial recurrent artery
  use Artery, Anterior Tibial, Left
  use Artery, Anterior Tibial, Right
Posterior ulnar recurrent artery
  use Artery, Ulnar, Left
  use Artery, Ulnar, Right
Posterior vagal trunk
  use Nerve, Vagus
PPN (peripheral parenteral nutrition)
  see Introduction of Nutritional Substance
Praxbind® (idarucizumab), Pradaxa® (dabigatran) reversal agent
  use Other Therapeutic Substance
Preauricular lymph node
  use Lymphatic, Head
Precava
  use Vena Cava, Superior
PRECICE intramedullary limb lengthening system
  use Internal Fixation Device, Intramedullary Limb Lengthening in 0PH
  use Internal Fixation Device, Intramedullary Limb Lengthening in 0QH
Precision TAVI™ Coronary Obstruction Module XXE3X68
Prepatellar bursa
  use Bursa and Ligament, Knee, Left
  use Bursa and Ligament, Knee, Right
Preputiotomy
  see Drainage, Male Reproductive System 0V9
Pressure support ventilation
  see Performance, Respiratory 5A19
PRESTIGE® Cervical Disc
  use Synthetic Substitute
Pretracheal fascia
  use Subcutaneous Tissue and Fascia, Neck, Left
  use Subcutaneous Tissue and Fascia, Neck, Right
Prevertebral fascia
  use Subcutaneous Tissue and Fascia, Neck, Left
  use Subcutaneous Tissue and Fascia, Neck, Right
PrimeAdvanced neurostimulator (SureScan)(MRI Safe)
  use Stimulator Generator, Multiple Array in 0JH
Princeps pollicis artery
  use Artery, Hand, Left
  use Artery, Hand, Right
Probing, duct
  Diagnostic
    see Inspection
  Dilation
    see Dilation
PROCEED™ Ventral Patch
  use Synthetic Substitute
Procerus muscle
  use Muscle, Facial
Proctectomy
  see Excision, Rectum 0DBP
  see Resection, Rectum 0DTP
Proctoclysis
  see Introduction of substance in or on, Gastrointestinal Tract, Lower 3E0H
Proctocolectomy
  see Excision, Gastrointestinal System 0DB
  see Resection, Gastrointestinal System 0DT

Proctocolpoplasty
  see Repair, Gastrointestinal System 0DQ
  see Supplement, Gastrointestinal System 0DU
Proctoperineoplasty
  see Repair, Gastrointestinal System 0DQ
  see Supplement, Gastrointestinal System 0DU
Proctoperineorrhaphy
  see Repair, Gastrointestinal System 0DQ
Proctopexy
  see Repair, Rectum 0DQP
  see Reposition, Rectum 0DSP
Proctoplasty
  see Repair, Rectum 0DQP
  see Supplement, Rectum 0DUP
Proctorrhaphy
  see Repair, Rectum 0DQP
Proctoscopy 0DJD8ZZ
Proctosigmoidectomy
  see Excision, Gastrointestinal System 0DB
  see Resection, Gastrointestinal System 0DT
Proctosigmoidoscopy 0DJD8ZZ
Proctostomy
  see Drainage, Rectum 0D9P
Proctotomy
  see Drainage, Rectum 0D9P
Prodisc-C
  use Synthetic Substitute
Prodisc-L
  use Synthetic Substitute
Production, atrial septal defect
  see Excision, Septum, Atrial 02B5
Profunda brachii
  use Artery, Brachial, Left
  use Artery, Brachial, Right
Profunda femoris (deep femoral) vein
  use Vein, Femoral, Left
  use Vein, Femoral, Right
PROLENE Polypropylene Hernia System (PHS)
  use Synthetic Substitute
Prolonged intermittent renal replacement therapy (PIRRT) 5A1D80Z
Pronator quadratus muscle
  use Muscle, Lower Arm and Wrist, Left
  use Muscle, Lower Arm and Wrist, Right
Pronator teres muscle
  use Muscle, Lower Arm and Wrist, Left
  use Muscle, Lower Arm and Wrist, Right
Prone positioning, intubated *see* Assistance, Respiratory 5A09
Prostatectomy
  see Excision, Prostate 0VB0
  see Resection, Prostate 0VT0
Prostatic artery
  use Internal Iliac Artery, Left
  use Internal Iliac Artery, Right
Prostatic urethra
  use Urethra
Prostatomy, prostatotomy
  see Drainage, Prostate 0V90
Protecta XT CRT-D
  use Cardiac Resynchronization Defibrillator Pulse Generator in 0JH
Protecta XT DR (XT VR)
  use Defibrillator Generator in 0JH

Protégé® RX Carotid Stent System
  use Intraluminal Device
Proximal radioulnar joint
  use Joint, Elbow, Left
  use Joint, Elbow, Right
Psoas muscle
  use Muscle, Hip, Left
  use Muscle, Hip, Right
PSV (pressure support ventilation)
  see Performance, Respiratory 5A19
Psychoanalysis GZ54ZZZ
Psychological Tests
  Cognitive Status GZ14ZZZ
  Developmental GZ10ZZZ
  Intellectual and Psychoeducational GZ12ZZZ
  Neurobehavioral Status GZ14ZZZ
  Neuropsychological GZ13ZZZ
  Personality and Behavioral GZ11ZZZ
Psychotherapy
  Family, Mental Health Services GZ72ZZZ
  Group
    GZHZZZZ
    Mental Health Services GZHZZZZ
  Individual
    see Psychotherapy, Individual, Mental Health Services
    for substance abuse
    12-Step HZ53ZZZ
    Behavioral HZ51ZZZ
    Cognitive HZ50ZZZ
    Cognitive-Behavioral HZ52ZZZ
    Confrontational HZ58ZZZ
    Interactive HZ55ZZZ
    Interpersonal HZ54ZZZ
    Motivational Enhancement HZ57ZZZ
    Psychoanalysis HZ5BZZZ
    Psychodynamic HZ5CZZZ
    Psychoeducation HZ56ZZZ
    Psychophysiological HZ5DZZZ
    Supportive HZ59ZZZ
  Mental Health Services
    Behavioral GZ51ZZZ
    Cognitive GZ52ZZZ
    Cognitive-Behavioral GZ58ZZZ
    Interactive GZ50ZZZ
    Interpersonal GZ53ZZZ
    Psychoanalysis GZ54ZZZ
    Psychodynamic GZ55ZZZ
    Psychophysiological GZ59ZZZ
    Supportive GZ56ZZZ
PTCA (percutaneous transluminal coronary angioplasty)
  see Dilation, Heart and Great Vessels 027
Pterygoid muscle
  use Muscle, Head
Pterygoid process
  use Bone, Sphenoid
Pterygopalatine (sphenopalatine) ganglion
  use Nerve, Head and Neck Sympathetic
Pubis
  use Bone, Pelvic, Left
  use Bone, Pelvic, Right
Pubofemoral ligament
  use Bursa and Ligament, Hip, Left
  use Bursa and Ligament, Hip, Right
Pudendal nerve
  use Nerve, Sacral Plexus

Pull-through, laparoscopic-assisted transanal
  see Excision, Gastrointestinal System 0DB
  see Resection, Gastrointestinal System 0DT

Pull-through, rectal
  see Resection, Rectum 0DTP

Pulmoaortic canal
  use Artery, Pulmonary, Left

Pulmonary annulus
  use Valve, Pulmonary

Pulmonary artery wedge monitoring
  see Monitoring, Arterial 4A13

Pulmonary plexus
  use Nerve, Thoracic Sympathetic
  use Nerve, Vagus

Pulmonic valve
  use Valve, Pulmonary

Pulpectomy
  see Excision, Mouth and Throat 0CB

Pulverization
  see Fragmentation

Pulvinar
  use Thalamus

Pump reservoir
  use Infusion Device, Pump in Subcutaneous Tissue and Fascia

Punch biopsy
  see Excision with qualifier Diagnostic

Puncture
  see Drainage

Puncture, lumbar
  see Drainage, Spinal Canal 009U

Pure-Vu® System XDPH8K7

Pyelography
  see Fluoroscopy, Urinary System BT1
  see Plain Radiography, Urinary System BT0

Pyeloileostomy, urinary diversion
  see Bypass, Urinary System 0T1

Pyeloplasty
  see Repair, Urinary System 0TQ
  see Replacement, Urinary System 0TR
  see Supplement, Urinary System 0TU

Pyeloplasty, dismembered
  see Repair, Kidney Pelvis

Pyelorrhaphy
  see Repair, Urinary System 0TQ

Pyeloscopy 0TJ58ZZ

Pyelostomy
  see Drainage, Urinary System 0T9
  see Bypass, Urinary System 0T1

Pyelotomy
  see Drainage, Urinary System 0T9

Pylorectomy
  see Excision, Stomach, Pylorus 0DB7
  see Resection, Stomach, Pylorus 0DT7

Pyloric antrum
  use Stomach, Pylorus

Pyloric canal
  use Stomach, Pylorus

Pyloric sphincter
  use Stomach, Pylorus

Pylorodiosis
  see Dilation, Stomach, Pylorus 0D77

Pylorogastrectomy
  see Excision, Gastrointestinal System 0DB
  see Resection, Gastrointestinal System 0DT

Pyloroplasty
  see Repair, Stomach, Pylorus 0DQ7
  see Supplement, Stomach, Pylorus 0DU7

Pyloroscopy 0DJ68ZZ

Pylorotomy
  see Drainage, Stomach, Pylorus 0D97

Pyramidalis muscle
  use Muscle, Abdomen, Left
  use Muscle, Abdomen, Right

Q

QAngio XA® 3D XXE3X58

QFR® (Quantitative Flow Ratio)
  analysis of coronary angiography XXE3X58

Quadrangular cartilage
  use Septum, Nasal

Quadrant resection of breast
  see Excision, Skin and Breast 0HB

Quadrate lobe
  use Liver

Quadratus femoris muscle
  use Muscle, Hip, Left
  use Muscle, Hip, Right

Quadratus lumborum muscle
  use Muscle, Trunk, Left
  use Muscle, Trunk, Right

Quadratus plantae muscle
  use Muscle, Foot, Left
  use Muscle, Foot, Right

Quadriceps (femoris)
  use Muscle, Upper Leg, Left
  use Muscle, Upper Leg, Right

Quantitative Flow Ratio Analysis, Coronary Artery Flow XXE3X58

Quarantine 8E0ZXY6

Quizartinib Antineoplastic XW0DXJ9

R

Radial artery arteriovenous fistula, using Thermal Resistance Energy X2K

Radial collateral carpal ligament
  use Bursa and Ligament, Wrist, Left
  use Bursa and Ligament, Wrist, Right

Radial collateral ligament
  use Bursa and Ligament, Elbow, Left
  use Bursa and Ligament, Elbow, Right

Radial notch
  use Ulna, Left
  use Ulna, Right

Radial recurrent artery
  use Artery, Radial, Left
  use Artery, Radial, Right

Radial vein
  use Vein, Brachial, Left
  use Vein, Brachial, Right

Radialis indicis
  use Artery, Hand, Left
  use Artery, Hand, Right

Radiation Therapy
  see Beam Radiation
  see Brachytherapy
  see Other Radiation
  see Stereotactic Radiosurgery

Radiation treatment
  see Radiation Therapy

Radiocarpal joint
  use Joint, Wrist, Left
  use Joint, Wrist, Right

Radiocarpal ligament
  use Bursa and Ligament, Wrist, Left
  use Bursa and Ligament, Wrist, Right

Radiography
  see Plain Radiography

Radiology, analog
  see Plain Radiography

Radiology, diagnostic
  see Imaging, Diagnostic

Radioulnar ligament
  use Bursa and Ligament, Wrist, Left
  use Bursa and Ligament, Wrist, Right

Range of motion testing
  see Motor Function Assessment, Rehabilitation F01

Rapid ASPECTS XXE0X07

REALIZE® Adjustable Gastric Band
  use Extraluminal Device

Reattachment
  Abdominal Wall 0WMF0ZZ
  Ampulla of Vater 0FMC
  Ankle Region
    Left 0YML0ZZ
    Right 0YMK0ZZ
  Arm
    Lower
      Left 0XMF0ZZ
      Right 0XMD0ZZ
    Upper
      Left 0XM90ZZ
      Right 0XM80ZZ
  Axilla
    Left 0XM50ZZ
    Right 0XM40ZZ
  Back
    Lower 0WML0ZZ
    Upper 0WMK0ZZ
  Bladder 0TMB
  Bladder Neck 0TMC
  Breast
    Bilateral 0HMVXZZ
    Left 0HMUXZZ
    Right 0HMTXZZ
  Bronchus
    Lingula 0BM90ZZ
    Lower Lobe
      Left 0BMB0ZZ
      Right 0BM60ZZ
    Main
      Left 0BM70ZZ
      Right 0BM30ZZ
    Middle Lobe, Right 0BM50ZZ
    Upper Lobe
      Left 0BM80ZZ
      Right 0BM40ZZ
  Bursa and Ligament
    Abdomen
      Left 0MMJ
      Right 0MMH
    Ankle
      Left 0MMR
      Right 0MMQ
    Elbow
      Left 0MM4
      Right 0MM3
    Foot
      Left 0MMT
      Right 0MMS
    Hand
      Left 0MM8
      Right 0MM7
    Head and Neck 0MM0
    Hip
      Left 0MMM
      Right 0MML
    Knee
      Left 0MMP
      Right 0MMN
    Lower Extremity
      Left 0MMW
      Right 0MMV
    Perineum 0MMK
    Rib(s) 0MMG
    Shoulder
      Left 0MM2
      Right 0MM1
    Spine
      Lower 0MMD
      Upper 0MMC
    Sternum 0MMF
    Upper Extremity
      Left 0MMB
      Right 0MM9

Reattachment *(continued)*
  Bursa and Ligament *(continued)*
    Wrist
      Left 0MM6
      Right 0MM5
  Buttock
    Left 0YM10ZZ
    Right 0YM00ZZ
  Carina 0BM20ZZ
  Cecum 0DMH
  Cervix 0UMC
  Chest Wall 0WM80ZZ
  Clitoris 0UMJXZZ
  Colon
    Ascending 0DMK
    Descending 0DMM
    Sigmoid 0DMN
    Transverse 0DML
  Cord
    Bilateral 0VMH
    Left 0VMG
    Right 0VMF
  Cul-de-sac 0UMF
  Diaphragm 0BMT0ZZ
  Duct
    Common Bile 0FM9
    Cystic 0FM8
    Hepatic
      Common 0FM7
      Left 0FM6
      Right 0FM5
    Pancreatic 0FMD
      Accessory 0FMF
  Duodenum 0DM9
  Ear
    Left 09M1XZZ
    Right 09M0XZZ
  Elbow Region
    Left 0XMC0ZZ
    Right 0XMB0ZZ
  Esophagus 0DM5
  Extremity
    Lower
      Left 0YMB0ZZ
      Right 0YM90ZZ
    Upper
      Left 0XM70ZZ
      Right 0XM60ZZ
  Eyelid
    Lower
      Left 08MRXZZ
      Right 08MQXZZ
    Upper
      Left 08MPXZZ
      Right 08MNXZZ
  Face 0WM20ZZ
  Fallopian Tube
    Left 0UM6
    Right 0UM5
  Fallopian Tubes, Bilateral 0UM7
  Femoral Region
    Left 0YM80ZZ
    Right 0YM70ZZ
  Finger
    Index
      Left 0XMP0ZZ
      Right 0XMN0ZZ
    Little
      Left 0XMW0ZZ
      Right 0XMV0ZZ
    Middle
      Left 0XMR0ZZ
      Right 0XMQ0ZZ
    Ring
      Left 0XMT0ZZ
      Right 0XMS0ZZ
  Foot
    Left 0YMN0ZZ
    Right 0YMM0ZZ
  Forequarter
    Left 0XM10ZZ
    Right 0XM00ZZ

Reattachment (continued)

Gallbladder 0FM4
Gland
  Left 0GM2
  Right 0GM3
Hand
  Left 0XMK0ZZ
  Right 0XMJ0ZZ
Hindquarter
  Bilateral 0YM40ZZ
  Left 0YM30ZZ
  Right 0YM20ZZ
Hymen 0UMK
Ileum 0DMB
Inguinal Region
  Left 0YM60ZZ
  Right 0YM50ZZ
Intestine
  Large 0DME
    Left 0DMG
    Right 0DMF
  Small 0DM8
Jaw
  Lower 0WM50ZZ
  Upper 0WM40ZZ
Jejunum 0DMA
Kidney
  Left 0TM1
  Right 0TM0
Kidney Pelvis
  Left 0TM4
  Right 0TM3
Kidneys, Bilateral 0TM2
Knee Region
  Left 0YMG0ZZ
  Right 0YMF0ZZ
Leg
  Lower
    Left 0YMJ0ZZ
    Right 0YMH0ZZ
  Upper
    Left 0YMD0ZZ
    Right 0YMC0ZZ
Lip
  Lower 0CM10ZZ
  Upper 0CM00ZZ
Liver 0FM0
  Left Lobe 0FM2
  Right Lobe 0FM1
Lung
  Left 0BML0ZZ
  Lower Lobe
    Left 0BMJ0ZZ
    Right 0BMF0ZZ
  Middle Lobe, Right 0BMD0ZZ
  Right 0BMK0ZZ
  Upper Lobe
    Left 0BMG0ZZ
    Right 0BMC0ZZ
Lung Lingula 0BMH0ZZ
Muscle
  Abdomen
    Left 0KML
    Right 0KMK
  Facial 0KM1
  Foot
    Left 0KMW
    Right 0KMV
  Hand
    Left 0KMD
    Right 0KMC
  Head 0KM0
  Hip
    Left 0KMP
    Right 0KMN
  Lower Arm and Wrist
    Left 0KMB
    Right 0KM9
  Lower Leg
    Left 0KMT
    Right 0KMS

Reattachment (continued)

Muscle (continued)
  Neck
    Left 0KM3
    Right 0KM2
  Perineum 0KMM
  Shoulder
    Left 0KM6
    Right 0KM5
  Thorax
    Left 0KMJ
    Right 0KMH
  Tongue, Palate, Pharynx
    0KM4
  Trunk
    Left 0KMG
    Right 0KMF
  Upper Arm
    Left 0KM8
    Right 0KM7
  Upper Leg
    Left 0KMR
    Right 0KMQ
Nasal Mucosa and Soft Tissue
  09MKXZZ
Neck 0WM60ZZ
Nipple
  Left 0HMXXZZ
  Right 0HMWXZZ
Ovary
  Bilateral 0UM2
  Left 0UM1
  Right 0UM0
Palate, Soft 0CM30ZZ
Pancreas 0FMG
Parathyroid Gland
  0GMR
  Inferior
    Left 0GMP
    Right 0GMN
  Multiple 0GMQ
  Superior
    Left 0GMM
    Right 0GML
Penis 0VMSXZZ
Perineum
  Female 0WMN0ZZ
  Male 0WMM0ZZ
Rectum 0DMP
Scrotum 0VM5XZZ
Shoulder Region
  Left 0XM30ZZ
  Right 0XM20ZZ
Skin
  Abdomen 0HM7XZZ
  Back 0HM6XZZ
  Buttock 0HM8XZZ
  Chest 0HM5XZZ
  Ear
    Left 0HM3XZZ
    Right 0HM2XZZ
  Face 0HM1XZZ
  Foot
    Left 0HMNXZZ
    Right 0HMMXZZ
  Hand
    Left 0HMGXZZ
    Right 0HMFXZZ
  Inguinal 0HMAXZZ
  Lower Arm
    Left 0HMEXZZ
    Right 0HMDXZZ
  Lower Leg
    Left 0HMLXZZ
    Right 0HMKXZZ
  Neck 0HM4XZZ
  Perineum 0HM9XZZ
  Scalp 0HM0XZZ
  Upper Arm
    Left 0HMCXZZ
    Right 0HMBXZZ

Reattachment (continued)

Skin (continued)
  Upper Leg
    Left 0HMJXZZ
    Right 0HMHXZZ
Stomach 0DM6
Tendon
  Abdomen
    Left 0LMG
    Right 0LMF
  Ankle
    Left 0LMT
    Right 0LMS
  Foot
    Left 0LMW
    Right 0LMV
  Hand
    Left 0LM8
    Right 0LM7
  Head and Neck
    0LM0
  Hip
    Left 0LMK
    Right 0LMJ
  Knee
    Left 0LMR
    Right 0LMQ
  Lower Arm and Wrist
    Left 0LM6
    Right 0LM5
  Lower Leg
    Left 0LMP
    Right 0LMN
  Perineum 0LMH
  Shoulder
    Left 0LM2
    Right 0LM1
  Thorax
    Left 0LMD
    Right 0LMC
  Trunk
    Left 0LMB
    Right 0LM9
  Upper Arm
    Left 0LM4
    Right 0LM3
  Upper Leg
    Left 0LMM
    Right 0LML
Testis
  Bilateral 0VMC
  Left 0VMB
  Right 0VM9
Thumb
  Left 0XMM0ZZ
  Right 0XML0ZZ
Thyroid Gland
  Left Lobe 0GMG
  Right Lobe 0GMH
Toe
  1st
    Left 0YMQ0ZZ
    Right 0YMP0ZZ
  2nd
    Left 0YMS0ZZ
    Right 0YMR0ZZ
  3rd
    Left 0YMU0ZZ
    Right 0YMT0ZZ
  4th
    Left 0YMW0ZZ
    Right 0YMV0ZZ
  5th
    Left 0YMY0ZZ
    Right 0YMX0ZZ
Tongue 0CM70ZZ
Tooth
  Lower 0CMX
  Upper 0CMW
Trachea 0BM10ZZ

Reattachment (continued)

Tunica Vaginalis
  Left 0VM7
  Right 0VM6
Ureter
  Left 0TM7
  Right 0TM6
Ureters, Bilateral 0TM8
Urethra 0TMD
Uterine Supporting Structure
  0UM4
Uterus 0UM9
Uvula 0CMN0ZZ
Vagina 0UMG
Vulva 0UMMXZZ
Wrist Region
  Left 0XMH0ZZ
  Right 0XMG0ZZ

REBOA (resuscitative endovascular balloon occlusion of the aorta)
  02LW3DJ
  04L03DJ

Rebound HRD® (Hernia Repair Device)
  use Synthetic Substitute

REBYOTA® use Broad Consortium Microbiota-based Live Biotherapeutic Suspension

RECELL® cell suspension autograft
  see Replacement, Skin and Breast 0HR

Recession
  see Repair
  see Reposition

Reclosure, disrupted abdominal wall
  0WQFXZZ

Reconstruction
  see Repair
  see Replacement
  see Supplement

Rectectomy
  see Excision, Rectum 0DBP
  see Resection, Rectum 0DTP

Rectocele repair
  see Repair, Subcutaneous Tissue and Fascia, Pelvic Region 0JQC

Rectopexy
  see Repair, Gastrointestinal System 0DQ
  see Reposition, Gastrointestinal System 0DS

Rectoplasty
  see Repair, Gastrointestinal System 0DQ
  see Supplement, Gastrointestinal System 0DU

Rectorrhaphy
  see Repair, Gastrointestinal System 0DQ

Rectoscopy 0DJD8ZZ

Rectosigmoid junction
  use Colon, Sigmoid

Rectosigmoidectomy
  see Excision, Gastrointestinal System 0DB
  see Resection, Gastrointestinal System 0DT

Rectostomy
  see Drainage, Rectum 0D9P

Rectotomy
  see Drainage, Rectum 0D9P

Rectus abdominis muscle
  use Muscle, Abdomen, Left
  use Muscle, Abdomen, Right

Rectus femoris muscle
  use Muscle, Upper Leg, Left
  use Muscle, Upper Leg, Right

Recurrent laryngeal nerve
  use Nerve, Vagus

Reducer® System
use Reduction Device in New
Technology
Reduction
Dislocation
see Reposition
Fracture
see Reposition
Intussusception, intestinal
see Reposition, Gastrointestinal
System 0DS
Mammoplasty
see Excision, Skin and Breast 0HB
Prolapse
see Reposition
Torsion
see Reposition
Volvulus, gastrointestinal
see Reposition, Gastrointestinal
System 0DS
Reduction Device, Coronary Sinus
X2V73Q7
Refusion
see Fusion
Rehabilitation
see Activities of Daily Living
Assessment, Rehabilitation F02
see Activities of Daily Living
Treatment, Rehabilitation F08
see Caregiver Training,
Rehabilitation F0F
see Cochlear Implant Treatment,
Rehabilitation F0B
see Device Fitting, Rehabilitation
F0D
see Hearing Treatment,
Rehabilitation F09
see Motor Function Assessment,
Rehabilitation F01
see Motor Treatment, Rehabilitation
F07
see Speech Assessment,
Rehabilitation F00
see Speech Treatment,
Rehabilitation F06
see Vestibular Treatment,
Rehabilitation F0C
Reimplantation
see Reattachment
see Reposition
see Transfer
Reinforcement
see Repair
see Supplement
Relaxation, scar tissue
see Release
Release
Acetabulum
Left 0QN5
Right 0QN4
Adenoids 0CNQ
Ampulla of Vater 0FNC
Anal Sphincter 0DNR
Anterior Chamber
Left 08N33ZZ
Right 08N23ZZ
Anus 0DNQ
Aorta
Abdominal 04N0
Thoracic
Ascending/Arch 02NX
Descending 02NW
Aortic Body 0GND
Appendix 0DNJ
Artery
Anterior Tibial
Left 04NQ
Right 04NP
Axillary
Left 03N6
Right 03N5

Release *(continued)*
Artery *(continued)*
Brachial
Left 03N8
Right 03N7
Celiac 04N1
Colic
Left 04N7
Middle 04N8
Right 04N6
Common Carotid
Left 03NJ
Right 03NH
Common Iliac
Left 04ND
Right 04NC
Coronary
Four or More Arteries 02N3
One Artery 02N0
Three Arteries 02N2
Two Arteries 02N1
External Carotid
Left 03NN
Right 03NM
External Iliac
Left 04NJ
Right 04NH
Face 03NR
Femoral
Left 04NL
Right 04NK
Foot
Left 04NW
Right 04NV
Gastric 04N2
Hand
Left 03NF
Right 03ND
Hepatic 04N3
Inferior Mesenteric
04NB
Innominate 03N2
Internal Carotid
Left 03NL
Right 03NK
Internal Iliac
Left 04NF
Right 04NE
Internal Mammary
Left 03N1
Right 03N0
Intracranial 03NG
Lower 04NY
Peroneal
Left 04NU
Right 04NT
Popliteal
Left 04NN
Right 04NM
Posterior Tibial
Left 04NS
Right 04NR
Pulmonary
Left 02NR
Right 02NQ
Pulmonary Trunk
02NP
Radial
Left 03NC
Right 03NB
Renal
Left 04NA
Right 04N9
Splenic 04N4
Subclavian
Left 03N4
Right 03N3
Superior Mesenteric 04N5
Temporal
Left 03NT
Right 03NS

Release *(continued)*
Artery *(continued)*
Thyroid
Left 03NV
Right 03NU
Ulnar
Left 03NA
Right 03N9
Upper 03NY
Vertebral
Left 03NQ
Right 03NP
Atrium
Left 02N7
Right 02N6
Auditory Ossicle
Left 09NA
Right 09N9
Basal Ganglia 00N8
Bladder 0TNB
Bladder Neck 0TNC
Bone
Ethmoid
Left 0NNG
Right 0NNF
Frontal 0NN1
Hyoid 0NNX
Lacrimal
Left 0NNJ
Right 0NNH
Nasal 0NNB
Occipital 0NN7
Palatine
Left 0NNL
Right 0NNK
Parietal
Left 0NN4
Right 0NN3
Pelvic
Left 0QN3
Right 0QN2
Sphenoid 0NNC
Temporal
Left 0NN6
Right 0NN5
Zygomatic
Left 0NNN
Right 0NNM
Brain 00N0
Breast
Bilateral 0HNV
Left 0HNU
Right 0HNT
Bronchus
Lingula 0BN9
Lower Lobe
Left 0BNB
Right 0BN6
Main
Left 0BN7
Right 0BN3
Middle Lobe, Right 0BN5
Upper Lobe
Left 0BN8
Right 0BN4
Buccal Mucosa 0CN4
Bursa and Ligament
Abdomen
Left 0MNJ
Right 0MNH
Ankle
Left 0MNR
Right 0MNQ
Elbow
Left 0MN4
Right 0MN3
Foot
Left 0MNT
Right 0MNS
Hand
Left 0MN8
Right 0MN7

Release *(continued)*
Bursa and Ligament *(continued)*
Head and Neck 0MN0
Hip
Left 0MNM
Right 0MNL
Knee
Left 0MNP
Right 0MNN
Lower Extremity
Left 0MNW
Right 0MNV
Perineum 0MNK
Rib(s) 0MNG
Shoulder
Left 0MN2
Right 0MN1
Spine
Lower 0MND
Upper 0MNC
Sternum 0MNF
Upper Extremity
Left 0MNB
Right 0MN9
Wrist
Left 0MN6
Right 0MN5
Carina 0BN2
Carotid Bodies, Bilateral 0GN8
Carotid Body
Left 0GN6
Right 0GN7
Carpal
Left 0PNN
Right 0PNM
Cecum 0DNH
Cerebellum 00NC
Cerebral Hemisphere 00N7
Cerebral Meninges 00N1
Cerebral Ventricle 00N6
Cervix 0UNC
Chordae Tendineae 02N9
Choroid
Left 08NB
Right 08NA
Cisterna Chyli 07NL
Clavicle
Left 0PNB
Right 0PN9
Clitoris 0UNJ
Coccygeal Glomus 0GNB
Coccyx 0QNS
Colon
Ascending 0DNK
Descending 0DNM
Sigmoid 0DNN
Transverse 0DNL
Conduction Mechanism 02N8
Conjunctiva
Left 08NTXZZ
Right 08NSXZZ
Cord
Bilateral 0VNH
Left 0VNG
Right 0VNF
Cornea
Left 08N9XZZ
Right 08N8XZZ
Cul-de-sac 0UNF
Diaphragm 0BNT
Disc
Cervical Vertebral 0RN3
Cervicothoracic Vertebral
0RN5
Lumbar Vertebral 0SN2
Lumbosacral 0SN4
Thoracic Vertebral 0RN9
Thoracolumbar Vertebral 0RNB
Duct
Common Bile 0FN9
Cystic 0FN8

Release *(continued)*
Duct *(continued)*
  Hepatic
    Common 0FN7
    Left 0FN6
    Right 0FN5
  Lacrimal
    Left 08NY
    Right 08NX
  Pancreatic 0FND
    Accessory 0FNF
  Parotid
    Left 0CNC
    Right 0CNB
Duodenum 0DN9
Dura Mater 00N2
Ear
  External
    Left 09N1
    Right 09N0
  External Auditory Canal
    Left 09N4
    Right 09N3
  Inner
    Left 09NE
    Right 09ND
  Middle
    Left 09N6
    Right 09N5
Epididymis
  Bilateral 0VNL
  Left 0VNK
  Right 0VNJ
Epiglottis 0CNR
Esophagogastric Junction
  0DN4
Esophagus 0DN5
  Lower 0DN3
  Middle 0DN2
  Upper 0DN1
Eustachian Tube
  Left 09NG
  Right 09NF
Eye
  Left 08N1XZZ
  Right 08N0XZZ
Eyelid
  Lower
    Left 08NR
    Right 08NQ
  Upper
    Left 08NP
    Right 08NN
Fallopian Tube
  Left 0UN6
  Right 0UN5
Fallopian Tubes, Bilateral
  0UN7
Femoral Shaft
  Left 0QN9
  Right 0QN8
Femur
  Lower
    Left 0QNC
    Right 0QNB
  Upper
    Left 0QN7
    Right 0QN6
Fibula
  Left 0QNK
  Right 0QNJ
Finger Nail 0HNQXZZ
Gallbladder 0FN4
Gingiva
  Lower 0CN6
  Upper 0CN5
Gland
  Adrenal
    Bilateral 0GN4
    Left 0GN2
    Right 0GN3

Release *(continued)*
  Glomus Jugulare 0GNC
  Lacrimal
    Left 08NW
    Right 08NV
  Minor Salivary 0CNJ
  Parotid
    Left 0CN9
    Right 0CN8
  Pituitary 0GN0
  Sublingual
    Left 0CNF
    Right 0CND
  Submaxillary
    Left 0CNH
    Right 0CNG
  Vestibular 0UNL
Glenoid Cavity
  Left 0PN8
  Right 0PN7
Humeral Head
  Left 0PND
  Right 0PNC
Humeral Shaft
  Left 0PNG
  Right 0PNF
Hymen 0UNK
Hypothalamus 00NA
Ileocecal Valve 0DNC
Ileum 0DNB
Intestine
  Large 0DNE
    Left 0DNG
    Right 0DNF
  Small 0DN8
Iris
  Left 08ND3
  Right 08NC3
Jejunum 0DNA
Joint
  Acromioclavicular
    Left 0RNH
    Right 0RNG
  Ankle
    Left 0SNG
    Right 0SNF
  Carpal
    Left 0RNR
    Right 0RNQ
  Carpometacarpal
    Left 0RNT
    Right 0RNS
  Cervical Vertebral 0RN1
  Cervicothoracic Vertebral
    0RN4
  Coccygeal 0SN6
  Elbow
    Left 0RNM
    Right 0RNL
  Finger Phalangeal
    Left 0RNX
    Right 0RNW
  Hip
    Left 0SNB
    Right 0SN9
  Knee
    Left 0SND
    Right 0SNC
  Lumbar Vertebral 0SN0
  Lumbosacral 0SN3
  Metacarpophalangeal
    Left 0RNV
    Right 0RNU
  Metatarsal-Phalangeal
    Left 0SNN
    Right 0SNM
  Occipital-cervical 0RN0
  Sacrococcygeal 0SN5
  Sacroiliac
    Left 0SN8
    Right 0SN7

Release *(continued)*
Joint *(continued)*
  Shoulder
    Left 0RNK
    Right 0RNJ
  Sternoclavicular
    Left 0RNF
    Right 0RNE
  Tarsal
    Left 0SNJ
    Right 0SNH
  Tarsometatarsal
    Left 0SNL
    Right 0SNK
  Temporomandibular
    Left 0RND
    Right 0RNC
  Thoracic Vertebral 0RN6
  Thoracolumbar Vertebral 0RNA
  Toe Phalangeal
    Left 0SNQ
    Right 0SNP
  Wrist
    Left 0RNP
    Right 0RNN
Kidney
  Left 0TN1
  Right 0TN0
Kidney Pelvis
  Left 0TN4
  Right 0TN3
Larynx 0CNS
Lens
  Left 08NK3ZZ
  Right 08NJ3ZZ
Lip
  Lower 0CN1
  Upper 0CN0
Liver 0FN0
  Left Lobe 0FN2
  Right Lobe 0FN1
Lung
  Bilateral 0BNM
  Left 0BNL
  Lower Lobe
    Left 0BNJ
    Right 0BNF
  Middle Lobe, Right 0BND
  Right 0BNK
  Upper Lobe
    Left 0BNG
    Right 0BNC
Lung Lingula 0BNH
Lymphatic
  Aortic 07ND
  Axillary
    Left 07N6
    Right 07N5
  Head 07N0
  Inguinal
    Left 07NJ
    Right 07NH
  Internal Mammary
    Left 07N9
    Right 07N8
  Lower Extremity
    Left 07NG
    Right 07NF
  Mesenteric 07NB
  Neck
    Left 07N2
    Right 07N1
  Pelvis 07NC
  Thoracic Duct 07NK
  Thorax 07N7
  Upper Extremity
    Left 07N4
    Right 07N3
Mandible
  Left 0NNV
  Right 0NNT

Release *(continued)*
Muscle *(continued)*
  Maxilla 0NNR
  Medulla Oblongata 00ND
  Mesentery 0DNV
  Metacarpal
    Left 0PNQ
    Right 0PNP
  Metatarsal
    Left 0QNP
    Right 0QNN
Muscle
  Abdomen
    Left 0KNL
    Right 0KNK
  Extraocular
    Left 08NM
    Right 08NL
  Facial 0KN1
  Foot
    Left 0KNW
    Right 0KNV
  Hand
    Left 0KND
    Right 0KNC
  Head 0KN0
  Hip
    Left 0KNP
    Right 0KNN
  Lower Arm and Wrist
    Left 0KNB
    Right 0KN9
  Lower Leg
    Left 0KNT
    Right 0KNS
  Neck
    Left 0KN3
    Right 0KN2
  Papillary 02ND
  Perineum 0KNM
  Shoulder
    Left 0KN6
    Right 0KN5
  Thorax
    Left 0KNJ
    Right 0KNH
  Tongue, Palate, Pharynx 0KN4
  Trunk
    Left 0KNG
    Right 0KNF
  Upper Arm
    Left 0KN8
    Right 0KN7
  Upper Leg
    Left 0KNR
    Right 0KNQ
Myocardial Bridge
  see Release, Artery, Coronary
Nasal Mucosa and Soft Tissue 09NK
Nasopharynx 09NN
Nerve
  Abdominal Sympathetic 01NM
  Abducens 00NL
  Accessory 00NR
  Acoustic 00NN
  Brachial Plexus 01N3
  Cervical 01N1
  Cervical Plexus 01N0
  Facial 00NM
  Femoral 01ND
  Glossopharyngeal 00NP
  Head and Neck Sympathetic 01NK
  Hypoglossal 00NS
  Lumbar 01NB
  Lumbar Plexus 01N9
  Lumbar Sympathetic 01NN
  Lumbosacral Plexus 01NA
  Median 01N5
  Oculomotor 00NH
  Olfactory 00NF
  Optic 00NG

61

Release *(continued)*

Nerve *(continued)*
Peroneal 01NH
Phrenic 01N2
Pudendal 01NC
Radial 01N6
Sacral 01NR
Sacral Plexus 01NQ
Sacral Sympathetic 01NP
Sciatic 01NF
Thoracic 01N8
Thoracic Sympathetic 01NL
Tibial 01NG
Trigeminal 00NK
Trochlear 00NJ
Ulnar 01N4
Vagus 00NQ
Nipple
Left 0HNX
Right 0HNW
Nose 09NKZZ
Omentum 0DNU
Orbit
Left 0NNQ
Right 0NNP
Ovary
Bilateral 0UN2
Left 0UN1
Right 0UN0
Palate
Hard 0CN2
Soft 0CN3
Pancreas 0FNG
Para-aortic Body 0GN9
Paraganglion Extremity 0GNF
Parathyroid Gland 0GNR
Inferior
Left 0GNP
Right 0GNN
Multiple 0GNQ
Superior
Left 0GNM
Right 0GNL
Patella
Left 0QNF
Right 0QND
Penis 0VNSZZ
Pericardium 02NN
Peritoneum 0DNW
Phalanx
Finger
Left 0PNV
Right 0PNT
Thumb
Left 0PNS
Right 0PNR
Toe
Left 0QNR
Right 0QNQ
Pharynx 0CNM
Pineal Body 0GN1
Pleura
Left 0BNP
Right 0BNN
Pons 00NB
Prepuce 0VNT
Prostate 0VN0
Radius
Left 0PNJ
Right 0PNH
Rectum 0DNP
Retina
Left 08NF3ZZ
Right 08NE3ZZ
Retinal Vessel
Left 08NH3ZZ
Right 08NG3ZZ
Ribs
1 to 2 0PN1
3 or More 0PN2
Sacrum 0QN1

Scapula
Left 0PN6
Right 0PN5
Sclera
Left 08N7XZZ
Right 08N6XZZ
Scrotum 0VN5
Septum
Atrial 02N5
Nasal 09NM
Ventricular 02NM
Sinus
Accessory 09NP
Ethmoid
Left 09NV
Right 09NU
Frontal
Left 09NT
Right 09NS
Mastoid
Left 09NC
Right 09NB
Maxillary
Left 09NR
Right 09NQ
Sphenoid
Left 09NX
Right 09NW
Skin
Abdomen 0HN7XZZ
Back 0HN6XZZ
Buttock 0HN8XZZ
Chest 0HN5XZZ
Ear
Left 0HN3XZZ
Right 0HN2XZZ
Face 0HN1XZZ
Foot
Left 0HNNXZZ
Right 0HNMXZZ
Hand
Left 0HNGXZZ
Right 0HNFXZZ
Inguinal 0HNAXZZ
Lower Arm
Left 0HNEXZZ
Right 0HNDXZZ
Lower Leg
Left 0HNLXZZ
Right 0HNKXZZ
Neck 0HN4XZZ
Perineum 0HN9XZZ
Scalp 0HN0XZZ
Upper Arm
Left 0HNCXZZ
Right 0HNBXZZ
Upper Leg
Left 0HNJXZZ
Right 0HNHXZZ
Spinal Cord
Cervical 00NW
Lumbar 00NY
Thoracic 00NX
Spinal Meninges 00NT
Spleen 07NP
Sternum 0PN0
Stomach 0DN6
Pylorus 0DN7
Subcutaneous Tissue and Fascia
Abdomen 0JN8
Back 0JN7
Buttock 0JN9
Chest 0JN6
Face 0JN1
Foot
Left 0JNR
Right 0JNQ
Hand
Left 0JNK
Right 0JNJ

Subcutaneous Tissue and Fascia
(continued)
Lower Arm
Left 0JNH
Right 0JNG
Lower Leg
Left 0JNP
Right 0JNN
Neck
Left 0JN5
Right 0JN4
Pelvic Region 0JNC
Perineum 0JNB
Scalp 0JN0
Upper Arm
Left 0JNF
Right 0JND
Upper Leg
Left 0JNM
Right 0JNL
Tarsal
Left 0QNM
Right 0QNL
Tendon
Abdomen
Left 0LNG
Right 0LNF
Ankle
Left 0LNT
Right 0LNS
Foot
Left 0LNW
Right 0LNV
Hand
Left 0LN8
Right 0LN7
Head and Neck 0LN0
Hip
Left 0LNK
Right 0LNJ
Knee
Left 0LNR
Right 0LNQ
Lower Arm and Wrist
Left 0LN6
Right 0LN5
Lower Leg
Left 0LNP
Right 0LNN
Perineum 0LNH
Shoulder
Left 0LN2
Right 0LN1
Thorax
Left 0LND
Right 0LNC
Trunk
Left 0LNB
Right 0LN9
Upper Arm
Left 0LN4
Right 0LN3
Upper Leg
Left 0LNM
Right 0LNL
Testis
Bilateral 0VNC
Left 0VNB
Right 0VN9
Thalamus 00N9
Thymus 07NM
Thyroid Gland 0GNK
Left Lobe 0GNG
Right Lobe 0GNH
Tibia
Left 0QNH
Right 0QNG
Toe Nail 0HNRXZZ
Tongue 0CN7
Tonsils 0CNP

Tooth
Lower 0CNX
Upper 0CNW
Trachea 0BN1
Tunica Vaginalis
Left 0VN7
Right 0VN6
Turbinate, Nasal 09NL
Tympanic Membrane
Left 09N8
Right 09N7
Ulna
Left 0PNL
Right 0PNK
Ureter
Left 0TN7
Right 0TN6
Urethra 0TND
Uterine Supporting Structure 0UN4
Uterus 0UN9
Uvula 0CNN
Vagina 0UNG
Valve
Aortic 02NF
Mitral 02NG
Pulmonary 02NH
Tricuspid 02NJ
Vas Deferens
Bilateral 0VNQ
Left 0VNP
Right 0VNN
Vein
Axillary
Left 05N8
Right 05N7
Azygos 05N0
Basilic
Left 05NC
Right 05NB
Brachial
Left 05NA
Right 05N9
Cephalic
Left 05NF
Right 05ND
Colic 06N7
Common Iliac
Left 06ND
Right 06NC
Coronary 02N4
Esophageal 06N3
External Iliac
Left 06NG
Right 06NF
External Jugular
Left 05NQ
Right 05NP
Face
Left 05NV
Right 05NT
Femoral
Left 06NN
Right 06NM
Foot
Left 06NV
Right 06NT
Gastric 06N2
Hand
Left 05NH
Right 05NG
Hemiazygos 05N1
Hepatic 06N4
Hypogastric
Left 06NJ
Right 06NH
Inferior Mesenteric 06N6
Innominate
Left 05N4
Right 05N3

Release (continued)
Vein (continued)
Internal Jugular
Left 05NN
Right 05NM
Intracranial 05NL
Lower 06NY
Portal 06N8
Pulmonary
Left 02NT
Right 02NS
Renal
Left 06NB
Right 06N9
Saphenous
Left 06NQ
Right 06NP
Splenic 06N1
Subclavian
Left 05N6
Right 05N5
Superior Mesenteric 06N5
Upper 05NY
Vertebral
Left 05NS
Right 05NR
Vena Cava
Inferior 06N0
Superior 02NV
Ventricle
Left 02NL
Right 02NK
Vertebra
Cervical 0PN3
Lumbar 0QN0
Thoracic 0PN4
Vesicle
Bilateral 0VN3
Left 0VN2
Right 0VN1
Vitreous
Left 08N53ZZ
Right 08N43ZZ
Vocal Cord
Left 0CNV
Right 0CNT
Vulva 0UNM
Relocation
see Reposition
Remdesivir Anti-infective XW0
Removal
Abdominal Wall 2W53X
Anorectal 2Y53X5
Arm
Lower
Left 2W5DX
Right 2W5CX
Upper
Left 2W5BX
Right 2W5AX
Back 2W55X
Chest Wall 2W54X
Ear 2Y52X5Z
Extremity
Lower
Left 2W5MX
Right 2W5LX
Upper
Left 2W59X
Right 2W58X
Face 2W51X
Finger
Left 2W5KX
Right 2W5JX
Foot
Left 2W5TX
Right 2W5SX
Genital Tract, Female 2Y54X5Z
Hand
Left 2W5FX
Right 2W5EX

Removal (continued)
Head 2W50X
Inguinal Region
Left 2W57X
Right 2W56X
Leg
Lower
Left 2W5RX
Right 2W5QX
Upper
Left 2W5PX
Right 2W5NX
Mouth and Pharynx 2Y50X5Z
Nasal 2Y51X5Z
Neck 2W52X
Thumb
Left 2W5HX
Right 2W5GX
Toe
Left 2W5VX
Right 2W5UX
Urethra 2Y55X5Z
Removal of device from
Abdominal Wall 0WPF
Acetabulum
Left 0QP5
Right 0QP4
Anal Sphincter 0DPR
Anus 0DPQ
Aorta, Thoracic, Descending
02PW3RZ
Artery
Lower 04PY
Upper 03PY
Back
Lower 0WPL
Upper 0WPK
Bladder 0TPB
Bone
Facial 0NPW
Lower 0QPY
Nasal 0NPB
Pelvic
Left 0QP3
Right 0QP2
Upper 0PPY
Bone Marrow 07PT
Brain 00P0
Breast
Left 0HPU
Right 0HPT
Bursa and Ligament
Lower 0MPY
Upper 0MPX
Carpal
Left 0PPN
Right 0PPM
Cavity, Cranial 0WP1
Cerebral Ventricle 00P6
Chest Wall 0WP8
Cisterna Chyli 07PL
Clavicle
Left 0PPB
Right 0PP9
Coccyx 0QPS
Diaphragm 0BPT
Disc
Cervical Vertebral 0RP3
Cervicothoracic Vertebral 0RP5
Lumbar Vertebral 0SP2
Lumbosacral 0SP4
Thoracic Vertebral 0RP9
Thoracolumbar Vertebral 0RPB
Duct
Hepatobiliary 0FPB
Pancreatic 0FPD
Ear
Inner
Left 09PE
Right 09PD
Left 09PJ
Right 09PH

Removal of device from (continued)
Epididymis and Spermatic Cord 0VPM
Esophagus 0DP5
Extremity
Lower
Left 0YPB
Right 0YP9
Upper
Left 0XP7
Right 0XP6
Eye
Left 08P1
Right 08P0
Face 0WP2
Fallopian Tube 0UP8
Femoral Shaft
Left 0QP9
Right 0QP8
Femur
Lower
Left 0QPC
Right 0QPB
Upper
Left 0QP7
Right 0QP6
Fibula
Left 0QPK
Right 0QPJ
Finger Nail 0HPQX
Gallbladder 0FP4
Gastrointestinal Tract 0WPP
Genitourinary Tract 0WPR
Gland
Adrenal 0GP5
Endocrine 0GPS
Pituitary 0GP0
Salivary 0CPA
Glenoid Cavity
Left 0PP8
Right 0PP7
Great Vessel 02PY
Hair 0HPSX
Head 0WP0
Heart 02PA
Humeral Head
Left 0PPD
Right 0PPC
Humeral Shaft
Left 0PPG
Right 0PPF
Intestinal Tract
Lower Intestinal Tract 0DPD
Upper Intestinal Tract 0DP0
Jaw
Lower 0WP5
Upper 0WP4
Joint
Acromioclavicular
Left 0RPH
Right 0RPG
Ankle
Left 0SPG
Right 0SPF
Carpal
Left 0RPR
Right 0RPQ
Carpometacarpal
Left 0RPT
Right 0RPS
Cervical Vertebral 0RP1
Cervicothoracic Vertebral 0RP4
Coccygeal 0SP6
Elbow
Left 0RPM
Right 0RPL
Finger Phalangeal
Left 0RPX
Right 0RPW
Hip
Left 0SPB
Acetabular Surface 0SPE
Femoral Surface 0SPS

Removal of device from (continued)
Joint (continued)
Hip (continued)
Right 0SP9
Acetabular Surface 0SPA
Femoral Surface 0SPR
Knee
Left 0SPD
Femoral Surface 0SPU
Tibial Surface 0SPW
Right 0SPC
Femoral Surface 0SPT
Tibial Surface 0SPV
Lumbar Vertebral 0SP0
Lumbosacral 0SP3
Metacarpophalangeal
Left 0RPV
Right 0RPU
Metatarsal-Phalangeal
Left 0SPN
Right 0SPM
Occipital-cervical 0RP0
Sacrococcygeal 0SP5
Sacroiliac
Left 0SP8
Right 0SP7
Shoulder
Left 0RPK
Right 0RPJ
Sternoclavicular
Left 0RPF
Right 0RPE
Tarsal
Left 0SPJ
Right 0SPH
Tarsometatarsal
Left 0SPL
Right 0SPK
Temporomandibular
Left 0RPD
Right 0RPC
Thoracic Vertebral 0RP6
Thoracolumbar Vertebral 0RPA
Toe Phalangeal
Left 0SPQ
Right 0SPP
Wrist
Left 0RPP
Right 0RPN
Kidney 0TP5
Larynx 0CPS
Lens
Left 08PK3
Right 08PJ3
Liver 0FP0
Lung
Left 0BPL
Right 0BPK
Lymphatic 07PN
Thoracic Duct 07PK
Mediastinum 0WPC
Mesentery 0DPV
Metacarpal
Left 0PPQ
Right 0PPP
Metatarsal
Left 0QPP
Right 0QPN
Mouth and Throat 0CPY
Muscle
Extraocular
Left 08PM
Right 08PL
Lower 0KPY
Upper 0KPX
Nasal Mucosa and Soft Tissue
09PK
Neck 0WP6
Nerve
Cranial 00PE
Peripheral 01PY

Removal of device from *(continued)*

Omentum 0DPU
Ovary 0UP3
Pancreas 0FPGZ
Parathyroid Gland 0GPR0
Patella
  Left 0QPF
  Right 0QPD
Pelvic Cavity 0WPJ
Penis 0VPS
Pericardial Cavity 0WPD
Perineum
  Female 0WPN
  Male 0WPM
Peritoneal Cavity 0WPG
Peritoneum 0DPW
Phalanx
  Finger
    Left 0PPV
    Right 0PPT
  Thumb
    Left 0PPS
    Right 0PPR
  Toe
    Left 0QPR
    Right 0QPQ
Pineal Body 0GP10
Pleura 0BPQ
Pleural Cavity
  Left 0WPB
  Right 0WP9
Products of Conception 10P0
Prostate and Seminal Vesicles
  0VP4
Radius
  Left 0PPJ
  Right 0PPH
Rectum 0DPP1
Respiratory Tract 0WPQZ
Retroperitoneum 0WPH
Ribs
  1 to 2 0PP1
  3 or More 0PP2
Sacrum 0QP1
Scapula
  Left 0PP6
  Right 0PP5
Scrotum and Tunica Vaginalis
  0VP8
Sinus 09PY0
Skin 0HPPX
Skull 0NP0
Spinal Canal 00PU
Spinal Cord 00PV
Spleen 07PP
Sternum 0PP0
Stomach 0DP6
Subcutaneous Tissue and
  Fascia
    Head and Neck 0JPS
    Lower Extremity 0JPW
    Trunk 0JPT
    Upper Extremity 0JPV
Tarsal
  Left 0QPM
  Right 0QPL
Tendon
  Lower 0LPY
  Upper 0LPX
Testis 0VPD
Thymus 07PM
Thyroid Gland 0GPK0
Tibia
  Left 0QPH
  Right 0QPG
Toe Nail 0HPRXZ
Trachea 0BP1
Tracheobronchial Tree 0BP0
Tympanic Membrane
  Left 09P80
  Right 09P70

Removal of device from *(continued)*

Ulna
  Left 0PPL
  Right 0PPK
Ureter 0TP9
Urethra 0TPD
Uterus and Cervix
  0UPD
Vagina and Cul-de-sac
  0UPH
Vas Deferens 0VPR
Vein
  Azygos 05P0
  Innominate
    Left 05P4
    Right 05P3
  Lower 06PY
  Upper 05PY
Vertebra
  Cervical 0PP3
  Lumbar 0QP0
  Thoracic 0PP4
Vulva 0UPM
Renal calyx
use Kidney
use Kidneys, Bilateral
use Kidney, Left
use Kidney, Right
Renal capsule
use Kidney
use Kidneys, Bilateral
use Kidney, Left
use Kidney, Right
Renal cortex
use Kidney
use Kidneys, Bilateral
use Kidney, Left
use Kidney, Right
Renal dialysis
see Performance, Urinary 5A1D
Renal nerve
use Abdominal Sympathetic
  Nerve
Renal plexus
use Nerve, Abdominal
  Sympathetic
Renal segment
use Kidney
use Kidneys, Bilateral
use Kidney, Left
use Kidney, Right
Renal segmental artery
use Artery, Renal, Left
use Artery, Renal, Right
Reopening, operative site
Control of bleeding
  see Control bleeding in
Inspection only
  see Inspection
Repair
Abdominal Wall 0WQF
Acetabulum
  Left 0QQ5
  Right 0QQ4
Adenoids 0CQQ
Ampulla of Vater 0FQC
Anal Sphincter 0DQR
Ankle Region
  Left 0YQL
  Right 0YQK
Anterior Chamber
  Left 08Q33
  Right 08Q23
Anus 0DQQ
Aorta
  Abdominal 04Q0
  Thoracic
    Ascending/Arch 02QX
    Descending 02QW
Aortic Body 0GQD
Appendix 0DQJ

Repair *(continued)*

Arm
  Lower
    Left 0XQF
    Right 0XQD
  Upper
    Left 0XQ9
    Right 0XQ8
Artery
  Anterior Tibial
    Left 04QQ
    Right 04QP
  Axillary
    Left 03Q6
    Right 03Q5
  Brachial
    Left 03Q8
    Right 03Q7
  Celiac 04Q1
  Colic
    Left 04Q7
    Middle 04Q8
    Right 04Q6
  Common Carotid
    Left 03QJ
    Right 03QH
  Common Iliac
    Left 04QD
    Right 04QC
  Coronary
    Four or More Arteries
      02Q3
    One Artery 02Q0
    Three Arteries
      02Q2
    Two Arteries 02Q1
  External Carotid
    Left 03QN
    Right 03QM
  External Iliac
    Left 04QJ
    Right 04QH
  Face 03QR
  Femoral
    Left 04QL
    Right 04QK
  Foot
    Left 04QW
    Right 04QV
  Gastric 04Q2
  Hand
    Left 03QF
    Right 03QD
  Hepatic 04Q3
  Inferior Mesenteric 04QB
  Innominate 03Q2
  Internal Carotid
    Left 03QL
    Right 03QK
  Internal Iliac
    Left 04QF
    Right 04QE
  Internal Mammary
    Left 03Q1
    Right 03Q0
  Intracranial 03QG
  Lower 04QY
  Peroneal
    Left 04QU
    Right 04QT
  Popliteal
    Left 04QN
    Right 04QM
  Posterior Tibial
    Left 04QS
    Right 04QR
  Pulmonary
    Left 02QR
    Right 02QQ
  Pulmonary Trunk
    02QP

Repair *(continued)*

Artery *(continued)*
  Radial
    Left 03QC
    Right 03QB
  Renal
    Left 04QA
    Right 04Q9
  Splenic 04Q4
  Subclavian
    Left 03Q4
    Right 03Q3
  Superior Mesenteric
    04Q5
  Temporal
    Left 03QT
    Right 03QS
  Thyroid
    Left 03QV
    Right 03QU
  Ulnar
    Left 03QA
    Right 03Q9
  Upper 03QY
  Vertebral
    Left 03QQ
    Right 03QP
Atrium
  Left 02Q7
  Right 02Q6
Auditory Ossicle
  Left 09QA
  Right 09Q9
Axilla
  Left 0XQ5
  Right 0XQ4
Back
  Lower 0WQL
  Upper 0WQK
Basal Ganglia 00Q8
Bladder 0TQB
Bladder Neck
  0TQC
Bone
  Ethmoid
    Left 0NQG
    Right 0NQF
  Frontal 0NQ1
  Hyoid 0NQX
  Lacrimal
    Left 0NQJ
    Right 0NQH
  Nasal 0NQB
  Occipital 0NQ7
  Palatine
    Left 0NQL
    Right 0NQK
  Parietal
    Left 0NQ4
    Right 0NQ3
  Pelvic
    Left 0QQ3
    Right 0QQ2
  Sphenoid 0NQC
  Temporal
    Left 0NQ6
    Right 0NQ
  Zygomatic
    Left 0NQN
    Right 0NQM
Brain 00Q0
Breast
  Bilateral 0HQV
  Left 0HQU
  Right 0HQT
  Supernumerary
    0HQY
Bronchus
  Lingula 0BQ9
  Lower Lobe
    Left 0BQB

Repair (continued)
Bronchus (continued)
  Lower Lobe (continued)
    Right 0BQ6
  Main
    Left 0BQ7
    Right 0BQ3
  Middle Lobe, Right
    0BQ5
  Upper Lobe
    Left 0BQ8
    Right 0BQ4
Buccal Mucosa 0CQ4
Bursa and Ligament
  Abdomen
    Left 0MQJ
    Right 0MQH
  Ankle
    Left 0MQR
    Right 0MQQ
  Elbow
    Left 0MQ4
    Right 0MQ3
  Foot
    Left 0MQT
    Right 0MQS
  Hand
    Left 0MQ8
    Right 0MQ7
  Head and Neck 0MQ0
  Hip
    Left 0MQM
    Right 0MQL
  Knee
    Left 0MQP
    Right 0MQN
  Lower Extremity
    Left 0MQW
    Right 0MQV
  Perineum 0MQK
  Rib(s) 0MQG
  Shoulder
    Left 0MQ2
    Right 0MQ1
  Spine
    Lower 0MQD
    Upper 0MQC
  Sternum 0MQF
  Upper Extremity
    Left 0MQB
    Right 0MQ9
  Wrist
    Left 0MQ6
    Right 0MQ5
Buttock
  Left 0YQ1
  Right 0YQ0
Carina 0BQ2
Carotid Bodies, Bilateral 0GQ8
Carotid Body
  Left 0GQ6
  Right 0GQ7
Carpal
  Left 0PQN
  Right 0PQM
Cecum 0DQH
Cerebellum 00QC
Cerebral Hemisphere
  00Q7
Cerebral Meninges 00Q1
Cerebral Ventricle 00Q6
Cervix 0UQC
Chest Wall 0WQ8
Chordae Tendineae 02Q9
Choroid
  Left 08QB
  Right 08QA
Cisterna Chyli 07QL
Clavicle
  Left 0PQB
  Right 0PQ9

Repair (continued)
Clitoris 0UQJ
Coccygeal Glomus
  0GQB
Coccyx 0QQS
Colon
  Ascending 0DQK
  Descending 0DQM
  Sigmoid 0DQN
  Transverse 0DQL
Conduction Mechanism
  02Q8
Conjunctiva
  Left 08QTXZZ
  Right 08QSXZZ
Cord
  Bilateral 0VQH
  Left 0VQG
  Right 0VQF
Cornea
  Left 08Q9XZZ
  Right 08Q8XZZ
Cul-de-sac 0UQF
Diaphragm 0BQT
Disc
  Cervical Vertebral
    0RQ3
  Cervicothoracic Vertebral
    0RQ5
  Lumbar Vertebral 0SQ2
  Lumbosacral 0SQ4
  Thoracic Vertebral
    0RQ9
  Thoracolumbar Vertebral
    0RQB
Duct
  Common Bile 0FQ9
  Cystic 0FQ8
  Hepatic
    Common 0FQ7
    Left 0FQ6
    Right 0FQ5
  Lacrimal
    Left 08QY
    Right 08QX
  Pancreatic 0FQD
    Accessory 0FQF
  Parotid
    Left 0CQC
    Right 0CQB
Duodenum 0DQ9
Dura Mater 00Q2
Ear
  External
    Bilateral 09Q2
    Left 09Q1
    Right 09Q0
  External Auditory
    Canal
      Left 09Q4
      Right 09Q3
  Inner
    Left 09QE
    Right 09QD
  Middle
    Left 09Q6
    Right 09Q5
Elbow Region
  Left 0XQC
  Right 0XQB
Epididymis
  Bilateral 0VQL
  Left 0VQK
  Right 0VQJ
Epiglottis 0CQR
Esophagogastric Junction
  0DQ4
Esophagus 0DQ5
  Lower 0DQ3
  Middle 0DQ2
  Upper 0DQ1

Repair (continued)
Eustachian Tube
  Left 09QG
  Right 09QF
Extremity
  Lower
    Left 0YQB
    Right 0YQ9
  Upper
    Left 0XQ7
    Right 0XQ6
Eye
  Left 08Q1XZZ
  Right 08Q0XZZ
Eyelid
  Lower
    Left 08QR
    Right 08QQ
  Upper
    Left 08QP
    Right 08QN
Face 0WQ2
Fallopian Tube
  Left 0UQ6
  Right 0UQ5
Fallopian Tubes, Bilateral
  0UQ7
Femoral Region
  Bilateral 0YQE
  Left 0YQ8
  Right 0YQ7
Femoral Shaft
  Left 0QQ9
  Right 0QQ8
Femur
  Lower
    Left 0QQC
    Right 0QQB
  Upper
    Left 0QQ7
    Right 0QQ6
Fibula
  Left 0QQK
  Right 0QQJ
Finger
  Index
    Left 0XQP
    Right 0XQN
  Little
    Left 0XQW
    Right 0XQV
  Middle
    Left 0XQR
    Right 0XQQ
  Ring
    Left 0XQT
    Right 0XQS
Finger Nail 0HQQXZZ
Floor of mouth
  see Repair, Oral Cavity and
    Throat 0WQ3
Foot
  Left 0YQN
  Right 0YQM
Gallbladder 0FQ4
Gingiva
  Lower 0CQ6
  Upper 0CQ5
Gland
  Adrenal
    Bilateral 0GQ4
    Left 0GQ2
    Right 0GQ3
  Lacrimal
    Left 08QW
    Right 08QV
  Minor Salivary 0CQJ
  Parotid
    Left 0CQ9
    Right 0CQ8
  Pituitary 0GQ0

Repair (continued)
Gland (continued)
  Sublingual
    Left 0CQF
    Right 0CQD
  Submaxillary
    Left 0CQH
    Right 0CQG
  Vestibular 0UQL
Glenoid Cavity
  Left 0PQ8
  Right 0PQ7
Glomus Jugulare
  0GQC
Hand
  Left 0XQK
  Right 0XQJ
Head 0WQ0
Heart 02QA
  Left 02QC
  Right 02QB
Humeral Head
  Left 0PQD
  Right 0PQC
Humeral Shaft
  Left 0PQG
  Right 0PQF
Hymen 0UQK
Hypothalamus 00QA
Ileocecal Valve 0DQC
Ileum 0DQB
Inguinal Region
  Bilateral 0YQA
  Left 0YQ6
  Right 0YQ5
Intestine
  Large 0DQE
    Left 0DQG
    Right 0DQF
  Small 0DQ8
Iris
  Left 08QD3ZZ
  Right 08QC3ZZ
Jaw
  Lower 0WQ5
  Upper 0WQ4
Jejunum 0DQA
Joint
  Acromioclavicular
    Left 0RQH
    Right 0RQG
  Ankle
    Left 0SQG
    Right 0SQF
  Carpal
    Left 0RQR
    Right 0RQQ
  Carpometacarpal
    Left 0RQT
    Right 0RQS
  Cervical Vertebral 0RQ1
  Cervicothoracic Vertebral
    0RQ4
  Coccygeal 0SQ6
  Elbow
    Left 0RQM
    Right 0RQL
  Finger Phalangeal
    Left 0RQX
    Right 0RQW
  Hip
    Left 0SQB
    Right 0SQ9
  Knee
    Left 0SQD
    Right 0SQC
  Lumbar Vertebral 0SQ0
  Lumbosacral 0SQ3
  Metacarpophalangeal
    Left 0RQV
    Right 0RQU

Repair *(continued)*

Joint *(continued)*
Metatarsal-Phalangeal
Left 0SQN
Right 0SQM
Occipital-cervical
0RQ0
Sacrococcygeal 0SQ5
Sacroiliac
Left 0SQ8
Right 0SQ7
Shoulder
Left 0RQK
Right 0RQJ
Sternoclavicular
Left 0RQF
Right 0RQE
Tarsal
Left 0SQJ
Right 0SQH
Tarsometatarsal
Left 0SQL
Right 0SQK
Temporomandibular
Left 0RQD
Right 0RQC
Thoracic Vertebral 0RQ6
Thoracolumbar Vertebral 0RQA
Toe Phalangeal
Left 0SQQ
Right 0SQP
Wrist
Left 0RQP
Right 0RQN
Kidney
Left 0TQ1
Right 0TQ0
Kidney Pelvis
Left 0TQ4
Right 0TQ3
Knee Region
Left 0YQG
Right 0YQF
Larynx 0CQS
Leg
Lower
Left 0YQJ
Right 0YQH
Upper
Left 0YQD
Right 0YQC
Lens
Left 08QK3ZZ
Right 08QJ3ZZ
Lip
Lower 0CQ1
Upper 0CQ0
Liver 0FQ0
Left Lobe 0FQ2
Right Lobe 0FQ1
Lung
Bilateral 0BQM
Left 0BQL
Lower Lobe
Left 0BQJ
Right 0BQF
Middle Lobe, Right 0BQD
Right 0BQK
Upper Lobe
Left 0BQG
Right 0BQC
Lung Lingula 0BQH
Lymphatic
Aortic 07QD
Axillary
Left 07Q6
Right 07Q5
Head 07Q0
Inguinal
Left 07QJ
Right 07QH

Repair *(continued)*

Lymphatic *(continued)*
Internal Mammary
Left 07Q9
Right 07Q8
Lower Extremity
Left 07QG
Right 07QF
Mesenteric 07QB
Neck
Left 07Q2
Right 07Q1
Pelvis 07QC
Thoracic Duct 07QK
Thorax 07Q7
Upper Extremity
Left 07Q4
Right 07Q3
Mandible
Left 0NQV
Right 0NQT
Maxilla 0NQR
Mediastinum 0WQC
Medulla Oblongata 00QD
Mesentery 0DQV
Metacarpal
Left 0PQQ
Right 0PQP
Metatarsal
Left 0QQP
Right 0QQN
Muscle
Abdomen
Left 0KQL
Right 0KQK
Extraocular
Left 08QM
Right 08QL
Facial 0KQ1
Foot
Left 0KQW
Right 0KQV
Hand
Left 0KQD
Right 0KQC
Head 0KQ0
Hip
Left 0KQP
Right 0KQN
Lower Arm and Wrist
Left 0KQB
Right 0KQ9
Lower Leg
Left 0KQT
Right 0KQS
Neck
Left 0KQ3
Right 0KQ2
Papillary 02QD
Perineum 0KQM
Shoulder
Left 0KQ6
Right 0KQ5
Thorax
Left 0KQJ
Right 0KQH
Tongue, Palate, Pharynx
0KQ4
Trunk
Left 0KQG
Right 0KQF
Upper Arm
Left 0KQ8
Right 0KQ7
Upper Leg
Left 0KQR
Right 0KQQ
Nasal Mucosa and Soft Tissue
09QK
Nasopharynx 09QN
Neck 0WQ6

Repair *(continued)*

Nerve
Abdominal Sympathetic
01QM
Abducens 00QL
Accessory 00QR
Acoustic 00QN
Brachial Plexus 01Q3
Cervical 01Q1
Cervical Plexus 01Q0
Facial 00QM
Femoral 01QD
Glossopharyngeal 00QP
Head and Neck Sympathetic
01QK
Hypoglossal 00QS
Lumbar 01QB
Lumbar Plexus 01Q9
Lumbar Sympathetic 01QN
Lumbosacral Plexus 01QA
Median 01Q5
Oculomotor 00QH
Olfactory 00QF
Optic 00QG
Peroneal 01QH
Phrenic 01Q2
Pudendal 01QC
Radial 01Q6
Sacral 01QR
Sacral Plexus 01QQ
Sacral Sympathetic 01QP
Sciatic 01QF
Thoracic 01Q8
Thoracic Sympathetic
01QL
Tibial 01QG
Trigeminal 00QK
Trochlear 00QJ
Ulnar 01Q4
Vagus 00QQ
Nipple
Left 0HQX
Right 0HQW
Omentum 0DQU
Oral Cavity and Throat
0WQ3
Orbit
Left 0NQQ
Right 0NQP
Ovary
Bilateral 0UQ2
Left 0UQ1
Right 0UQ0
Palate
Hard 0CQ2
Soft 0CQ3
Pancreas 0FQG
Para-aortic Body 0GQ9
Paraganglion Extremity
0GQF
Parathyroid Gland 0GQR
Inferior
Left 0GQP
Right 0GQN
Multiple 0GQQ
Superior
Left 0GQM
Right 0GQL
Patella
Left 0QQF
Right 0QQD
Penis 0VQS
Pericardium 02QN
Perineum
Female 0WQN
Male 0WQM
Peritoneum 0DQW
Phalanx
Finger
Left 0PQV
Right 0PQT

Repair *(continued)*

Phalanx *(continued)*
Thumb
Left 0PQS
Right 0PQR
Toe
Left 0QQR
Right 0QQQ
Pharynx 0CQM
Pineal Body 0GQ1
Pleura
Left 0BQP
Right 0BQN
Pons 00QB
Prepuce 0VQT
Products of Conception
10Q0
Prostate 0VQ0
Radius
Left 0PQJ
Right 0PQH
Rectum 0DQP
Retina
Left 08QF3ZZ
Right 08QE3ZZ
Retinal Vessel
Left 08QH3ZZ
Right 08QG3ZZ
Ribs
1 to 2 0PQ1
3 or More 0PQ2
Sacrum 0QQ1
Scapula
Left 0PQ6
Right 0PQ5
Sclera
Left 08Q7XZZ
Right 08Q6XZZ
Scrotum 0VQ5
Septum
Atrial 02Q5
Nasal 09QM
Ventricular 02QM
Shoulder Region
Left 0XQ3
Right 0XQ2
Sinus
Accessory 09QP
Ethmoid
Left 09QV
Right 09QU
Frontal
Left 09QT
Right 09QS
Mastoid
Left 09QC
Right 09QB
Maxillary
Left 09QR
Right 09QQ
Sphenoid
Left 09QX
Right 09QW
Skin
Abdomen 0HQ7XZZ
Back 0HQ6XZZ
Buttock 0HQ8XZZ
Chest 0HQ5XZZ
Ear
Left 0HQ3XZZ
Right 0HQ2XZZ
Face 0HQ1XZZ
Foot
Left 0HQNXZZ
Right 0HQMXZZ
Hand
Left 0HQGXZZ
Right 0HQFXZZ
Inguinal 0HQAXZZ
Lower Arm

Repair *(continued)*
Skin *(continued)*
  Lower Arm *(continued)*
    Left 0HQEXZZ
    Right 0HQDXZZ
  Lower Leg
    Left 0HQLXZZ
    Right 0HQKXZZ
  Neck 0HQ4XZZ
  Perineum 0HQ9XZZ
  Scalp 0HQ0XZZ
  Upper Arm
    Left 0HQCXZZ
    Right 0HQBXZZ
  Upper Leg
    Left 0HQJXZZ
    Right 0HQHXZZ
Skull 0NQ0
Spinal Cord
  Cervical 00QW
  Lumbar 00QY
  Thoracic 00QX
Spinal Meninges 00QT
Spleen 07QP
Sternum 0PQ0
Stomach 0DQ6
  Pylorus 0DQ7
Subcutaneous Tissue and Fascia
  Abdomen 0JQ8
  Back 0JQ7
  Buttock 0JQ9
  Chest 0JQ6
  Face 0JQ1
  Foot
    Left 0JQR
    Right 0JQQ
  Hand
    Left 0JQK
    Right 0JQJ
  Lower Arm
    Left 0JQH
    Right 0JQG
  Lower Leg
    Left 0JQP
    Right 0JQN
  Neck
    Left 0JQ5
    Right 0JQ4
  Pelvic Region 0JQC
  Perineum 0JQB
  Scalp 0JQ0
  Upper Arm
    Left 0JQF
    Right 0JQD
  Upper Leg
    Left 0JQM
    Right 0JQL
Tarsal
  Left 0QQM
  Right 0QQL
Tendon
  Abdomen
    Left 0LQG
    Right 0LQF
  Ankle
    Left 0LQT
    Right 0LQS
  Foot
    Left 0LQW
    Right 0LQV
  Hand
    Left 0LQ8
    Right 0LQ7
  Head and Neck
    0LQ0
  Hip
    Left 0LQK
    Right 0LQJ
  Knee
    Left 0LQR
    Right 0LQQ

Repair *(continued)*
Tendon *(continued)*
  Lower Arm and Wrist
    Left 0LQ6
    Right 0LQ5
  Lower Leg
    Left 0LQP
    Right 0LQN
  Perineum 0LQH
  Shoulder
    Left 0LQ2
    Right 0LQ1
  Thorax
    Left 0LQD
    Right 0LQC
  Trunk
    Left 0LQB
    Right 0LQ9
  Upper Arm
    Left 0LQ4
    Right 0LQ3
  Upper Leg
    Left 0LQM
    Right 0LQL
Testis
  Bilateral 0VQC
  Left 0VQB
  Right 0VQ9
Thalamus 00Q9
Thumb
  Left 0XQM
  Right 0XQL
Thymus 07QM
Thyroid Gland 0GQK
  Left Lobe 0GQG
  Right Lobe 0GQH
Thyroid Gland Isthmus
  0GQJ
Tibia
  Left 0QQH
  Right 0QQG
Toe
  1st
    Left 0YQQ
    Right 0YQP
  2nd
    Left 0YQS
    Right 0YQR
  3rd
    Left 0YQU
    Right 0YQT
  4th
    Left 0YQW
    Right 0YQV
  5th
    Left 0YQY
    Right 0YQX
Toe Nail 0HQRXZZ
Tongue 0CQ7
Tonsils 0CQP
Tooth
  Lower 0CQX
  Upper 0CQW
Trachea 0BQ1
Tunica Vaginalis
  Left 0VQ7
  Right 0VQ6
Turbinate, Nasal
  09QL
Tympanic Membrane
  Left 09Q8
  Right 09Q7
Ulna
  Left 0PQL
  Right 0PQK
Ureter
  Left 0TQ7
  Right 0TQ6
Urethra 0TQD
Uterine Supporting Structure
  0UQ4

Repair *(continued)*
Uterus 0UQ9
Uvula 0CQN
Vagina 0UQG
Valve
  Aortic 02QF
  Mitral 02QG
  Pulmonary 02QH
  Tricuspid 02QJ
Vas Deferens
  Bilateral 0VQQ
  Left 0VQP
  Right 0VQN
Vein
  Axillary
    Left 05Q8
    Right 05Q7
  Azygos 05Q0
  Basilic
    Left 05QC
    Right 05QB
  Brachial
    Left 05QA
    Right 05Q9
  Cephalic
    Left 05QF
    Right 05QD
  Colic 06Q7
  Common Iliac
    Left 06QD
    Right 06QC
  Coronary 02Q4
  Esophageal 06Q3
  External Iliac
    Left 06QG
    Right 06QF
  External Jugular
    Left 05QQ
    Right 05QP
  Face
    Left 05QV
    Right 05QT
  Femoral
    Left 06QN
    Right 06QM
  Foot
    Left 06QV
    Right 06QT
  Gastric 06Q2
  Hand
    Left 05QH
    Right 05QG
  Hemiazygos 05Q1
  Hepatic 06Q4
  Hypogastric
    Left 06QJ
    Right 06QH
  Inferior Mesenteric
    06Q6
  Innominate
    Left 05Q4
    Right 05Q3
  Internal Jugular
    Left 05QN
    Right 05QM
  Intracranial 05QL
  Lower 06QY
  Portal 06Q8
  Pulmonary
    Left 02QT
    Right 02QS
  Renal
    Left 06QB
    Right 06Q9
  Saphenous
    Left 06QQ
    Right 06QP
  Splenic 06Q1
  Subclavian
    Left 05Q6
    Right 05Q5

Repair *(continued)*
Vein *(continued)*
  Superior Mesenteric 06Q5
  Upper 05QY
  Vertebral
    Left 05QS
    Right 05QR
Vena Cava
  Inferior 06Q0
  Superior 02QV
Ventricle
  Left 02QL
  Right 02QK
Vertebra
  Cervical 0PQ3
  Lumbar 0QQ0
  Thoracic 0PQ4
Vesicle
  Bilateral 0VQ3
  Left 0VQ2
  Right 0VQ1
Vitreous
  Left 08Q53ZZ
  Right 08Q43ZZ
Vocal Cord
  Left 0CQV
  Right 0CQT
Vulva 0UQM
Wrist Region
  Left 0XQH
  Right 0XQG
Repair, obstetric laceration,
  periurethral 0UQMXZZ
Replacement
Acetabulum
  Left 0QR5
  Right 0QR4
Ampulla of Vater 0FRC
Anal Sphincter 0DRR
Aorta
  Abdominal 04R0
  Thoracic
    Ascending/Arch
      02RX
    Descending
      02RW
Artery
  Anterior Tibial
    Left 04RQ
    Right 04RP
  Axillary
    Left 03R6
    Right 03R5
  Brachial
    Left 03R8
    Right 03R7
  Celiac 04R1
  Colic
    Left 04R7
    Middle 04R8
    Right 04R6
  Common Carotid
    Left 03RJ
    Right 03RH
  Common Iliac
    Left 04RD
    Right 04RC
  External Carotid
    Left 03RN
    Right 03RM
  External Iliac
    Left 04RJ
    Right 04RH
  Face 03RR
  Femoral
    Left 04RL
    Right 04RK
  Foot
    Left 04RW
    Right 04RV
  Gastric 04R2

Replacement (*continued*)

Artery (*continued*)
Hand
Left 03RF
Right 03RD
Hepatic 04R3
Inferior Mesenteric
04R B
Innominate 03R2
Internal Carotid
Left 03RL
Right 03RK
Internal Iliac
Left 04RF
Right 04RE
Internal Mammary
Left 03R1
Right 03R0
Intracranial 03RG
Lower 04RY
Peroneal
Left 04RU
Right 04RT
Popliteal
Left 04RN
Right 04RM
Posterior Tibial
Left 04RS
Right 04RR
Pulmonary
Left 02RR
Right 02RQ
Pulmonary Trunk
02RP
Radial
Left 03RC
Right 03RB
Renal
Left 04RA
Right 04R9
Splenic 04R4
Subclavian
Left 03R4
Right 03R3
Superior Mesenteric
04R5
Temporal
Left 03RT
Right 03RS
Thyroid
Left 03RV
Right 03RU
Ulnar
Left 03RA
Right 03R9
Upper 03RY
Vertebral
Left 03RQ
Right 03RP
Atrium
Left 02R
Right 02R6
Auditory Ossicle
Left 09RA0
Right 09R90
Bladder 0TRB
Bladder Neck 0TRC
Bone
Ethmoid
Left 0NRG
Right 0NRF
Frontal 0NR1
Hyoid 0NRX
Lacrimal
Left 0NRJ
Right 0NRH
Nasal 0NRB
Occipital 0NR7
Palatine
Left 0NRL
Right 0NRK

Replacement (*continued*)

Bone (*continued*)
Parietal
Left 0NR4
Right 0NR3
Pelvic
Left 0QR3
Right 0QR2
Sphenoid 0NRC
Temporal
Left 0NR6
Right 0NR5
Zygomatic
Left 0NRN
Right 0NRM
Breast
Bilateral 0HRV
Left 0HRU
Right 0HRT
Bronchus
Lingula 0BR9
Lower Lobe
Left 0BRB
Right 0BR6
Main
Left 0BR7
Right 0BR3
Middle Lobe, Right
0BR5
Upper Lobe
Left 0BR8
Right 0BR4
Buccal Mucosa 0CR4
Bursa and Ligament
Abdomen
Left 0MRJ
Right 0MRH
Ankle
Left 0MRR
Right 0MRQ
Elbow
Left 0MR4
Right 0MR3
Foot
Left 0MRT
Right 0MRS
Hand
Left 0MR8
Right 0MR7
Head and Neck 0MR0
Hip
Left 0MRM
Right 0MRL
Knee
Left 0MRP
Right 0MRN
Lower Extremity
Left 0MRW
Right 0MRV
Perineum 0MRK
Rib(s) 0MRG
Shoulder
Left 0MR2
Right 0MR1
Spine
Lower 0MRD
Upper 0MRC
Sternum 0MRF
Upper Extremity
Left 0MRB
Right 0MR9
Wrist
Left 0MR6
Right 0MR5
Carina 0BR2
Carpal
Left 0PRN
Right 0PRM
Cerebral Meninges
00R1
Cerebral Ventricle 00R6

Replacement (*continued*)

Chordae Tendineae 02R9
Choroid
Left 08RB
Right 08RA
Clavicle
Left 0PRB
Right 0PR9
Coccyx 0QRS
Conjunctiva
Left 08RTX
Right 08RSX
Cornea
Left 08R9
Right 08R8
Diaphragm 0BRT
Disc
Cervical Vertebral 0RR30
Cervicothoracic Vertebral
0RR50
Lumbar Vertebral 0SR20
Lumbosacral 0SR40
Thoracic Vertebral 0RR90
Thoracolumbar Vertebral
0RRB0
Duct
Common Bile 0FR9
Cystic 0FR8
Hepatic
Common 0FR7
Left 0FR6
Right 0FR5
Lacrimal
Left 08RY
Right 08RX
Pancreatic 0FRD
Accessory 0FRF
Parotid
Left 0CRC
Right 0CRB
Dura Mater 00R2
Ear
External
Bilateral 09R2
Left 09R1
Right 09R0
Inner
Left 09RE0
Right 09RD0
Middle
Left 09R60
Right 09R50
Epiglottis 0CRR
Esophagus 0DR5
Eye
Left 08R1
Right 08R0
Eyelid
Lower
Left 08RR
Right 08RQ
Upper
Left 08RP
Right 08RN
Femoral Shaft
Left 0QR9
Right 0QR8
Femur
Lower
Left 0QRC
Right 0QRB
Upper
Left 0QR7
Right 0QR6
Fibula
Left 0QRK
Right 0QRJ
Finger Nail 0HRQX
Gingiva
Lower 0CR6
Upper 0CR5

Replacement (*continued*)

Glenoid Cavity
Left 0PR8
Right 0PR7
Hair 0HRSX
Heart 02RA0
Humeral Head
Left 0PRD
Right 0PRC
Humeral Shaft
Left 0PRG
Right 0PRF
Iris
Left 08RD3
Right 08RC3
Joint
Acromioclavicular
Left 0RRH0
Right 0RRG0
Ankle
Left 0SRG
Right 0SRF
Carpal
Left 0RRR0
Right 0RRQ0
Carpometacarpal
Left 0RRT0
Right 0RRS0
Cervical Vertebral 0RR10
Cervicothoracic Vertebral
0RR40
Coccygeal 0SR60
Elbow
Left 0RRM0
Right 0RRL0
Finger Phalangeal
Left 0RRX0
Right 0RRW0
Hip
Left 0SRB
Acetabular Surface 0SRE
Femoral Surface 0SRS
Right 0SR9
Acetabular Surface
0SRA
Femoral Surface 0SRR
Knee
Left 0SRD
Femoral Surface 0SRU
Tibial Surface 0SRW
Right 0SRC
Femoral Surface 0SRT
Tibial Surface 0SRV
Lumbar Vertebral 0SR00
Lumbosacral 0SR30
Metacarpophalangeal
Left 0RRV0
Right 0RRU0
Metatarsal-Phalangeal
Left 0SRN0
Right 0SRM0
Occipital-cervical 0RR00
Sacrococcygeal 0SR50
Sacroiliac
Left 0SR80
Right 0SR70
Shoulder
Left 0RRK
Right 0RRJ
Sternoclavicular
Left 0RRF0
Right 0RRE0
Tarsal
Left 0SRJ0
Right 0SRH0
Tarsometatarsal
Left 0SRL0
Right 0SRK0
Temporomandibular
Left 0RRD0
Right 0RRC0

Replacement *(continued)*

Joint *(continued)*
  Thoracic Vertebral
    0RR60
  Thoracolumbar Vertebral
    0RRA0
  Toe Phalangeal
    Left 0SRQ0
    Right 0SRP0
  Wrist
    Left 0RRP0
    Right 0RRN0
Kidney Pelvis
  Left 0TR4
  Right 0TR3
Larynx 0CRS
Lens
  Left 08RK30Z
  Right 08RJ30Z
Lip
  Lower 0CR1
  Upper 0CR0
Mandible
  Left 0NRV
  Right 0NRT
Maxilla 0NRR
Mesentery 0DRV
Metacarpal
  Left 0PRQ
  Right 0PRP
Metatarsal
  Left 0QRP
  Right 0QR
Muscle
  Abdomen
    Left 0KRL
    Right 0KRK
  Facial 0KR1
  Foot
    Left 0KRW
    Right 0KRV
  Hand
    Left 0KRD
    Right 0KRC
  Head 0KR0
  Hip
    Left 0KRP
    Right 0KRN
  Lower Arm and Wrist
    Left 0KRB
    Right 0KR9
  Lower Leg
    Left 0KRT
    Right 0KRS
  Neck
    Left 0KR3
    Right 0KR2
  Papillary 02RD
  Perineum 0KRM
  Shoulder
    Left 0KR6
    Right 0KR5
  Thorax
    Left 0KRJ
    Right 0KRH
  Tongue, Palate, Pharynx
    0KR4
  Trunk
    Left 0KRG
    Right 0KRF
  Upper Arm
    Left 0KR8
    Right 0KR7
  Upper Leg
    Left 0KRR
    Right 0KRQ
Nasal Mucosa and Soft Tissue
  09RK
Nasopharynx 09RN
Nerve
  Abducens 00RL

Replacement *(continued)*

Nerve *(continued)*
  Accessory 00RR
  Acoustic 00RN
  Cervical 01R1
  Facial 00RM
  Femoral 01RD
  Glossopharyngeal 00RP
  Hypoglossal 00RS
  Lumbar 01RB
  Median 01R5
  Oculomotor 00RH
  Olfactory 00RF
  Optic 00RG
  Peroneal 01RH
  Phrenic 01R2
  Pudendal 01RC
  Radial 01R6
  Sacral 01RR
  Sciatic 01RF
  Thoracic 01R8
  Tibial 01RG
  Trigeminal 00RK
  Trochlear 00RJ
  Ulnar 01R4
  Vagus 00RQ
Nipple
  Left 0HRX
  Right 0HRW
Omentum 0DRU
Orbit
  Left 0NRQ
  Right 0NRP
Palate
  Hard 0CR2
  Soft 0CR3
Patella
  Left 0QRF
  Right 0QRD
Pericardium 02RN
Peritoneum 0DRW
Phalanx
  Finger
    Left 0PRV
    Right 0PRT
  Thumb
    Left 0PRS
    Right 0PRR
  Toe
    Left 0QRR
    Right 0QRQ
Pharynx 0CRM
Radius
  Left 0PRJ
  Right 0PRH
Retinal Vessel
  Left 08RH3
  Right 08RG3
Ribs
  1 to 2 0PR1
  3 or More 0PR2
Sacrum 0QR1
Scapula
  Left 0PR6
  Right 0PR5
Sclera
  Left 08R7X
  Right 08R6X
Septum
  Atrial 02R5
  Nasal 09RM
  Ventricular 02RM
Skin
  Abdomen 0HR7
  Back 0HR6
  Buttock 0HR8
  Chest 0HR5
  Ear
    Left 0HR3
    Right 0HR2
  Face 0HR1

Replacement *(continued)*

Skin *(continued)*
  Foot
    Left 0HRN
    Right 0HRM
  Hand
    Left 0HRG
    Right 0HRF
  Inguinal 0HRA
  Lower Arm
    Left 0HRE
    Right 0HRD
  Lower Leg
    Left 0HRL
    Right 0HRK
  Neck 0HR4
  Perineum 0HR9
  Scalp 0HR0
  Upper Arm
    Left 0HRC
    Right 0HRB
  Upper Leg
    Left 0HRJ
    Right 0HRH
Skull 0NR0
Spinal Meninges 00RT
Sternum 0PR0
Subcutaneous Tissue and Fascia
  Abdomen 0JR8
  Back 0JR7
  Buttock 0JR9
  Chest 0JR6
  Face 0JR1
  Foot
    Left 0JRR
    Right 0JRQ
  Hand
    Left 0JRK
    Right 0JRJ
  Lower Arm
    Left 0JRH
    Right 0JRG
  Lower Leg
    Left 0JRP
    Right 0JRN
  Neck
    Left 0JR5
    Right 0JR4
  Pelvic Region 0JRC
  Perineum 0JRB
  Scalp 0JR0
  Upper Arm
    Left 0JRF
    Right 0JRD
  Upper Leg
    Left 0JRM
    Right 0JRL
Tarsal
  Left 0QRM
  Right 0QRL
Tendon
  Abdomen
    Left 0LRG
    Right 0LRF
  Ankle
    Left 0LRT
    Right 0LRS
  Foot
    Left 0LRW
    Right 0LRV
  Hand
    Left 0LR8
    Right 0LR7
  Head and Neck
    0LR0
  Hip
    Left 0LRK
    Right 0LRJ
  Knee
    Left 0LRR
    Right 0LRQ

Replacement *(continued)*

Tendon *(continued)*
  Lower Arm and Wrist
    Left 0LR6
    Right 0LR5
  Lower Leg
    Left 0LRP
    Right 0LRN
  Perineum 0LRH
  Shoulder
    Left 0LR2
    Right 0LR1
  Thorax
    Left 0LRD
    Right 0LRC
  Trunk
    Left 0LRB
    Right 0LR9
  Upper Arm
    Left 0LR4
    Right 0LR3
  Upper Leg
    Left 0LRM
    Right 0LRL
Testis
  Bilateral 0VRC0J
  Left 0VRB0J
  Right 0VR90J
Thumb
  Left 0XRM
  Right 0XRL
Tibia
  Left 0QRH
  Right 0QRG
Toe Nail 0HRRX
Tongue 0CR7
Tooth
  Lower 0CRX
  Upper 0CRW
Trachea 0BR1
Turbinate, Nasal
  09RL
Tympanic Membrane
  Left 09R8
  Right 09R7
Ulna
  Left 0PRL
  Right 0PRK
Ureter
  Left 0TR7
  Right 0TR6
Urethra 0TRD
Uvula 0CRN
Valve
  Aortic 02RF
  Mitral 02RG
  Pulmonary 02RH
  Tricuspid 02RJ
Vein
  Axillary
    Left 05R8
    Right 05R7
  Azygos 05R0
  Basilic
    Left 05RC
    Right 05RB
  Brachial
    Left 05RA
    Right 05R9
  Cephalic
    Left 05RF
    Right 05RD
  Colic 06R7
  Common Iliac
    Left 06RD
    Right 06RC
  Esophageal 06R3
  External Iliac
    Left 06RG
    Right 06RF

Replacement–Reposition

Replacement (continued)
  Vein (continued)
    External Jugular
      Left 05RQ
      Right 05RP
    Face
      Left 05RV
      Right 05RT
    Femoral
      Left 06RN
      Right 06RM
    Foot
      Left 06RV
      Right 06RT
    Gastric 06R2
    Hand
      Left 05RH
      Right 05RG
    Hemiazygos 05R1
    Hepatic 06R4
    Hypogastric
      Left 06RJ
      Right 06RH
    Inferior Mesenteric 06R6
    Innominate
      Left 05R4
      Right 05R3
    Internal Jugular
      Left 05RN
      Right 05RM
    Intracranial 05RL
    Lower 06RY
    Portal 06R8
    Pulmonary
      Left 02RT
      Right 02RS
    Renal
      Left 06RB
      Right 06R9
    Saphenous
      Left 06RQ
      Right 06RP
    Splenic 06R1
    Subclavian
      Left 05R6
      Right 05R5
    Superior Mesenteric 06R5
    Upper 05RY
    Vertebral
      Left 05RS
      Right 05RR
  Vena Cava
    Inferior 06R0
    Superior 02RV
  Ventricle
    Left 02RL
    Right 02RK
  Vertebra
    Cervical 0PR3
    Lumbar 0QR0
    Thoracic 0PR4
  Vitreous
    Left 08R53
    Right 08R43
  Vocal Cord
    Left 0CRV
    Right 0CRT
Replacement, hip
  Partial or total
    see Replacement, Lower Joints
    0SR
  Resurfacing only
    see Supplement, Lower Joints
    0SU
Replacement, knee
  Meniscus implant only see New
    Technology, Joints XRR
  Partial or total see Replacement,
    Lower Joints 0SR
Replantation
  see Reposition

Replantation, scalp
  see Reattachment, Skin, Scalp
  0HM0
Reposition
  Acetabulum
    Left 0QS5
    Right 0QS4
  Ampulla of Vater 0FSC
  Anus 0DSQ
  Aorta
    Abdominal 04S0
    Thoracic
      Ascending/Arch 02SX0ZZ
      Descending 02SW0ZZ
  Artery
    Anterior Tibial
      Left 04SQ
      Right 04SP
    Axillary
      Left 03S6
      Right 03S5
    Brachial
      Left 03S8
      Right 03S7
    Celiac 04S1
    Colic
      Left 04S7
      Middle 04S8
      Right 04S6
    Common Carotid
      Left 03SJ
      Right 03SH
    Common Iliac
      Left 04SD
      Right 04SC
    Coronary
      One Artery 02S00ZZ
      Two Arteries 02S10ZZ
    External Carotid
      Left 03SN
      Right 03SM
    External Iliac
      Left 04SJ
      Right 04SH
    Face 03SR
    Femoral
      Left 04SL
      Right 04SK
    Foot
      Left 04SW
      Right 04SV
    Gastric 04S2
    Hand
      Left 03SF
      Right 03SD
    Hepatic 04S3
    Inferior Mesenteric
      04SB
    Innominate 03S2
    Internal Carotid
      Left 03SL
      Right 03SK
    Internal Iliac
      Left 04SF
      Right 04SE
    Internal Mammary
      Left 03S1
      Right 03S0
    Intracranial 03SG
    Lower 04SY
    Peroneal
      Left 04SU
      Right 04ST
    Popliteal
      Left 04SN
      Right 04SM
    Posterior Tibial
      Left 04SS
      Right 04SR
    Pulmonary
      Left 02SR0ZZ

Reposition (continued)
  Artery (continued)
    Pulmonary (continued)
      Right 02SQ0ZZ
    Pulmonary Trunk
      02SP0ZZ
    Radial
      Left 03SC
      Right 03SB
    Renal
      Left 04SA
      Right 04S9
    Splenic 04S4
    Subclavian
      Left 03S4
      Right 03S3
    Superior Mesenteric
      04S5
    Temporal
      Left 03ST
      Right 03SS
    Thyroid
      Left 03SV
      Right 03SU
    Ulnar
      Left 03SA
      Right 03S9
    Upper 03SY
    Vertebral
      Left 03SQ
      Right 03SP
  Auditory Ossicle
    Left 09SA
    Right 09S9
  Bladder 0TSB
  Bladder Neck
    0TSC
  Bone
    Ethmoid
      Left 0NSG
      Right 0NSF
    Frontal 0NS1
    Hyoid 0NSX
    Lacrimal
      Left 0NSJ
      Right 0NSH
    Nasal 0NSB
    Occipital 0NS7
    Palatine
      Left 0NSL
      Right 0NSK
    Parietal
      Left 0NS4
      Right 0NS3
    Pelvic
      Left 0QS3
      Right 0QS2
    Sphenoid 0NSC
    Temporal
      Left 0NS6
      Right 0NS5
    Zygomatic
      Left 0NSN
      Right 0NSM
  Breast
    Bilateral 0HSV0ZZ
    Left 0HSU0ZZ
    Right 0HST0ZZ
  Bronchus
    Lingula 0BS90ZZ
    Lower Lobe
      Left 0BSB0ZZ
      Right 0BS60ZZ
    Main
      Left 0BS70ZZ
      Right 0BS30ZZ
    Middle Lobe, Right
      0BS50ZZ
    Upper Lobe
      Left 0BS80ZZ
      Right 0BS40ZZ

Reposition (continued)
  Bursa and Ligament
    Abdomen
      Left 0MSJ
      Right 0MSH
    Ankle
      Left 0MSR
      Right 0MSQ
    Elbow
      Left 0MS4
      Right 0MS3
    Foot
      Left 0MST
      Right 0MSS
    Hand
      Left 0MS8
      Right 0MS7
    Head and Neck
      0MS0
    Hip
      Left 0MSM
      Right 0MSL
    Knee
      Left 0MSP
      Right 0MSN
    Lower Extremity
      Left 0MSW
      Right 0MSV
    Perineum 0MSK
    Rib(s) 0MSG
    Shoulder
      Left 0MS2
      Right 0MS1
    Spine
      Lower 0MSD
      Upper 0MSC
    Sternum 0MSF
    Upper Extremity
      Left 0MSB
      Right 0MS9
    Wrist
      Left 0MS6
      Right 0MS5
  Carina 0BS20ZZ
  Carpal
    Left 0PSN
    Right 0PSM
  Cecum 0DSH
  Cervix 0USC
  Clavicle
    Left 0PSB
    Right 0PS9
  Coccyx 0QSS
  Colon
    Ascending 0DSK
    Descending 0DSM
    Sigmoid 0DSN
    Transverse 0DSL
  Cord
    Bilateral 0VSH
    Left 0VSG
    Right 0VSF
  Cul-de-sac 0USF
  Diaphragm 0BST0ZZ
  Duct
    Common Bile
      0FS9
    Cystic 0FS8
    Hepatic
      Common 0FS7
      Left 0FS6
      Right 0FS5
    Lacrimal
      Left 08SY
      Right 08SX
    Pancreatic 0FSD
      Accessory 0FSF
    Parotid
      Left 0CSC
      Right 0CSB
  Duodenum 0DS9ZZ

70

Reposition *(continued)*
Ear
   Bilateral 09S2ZZ
   Left 09S1ZZ
   Right 09S0ZZ
Epiglottis 0CSR
Esophagus 0DS5ZZ
Eustachian Tube
   Left 09SG
   Right 09SF
Eyelid
  Lower
    Left 08SR
    Right 08SQ
  Upper
    Left 08SP
    Right 08SN
Fallopian Tube
   Left 0US6
   Right 0US5
Fallopian Tubes, Bilateral
   0US7
Femoral Shaft
   Left 0QS9
   Right 0QS8
Femur
  Lower
    Left 0QSC
    Right 0QSB
  Upper
    Left 0QS7
    Right 0QS6
Fibula
   Left 0QSK
   Right 0QSJ
Gallbladder 0FS4
Gland
  Adrenal
    Left 0GS2
    Right 0GS3
  Lacrimal
    Left 08SW
    Right 08SV
Glenoid Cavity
   Left 0PS8
   Right 0PS7
Hair 0HSSXZZ
Humeral Head
   Left 0PSD
   Right 0PSC
Humeral Shaft
   Left 0PSG
   Right 0PSF
Ileum 0DSB
Intestine
  Large 0DSE
  Small 0DS8
Iris
   Left 08SD3ZZ
   Right 08SC3ZZ
Jejunum 0DSAZZ
Joint
  Acromioclavicular
    Left 0RSHZ
    Right 0RSGZ
  Ankle
    Left 0SSG
    Right 0SSF
  Carpal
    Left 0RSR
    Right 0RSQ
  Carpometacarpal
    Left 0RST
    Right 0RSS
  Cervical Vertebral 0RS1
  Cervicothoracic Vertebral
    0RS4
  Coccygeal 0SS6
  Elbow
    Left 0RSM
    Right 0RSL

Reposition *(continued)*
Joint *(continued)*
  Finger Phalangeal
    Left 0RSX
    Right 0RSW
  Hip
    Left 0SSB
    Right 0SS9
  Knee
    Left 0SSD
    Right 0SSC
  Lumbar Vertebral 0SS0
  Lumbosacral 0SS3
  Metacarpophalangeal
    Left 0RSV
    Right 0RSU
  Metatarsal-Phalangeal
    Left 0SSN
    Right 0SSM
  Occipital-cervical 0RS0
  Sacrococcygeal 0SS5
  Sacroiliac
    Left 0SS8
    Right 0SS7
  Shoulder
    Left 0RSK
    Right 0RSJ
  Sternoclavicular
    Left 0RSF
    Right 0RSE
  Tarsal
    Left 0SSJ
    Right 0SSH
  Tarsometatarsal
    Left 0SSL
    Right 0SSK
  Temporomandibular
    Left 0RSD
    Right 0RSC
  Thoracic Vertebral 0RS6
  Thoracolumbar Vertebral 0RSA
  Toe Phalangeal
    Left 0SSQ
    Right 0SSP
  Wrist
    Left 0RSP
    Right 0RSN
Kidney
   Left 0TS1
   Right 0TS0
Kidney Pelvis
   Left 0TS4
   Right 0TS3
Kidneys, Bilateral 0TS2
Larynx 0CSS
Lens
   Left 08SK3ZZ
   Right 08SJ3ZZ
Lip
  Lower 0CS1
  Upper 0CS0
Liver 0FS0
Lung
   Left 0BSL0ZZ
  Lower Lobe
    Left 0BSJ0ZZ
    Right 0BSF0ZZ
  Middle Lobe, Right 0BSD0ZZ
   Right 0BSK0ZZ
  Upper Lobe
    Left 0BSG0ZZ
    Right 0BSC0ZZ
Lung Lingula 0BSH0ZZ
Mandible
   Left 0NSV
   Right 0NST
Maxilla 0NSR
Metacarpal
   Left 0PSQ
   Right 0PSP
Metatarsal
   Left 0QSP

Reposition *(continued)*
Metatarsal *(continued)*
   Right 0QSN
Muscle
  Abdomen
    Left 0KSL
    Right 0KSK
  Extraocular
    Left 08SM
    Right 08SL
  Facial 0KS1
  Foot
    Left 0KSW
    Right 0KSV
  Hand
    Left 0KSD
    Right 0KSC
  Head 0KS0
  Hip
    Left 0KSP
    Right 0KSN
  Lower Arm and Wrist
    Left 0KSB
    Right 0KS9
  Lower Leg
    Left 0KST
    Right 0KSS
  Neck
    Left 0KS3
    Right 0KS2
  Perineum 0KSM
  Shoulder
    Left 0KS6
    Right 0KS5
  Thorax
    Left 0KSJ
    Right 0KSH
  Tongue, Palate, Pharynx 0KS4
  Trunk
    Left 0KSG
    Right 0KSF
  Upper Arm
    Left 0KS8
    Right 0KS7
  Upper Leg
    Left 0KSR
    Right 0KSQ
Nasal Mucosa and Soft Tissue 09SK
Nerve
  Abducens 00SL
  Accessory 00SR
  Acoustic 00SN
  Brachial Plexus 01S3
  Cervical 01S1
  Cervical Plexus 01S0
  Facial 00SM
  Femoral 01SD
  Glossopharyngeal 00SP
  Hypoglossal 00SS
  Lumbar 01SB
  Lumbar Plexus 01S9
  Lumbosacral Plexus 01SA
  Median 01S5
  Oculomotor 00SH
  Olfactory 00SF
  Optic 00SG
  Peroneal 01SH
  Phrenic 01S2
  Pudendal 01SC
  Radial 01S6
  Sacral 01SR
  Sacral Plexus 01SQ
  Sciatic 01SF
  Thoracic 01S8
  Tibial 01SG
  Trigeminal 00SK
  Trochlear 00SJ
  Ulnar 01S4
  Vagus 00SQ
Nipple
  Left 0HSXXZZ

Reposition *(continued)*
Nipple *(continued)*
   Right 0HSWXZZ
Orbit
   Left 0NSQ
   Right 0NSP
Ovary
  Bilateral 0US2
  Left 0US1
  Right 0US0
Palate
  Hard 0CS2
  Soft 0CS3
Pancreas 0FSG
Parathyroid Gland 0GSR
  Inferior
    Left 0GSP
    Right 0GSN
  Multiple 0GSQ
  Superior
    Left 0GSM
    Right 0GSL
Patella
   Left 0QSF
   Right 0QSD
Phalanx
  Finger
    Left 0PSV
    Right 0PST
  Thumb
    Left 0PSS
    Right 0PSR
  Toe
    Left 0QSR
    Right 0QSQ
Products of Conception 10S0
  Ectopic 10S2
Radius
   Left 0PSJ
   Right 0PSH
Rectum 0DSP
Retinal Vessel
   Left 08SH3ZZ
   Right 08SG3ZZ
Ribs
  1 to 2 0PS1
  3 or More 0PS2
Sacrum 0QS1
Scapula
   Left 0PS6
   Right 0PS5
Septum, Nasal 09SM
Sesamoid Bone(s) 1st Toe
   see Reposition, Metatarsal, Right
    0QSN
   see Reposition, Metatarsal, Left
    0QSP
Skull 0NS0
Spinal Cord
  Cervical 00SW
  Lumbar 00SY
  Thoracic 00SX
Spleen 07SP0ZZ
Sternum 0PS0
Stomach 0DS6
Tarsal
   Left 0QSM
   Right 0QSL
Tendon
  Abdomen
    Left 0LSG
    Right 0LSF
  Ankle
    Left 0LST
    Right 0LSS
  Foot
    Left 0LSW
    Right 0LSV
  Hand
    Left 0LS8
    Right 0LS7

Reposition *(continued)*

Tendon *(continued)*
Head and Neck 0LS0
Hip
Left 0LSK
Right 0LSJ
Knee
Left 0LSR
Right 0LSQ
Lower Arm and
Wrist
Left 0LS6
Right 0LS5
Lower Leg
Left 0LSP
Right 0LSN
Perineum 0LSH
Shoulder
Left 0LS2
Right 0LS1
Thorax
Left 0LSD
Right 0LSC
Trunk
Left 0LSB
Right 0LS9
Upper Arm
Left 0LS4
Right 0LS3
Upper Leg
Left 0LSM
Right 0LSL
Testis
Bilateral 0VSC
Left 0VSB
Right 0VS9
Thymus 07SM0ZZ
Thyroid Gland
Left Lobe 0GSG
Right Lobe
0GSH
Tibia
Left 0QSH
Right 0QSG
Tongue 0CS7
Tooth
Lower 0CSX
Upper 0CSW
Trachea 0BS10ZZ
Turbinate, Nasal 09SL
Tympanic Membrane
Left 09S8
Right 09S7
Ulna
Left 0PSL
Right 0PSK
Ureter
Left 0TS7
Right 0TS6
Ureters, Bilateral
0TS8
Urethra 0TSD
Uterine Supporting Structure
0US4
Uterus 0US9
Uvula 0CSN
Vagina 0USG
Vein
Axillary
Left 05S8
Right 05S7
Azygos 05S0
Basilic
Left 05SC
Right 05SB
Brachial
Left 05SA
Right 05S9
Cephalic
Left 05SF
Right 05SD

Reposition *(continued)*

Vein *(continued)*
Colic 06S7
Common Iliac
Left 06SD
Right 06SC
Esophageal 06S3
External Iliac
Left 06SG
Right 06SF
External Jugular
Left 05SQ
Right 05SP
Face
Left 05SV
Right 05ST
Femoral
Left 06SN
Right 06SM
Foot
Left 06SV
Right 06ST
Gastric 06S2
Hand
Left 05SH
Right 05SG
Hemiazygos 05S1
Hepatic 06S4
Hypogastric
Left 06SJ
Right 06SH
Inferior Mesenteric
06S6
Innominate
Left 05S4
Right 05S3
Internal Jugular
Left 05SN
Right 05SM
Intracranial 05SL
Lower 06SY
Portal 06S8
Pulmonary
Left 02ST0ZZ
Right 02SS0ZZ
Renal
Left 06SB
Right 06S9
Saphenous
Left 06SQ
Right 06SP
Splenic 06S1
Subclavian
Left 05S6
Right 05S5
Superior Mesenteric 06S5
Upper 05SY
Vertebral
Left 05SS
Right 05SR
Vena Cava
Inferior 06S0
Superior 02SV0ZZ
Vertebra
Cervical 0PS3
Magnetically Controlled
Growth Rod(s) XNS3
Lumbar 0QS0
Magnetically Controlled
Growth Rod(s) XNS0
Posterior (Dynamic)
Distraction Device XNS0
Thoracic 0PS4
Magnetically
Controlled Growth Rod(s)
XNS4
Posterior (Dynamic)
Distraction Device XNS4
Vocal Cord
Left 0CSV
Right 0CST

Resection

Acetabulum
Left 0QT50ZZ
Right 0QT40ZZ
Adenoids 0CTQ
Ampulla of Vater 0FTC
Anal Sphincter 0DTR
Anus 0DTQ
Aortic Body 0GTD
Appendix 0DTJ
Auditory Ossicle
Left 09TA
Right 09T9
Bladder 0TTB
Bladder Neck 0TTC
Bone
Ethmoid
Left 0NTG0ZZ
Right 0NTF0ZZ
Frontal 0NT10ZZ
Hyoid 0NTX0ZZ
Lacrimal
Left 0NTJ0ZZ
Right 0NTH0ZZ
Nasal 0NTB0ZZ
Occipital 0NT70ZZ
Palatine
Left 0NTL0ZZ
Right 0NTK0ZZ
Parietal
Left 0NT40ZZ
Right 0NT30ZZ
Pelvic
Left 0QT30ZZ
Right 0QT20ZZ
Sphenoid 0NTC0ZZ
Temporal
Left 0NT60ZZ
Right 0NT50ZZ
Zygomatic
Left 0NTN0ZZ
Right 0NTM0ZZ
Breast
Bilateral 0HTV0ZZ
Left 0HTU0ZZ
Right 0HTT0ZZ
Supernumerary
0HTY0ZZ
Bronchus
Lingula 0BT9
Lower Lobe
Left 0BTB
Right 0BT6
Main
Left 0BT7
Right 0BT3
Middle Lobe, Right
0BT5
Upper Lobe
Left 0BT8
Right 0BT4
Bursa and Ligament
Abdomen
Left 0MTJ
Right 0MTH
Ankle
Left 0MTR
Right 0MTQ
Elbow
Left 0MT4
Right 0MT3
Foot
Left 0MTT
Right 0MTS
Hand
Left 0MT8
Right 0MT7
Head and Neck 0MT0
Hip
Left 0MTM
Right 0MTL

Resection *(continued)*

Bursa and Ligament *(continued)*
Knee
Left 0MTP
Right 0MTN
Lower Extremity
Left 0MTW
Right 0MTV
Perineum 0MTK
Rib(s) 0MTG
Shoulder
Left 0MT2
Right 0MT1
Spine
Lower 0MTD
Upper 0MTC
Sternum 0MTF
Upper Extremity
Left 0MTB
Right 0MT9
Wrist
Left 0MT6
Right 0MT5
Carina 0BT2
Carotid Bodies, Bilateral 0GT8
Carotid Body
Left 0GT6
Right 0GT7
Carpal
Left 0PTN0ZZ
Right 0PTM0ZZ
Cecum 0DTH
Cerebral Hemisphere 00T7
Cervix 0UTC
Chordae Tendineae 02T9
Cisterna Chyli 07TL
Clavicle
Left 0PTB0ZZ
Right 0PT90ZZ
Clitoris 0UTJ
Coccygeal Glomus 0GTB
Coccyx 0QTS0ZZ
Colon
Ascending 0DTK
Descending 0DTM
Sigmoid 0DTN
Transverse 0DTL
Conduction Mechanism 02T8
Cord
Bilateral 0VTH
Left 0VTG
Right 0VTF
Cornea
Left 08T9XZZ
Right 08T8XZZ
Cul-de-sac 0UTF
Diaphragm 0BTT
Disc
Cervical Vertebral 0RT30ZZ
Cervicothoracic Vertebral
0RT50ZZ
Lumbar Vertebral 0ST20ZZ
Lumbosacral 0ST40ZZ
Thoracic Vertebral 0RT90ZZ
Thoracolumbar Vertebral
0RTB0ZZ
Duct
Common Bile 0FT9
Cystic 0FT8
Hepatic
Common 0FT7
Left 0FT6
Right 0FT5
Lacrimal
Left 08TY
Right 08TX
Pancreatic 0FTD
Accessory 0FTF
Parotid
Left 0CTC0ZZ
Right 0CTB0ZZ

Resection *(continued)*
Duodenum 0DT9
Ear
  External
    Left 09T1
    Right 09T0
  Inner
    Left 09TE
    Right 09TD
  Middle
    Left 09T6
    Right 09T5
Epididymis
  Bilateral 0VTL
  Left 0VTK
  Right 0VTJ
Epiglottis 0CTR
Esophagogastric Junction 0DT4
Esophagus 0DT5
  Lower 0DT3
  Middle 0DT2
  Upper 0DT1
Eustachian Tube
  Left 09TG
  Right 09TF
Eye
  Left 08T1XZZ
  Right 08T0XZZ
Eyelid
  Lower
    Left 08TR
    Right 08TQ
  Upper
    Left 08TP
    Right 08TN
Fallopian Tube
  Left 0UT6
  Right 0UT5
Fallopian Tubes, Bilateral 0UT7
Femoral Shaft
  Left 0QT90ZZ
  Right 0QT80ZZ
Femur
  Lower
    Left 0QTC0ZZ
    Right 0QTB0ZZ
  Upper
    Left 0QT70ZZ
    Right 0QT60ZZ
Fibula
  Left 0QTK0ZZ
  Right 0QTJ0ZZ
Finger Nail 0HTQXZZ
Gallbladder 0FT4
Gland
  Adrenal
    Bilateral 0GT4
    Left 0GT2
    Right 0GT3
  Lacrimal
    Left 08TW
    Right 08TV
  Minor Salivary 0CTJ0ZZ
  Parotid
    Left 0CT90ZZ
    Right 0CT80ZZ
  Pituitary 0GT0
  Sublingual
    Left 0CTF0ZZ
    Right 0CTD0ZZ
  Submaxillary
    Left 0CTH0ZZ
    Right 0CTG0ZZ
  Vestibular 0UTL
Glenoid Cavity
  Left 0PT80ZZ
  Right 0PT70ZZ
Glomus Jugulare 0GTC
Humeral Head
  Left 0PTD0ZZ
  Right 0PTC0ZZ

Resection *(continued)*
Humeral Shaft
  Left 0PTG0ZZ
  Right 0PTF0ZZ
Hymen 0UTK
Ileocecal Valve
  0DTC
Ileum 0DTB
Intestine
  Large 0DTE
    Left 0DTG
    Right 0DTF
  Small 0DT8
Iris
  Left 08TD3ZZ
  Right 08TC3ZZ
Jejunum 0DTA
Joint
  Acromioclavicular
    Left 0RTH0ZZ
    Right 0RTG0ZZ
  Ankle
    Left 0STG0ZZ
    Right 0STF0ZZ
  Carpal
    Left 0RTR0ZZ
    Right 0RTQ0ZZ
  Carpometacarpal
    Left 0RTT0ZZ
    Right 0RTS0ZZ
  Cervicothoracic Vertebral
    0RT40ZZ
  Coccygeal
    0ST60ZZ
  Elbow
    Left 0RTM0ZZ
    Right 0RTL0ZZ
  Finger Phalangeal
    Left 0RTX0ZZ
    Right 0RTW0ZZ
  Hip
    Left 0STB0ZZ
    Right 0ST90ZZ
  Knee
    Left 0STD0ZZ
    Right 0STC0ZZ
  Metacarpophalangeal
    Left 0RTV0ZZ
    Right 0RTU0ZZ
  Metatarsal-Phalangeal
    Left 0STN0ZZ
    Right 0STM0ZZ
  Sacrococcygeal
    0ST50ZZ
  Sacroiliac
    Left 0ST80ZZ
    Right 0ST70ZZ
  Shoulder
    Left 0RTK0ZZ
    Right 0RTJ0ZZ
  Sternoclavicular
    Left 0RTF0ZZ
    Right 0RTE0ZZ
  Tarsal
    Left 0STJ0ZZ
    Right 0STH0ZZ
  Tarsometatarsal
    Left 0STL0ZZ
    Right 0STK0ZZ
  Temporomandibular
    Left 0RTD0ZZ
    Right 0RTC0ZZ
  Toe Phalangeal
    Left 0STQ0ZZ
    Right 0STP0ZZ
  Wrist
    Left 0RTP0ZZ
    Right 0RTN0ZZ
Kidney
  Left 0TT1
  Right 0TT0

Resection *(continued)*
Kidney Pelvis
  Left 0TT4
  Right 0TT3
Kidneys, Bilateral
  0TT2
Larynx 0CTS
Lens
  Left 08TK3ZZ
  Right 08TJ3ZZ
Lip
  Lower 0CT1
  Upper 0CT0
Liver 0FT0
  Left Lobe 0FT2
  Right Lobe 0FT1
Lung
  Bilateral 0BTM
  Left 0BTL
  Lower Lobe
    Left 0BTJ
    Right 0BTF
  Middle Lobe, Right 0BTD
  Right 0BTK
  Upper Lobe
    Left 0BTG
    Right 0BTC
Lung Lingula 0BTH
Lymphatic
  Aortic 07TD
  Axillary
    Left 07T6
    Right 07T5
  Head 07T0
  Inguinal
    Left 07TJ
    Right 07TH
  Internal Mammary
    Left 07T9
    Right 07T8
  Lower Extremity
    Left 07TG
    Right 07TF
  Mesenteric 07TB
  Neck
    Left 07T2
    Right 07T1
  Pelvis 07TC
  Thoracic Duct 07TK
  Thorax 07T7
  Upper Extremity
    Left 07T4
    Right 07T3
Mandible
  Left 0NTV0ZZ
  Right 0NTT0ZZ
Maxilla 0NTR0ZZ
Metacarpal
  Left 0PTQ0ZZ
  Right 0PTP0ZZ
Metatarsal
  Left 0QTP0ZZ
  Right 0QTN0ZZ
Muscle
  Abdomen
    Left 0KTL
    Right 0KTK
  Extraocular
    Left 08TM
    Right 08TL
  Facial 0KT1
  Foot
    Left 0KTW
    Right 0KTV
  Hand
    Left 0KTD
    Right 0KTC
  Head 0KT0
  Hip
    Left 0KTP
    Right 0KTN

Resection *(continued)*
Muscle *(continued)*
  Lower Arm and Wrist
    Left 0KTB
    Right 0KT9
  Lower Leg
    Left 0KTT
    Right 0KTS
  Neck
    Left 0KT3
    Right 0KT2
  Papillary 02TD
  Perineum 0KTM
  Shoulder
    Left 0KT6
    Right 0KT5
  Thorax
    Left 0KTJ
    Right 0KTH
  Tongue, Palate, Pharynx
    0KT4
  Trunk
    Left 0KTG
    Right 0KTF
  Upper Arm
    Left 0KT8
    Right 0KT7
  Upper Leg
    Left 0KTR
    Right 0KTQ
Nasal Mucosa and Soft Tissue
  09TK
Nasopharynx 09TN
Nipple
  Left 0HTXXZZ
  Right 0HTWXZZ
Omentum 0DTU
Orbit
  Left 0NTQ0ZZ
  Right 0NTP0ZZ
Ovary
  Bilateral 0UT2
  Left 0UT1
  Right 0UT0
Palate
  Hard 0CT2
  Soft 0CT3
Pancreas 0FTG
Para-aortic Body 0GT9
Paraganglion Extremity 0GTF
Parathyroid Gland 0GTR
  Inferior
    Left 0GTP
    Right 0GTN
  Multiple 0GTQ
  Superior
    Left 0GTM
    Right 0GTL
Patella
  Left 0QTF0ZZ
  Right 0QTD0ZZ
Penis 0VTS
Pericardium 02TN
Phalanx
  Finger
    Left 0PTV0ZZ
    Right 0PTT0ZZ
  Thumb
    Left 0PTS0ZZ
    Right 0PTR0ZZ
  Toe
    Left 0QTR0ZZ
    Right 0QTQ0ZZ
Pharynx 0CTM
Pineal Body 0GT1
Prepuce 0VTT
Products of Conception, Ectopic 10T2
Prostate 0VT0
Radius
  Left 0PTJ0ZZ
  Right 0PTH0ZZ

Resection (continued)
Rectum 0DTP
Ribs
  1 to 2 0PT10ZZ
  3 or More 0PT20ZZ
Scapula
  Left 0PT60ZZ
  Right 0PT50ZZ
Scrotum 0VT5
Septum
  Atrial 02T5
  Nasal 09TM
  Ventricular 02TM
Sinus
  Accessory 09TP
  Ethmoid
    Left 09TV
    Right 09TU
  Frontal
    Left 09TT
    Right 09TS
  Mastoid
    Left 09TC
    Right 09TB
  Maxillary
    Left 09TR
    Right 09TQ
  Sphenoid
    Left 09TX
    Right 09TW
Spleen 07TP
Sternum 0PT00ZZ
Stomach 0DT6
  Pylorus 0DT7
Tarsal
  Left 0QTM0ZZ
  Right 0QTL0ZZ
Tendon
  Abdomen
    Left 0LTG
    Right 0LTF
  Ankle
    Left 0LTT
    Right 0LTS
  Foot
    Left 0LTW
    Right 0LTV
  Hand
    Left 0LT8
    Right 0LT7
  Head and Neck
    0LT0
  Hip
    Left 0LTK
    Right 0LTJ
  Knee
    Left 0LTR
    Right 0LTQ
  Lower Arm and
    Wrist
    Left 0LT6
    Right 0LT5
  Lower Leg
    Left 0LTP
    Right 0LTN
  Perineum 0LTH
  Shoulder
    Left 0LT2
    Right 0LT1
  Thorax
    Left 0LTD
    Right 0LTC
  Trunk
    Left 0LTB
    Right 0LT9
  Upper Arm
    Left 0LT4
    Right 0LT3
  Upper Leg
    Left 0LTM
    Right 0LTL

Resection (continued)
Testis
  Bilateral 0VTC
  Left 0VTB
  Right 0VT9
Thymus 07TM
Thyroid Gland 0GTK
  Left Lobe 0GTG
  Right Lobe 0GTH
Thyroid Gland Isthmus 0GTJ
Tibia
  Left 0QTH0ZZ
  Right 0QTG0ZZ
Toe Nail 0HTRXZZ
Tongue 0CT7
Tonsils 0CTP
Tooth
  Lower 0CTX0Z
  Upper 0CTW0Z
Trachea 0BT1
Tunica Vaginalis
  Left 0VT7
  Right 0VT6
Turbinate, Nasal 09TL
Tympanic Membrane
  Left 09T8
  Right 09T7
Ulna
  Left 0PTL0ZZ
  Right 0PTK0ZZ
Ureter
  Left 0TT7
  Right 0TT6
Urethra 0TTD
Uterine Supporting Structure
  0UT4
Uterus 0UT9
Uvula 0CTN
Vagina 0UTG
Valve, Pulmonary 02TH
Vas Deferens
  Bilateral 0VTQ
  Left 0VTP
  Right 0VTN
Vesicle
  Bilateral 0VT3
  Left 0VT2
  Right 0VT1
Vitreous
  Left 08T53ZZ
  Right 08T43ZZ
Vocal Cord
  Left 0CTV
  Right 0CTT
Vulva 0UTM
Resection, Left ventricular
** outflow tract obstruction**
** (LVOT)**
see Dilation, Ventricle,
  Left 027L
Resection, Subaortic membrane
** (Left ventricular outflow tract**
** obstruction)**
see Dilation, Ventricle, Left 027L
Restoration, Cardiac, Single,
** Rhythm 5A2204Z**
RestoreAdvanced neurostimulator
** (SureScan)(MRI Safe)**
use Stimulator Generator, Multiple
  Array Rechargeable in 0JH
RestoreSensor neurostimulator
** (SureScan)(MRI Safe)**
use Stimulator Generator, Multiple
  Array Rechargeable in 0JH
RestoreUltra neurostimulator
** (SureScan)(MRI Safe)**
use Stimulator Generator, Multiple
  Array Rechargeable in 0JH
Restriction
Ampulla of Vater 0FVC
Anus 0DVQ

Restriction (continued)
Aorta
  Abdominal 04V0
    Intraluminal Device, Branched
      or Fenestrated 04V0
  Thoracic
    Ascending/Arch, Intraluminal
      Device, Branched or
      Fenestrated 02VX
    Descending, Intraluminal
      Device, Branched or
      Fenestrated 02VW
Artery
  Anterior Tibial
    Left 04VQ
    Right 04VP
  Axillary
    Left 03V6
    Right 03V5
  Brachial
    Left 03V8
    Right 03V7
  Celiac 04V1
  Colic
    Left 04V7
    Middle 04V8
    Right 04V6
  Common Carotid
    Left 03VJ
    Right 03VH
  Common Iliac
    Left 04VD
    Right 04VC
  External Carotid
    Left 03VN
    Right 03VM
  External Iliac
    Left 04VJ
    Right, 04VHZ
  Face 03VR
  Femoral
    Left 04VL
    Right 04VK
  Foot
    Left 04VW
    Right 04VV
  Gastric 04V2
  Hand
    Left 03VF
    Right 03VD
  Hepatic 04V3
  Inferior Mesenteric
    04VB
  Innominate 03V2
  Internal Carotid
    Left 03VL
    Right 03VK
  Internal Iliac
    Left 04VF
    Right 04VE
  Internal Mammary
    Left 03V1
    Right 03V0
  Intracranial 03VG
  Lower 04VY
  Peroneal
    Left 04VU
    Right 04VT
  Popliteal
    Left 04VN
    Right 04VM
  Posterior Tibial
    Left 04VS
    Right 04VR
  Pulmonary
    Left 02VR
    Right 02VQ
  Pulmonary Trunk 02VP
  Radial
    Left 03VC
    Right 03VB

Restriction (continued)
Artery (continued)
  Renal
    Left 04VA
    Right 04V9
  Splenic 04V4
  Subclavian
    Left 03V4
    Right 03V3
  Superior Mesenteric 04V5
  Temporal
    Left 03VT
    Right 03VS
  Thyroid
    Left 03VV
    Right 03VU
  Ulnar
    Left 03VA
    Right 03V9
  Upper 03VY
  Vertebral
    Left 03VQ
    Right 03VP
Bladder 0TVB
Bladder Neck 0TVC
Bronchus
  Lingula 0BV9
  Lower Lobe
    Left 0BVB
    Right 0BV6
  Main
    Left 0BV7
    Right 0BV3
  Middle Lobe, Right
    0BV5
  Upper Lobe
    Left 0BV8
    Right 0BV4
Carina 0BV2
Cecum 0DVH
Cervix 0UVC
Cisterna Chyli 07VL
Colon
  Ascending 0DVK
  Descending 0DVM
  Sigmoid 0DVN
  Transverse 0DVL
Duct
  Common Bile
    0FV9
  Cystic 0FV8
  Hepatic
    Common 0FV7
    Left 0FV6
    Right 0FV5
  Lacrimal
    Left 08VY
    Right 08VX
  Pancreatic 0FVD
    Accessory 0FVF
  Parotid
    Left 0CVC
    Right 0CVB
Duodenum 0DV9
Esophagogastric Junction
  0DV4
Esophagus 0DV5
  Lower 0DV3
  Middle 0DV2
  Upper 0DV1
Heart 02VA
Ileocecal Valve 0DVC
Ileum 0DVB
Intestine
  Large 0DVE
    Left 0DVG
    Right 0DVF
  Small 0DV8
Jejunum 0DVA
Kidney Pelvis
  Left 0TV4

Restriction *(continued)*
Kidney Pelvis *(continued)*
Right 0TV3
Lymphatic
Aortic 07VD
Axillary
Left 07V6
Right 07V5
Head 07V0
Inguinal
Left 07VJ
Right 07VH
Internal Mammary
Left 07V9
Right 07V8
Lower Extremity
Left 07VG
Right 07VF
Mesenteric 07VB
Neck
Left 07V2
Right 07V1
Pelvis 07VC
Thoracic Duct 07VK
Thorax 07V7
Upper Extremity
Left 07V4
Right 07V3
Rectum 0DVP
Stomach 0DV6
Pylorus 0DV7
Trachea 0BV1
Ureter
Left 0TV7
Right 0TV6
Urethra 0TVD
Valve, Mitral 02VG
Vein
Axillary
Left 05V8
Right 05V7
Azygos 05V0
Basilic
Left 05VC
Right 05VB
Brachial
Left 05VA
Right 05V9
Cephalic
Left 05VF
Right 05VD
Colic 06V7Z
Common Iliac
Left 06VD
Right 06VC
Esophageal 06V3
External Iliac
Left 06VG
Right 06VF
External Jugular
Left 05VQ
Right 05VP
Face
Left 05VV
Right 05VT
Femoral
Left 06VN
Right 06VM
Foot
Left 06VV
Right 06VT
Gastric 06V2
Hand
Left 05VH
Right 05VG
Hemiazygos 05V1
Hepatic 06V4
Hypogastric
Left 06VJ
Right 06VH

Resuscitation *(continued)*
Vein *(continued)*
Inferior Mesenteric 06V6
Innominate
Left 05V4
Right 05V3
Internal Jugular
Left 05VN
Right 05VM
Intracranial 05VL
Lower 06VY
Portal 06V8
Pulmonary
Left 02VT
Right 02VS
Renal
Left 06VB
Right 06V9
Saphenous
Left 06VQ
Right 06VP
Splenic 06V1
Subclavian
Left 05V6
Right 05V5
Superior Mesenteric 06V5
Upper 05VY
Vertebral
Left 05VS
Right 05VR
Vena Cava
Inferior 06V0
Superior 02VV
Ventricle, Left 02VL
Resurfacing Device
Removal of device from
Left 0SPB0BZ
Right 0SP90BZ
Revision of device in
Left 0SWB0BZ
Right 0SW90BZ
Supplement
Left 0SUB0BZ
Acetabular Surface 0SUE0BZ
Femoral Surface 0SUS0BZ
Right 0SU90BZ
Acetabular Surface 0SUA0BZ
Femoral Surface 0SUR0BZ
Resuscitation
Cardiopulmonary
see Assistance, Cardiac 5A02
Cardioversion 5A2204Z
Defibrillation 5A2204Z
Endotracheal intubation
see Insertion of device in, Trachea 0BH1
External chest compression, manual 5A12012
External chest compression, mechanical 5A1221J
Pulmonary 5A19054
Resuscitative endovascular balloon occlusion of the aorta (REBOA)
02LW3DJ
04L03DJ
Resuture, Heart valve prosthesis
see Revision of device in, Heart and Great Vessels 02W
Retained placenta, manual removal
see Extraction, Products of Conception, Retained 10D1
RETHYMIC® *use* Engineered Allogeneic Thymus Tissue
Retraining
Cardiac
see Motor Treatment, Rehabilitation F07
Vocational
see Activities of Daily Living Treatment, Rehabilitation F08

Retrogasserian rhizotomy
see Division, Nerve, Trigeminal 008K
Retroperitoneal cavity
use Retroperitoneum
Retroperitoneal lymph node
use Lymphatic, Aortic
Retroperitoneal space
use Retroperitoneum
Retropharyngeal lymph node
use Lymphatic, Neck, Left
use Lymphatic, Neck, Right
Retropharyngeal space *use* Neck
Retropubic space
use Pelvic Cavity
Reveal (LINQ) (DX)(XT)
use Monitoring Device
Reverse® Shoulder Prosthesis
use Synthetic Substitute, Reverse Ball and Socket in 0RR
Reverse total shoulder replacement
see Replacement, Upper Joints 0RR
Revision
Correcting a portion of existing device
see Revision of device in
Removal of device without replacement
see Removal of device from
Replacement of existing device
see Removal of device from
see Root operation to place new device, e.g., Insertion, Replacement, Supplement
Revision of device in
Abdominal Wall 0WWF
Acetabulum
Left 0QW5
Right 0QW4
Anal Sphincter 0DWR
Anus 0DWQ
Aorta, Thoracic, Descending 02WW3RZ
Artery
Lower 04WY
Upper 03WYM
Auditory Ossicle
Left 09WA
Right 09W9
Back
Lower 0WWL
Upper 0WWK
Bladder 0TWB
Bone
Facial 0NWW
Lower 0QWY
Nasal 0NWB
Pelvic
Left 0QW3
Right 0QW2
Upper 0PWY
Bone Marrow 07WT
Brain 00W0
Breast
Left 0HWU
Right 0HWT
Bursa and Ligament
Lower 0MWY
Upper 0MWX
Carpal
Left 0PWN
Right 0PWM
Cavity, Cranial 0WW1
Cerebral Ventricle 00W6
Chest Wall 0WW8
Cisterna Chyli 07WL
Clavicle
Left 0PWB
Right 0PW9
Coccyx 0QWS
Diaphragm 0BWTM

Revision of device in *(continued)*
Disc
Cervical Vertebral 0RW3
Cervicothoracic Vertebral 0RW5
Lumbar Vertebral 0SW2
Lumbosacral 0SW4
Thoracic Vertebral 0RW9
Thoracolumbar Vertebral 0RWB
Duct
Hepatobiliary 0FWB
Pancreatic 0FWD
Ear
Inner
Left 09WE
Right 09WD
Left 09WJ
Right 09WH
Epididymis and Spermatic Cord 0VWM
Esophagus 0DW5D
Extremity
Lower
Left 0YWB
Right 0YW9
Upper
Left 0XW7
Right 0XW6
Eye
Left 08W1
Right 08W0
Face 0WW2
Fallopian Tube 0UW8
Femoral Shaft
Left 0QW9
Right 0QW8
Femur
Lower
Left 0QWC
Right 0QWB
Upper
Left 0QW7
Right 0QW6
Fibula
Left 0QWK
Right 0QWJ
Finger Nail 0HWQX
Gallbladder 0FW4
Gastrointestinal Tract 0WWP
Genitourinary Tract 0WWR
Gland
Adrenal 0GW50
Endocrine 0GWS
Pituitary 0GW00
Salivary 0CWA
Glenoid Cavity
Left 0PW8
Right 0PW7
Great Vessel 02WY
Hair 0HWSX
Head 0WW0
Heart 02WA
Humeral Head
Left 0PWD
Right 0PWC
Humeral Shaft
Left 0PWG
Right 0PWF
Intestinal Tract
Lower Intestinal Tract 0DWD
Upper Intestinal Tract 0DW0
Intestine
Large 0DWE
Small 0DW8
Jaw
Lower 0WW5
Upper 0WW4

Revision of device in *(continued)*
Joint
  Acromioclavicular
    Left 0RWH
    Right 0RWG
  Ankle
    Left 0SWG
    Right 0SWF
  Carpal
    Left 0RWR
    Right 0RWQ
  Carpometacarpal
    Left 0RWT
    Right 0RWS
  Cervical Vertebral 0RW1
  Cervicothoracic Vertebral
    0RW4
  Coccygeal 0SW6
  Elbow
    Left 0RWM
    Right 0RWL
  Finger Phalangeal
    Left 0RWX
    Right 0RWW
  Hip
    Left 0SWB
      Acetabluar Surface 0SWE
      Femoral Surface 0SWS
    Right 0SW9
      Acetabluar Surface 0SWA
      Femoral Surface 0SWR
  Knee
    Left 0SWD
      Femoral Surface 0SWU
      Tibial Surface 0SWW
    Right 0SWC
      Femoral Surface 0SWT
      Tibial Surface 0SWV
  Lumbar Vertebral 0SW0
  Lumbosacral 0SW3
  Metacarpophalangeal
    Left 0RWV
    Right 0RWU
  Metatarsal-Phalangeal
    Left 0SWN
    Right 0SWM
  Occipital-cervical 0RW0
  Sacrococcygeal 0SW5
  Sacroiliac
    Left 0SW8
    Right 0SW7
  Shoulder
    Left 0RWK
    Right 0RWJ
  Sternoclavicular
    Left 0RWF
    Right 0RWE
  Tarsal
    Left 0SWJ
    Right 0SWH
  Tarsometatarsal
    Left 0SWL
    Right 0SWK
  Temporomandibular
    Left 0RWD
    Right 0RWC
  Thoracic Vertebral 0RW6
  Thoracolumbar Vertebral
    0RWA
  Toe Phalangeal
    Left 0SWQ
    Right 0SWP
  Wrist
    Left 0RWP
    Right 0RWN
Kidney 0TW5
Larynx 0CWS
Lens
  Left 08WKJ
  Right 08WJ
Liver 0FW0

Revision of device in *(continued)*
Lung
  Left 0BWL
  Right 0BWK
Lymphatic 07WN
  Thoracic Duct 07WK
Mediastinum 0WWC
Mesentery 0DWV
Metacarpal
  Left 0PWQ
  Right 0PWP
Metatarsal
  Left 0QWP
  Right 0QWN
Mouth and Throat 0CWY
Muscle
  Extraocular
    Left 08WM
    Right 08WL
  Lower 0KWY
  Upper 0KWX
Nasal Mucosa and Soft Tissue
  09WK
Neck 0WW6
Nerve
  Cranial 00WE
  Peripheral 01WY
Omentum 0DWU
Ovary 0UW3
Pancreas 0FWG
Parathyroid Gland 0GWR
Patella
  Left 0QWF
  Right 0QWD
Pelvic Cavity 0WWJ
Penis 0VWS
Pericardial Cavity 0WWD
Perineum
  Female 0WWN
  Male 0WWM
Peritoneal Cavity 0WWG
Peritoneum 0DWW
Phalanx
  Finger
    Left 0PWV
    Right 0PWT
  Thumb
    Left 0PWS
    Right 0PWR
  Toe
    Left 0QWR
    Right 0QWQ
Pineal Body 0GW10
Pleura 0BWQ
Pleural Cavity
  Left 0WWB
  Right 0WW9
Prostate and Seminal Vesicles
  0VW4
Radius
  Left 0PWJ
  Right 0PWH
Respiratory Tract 0WWQ
Retroperitoneum 0WWH
Ribs
  1 to 2 0PW1
  3 or More 0PW2
Sacrum 0QW1
Scapula
  Left 0PW6
  Right 0PW5
Scrotum and Tunica Vaginalis
  0VW8
Septum
  Atrial 02W5
  Ventricular 02WM
Sinus 09WY0
Skin 0HWPX
Skull 0NW0
Spinal Canal 00WU
Spinal Cord 00WV

Revision of device in *(continued)*
Spleen 07WP
Sternum 0PW0
Stomach 0DW6
Subcutaneous Tissue
  and Fascia
    Head and Neck 0JWS
    Lower Extremity 0JWW
    Trunk 0JWT
    Upper Extremity 0JWV
Tarsal
  Left 0QWM
  Right 0QWL
Tendon
  Lower 0LWY
  Upper 0LWX
Testis 0VWD
Thymus 07WM
Thyroid Gland 0GWK0
Tibia
  Left 0QWH
  Right 0QWG
Toe Nail 0HWRX
Trachea 0BW1F
Tracheobronchial Tree
  0BW0
Tympanic Membrane
  Left 09W8
  Right 09W7
Ulna
  Left 0PWL
  Right 0PWK
Ureter 0TW9M
Urethra 0TWD
Uterus and Cervix
  0UWD
Vagina and Cul-de-sac 0UWH
Valve
  Aortic 02WF
  Mitral 02WG
  Pulmonary 02WH
  Tricuspid 02WJ
Vas Deferens 0VWR
Vein
  Azygos 05W0
  Innominate
    Left 05W4
    Right 05W3
  Lower 06WY
  Upper 05WY
Vertebra
  Cervical 0PW3
  Lumbar 0QW0
  Thoracic 0PW4
Vulva 0UWM
Revo MRI™ SureScan®
  pacemaker
  use Pacemaker, Dual Chamber
    in 0JH
Rezafungin XW0
rhBMP-2
  use Recombinant Bone
    Morphogenetic Protein
Rheos® System device
  use Stimulator Generator in
    Subcutaneous Tissue and
    Fascia
Rheos® System lead
  use Stimulator Lead in Upper
    Arteries
Rhinopharynx
  use Nasopharynx
Rhinoplasty
  see Alteration, Nasal Mucosa and
    Soft Tissue 090K
  see Repair, Nasal Mucosa and Soft
    Tissue 09QK
  see Replacement, Nasal Mucosa and
    Soft Tissue 09RK
  see Supplement, Nasal Mucosa and
    Soft Tissue 09UK

Rhinorrhaphy
  see Repair, Nasal Mucosa and Soft
    Tissue 09QK
Rhinoscopy 09JKXZZ
Rhizotomy
  see Division, Central Nervous
    System and Cranial Nerves 008
  see Division, Peripheral Nervous
    System 018
Rhomboid major muscle
  use Muscle, Trunk, Left
  use Muscle, Trunk, Right
Rhomboid minor muscle
  use Muscle, Trunk, Left
  use Muscle, Trunk, Right
Rhythm electrocardiogram
  see Measurement, Cardiac 4A02
Rhytidectomy
  see Alteration, Face 0W02
Right ascending lumbar vein
  use Vein, Azygos
Right atrioventricular valve
  use Valve, Tricuspid
Right auricular appendix
  use Atrium, Right
Right colic vein
  use Vein, Colic
Right coronary sulcus
  use Heart, Right
Right gastric artery
  use Artery, Gastric
Right gastroepiploic vein
  use Vein, Superior Mesenteric
Right inferior phrenic vein
  use Vena Cava, Inferior
Right inferior pulmonary vein
  use Vein, Pulmonary, Right
Right jugular trunk
  use Lymphatic, Neck, Right
Right lateral ventricle
  use Cerebral Ventricle
Right lymphatic duct
  use Lymphatic, Neck, Right
Right ovarian vein
  use Vena Cava, Inferior
Right second lumbar vein
  use Vena Cava, Inferior
Right subclavian trunk
  use Lymphatic, Neck, Right
Right subcostal vein
  use Vein, Azygos
Right superior pulmonary vein
  use Vein, Pulmonary, Right
Right suprarenal vein
  use Vena Cava, Inferior
Right testicular vein
  use Vena Cava, Inferior
Rima glottidis
  use Larynx
Risorius muscle
  use Muscle, Facial
RNS System lead
  use Neurostimulator Lead in Central
    Nervous System and Cranial
    Nerves
RNS system neurostimulator
  generator
  use Neurostimulator Generator in
    Head and Facial Bones
Robotic Assisted Procedure
  Extremity
    Lower 8E0Y
    Upper 8E0X
  Head and Neck Region 8E09
  Trunk Region 8E0W
Rotation of fetal head
  Forceps 10S07ZZ
  Manual 10S0XZZ
Round ligament of uterus
  use Uterine Supporting Structure

Round window
use Ear, Inner, Left
use Ear, Inner, Right
Roux-en-Y operation
see Bypass, Gastrointestinal System 0D1
see Bypass, Hepatobiliary System and Pancreas 0F1
Rupture
Adhesions
see Release
Fluid collection
see Drainage
Ruxolitinib XW0DXT5
RYBREVANT™ *use* Amivantamab Monoclonal Antibody

S

S-ICD™ lead
use SubcutaneousDifibrillator Lead in Subcutaneous Tissue and Fascia
Sabizabulin XW0
Sacral ganglion
use Nerve, Sacral Sympathetic
Sacral lymph node
use Lymphatic, Pelvis
Sacral nerve modulation (SNM) lead
use Stimulator Lead in Urinary System
Sacral neuromodulation lead
use Stimulator Lead in Urinary System
Sacral splanchnic nerve
use Nerve, Sacral Sympathetic
Sacrectomy
see Excision, Lower Bones 0QB
Sacrococcygeal ligament
use Bursa and Ligament, Lower Spine
Sacrococcygeal symphysis
use Joint, Sacrococcygeal
Sacroiliac ligament
use Bursa and Ligament, Lower Spine
Sacrospinous ligament
use Bursa and Ligament, Lower Spine
Sacrotuberous ligament
use Bursa and Ligament, Lower Spine
Salpingectomy
see Excision, Female Reproductive System 0UB
see Resection, Female Reproductive System 0UT
Salpingolysis
see Release, Female Reproductive System 0UN
Salpingopexy
see Repair, Female Reproductive System 0UQ
see Reposition, Female Reproductive System 0US
Salpingopharyngeus muscle
use Muscle, Tongue, Palate, Pharynx
Salpingoplasty
see Repair, Female Reproductive System 0UQ
see Supplement, Female Reproductive System 0UU
Salpingorrhaphy
see Repair, Female Reproductive System 0UQ
Salpingoscopy 0UJ88ZZ
Salpingostomy
see Drainage, Female Reproductive System 0U9
Salpingotomy
see Drainage, Female Reproductive System 0U9

Salpinx
use Fallopian Tube, Left
use Fallopian Tube, Right
Saphenous nerve
use Nerve, Femoral
SAPIEN transcatheter aortic valve
use Zooplastic Tissue in Heart and Great Vessels
Sarilumab XW0
SARS-CoV-2 Antibody Detection, Serum/Plasma Nanoparticle Fluorescence XXE5XV7
SARS-CoV-2 Polymerase Chain Reaction, Nasopharyngeal Fluid XXE97U7
Sartorius muscle
use Muscle, Upper Leg, Left
use Muscle, Upper Leg, Right
Satralizumab-mwge XW01397
SAVAL below-the-knee (BTK) drug-eluting stent system
use Intraluminal Device, Sustained Release Drug-eluting in New Technology
use Intraluminal Device, Sustained Release Drug-eluting, Four or More in New Technology
use Intraluminal Device, Sustained Release Drug-eluting, Three in New Technology
use Intraluminal Device, Sustained Release Drug-eluting, Two in New Technology
Scalene muscle
use Muscle, Neck, Left
use Muscle, Neck, Right
Scan
Computerized Tomography (CT)
see Computerized Tomography (CT Scan)
Radioisotope
see Planar Nuclear Medicine Imaging
Scaphoid bone
use Carpal, Left
use Carpal, Right
Scapholunate ligament
use Bursa and Ligament, Wrist, Left
use Bursa and Ligament, Wrist, Right
Scaphotrapezium ligament
use Bursa and Ligament, Hand, Left
use Bursa and Ligament, Hand, Right
Scapulectomy
see Excision, Upper Bones 0PB
see Resection, Upper Bones 0PT
Scapulopexy
see Repair, Upper Bones 0PQ
see Reposition, Upper Bones 0PS
Scarpa's (vestibular) ganglion
use Nerve, Acoustic
Sclerectomy
see Excision, Eye 08B
Sclerotherapy, mechanical
see Destruction
Sclerotherapy, via injection of sclerosing agent
see Introduction, Destructive Agent
Sclerotomy
see Drainage, Eye 089
Scrotectomy
see Excision, Male Reproductive System 0VB
see Resection, Male Reproductive System 0VT
Scrotoplasty
see Repair, Male Reproductive System 0VQ
see Supplement, Male Reproductive System 0VU

Scrotorrhaphy
see Repair, Male Reproductive System 0VQ
Scrototomy
see Drainage, Male Reproductive System 0V9
Sebaceous gland
use Skin
Second cranial nerve
use Nerve, Optic
Section, cesarean
see Extraction, Pregnancy 10D
Secura (DR) (VR)
use Defibrillator Generator in 0JH
Sella Turcica
use Bone, Sphenoid
Selux Rapid AST Platform XXE5XY9
Semicircular canal
use Ear, Inner, Left
use Ear, Inner, Right
Semimembranosus muscle
use Muscle, Upper Leg, Left
use Muscle, Upper Leg, Right
Semitendinosus muscle
use Muscle, Upper Leg, Left
use Muscle, Upper Leg, Right
Sentinel™ Cerebral Protection System (CPS) X2A5312
Seprafilm
use Adhesion Barrier
Septal cartilage
use Septum, Nasal
Septectomy
see Excision, Ear, Nose, Sinus 09B
see Excision, Heart and Great Vessels 02B
see Resection, Ear, Nose, Sinus 09T
see Resection, Heart and Great Vessels 02T
SeptiCyte® RAPID XXE5X38
Septoplasty
see Repair, Ear, Nose, Sinus 09Q
see Repair, Heart and Great Vessels 02Q
see Replacement, Ear, Nose, Sinus 09R
see Replacement, Heart and Great Vessels 02R
see Reposition, Ear, Nose, Sinus 09S
see Supplement, Ear, Nose, Sinus 09U
see Supplement, Heart and Great Vessels 02U
Septostomy, balloon atrial 02163Z7
Septotomy
see Drainage, Ear, Nose, Sinus 099
Sequestrectomy, bone
see Extirpation
SER-109 XW0DXN9
Serratus anterior muscle
use Muscle, Thorax, Left
use Muscle, Thorax, Right
Serratus posterior muscle
use Muscle, Trunk, Left
use Muscle, Trunk, Right
Seventh cranial nerve
use Nerve, Facial
Sheffield hybrid external fixator
use External Fixation Device, Hybrid in 0PH
use External Fixation Device, Hybrid in 0PS
use External Fixation Device, Hybrid in 0QH
use External Fixation Device, Hybrid in 0QS
Sheffield ring external fixator
use External Fixation Device, Ring in 0PH

use External Fixation Device, Ring in 0PS
use External Fixation Device, Ring in 0QH
use External Fixation Device, Ring in 0QS
Shirodkar cervical cerclage 0UVC7ZZ
Shockwave Intravascular Lithotripsy (Shockwave IVL)
see Fragmentation
Shock Wave Therapy, Musculoskeletal 6A93
Short gastric artery
use Artery, Splenic
Shortening
see Excision
see Repair
see Reposition
Shunt creation
see Bypass
Sialoadenectomy
Complete
see Resection, Mouth and Throat 0CT
Partial
see Excision, Mouth and Throat 0CB
Sialodochoplasty
see Repair, Mouth and Throat 0CQ
see Replacement, Mouth and Throat 0CR
see Supplement, Mouth and Throat 0CU
Sialoectomy
see Excision, Mouth and Throat 0CB
see Resection, Mouth and Throat 0CT
Sialography
see Plain Radiography, Ear, Nose, Mouth and Throat B90
Sialolithotomy
see Extirpation, Mouth and Throat 0CC
Sigmoid artery
use Artery, Inferior Mesenteric
Sigmoid flexure
use Colon, Sigmoid
Sigmoid vein
use Vein, Inferior Mesenteric
Sigmoidectomy
see Excision, Gastrointestinal System 0DB
see Resection, Gastrointestinal System 0DT
Sigmoidorrhaphy
see Repair, Gastrointestinal System 0DQ
Sigmoidoscopy 0DJD8ZZ
Sigmoidotomy
see Drainage, Gastrointestinal System 0D9
Single lead pacemaker (atrium) (ventricle)
use Pacemaker, Single Chamber in 0JH
Single lead rate responsive pacemaker (atrium)(ventricle)
use Pacemaker, Single Chamber Rate Responsive in 0JH
Single-use Duodenoscope XFJ
Single-use Oversleeve with Intraoperative Colonic Irrigation XDPH8K7
Sinoatrial node
use Conduction Mechanism
Sinogram
Abdominal Wall
see Fluoroscopy, Abdomen and Pelvis BW11

Sinogram *(continued)*
 Chest Wall
  see Plain Radiography, Chest
   BW03
 Retroperitoneum
  see Fluoroscopy, Abdomen and
   Pelvis BW11
Sinusectomy
 see Excision, Ear, Nose, Sinus 09B
 see Resection, Ear, Nose, Sinus 09T
Sinusoscopy 09JY4ZZ
Sinusotomy
 see Drainage, Ear, Nose, Sinus 099
Sinus venosus
 use Atrium, Right
Sirolimus-eluting coronary stent
 use Intraluminal Device, Drug-
  eluting in Heart and Great
  Vessels
Sixth cranial nerve
 use Nerve, Abducens
Size reduction, breast
 see Excision, Skin and Breast 0HB
SJM Biocor® Stented Valve
 System
 use Zooplastic Tissue in Heart and
  Great Vessels
Skene's (paraurethral) gland
 use Gland, Vestibular
Sling
 Fascial, orbicularis muscle
  (mouth)
  see Supplement, Muscle, Facial
   0KU1
 Levator muscle, for urethral
  suspension
  see Reposition, Bladder Neck
   0TSC
 Pubococcygeal, for urethral
  suspension
  see Reposition, Bladder Neck
   0TSC
 Rectum
  see Reposition, Rectum 0DSP
Small bowel series
 see Fluoroscopy, Bowel, Small
  BD13
Small saphenous vein
 use Vein, Saphenous, Left
 use Vein, Saphenous, Right
Snapshot_NIR 8E02XDZ
Snaring, polyp, colon
 see Excision, Gastrointestinal
  System 0DB
Solar (celiac) plexus
 use Nerve, Abdominal Sympathetic
Soleus muscle
 use Muscle, Lower Leg, Left
 use Muscle, Lower Leg, Right
Soliris®
 see Eculizumab
Space of Retzius
 use Pelvic Cavity
Spacer
 Insertion of device in
  Disc
   Lumbar Vertebral 0SH2
   Lumbosacral 0SH4
  Joint
   Acromioclavicular
    Left 0RHH
    Right 0RHG
   Ankle
    Left 0SHG
    Right 0SHF
   Carpal
    Left 0RHR
    Right 0RHQ
   Carpometacarpal
    Left 0RHT
    Right 0RHS

Spacer *(continued)*
 Insertion of device in *(continued)*
  Joint *(continued)*
   Cervical Vertebral 0RH1
   Cervicothoracic Vertebral
    0RH4
   Coccygeal 0SH6
   Elbow
    Left 0RHM
    Right 0RHL
   Finger Phalangeal
    Left 0RHX
    Right 0RHW
   Hip
    Left 0SHB
    Right 0SH9
   Knee
    Left 0SHD
    Right 0SHC
   Lumbar Vertebral 0SH0
   Lumbosacral 0SH3
   Metacarpophalangeal
    Left 0RHV
    Right 0RHU
   Metatarsal-Phalangeal
    Left 0SHN
    Right 0SHM
   Occipital-cervical 0RH0
   Sacrococcygeal 0SH5
   Sacroiliac
    Left 0SH8
    Right 0SH7
   Shoulder
    Left 0RHK
    Right 0RHJ
   Sternoclavicular
    Left 0RHF
    Right 0RHE
   Tarsal
    Left 0SHJ
    Right 0SHH
   Tarsometatarsal
    Left 0SHL
    Right 0SHK
   Temporomandibular
    Left 0RHD
    Right 0RHC
   Thoracic Vertebral 0RH6
   Thoracolumbar Vertebral
    0RHA
   Toe Phalangeal
    Left 0SHQ
    Right 0SHP
   Wrist
    Left 0RHP
    Right 0RHN
 Removal of device from
  Acromioclavicular
   Left 0RPH
   Right 0RPG
  Ankle
   Left 0SPG
   Right 0SPF
  Carpal
   Left 0RPR
   Right 0RPQ
  Carpometacarpal
   Left 0RPT
   Right 0RPS
  Cervical Vertebral 0RP1
  Cervicothoracic Vertebral 0RP4
  Coccygeal 0SP6
  Elbow
   Left 0RPM
   Right 0RPL
  Finger Phalangeal
   Left 0RPX
   Right 0RPW
  Hip
   Left 0SPB
   Right 0SP9

Spacer *(continued)*
 Removal of device from *(continued)*
  Knee
   Left 0SPD
   Right 0SPC
  Lumbar Vertebral 0SP0
  Lumbosacral 0SP3
  Metacarpophalangeal
   Left 0RPV
   Right 0RPU
  Metatarsal-Phalangeal
   Left 0SPN
   Right 0SPM
  Occipital-cervical 0RP0
  Sacrococcygeal 0SP5
  Sacroiliac
   Left 0SP8
   Right 0SP7
  Shoulder
   Left 0RPK
   Right 0RPJ
  Sternoclavicular
   Left 0RPF
   Right 0RPE
  Tarsal
   Left 0SPJ
   Right 0SPH
  Tarsometatarsal
   Left 0SPL
   Right 0SPK
  Temporomandibular
   Left 0RPD
   Right 0RPC
  Thoracic Vertebral 0RP6
  Thoracolumbar Vertebral
   0RPA
  Toe Phalangeal
   Left 0SPQ
   Right 0SPP
  Wrist
   Left 0RPP
   Right 0RPN
 Revision of device in
  Acromioclavicular
   Left 0RWH
   Right 0RWG
  Ankle
   Left 0SWG
   Right 0SWF
  Carpal
   Left 0RWR
   Right 0RWQ
  Carpometacarpal
   Left 0RWT
   Right 0RWS
  Cervical Vertebral 0RW1
  Cervicothoracic Vertebral
   0RW4
  Coccygeal 0SW6
  Elbow
   Left 0RWM
   Right 0RWL
  Finger Phalangeal
   Left 0RWX
   Right 0RWW
  Hip
   Left 0SWB
   Right 0SW9
  Knee
   Left 0SWD
   Right 0SWC
  Lumbar Vertebral 0SW0
  Lumbosacral 0SW3
  Metacarpophalangeal
   Left 0RWV
   Right 0RWU
  Metatarsal-Phalangeal
   Left 0SWN
   Right 0SWM
  Occipital-cervical 0RW0
  Sacrococcygeal 0SW5

Spacer *(continued)*
 Revision of device in *(continued)*
  Sacroiliac
   Left 0SW8
   Right 0SW7
  Shoulder
   Left 0RWK
   Right 0RWJ
  Sternoclavicular
   Left 0RWF
   Right 0RWE
  Tarsal
   Left 0SWJ
   Right 0SWH
  Tarsometatarsal
   Left 0SWL
   Right 0SWK
  Temporomandibular
   Left 0RWD
   Right 0RWC
  Thoracic Vertebral 0RW6
  Thoracolumbar Vertebral 0RWA
  Toe Phalangeal
   Left 0SWQ
   Right 0SWP
  Wrist
   Left 0RWP
   Right 0RWN
Spacer, Articulating (Antibiotic)
 use Articulating Spacer in Lower
  Joints
Spacer, Static (Antibiotic)
 use Spacer in Lower Joints
Spectroscopy
 Intravascular Near Infrared 8E023DZ
 Near Infrared
  see Physiological Systems and
   Anatomical Regions 8E0
Speech Assessment F00
Speech therapy
 see Speech Treatment,
  Rehabilitation F06
Speech Treatment F06
Spesolimab Monoclonal Antibody XW0
Sphenoidectomy
 see Excision, Ear, Nose, Sinus 09B
 see Excision, Head and Facial
  Bones 0NB
 see Resection, Ear, Nose, Sinus 09T
 see Resection, Head and Facial
  Bones 0NT
Sphenoidotomy
 see Drainage, Ear, Nose, Sinus 099
Sphenomandibular ligament
 use Bursa and Ligament, Head and
  Neck
Sphenopalatine (pterygopalatine)
 ganglion
 use Nerve, Head and Neck
  Sympathetic
Sphincterorrhaphy, anal
 see Repair, Anal Sphincter 0DQR
Sphincterotomy, anal
 see Division, Anal Sphincter 0D8R
 see Drainage, Anal Sphincter 0D9R
SPIKEVAX™
 use COVID-19 Vaccine
 use COVID-19 Vaccine Booster
 use COVID-19 Vaccine Dose 1
 use COVID-19 Vaccine Dose 2
 use COVID-19 Vaccine Dose 3
Spinal cord neurostimulator lead
 use Neurostimulator Lead in Central
  Nervous System and Cranial
  Nerves
Spinal growth rod(s), magnetically
 controlled
 use Magnetically Controlled Growth
  Rod(s) in New Technology
Spinal nerve, cervical
 use Nerve, Cervical

Spinal nerve, lumbar
  use Nerve, Lumbar
Spinal nerve, sacral
  use Nerve, Sacral
Spinal nerve, thoracic
  use Nerve, Thoracic
Spinal Stabilization Device
  Facet Replacement
    Cervical Vertebral 0RH1
    Cervicothoracic Vertebral 0RH4
    Lumbar Vertebral 0SH0
    Lumbosacral 0SH3
    Occipital-cervical 0RH0
    Thoracic Vertebral 0RH6
    Thoracolumbar Vertebral 0RHA
  Interspinous Process
    Cervical Vertebral 0RH1
    Cervicothoracic Vertebral 0RH4
    Lumbar Vertebral 0SH0
    Lumbosacral 0SH3
    Occipital-cervical 0RH0
    Thoracic Vertebral 0RH6
    Thoracolumbar Vertebral 0RHA
  Pedicle-Based
    Cervical Vertebral 0RH1
    Cervicothoracic Vertebral 0RH4
    Lumbar Vertebral 0SH0
    Lumbosacral 0SH3
    Occipital-cervical 0RH0
    Thoracic Vertebral 0RH6
    Thoracolumbar Vertebral 0RHA
SpineJack® system
  use Synthetic Substitute,
    Mechanically Expandable
    (Paired) in New Technology
Spinous process
  use Vertebra, Cervical
  use Vertebra, Lumbar
  use Vertebra, Thoracic
Spiral ganglion
  use Nerve, Acoustic
Spiration IBV™ Valve System
  use Intraluminal Device,
    Endobronchial Valve in
    Respiratory System
Splenectomy
  see Excision, Lymphatic and Hemic
    Systems 07B
  see Resection, Lymphatic and
    Hemic Systems 07T
Splenic flexure
  use Colon, Transverse
Splenic plexus
  use Nerve, Abdominal Sympathetic
Splenius capitis muscle
  use Muscle, Head
Splenius cervicis muscle
  use Muscle, Neck, Left
  use Muscle, Neck, Right
Splenolysis
  see Release, Lymphatic and Hemic
    Systems 07N
Splenopexy
  see Repair, Lymphatic and Hemic
    Systems 07Q
  see Reposition, Lymphatic and
    Hemic Systems 07S
Splenoplasty
  see Repair, Lymphatic and Hemic
    Systems 07Q
Splenorrhaphy
  see Repair, Lymphatic and Hemic
    Systems 07Q
Splenotomy
  see Drainage, Lymphatic and Hemic
    Systems 079
Splinting, musculoskeletal
  see Immobilization, Anatomical
    Regions 2W3
SPRAVATO™
  use Esketamine Hydrochloride

SPY system intravascular
  fluorescence angiography
  see Monitoring, Physiological
    Systems 4A1
SPY PINPOINT fluorescence
  imaging system
  see Monitoring, Physiological
    Systems 4A1
  see Other Imaging, Hepatobiliary
    System and Pancreas BF5
SPY system intraoperative
  fluorescence cholangiography
  see Other Imaging, Hepatobiliary
    System and Pancreas BF5
SSO2 (Supersaturated Oxygen)
  therapy, cardiac intra-arterial
  5A0222C
Staged hepatectomy
  see Division, Hepatobiliary System
    and Pancreas 0F8
  see Resection, Hepatobiliary
    System and Pancreas 0FT
Stapedectomy
  see Excision, Ear, Nose, Sinus
    09B
  see Resection, Ear, Nose, Sinus
    09T
Stapediolysis
  see Release, Ear, Nose, Sinus 09N
Stapedioplasty
  see Repair, Ear, Nose, Sinus 09Q
  see Replacement, Ear, Nose, Sinus
    09R
  see Supplement, Ear, Nose, Sinus 09U
Stapedotomy
  see Drainage, Ear, Nose, Sinus 099
Stapes
  use Auditory Ossicle, Left
  use Auditory Ossicle, Right
Static Spacer (Antibiotic)
  use Spacer in Lower Joints
STELARA®
  use Other New Technology
    Therapeutic Substance
Stellate ganglion
  use Nerve, Head and Neck
    Sympathetic
Stem cell transplant
  see Transfusion, Circulatory 302
Stensen's duct
  use Duct, Parotid, Left
  use Duct, Parotid, Right
Stent retriever thrombectomy
  see Extirpation, Upper Arteries 03C
Stent, intraluminal (cardiovascular)
  (gastrointestinal)(hepatobiliary)
  (urinary)
  use Intraluminal Device
Stented tissue valve
  use Zooplastic Tissue in Heart and
    Great Vessels
Stereotactic Radiosurgery
  Abdomen DW23
  Adrenal Gland DG22
  Bile Ducts DF22
  Bladder DT22
  Bone Marrow D720
  Brain D020
  Brain Stem D021
  Breast
    Left DM20
    Right DM21
  Bronchus DB21
  Cervix DU21
  Chest DW22
  Chest Wall DB27
  Colon DD25
  Diaphragm DB28
  Duodenum DD22
  Ear D920
  Esophagus DD20

Stereotactic
  Radiosurgery (continued)
  Eye D820
  Gallbladder DF21
  Gamma Beam
    Abdomen DW23JZZ
    Adrenal Gland DG22JZZ
    Bile Ducts DF22JZZ
    Bladder DT22JZZ
    Bone Marrow D720JZZ
    Brain D020JZZ
    Brain Stem D021JZZ
    Breast
      Left DM20JZZ
      Right DM21JZZ
    Bronchus DB21JZZ
    Cervix DU21JZZ
    Chest DW22JZZ
    Chest Wall DB27JZZ
    Colon DD25JZZ
    Diaphragm DB28JZZ
    Duodenum DD22JZZ
    Ear D920JZZ
    Esophagus DD20JZZ
    Eye D820JZZ
    Gallbladder DF21JZZ
    Gland
      Adrenal DG22JZZ
      Parathyroid DG24JZZ
      Pituitary DG20JZZ
      Thyroid DG25JZZ
    Glands, Salivary D926JZZ
    Head and Neck DW21JZZ
    Ileum DD24JZZ
    Jejunum DD23JZZ
    Kidney DT20JZZ
    Larynx D92BJZZ
    Liver DF20JZZ
    Lung DB22JZZ
    Lymphatics
      Abdomen D726JZZ
      Axillary D724JZZ
      Inguinal D728JZZ
      Neck D723JZZ
      Pelvis D727JZZ
      Thorax D725JZZ
    Mediastinum DB26JZZ
    Mouth D924JZZ
    Nasopharynx D92DJZZ
    Neck and Head DW21JZZ
    Nerve, Peripheral D027JZZ
    Nose D921JZZ
    Ovary DU20JZZ
    Palate
      Hard D928JZZ
      Soft D929JZZ
    Pancreas DF23JZZ
    Parathyroid Gland DG24JZZ
    Pelvic Region DW26JZZ
    Pharynx D92CJZZ
    Pineal Body DG21JZZ
    Pituitary Gland DG20JZZ
    Pleura DB25JZZ
    Prostate DV20JZZ
    Rectum DD27JZZ
    Sinuses D927JZZ
    Spinal Cord D026JZZ
    Spleen D722JZZ
    Stomach DD21JZZ
    Testis DV21JZZ
    Thymus D721JZZ
    Thyroid Gland DG25JZZ
    Tongue D925JZZ
    Trachea DB20JZZ
    Ureter DT21JZZ
    Urethra DT23JZZ
    Uterus DU22JZZ
  Gland
    Adrenal DG22
    Parathyroid DG24
    Pituitary DG20

Stereotactic
  Radiosurgery (continued)
  Gland (continued)
    Thyroid DG25
  Glands, Salivary D926
  Head and Neck DW21
  Ileum DD24
  Jejunum DD23
  Kidney DT20
  Larynx D92B
  Liver DF20
  Lung DB22
  Lymphatics
    Abdomen D726
    Axillary D724
    Inguinal D728
    Neck D723
    Pelvis D727
    Thorax D725
  Mediastinum DB26
  Mouth D924
  Nasopharynx D92D
  Neck and Head DW21
  Nerve, Peripheral D027
  Nose D921
  Other Photon
    Abdomen DW23DZZ
    Adrenal Gland DG22DZZ
    Bile Ducts DF22DZZ
    Bladder DT22DZZ
    Bone Marrow D720DZZ
    Brain D020DZZ
    Brain Stem D021DZZ
    Breast
      Left DM20DZZ
      Right DM21DZZ
    Bronchus DB21DZZ
    Cervix DU21DZZ
    Chest DW22DZZ
    Chest Wall DB27DZZ
    Colon DD25DZZ
    Diaphragm DB28DZZ
    Duodenum DD22DZZ
    Ear D920DZZ
    Esophagus DD20DZZ
    Eye D820DZZ
    Gallbladder DF21DZZ
    Gland
      Adrenal DG22DZZ
      Parathyroid DG24DZZ
      Pituitary DG20DZZ
      Thyroid DG25DZZ
    Glands, Salivary D926DZZ
    Head and Neck DW21DZZ
    Ileum DD24DZZ
    Jejunum DD23DZZ
    Kidney DT20DZZ
    Larynx D92BDZZ
    Liver DF20DZZ
    Lung DB22DZZ
    Lymphatics
      Abdomen D726DZZ
      Axillary D724DZZ
      Inguinal D728DZZ
      Neck D723DZZ
      Pelvis D727DZZ
      Thorax D725DZZ
    Mediastinum DB26DZZ
    Mouth D924DZZ
    Nasopharynx D92DDZZ
    Neck and Head DW21DZZ
    Nerve, Peripheral D027DZZ
    Nose D921DZZ
    Ovary DU20DZZ
    Palate
      Hard D928DZZ
      Soft D929DZZ
    Pancreas DF23DZZ
    Parathyroid Gland DG24DZZ
    Pelvic Region DW26DZZ
    Pharynx D92CDZZ

79

Stereotactic
  Radiosurgery *(continued)*
    Other Photon *(continued)*
      Pineal Body DG21DZZ
      Pituitary Gland DG20DZZ
      Pleura DB25DZZ
      Prostate DV20DZZ
      Rectum DD27DZZ
      Sinuses D927DZZ
      Spinal Cord D026DZZ
      Spleen D722DZZ
      Stomach DD21DZZ
      Testis DV21DZZ
      Thymus D721DZZ
      Thyroid Gland DG25DZZ
      Tongue D925DZZ
      Trachea DB20DZZ
      Ureter DT21DZZ
      Urethra DT23DZZ
      Uterus DU22DZZ
    Ovary DU20
    Palate
      Hard D928
      Soft D929
    Pancreas DF23
    Parathyroid Gland DG24
    Particulate
      Abdomen DW23HZZ
      Adrenal Gland DG22HZZ
      Bile Ducts DF22HZZ
      Bladder DT22HZZ
      Bone Marrow D720HZZ
      Brain D020HZZ
      Brain Stem D021HZZ
      Breast
        Left DM20HZZ
        Right DM21HZZ
      Bronchus DB21HZZ
      Cervix DU21HZZ
      Chest DW22HZZ
      Chest Wall DB27HZZ
      Colon DD25HZZ
      Diaphragm DB28HZZ
      Duodenum DD22HZZ
      Ear D920HZZ
      Esophagus DD20HZZ
      Eye D820HZZ
      Gallbladder DF21HZZ
      Gland
        Adrenal DG22HZZ
        Parathyroid DG24HZZ
        Pituitary DG20HZZ
        Thyroid DG25HZZ
      Glands, Salivary D926HZZ
      Head and Neck DW21HZZ
      Ileum DD24HZZ
      Jejunum DD23HZZ
      Kidney DT20HZZ
      Larynx D92BHZZ
      Liver DF20HZZ
      Lung DB22HZZ
      Lymphatics
        Abdomen D726HZZ
        Axillary D724HZZ
        Inguinal D728HZZ
        Neck D723HZZ
        Pelvis D727HZZ
        Thorax D725HZZ
      Mediastinum DB26HZZ
      Mouth D924HZZ
      Nasopharynx D92DHZZ
      Neck and Head DW21HZZ
      Nerve, Peripheral D027HZZ
      Nose D921HZZ
      Ovary DU20HZZ
      Palate
        Hard D928HZZ
        Soft D929HZZ
      Pancreas DF23HZZ
      Parathyroid Gland DG24HZZ
      Pelvic Region DW26HZZ

Stereotactic
  Radiosurgery *(continued)*
    Particulate *(continued)*
      Pharynx D92CHZZ
      Pineal Body DG21HZZ
      Pituitary Gland DG20HZZ
      Pleura DB25HZZ
      Prostate DV20HZZ
      Rectum DD27HZZ
      Sinuses D927HZZ
      Spinal Cord D026HZZ
      Spleen D722HZZ
      Stomach DD21HZZ
      Testis DV21HZZ
      Thymus D721HZZ
      Thyroid Gland DG25HZZ
      Tongue D925HZZ
      Trachea DB20HZZ
      Ureter DT21HZZ
      Urethra DT23HZZ
      Uterus DU22HZZ
    Pelvic Region DW26
    Pharynx D92C
    Pineal Body DG21
    Pituitary Gland DG20
    Pleura DB25
    Prostate DV20
    Rectum DD27
    Sinuses D927
    Spinal Cord D026
    Spleen D722
    Stomach DD21
    Testis DV21
    Thymus D721
    Thyroid Gland DG25
    Tongue D925
    Trachea SB20
    Ureter DT21
    Urethra DT23
    Uterus DU22

Steripath® Micro™ Blood Collection System XXE5XR7
Sternoclavicular ligament
  use Bursa and Ligament, Shoulder, Left
  use Bursa and Ligament, Shoulder, Right
Sternocleidomastoid artery
  use Artery, Thyroid, Left
  use Artery, Thyroid, Right
Sternocleidomastoid muscle
  use Muscle, Neck, Left
  use Muscle, Neck, Right
Sternocostal ligament
  use Sternum Bursa and Ligament
Sternotomy
  see Division, Sternum 0P80
  see Drainage, Sternum 0P90
Stimulation, cardiac
  Cardioversion 5A2204Z
  Electrophysiologic testing
    see Measurement, Cardiac 4A02
Stimulator Generator
  Insertion of device in
    Abdomen 0JH8
    Back 0JH7
    Chest 0JH6
  Multiple Array
    Abdomen 0JH8
    Back 0JH7
    Chest 0JH6
  Multiple Array Rechargeable
    Abdomen 0JH8
    Back 0JH7
    Chest 0JH6
  Removal of device from,
    Subcutaneous Tissue and Fascia, Trunk 0JPT
  Revision of device in, Subcutaneous Tissue and Fascia, Trunk 0JWT

Stimulator Generator *(continued)*
  Single Array
    Abdomen 0JH8
    Back 0JH7
    Chest 0JH6
  Single Array Rechargeable
    Abdomen 0JH8
    Back 0JH7
    Chest 0JH6
Stimulator Lead
  Insertion of device in
    Anal Sphincter 0DHR
    Artery
      Left 03HL
      Right 03HK
    Bladder 0THB
    Muscle
      Lower 0KHY
      Upper 0KHX
    Stomach 0DH6
    Ureter 0TH9
  Removal of device from
    Anal Sphincter 0DPR
    Artery, Upper 03PY
    Bladder 0TPB
    Muscle
      Lower 0KPY
      Upper 0KPX
    Stomach 0DP6
    Ureter 0TP9
  Revision of device in
    Anal Sphincter 0DWR
    Artery, Upper 03WY
    Bladder 0TWB
    Muscle
      Lower 0KWY
      Upper 0KWX
    Stomach 0DW6
    Ureter 0TW9
Stoma
  Excision
    Abdominal Wall 0WBFXZ2
    Neck 0WB6XZ2
  Repair
    Abdominal Wall 0WQFXZ2
    Neck 0WQ6XZ2
Stomatoplasty
  see Repair, Mouth and Throat 0CQ
  see Replacement, Mouth and Throat 0CR
  see Supplement, Mouth and Throat 0CU
Stomatorrhaphy
  see Repair, Mouth and Throat 0CQ
StrataGraft®
  use Bioengineered Allogeneic Construct
Stratos LV
  use Cardiac Resynchronization Pacemaker Pulse Generator in 0JH
Stress test
  4A02XM4
  4A12XM4
Stripping
  see Extraction
Study
  Electrophysiologic stimulation, cardiac
    see Measurement, Cardiac 4A02
  Ocular motility 4A07X7Z
  Pulmonary airway flow measurement
    see Measurement, Respiratory 4A09
  Visual acuity 4A07X0Z
Styloglossus muscle
  use Muscle, Tongue, Palate, Pharynx
Stylomandibular ligament
  use Bursa and Ligament, Head and Neck

Stylopharyngeus muscle
  use Muscle, Tongue, Palate, Pharynx
Subacromial bursa
  use Bursa and Ligament, Shoulder, Left
  use Bursa and Ligament, Shoulder, Right
Subaortic (common iliac) lymph node
  use Lymphatic, Pelvis
Subarachnoid space, spinal
  use Spinal Canal
Subclavicular (apical) lymph node
  use Lymphatic, Axillary, Left
  use Lymphatic, Axillary, Right
Subclavius muscle
  use Muscle, Thorax, Left
  use Muscle, Thorax, Right
Subclavius nerve
  use Nerve, Brachial Plexus
Subcostal artery
  use Upper Artery
Subcostal muscle
  use Muscle, Thorax, Left
  use Muscle, Thorax, Right
Subcostal nerve
  use Nerve, Thoracic
Subcutaneous injection reservoir, port
  use Vascular Access Device, Totally Implantable in Subcutaneous Tissue and Fascia
Subcutaneous Defibrillator Lead
  Insertion of device in, Subcutaneous Tissue and Fascia, Chest 0JH6
  Removal of device from, Subcutaneous Tissue and Fascia, Trunk 0JPT
  Revision of device in, Subcutaneous Tissue and Fascia, Trunk 0JWT
Subcutaneous injection reservoir, pump
  use Infusion Device, Pump in Subcutaneous Tissue and Fascia
Subdermal progesterone implant
  use Contraceptive Device in Subcutaneous Tissue and Fascia
Subdural space, spinal
  use Spinal Canal
Submandibular ganglion
  use Nerve, Facial
  use Nerve, Head and Neck Sympathetic
Submandibular gland
  use Gland, Submaxillary, Left
  use Gland, Submaxillary, Right
Submandibular lymph node
  use Lymphatic, Head
Submandibular space
  use Subcutaneous Tissue and Fascia, Face
Submaxillary ganglion
  use Nerve, Head and Neck Sympathetic
Submaxillary lymph node
  use Lymphatic, Head
Submental artery
  use Artery, Face
Submental lymph node
  use Lymphatic, Head
Submucous (Meissner's) plexus
  use Nerve, Abdominal Sympathetic
Suboccipital nerve
  use Nerve, Cervical
Suboccipital venous plexus
  use Vein, Vertebral, Left
  use Vein, Vertebral, Right

Subparotid lymph node
use Lymphatic, Head
Subscapular (posterior) lymph node
use Lymphatic, Axillary, Left
use Lymphatic, Axillary, Right
Subscapular aponeurosis
use Subcutaneous Tissue and Fascia, Upper Arm, Left
use Subcutaneous Tissue and Fascia, Upper Arm, Right
Subscapular artery
use Artery, Axillary, Left
use Artery, Axillary, Right
Subscapularis muscle
use Muscle, Shoulder, Left
use Muscle, Shoulder, Right
Substance Abuse Treatment
Counseling
  Family, for substance abuse, Other Family Counseling HZ63ZZZ
  Group
    12-Step HZ43ZZZ
    Behavioral HZ41ZZZ
    Cognitive HZ40ZZZ
    Cognitive-Behavioral HZ42ZZZ
    Confrontational HZ48ZZZ
    Continuing Care HZ49ZZZ
    Infectious Disease
      Post-Test HZ4CZZZ
      Pre-Test HZ4CZZZ
    Interpersonal HZ44ZZZ
    Motivational Enhancement HZ47ZZZ
    Psychoeducation HZ46ZZZ
    Spiritual HZ4BZZZ
    Vocational HZ45ZZZ
  Individual
    12-Step HZ33ZZZ
    Behavioral HZ31ZZZ
    Cognitive HZ30ZZZ
    Cognitive-Behavioral HZ32ZZZ
    Confrontational HZ38ZZZ
    Continuing Care HZ39ZZZ
    Infectious Disease
      Post-Test HZ3CZZZ
      Pre-Test HZ3CZZZ
    Interpersonal HZ34ZZZ
    Motivational Enhancement HZ37ZZZ
    Psychoeducation HZ36ZZZ
    Spiritual HZ3BZZZ
    Vocational HZ35ZZZ
  Detoxification Services, for substance abuse HZ2ZZZZ
  Medication Management
    Antabuse HZ83ZZZ
    Bupropion HZ87ZZZ
    Clonidine HZ86ZZZ
    Levo-alpha-acetyl-methadol (LAAM) HZ82ZZZ
    Methadone Maintenance HZ81ZZZ
    Naloxone HZ85ZZZ
    Naltrexone HZ84ZZZ
    Nicotine Replacement HZ80ZZZ
    Other Replacement Medication HZ89ZZZ
    Psychiatric Medication HZ88ZZZ
  Pharmacotherapy
    Antabuse HZ93ZZZ
    Bupropion HZ97ZZZ
    Clonidine HZ96ZZZ
    Levo-alpha-acetyl-methadol (LAAM) HZ92ZZZ
    Methadone Maintenance HZ91ZZZ
    Naloxone HZ95ZZZ
    Naltrexone HZ94ZZZ
    Nicotine Replacement HZ90ZZZ

Substance Abuse Treatment *(continued)*
  Pharmacotherapy *(continued)*
    Psychiatric Medication HZ98ZZZ
    Replacement Medication, Other HZ99ZZZ
  Psychotherapy
    12-Step HZ53ZZZ
    Behavioral HZ51ZZZ
    Cognitive HZ50ZZZ
    Cognitive-Behavioral HZ52ZZZ
    Confrontational HZ58ZZZ
    Interactive HZ55ZZZ
    Interpersonal HZ54ZZZ
    Motivational Enhancement HZ57ZZZ
    Psychoanalysis HZ5BZZZ
    Psychodynamic HZ5CZZZ
    Psychoeducation HZ56ZZZ
    Psychophysiological HZ5DZZZ
    Supportive HZ59ZZZ
Substantia nigra
use Basal Ganglia
Subtalar (talocalcaneal) joint
use Joint, Tarsal, Left
use Joint, Tarsal, Right
Subtalar ligament
use Bursa and Ligament, Foot, Left
use Bursa and Ligament, Foot, Right
Subthalamic nucleus
use Basal Ganglia
Suction curettage (D&C), nonobstetric
see Extraction, Endometrium 0UDB
Suction curettage, obstetric post-delivery
see Extraction, Products of Conception, Retained 10D1
SUL-DUR *use* Sulbactam-Durlobactam
Sulbactam-Durlobactam XW0
Superficial circumflex iliac vein
use Vein, Saphenous, Left
use Vein, Saphenous, Right
Superficial epigastric artery
use Artery, Femoral, Left
use Artery, Femoral, Right
Superficial epigastric vein
use Vein, Saphenous, Left
use Vein, Saphenous, Right
Superficial Inferior Epigastric Artery Flap
  Replacement
    Bilateral 0HRV078
    Left 0HRU078
    Right 0HRT078
  Transfer
    Left 0KXG
    Right 0KXF
Superficial palmar arch
use Artery, Hand, Left
use Artery, Hand, Right
Superficial palmar venous arch
use Vein, Hand, Left
use Vein, Hand, Right
Superficial temporal artery
use Artery, Temporal, Left
use Artery, Temporal, Right
Superficial transverse perineal muscle
use Muscle, Perineum
Superior cardiac nerve
use Nerve, Thoracic Sympathetic
Superior cerebellar vein
use Vein, Intracranial
Superior cerebral vein
use Vein, Intracranial
Superior clunic (cluneal) nerve
use Nerve, Lumbar

Superior epigastric artery
use Artery, Internal Mammary, Left
use Artery, Internal Mammary, Right
Superior genicular artery
use Artery, Popliteal, Left
use Artery, Popliteal, Right
Superior gluteal artery
use Artery, Internal Iliac, Left
use Artery, Internal Iliac, Right
Superior gluteal nerve
use Nerve, Lumbar Plexus
Superior hypogastric plexus
use Nerve, Abdominal Sympathetic
Superior labial artery
use Artery, Face
Superior laryngeal artery
use Artery, Thyroid, Left
use Artery, Thyroid, Right
Superior laryngeal nerve
use Nerve, Vagus
Superior longitudinal muscle
use Muscle, Tongue, Palate, Pharynx
Superior mesenteric ganglion
use Nerve, Abdominal Sympathetic
Superior mesenteric lymph node
use Lymphatic, Mesenteric
Superior mesenteric plexus
use Nerve, Abdominal Sympathetic
Superior oblique muscle
use Muscle, Extraocular, Left
use Muscle, Extraocular, Right
Superior olivary nucleus
use Pons
Superior rectal artery
use Artery, Inferior Mesenteric
Superior rectal vein
use Vein, Inferior Mesenteric
Superior rectus muscle
use Muscle, Extraocular, Left
use Muscle, Extraocular, Right
Superior tarsal plate
use Eyelid, Upper, Left
use Eyelid, Upper, Right
Superior thoracic artery
use Artery, Axillary, Left
use Artery, Axillary, Right
Superior thyroid artery
use External Carotid Artery, Left
use External Carotid Artery, Right
use Thyroid, Left
use Thyroid, Right
Superior turbinate
use Turbinate, Nasal
Superior ulnar collateral artery
use Artery, Brachial, Left
use Artery, Brachial, Right
Superior vesical artery
use Internal Iliac Artery, Left
use Internal Iliac Artery, Right
Supersaturated Oxygen (SSO2) therapy, cardiac intra-arterial 5A0222C
Supplement
  Abdominal Wall 0WUF
  Acetabulum
    Left 0QU5
    Right 0QU4
  Ampulla of Vater 0FUC
  Anal Sphincter 0DUR
  Ankle Region
    Left 0YUL
    Right 0YUK
  Anus 0DUQ
  Aorta
    Abdominal 04U0
    Thoracic
      Ascending/Arch 02UX
      Descending 02UW
  Arm
    Lower
      Left 0XUF
      Right 0XUD

Supplement *(continued)*
  Arm *(continued)*
    Upper
      Left 0XU9
      Right 0XU8
  Arteriovenous Fistula, Extraluminal Support Device X2U
  Artery
    Anterior Tibial
      Left 04UQ
      Right 04UP
    Axillary
      Left 03U6
      Right 03U5
    Brachial
      Left 03U8
      Right 03U7
    Celiac 04U1
    Colic
      Left 04U7
      Middle 04U8
      Right 04U6
    Common Carotid
      Left 03UJ
      Right 03UH
    Common Iliac
      Left 04UD
      Right 04UC
    Coronary
      Four or More Arteries 02U3
      One Artery 02U0
      Three Arteries 02U2
      Two Arteries 02U1
    External Carotid
      Left 03UN
      Right 03UM
    External Iliac
      Left 04UJ
      Right 04UH
    Face 03UR
    Femoral
      Left 04UL
      Right 04UK
    Foot
      Left 04UW
      Right 04UV
    Gastric 04U2
    Hand
      Left 03UF
      Right 03UD
    Hepatic 04U3
    Inferior Mesenteric 04UB
    Innominate 03U2
    Internal Carotid
      Left 03UL
      Right 03UK
    Internal Iliac
      Left 04UF
      Right 04UE
    Internal Mammary
      Left 03U1
      Right 03U0
    Intracranial 03UG
    Lower 04UY
    Peroneal
      Left 04UU
      Right 04UT
    Popliteal
      Left 04UN
      Right 04UM
    Posterior Tibial
      Left 04US
      Right 04UR
    Pulmonary
      Left 02UR
      Right 02UQ
    Pulmonary Trunk 02UP
    Radial
      Left 03UC
      Right 03UB

Supplement (continued)

Artery (continued)
  Renal
    Left 04UA
    Right 04U9
  Splenic 04U4
  Subclavian
    Left 03U4
    Right 03U3
  Superior Mesenteric 04U5
  Temporal
    Left 03UT
    Right 03US
  Thyroid
    Left 03UV
    Right 03UU
  Ulnar
    Left 03UA
    Right 03U9
  Upper 03UY
  Vertebral
    Left 03UQ
    Right 03UP
Atrium
  Left 02U7
  Right 02U6
Auditory Ossicle
  Left 09UA
  Right 09U9
Axilla
  Left 0XU5
  Right 0XU4
Back
  Lower 0WUL
  Upper 0WUK
Bladder 0TUB
Bladder Neck 0TUC
Bone
  Ethmoid
    Left 0NUG
    Right 0NUF
  Frontal 0NU1
  Hyoid 0NUX
  Lacrimal
    Left 0NUJ
    Right 0NUH
  Nasal 0NUB
  Occipital 0NU7
  Palatine
    Left 0NUL
    Right 0NUK
  Parietal
    Left 0NU4
    Right 0NU3
  Pelvic
    Left 0QU3
    Right 0QU2
  Sphenoid 0NUC
  Temporal
    Left 0NU6
    Right 0NU5
  Zygomatic
    Left 0NUN
    Right 0NUM
Breast
  Bilateral 0HUV
  Left 0HUU
  Right 0HUT
Bronchus
  Lingula 0BU9
  Lower Lobe
    Left 0BUB
    Right 0BU6
  Main
    Left 0BU7
    Right 0BU3
  Middle Lobe, Right 0BU5
  Upper Lobe
    Left 0BU8
    Right 0BU4
Buccal Mucosa 0CU4

Supplement (continued)

Bursa and Ligament
  Abdomen
    Left 0MUJ
    Right 0MUH
  Ankle
    Left 0MUR
    Right 0MUQ
  Elbow
    Left 0MU4
    Right 0MU3
  Foot
    Left 0MUT
    Right 0MUS
  Hand
    Left 0MU8
    Right 0MU7
  Head and Neck 0MU0
  Hip
    Left 0MUM
    Right 0MUL
  Knee
    Left 0MUP
    Right 0MUN
  Lower Extremity
    Left 0MUW
    Right 0MUV
  Perineum 0MUK
  Rib(s) 0MUC
  Shoulder
    Left 0MU2
    Right 0MU1
  Spine
    Lower 0MUD
    Posterior Vertebral Tether
      XKU
    Upper 0MUC
  Sternum 0MUF
  Upper Extremity
    Left 0MUB
    Right 0MU9
  Wrist
    Left 0MU6
    Right 0MU5
Buttock
  Left 0YU1
  Right 0YU0
Carina 0BU2
Carpal
  Left 0PUN
  Right 0PUM
Cecum 0DUH
Cerebral Meninges 00U1
Cerebral Ventricle 00U6
Chest Wall 0WU8
Chordae Tendineae 02U9
Cisterna Chyli 07UL
Clavicle
  Left 0PUB
  Right 0PU9
Clitoris 0UUJ
Coccyx 0QUS
Colon
  Ascending 0DUK
  Descending 0DUM
  Sigmoid 0DUN
  Transverse 0DUL
Cord
  Bilateral 0VUH
  Left 0VUG
  Right 0VUF
Cornea
  Left 08U9
  Right 08U8
Coronary Artery/Arteries, Vein
  Graft Extraluminal Support
  Device(s) X2U4079
Cul-de-sac 0UUF
Diaphragm 0BUT
Disc
  Cervical Vertebral 0RU3

Supplement (continued)

  Cervicothoracic Vertebral 0RU5
  Lumbar Vertebral 0SU2
  Lumbosacral 0SU4
  Thoracic Vertebral 0RU9
  Thoracolumbar Vertebral 0RUB
Duct
  Common Bile 0FU9
  Cystic 0FU8
  Hepatic
    Common 0FU7
    Left 0FU6
    Right 0FU5
  Lacrimal
    Left 08UY
    Right 08UX
  Pancreatic 0FUD
    Accessory
    0FUF
Duodenum 0DU9
Dura Mater 00U2
Ear
  External
    Bilateral 09U2
    Left 09U1
    Right 09U0
  Inner
    Left 09UE
    Right 09UD
  Middle
    Left 09U6
    Right 09U5
Elbow Region
  Left 0XUC
  Right 0XUB
Epididymis
  Bilateral 0VUL
  Left 0VUK
  Right 0VUJ
Epiglottis 0CUR
Esophagogastric Junction 0DU4
Esophagus 0DU5
  Lower 0DU3
  Middle 0DU2
  Upper 0DU1
Extremity
  Lower
    Left 0YUB
    Right 0YU9
  Upper
    Left 0XU7
    Right 0XU6
Eye
  Left 08U1
  Right 08U0
Eyelid
  Lower
    Left 08UR
    Right 08UQ
  Upper
    Left 08UP
    Right 08UN
Face 0WU2
Fallopian Tube
  Left 0UU6
  Right 0UU5
Fallopian Tubes, Bilateral 0UU7
Femoral Region
  Bilateral 0YUE
  Left 0YU8
  Right 0YU7
Femoral Shaft
  Left 0QU9
  Right 0QU8
Femur
  Lower
    Left 0QUC
    Right 0QUB
  Upper
    Left 0QU7
    Right 0QU6

Supplement (continued)

Fibula
  Left 0QUK
  Right 0QUJ
Finger
  Index
    Left 0XUP
    Right 0XUN
  Little
    Left 0XUW
    Right 0XUV
  Middle
    Left 0XUR
    Right 0XUQ
  Ring
    Left 0XUT
    Right 0XUS
Foot
  Left 0YUN
  Right 0YUM
Gingiva
  Lower 0CU6
  Upper 0CU5
Glenoid Cavity
  Left 0PU8
  Right 0PU7
Hand
  Left 0XUK
  Right 0XUJ
Head 0WU0
Heart 02UA
Humeral Head
  Left 0PUD
  Right 0PUC
Humeral Shaft
  Left 0PUG
  Right 0PUF
Hymen 0UUK
Ileocecal Valve 0DUC
Ileum 0DUB
Inguinal Region
  Bilateral 0YUA
  Left 0YU6
  Right 0YU5
Intestine
  Large 0DUE
    Left 0DUG
    Right 0DUF
  Small 0DU8
Iris
  Left 08UD
  Right 08UC
Jaw
  Lower 0WU5
  Upper 0WU4
Jejunum 0DUA
Joint
  Acromioclavicular
    Left 0RUH
    Right 0RUG
  Ankle
    Left 0SUG
    Right 0SUF
  Carpal
    Left 0RUR
    Right 0RUQ
  Carpometacarpal
    Left 0RUT
    Right 0RUS
  Cervical Vertebral 0RU1
  Cervicothoracic Vertebral
    0RU4
  Coccygeal 0SU6
  Elbow
    Left 0RUM
    Right 0RUL
  Finger Phalangeal
    Left 0RUX
    Right 0RUW
  Hip
    Left 0SUB

Supplement *(continued)*

Joint *(continued)*
Hip *(continued)*
Acetabular Surface 0SUE
Femoral Surface 0SUS
Right 0SU9
Acetabular Surface 0SUA
Femoral Surface 0SUR
Knee
Left 0SUD
Femoral Surface 0SUU09Z
Tibial Surface 0SUW09Z
Right 0SUC
Femoral Surface 0SUT09Z
Tibial Surface
0SUV09Z
Lumbar Vertebral 0SU0
Lumbosacral 0SU3
Metacarpophalangeal
Left 0RUV
Right 0RUU
Metatarsal-Phalangeal
Left 0SUN
Right 0SUM
Occipital-cervical 0RU0
Sacrococcygeal 0SU5
Sacroiliac
Left 0SU8
Right 0SU7
Shoulder
Left 0RUK
Right 0RUJ
Sternoclavicular
Left 0RUF
Right 0RUE
Tarsal
Left 0SUJ
Right 0SUH
Tarsometatarsal
Left 0SUL
Right 0SUK
Temporomandibular
Left 0RUD
Right 0RUC
Thoracic Vertebral 0RU6
Thoracolumbar Vertebral 0RUA
Toe Phalangeal
Left 0SUQ
Right 0SUP
Wrist
Left 0RUP
Right 0RUN
Kidney Pelvis
Left 0TU4
Right 0TU3
Knee Region
Left 0YUG
Right 0YUF
Larynx 0CUS
Leg
Lower
Left 0YUJ
Right 0YUH
Upper
Left 0YUD
Right 0YUC
Lip
Lower 0CU1
Upper 0CU0
Lymphatic
Aortic 07UD
Axillary
Left 07U6
Right 07U5
Head 07U0
Inguinal
Left 07UJ
Right 07UH
Internal Mammary
Left 07U9
Right 07U8

Supplement *(continued)*

Lymphatic *(continued)*
Lower Extremity
Left 07UG
Right 07UF
Mesenteric 07UB
Neck
Left 07U2
Right 07U1
Pelvis 07UC
Thoracic Duct
07UK
Thorax 07U7
Upper Extremity
Left 07U4
Right 07U3
Mandible
Left 0NUV
Right 0NUT
Maxilla 0NUR
Mediastinum 0WUC
Mesentery 0DUV
Metacarpal
Left 0PUQ
Right 0PUP
Metatarsal
Left 0QUP
Right 0QUN
Muscle
Abdomen
Left 0KUL
Right 0KUK
Extraocular
Left 08UM
Right 08UL
Facial 0KU1
Foot
Left 0KUW
Right 0KUV
Hand
Left 0KUD
Right 0KUC
Head 0KU0
Hip
Left 0KUP
Right 0KUN
Lower Arm and Wrist
Left 0KUB
Right 0KU9
Lower Leg
Left 0KUT
Right 0KUS
Neck
Left 0KU3
Right 0KU2
Papillary 02UD
Perineum 0KUM
Shoulder
Left 0KU6
Right 0KU5
Thorax
Left 0KUJ
Right 0KUH
Tongue, Palate, Pharynx
0KU4
Trunk
Left 0KUG
Right 0KUF
Upper Arm
Left 0KU8
Right 0KU7
Upper Leg
Left 0KUR
Right 0KUQ
Nasal Mucosa and Soft Tissue
09UK
Nasopharynx 09UN
Neck 0WU6
Nerve
Abducens 00UL
Accessory 00UR

Supplement *(continued)*

Nerve *(continued)*
Acoustic 00UN
Cervical 01U1
Facial 00UM
Femoral 01UD
Glossopharyngeal 00UP
Hypoglossal 00US
Lumbar 01UB
Median 01U5
Oculomotor 00UH
Olfactory 00UF
Optic 00UG
Peroneal 01UH
Phrenic 01U2
Pudendal 01UC
Radial 01U6
Sacral 01UR
Sciatic 01UF
Thoracic 01U8
Tibial 01UG
Trigeminal 00UK
Trochlear 00UJ
Ulnar 01U4
Vagus 00UQ
Nipple
Left 0HUX
Right 0HUW
Omentum 0DUU
Orbit
Left 0NUQ
Right 0NUP
Palate
Hard 0CU2
Soft 0CU3
Patella
Left 0QUF
Right 0QUD
Penis 0VUS
Pericardium 02UN
Perineum
Female 0WUN
Male 0WUM
Peritoneum 0DUW
Phalanx
Finger
Left 0PUV
Right 0PUT
Thumb
Left 0PUS
Right 0PUR
Toe
Left 0QUR
Right 0QUQ
Pharynx 0CUM
Prepuce 0VUT
Radius
Left 0PUJ
Right 0PUH
Rectum 0DUP
Retina
Left 08UF
Right 08UE
Retinal Vessel
Left 08UH
Right 08UG
Ribs
1 to 2 0PU1
3 or More 0PU2
Sacrum 0QU1
Scapula
Left 0PU6
Right 0PU5
Scrotum 0VU5
Septum
Atrial 02U5
Nasal 09UM
Ventricular 02UM
Shoulder Region
Left 0XU3
Right 0XU2

Supplement *(continued)*

Sinus
Accessory 09UP
Ethmoid
Left 09UV
Right 09UU
Frontal
Left 09UT
Right 09US
Mastoid
Left 09UC
Right 09UB
Maxillary
Left 09UR
Right 09UQ
Sphenoid
Left 09UX
Right 09UW
Skull 0NU0
Spinal Meninges 00UT
Sternum 0PU0
Stomach 0DU6
Pylorus 0DU7
Subcutaneous Tissue and Fascia
Abdomen 0JU8
Back 0JU7
Buttock 0JU9
Chest 0JU6
Face 0JU1
Foot
Left 0JUR
Right 0JUQ
Hand
Left 0JUK
Right 0JUJ
Lower Arm
Left 0JUH
Right 0JUG
Lower Leg
Left 0JUP
Right 0JUN
Neck
Left 0JU5
Right 0JU4
Pelvic Region 0JUC
Perineum 0JUB
Scalp 0JU0
Upper Arm
Left 0JUF
Right 0JUD
Upper Leg
Left 0JUM
Right 0JUL
Tarsal
Left 0QUM
Right 0QUL
Tendon
Abdomen
Left 0LUG
Right 0LUF
Ankle
Left 0LUT
Right 0LUS
Foot
Left 0LUW
Right 0LUV
Hand
Left 0LU8
Right 0LU7
Head and Neck
0LU0
Hip
Left 0LUK
Right 0LUJ
Knee
Left 0LUR
Right 0LUQ
Lower Arm and
Wrist
Left 0LU6
Right 0LU5

Supplement (*continued*)
  Tendon (*continued*)
    Lower Leg
      Left 0LUP
      Right 0LUN
    Perineum 0LUH
    Shoulder
      Left 0LU2
      Right 0LU1
    Thorax
      Left 0LUD
      Right 0LUC
    Trunk
      Left 0LUB
      Right 0LU9
    Upper Arm
      Left 0LU4
      Right 0LU3
    Upper Leg
      Left 0LUM
      Right 0LUL
  Testis
    Bilateral 0VUC0
    Left 0VUB0
    Right 0VU90
  Thumb
    Left 0XUM
    Right 0XUL
  Tibia
    Left 0QUH
    Right 0QUG
  Toe
    1st
      Left 0YUQ
      Right 0YUP
    2nd
      Left 0YUS
      Right 0YUR
    3rd
      Left 0YUU
      Right 0YUT
    4th
      Left 0YUW
      Right 0YUV
    5th
      Left 0YUY
      Right 0YUX
  Tongue 0CU7
  Trachea 0BU1
  Tunica Vaginalis
    Left 0VU7
    Right 0VU6
  Turbinate, Nasal 09UL
  Tympanic Membrane
    Left 09U8
    Right 09U7
  Ulna
    Left 0PUL
    Right 0PUK
  Ureter
    Left 0TU7
    Right 0TU6
  Urethra 0TUD
  Uterine Supporting Structure
    0UU4
  Uvula 0CUN
  Vagina 0UUG
  Valve
    Aortic 02UF
    Mitral 02UG
    Pulmonary 02UH
    Tricuspid 02UJ
  Vas Deferens
    Bilateral 0VUQ
    Left 0VUP
    Right 0VUN
  Vein
    Axillary
      Left 05U8
      Right 05U7
    Azygos 05U0

Supplement (*continued*)
  Vein (*continued*)
    Basilic
      Left 05UC
      Right 05UB
    Brachial
      Left 05UA
      Right 05U9
    Cephalic
      Left 05UF
      Right 05UD
    Colic 06U7
    Common Iliac
      Left 06UD
      Right 06UC
    Esophageal 06U3
    External Iliac
      Left 06UG
      Right 06UF
    External Jugular
      Left 05UQ
      Right 05UP
    Face
      Left 05UV
      Right 05UT
    Femoral
      Left 06UN
      Right 06UM
    Foot
      Left 06UV
      Right 06UT
    Gastric 06U2
    Hand
      Left 05UH
      Right 05UG
    Hemiazygos 05U1
    Hepatic 06U4
    Hypogastric
      Left 06UJ
      Right 06UH
    Inferior Mesenteric 06U6
    Innominate
      Left 05U4
      Right 05U3
    Internal Jugular
      Left 05UN
      Right 05UM
    Intracranial 05UL
    Lower 06UY
    Portal 06U8
    Pulmonary
      Left 02UT
      Right 02US
    Renal
      Left 06UB
      Right 06U9
    Saphenous
      Left 06UQ
      Right 06UP
    Splenic 06U1
    Subclavian
      Left 05U6
      Right 05U5
    Superior Mesenteric
      06U5
    Upper 05UY
    Vertebral
      Left 05US
      Right 05UR
    Vena Cava
      Inferior 06U0
      Superior 02UV
    Ventricle
      Left 02UL
      Right 02UK
    Vertebra
      Cervical 0PU3
      Lumbar 0QU0
        Mechanically Expandable
          (Paired) Synthetic
          Substitute XNU0356

Supplement (*continued*)
  Vertebra (*continued*)
    Thoracic 0PU4
      Mechanically Expandable
        (Paired) Synthetic
        Substitute XNU4356
  Vesicle
    Bilateral 0VU3
    Left 0VU2
    Right 0VU1
  Vocal Cord
    Left 0CUV
    Right 0CUT
  Vulva 0UUM
  Wrist Region
    Left 0XUH
    Right 0XUG
Supraclavicular (Virchow's) lymph node
  use Lymphatic, Neck, Left
  use Lymphatic, Neck, Right
Supraclavicular nerve
  use Nerve, Cervical Plexus
Suprahyoid lymph node
  use Lymphatic, Head
Suprahyoid muscle
  use Muscle, Neck, Left
  use Muscle, Neck, Right
Suprainguinal lymph node
  use Lymphatic, Pelvis
Supraorbital vein
  use Vein, Face, Left
  use Vein, Face, Right
Suprarenal gland
  use Gland, Adrenal
  use Gland, Adrenal, Bilateral
  use Gland, Adrenal, Left
  use Gland, Adrenal, Right
Suprarenal plexus
  use Nerve, Abdominal Sympathetic
Suprascapular nerve
  use Nerve, Brachial Plexus
Supraspinatus fascia
  use Subcutaneous Tissue and Fascia,
    Upper Arm, Left
  use Subcutaneous Tissue and Fascia,
    Upper Arm, Right
Supraspinatus muscle
  use Muscle, Shoulder, Left
  use Muscle, Shoulder, Right
Supraspinous ligament
  use Bursa and Ligament, Lower Spine
  use Bursa and Ligament, Upper Spine
Suprasternal notch
  use Sternum
Supratrochlear lymph node
  use Lymphatic, Upper Extremity, Left
  use Lymphatic, Upper Extremity,
    Right
Sural artery
  use Artery, Popliteal, Left
  use Artery, Popliteal, Right
Surpass Streamline™ Flow Diverter
  use Intraluminal Device, Flow
    Diverter in 03V
Suspension
  Bladder Neck
    see Reposition, Bladder Neck
      0TSC
  Kidney
    see Reposition, Urinary System
      0TS
  Urethra
    see Reposition, Urinary System
      0TS
  Urethrovesical
    see Reposition, Bladder Neck
      0TSC
  Uterus
    see Reposition, Uterus 0US9

Suspension (*continued*)
  Uterus (*continued*)
    Vagina
      see Reposition, Vagina 0USG
Sustained Release Drug-eluting Intraluminal Device
  Dilation
    Anterior Tibial
      Left X27Q385
      Right X27P385
    Femoral
      Left X27J385
      Right X27H385
    Peroneal
      Left X27U385
      Right X27T385
    Popliteal
      Left Distal X27N385
      Left Proximal X27L385
      Right Distal X27M385
      Right Proximal X27K385
    Posterior Tibial
      Left X27S385
      Right X27R385
  Four or More
    Anterior Tibial
      Left X27Q3C5
      Right X27P3C5
    Femoral
      Left X27J3C5
      Right X27H3C5
    Peroneal
      Left X27U3C5
      Right X27T3C5
    Popliteal
      Left Distal X27N3C5
      Left Proximal X27L3C5
      Right Distal X27M3C5
      Right Proximal X27K3C5
    Posterior Tibial
      Left X27S3C5
      Right X27R3C5
  Three
    Anterior Tibial
      Left X27Q3B5
      Right X27P3B5
    Femoral
      Left X27J3B5
      Right X27H3B5
    Peroneal
      Left X27U3B5
      Right X27T3B5
    Popliteal
      Left Distal X27N3B5
      Left Proximal X27L3B5
      Right Distal X27M3B5
      Right Proximal X27K3B5
    Posterior Tibial
      Left X27S3B5
      Right X27R3B5
  Two
    Anterior Tibial
      Left X27Q395
      Right X27P395
    Femoral
      Left X27J395
      Right X27H395
    Peroneal
      Left X27U395
      Right X27T395
    Popliteal
      Left Distal X27N395
      Left Proximal X27L395
      Right Distal X27M395
      Right Proximal X27K395
    Posterior Tibial
      Left X27S395
      Right X27R395
Suture
  Laceration repair
    see Repair

Suture *(continued)*
  Ligation
    see Occlusion
Suture Removal
  Extremity
    Lower 8E0YXY8
    Upper 8E0XXY8
  Head and Neck Region 8E09XY8
  Trunk Region 8E0WXY8
Sutureless valve, Perceval
  (rapid deployment technique) *see*
    Replacement, Valve, Aortic 02RF
Sweat gland
  use Skin
Sympathectomy
  see Excision, Peripheral Nervous
    System 01B
SynCardia Total Artificial Heart
  use Synthetic Substitute
**SynCardia (temporary) total
  artificial heart (TAH)** *use*
    Synthetic Substitute, Pneumatic
    in 02R
Synchra CRT-P
  use Cardiac Resynchronization
    Pacemaker Pulse Generator in 0JH
SynchroMed pump
  use Infusion Device, Pump in
    Subcutaneous Tissue and Fascia
Synechiotomy, iris
  see Release, Eye 08N
Synovectomy
  Lower joint
    see Excision, Lower Joints 0SB
  Upper joint
    see Excision, Upper Joints 0RB
Systemic Nuclear Medicine Therapy
  Abdomen CW70
  Anatomical Regions, Multiple
    CW7YYZZ
  Chest CW73
  Thyroid CW7G
  Whole Body CW7N

T

tab-cel® *use* Tabelecleucel
  Immunotherapy
Tabelecleucel Immunotherapy XW0
Tagraxofusp-erzs Antineoplastic
  XW0
Takedown
  Arteriovenous shunt
    see Removal of device from,
      Upper Arteries 03P
  Arteriovenous shunt, with creation
    of new shunt
    see Bypass, Upper Arteries 031
  Stoma
    see Excision
    see Reposition
Talent® Converter
  use Intraluminal Device
Talent® Occluder
  use Intraluminal Device
**Talent® Stent Graft (abdominal)
  (thoracic)**
  use Intraluminal Device
Talocalcaneal (subtalar) joint
  use Joint, Tarsal, Left
  use Joint, Tarsal, Right
Talocalcaneal ligament
  use Bursa and Ligament, Foot,
    Left
  use Bursa and Ligament, Foot,
    Right
Talocalcaneonavicular joint
  use Joint, Tarsal, Left
  use Joint, Tarsal, Right
Talocalcaneonavicular ligament
  use Bursa and Ligament, Foot, Left

**Talocalcaneonavicular
  ligament** *(continued)*
  use Bursa and Ligament, Foot, Right
Talocrural joint
  use Joint, Ankle, Left
  use Joint, Ankle, Right
Talofibular ligament
  use Bursa and Ligament, Ankle, Left
  use Bursa and Ligament, Ankle, Right
Talus bone
  use Tarsal, Left
  use Tarsal, Right
TandemHeart® System
  use Short-term External Heart
    Assist System in Heart and Great
    Vessels
Tarsectomy
  see Excision, Lower Bones 0QB
  see Resection, Lower Bones 0QT
Tarsometatarsal ligament
  use Bursa and Ligament, Foot, Left
  use Bursa and Ligament, Foot, Right
Tarsorrhaphy
  see Repair, Eye 08Q
Tattooing
  Cornea 3E0CXMZ
  Skin
    see Introduction of substance in
      or on, Skin 3E00
**Taurolidine Anti-infective and Heparin
  Anticoagulant** XY0YX28
**TAXUS® Liberté® Paclitaxel-eluting
  Coronary Stent System**
  use Intraluminal Device, Drug-
    eluting in Heart and Great Vessels
**TBNA (transbronchial needle
  aspiration)**
  Fluid or gas
    see Drainage, Respiratory
      System 0B9
  Tissue biopsy
    see Extraction, Respiratory
      System 0BD
Tecartus™
  use Brexucabtagene Autoleucel
    Immunotherapy
TECENTRIQ®
  use Atezolizumab Antineoplastic
Teclistamab Antineoplastic
  XW01348
Telemetry 4A12X4Z
  Ambulatory 4A12X45
Temperature gradient study
  4A0ZXKZ
Temporal lobe
  use Cerebral Hemisphere
Temporalis muscle
  use Muscle, Head
Temporoparietalis muscle
  use Muscle, Head
Tendolysis
  see Release, Tendons 0LN
Tendonectomy
  see Excision, Tendons 0LB
  see Resection, Tendons 0LT
Tendonoplasty, tenoplasty
  see Repair, Tendons 0LQ
  see Replacement, Tendons 0LR
  see Supplement, Tendons 0LU
Tendorrhaphy
  see Repair, Tendons 0LQ
Tendototomy
  see Division, Tendons 0L8
  see Drainage, Tendons 0L9
Tenectomy, tenonectomy
  see Excision, Tendons 0LB
  see Resection, Tendons 0LT
Tenolysis
  see Release, Tendons 0LN
Tenontorrhaphy
  see Repair, Tendons 0LQ

Tenontotomy
  see Division, Tendons 0L8
  see Drainage, Tendons 0L9
Tenorrhaphy
  see Repair, Tendons 0LQ
Tenosynovectomy
  see Excision, Tendons 0LB
  see Resection, Tendons 0LT
Tenotomy
  see Division, Tendons 0L8
  see Drainage, Tendons 0L9
Tensor fasciae latae muscle
  use Muscle, Hip, Left
  use Muscle, Hip, Right
Tensor veli palatini muscle
  use Muscle, Tongue, Palate,
    Pharynx
Tenth cranial nerve
  use Nerve, Vagus
Tentorium cerebelli
  use Dura Mater
Teres major muscle
  use Muscle, Shoulder, Left
  use Muscle, Shoulder, Right
Teres minor muscle
  use Muscle, Shoulder, Left
  use Muscle, Shoulder, Right
Terlipressin XW0
TERLIVAZ®
  use Terlipressin
Termination of pregnancy
  Aspiration curettage 10A07ZZ
  Dilation and curettage 10A07ZZ
  Hysterotomy 10A00ZZ
  Intra-amniotic injection
    10A03ZZ
  Laminaria 10A07ZW
  Vacuum 10A07Z6
Testectomy
  see Excision, Male Reproductive
    System 0VB
  see Resection, Male Reproductive
    System 0VT
Testicular artery
  use Aorta, Abdominal
Testing
  Glaucoma 4A07XBZ
  Hearing
    see Hearing Assessment,
      Diagnostic Audiology F13
  Mental health
    see Psychological Tests
  Muscle function, electromyography
    (EMG)
    see Measurement,
      Musculoskeletal 4A0F
  Muscle function, manual
    see Motor Function Assessment,
      Rehabilitation F01
  Neurophysiologic monitoring, intra-
    operative
    see Monitoring, Physiological
      Systems 4A1
  Range of motion
    see Motor Function Assessment,
      Rehabilitation F01
  Vestibular function
    see Vestibular Assessment,
      Diagnostic Audiology F15
Thalamectomy
  see Excision, Thalamus 00B9
Thalamotomy
  see Drainage, Thalamus 0099
Thenar muscle
  use Muscle, Hand, Left
  use Muscle, Hand, Right
Therapeutic Massage
  Musculoskeletal System 8E0KX1Z
  Reproductive System
    Prostate 8E0VX1C
    Rectum 8E0VX1D

Therapeutic occlusion coil(s)
  use Intraluminal Device
Thermography 4A0ZXKZ
Thermotherapy, prostate
  see Destruction, Prostate 0V50
Third cranial nerve
  use Nerve, Oculomotor
Third occipital nerve
  use Nerve, Cervical
Third ventricle
  use Cerebral Ventricle
Thoracectomy
  see Excision, Anatomical Regions,
    General 0WB
Thoracentesis
  see Drainage, Anatomical Regions,
    General 0W9
Thoracic aortic plexus
  use Nerve, Thoracic Sympathetic
Thoracic esophagus
  use Esophagus, Middle
Thoracic facet joint
  use Joint, Thoracic Vertebral
Thoracic ganglion
  use Nerve, Thoracic Sympathetic
Thoracoacromial artery
  use Artery, Axillary, Left
  use Artery, Axillary, Right
Thoracocentesis
  see Drainage, Anatomical Regions,
    General 0W9
Thoracolumbar facet joint
  use Joint, Thoracolumbar Vertebral
Thoracoplasty
  see Repair, Anatomical Regions,
    General 0WQ
  see Supplement, Anatomical
    Regions, General 0WU
Thoracostomy tube
  use Drainage Device
Thoracostomy, for lung collapse
  see Drainage, Respiratory System
    0B9
Thoracotomy
  see Drainage, Anatomical Regions,
    General 0W9
Thoraflex™ Hybrid device *use*
  Branched Synthetic Substitute
    with Intraluminal Device in New
    Technology
**Thoratec IVAD (Implantable
  Ventricular Assist Device)**
  use Implantable Heart Assist System
    in Heart and Great Vessels
**Thoratec Paracorporeal Ventricular
  Assist Device**
  use Short-term External Heart
    Assist System in Heart and Great
    Vessels
Thrombectomy
  see Extirpation
Thrombolysis, Ultrasound assisted
  see Fragmentation, Artery
Thymectomy
  see Excision, Lymphatic and Hemic
    Systems 07B
  see Resection, Lymphatic and
    Hemic Systems 07T
Thymopexy
  see Repair, Lymphatic and Hemic
    Systems 07Q
  see Reposition, Lymphatic and
    Hemic Systems 07S
Thymus gland
  use Thymus
Thyroarytenoid muscle
  use Muscle, Neck, Left
  use Muscle, Neck, Right
Thyrocervical trunk
  use Artery, Thyroid, Left
  use Artery, Thyroid, Right

Thyroid cartilage
use Larynx
Thyroidectomy
see Excision, Endocrine System 0GB
see Resection, Endocrine System 0GT
Thyroidorrhaphy
see Repair, Endocrine System 0GQ
Thyroidoscopy 0GJK4ZZ
Thyroidotomy
see Drainage, Endocrine System 0G9
Tibial Extension with Motion Sensors, Insertion XNH
Tibial insert
use Liner in Lower Joints
Tibial sesamoid
use Metatarsal, Left
use Metatarsal, Right
Tibialis anterior muscle
use Muscle, Lower Leg, Left
use Muscle, Lower Leg, Right
Tibialis posterior muscle
use Muscle, Lower Leg, Left
use Muscle, Lower Leg, Right
Tibiofemoral joint
use Joint, Knee, Left
use Joint, Knee, Left, Tibial Surface
use Joint, Knee, Right
use Joint, Knee, Right, Tibial Surface
Tibioperoneal trunk
use Popliteal Artery, Left
use Popliteal Artery, Right
Tisagenlecleucel
use Tisagenlecleucel Immunotherapy
Tisagenlecleucel Immunotherapy XW0
Tissue bank graft
use Nonautologous Tissue Substitute
Tissue Expander
Insertion of device in
Breast
Bilateral 0HHV
Left 0HHU
Right 0HHT
Nipple
Left 0HHX
Right 0HHW
Subcutaneous Tissue and Fascia
Abdomen 0JH8
Back 0JH7
Buttock 0JH9
Chest 0JH6
Face 0JH1
Foot
Left 0JHR
Right 0JHQ
Hand
Left 0JHK
Right 0JHJ
Lower Arm
Left 0JHH
Right 0JHG
Lower Leg
Left 0JHP
Right 0JHN
Neck
Left 0JH5
Right 0JH4
Pelvic Region 0JHC
Perineum 0JHB
Scalp 0JH0
Upper Arm
Left 0JHF
Right 0JHD
Upper Leg
Left 0JHM
Right 0JHL

Tissue Expander *(continued)*
Insertion of device in *(continued)*
Subcutaneous Tissue and Fascia *(continued)*
Left 0HPU
Right 0HPT
Subcutaneous Tissue and Fascia
Head and Neck 0JPS
Lower Extremity 0JPW
Trunk 0JPT
Upper Extremity 0JPV
Revision of device in
Breast
Left 0HWU
Right 0HWT
Subcutaneous Tissue and Fascia
Head and Neck 0JWS
Lower Extremity 0JWW
Trunk 0JWT
Upper Extremity 0JWV
Tissue expander (inflatable)(injectable)
use Tissue Expander in Skin and Breast
use Tissue Expander in Subcutaneous Tissue and Fascia
Tissue Plasminogen Activator (tPA) (r-tPA)
use Thrombolytic Other
Titan Endoskeleton™
use Interbody Fusion Device in Lower Joints
use Interbody Fusion Device in Upper Joints
Titanium Sternal Fixation System (TSFS)
use Internal Fixation Device, Rigid Plate in 0PS
use Internal Fixation Device, Rigid Plate in 0PH
Tixagevimab and Cilgavimab Monoclonal Antibody XW023X7
Tocilizumab XW0
Tomographic (Tomo) Nuclear Medicine Imaging
Abdomen CW20
Abdomen and Chest CW24
Abdomen and Pelvis CW21
Anatomical Regions, Multiple CW2YYZZ
Bladder, Kidneys and Ureters CT23
Brain C020
Breast CH2YYZZ
Bilateral CH22
Left CH21
Right CH20
Bronchi and Lungs CB22
Central Nervous System C02YYZZ
Cerebrospinal Fluid C025
Chest CW23
Chest and Abdomen CW24
Chest and Neck CW26
Digestive System CD2YYZZ
Endocrine System CG2YYZZ
Extremity
Lower CW2D
Bilateral CP2F
Left CP2D
Right CP2C
Upper CW2M
Bilateral CP2B
Left CP29
Right CP28
Gallbladder CF24
Gastrointestinal Tract CD27
Gland, Parathyroid CG21
Head and Neck CW2B
Heart C22YYZZ
Right and Left C226
Hepatobiliary System and Pancreas CF2YYZZ
Kidneys, Ureters and Bladder CT23

Tomographic (Tomo) Nuclear Medicine Imaging *(continued)*
Liver CF25
Liver and Spleen CF26
Lungs and Bronchi CB22
Lymphatics and Hematologic System C72YYZZ
Musculoskeletal System, Other CP2YYZZ
Myocardium C22G
Neck and Chest CW26
Neck and Head CW2B
Pancreas and Hepatobiliary System CF2YYZZ
Pelvic Region CW2J
Pelvis CP26
Pelvis and Abdomen CW21
Pelvis and Spine CP27
Respiratory System CB2YYZZ
Skin CH2YYZZ
Skull CP21
Skull and Cervical Spine CP23
Spine
Cervical CP22
Cervical and Skull CP23
Lumbar CP2H
Thoracic CP2G
Thoracolumbar CP2J
Spine and Pelvis CP27
Spleen C722
Spleen and Liver CF26
Subcutaneous Tissue CH2YYZZ
Thorax CP24
Ureters, Kidneys and Bladder CT23
Urinary System CT2YYZZ
Tomography, computerized
see Computerized Tomography (CT Scan)
Tongue, base of
use Pharynx
Tonometry 4A07XBZ
Tonsillectomy
see Excision, Mouth and Throat 0CB
see Resection, Mouth and Throat 0CT
Tonsillotomy
see Drainage, Mouth and Throat 0C9
TOPS™ System *use* Posterior Spinal Motion Preservation Device in New Technology
Total Ankle Talar Replacement™ (TATR) *use* Synthetic Substitute, Talar Prosthesis in New Technology
Total Anomalous Pulmonary Venous Return (TAPVR) repair
see Bypass, Atrium, Left 0217
see Bypass, Vena Cava, Superior 021V
Total artificial (replacement) heart
use Synthetic Substitute
Total parenteral nutrition (TPN)
see Introduction of Nutritional Substance
Tourniquet, External
see Compression, Anatomical Regions 2W1
Trachectomy
see Excision, Trachea 0BB1
see Resection, Trachea 0BT1
Trachelectomy
see Excision, Cervix 0UBC
see Resection, Cervix 0UTC
Trachelopexy
see Repair, Cervix 0UQC
see Reposition, Cervix 0USC
Tracheloplasty
see Repair, Cervix 0UQC
Trachelorrhaphy
see Repair, Cervix 0UQC
Trachelotomy
see Drainage, Cervix 0U9C

Tracheobronchial lymph node
use Lymphatic, Thorax
Tracheoesophageal fistulization 0B110D6
Tracheolysis
see Release, Respiratory System 0BN
Tracheoplasty
see Repair, Respiratory System 0BQ
see Supplement, Respiratory System 0BU
Tracheorrhaphy
see Repair, Respiratory System 0BQ
Tracheoscopy 0BJ18ZZ
Tracheostomy
see Bypass, Respiratory System 0B1
Tracheostomy Device
Bypass, Trachea 0B11
Change device in, Trachea 0B21XFZ
Removal of device from, Trachea 0BP1
Revision of device in, Trachea 0BW1
Tracheostomy tube
use Tracheostomy Device in Respiratory System
Tracheotomy
see Drainage, Respiratory System 0B9
Traction
Abdominal Wall 2W63X
Arm
Lower
Left 2W6DX
Right 2W6CX
Upper
Left 2W6BX
Right 2W6AX
Back 2W65X
Chest Wall 2W64X
Extremity
Lower
Left 2W6MX
Right 2W6LX
Upper
Left 2W69X
Right 2W68X
Face 2W61X
Finger
Left 2W6KX
Right 2W6JX
Foot
Left 2W6TX
Right 2W6SX
Hand
Left 2W6FXZ
Right 2W6EXZ
Head 2W60X
Inguinal Region
Left 2W67X
Right 2W66X
Leg
Lower
Left 2W6RX
Right 2W6QX
Upper
Left 2W6PX
Right 2W6NX
Neck 2W62X
Thumb
Left 2W6HX
Right 2W6GX
Toe
Left 2W6VX
Right 2W6UX
Tractotomy
see Division, Central Nervous System and Cranial Nerves 008
Tragus
use Ear, External, Bilateral
use Ear, External, Left
use Ear, External, Right

Training, caregiver
see Caregiver Training
TRAM (transverse rectus abdominis myocutaneous) flap reconstruction
Free
see Replacement, Skin and Breast 0HR
Pedicled
see Transfer, Muscles 0KX
Transcatheter Pulmonary Valve (TPV) placement
In conduit 02RH38L
Native site 02RH38M
Transdermal Glomerular Filtration Rate (GFR) Measurement System XT25XE5
Transection
see Division
Transfer
Buccal Mucosa 0CX4
Bursa and Ligament
Abdomen
Left 0MXJ
Right 0MXH
Ankle
Left 0MXR
Right 0MXQ
Elbow
Left 0MX4
Right 0MX3
Foot
Left 0MXT
Right 0MXS
Hand
Left 0MX8
Right 0MX7
Head and Neck 0MX0
Hip
Left 0MXM
Right 0MXL
Knee
Left 0MXP
Right 0MXN
Lower Extremity
Left 0MXW
Right 0MXV
Perineum 0MXK
Rib(s) 0MXG
Shoulder
Left 0MX2
Right 0MX1
Spine
Lower 0MXD
Upper 0MXC
Sternum 0MXF
Upper Extremity
Left 0MXB
Right 0MX9
Wrist
Left 0MX6
Right 0MX5
Finger
Left 0XXP0ZM
Right 0XXN0ZL
Gingiva
Lower 0CX6
Upper 0CX5
Immunotherapy
see New Technology, Anatomical Regions XW2
Intestine
Large 0DXE
Small 0DX8
Lip
Lower 0CX1
Upper 0CX0
Muscle
Abdomen
Left 0KXL
Right 0KXK

Transfer *(continued)*
Muscle *(continued)*
Extraocular
Left 08XM
Right 08XL
Facial 0KX1
Foot
Left 0KXW
Right 0KXV
Hand
Left 0KXD
Right 0KXC
Head 0KX0
Hip
Left 0KXP
Right 0KXN
Lower Arm and Wrist
Left 0KXB
Right 0KX9
Lower Leg
Left 0KXT
Right 0KXS
Neck
Left 0KX3
Right 0KX2
Perineum 0KXM
Shoulder
Left 0KX6
Right 0KX5
Thorax
Left 0KXJ
Right 0KXH
Tongue, Palate, Pharynx 0KX4
Trunk
Left 0KXG
Right 0KXF
Upper Arm
Left 0KX8
Right 0KX7
Upper Leg
Left 0KXR
Right 0KXQ
Nerve
Abducens 00XL
Accessory 00XR
Acoustic 00XN
Cervical 01X1
Facial 00XM
Femoral 01XD
Glossopharyngeal 00XP
Hypoglossal 00XS
Lumbar 01XB
Median 01X5
Oculomotor 00XH
Olfactory 00XF
Optic 00XG
Peroneal 01XH
Phrenic 01X2
Pudendal 01XC
Radial 01X6
Sciatic 01XF
Thoracic 01X8
Tibial 01XG
Trigeminal 00XK
Trochlear 00XJ
Ulnar 01X4
Vagus 00XQ
Palate, Soft 0CX3
Prepuce 0VXT
Skin
Abdomen 0HX7XZZ
Back 0HX6XZZ
Buttock 0HX8XZZ
Chest 0HX5XZZ
Ear
Left 0HX3XZZ
Right 0HX2XZZ
Face 0HX1XZZ
Foot
Left 0HXNXZZ
Right 0HXMXZZ

Transfer *(continued)*
Skin *(continued)*
Hand
Left 0HXGXZZ
Right 0HXFXZZ
Inguinal 0HXAXZZ
Lower Arm
Left 0HXEXZZ
Right 0HXDXZZ
Lower Leg
Left 0HXLXZZ
Right 0HXKXZZ
Neck 0HX4XZZ
Perineum 0HX9XZZ
Scalp 0HX0XZZ
Upper Arm
Left 0HXCXZZ
Right 0HXBXZZ
Upper Leg
Left 0HXJXZZ
Right 0HXHXZZ
Stomach 0DX6
Subcutaneous Tissue and Fascia
Abdomen 0JX8
Back 0JX7
Buttock 0JX9
Chest 0JX6
Face 0JX1
Foot
Left 0JXR
Right 0JXQ
Hand
Left 0JXK
Right 0JXJ
Lower Arm
Left 0JXH
Right 0JXG
Lower Leg
Left 0JXP
Right 0JXN
Neck
Left 0JX5
Right 0JX4
Pelvic Region 0JXC
Perineum 0JXB
Scalp 0JX0
Upper Arm
Left 0JXF
Right 0JXD
Upper Leg
Left 0JXM
Right 0JXL
Tendon
Abdomen
Left 0LXG
Right 0LXF
Ankle
Left 0LXT
Right 0LXS
Foot
Left 0LXW
Right 0LXV
Hand
Left 0LX8
Right 0LX7
Head and Neck 0LX0
Hip
Left 0LXK
Right 0LXJ
Knee
Left 0LXR
Right 0LXQ
Lower Arm and Wrist
Left 0LX6
Right 0LX5
Lower Leg
Left 0LXP
Right 0LXN
Perineum 0LXH
Shoulder
Left 0LX2
Right 0LX1

Transfer *(continued)*
Tendon *(continued)*
Thorax
Left 0LXD
Right 0LXC
Trunk
Left 0LXB
Right 0LX9
Upper Arm
Left 0LX4
Right 0LX3
Upper Leg
Left 0LXM
Right 0LXL
Tongue 0CX7
Transfusion
Bone Marrow
Blood
Platelets 302A3R
Red Cells 302A3N
Frozen 302A3P
Whole 302A3H
Plasma
Fresh 302A3L
Frozen 302A3K
Serum Albumin 302A3J
New Technology
see New Technology, Anatomical Regions XW1
Products of Conception
Antihemophilic Factors 3027
Blood
Platelets 3027
Red Cells 3027
Frozen 3027
White Cells 3027
Whole 3027
Factor IX 3027
Fibrinogen 3027
Globulin 3027
Plasma
Fresh 3027
Frozen 3027
Plasma Cryoprecipitate 3027
Serum Albumin 3027
Vein
4-Factor Prothrombin Complex Concentrate 30283B1
Central
Antihemophilic Factors 30243V
Blood
Platelets 30243R
Red Cells 30243N
Frozen 30243P
White Cells 30243Q
Whole 30243H
Bone Marrow 30243G
Factor IX 30243W
Fibrinogen 30243T
Globulin 30243S
Hematopoietic Stem/Progenitor Cells (HSPC), Genetically Modified 30243C0
Pathogen Reduced Cryoprecipitated Fibrinogen Complex 30243D1
Plasma
Fresh 30243L
Frozen 30243K
Plasma Cryoprecipitate 30243M
Serum Albumin 30243J
Stem Cells
Cord Blood 30243X
Embryonic 30243AZ
Hematopoietic 30243Y
T-cell Depleted Hematopoietic 30243U
Peripheral
Antihemophilic Factors 30233V

Transfusion *(continued)*
Vein *(continued)*
Peripheral *(continued)*
Blood
Platelets 30233R
Red Cells 30233N
Frozen 30233P
White Cells 30233Q
Whole 30233H
Bone Marrow 30233G
Factor IX 30233W
Fibrinogen 30233T
Globulin 30233S
Hematopoietic Stem/
Progenitor Cells (HSPC),
Genetically Modified
30233C0
Pathogen Reduced
Cryoprecipitated Fibrinogen
Complex 30233D1
Plasma
Fresh 30233L
Frozen 30233K
Plasma Cryoprecipitate
30233M
Serum Albumin 30233J
Stem Cells
Cord Blood 30233X
Embryonic 30233AZ
Hematopoietic 30233Y
T-cell Depleted
Hematopoietic 30233U

Transplant
see Transplantation
Transplantation
Bone marrow
see Transfusion, Circulatory 302
Esophagus 0DY50Z
Face 0WY20Z
Hand
Left 0XYK0Z
Right 0XYJ0Z
Heart 02YA0Z
Hematopoietic cell
see Transfusion, Circulatory 302
Intestine
Large 0DYE0Z
Small 0DY80Z
Kidney
Left 0TY10Z
Right 0TY00Z
Liver 0FY00Z
Lung
Bilateral 0BYM0Z
Left 0BYL0Z
Lower Lobe
Left 0BYJ0Z
Right 0BYF0Z
Middle Lobe, Right 0BYD0Z
Right 0BYK0Z
Upper Lobe
Left 0BYG0Z
Right 0BYC0Z
Lung Lingula 0BYH0Z
Ovary
Left 0UY10Z
Right 0UY00Z
Pancreas 0FYG0Z
Penis 0VYS0Z
Products of Conception 10Y0
Scrotum 0VY50Z
Spleen 07YP0Z
Stem cell
see Transfusion, Circulatory 302
Stomach 0DY60Z
Thymus 07YM0Z
Uterus 0UY90Z
Transposition
see Bypass
see Reposition
see Transfer

Transversalis fascia
use Subcutaneous Tissue and Fascia,
Trunk
Transverse acetabular ligament
use Bursa and Ligament, Hip,
Left
use Bursa and Ligament, Hip,
Right
Transverse (cutaneous) cervical
nerve
use Nerve, Cervical Plexus
Transverse facial artery
use Artery, Temporal, Left
use Artery, Temporal, Right
Transverse foramen
use Cervical Vertebra
Transverse humeral ligament
use Bursa and Ligament, Shoulder,
Left
use Bursa and Ligament, Shoulder,
Right
Transverse ligament of atlas
use Bursa and Ligament, Head and
Neck
Transverse process
use Cervical Vertebra
use Thoracic Vertebra
use Lumbar Vertebra
Transverse Rectus Abdominis
Myocutaneous Flap
Replacement
Bilateral 0HRV076
Left 0HRU076
Right 0HRT076
Transfer
Left 0KXL
Right 0KXK
Transverse scapular ligament
use Bursa and Ligament, Shoulder,
Left
use Bursa and Ligament, Shoulder,
Right
Transverse thoracis muscle
use Muscle, Thorax, Left
use Muscle, Thorax, Right
Transversospinalis muscle
use Muscle, Trunk, Left
use Muscle, Trunk, Right
Transversus abdominis muscle
use Muscle, Abdomen, Left
use Muscle, Abdomen, Right
Trapezium bone
use Carpal, Left
use Carpal, Right
Trapezius muscle
use Muscle, Trunk, Left
use Muscle, Trunk, Right
Trapezoid bone
use Carpal, Left
use Carpal, Right
Treosulfan XW0
Triceps brachii muscle
use Muscle, Upper Arm, Left
use Muscle, Upper Arm, Right
Tricuspid annulus
use Valve, Tricuspid
TricValve® Transcatheter Bicaval
Valve System *use* Intraluminal
Device, Bioprosthetic Valve in
New Technology.
Trifacial nerve
use Nerve, Trigeminal
Trifecta™ Valve (aortic)
use Zooplastic Tissue in Heart and
Great Vessels
Trigone of bladder
use Bladder
TriGuard 3™ CEPD (cerebral
embolic protection device)
X2A6325
Trilaciclib XW0

Trimming, excisional
see Excision
Triquetral bone
use Carpal, Left
use Carpal, Right
Trochanteric bursa
use Bursa and Ligament, Hip,
Left
use Bursa and Ligament, Hip,
Right
TUMT (Transurethral microwave
thermotherapy of prostate)
0V507ZZ
TUNA (transurethral needle
ablation of prostate) 0V507ZZ
Tunneled central venous catheter
use Vascular Access Device
Tunneled in Subcutaneous Tissue
and Fascia
Tunneled spinal (intrathecal)
catheter
use Infusion Device
Turbinectomy
see Excision, Ear, Nose, Sinus 09B
see Resection, Ear, Nose, Sinus 09T
Turbinoplasty
see Repair, Ear, Nose, Sinus 09Q
see Replacement, Ear, Nose, Sinus
09R
see Supplement, Ear, Nose, Sinus 09U
Turbinotomy
see Division, Ear, Nose, Sinus 098
see Drainage, Ear, Nose, Sinus 099
TURP (transurethral resection of
prostate)
see Excision, Prostate 0VB0
see Resection, Prostate 0VT0
Twelfth cranial nerve
use Nerve, Hypoglossal
Two lead pacemaker
use Pacemaker, Dual Chamber in
0JH
Tympanic cavity
use Ear, Middle, Left
use Ear, Middle, Right
Tympanic nerve
use Nerve, Glossopharyngeal
Tympanic part of temoporal bone
use Bone, Temporal, Left
use Bone, Temporal, Right
Tympanogram
see Hearing Assessment, Diagnostic
Audiology F13
Tympanoplasty
see Repair, Ear, Nose, Sinus 09Q
see Replacement, Ear, Nose, Sinus
09R
see Supplement, Ear, Nose, Sinus
09U
Tympanosympathectomy
see Excision, Nerve, Head and Neck
Sympathetic 01BK
Tympanotomy
see Drainage, Ear, Nose, Sinus 099
TYRX Antibacterial Envelope
use Anti-infective Envelope

U

Ulnar collateral carpal ligament
use Bursa and Ligament, Wrist, Left
use Bursa and Ligament, Wrist,
Right
Ulnar collateral ligament
use Bursa and Ligament, Elbow,
Left
use Bursa and Ligament, Elbow,
Right
Ulnar notch
use Radius, Left
use Radius, Right

Ulnar vein
use Vein, Brachial, Left
use Vein, Brachial, Right
Ultrafiltration
Hemodialysis
see Performance, Urinary 5A1D
Therapeutic plasmapheresis
see Pheresis, Circulatory 6A55
Ultraflex™ Precision Colonic Stent
System
use Intraluminal Device
ULTRAPRO Hernia System (UHS)
use Synthetic Substitute
ULTRAPRO Partially Absorbable
Lightweight Mesh
use Synthetic Substitute
ULTRAPRO Plug
use Synthetic Substitute
Ultrasonic osteogenic stimulator
use Bone Growth Stimulator in
Head and Facial Bones
use Bone Growth Stimulator in
Lower Bones
use Bone Growth Stimulator in
Upper Bones
Ultrasonography
Abdomen BW40ZZZ
Abdomen and Pelvis BW41ZZZ
Abdominal Wall BH49ZZZ
Aorta
Abdominal, Intravascular
B440ZZ3
Thoracic, Intravascular B340ZZ3
Appendix BD48ZZZ
Artery
Brachiocephalic-Subclavian,
Right, Intravascular B341ZZ3
Celiac and Mesenteric,
Intravascular B44KZZ3
Common Carotid
Bilateral, Intravascular
B345ZZ3
Left, Intravascular B344ZZ3
Right, Intravascular B343ZZ3
Coronary
Multiple B241YZZ
Intravascular B241ZZ3
Transesophageal B241ZZ4
Single B240YZZ
Intravascular B240ZZ3
Transesophageal B240ZZ4
Femoral, Intravascular B44LZZ3
Inferior Mesenteric, Intravascular
B445ZZ3
Internal Carotid
Bilateral, Intravascular
B348ZZ3
Left, Intravascular B347ZZ3
Right, Intravascular B346ZZ3
Intra-Abdominal, Other,
Intravascular B44BZZ3
Intracranial, Intravascular
B34RZZ3
Lower Extremity
Bilateral, Intravascular
B44HZZ3
Left, Intravascular B44GZZ3
Right, Intravascular B44FZZ3
Mesenteric and Celiac,
Intravascular B44KZZ3
Ophthalmic, Intravascular
B34VZZ3
Penile, Intravascular B44NZZ3
Pulmonary
Left, Intravascular B34TZZ3
Right, Intravascular B34SZZ3
Renal
Bilateral, Intravascular
B448ZZ3
Left, Intravascular B447ZZ3
Right, Intravascular B446ZZ3

Ultrasonography (continued)
Artery (continued)
Subclavian, Left, Intravascular
B342ZZ3
Superior Mesenteric, Intravascular
B444ZZ3
Upper Extremity
Bilateral, Intravascular
B34KZZ3
Left, Intravascular B34JZZ3
Right, Intravascular B34HZZ3
Bile Duct BF40ZZZ
Bile Duct and Gallbladder
BF43ZZZ
Bladder BT40ZZZ
and Kidney BT4JZZZ
Brain B040ZZZ
Breast
Bilateral BH42ZZZ
Left BH41ZZZ
Right BH40ZZZ
Chest Wall BH4BZZZ
Coccyx BR4FZZZ
Connective Tissue
Lower Extremity BL41ZZZ
Upper Extremity BL40ZZZ
Duodenum BD49ZZZ
Elbow
Left, Densitometry BP4HZZ1
Right, Densitometry BP4GZZ1
Esophagus BD41ZZZ
Extremity
Lower BH48ZZZ
Upper BH47ZZZ
Eye
Bilateral B847ZZZ
Left B846ZZZ
Right B845ZZZ
Fallopian Tube
Bilateral BU42
Left BU41
Right BU40
Fetal Umbilical Cord BY47ZZZ
Fetus
First Trimester, Multiple
Gestation BY4BZZZ
Second Trimester, Multiple
Gestation BY4DZZZ
Single
First Trimester BY49ZZZ
Second Trimester
BY4CZZZ
Third Trimester BY4FZZZ
Third Trimester, Multiple
Gestation BY4GZZZ
Gallbladder BF42ZZZ
Gallbladder and Bile Duct
BF43ZZZ
Gastrointestinal Tract BD47ZZZ
Gland
Adrenal
Bilateral BG42ZZZ
Left BG41ZZZ
Right BG40ZZZ
Parathyroid BG43ZZZ
Thyroid BG44ZZZ
Hand
Left, Densitometry BP4PZZ1
Right, Densitometry BP4NZZ1
Head and Neck BH4CZZZ
Heart
Left B245YZZ
Intravascular B245ZZ3
Transesophageal B245ZZ4
Pediatric B24DYZZ
Intravascular B24DZZ3
Transesophageal
B24DZZ4
Right B244YZZ
Intravascular B244ZZ3
Transesophageal B244ZZ4

Ultrasonography (continued)
Hip (continued)
Right and Left B246YZZ
Intravascular B246ZZ3
Transesophageal B246ZZ4
Heart with Aorta B24BYZZ
Intravascular B24BZZ3
Transesophageal B24BZZ4
Hepatobiliary System, All
BF4CZZZ
Hip
Bilateral BQ42ZZZ
Left BQ41ZZZ
Right BQ40ZZZ
Kidney
and Bladder BT4JZZZ
Bilateral BT43ZZZ
Left BT42ZZZ
Right BT41ZZZ
Transplant BT49ZZZ
Knee
Bilateral BQ49ZZZ
Left BQ48ZZZ
Right BQ47ZZZ
Liver BF45ZZZ
Liver and Spleen BF46ZZZ
Mediastinum BB4CZZZ
Neck BW4FZZZ
Ovary
Bilateral BU45
Left BU44
Right BU43
Ovary and Uterus BU4C
Pancreas BF47ZZZ
Pelvic Region BW4GZZZ
Pelvis and Abdomen BW41ZZZ
Penis BV4BZZZ
Pericardium B24CYZZ
Intravascular B24CZZ3
Transesophageal B24CZZ4
Placenta BY48ZZZ
Pleura BB4BZZZ
Prostate and Seminal Vesicle
BV49ZZZ
Rectum BD4CZZZ
Sacrum BR4FZZZ
Scrotum BV44ZZZ
Seminal Vesicle and Prostate
BV49ZZZ
Shoulder
Left, Densitometry BP49ZZ1
Right, Densitometry BP48ZZ1
Spinal Cord B04BZZZ
Spine
Cervical BR40ZZZ
Lumbar BR49ZZZ
Thoracic BR47ZZZ
Spleen and Liver BF46ZZZ
Stomach BD42ZZZ
Tendon
Lower Extremity BL43ZZZ
Upper Extremity BL42ZZZ
Ureter
Bilateral BT48ZZZ
Left BT47ZZZ
Right BT46ZZZ
Urethra BT45ZZZ
Uterus BU46
Uterus and Ovary BU4C
Vein
Jugular
Left, Intravascular
B544ZZ3
Right, Intravascular
B543ZZ3
Lower Extremity
Bilateral, Intravascular
B54DZZ3
Left, Intravascular B54CZZ3
Right, Intravascular B54BZZ3
Portal, Intravascular B54TZZ3

Ultrasonography (continued)
Vein (continued)
Renal
Bilateral, Intravascular
B54LZZ3
Left, Intravascular
B54KZZ3
Right, Intravascular B54JZZ3
Spanchnic, Intravascular
B54TZZ3
Subclavian
Left, Intravascular B547ZZ3
Right, Intravascular B546ZZ3
Upper Extremity
Bilateral, Intravascular
B54PZZ3
Left, Intravascular B54NZZ3
Right, Intravascular
B54MZZ3
Vena Cava
Inferior, Intravascular B549ZZ3
Superior, Intravascular
B548ZZ3
Wrist
Left, Densitometry BP4MZZ1
Right, Densitometry BP4LZZ1
**Ultrasound Ablation, Destruction,
Renal Sympathetic Nerve(s)**
X051329
Ultrasound bone healing system
use Bone Growth Stimulator in
Head and Facial Bones
use Bone Growth Stimulator in
Lower Bones
use Bone Growth Stimulator in
Upper Bones
**Ultrasound Penetrable Synthetic
Substitute, Skull** XNR80D9
Ultrasound Therapy
Heart 6A75
No Qualifier 6A75
Vessels
Head and Neck 6A75
Other 6A75
Peripheral 6A75
Ultraviolet Light Therapy, Skin
6A80
Umbilical artery
use Artery, Internal Iliac, Left
use Artery, Internal Iliac, Right
use Artery, Lower
Uniplanar external fixator
use External Fixation Device,
Monoplanar in 0PH
use External Fixation Device,
Monoplanar in 0PS
use External Fixation Device,
Monoplanar in 0QH
use External Fixation Device,
Monoplanar in 0QS
UPLIZNA® use Inebilizumab-cdon
Upper GI series
see Fluoroscopy, Gastrointestinal,
Upper BD15
Ureteral orifice
use Ureter
use Ureter, Left
use Ureter, Right
use Ureters, Bilateral
Ureterectomy
see Excision, Urinary System 0TB
see Resection, Urinary System
0TT
Ureterocolostomy
see Bypass, Urinary System 0T1
Ureterocystostomy
see Bypass, Urinary System 0T1
Ureteroenterostomy
see Bypass, Urinary System 0T1
Ureteroileostomy
see Bypass, Urinary System 0T1

Ureterolithotomy
see Extirpation, Urinary System
0TC
Ureterolysis
see Release, Urinary System 0TN
Ureteroneocystostomy
see Bypass, Urinary System 0T1
see Reposition, Urinary System 0TS
Ureteropelvic junction (UPJ)
use Kidney Pelvis, Left
use Kidney Pelvis, Right
Ureteropexy
see Repair, Urinary System 0TQ
see Reposition, Urinary System 0TS
Ureteroplasty
see Repair, Urinary System 0TQ
see Replacement, Urinary System
0TR
see Supplement, Urinary System
0TU
Ureteroplication
see Restriction, Urinary System 0TV
Ureteropyelography
see Fluoroscopy, Urinary System
BT1
Ureterorrhaphy
see Repair, Urinary System 0TQ
Ureteroscopy 0TJ98ZZ
Ureterostomy
see Bypass, Urinary System 0T1
see Drainage, Urinary
System 0T9
Ureterotomy
see Drainage, Urinary
System 0T9
Ureteroureterostomy
see Bypass, Urinary System 0T1
Ureterovesical orifice
use Ureter
use Ureters, Bilateral
use Ureter, Left
use Ureter, Right
Urethral catheterization, indwelling
0T9B70Z
Urethrectomy
see Excision, Urethra 0TBD
see Resection, Urethra 0TTD
Urethrolithotomy
see Extirpation, Urethra 0TCD
Urethrolysis
see Release, Urethra 0TND
Urethropexy
see Repair, Urethra 0TQD
see Reposition, Urethra 0TSD
Urethroplasty
see Repair, Urethra 0TQD
see Replacement, Urethra 0TRD
see Supplement, Urethra 0TUD
Urethrorrhaphy
see Repair, Urethra 0TQD
Urethroscopy 0TJD8ZZ
Urethrotomy
see Drainage, Urethra 0T9D
Uridine Triacetate XW0DX82
**Urinary incontinence stimulator
lead**
use Stimulator Lead in Urinary
System
Urography
see Fluoroscopy, Urinary System
BT1
Ustekinumab
use Other New Technology
Therapeutic Substance
Uterine Artery
use Artery, Internal Iliac, Left
use Artery, Internal Iliac, Right
**Uterine artery embolization
(UAE)**
see Occlusion, Lower
Arteries 04L

Uterine cornu
 use Uterus
Uterine tube
 use Fallopian Tube, Left
 use Fallopian Tube, Right
Uterine vein
 use Vein, Hypogastric, Left
 use Vein, Hypogastric, Right
Uvulectomy
 see Excision, Uvula 0CBN
 see Resection, Uvula 0CTN
Uvulorrhaphy
 see Repair, Uvula 0CQN
Uvulotomy
 see Drainage, Uvula 0C9N

V

V-Wave Interatrial Shunt System
 use Synthetic Substitute
Vabomere™
 use Meropenem-vaboractam Anti-
 infective
Vaccination
 see Introduction of Serum, Toxoid,
 and Vaccine
Vacuum extraction, obstetric
 10D07Z6
Vaginal artery
 use Artery, Internal Iliac, Left
 use Artery, Internal Iliac, Right
Vaginal pessary
 use Intraluminal Device, Pessary
 in Female Reproductive
 System
Vaginal vein
 use Vein, Hypogastric, Left
 use Vein, Hypogastric, Right
Vaginectomy
 see Excision, Vagina 0UBG
 see Resection, Vagina
 0UTG
Vaginofixation
 see Repair, Vagina 0UQG
 see Reposition, Vagina 0USG
Vaginoplasty
 see Repair, Vagina 0UQG
 see Supplement, Vagina 0UUG
Vaginorrhaphy
 see Repair, Vagina 0UQG
Vaginoscopy 0UJH8ZZ
Vaginotomy
 see Drainage, Female Reproductive
 System 0U9
Vagotomy
 see Division, Nerve, Vagus 008Q
Valiant Thoracic Stent Graft
 use Intraluminal Device
Valvotomy, valvulotomy
 see Division, Heart and Great
 Vessels 028
 see Release, Heart and Great Vessels
 02N
Valvuloplasty
 see Repair, Heart and Great Vessels
 02Q
 see Replacement, Heart and Great
 Vessels 02R
 see Supplement, Heart and Great
 Vessels 02U
Valvuloplasty, Alfieri Stitch
 see Restriction, Valve, Mitral
 02VG
Vanta™ PC neurostimulator *use*
 Stimulator Generator, Multiple
 Array in 0JH
Vascular Access Device
 Totally Implantable
 Insertion of device in
 Abdomen 0JH8
 Chest 0JH6

Vascular Access Device *(continued)*
 Totally Implantable *(continued)*
 Insertion of device in *(continued)*
 Lower Arm
 Left 0JHH
 Right 0JHG
 Lower Leg
 Left 0JHP
 Right 0JHN
 Upper Arm
 Left 0JHF
 Right 0JHD
 Upper Leg
 Left 0JHM
 Right 0JHL
 Removal of device from
 Lower Extremity 0JPW
 Trunk 0JPT
 Upper Extremity 0JPV
 Revision of device in
 Lower Extremity 0JWW
 Trunk 0JWT
 Upper Extremity 0JWV
 Tunneled
 Insertion of device in
 Abdomen 0JH8
 Chest 0JH6
 Lower Arm
 Left 0JHH
 Right 0JHG
 Lower Leg
 Left 0JHP
 Right 0JHN
 Upper Arm
 Left 0JHF
 Right 0JHD
 Upper Leg
 Left 0JHM
 Right 0JHL
 Removal of device from
 Lower Extremity 0JPW
 Trunk 0JPT
 Upper Extremity 0JPV
 Revision of device in
 Lower Extremity 0JWW
 Trunk 0JWT
 Upper Extremity 0JWV
Vasectomy
 see Excision, Male Reproductive
 System 0VB
Vasography
 see Fluoroscopy, Male Reproductive
 System BV1
 see Plain Radiography, Male
 Reproductive System BV0
Vasoligation
 see Occlusion, Male Reproductive
 System 0VL
Vasorrhaphy
 see Repair, Male Reproductive
 System 0VQ
Vasostomy
 see Bypass, Male Reproductive
 System 0V1
Vasotomy
 Drainage
 see Drainage, Male Reproductive
 System 0V9
 see Occlusion, Male
 Reproductive System 0VL
 With ligation
Vasovasostomy
 see Repair, Male Reproductive
 System 0VQ
VasQ™ External Support device
 use Synthetic Substitute,
 Extraluminal Support Device in
 New Technology
Vastus intermedius muscle
 use Muscle, Upper Leg, Left
 use Muscle, Upper Leg, Right

Vastus lateralis muscle
 use Muscle, Upper Leg, Left
 use Muscle, Upper Leg, Right
Vastus medialis muscle
 use Muscle, Upper Leg, Left
 use Muscle, Upper Leg, Right
VCG (vectorcardiogram)
 see Measurement, Cardiac 4A02
Vectra® Vascular Access Graft
 use Vascular Access Device,
 Tunneled in Subcutaneous Tissue
 and Fascia
**Vein Graft Extraluminal Support
 Device(s), Supplement, Coronary
 Artery/Arteries** X2U4079
Veklury *use* Remdesivir
 Anti-infective
Venclexta®
 use Venetoclax Antineoplastic
Venetoclax Antineoplastic
 XW0DXR5
Venectomy
 see Excision, Lower Veins 06B
 see Excision, Upper Veins 05B
Venography
 see Fluoroscopy, Veins B51
 see Plain Radiography, Veins B50
Venorrhaphy
 see Repair, Lower Veins 06Q
 see Repair, Upper Veins 05Q
Venotripsy
 see Occlusion, Lower Veins 06L
 see Occlusion, Upper Veins 05L
VenoValve® *use* Intraluminal Device,
 Bioprosthetic Valve in New
 Technology
Ventricular fold
 use Larynx
Ventriculoatriostomy
 see Bypass, Central Nervous System
 and Cranial Nerves 001
Ventriculocisternostomy
 see Bypass, Central Nervous System
 and Cranial Nerves 001
Ventriculogram, cardiac
 Combined left and right heart
 see Fluoroscopy, Heart, Right and
 Left B216
 Left ventricle
 see Fluoroscopy, Heart, Left
 B215
 Right ventricle
 see Fluoroscopy, Heart, Right
 B214
**Ventriculopuncture, through
 previously implanted
 catheter** 8C01X6J
Ventriculoscopy 00J04ZZ
Ventriculostomy
 External drainage
 see Drainage, Cerebral Ventricle
 0096
 Internal shunt
 see Bypass, Cerebral Ventricle
 0016
Ventriculovenostomy
 see Bypass, Cerebral Ventricle 0016
Ventrio™ Hernia Patch
 use Synthetic Substitute
VEP (visual evoked potential)
 4A07X0Z
Vermiform appendix
 use Appendix
Vermilion border
 use Lip, Lower
 use Lip, Upper
Versa
 use Pacemaker, Dual Chamber in 0JH
Version, obstetric
 External 10S0XZZ
 Internal 10S07ZZ

Vertebral arch
 use Vertebra, Cervical
 use Vertebra, Lumbar
 use Vertebra, Thoracic
**Vertebral artery, intracranial
 portion** *use* Intracranial Artery
Vertebral body
 use Cervical Vertebra
 use Thoracic Vertebra
 use Lumbar Vertebra
Vertebral canal
 use Spinal Canal
Vertebral foramen
 use Vertebra, Cervical
 use Vertebra, Lumbar
 use Vertebra, Thoracic
Vertebral lamina
 use Vertebra, Cervical
 use Vertebra, Lumbar
 use Vertebra, Thoracic
Vertebral pedicle
 use Vertebra, Cervical
 use Vertebra, Lumbar
 use Vertebra, Thoracic
Vesical vein
 use Vein, Hypogastric, Left
 use Vein, Hypogastric, Right
Vesicotomy
 see Drainage, Urinary System
 0T9
Vesiculectomy
 see Excision, Male Reproductive
 System 0VB
 see Resection, Male Reproductive
 System 0VT
Vesiculogram, seminal
 see Plain Radiography, Male
 Reproductive System BV0
Vesiculotomy
 see Drainage, Male Reproductive
 System 0V9
**VEST™ Venous External
 Support device** *use* Vein Graft
 Extraluminal Support Device(s)
 in New Technology
Vestibular (Scarpa's) ganglion
 use Nerve, Acoustic
Vestibular Assessment F15Z
Vestibular nerve
 use Nerve, Acoustic
Vestibular Treatment F0C
Vestibulocochlear nerve
 use Nerve, Acoustic
**VH-IVUS (virtual histology
 intravascular ultrasound)**
 see Ultrasonography, Heart B24
**Virchow's (supraclavicular) lymph
 node**
 use Lymphatic, Neck, Left
 use Lymphatic, Neck, Right
Virtuoso (II) (DR) (VR)
 use Defibrillator Generator
 in 0JH
Vistogard®
 use Uridine Triacetate
**Visualase™ MRI-Guided Laser
 Ablation System** *see* Destruction
Vitrectomy
 see Excision, Eye 08B
 see Resection, Eye 08T
Vitreous body
 use Vitreous, Left
 use Vitreous, Right
Viva (XT)(S)
 use Cardiac Resynchronization
 Defibrillator Pulse Generator in
 0JH
Vivistim® Paired VNS System Lead
 use Neurostimulator Lead with
 Paired Stimulation System in
 New Technology

Vocal fold
　use Vocal Cord, Left
　use Vocal Cord, Right
Vocational
　Assessment
　Retraining
　　see Activities of Daily Living Assessment, Rehabilitation F02
　　see Activities of Daily Living Treatment, Rehabilitation F08
Volar (palmar) digital vein
　use Vein, Hand, Left
　use Vein, Hand, Right
Volar (palmar) metacarpal vein
　use Vein, Hand, Left
　use Vein, Hand, Right
Vomer bone
　use Septum, Nasal
Vomer of nasal septum
　use Bone, Nasal
Voraxaze
　Glucarpidase
Vulvectomy
　see Excision, Female Reproductive System 0UB
　see Resection, Female Reproductive System 0UT
VYXEOS™
　use Cytarabine and Daunorubicin Liposome Antineoplastic

W

WALLSTENT® Endoprosthesis
　use Intraluminal Device
Washing
　see Irrigation
WavelinQ EndoAVF system
　Radial Artery, Left 031C
　Radial Artery, Right 031B
　Ulnar Artery, Left 031A

WavelinQ EndoAVF system
　(continued)
　Ulnar Artery, Right 0319
Wedge resection, pulmonary
　see Excision, Respiratory System 0BB
Whole Blood Nucleic Acid-base Microbial Detection XXE5XM5
Whole Blood Reverse Transcription and Quantitative Real-time Polymerase Chain Reaction XXE5X38
Window
　see Drainage
Wiring, dental 2W31X9Z

X

X-ray
　see Plain Radiography
X-Spine Axle Cage
　use Spinal Stabilization Device, Interspinous Process in 0RH
　use Spinal Stabilization Device, Interspinous Process in 0SH
X-STOP® Spacer
　use Spinal Stabilization Device, Interspinous Process in 0RH
　use Spinal Stabilization Device, Interspinous Process in 0SH
Xact Carotid Stent System
　use Intraluminal Device
XENLETA™
　use Lefamulin Anti-infective
Xenograft
　use Zooplastic Tissue in Heart and Great Vessels
XENOVIEW™ BB34Z3Z
XIENCE Everolimus Eluting Coronary Stent System
　use Intraluminal Device, Drug-eluting in Heart and Great Vessels

Xiphoid process
　use Sternum
XLIF® System
　use Interbody Fusion Device in Lower Joints
XOSPATA®
　use Gilteritinib Antineoplastic

Y

Yescarta®
　use Axicabtagene Ciloleucel Immunotherapy
Yoga Therapy 8E0ZXY4

Z

Z-plasty, skin for scar contracture
　see Release, Skin and Breast 0HN
Zenith AAA Endovascular Graft
　use Intraluminal Device
Zenith® Fenestrated AAA Endovascular Graft
　use Intraluminal Device, Branched or Fenestrated, One or Two Arteries in 04V
　use Intraluminal Device, Branched or Fenestrated, Three or More Arteries in 04V
Zenith Flex® AAA Endovascular Graft
　use Intraluminal Device
Zenith TX2® TAA Endovascular Graft
　use Intraluminal Device
Zenith® Renu™ AAA Ancillary Graft
　use Intraluminal Device

ZEPZELCA™ *use* Lurbinectedin
ZERBAXA®
　use Ceftolozane/Tazobactam Anti-infective
Zilver® PTX® (paclitaxel) Drug-Eluting Peripheral Stent
　use Intraluminal Device, Drug-eluting in Lower Arteries
　use Intraluminal Device, Drug-eluting in Upper Arteries
Zimmer® NexGen® LPS Mobile Bearing Knee
　use Synthetic Substitute
Zimmer® NexGen® LPS-Flex Mobile Knee
　use Synthetic Substitute
ZINPLAVA™ infusion *see* Introduction with qualifier Other Therapeutic Monoclonal Antibody
Zonule of Zinn
　use Lens, Left
　use Lens, Right
Zotarolimus-eluting coronary stent
　use Intraluminal Device, Drug-eluting in Heart and Great Vessels
ZULRESSO™
　use Brexanolone
Zygomatic process of frontal bone
　use Bone, Frontal
Zygomatic process of temporal bone
　use Bone, Temporal, Left
　use Bone, Temporal, Right
Zygomaticus muscle
　use Muscle, Facial
ZYNTEGLO® *use* Betibeglogene Autotemcel
Zyvox
　use Oxazolidinones

Medical and Surgical (001–0YW)

Within each section of ICD-10-PCS the characters have different meanings. The seven character meanings for the Medical and Surgical section are illustrated here through the procedure example of *Percutaneous needle core biopsy of the right kidney*.

Section	Body System	Root Operation	Body Part	Approach	Device	Qualifier
Med/Surg	Urinary	Excision	Kidney, Right	Percutaneous	None	Diagnostic
0	T	B	0	3	Z	X

Section (Character 1)

All Medical and Surgical procedure codes have a first character value of 0.

Body System (Character 2)

The alphanumeric character for the body system is placed in the second position. The following are the body systems applicable to the Medical and Surgical section.

Character Value	Character Value Description
0	Central Nervous System and Cranial Nerves
1	Peripheral Nervous System
2	Heart and Great Vessels
3	Upper Arteries
4	Lower Arteries
5	Upper Veins
6	Lower Veins
7	Lymphatic and Hemic Systems
8	Eye
9	Ear, Nose, Sinus
B	Respiratory System
C	Mouth and Throat
D	Gastrointestinal System
F	Hepatobiliary System and Pancreas
G	Endocrine System
H	Skin and Breast
J	Subcutaneous Tissue and Fascia
K	Muscles
L	Tendons
M	Bursae and Ligaments
N	Head and Facial Bones
P	Upper Bones
Q	Lower Bones
R	Upper Joints
S	Lower Joints
T	Urinary System
U	Female Reproductive System
V	Male Reproductive System
W	Anatomical Regions, General
X	Anatomical Regions, Upper Extremities
Y	Anatomical Regions, Lower Extremities

Root Operations (Character 3)

The alphanumeric character value for root operations is placed in the third position. Listed below are the root operations applicable to the Medical and Surgical section with their associated meaning.

Character Value	Root Operation	Root Operation Definition
0	Alteration	Modifying the anatomic structure of a body part without affecting the function of the body part
1	Bypass	Altering the route of passage of the contents of a tubular body part
2	Change	Taking out or off a device from a body part and putting back an identical or similar device in or on the same body part without cutting or puncturing the skin or a mucous membrane
3	Control	Stopping, or attempting to stop, postprocedural or other acute bleeding
4	Creation	Making a new genital structure that does not take over the function of a body part
5	Destruction	Physical eradication of all or a portion of a body part by the direct use of energy, force, or a destructive agent
6	Detachment	Cutting off all or a portion of the upper or lower extremities
7	Dilation	Expanding an orifice or the lumen of a tubular body part
8	Division	Cutting into a body part, without draining fluids and/or gases from the body part, in order to separate or transect a body part
9	Drainage	Taking or letting out fluids and/or gases from a body part
B	Excision	Cutting out or off, without replacement, a portion of a body part
C	Extirpation	Taking or cutting out solid matter from a body part
D	Extraction	Pulling or stripping out or off all or a portion of a body part by the use of force
F	Fragmentation	Breaking solid matter in a body part into pieces
G	Fusion	Joining together portions of an articular body part rendering the articular body part immobile
H	Insertion	Putting in a nonbiological appliance that monitors, assists, performs, or prevents a physiological function but does not physically take the place of a body part
J	Inspection	Visually and/or manually exploring a body part
K	Map	Locating the route of passage of electrical impulses and/or locating functional areas in a body part
L	Occlusion	Completely closing an orifice or the lumen of a tubular body part
M	Reattachment	Putting back in or on all or a portion of a separated body part to its normal location or other suitable location
N	Release	Freeing a body part from an abnormal physical constraint by cutting or by the use of force
P	Removal	Taking out or off a device from a body part
Q	Repair	Restoring, to the extent possible, a body part to its normal anatomic structure and function
R	Replacement	Putting in or on biological or synthetic material that physically takes the place and/or function of all or a portion of a body part
S	Reposition	Moving to its normal location, or other suitable location, all or a portion of a body part
T	Resection	Cutting out or off, without replacement, all of a body part
V	Restriction	Partially closing an orifice or the lumen of a tubular body part
W	Revision	Correcting, to the extent possible, a portion of a malfunctioning device or the position of a displaced device
U	Supplement	Putting in or on biological or synthetic material that physically reinforces and/or augments the function of a portion of a body part
X	Transfer	Moving, without taking out, all or a portion of a body part to another location to take over the function of all or a portion of a body part
Y	Transplantation	Putting in or on all or a portion of a living body part taken from another individual or animal to physically take the place and/or function of all or a portion of a similar body part

Body Part (Character 4)

For each body system the applicable body part character values will be available for procedure code construction. An example of a body part for this section is the Large Intestines.

Approach (Character 5)

The approach is the technique used to reach the procedure site. The following are the approach character values for the Medical and Surgical section with the associated definitions.

Character Value	Approach	Approach Definition
0	Open	Cutting through the skin or mucous membrane and any other body layers necessary to expose the site of the procedure
3	Percutaneous	Entry, by puncture or minor incision, of instrumentation through the skin or mucous membrane and any other body layers necessary to reach the site of the procedure
4	Percutaneous Endoscopic	Entry, by puncture or minor incision, of instrumentation through the skin or mucous membrane and any other body layers necessary to reach and visualize the site of the procedure
7	Via Natural or Artificial Opening	Entry of instrumentation through a natural or artificial external opening to reach the site of the procedure
8	Via Natural or Artificial Opening Endoscopic	Entry of instrumentation through a natural or artificial external opening to reach and visualize the site of the procedure
F	Via Natural or Artificial Opening Percutaneous Endoscopic	Entry of instrumentation through a natural or artificial external opening to reach and visualize the site of the procedure, and entry, by puncture or minor incision, of instrumentation through the skin or mucous membrane and any other body layers necessary to aid in the performance of the procedure
X	External	Procedures performed directly on the skin or mucous membrane and procedures performed indirectly by the application of external force through the skin or mucous membrane

Device (Character 6)

Depending on the procedure performed there may or may not be a device used. There are several types of devices included in the Medical and Surgical section that fall into one of the four following categories.

- Electronic Appliances
- Grafts and Prostheses
- Implants
- Simple or Mechanical Appliances

When a device is not utilized during the procedure, the character value of Z should be reported.

If a coder is unsure of which option to select for the device utilized during the procedure, Appendix E can be used to guide the selection. For example, if the coder is in Table 02R (replacement of heart and great vessels) the coder can locate the device categories in Appendix E (Autologous Tissue Substitute, Zooplastic Tissue, Synthetic Substitute, and Nonautologous Tissue Substitue). For each of these categories brand name devices and other devices are listed. The coder should select the category in which the device utilized during the procedure is listed.

Qualifier (Character 7)

The qualifier represents an additional attribute for the procedure when applicable. In the preceding example of *Percutaneous needle core biopsy of the right kidney*, the qualifier of X was used to report that the biopsy procedure was diagnostic in nature. If there is no qualifier for a procedure, the Z character value should be reported.

Important Definitions for the Medical and Surgical Section

Medical Surgical Root Operation	Qualifier	Definition
Detachment of Upper and Lower Extremities (0X6 and 0Y6) Arms and Legs	1 – High	Amputation at the proximal portion of the shaft of the humerus or femur
	2 – Mid	Amputation at the middle portion of the shaft of the humerus or femur
	3 – Low	Amputation at the distal portion of the shaft of the humerus or femur
Detachment of Upper and Lower Extremities (0X6 and 0Y6) Fingers, Thumbs, and Toes	0 – Complete	Amputation at the metacarpophalangeal/metatarsal-phalangeal joint
	1 – High	Amputation anywhere along the proximal phalanx
	2 – Mid	Amputation through the proximal interphalangeal joint or anywhere along the middle phalanx
	3 – Low	Amputation through the distal interphalangeal joint or anywhere along the distal phalanx
Transplantation	0 – Allogeneic	Being genetically different although belonging to or obtained from the same species*
	1 – Syngeneic	Genetically identical or closely related, so as to allow tissue transplant; immunologically compatible*
	2 – Zooplastic	Surgical transfer of tissue from an animal to a human*

*Taken from The Free Dictionary by Farlex at www.thefreedictionary.com

Official Coding Guidelines for the Medical and Surgical Section

Medical and Surgical Section Guidelines (section 0)

B2. Body System

General guidelines

B2.1a The procedure codes in Anatomical Regions, General, Anatomical Regions, Upper Extremities and Anatomical Regions, Lower Extremities can be used when the procedure is performed on an anatomical region rather than a specific body part, or on the rare occasion when no information is available to support assignment of a code to a specific body part.

Examples: Chest tube drainage of the pleural cavity is coded to the root operation Drainage found in the body system Anatomical Regions, General. Suture repair of the abdominal wall is coded to the root operation Repair in the body system Anatomical Regions, General. Amputation of the foot is coded to the root operation Detachment in the body system Anatomical Regions, Lower Extremities.

B2.1b Where the general body part values "upper" and "lower" are provided as an option in the Upper Arteries, Lower Arteries, Upper Veins, Lower Veins, Muscles and Tendons body systems, "upper" or "lower" specifies body parts located above or below the diaphragm respectively.

Example: Vein body parts above the diaphragm are found in the Upper Veins body system; vein body parts below the diaphragm are found in the Lower Veins body system.

B3. Root Operation

General guidelines

B3.1a In order to determine the appropriate root operation, the full definition of the root operation as contained in the PCS Tables must be applied.

B3.1b Components of a procedure specified in the root operation definition or explanation as integral to that root operation are not coded separately. Procedural steps necessary to reach the operative site and close the operative site, including anastomosis of a tubular body part, are also not coded separately.

Examples: Resection of a joint as part of a joint replacement procedure is included in the root operation definition of Replacement and is not coded separately. Laparotomy performed to reach the site of an open liver biopsy is not coded separately. In a resection of sigmoid colon with anastomosis of descending colon to rectum, the anastomosis is not coded separately.

Multiple procedures

B3.2 During the same operative episode, multiple procedures are coded if:

a. The same root operation is performed on different body parts as defined by distinct values of the body part character.

Examples: Diagnostic excision of liver and pancreas are coded separately. Excision of lesion in the ascending colon and excision of lesion in the transverse colon are coded separately.

b. The same root operation is repeated at different body sites that are included in the same body part value.

Examples: Excision of the sartorius muscle and excision of the gracilis muscle are both included in the upper leg muscle body part value, and multiple procedures are coded. Extraction of multiple toenails are coded separately.

c. Multiple root operations with distinct objectives are performed on the same body part.

Example: Destruction of sigmoid lesion and bypass of sigmoid colon are coded separately.

d. The intended root operation is attempted using one approach but is converted to a different approach.

Example: Laparoscopic cholecystectomy converted to an open cholecystectomy is coded as percutaneous endoscopic Inspection and open Resection.

Discontinued or incomplete procedures

B3.3 If the intended procedure is discontinued or otherwise not complete, code the procedure to the root operation performed. If a procedure is discontinued before any other root operation is performed, code the root operation Inspection of the body part or anatomical region inspected.

Example: A planned aortic valve replacement procedure is discontinued after the initial thoracotomy and before any incision is made in the heart muscle, when the patient becomes hemodynamically unstable. This procedure is coded as an open Inspection of the mediastinum.

Biopsy procedures

B3.4a Biopsy procedures are coded using the root operations Excision, Extraction, or Drainage and the qualifier Diagnostic.

Examples: Fine needle aspiration biopsy of lung is coded to the root operation Drainage with the qualifier Diagnostic. Biopsy of bone marrow is coded to the root operation Extraction with the qualifier Diagnostic. Lymph node sampling for biopsy is coded to the root operation Excision with the qualifier Diagnostic.

Biopsy followed by more definitive treatment

B3.4b If a diagnostic Excision, Extraction, or Drainage procedure (biopsy) is followed by a more definitive procedure, such as Destruction, Excision or Resection at the same procedure site, both the biopsy and the more definitive treatment are coded.

Example: Biopsy of breast followed by partial mastectomy at the same procedure site, both the biopsy and the partial mastectomy procedure are coded.

Overlapping body layers

B3.5 If root operations Excision, Extraction, Repair or Inspection are performed on overlapping layers of the musculoskeletal system, the body part specifying the deepest layer is coded.

Example: Excisional debridement that includes skin and subcutaneous tissue and muscle is coded to the muscle body part.

Bypass procedures

B3.6a Bypass procedures are coded by identifying the body part bypassed "from" and the body part bypassed "to." The fourth character body part specifies the body part bypassed from, and the qualifier specifies the body part bypassed to.

Example: Bypass from stomach to jejunum, stomach is the body part and jejunum is the qualifier.

B3.6b Coronary artery bypass procedures are coded differently than other bypass procedures as described in the previous guideline. Rather than identifying the body part bypassed from, the body part identifies the number of coronary artery sites bypassed to, and the qualifier specifies the vessel bypassed from.

Example: Aortocoronary artery bypass of the left anterior descending coronary artery and the obtuse marginal coronary artery is classified in the body part axis of classification as two coronary arteries and the qualifier specifies the aorta as the body part bypassed from.

B3.6c If multiple coronary arteries are bypassed, a separate procedure is coded for each coronary artery that uses a different device and/or qualifier.

Example: Aortocoronary artery bypass and internal mammary coronary artery bypass are coded separately.

Control vs. more definitive root operations

B3.7 The root operation Control is defined as, "Stopping, or attempting to stop, postprocedural or other acute bleeding." Control is the root operation coded when the procedure performed to achieve hemostasis, beyond what would be considered integral to a procedure, utilizes techniques (e.g. cautery, application of substances or pressure, suturing or ligation or clipping of bleeding points at the site) that are not described by a more specific root operation definition, such as Bypass, Detachment, Excision, Extraction, Reposition, Replacement, or Resection. If a more specific root operation definition applies to the procedure performed, then the more specific root operation is coded instead of Control.

Examples: Silver nitrate cautery to treat acute nasal bleeding is coded to the root operation Control. Liquid embolization of the right internal iliac artery to treat acute hematoma by stopping blood flow is coded to the root operation Occlusion. Suctioning of residual blood to achieve hemostasis during a transbronchial cryobiopsy is considered integral to the cryobiopsy procedure and is not coded separately.

Excision vs. Resection

B3.8 PCS contains specific body parts for anatomical subdivisions of a body part, such as lobes of the lungs or liver and regions of the intestine. Resection of the specific body part is coded whenever all of the body part is cut out or off, rather than coding Excision of a less specific body part.

Example: Left upper lung lobectomy is coded to Resection of Upper Lung Lobe, Left rather than Excision of Lung, Left.

Excision for graft

B3.9 If an autograft is obtained from a different procedure site in order to complete the objective of the procedure, a separate procedure is coded, except when the seventh character qualifier value in the ICD-10-PCS table fully specifies the site from which the autograft was obtained.

Examples: Coronary bypass with excision of saphenous vein graft, excision of saphenous vein is coded separately. Replacement of breast with autologous deep inferior epigastric artery perforator (DIEP) flap, excision of the DIEP flap is not coded separately. The seventh character qualifier value Deep Inferior Epigastric Artery Perforator Flap in the Replacement table fully specifies the site of the autograft harvest.

Fusion procedures of the spine

B3.10a The body part coded for a spinal vertebral joint(s) rendered immobile by a spinal fusion procedure is classified by the level of the spine (e.g. thoracic). There are distinct body part values for a single vertebral joint and for multiple vertebral joints at each spinal level.

Example: Body part values specify Lumbar Vertebral Joint, Lumbar Vertebral Joints, 2 or More and Lumbosacral Vertebral Joint.

B3.10b If multiple vertebral joints are fused, a separate procedure is coded for each vertebral joint that uses a different device and/or qualifier.

Example: Fusion of lumbar vertebral joint, posterior approach, anterior column and fusion of lumbar vertebral joint, posterior approach, posterior column are coded separately.

B3.10c Combinations of devices and materials are often used on a vertebral joint to render the joint immobile. When combinations of devices are used on the same vertebral joint, the device value coded for the procedure is as follows:

- If an interbody fusion device is used to render the joint immobile (containing bone graft or bone graft substitute), the procedure is coded with the device value Interbody Fusion Device
- If bone graft is the only device used to render the joint immobile, the procedure is coded with the device value Nonautologous Tissue Substitute or Autologous Tissue Substitute
- If a mixture of autologous and nonautologous bone graft (with or without biological or synthetic extenders or binders) is used to render the joint immobile, code the procedure with the device value Autologous Tissue Substitute

Examples: Fusion of a vertebral joint using a cage style interbody fusion device containing morsellized bone graft is coded to the device Interbody Fusion Device. Fusion of a vertebral joint using a bone dowel interbody fusion device made of cadaver bone and packed with a mixture of local morsellized bone and demineralized bone matrix is coded to the device Interbody Fusion Device. Fusion of a vertebral joint using both autologous bone graft and bone bank bone graft is coded to the device Autologous Tissue Substitute.

Inspection procedures

B3.11a Inspection of a body part(s) performed in order to achieve the objective of a procedure is not coded separately.

Example: Fiberoptic bronchoscopy performed for irrigation of bronchus, only the irrigation procedure is coded.

B3.11b If multiple tubular body parts are inspected, the most distal body part inspected is coded. If multiple non-tubular body parts in a region are inspected, the body part that specifies the entire area inspected is coded.

Examples: Cystoureteroscopy with inspection of bladder and ureters is coded to the ureter body part value. Exploratory laparotomy with general inspection of abdominal contents is coded to the peritoneal cavity body part value.

B3.11c When both an Inspection procedure and another procedure are performed on the same body part during the same episode, if the Inspection procedure is performed using a different approach than the other procedure, the Inspection procedure is coded separately.

Example: Endoscopic Inspection of the duodenum is coded separately when open Excision of the duodenum is performed during the same procedural episode.

Occlusion vs. Restriction for vessel embolization procedures

B3.12 If the objective of an embolization procedure is to completely close a vessel, the root operation Occlusion is coded. If the objective of an embolization procedure is to narrow the lumen of a vessel, the root operation Restriction is coded.

Examples: Tumor embolization is coded to the root operation Occlusion, because the objective of the procedure is to cut off the blood supply to the vessel. Embolization of a cerebral aneurysm is coded to the root operation Restriction, because the objective of the procedure is not to close off the vessel entirely, but to narrow the lumen of the vessel at the site of the aneurysm where it is abnormally wide.

Release procedures

B3.13 In the root operation Release, the body part value coded is the body part being freed and not the tissue being manipulated or cut to free the body part.

Example: Lysis of intestinal adhesions is coded to the specific intestine body part value.

Release vs. Division

B3.14 If the sole objective of the procedure is freeing a body part without cutting the body part, the root operation is Release. If the sole objective of the procedure is separating or transecting a body part, the root operation is Division.

Example: Freeing a nerve root from surrounding scar tissue to relieve pain is coded to the root operation Release. Severing a nerve root to relieve pain is coded to the root operation Division.

Reposition for fracture treatment

B3.15 Reduction of a displaced fracture is coded to the root operation Reposition and the application of a cast or splint in conjunction with the Reposition procedure is not coded separately. Treatment of a nondisplaced fracture is coded to the procedure performed.

Examples: Putting a pin in a nondisplaced fracture is coded to the root operation Insertion. Casting of a nondisplaced fracture is coded to the root operation Immobilization in the Placement section.

Transplantation vs. Administration

B3.16 Putting in a mature and functioning living body part taken from another individual or animal is coded to the root operation Transplantation. Putting in autologous or nonautologous cells is coded to the Administration section.

Example: Putting in autologous or nonautologous bone marrow, pancreatic islet cells or stem cells is coded to the Administration section.

Transfer procedures using multiple tissue layers

B3.17 The root operation Transfer contains qualifiers that can be used to specify when a transfer flap is composed of more than one tissue layer, such as a musculocutaneous flap. For procedures involving transfer of multiple tissue layers including skin, subcutaneous tissue, fascia or muscle, the procedure is coded to the body part value that describes the deepest tissue layer in the flap, and the qualifier can be used to describe the other tissue layer(s) in the transfer flap.

Example: A musculocutaneous flap transfer is coded to the appropriate body part value in the body system Muscles, and the qualifier is used to describe the additional tissue layer(s) in the transfer flap.

Excision/Resection followed by replacement

B3.18 If an Excision or Resection of a body part is followed by a Replacement procedure, code both procedures to identify each distinct objective, except when the Excision or Resection is considered integral and preparatory for the Replacement procedure.

Examples: Mastectomy followed by reconstruction, both Resection and Replacement of the breast are coded to fully capture the distinct objectives of the procedures performed. Maxillectomy with obturator reconstruction, both Excision and Replacement of the maxilla are coded to fully capture the distinct objectives of the procedures performed. Excisional debridement of tendon with skin graft, both the Excision of the tendon and the Replacement of the skin with a graft are coded to fully capture the distinct objectives of the procedures performed. Esophagectomy followed by reconstruction with colonic interposition, both the Resection and the Transfer of the large intestine to function as the esophagus are coded to fully capture the distinct objectives of the procedures performed.

Examples: Resection of a joint as part of a joint replacement procedure is considered integral and preparatory for the Replacement of the joint and the Resection is not coded separately. Resection of a valve as part of a valve replacement procedure is considered integral and preparatory for the valve Replacement and the Resection is not coded separately.

Detachment procedures of extremities

B3.19 The root operation Detachment contains qualifiers that can be used to specify the level where the extremity was amputated. These qualifiers are dependent on the body part value in the "upper extremities" and "lower extremities" body systems. For procedures involving detachment of all or part of the upper or lower extremities, the procedure is coded to the body part value that describes the site of the detachment.

Example: An amputation at the proximal portion of the shaft of the tibia and fibula is coded to the Lower leg body part value in the body system Anatomical Regions, Lower Extremities, and the qualifier High is used to specify the level where the extremity was detached.

The following definitions were developed for the Detachment qualifiers.

Body Part	Qualifier	Definition
Upper arm and upper leg	1	High: Amputation at the proximal portion of the shaft of the humerus or femur
	2	Mid: Amputation at the middle portion of the shaft of the humerus or femur
	3	Low: Amputation at the distal portion of the shaft of the humerus or femur
Lower arm and lower leg	1	High: Amputation at the proximal portion of the shaft of the radius/ulna or tibia/fibula
	2	Mid: Amputation at the middle portion of the shaft of the radius/ulna or tibia/fibula
	3	Low: Amputation at the distal portion of the shaft of the radius/ulna or tibia/fibula
Hand and Foot	0	Complete*
	4	Complete 1st Ray
	5	Complete 2nd Ray
	6	Complete 3rd Ray
	7	Complete 4th Ray
	8	Complete 5th Ray
	9	Partial 1st Ray
	B	Partial 2nd Ray
	C	Partial 3rd Ray
	D	Partial 4th Ray

Body Part	Qualifier	Definition
	F	Partial 5th Ray
Thumb, finger, or toe	0	Complete: Amputation at the metacarpophalangeal/metatarsal-phalangeal joint
	1	High: Amputation anywhere along the proximal phalanx
	2	Mid: Amputation through the proximal interphalangeal joint or anywhere along the middle phalanx
	3	Low: Amputation through the distal interphalangeal joint or anywhere along the distal phalanx

* When coding amputation of Hand and Foot, the following definitions are followed:
-Complete: Amputation through the carpometacarpal joint of the hand, or through the tarsal-metatarsal joint of the foot.
-Partial: Amputation anywhere along the shaft or head of the metacarpal bone of the hand, or of the metatarsal bone of the foot.

B4. Body Part

General guidelines

B4.1a If a procedure is performed on a portion of a body part that does not have a separate body part value, code the body part value corresponding to the whole body part.

Example: A procedure performed on the alveolar process of the mandible is coded to the mandible body part.

B4.1b If the prefix "peri" is combined with a body part to identify the site of the procedure, and the site of the procedure is not further specified, then the procedure is coded to the body part named. This guideline applies only when a more specific body part value is not available.

Examples: A procedure site identified as perirenal is coded to the kidney body part when the site of the procedure is not further specified. A procedure site described in the documentation as peri-urethral tissue, and the documentation also indicates that it is the vulvar tissue and not the urethral tissue that is the site of the procedure, then the procedure is coded to the vulva body part. A procedure site documented as involving the periosteum is coded to the corresponding bone body part.

B4.1c If a single vascular procedure is performed on a continuous section of an arterial or venous body part, code the body part value corresponding to the anatomically most proximal (closest to the heart) portion of the arterial or venous body part.

Examples: A procedure performed on a continuous section of artery from the femoral artery to the external iliac artery with the point of entry at the femoral artery is coded to the external iliac body part. A procedure performed on a continuous section of artery from the femoral artery to the external iliac artery with the point of entry at the external iliac artery is also coded to the external iliac artery body part.

Branches of body parts

B4.2 Where a specific branch of a body part does not have its own body part value in PCS, the body part is typically coded to the closest proximal branch that has a specific body part value. In the cardiovascular body systems, if a general body part is available in the correct root operation table, and coding to a proximal branch would require assigning a code in a different body system, the procedure is coded using the general body part value.

Examples: A procedure performed on the mandibular branch of the trigeminal nerve is coded to the trigeminal nerve body part value. Occlusion of the bronchial artery is coded to the body part value Upper Artery in the body system Upper Arteries, and not to the body part value Thoracic Aorta, Descending in the body system Heart and Great Vessels.

Bilateral body part values

B4.3 Bilateral body part values are available for a limited number of body parts. If the identical procedure is performed on contralateral body parts, and a bilateral body part value exists for that body part, a single procedure is coded using the bilateral body part value. If no bilateral body part value exists, each procedure is coded separately using the appropriate body part value.

Examples: The identical procedure performed on both fallopian tubes is coded once using the body part value Fallopian Tube, Bilateral. The identical procedure performed on both knee joints is coded twice using the body part values Knee Joint, Right and Knee Joint, Left.

Coronary arteries

B4.4 The coronary arteries are classified as a single body part that is further specified by number of arteries treated. One procedure code specifying multiple arteries is used when the same procedure is performed, including the same device and qualifier values.

Examples: Angioplasty of two distinct coronary arteries with placement of two stents is coded as Dilation of Coronary Artery, Two Arteries, with Two Intraluminal Devices. Angioplasty of two distinct coronary arteries, one with stent placed and one without, is coded separately as Dilation of Coronary Artery, One Artery with Intraluminal Device, and Dilation of Coronary Artery, One Artery with no device.

Tendons, ligaments, bursae and fascia near a joint

B4.5 Procedures performed on tendons, ligaments, bursae and fascia supporting a joint are coded to the body part in the respective body system that is the focus of the procedure. Procedures performed on joint structures themselves are coded to the body part in the joint body systems.

Examples: Repair of the anterior cruciate ligament of the knee is coded to the knee bursae and ligament body part in the Bursae and Ligaments body system. Knee arthroscopy with shaving of articular cartilage is coded to the knee joint body part in the Lower Joints body system.

Skin, subcutaneous tissue and fascia overlying a joint

B4.6 If a procedure is performed on the skin, subcutaneous tissue or fascia overlying a joint, the procedure is coded to the following body part:

- Shoulder is coded to Upper Arm
- Elbow is coded to Lower Arm
- Wrist is coded to Lower Arm
- Hip is coded to Upper Leg
- Knee is coded to Lower Leg
- Ankle is coded to Foot

Fingers and toes

B4.7 If a body system does not contain a separate body part value for fingers, procedures performed on the fingers are coded to the body part value for the hand. If a body system does not contain a separate body part value for toes, procedures performed on the toes are coded to the body part value for the foot.

Example: Excision of finger muscle is coded to one of the hand muscle body part values in the Muscles body system.

Upper and lower intestinal tract

B4.8 In the Gastrointestinal body system, the general body part values Upper Intestinal Tract and Lower Intestinal Tract are provided as an option for the root operations such as Change, Insertion, Inspection, Removal and Revision. Upper Intestinal Tract includes the portion of the gastrointestinal tract from the esophagus down to and including the duodenum, and Lower Intestinal Tract includes the portion of the gastrointestinal tract from the jejunum down to and including the rectum and anus.

Example: In the root operation Change table, change of a device in the jejunum is coded using the body part Lower Intestinal Tract.

B5. Approach

Open approach with percutaneous endoscopic assistance

B5.2a Procedures performed using the open approach with percutaneous endoscopic assistance are coded to the approach Open.

Example: Laparoscopic-assisted sigmoidectomy is coded to the approach Open.

Percutaneous endoscopic approach with hand-assistance or extension of incision

B5.2b Procedures performed using the percutaneous endoscopic approach, with hand-assistance, or with incision or extension of an incision to assist in the removal of all or a portion of a body part or to anastomose a tubular body part with or without the temporary exteriorization of a body structure are coded to the approach value Percutaneous Endoscopic.

Examples: Hand-assisted laparoscopic sigmoid colon resection with exteriorization of a segment of the colon for removal of specimen with return of colon back into abdominal cavity is coded to the approach value percutaneous endoscopic. Laparoscopic sigmoid colectomy with extension of stapling port for removal of specimen and direct anastomosis is coded to the approach value Percutaneous Endoscopic. Laparoscopic nephrectomy with midline incision for removing the resected kidney is coded to the approach value Percutaneous Endoscopic. Robotic-assisted laparoscopic prostatectomy with extension of incision for removal of the resected prostate is coded to the approach value Percutaneous Endoscopic.

External approach

B5.3a Procedures performed within an orifice on structures that are visible without the aid of any instrumentation are coded to the approach External.

Example: Resection of tonsils is coded to the approach External.

B5.3b Procedures performed indirectly by the application of external force through the intervening body layers are coded to the approach External.

Example: Closed reduction of fracture is coded to the approach External.

Percutaneous procedure via device

B5.4 Procedures performed percutaneously via a device placed for the procedure are coded to the approach Percutaneous.

Example: Fragmentation of kidney stone performed via percutaneous nephrostomy is coded to the approach Percutaneous.

B6. Device

General guidelines

B6.1a A device is coded only if a device remains after the procedure is completed. If no device remains, the device value No Device is coded. In limited root operations, the classification provides the qualifier values Temporary and Intraoperative, for specific procedures involving clinically significant devices, where the purpose of the device is to be utilized for a brief duration during the procedure or current inpatient stay. If a device that is intended to remain after the procedure is completed requires removal before the end of the operative episode in which it was inserted, both the insertion and removal of the device should be coded.

B6.1b Materials such as sutures, ligatures, radiological markers and temporary post-operative wound drains are considered integral to the performance of a procedure and are not coded as devices.

B6.1c Procedures performed on a device only and not on a body part are specified in the root operations Change, Irrigation, Removal and Revision, and are coded to the procedure performed.

Example: Irrigation of percutaneous nephrostomy tube is coded to the root operation Irrigation of indwelling device in the Administration section.

Drainage device

B6.2 A separate procedure to put in a drainage device is coded to the root operation Drainage with the device value Drainage Device.

Coding Guidelines Reference

Coding Guidelines References

The tables below link ICD-10-PCS coding guidelines to Medical and Surgical section root operations, specific body system tables, and body systems. The guidelines identified in each table are provided in order to remind users to reference the coding guidelines prior to code reporting. The tables provide coding guideline references at the body system and root operation level. It is imperative to review the ICD-10-PCS coding guidelines to ensure the procedure code being reported is accurate and complete.

Root Operation References

Root Operation	Character Value	Coding Guideline(s)
Bypass	1	B3.6a
Change	2	B6.1c
Control	3	B3.7
Detachment	6	B3.19
Division	8	B3.14
Drainage	9	B3.4a, B3.4b, B6.2
Excision	B	B3.4a, B3.4b, B3.8, B3.9, B3.18
Extraction	D	B3.4a, B3.4b
Inspection	J	B3.11a, B3.11b, B3.11c
Occlusion	L	B3.12
Release	N	B3.13, B3.14
Removal	P	B6.1c
Replacement	R	B3.18
Resection	T	B3.8, B3.18
Restriction	V	B3.12
Revision	W	B6.1c
Transplantation	Y	B3.16

Table References

Table	Body System	Root Operation	Coding Guideline(s)
021	Heart and Great Vessels	Bypass	B3.6b, B3.6c, B4.4
027	Heart and Great Vessels	Dilation	B4.4
02C	Heart and Great Vessels	Extirpation	B4.4

Continued →

101

Table	Body System	Root Operation	Coding Guideline(s)
02Q	Heart and Great Vessels	Repair	B4.4
0HB	Skin and Breast	Excision	B3.5
0HJ	Skin and Breast	Inspection	B3.5
0HQ	Skin and Breast	Repair	B3.5
0HX	Skin and Breast	Transfer	B3.17
0JB	Subcutaneous Tissue and Fascia	Excision	B3.5
0JJ	Subcutaneous Tissue and Fascia	Inspection	B3.5
0JQ	Subcutaneous Tissue and Fascia	Repair	B3.5
0JX	Subcutaneous Tissue and Fascia	Transfer	B3.17
0KB	Muscles	Excision	B3.5
0KJ	Muscles	Inspection	B3.5
0KQ	Muscles	Repair	B3.5
0KX	Muscles	Transfer	B3.17
0LB	Tendons	Excision	B3.5
0LJ	Tendons	Inspection	B3.5
0LQ	Tendons	Repair	B3.5
0MB	Bursae and Ligaments	Excision	B3.5
0MJ	Bursae and Ligaments	Inspection	B3.5
0MQ	Bursae and Ligaments	Repair	B3.5
0NB	Head and Facial Bones	Excision	B3.5
0NJ	Head and Facial Bones	Inspection	B3.5
0NQ	Head and Facial Bones	Repair	B3.5
0NS	Head and Facial Bones	Reposition	B3.15
0PB	Upper Bones	Excision	B3.5
0PJ	Upper Bones	Inspection	B3.5
0PQ	Upper Bones	Repair	B3.5
0PS	Upper Bones	Reposition	B3.15
0QB	Lower Bones	Excision	B3.5
0QJ	Lower Bones	Inspection	B3.5
0QQ	Lower Bones	Repair	B3.5
0QS	Lower Bones	Reposition	B3.15
0RB	Upper Joints	Excision	B3.5
0RG	Upper Joints	Fusion	B3.10a, B3.10b, B3.10c
0RJ	Upper Joints	Inspection	B3.5
0RQ	Upper Joints	Repair	B3.5
0SB	Lower Joints	Excision	B3.5
0SG	Lower Joints	Fusion	B3.10a, B3.10b, B3.10c
0SJ	Lower Joints	Inspection	B3.5
0SQ	Lower Joints	Repair	B3.5
0UD	Female Reproductive System	Extraction	C2

Body System References

Body System	Character Value	Coding Guideline(s)
Gastrointestinal System	D	B4.8
Subcutaneous Tissue and Fascia	J	B4.5, B4.6
Tendons	L	B4.5
Bursae and Ligaments	M	B4.5
Upper Joints	R	B4.5
Lower Joints	S	B4.5

Central Nervous System and Cranial Nerves

103

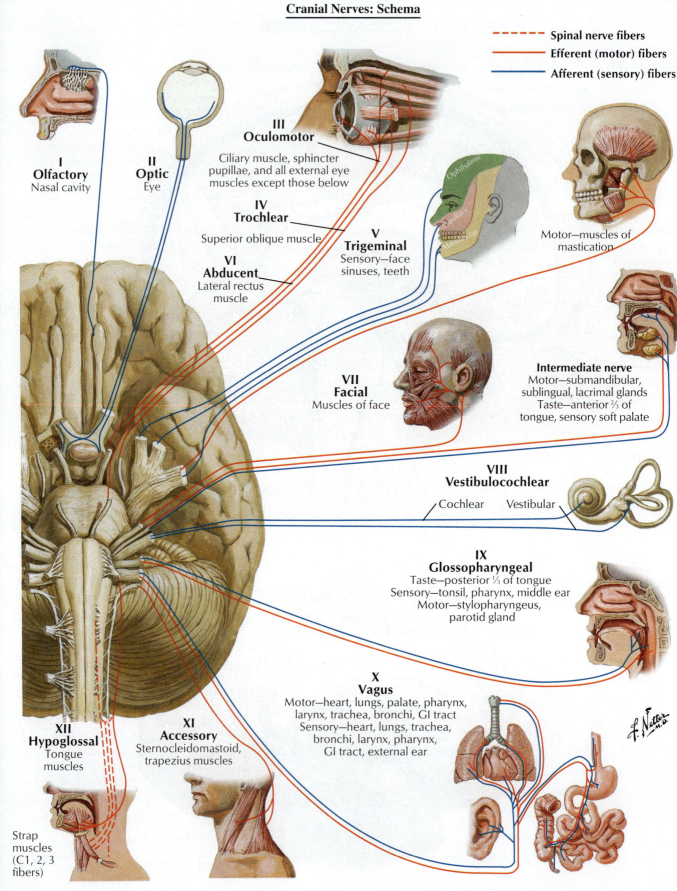

Schematic Reconstruction of Hypothalamus (Three Dimensional)

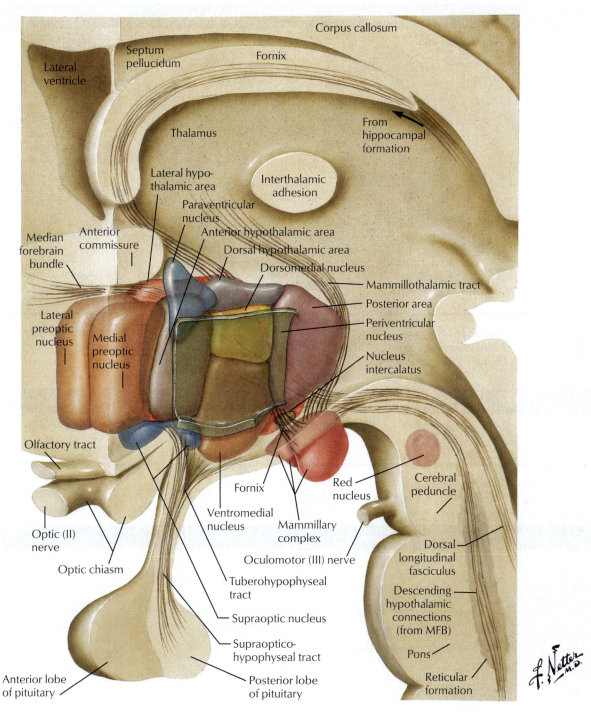

105

Central Nervous System and Cranial Nerves Tables 001–00X

Section	0	Medical and Surgical
Body System	0	Central Nervous System and Cranial Nerves
Operation	1	Bypass: Altering the route of passage of the contents of a tubular body part

Body Part (4th)	Approach (5th)	Device (6th)	Qualifier (7th)
6 Cerebral Ventricle	0 Open 3 Percutaneous 4 Percutaneous Endoscopic	7 Autologous Tissue Substitute J Synthetic Substitute K Nonautologous Tissue Substitute	0 Nasopharynx 1 Mastoid Sinus 2 Atrium 3 Blood Vessel 4 Pleural Cavity 5 Intestine 6 Peritoneal Cavity 7 Urinary Tract 8 Bone Marrow A Subgaleal Space B Cerebral Cisterns
6 Cerebral Ventricle	0 Open 3 Percutaneous 4 Percutaneous Endoscopic	Z No Device	B Cerebral Cisterns
U Spinal Canal	0 Open 3 Percutaneous 4 Percutaneous Endoscopic	7 Autologous Tissue Substitute J Synthetic Substitute K Nonautologous Tissue Substitute	2 Atrium 4 Pleural Cavity 6 Peritoneal Cavity 7 Urinary Tract 9 Fallopian Tube

Section	0	Medical and Surgical
Body System	0	Central Nervous System and Cranial Nerves
Operation	2	Change: Taking out or off a device from a body part and putting back an identical or similar device in or on the same body part without cutting or puncturing the skin or a mucous membrane

Body Part (4th)	Approach (5th)	Device (6th)	Qualifier (7th)
0 Brain E Cranial Nerve U Spinal Canal	X External	0 Drainage Device Y Other Device	Z No Qualifier

Section	0	Medical and Surgical
Body System	0	Central Nervous System and Cranial Nerves
Operation	5	Destruction: Physical eradication of all or a portion of a body part by the direct use of energy, force, or a destructive agent

Body Part (4th)	Approach (5th)	Device (6th)	Qualifier (7th)
0 Brain W Cervical Spinal Cord X Thoracic Spinal Cord Y Lumbar Spinal Cord	0 Open 3 Percutaneous 4 Percutaneous Endoscopic	Z No Device	3 Laser interstitial Thermal Therapy Z No Qualifier
1 Cerebral Meninges 2 Dura Mater 6 Cerebral Ventricle 7 Cerebral Hemisphere 8 Basal Ganglia 9 Thalamus A Hypothalamus B Pons C Cerebellum D Medulla Oblongata F Olfactory Nerve G Optic Nerve H Oculomotor Nerve J Trochlear Nerve K Trigeminal Nerve L Abducens Nerve M Facial Nerve N Acoustic Nerve P Glossopharyngeal Nerve Q Vagus Nerve R Accessory Nerve S Hypoglossal Nerve T Spinal Meninges	0 Open 3 Percutaneous 4 Percutaneous Endoscopic	Z No Device	Z No Qualifier

Section	0	Medical and Surgical
Body System	0	Central Nervous System and Cranial Nerves
Operation	7	Dilation: Expanding an orifice or the lumen of a tubular body part

Body Part (4th)	Approach (5th)	Device (6th)	Qualifier (7th)
6 Cerebral Ventricle	0 Open 3 Percutaneous 4 Percutaneous Endoscopic	Z No Device	Z No Qualifier

Section	0	Medical and Surgical
Body System	0	Central Nervous System and Cranial Nerves
Operation	8	Division: Cutting into a body part, without draining fluids and/or gases from the body part, in order to separate or transect a body part

Body Part (4th)	Approach (5th)	Device (6th)	Qualifier (7th)
0 Brain 7 Cerebral Hemisphere 8 Basal Ganglia F Olfactory Nerve G Optic Nerve H Oculomotor Nerve J Trochlear Nerve K Trigeminal Nerve L Abducens Nerve M Facial Nerve N Acoustic Nerve P Glossopharyngeal Nerve Q Vagus Nerve R Accessory Nerve S Hypoglossal Nerve W Cervical Spinal Cord X Thoracic Spinal Cord Y Lumbar Spinal Cord	0 Open 3 Percutaneous 4 Percutaneous Endoscopic	Z No Device	Z No Qualifier

Section	0	Medical and Surgical
Body System	0	Central Nervous System and Cranial Nerves
Operation	9	Drainage: Taking or letting out fluids and/or gases from a body part

Body Part (4th)	Approach (5th)	Device (6th)	Qualifier (7th)
0 Brain 1 Cerebral Meninges 2 Dura Mater 3 Epidural Space, Intracranial 4 Subdural Space, Intracranial 5 Subarachnoid Space, Intracranial 6 Cerebral Ventricle 7 Cerebral Hemisphere 8 Basal Ganglia 9 Thalamus A Hypothalamus B Pons C Cerebellum D Medulla Oblongata F Olfactory Nerve G Optic Nerve H Oculomotor Nerve J Trochlear Nerve K Trigeminal Nerve L Abducens Nerve M Facial Nerve N Acoustic Nerve P Glossopharyngeal Nerve Q Vagus Nerve R Accessory Nerve S Hypoglossal Nerve T Spinal Meninges U Spinal Canal W Cervical Spinal Cord X Thoracic Spinal Cord Y Lumbar Spinal Cord	0 Open 3 Percutaneous 4 Percutaneous Endoscopic	0 Drainage Device	Z No Qualifier

Continued ➞

Section	0	Medical and Surgical
Body System	0	Central Nervous System and Cranial Nerves
Operation	9	Drainage: Taking or letting out fluids and/or gases from a body part

009 Continued

Body Part (4th)	Approach (5th)	Device (6th)	Qualifier (7th)
0 Brain	0 Open	Z No Device	X Diagnostic
1 Cerebral Meninges	3 Percutaneous		Z No Qualifier
2 Dura Mater	4 Percutaneous Endoscopic		
3 Epidural Space, Intracranial			
4 Subdural Space, Intracranial			
5 Subarachnoid Space, Intracranial			
6 Cerebral Ventricle			
7 Cerebral Hemisphere			
8 Basal Ganglia			
9 Thalamus			
A Hypothalamus			
B Pons			
C Cerebellum			
D Medulla Oblongata			
F Olfactory Nerve			
G Optic Nerve			
H Oculomotor Nerve			
J Trochlear Nerve			
K Trigeminal Nerve			
L Abducens Nerve			
M Facial Nerve			
N Acoustic Nerve			
P Glossopharyngeal Nerve			
Q Vagus Nerve			
R Accessory Nerve			
S Hypoglossal Nerve			
T Spinal Meninges			
U Spinal Canal			
W Cervical Spinal Cord			
X Thoracic Spinal Cord			
Y Lumbar Spinal Cord			

Section	0	Medical and Surgical
Body System	0	Central Nervous System and Cranial Nerves
Operation	B	Excision: Cutting out or off, without replacement, a portion of a body part

Body Part (4th)	Approach (5th)	Device (6th)	Qualifier (7th)
0 Brain	0 Open	Z No Device	X Diagnostic
1 Cerebral Meninges	3 Percutaneous		Z No Qualifier
2 Dura Mater	4 Percutaneous Endoscopic		
6 Cerebral Ventricle			
7 Cerebral Hemisphere			
8 Basal Ganglia			
9 Thalamus			
A Hypothalamus			
B Pons			
C Cerebellum			
D Medulla Oblongata			
F Olfactory Nerve			
G Optic Nerve			
H Oculomotor Nerve			
J Trochlear Nerve			
K Trigeminal Nerve			
L Abducens Nerve			
M Facial Nerve			
N Acoustic Nerve			
P Glossopharyngeal Nerve			
Q Vagus Nerve			
R Accessory Nerve			
S Hypoglossal Nerve			
T Spinal Meninges			
W Cervical Spinal Cord			
X Thoracic Spinal Cord			
Y Lumbar Spinal Cord			

Section	0	Medical and Surgical
Body System	0	Central Nervous System and Cranial Nerves
Operation	C	Extirpation: Taking or cutting out solid matter from a body part

Body Part (4th)	Approach (5th)	Device (6th)	Qualifier (7th)
0 Brain	0 Open	Z No Device	Z No Qualifier
1 Cerebral Meninges	3 Percutaneous		
2 Dura Mater	4 Percutaneous Endoscopic		
3 Epidural Space, Intracranial			
4 Subdural Space, Intracranial			
5 Subarachnoid Space, Intracranial			
6 Cerebral Ventricle			
7 Cerebral Hemisphere			
8 Basal Ganglia			
9 Thalamus			
A Hypothalamus			
B Pons			
C Cerebellum			
D Medulla Oblongata			
F Olfactory Nerve			
G Optic Nerve			
H Oculomotor Nerve			
J Trochlear Nerve			
K Trigeminal Nerve			
L Abducens Nerve			
M Facial Nerve			
N Acoustic Nerve			
P Glossopharyngeal Nerve			
Q Vagus Nerve			
R Accessory Nerve			
S Hypoglossal Nerve			
T Spinal Meninges			
U Spinal Canal			
W Cervical Spinal Cord			
X Thoracic Spinal Cord			
Y Lumbar Spinal Cord			

Section	0	Medical and Surgical
Body System	0	Central Nervous System and Cranial Nerves
Operation	D	Extraction: Pulling or stripping out or off all or a portion of a body part by the use of force

Body Part (4th)	Approach (5th)	Device (6th)	Qualifier (7th)
0 Brain	0 Open	Z No Device	Z No Qualifier
1 Cerebral Meninges	3 Percutaneous		
2 Dura Mater	4 Percutaneous Endoscopic		
7 Cerebral Hemisphere			
C Cerebellum			
F Olfactory Nerve			
G Optic Nerve			
H Oculomotor Nerve			
J Trochlear Nerve			
K Trigeminal Nerve			
L Abducens Nerve			
M Facial Nerve			
N Acoustic Nerve			
P Glossopharyngeal Nerve			
Q Vagus Nerve			
R Accessory Nerve			
S Hypoglossal Nerve			
T Spinal Meninges			

Section 0 **Medical and Surgical**
Body System 0 **Central Nervous System and Cranial Nerves**
Operation F **Fragmentation:** Breaking solid matter in a body part into pieces

Body Part (4th)	Approach (5th)	Device (6th)	Qualifier (7th)
3 Epidural Space, Intracranial 4 Subdural Space, Intracranial 5 Subarachnoid Space, Intracranial 6 Cerebral Ventricle U Spinal Canal	0 Open 3 Percutaneous 4 Percutaneous Endoscopic X External	Z No Device	Z No Qualifier

Section 0 **Medical and Surgical**
Body System 0 **Central Nervous System and Cranial Nerves**
Operation H **Insertion:** Putting in a nonbiological appliance that monitors, assists, performs, or prevents a physiological function but does not physically take the place of a body part

Body Part (4th)	Approach (5th)	Device (6th)	Qualifier (7th)
0 Brain	0 Open	1 Radioactive Element 2 Monitoring Device 3 Infusion Device 4 Radioactive Element, Cesium-131 Collagen Implant M Neurostimulator Lead Y Other Device	Z No Qualifier
0 Brain	3 Percutaneous 4 Percutaneous Endoscopic	1 Radioactive Element 2 Monitoring Device 3 Infusion Device M Neurostimulator Lead Y Other Device	Z No Qualifier
6 Cerebral Ventricle E Cranial Nerve U Spinal Canal V Spinal Cord	0 Open 3 Percutaneous 4 Percutaneous Endoscopic	1 Radioactive Element 2 Monitoring Device 3 Infusion Device M Neurostimulator Lead Y Other Device	Z No Qualifier

Section 0 **Medical and Surgical**
Body System 0 **Central Nervous System and Cranial Nerves**
Operation J **Inspection:** Visually and/or manually exploring a body part

Body Part (4th)	Approach (5th)	Device (6th)	Qualifier (7th)
0 Brain E Cranial Nerve U Spinal Canal V Spinal Cord	0 Open 3 Percutaneous 4 Percutaneous Endoscopic	Z No Device	Z No Qualifier

Section 0 **Medical and Surgical**
Body System 0 **Central Nervous System and Cranial Nerves**
Operation K **Map:** Locating the route of passage of electrical impulses and/or locating functional areas in a body part

Body Part (4th)	Approach (5th)	Device (6th)	Qualifier (7th)
0 Brain 7 Cerebral Hemisphere 8 Basal Ganglia 9 Thalamus A Hypothalamus B Pons C Cerebellum D Medulla Oblongata	0 Open 3 Percutaneous 4 Percutaneous Endoscopic	Z No Device	Z No Qualifier

Section	0	Medical and Surgical
Body System	0	Central Nervous System and Cranial Nerves
Operation	N	Release: Freeing a body part from an abnormal physical constraint by cutting or by the use of force

Body Part (4th)	Approach (5th)	Device (6th)	Qualifier (7th)
0 Brain 1 Cerebral Meninges 2 Dura Mater 6 Cerebral Ventricle 7 Cerebral Hemisphere 8 Basal Ganglia 9 Thalamus A Hypothalamus B Pons C Cerebellum D Medulla Oblongata F Olfactory Nerve G Optic Nerve H Oculomotor Nerve J Trochlear Nerve K Trigeminal Nerve L Abducens Nerve M Facial Nerve N Acoustic Nerve P Glossopharyngeal Nerve Q Vagus Nerve R Accessory Nerve S Hypoglossal Nerve T Spinal Meninges W Cervical Spinal Cord X Thoracic Spinal Cord Y Lumbar Spinal Cord	0 Open 3 Percutaneous 4 Percutaneous Endoscopic	Z No Device	Z No Qualifier

Section	0	Medical and Surgical
Body System	0	Central Nervous System and Cranial Nerves
Operation	P	Removal: Taking out or off a device from a body part

Body Part (4th)	Approach (5th)	Device (6th)	Qualifier (7th)
0 Brain V Spinal Cord	0 Open 3 Percutaneous 4 Percutaneous Endoscopic	0 Drainage Device 2 Monitoring Device 3 Infusion Device 7 Autologous Tissue Substitute J Synthetic Substitute K Nonautologous Tissue Substitute M Neurostimulator Lead Y Other Device	Z No Qualifier
0 Brain V Spinal Cord	X External	0 Drainage Device 2 Monitoring Device 3 Infusion Device M Neurostimulator Lead	Z No Qualifier
6 Cerebral Ventricle U Spinal Canal	0 Open 3 Percutaneous 4 Percutaneous Endoscopic	0 Drainage Device 2 Monitoring Device 3 Infusion Device J Synthetic Substitute M Neurostimulator Lead Y Other Device	Z No Qualifier
6 Cerebral Ventricle U Spinal Canal	X External	0 Drainage Device 2 Monitoring Device 3 Infusion Device M Neurostimulator Lead	Z No Qualifier

Continued ➡

Section	0	Medical and Surgical
Body System	0	Central Nervous System and Cranial Nerves
Operation	P	**Removal:** Taking out or off a device from a body part

00P Continued

Body Part (4th)	Approach (5th)	Device (6th)	Qualifier (7th)
E Cranial Nerve	0 Open 3 Percutaneous 4 Percutaneous Endoscopic	0 Drainage Device 2 Monitoring Device 3 Infusion Device 7 Autologous Tissue Substitute M Neurostimulator Lead Y Other Device	Z No Qualifier
E Cranial Nerve	X External	0 Drainage Device 2 Monitoring Device 3 Infusion Device M Neurostimulator Lead	Z No Qualifier

Section	0	Medical and Surgical
Body System	0	Central Nervous System and Cranial Nerves
Operation	Q	**Repair:** Restoring, to the extent possible, a body part to its normal anatomic structure and function

Body Part (4th)	Approach (5th)	Device (6th)	Qualifier (7th)
0 Brain 1 Cerebral Meninges 2 Dura Mater 6 Cerebral Ventricle 7 Cerebral Hemisphere 8 Basal Ganglia 9 Thalamus A Hypothalamus B Pons C Cerebellum D Medulla Oblongata F Olfactory Nerve G Optic Nerve H Oculomotor Nerve J Trochlear Nerve K Trigeminal Nerve L Abducens Nerve M Facial Nerve N Acoustic Nerve P Glossopharyngeal Nerve Q Vagus Nerve R Accessory Nerve S Hypoglossal Nerve T Spinal Meninges W Cervical Spinal Cord X Thoracic Spinal Cord Y Lumbar Spinal Cord	0 Open 3 Percutaneous 4 Percutaneous Endoscopic	Z No Device	Z No Qualifier

Section	0	Medical and Surgical
Body System	0	Central Nervous System and Cranial Nerves
Operation	R	Replacement: Putting in or on biological or synthetic material that physically takes the place and/or function of all or a portion of a body part

Body Part (4th)	Approach (5th)	Device (6th)	Qualifier (7th)
1 Cerebral Meninges 2 Dura Mater 6 Cerebral Ventricle F Olfactory Nerve G Optic Nerve H Oculomotor Nerve J Trochlear Nerve K Trigeminal Nerve L Abducens Nerve M Facial Nerve N Acoustic Nerve P Glossopharyngeal Nerve Q Vagus Nerve R Accessory Nerve S Hypoglossal Nerve T Spinal Meninges	0 Open 4 Percutaneous Endoscopic	7 Autologous Tissue Substitute J Synthetic Substitute K Nonautologous Tissue Substitute	Z No Qualifier

Section	0	Medical and Surgical
Body System	0	Central Nervous System and Cranial Nerves
Operation	S	Reposition: Moving to its normal location, or other suitable location, all or a portion of a body part

Body Part (4th)	Approach (5th)	Device (6th)	Qualifier (7th)
F Olfactory Nerve G Optic Nerve H Oculomotor Nerve J Trochlear Nerve K Trigeminal Nerve L Abducens Nerve M Facial Nerve N Acoustic Nerve P Glossopharyngeal Nerve Q Vagus Nerve R Accessory Nerve S Hypoglossal Nerve W Cervical Spinal Cord X Thoracic Spinal Cord Y Lumbar Spinal Cord	0 Open 3 Percutaneous 4 Percutaneous Endoscopic	Z No Device	Z No Qualifier

Section	0	Medical and Surgical
Body System	0	Central Nervous System and Cranial Nerves
Operation	T	Resection: Cutting out or off, without replacement, all of a body part

Body Part (4th)	Approach (5th)	Device (6th)	Qualifier (7th)
7 Cerebral Hemisphere	0 Open 3 Percutaneous 4 Percutaneous Endoscopic	Z No Device	Z No Qualifier

00U–00W

Medical and Surgical, Central Nervous System and Cranial Nerves Tables

Section	0	Medical and Surgical
Body System	0	Central Nervous System and Cranial Nerves
Operation	U	Supplement: Putting in or on biological or synthetic material that physically reinforces and/or augments the function of a portion of a body part

Body Part (4th)	Approach (5th)	Device (6th)	Qualifier (7th)
1 Cerebral Meninges 2 Dura Mater 6 Cerebral Ventricle F Olfactory Nerve G Optic Nerve H Oculomotor Nerve J Trochlear Nerve K Trigeminal Nerve L Abducens Nerve M Facial Nerve N Acoustic Nerve P Glossopharyngeal Nerve Q Vagus Nerve R Accessory Nerve S Hypoglossal Nerve T Spinal Meninges	0 Open 3 Percutaneous 4 Percutaneous Endoscopic	7 Autologous Tissue Substitute J Synthetic Substitute K Nonautologous Tissue Substitute	Z No Qualifier

Section	0	Medical and Surgical
Body System	0	Central Nervous System and Cranial Nerves
Operation	W	Revision: Correcting, to the extent possible, a portion of a malfunctioning device or the position of a displaced device

Body Part (4th)	Approach (5th)	Device (6th)	Qualifier (7th)
0 Brain V Spinal Cord	0 Open 3 Percutaneous 4 Percutaneous Endoscopic	0 Drainage Device 2 Monitoring Device 3 Infusion Device 7 Autologous Tissue Substitute J Synthetic Substitute K Nonautologous Tissue Substitute M Neurostimulator Lead Y Other Device	Z No Qualifier
0 Brain V Spinal Cord	X External	0 Drainage Device 2 Monitoring Device 3 Infusion Device 7 Autologous Tissue Substitute J Synthetic Substitute K Nonautologous Tissue Substitute M Neurostimulator Lead	Z No Qualifier
6 Cerebral Ventricle U Spinal Canal	0 Open 3 Percutaneous 4 Percutaneous Endoscopic	0 Drainage Device 2 Monitoring Device 3 Infusion Device J Synthetic Substitute M Neurostimulator Lead Y Other Device	Z No Qualifier
6 Cerebral Ventricle U Spinal Canal	X External	0 Drainage Device 2 Monitoring Device 3 Infusion Device J Synthetic Substitute M Neurostimulator Lead	Z No Qualifier

Continued →

Section	0	Medical and Surgical				
Body System	0	Central Nervous System and Cranial Nerves				
Operation	W	Revision: Correcting, to the extent possible, a portion of a malfunctioning device or the position of a displaced device				

00W Continued

Body Part (4th)	Approach (5th)	Device (6th)	Qualifier (7th)
E Cranial Nerve	0 Open 3 Percutaneous 4 Percutaneous Endoscopic	0 Drainage Device 2 Monitoring Device 3 Infusion Device 7 Autologous Tissue Substitute M Neurostimulator Lead Y Other Device	Z No Qualifier
E Cranial Nerve	X External	0 Drainage Device 2 Monitoring Device 3 Infusion Device 7 Autologous Tissue Substitute M Neurostimulator Lead	Z No Qualifier

Section	0	Medical and Surgical				
Body System	0	Central Nervous System and Cranial Nerves				
Operation	X	Transfer: Moving, without taking out, all or a portion of a body part to another location to take over the function of all or a portion of a body part				

Body Part (4th)	Approach (5th)	Device (6th)	Qualifier (7th)
F Olfactory Nerve G Optic Nerve H Oculomotor Nerve J Trochlear Nerve K Trigeminal Nerve L Abducens Nerve M Facial Nerve N Acoustic Nerve P Glossopharyngeal Nerve Q Vagus Nerve R Accessory Nerve S Hypoglossal Nerve	0 Open 4 Percutaneous Endoscopic	Z No Device	F Olfactory Nerve G Optic Nerve H Oculomotor Nerve J Trochlear Nerve K Trigeminal Nerve L Abducens Nerve M Facial Nerve N Acoustic Nerve P Glossopharyngeal Nerve Q Vagus Nerve R Accessory Nerve S Hypoglossal Nerve

AHA Coding Clinic

00163J6 Bypass Cerebral Ventricle to Peritoneal Cavity with Synthetic Substitute, Percutaneous Approach—AHA CC: 2Q, 2013, 36-37; 2Q, 2021, 19-20

00163JA Bypass Cerebral Ventricle to Subgaleal Space with Synthetic Substitute, Percutaneous Approach—AHA CC: 4Q, 2019, 22

001U0J2 Bypass Spinal Canal to Atrium with Synthetic Substitute, Open Approach—AHA CC: 4Q, 2018, 86

005C0ZZ Destruction of Cerebellum, Open Approach—AHA CC: 3Q, 2021, 16-17

005K3ZZ Destruction of Trigeminal Nerve, Percutaneous Approach—AHA CC: 1Q, 2022, 50

005W0ZZ Destruction of Cervical Spinal Cord, Open Approach—AHA CC: 2Q, 2021, 17-18

005X0ZZ Destruction of Thoracic Spinal Cord, Open Approach—AHA CC: 2Q, 2021, 17-18

00764AA Dilation of Cerebral Ventricle, Percutaneous Endoscopic Approach—AHA CC: 4Q, 2017, 40-41

009430Z Drainage of Intracranial Subdural Space with Drainage Device, Percutaneous Approach—AHA CC: 3Q, 2015, 11-12

009630Z Drainage of Cerebral Ventricle with Drainage Device, Percutaneous Approach—AHA CC: 3Q, 2015, 12-13

009U00Z Drainage of Spinal Canal with Drainage Device, Open Approach—AHA CC: 4Q, 2018, 85

009U3ZX Drainage of Spinal Canal, Percutaneous Approach, Diagnostic—AHA CC: 1Q, 2014, 8

009W00Z Drainage of Cervical Spinal Cord with Drainage Device, Open Approach—AHA CC: 2Q, 2015, 30

00B00ZX Excision of Brain, Open Approach, Diagnostic—AHA CC: 1Q, 2015, 12-13

00B70ZZ Excision of Cerebral Hemisphere, Open Approach—AHA CC: 4Q, 2014, 34-35; 2Q, 2016, 18

00BC0ZZ Excision of Cerebellum, Open Approach—AHA CC: 3Q, 2021, 16-17

00BM0ZZ Excision of Facial Nerve, Open Approach—AHA CC: 2Q, 2016, 12-14

00BR0ZZ Excision of Accessory Nerve, Open Approach—AHA CC: 2Q, 2016, 12-14

00BS0ZZ Excision of Hypoglossal Nerve, Open Approach—AHA CC: 2Q, 2016, 12-14

00BY0ZZ Excision of Lumbar Spinal Cord, Open Approach—AHA CC: 3Q, 2014, 24

00C00ZZ Extirpation of Matter from Brain, Open Approach—AHA CC: 1Q, 2015, 12-13; 4Q, 2016, 27-28

00C04ZZ Extirpation of Matter from Brain, Percutaneous Endoscopic Approach—AHA CC: 2Q, 2019, 36-37

00C40ZZ Extirpation of Matter from Intracranial Subdural Space, Open Approach—AHA CC: 3Q, 2015, 10-11; 2Q, 2016, 29; 3Q, 2019, 4-5

00C74ZZ Extirpation of Matter from Cerebral Hemisphere, Percutaneous Endoscopic Approach—AHA CC: 3Q, 2015, 13

00CU0ZZ Extirpation of Matter from Spinal Canal, Open Approach—AHA CC: 4Q, 2017, 48

00D00ZZ Extraction of Brain, Open Approach—AHA CC: 4Q, 2021, 38-40

00D20ZZ Extraction of Dura Mater, Open Approach—AHA CC: 3Q, 2015, 13-14

00D70ZZ Extraction of Cerebral Hemisphere, Open Approach—AHA CC: 4Q, 2021, 38-40

00H633Z Insertion of Infusion Device into Cerebral Ventricle, Percutaneous Approach—AHA CC: 2Q, 2020, 15-16

00HU03Z Insertion of Infusion Device into Spinal Canal, Open Approach—AHA CC: 2Q, 2020, 16-17

00HU33Z Insertion of Infusion Device into Spinal Canal, Percutaneous Approach—AHA CC: 3Q, 2014, 19-20

00J00ZZ Inspection of Brain, Open Approach—AHA CC: 2Q, 2019, 36-37

00J04ZZ Inspection of Brain, Percutaneous Endoscopic Approach—AHA CC: 2Q, 2021, 19-20

00JU3ZZ Inspection of Spinal Canal, Percutaneous Approach—AHA CC: 1Q, 2017, 50

00N00ZZ Release Brain, Open Approach—AHA CC: 2Q, 2016, 29

00N70ZZ Release Cerebral Hemisphere, Open Approach—AHA CC: 3Q, 2018, 30

00NC0ZZ Release Cerebellum, Open Approach—AHA CC: 3Q, 2017, 10-11

00NM4ZZ Release Facial Nerve, Percutaneous Endoscopic Approach—AHA CC: 4Q, 2018, 10

00NW0ZZ Release Cervical Spinal Cord, Open Approach—AHA CC: 2Q, 2015, 20-22; 2Q, 2017, 23-24

00NW3ZZ Release Cervical Spinal Cord, Percutaneous Approach—AHA CC: 2Q, 2019, 19-20

00NY0ZZ Release Lumbar Spinal Cord, Open Approach—AHA CC: 3Q, 2014, 24; 1Q, 2019, 28-29

00PU03Z Removal of Infusion Device from Spinal Canal, Open Approach—AHA CC: 3Q, 2014, 19-20

00Q20ZZ Repair Dura Mater, Open Approach—AHA CC: 3Q, 2013, 25; 3Q, 2014, 7-8

00SM0ZZ Reposition Facial Nerve, Open Approach—AHA CC: 4Q, 2014, 35

00U20KZ Supplement Dura Mater with Nonautologous Tissue Substitute, Open Approach—AHA CC: 3Q, 2017, 10-11; 1Q, 2018, 9; 3Q, 2021, 16-17

00UT0KZ Supplement Spinal Meninges with Nonautologous Tissue Substitute, Open Approach—AHA CC: 3Q, 2014, 24

Peripheral Nervous System

Spinal Column

Peripheral Nervous System Tables 012–01X

Section	0	Medical and Surgical
Body System	1	Peripheral Nervous System
Operation	2	**Change:** Taking out or off a device from a body part and putting back an identical or similar device in or on the same body part without cutting or puncturing the skin or a mucous membrane

Body Part (4th)	Approach (5th)	Device (6th)	Qualifier (7th)
Y Peripheral Nerve	X External	0 Drainage Device Y Other Device	Z No Qualifier

Section	0	Medical and Surgical
Body System	1	Peripheral Nervous System
Operation	5	**Destruction:** Physical eradication of all or a portion of a body part by the direct use of energy, force, or a destructive agent

Body Part (4th)	Approach (5th)	Device (6th)	Qualifier (7th)
0 Cervical Plexus 1 Cervical Nerve 2 Phrenic Nerve 3 Brachial Plexus 4 Ulnar Nerve 5 Median Nerve 6 Radial Nerve 8 Thoracic Nerve 9 Lumbar Plexus A Lumbosacral Plexus B Lumbar Nerve C Pudendal Nerve D Femoral Nerve F Sciatic Nerve G Tibial Nerve H Peroneal Nerve K Head and Neck Sympathetic Nerve L Thoracic Sympathetic Nerve M Abdominal Sympathetic Nerve N Lumbar Sympathetic Nerve P Sacral Sympathetic Nerve Q Sacral Plexus R Sacral Nerve	0 Open 3 Percutaneous 4 Percutaneous Endoscopic	Z No Device	Z No Qualifier

Section 0 **Medical and Surgical**
Body System 1 **Peripheral Nervous System**
Operation 8 **Division:** Cutting into a body part, without draining fluids and/or gases from the body part, in order to separate or transect a body part

Body Part (4th)	Approach (5th)	Device (6th)	Qualifier (7th)
0 Cervical Plexus	0 Open	Z No Device	Z No Qualifier
1 Cervical Nerve	3 Percutaneous		
2 Phrenic Nerve	4 Percutaneous		
3 Brachial Plexus	Endoscopic		
4 Ulnar Nerve			
5 Median Nerve			
6 Radial Nerve			
8 Thoracic Nerve			
9 Lumbar Plexus			
A Lumbosacral Plexus			
B Lumbar Nerve			
C Pudendal Nerve			
D Femoral Nerve			
F Sciatic Nerve			
G Tibial Nerve			
H Peroneal Nerve			
K Head and Neck Sympathetic Nerve			
L Thoracic Sympathetic Nerve			
M Abdominal Sympathetic Nerve			
N Lumbar Sympathetic Nerve			
P Sacral Sympathetic Nerve			
Q Sacral Plexus			
R Sacral Nerve			

Section 0 **Medical and Surgical**
Body System 1 **Peripheral Nervous System**
Operation 9 **Drainage:** Taking or letting out fluids and/or gases from a body part

Body Part (4th)	Approach (5th)	Device (6th)	Qualifier (7th)
0 Cervical Plexus	0 Open	0 Drainage Device	Z No Qualifier
1 Cervical Nerve	3 Percutaneous		
2 Phrenic Nerve	4 Percutaneous		
3 Brachial Plexus	Endoscopic		
4 Ulnar Nerve			
5 Median Nerve			
6 Radial Nerve			
8 Thoracic Nerve			
9 Lumbar Plexus			
A Lumbosacral Plexus			
B Lumbar Nerve			
C Pudendal Nerve			
D Femoral Nerve			
F Sciatic Nerve			
G Tibial Nerve			
H Peroneal Nerve			
K Head and Neck Sympathetic Nerve			
L Thoracic Sympathetic Nerve			
M Abdominal Sympathetic Nerve			
N Lumbar Sympathetic Nerve			
P Sacral Sympathetic Nerve			
Q Sacral Plexus			
R Sacral Nerve			

Continued ➞

Section	0	Medical and Surgical
Body System	1	Peripheral Nervous System
Operation	9	Drainage: Taking or letting out fluids and/or gases from a body part

019 Continued

Body Part (4th)	Approach (5th)	Device (6th)	Qualifier (7th)
0 Cervical Plexus	0 Open	Z No Device	X Diagnostic
1 Cervical Nerve	3 Percutaneous		Z No Qualifier
2 Phrenic Nerve	4 Percutaneous		
3 Brachial Plexus	Endoscopic		
4 Ulnar Nerve			
5 Median Nerve			
6 Radial Nerve			
8 Thoracic Nerve			
9 Lumbar Plexus			
A Lumbosacral Plexus			
B Lumbar Nerve			
C Pudendal Nerve			
D Femoral Nerve			
F Sciatic Nerve			
G Tibial Nerve			
H Peroneal Nerve			
K Head and Neck Sympathetic Nerve			
L Thoracic Sympathetic Nerve			
M Abdominal Sympathetic Nerve			
N Lumbar Sympathetic Nerve			
P Sacral Sympathetic Nerve			
Q Sacral Plexus			
R Sacral Nerve			

Section	0	Medical and Surgical
Body System	1	Peripheral Nervous System
Operation	B	Excision: Cutting out or off, without replacement, a portion of a body part

Body Part (4th)	Approach (5th)	Device (6th)	Qualifier (7th)
0 Cervical Plexus	0 Open	Z No Device	X Diagnostic
1 Cervical Nerve	3 Percutaneous		Z No Qualifier
2 Phrenic Nerve	4 Percutaneous		
3 Brachial Plexus	Endoscopic		
4 Ulnar Nerve			
5 Median Nerve			
6 Radial Nerve			
8 Thoracic Nerve			
9 Lumbar Plexus			
A Lumbosacral Plexus			
B Lumbar Nerve			
C Pudendal Nerve			
D Femoral Nerve			
F Sciatic Nerve			
G Tibial Nerve			
H Peroneal Nerve			
K Head and Neck Sympathetic Nerve			
L Thoracic Sympathetic Nerve			
M Abdominal Sympathetic Nerve			
N Lumbar Sympathetic Nerve			
P Sacral Sympathetic Nerve			
Q Sacral Plexus			
R Sacral Nerve			

Section   0   **Medical and Surgical**
Body System   1   **Peripheral Nervous System**
Operation   C   **Extirpation:** Taking or cutting out solid matter from a body part

Body Part (4th)	Approach (5th)	Device (6th)	Qualifier (7th)
0 Cervical Plexus 1 Cervical Nerve 2 Phrenic Nerve 3 Brachial Plexus 4 Ulnar Nerve 5 Median Nerve 6 Radial Nerve 8 Thoracic Nerve 9 Lumbar Plexus A Lumbosacral Plexus B Lumbar Nerve C Pudendal Nerve D Femoral Nerve F Sciatic Nerve G Tibial Nerve H Peroneal Nerve K Head and Neck Sympathetic Nerve L Thoracic Sympathetic Nerve M Abdominal Sympathetic Nerve N Lumbar Sympathetic Nerve P Sacral Sympathetic Nerve Q Sacral Plexus R Sacral Nerve	0 Open 3 Percutaneous 4 Percutaneous Endoscopic	Z No Device	Z No Qualifier

Section   0   **Medical and Surgical**
Body System   1   **Peripheral Nervous System**
Operation   D   **Extraction:** Pulling or stripping out or off all or a portion of a body part by the use of force

Body Part (4th)	Approach (5th)	Device (6th)	Qualifier (7th)
0 Cervical Plexus 1 Cervical Nerve 2 Phrenic Nerve 3 Brachial Plexus 4 Ulnar Nerve 5 Median Nerve 6 Radial Nerve 8 Thoracic Nerve 9 Lumbar Plexus A Lumbosacral Plexus B Lumbar Nerve C Pudendal Nerve D Femoral Nerve F Sciatic Nerve G Tibial Nerve H Peroneal Nerve K Head and Neck Sympathetic Nerve L Thoracic Sympathetic Nerve M Abdominal Sympathetic Nerve N Lumbar Sympathetic Nerve P Sacral Sympathetic Nerve Q Sacral Plexus R Sacral Nerve	0 Open 3 Percutaneous 4 Percutaneous Endoscopic	Z No Device	Z No Qualifier

Section	0	Medical and Surgical
Body System	1	Peripheral Nervous System
Operation	H	**Insertion:** Putting in a nonbiological appliance that monitors, assists, performs, or prevents a physiological function but does not physically take the place of a body part

Body Part (4th)	Approach (5th)	Device (6th)	Qualifier (7th)
Y Peripheral Nerve	0 Open 3 Percutaneous 4 Percutaneous Endoscopic	1 Radioactive Element 2 Monitoring Device M Neurostimulator Lead Y Other Device	Z No Qualifier

Section	0	Medical and Surgical
Body System	1	Peripheral Nervous System
Operation	J	**Inspection:** Visually and/or manually exploring a body part

Body Part (4th)	Approach (5th)	Device (6th)	Qualifier (7th)
Y Peripheral Nerve	0 Open 3 Percutaneous 4 Percutaneous Endoscopic	Z No Device	Z No Qualifier

Section	0	Medical and Surgical
Body System	1	Peripheral Nervous System
Operation	N	**Release:** Freeing a body part from an abnormal physical constraint by cutting or by the use of force

Body Part (4th)	Approach (5th)	Device (6th)	Qualifier (7th)
0 Cervical Plexus 1 Cervical Nerve 2 Phrenic Nerve 3 Brachial Plexus 4 Ulnar Nerve 5 Median Nerve 6 Radial Nerve 8 Thoracic Nerve 9 Lumbar Plexus A Lumbosacral Plexus B Lumbar Nerve C Pudendal Nerve D Femoral Nerve F Sciatic Nerve G Tibial Nerve H Peroneal Nerve K Head and Neck Sympathetic Nerve L Thoracic Sympathetic Nerve M Abdominal Sympathetic Nerve N Lumbar Sympathetic Nerve P Sacral Sympathetic Nerve Q Sacral Plexus R Sacral Nerve	0 Open 3 Percutaneous 4 Percutaneous Endoscopic	Z No Device	Z No Qualifier

Section	0	Medical and Surgical
Body System	1	Peripheral Nervous System
Operation	P	**Removal:** Taking out or off a device from a body part

Body Part (4th)	Approach (5th)	Device (6th)	Qualifier (7th)
Y Peripheral Nerve	0 Open 3 Percutaneous 4 Percutaneous Endoscopic	0 Drainage Device 2 Monitoring Device 7 Autologous Tissue Substitute M Neurostimulator Lead Y Other Device	Z No Qualifier
Y Peripheral Nerve	X External	0 Drainage Device 2 Monitoring Device M Neurostimulator Lead	Z No Qualifier

01Q–01R

Medical and Surgical, Peripheral Nervous System Tables

Section	0	Medical and Surgical
Body System	1	Peripheral Nervous System
Operation	Q	**Repair:** Restoring, to the extent possible, a body part to its normal anatomic structure and function

Body Part (4th)	Approach (5th)	Device (6th)	Qualifier (7th)
0 Cervical Plexus	0 Open	Z No Device	Z No Qualifier
1 Cervical Nerve	3 Percutaneous		
2 Phrenic Nerve	4 Percutaneous		
3 Brachial Plexus	Endoscopic		
4 Ulnar Nerve			
5 Median Nerve			
6 Radial Nerve			
8 Thoracic Nerve			
9 Lumbar Plexus			
A Lumbosacral Plexus			
B Lumbar Nerve			
C Pudendal Nerve			
D Femoral Nerve			
F Sciatic Nerve			
G Tibial Nerve			
H Peroneal Nerve			
K Head and Neck Sympathetic Nerve			
L Thoracic Sympathetic Nerve			
M Abdominal Sympathetic Nerve			
N Lumbar Sympathetic Nerve			
P Sacral Sympathetic Nerve			
Q Sacral Plexus			
R Sacral Nerve			

Section	0	Medical and Surgical
Body System	1	Peripheral Nervous System
Operation	R	**Replacement:** Putting in or on biological or synthetic material that physically takes the place and/or function of all or a portion of a body part

Body Part (4th)	Approach (5th)	Device (6th)	Qualifier (7th)
1 Cervical Nerve	0 Open	7 Autologous Tissue Substitute	Z No Qualifier
2 Phrenic Nerve	4 Percutaneous Endoscopic	J Synthetic Substitute	
4 Ulnar Nerve		K Nonautologous Tissue Substitute	
5 Median Nerve			
6 Radial Nerve			
8 Thoracic Nerve			
B Lumbar Nerve			
C Pudendal Nerve			
D Femoral Nerve			
F Sciatic Nerve			
G Tibial Nerve			
H Peroneal Nerve			
R Sacral Nerve			

124

Section	0	Medical and Surgical
Body System	1	Peripheral Nervous System
Operation	S	Reposition: Moving to its normal location, or other suitable location, all or a portion of a body part

Body Part (4th)	Approach (5th)	Device (6th)	Qualifier (7th)
0 Cervical Plexus	0 Open	Z No Device	Z No Qualifier
1 Cervical Nerve	3 Percutaneous		
2 Phrenic Nerve	4 Percutaneous		
3 Brachial Plexus	Endoscopic		
4 Ulnar Nerve			
5 Median Nerve			
6 Radial Nerve			
8 Thoracic Nerve			
9 Lumbar Plexus			
A Lumbosacral Plexus			
B Lumbar Nerve			
C Pudendal Nerve			
D Femoral Nerve			
F Sciatic Nerve			
G Tibial Nerve			
H Peroneal Nerve			
Q Sacral Plexus			
R Sacral Nerve			

Section	0	Medical and Surgical
Body System	1	Peripheral Nervous System
Operation	U	Supplement: Putting in or on biological or synthetic material that physically reinforces and/or augments the function of a portion of a body part

Body Part (4th)	Approach (5th)	Device (6th)	Qualifier (7th)
1 Cervical Nerve	0 Open	7 Autologous Tissue Substitute	Z No Qualifier
2 Phrenic Nerve	3 Percutaneous	J Synthetic Substitute	
4 Ulnar Nerve	4 Percutaneous Endoscopic	K Nonautologous Tissue	
5 Median Nerve		Substitute	
6 Radial Nerve			
8 Thoracic Nerve			
B Lumbar Nerve			
C Pudendal Nerve			
D Femoral Nerve			
F Sciatic Nerve			
G Tibial Nerve			
H Peroneal Nerve			
R Sacral Nerve			

Section	0	Medical and Surgical
Body System	1	Peripheral Nervous System
Operation	W	Revision: Correcting, to the extent possible, a portion of a malfunctioning device or the position of a displaced device

Body Part (4th)	Approach (5th)	Device (6th)	Qualifier (7th)
Y Peripheral Nerve	0 Open	0 Drainage Device	Z No Qualifier
	3 Percutaneous	2 Monitoring Device	
	4 Percutaneous Endoscopic	7 Autologous Tissue Substitute	
		M Neurostimulator Lead	
		Y Other Device	
Y Peripheral Nerve	X External	0 Drainage Device	Z No Qualifier
		2 Monitoring Device	
		7 Autologous Tissue Substitute	
		M Neurostimulator Lead	

Section   **0**   **Medical and Surgical**
Body System   **1**   **Peripheral Nervous System**
Operation   **X**   **Transfer:** Moving, without taking out, all or a portion of a body part to another location to take over the function of all or a portion of a body part

Body Part (4ᵗʰ)	Approach (5ᵗʰ)	Device (6ᵗʰ)	Qualifier (7ᵗʰ)
1 Cervical Nerve 2 Phrenic Nerve	0 Open 4 Percutaneous Endoscopic	Z No Device	1 Cervical Nerve 2 Phrenic Nerve
4 Ulnar Nerve 5 Median Nerve 6 Radial Nerve	0 Open 4 Percutaneous Endoscopic	Z No Device	4 Ulnar Nerve 5 Median Nerve 6 Radial Nerve
8 Thoracic Nerve	0 Open 4 Percutaneous Endoscopic	Z No Device	8 Thoracic Nerve
B Lumbar Nerve C Pudendal Nerve	0 Open 4 Percutaneous Endoscopic	Z No Device	B Lumbar Nerve C Perineal Nerve
D Femoral Nerve F Sciatic Nerve G Tibial Nerve H Peroneal Nerve	0 Open 4 Percutaneous Endoscopic	Z No Device	D Femoral Nerve F Sciatic Nerve G Tibial Nerve H Peroneal Nerve

AHA Coding Clinic

01BL0ZZ Excision of Thoracic Sympathetic Nerve, Open Approach—AHA CC: 2Q, 2017, 19-20

01N10ZZ Release Cervical Nerve, Open Approach—AHA CC: 2Q, 2016, 17

01N30ZZ Release Brachial Plexus, Open Approach—AHA CC: 2Q, 2016, 23

01N50ZZ Release Median Nerve, Open Approach—AHA CC: 3Q, 2014, 33-34

01NB0ZZ Release Lumbar Nerve, Open Approach—AHA CC: 2Q, 2015, 34; 2Q, 2016, 16; 2Q, 2018, 22-23; 1Q, 2019, 28-29

01NR0ZZ Release Sacral Nerve, Open Approach—AHA CC: 1Q, 2019, 28-29

01S30ZZ Reposition Brachial Plexus, Open Approach—AHA CC: 3Q, 2021, 19-20

01S40ZZ Reposition Ulnar Nerve, Open Approach—AHA CC: 3Q, 2021, 19-20

01S50ZZ Reposition Median Nerve, Open Approach—AHA CC: 3Q, 2021, 19-20

01S60ZZ Reposition Radial Nerve, Open Approach—AHA CC: 3Q, 2021, 19-20

01U50KZ Supplement Median Nerve with Nonautologous Tissue Substitute, Open Approach—AHA CC: 4Q, 2017, 62

01U80KZ Supplement Thoracic Nerve with Nonautologous Tissue Substitute, Open Approach—AHA CC: 3Q, 2019, 32-33

Heart and Great Vessels

Atria, Ventricles and Interventricular Septum

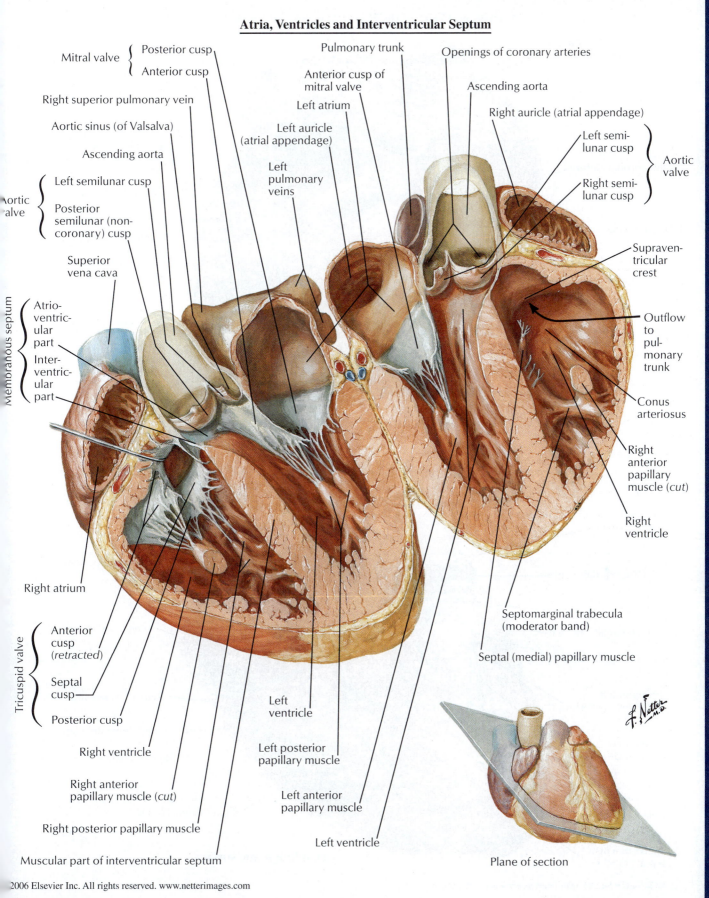

Arteries and Veins of the Heart; Arteries and Cardiac Veins

Sternocostal surface

Diaphragmatic surface

Right Coronary Artery – Segmental Replacement

Right coronary-artery segmental replacement

A. Diseased segment of right coronary artery widely exposed, clamped, and incised; portion between broken lines to be excised

B. Segment of saphenous vein being sutured to proximal end of transected coronary artery

C. Lower end of saphenous graft sutured to distal portion of artery; blood and air allowed to escape by loosening distal clamp prior to final closure

Right coronary-artery bypass

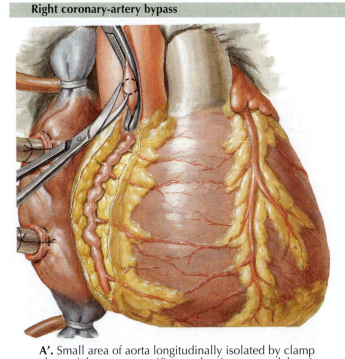

A'. Small area of aorta longitudinally isolated by clamp above right coronary orifice, and ostium created therein

B'. Segment of saphenous vein implanted into new aortic ostium and anastomosed to end of divided right coronary artery distal to diseased area; proximal end of artery ligated

Heart and Great Vessels Tables 021–02Y

Section	0	Medical and Surgical
Body System	2	Heart and Great Vessels
Operation	1	Bypass: Altering the route of passage of the contents of a tubular body part

Body Part (4th)	Approach (5th)	Device (6th)	Qualifier (7th)
0 Coronary Artery, One Artery 1 Coronary Artery, Two Arteries 2 Coronary Artery, Three Arteries 3 Coronary Artery, Four or More Arteries	0 Open	8 Zooplastic Tissue 9 Autologous Venous Tissue A Autologous Arterial Tissue J Synthetic Substitute K Nonautologous Tissue Substitute	3 Coronary Artery 8 Internal Mammary, Right 9 Internal Mammary, Left C Thoracic Artery F Abdominal Artery W Aorta
0 Coronary Artery, One Artery 1 Coronary Artery, Two Arteries 2 Coronary Artery, Three Arteries 3 Coronary Artery, Four or More Arteries	0 Open	Z No Device	3 Coronary Artery 8 Internal Mammary, Right 9 Internal Mammary, Left C Thoracic Artery F Abdominal Artery
0 Coronary Artery, One Artery 1 Coronary Artery, Two Arteries 2 Coronary Artery, Three Arteries 3 Coronary Artery, Four or More Arteries	3 Percutaneous	4 Intraluminal Device, Drug-eluting D Intraluminal Device	4 Coronary Vein
0 Coronary Artery, One Artery 1 Coronary Artery, Two Arteries 2 Coronary Artery, Three Arteries 3 Coronary Artery, Four or More Arteries	4 Percutaneous Endoscopic	4 Intraluminal Device, Drug-eluting D Intraluminal Device	4 Coronary Vein
0 Coronary Artery, One Artery 1 Coronary Artery, Two Arteries 2 Coronary Artery, Three Arteries 3 Coronary Artery, Four or More Arteries	4 Percutaneous Endoscopic	8 Zooplastic Tissue 9 Autologous Venous Tissue A Autologous Arterial Tissue J Synthetic Substitute K Nonautologous Tissue Substitute	3 Coronary Artery 8 Internal Mammary, Right 9 Internal Mammary, Left C Thoracic Artery F Abdominal Artery W Aorta
0 Coronary Artery, One Artery 1 Coronary Artery, Two Arteries 2 Coronary Artery, Three Arteries 3 Coronary Artery, Four or More Arteries	4 Percutaneous Endoscopic	Z No Device	3 Coronary Artery 8 Internal Mammary, Right 9 Internal Mammary, Left C Thoracic Artery F Abdominal Artery
6 Atrium, Right	0 Open 4 Percutaneous Endoscopic	8 Zooplastic Tissue 9 Autologous Venous Tissue A Autologous Arterial Tissue J Synthetic Substitute K Nonautologous Tissue Substitute	P Pulmonary Trunk Q Pulmonary Artery, Right R Pulmonary Artery, Left
6 Atrium, Right	0 Open 4 Percutaneous Endoscopic	Z No Device	7 Atrium, Left P Pulmonary Trunk Q Pulmonary Artery, Right R Pulmonary Artery, Left
6 Atrium, Right	3 Percutaneous	Z No Device	7 Atrium, Left
7 Atrium, Left	0 Open 4 Percutaneous Endoscopic	8 Zooplastic Tissue 9 Autologous Venous Tissue A Autologous Arterial Tissue J Synthetic Substitute K Nonautologous Tissue Substitute Z No Device	P Pulmonary Trunk Q Pulmonary Artery, Right R Pulmonary Artery, Left S Pulmonary Vein, Right T Pulmonary Vein, Left U Pulmonary Vein, Confluence
7 Atrium	3 Percutaneous	J Synthetic Substitute	6 Atrium, Right
K Ventricle, Right L Ventricle, Left	0 Open 4 Percutaneous Endoscopic	8 Zooplastic Tissue 9 Autologous Venous Tissue A Autologous Arterial Tissue J Synthetic Substitute K Nonautologous Tissue Substitute	P Pulmonary Trunk Q Pulmonary Artery, Right R Pulmonary Artery, Left

Continued →

Section	0	Medical and Surgical
Body System	2	Heart and Great Vessels
Operation	1	Bypass: Altering the route of passage of the contents of a tubular body part

021 Continued

Body Part (4th)	Approach (5th)	Device (6th)	Qualifier (7th)
K Ventricle, Right L Ventricle, Left	0 Open 4 Percutaneous Endoscopic	Z No Device	5 Coronary Circulation 8 Internal Mammary, Right 9 Internal Mammary, Left C Thoracic Artery F Abdominal Artery P Pulmonary Trunk Q Pulmonary Artery, Right R Pulmonary Artery, Left W Aorta
P Pulmonary Trunk Q Right Pulmonary Artery R Left Pulmonary Artery	0 Open 4 Percutaneous Endoscopic	8 Zooplastic Tissue 9 Autologous Venous Tissue A Autologous Arterial Tissue J Synthetic Substitute K Nonautologous Tissue Substitute	A Innominate Artery B Subclavin D Carotid
V Superior Vena Cava	0 Open 4 Percutaneous Endoscopic	8 Zooplastic Tissue 9 Autologous Venous Tissue A Autologous Arterial Tissue J Synthetic Substitute K Nonautologous Tissue Substitute Z No Device	P Pulmonary Trunk Q Pulmonary Artery, Right R Pulmonary Artery, Left S Pulmonary Vein, Right T Pulmonary Vein, Left U Pulmonary Vein, Confluence
W Thoracic Aorta, Descending	0 Open	8 Zooplastic Tissue 9 Autologous Venous Tissue A Autologous Arterial Tissue J Synthetic Substitute K Nonautologous Tissue Substitute	A Innominate Artery B Subclavian D Carotid F Abdominal Artery G Axillary Artery H Brachial Artery P Pulmonary Trunk Q Pulmonary Artery, Right R Pulmonary Artery, Left V Lower Extremity Artery
W Thoracic Aorta, Descending	0 Open	Z No Device	A Innominate Artery B Subclavian D Carotid P Pulmonary Trunk Q Pulmonary Artery, Right R Pulmonary Artery, Left
W Thoracic Aorta, Descending	4 Percutaneous Endoscopic	8 Zooplastic Tissue 9 Autologous Venous Tissue A Autologous Arterial Tissue J Synthetic Substitute K Nonautologous Tissue Substitute Z No Device	A Innominate Artery B Subclavian D Carotid P Pulmonary Trunk Q Pulmonary Artery, Right R Pulmonary Artery, Left
X Thoracic Aorta, Ascending/Arch	0 Open 4 Percutaneous Endoscopic	8 Zooplastic Tissue 9 Autologous Venous Tissue A Autologous Arterial Tissue J Synthetic Substitute K Nonautologous Tissue Substitute Z No Device	A Innominate Artery B Subclavian D Carotid P Pulmonary Trunk Q Pulmonary Artery, Right R Pulmonary Artery, Left

Section	0	Medical and Surgical
Body System	2	Heart and Great Vessels
Operation	4	Creation: Putting in or on biological or synthetic material to form a new body part that to the extent possible replicates the anatomic structure or function of an absent body part

Body Part (4th)	Approach (5th)	Device (6th)	Qualifier (7th)
F Aortic Valve	0 Open	7 Autologous Tissue Substitute 8 Zooplastic Tissue J Synthetic Substitute K Nonautologous Tissue Substitute	J Truncal Valve
G Mitral Valve J Tricuspid Valve	0 Open	7 Autologous Tissue Substitute 8 Zooplastic Tissue J Synthetic Substitute K Nonautologous Tissue Substitute	2 Common Atrioventricular Valve

Section	0	Medical and Surgical
Body System	2	Heart and Great Vessels
Operation	5	Destruction: Physical eradication of all or a portion of a body part by the direct use of energy, force, or a destructive agent

Body Part (4th)	Approach (5th)	Device (6th)	Qualifier (7th)
4 Coronary Vein 5 Atrial Septum 6 Atrium, Right 8 Conduction Mechanism 9 Chordae Tendineae D Papillary Muscle F Aortic Valve G Mitral Valve H Pulmonary Valve J Tricuspid Valve K Ventricle, Right L Ventricle, Left M Ventricular Septum N Pericardium P Pulmonary Trunk Q Pulmonary Artery, Right R Pulmonary Artery, Left S Pulmonary Vein, Right T Pulmonary Vein, Left V Superior Vena Cava W Thoracic Aorta, Descending X Thoracic Aorta, Ascending/Arch	0 Open 3 Percutaneous 4 Percutaneous Endoscopic	Z No Device	Z No Qualifier
7 Atrium, Left	0 Open 3 Percutaneous 4 Percutaneous Endoscopic	Z No Device	K Left Atrial Appendage Z No Qualifier

Section	0	Medical and Surgical
Body System	2	Heart and Great Vessels
Operation	7	Dilation: Expanding an orifice or the lumen of a tubular body part

Body Part (4th)	Approach (5th)	Device (6th)	Qualifier (7th)
0 Coronary Artery, One Artery 1 Coronary Artery, Two Arteries 2 Coronary Artery, Three Arteries 3 Coronary Artery, Four or More Arteries	0 Open 3 Percutaneous 4 Percutaneous Endoscopic	4 Intraluminal Device, Drug-eluting 5 Intraluminal Device, Drug-eluting, Two 6 Intraluminal Device, Drug-eluting, Three 7 Intraluminal Device, Drug-eluting, Four or More D Intraluminal Device E Intraluminal Devices, Two F Intraluminal Devices, Three G Intraluminal Devices, Four or More T Intraluminal Device, Radioactive Z No Device	6 Bifurcation Z No Qualifier
F Aortic Valve G Mitral Valve H Pulmonary Valve J Tricuspid Valve K Ventricle, Right L Ventricle, Left P Pulmonary Trunk Q Pulmonary Artery, Right S Pulmonary Vein, Right T Pulmonary Vein, Left V Superior Vena Cava W Thoracic Aorta, Descending X Thoracic Aorta, Ascending/Arch	0 Open 3 Percutaneous 4 Percutaneous Endoscopic	4 Intraluminal Device, Drug-eluting D Intraluminal Device Z No Device	Z No Qualifier
R Pulmonary Artery, Left	0 Open 3 Percutaneous 4 Percutaneous Endoscopic	4 Intraluminal Device, Drug-eluting D Intraluminal Device Z No Device	T Ductus Arteriosus Z No Qualifier

Section	0	Medical and Surgical
Body System	2	Heart and Great Vessels
Operation	8	Division: Cutting into a body part, without draining fluids and/or gases from the body part, in order to separate or transect a body part

Body Part (4th)	Approach (5th)	Device (6th)	Qualifier (7th)
8 Conduction Mechanism 9 Chordae Tendineae D Papillary Muscle	0 Open 3 Percutaneous 4 Percutaneous Endoscopic	Z No Device	Z No Qualifier

Section	0	Medical and Surgical
Body System	2	Heart and Great Vessels
Operation	B	Excision: Cutting out or off, without replacement, a portion of a body part

Body Part (4th)	Approach (5th)	Device (6th)	Qualifier (7th)
4 Coronary Vein 5 Atrial Septum 6 Atrium, Right 8 Conduction Mechanism 9 Chordae Tendineae D Papillary Muscle F Aortic Valve G Mitral Valve H Pulmonary Valve J Tricuspid Valve K Ventricle, Right L Ventricle, Left M Ventricular Septum N Pericardium P Pulmonary Trunk Q Pulmonary Artery, Right R Pulmonary Artery, Left S Pulmonary Vein, Right T Pulmonary Vein, Left V Superior Vena Cava W Thoracic Aorta, Descending X Thoracic Aorta, Ascending/Arch	0 Open 3 Percutaneous 4 Percutaneous Endoscopic	Z No Device	X Diagnostic Z No Qualifier
7 Atrium, Left	0 Open 3 Percutaneous 4 Percutaneous Endoscopic	Z No Device	K Left Atrial Appendage X Diagnostic Z No Qualifier

Section	0	Medical and Surgical
Body System	2	Heart and Great Vessels
Operation	C	Extirpation: Taking or cutting out solid matter from a body part

Body Part (4th)	Approach (5th)	Device (6th)	Qualifier (7th)
0 Coronary Artery, One Artery 1 Coronary Artery, Two Arteries 2 Coronary Artery, Three Arteries 3 Coronary Artery, Four or More Arteries	0 Open 4 Percutaneous Endoscopic	Z No Device	6 Bifurcation Z No Qualifier
0 Coronary Artery, One Artery 1 Coronary Artery, Two Arteries 2 Coronary Artery, Three Arteries 3 Coronary Artery, Four or More Arteries	3 Percutaneous	Z No Device	6 Bifurcation 7 Orbital Atherectomy Technique Z No Qualifier

Continued →

Section	0	Medical and Surgical
Body System	2	Heart and Great Vessels
Operation	C	**Extirpation:** Taking or cutting out solid matter from a body part

Body Part (4th)	Approach (5th)	Device (6th)	Qualifier (7th)
4 Coronary Vein 5 Atrial Septum 6 Atrium, Right 7 Atrium, Left 8 Conduction Mechanism 9 Chordae Tendineae D Papillary Muscle F Aortic Valve G Mitral Valve H Pulmonary Valve J Tricuspid Valve K Ventricle, Right L Ventricle, Left M Ventricular Septum N Pericardium P Pulmonary Trunk Q Pulmonary Artery, Right R Pulmonary Artery, Left S Pulmonary Vein, Right T Pulmonary Vein, Left V Superior Vena Cava W Thoracic Aorta, Descending X Thoracic Aorta, Ascending/Arch	0 Open 3 Percutaneous 4 Percutaneous Endoscopic	Z No Device	Z No Qualifier

Section	0	Medical and Surgical
Body System	2	Heart and Great Vessels
Operation	F	**Fragmentation:** Breaking solid matter in a body part into pieces

Body Part (4th)	Approach (5th)	Device (6th)	Qualifier (7th)
0 Coronary Artery, One Artery 1 Coronary Artery, Two Arteries 2 Coronary Artery, Three Arteries 3 Coronary Artery, Four or More Arteries	3 Percutaneous	Z No Device	Z No Qualifier
N Pericardium	0 Open 3 Percutaneous 4 Percutaneous Endoscopic X External	Z No Device	Z No Qualifier
P Pulmonary Trunk Q Pulmonary Artery, Right R Pulmonary Artery, Left S Pulmonary Vein, Right T Pulmonary Vein, Left	3 Percutaneous	Z No Device	0 Ultrasonic Z No Qualifier

Section	0	Medical and Surgical
Body System	2	Heart and Great Vessels
Operation	H	**Insertion:** Putting in a nonbiological appliance that monitors, assists, performs, or prevents a physiological function but does not physically take the place of a body part

Body Part (4th)	Approach (5th)	Device (6th)	Qualifier (7th)
0 Coronary Artery, One Artery 1 Coronary Artery, Two Arteries 2 Coronary Artery, Three Arteries 3 Coronary Artery, Four or More Arteries	0 Open 3 Percutaneous 4 Percutaneous Endoscopic	D Intraluminal Device Y Other Device	Z No Qualifier

Continued →

Section	0	Medical and Surgical
Body System	2	Heart and Great Vessels
Operation	H	Insertion: Putting in a nonbiological appliance that monitors, assists, performs, or prevents a physiological function but does not physically take the place of a body part

02H Continued

Body Part (4th)	Approach (5th)	Device (6th)	Qualifier (7th)
4 Coronary Vein 6 Atrium, Right 7 Atrium, Left K Ventricle, Right L Ventricle, Left	0 Open 3 Percutaneous 4 Percutaneous Endoscopic	0 Monitoring Device, Pressure Sensor 2 Monitoring Device 3 Infusion Device D Intraluminal Device J Cardiac Lead, Pacemaker K Cardiac Lead, Defibrillator M Cardiac Lead N Intracardiac Pacemaker Y Other Device	Z No Qualifier
A Heart	0 Open 3 Percutaneous 4 Percutaneous Endoscopic	Q Implantable Heart Assist System Y Other Device	Z No Qualifier
A Heart	0 Open 3 Percutaneous 4 Percutaneous Endoscopic	R Short-term External Heart Assist System	J Intraoperative S Biventricular Z No Qualifier
N Pericardium	0 Open 3 Percutaneous 4 Percutaneous Endoscopic	0 Monitoring Device, Pressure Sensor 2 Monitoring Device J Cardiac Lead, Pacemaker K Cardiac Lead, Defibrillator M Cardiac Lead Y Other Device	Z No Qualifier
P Pulmonary Trunk Q Pulmonary Artery, Right R Pulmonary Artery, Left S Pulmonary Vein, Right T Pulmonary Vein, Left V Superior Vena Cava	0 Open 3 Percutaneous 4 Percutaneous Endoscopic	0 Monitoring Device, Pressure Sensor 2 Monitoring Device 3 Infusion Device D Intraluminal Device Y Other Device	Z No Qualifier
W Thoracic Aorta, Descending	0 Open 4 Percutaneous Endoscopic	0 Monitoring Device, Pressure Sensor 2 Monitoring Device 3 Infusion Device D Intraluminal Device Y Other Device	Z No Qualifier
W Thoracic Aorta, Descending	3 Percutaneous	0 Monitoring Device, Pressure Sensor 2 Monitoring Device 3 Infusion Device D Intraluminal Device R Short-term External Heart Assist System Y Other Device	Z No Qualifier
X Thoracic Aorta, Ascending/Arch	0 Open 3 Percutaneous 4 Percutaneous Endoscopic	0 Monitoring Device, Pressure Sensor 2 Monitoring Device 3 Infusion Device D Intraluminal Device	Z No Qualifier

Section	0	Medical and Surgical
Body System	2	Heart and Great Vessels
Operation	J	Inspection: Visually and/or manually exploring a body part

Body Part (4th)	Approach (5th)	Device (6th)	Qualifier (7th)
A Heart Y Great Vessel	0 Open 3 Percutaneous 4 Percutaneous Endoscopic	Z No Device	Z No Qualifier

02K–02N

Medical and Surgical, Heart and Great Vessels Tables

Section	0	Medical and Surgical
Body System	2	Heart and Great Vessels
Operation	K	Map: Locating the route of passage of electrical impulses and/or locating functional areas in a body part

Body Part (4th)	Approach (5th)	Device (6th)	Qualifier (7th)
8 Conduction Mechanism	0 Open 3 Percutaneous 4 Percutaneous Endoscopic	Z No Device	Z No Qualifier

Section	0	Medical and Surgical
Body System	2	Heart and Great Vessels
Operation	L	Occlusion: Completely closing an orifice or the lumen of a tubular body part

Body Part (4th)	Approach (5th)	Device (6th)	Qualifier (7th)
7 Atrium, Left	0 Open 3 Percutaneous 4 Percutaneous Endoscopic	C Extraluminal Device D Intraluminal Device Z No Device	K Left Atrial Appendage
H Pulmonary Valve P Pulmonary Trunk Q Pulmonary Artery, Right S Pulmonary Vein, Right T Pulmonary Vein, Left V Superior Vena Cava	0 Open 3 Percutaneous 4 Percutaneous Endoscopic	C Extraluminal Device D Intraluminal Device Z No Device	Z No Qualifier
R Pulmonary Artery, Left	0 Open 3 Percutaneous 4 Percutaneous Endoscopic	C Extraluminal Device D Intraluminal Device Z No Device	T Ductus Arteriosus Z No Qualifier
W Thoracic Aorta, Descending	0 Open 3 Percutaneous	D Intraluminal Device	J Temporary

Section	0	Medical and Surgical
Body System	2	Heart and Great Vessels
Operation	N	Release: Freeing a body part from an abnormal physical constraint by cutting or by the use of force

Body Part (4th)	Approach (5th)	Device (6th)	Qualifier (7th)
0 Coronary Artery, One Artery 1 Coronary Artery, Two Arteries 2 Coronary Artery, Three Arteries 3 Coronary Artery, Four or More Arteries 4 Coronary Vein 5 Atrial Septum 6 Atrium, Right 7 Atrium, Left 8 Conduction Mechanism 9 Chordae Tendineae D Papillary Muscle F Aortic Valve G Mitral Valve H Pulmonary Valve J Tricuspid Valve K Ventricle, Right L Ventricle, Left M Ventricular Septum N Pericardium P Pulmonary Trunk Q Pulmonary Artery, Right R Pulmonary Artery, Left S Pulmonary Vein, Right T Pulmonary Vein, Left V Superior Vena Cava W Thoracic Aorta, Descending X Thoracic Aorta, Ascending/ Arch	0 Open 3 Percutaneous 4 Percutaneous Endoscopic	Z No Device	Z No Qualifier

136

Section	0	Medical and Surgical
Body System	2	Heart and Great Vessels
Operation	P	Removal: Taking out or off a device from a body part

02P–02Q

Body Part (4th)	Approach (5th)	Device (6th)	Qualifier (7th)
A Heart	0 Open 3 Percutaneous 4 Percutaneous Endoscopic	2 Monitoring Device 3 Infusion Device 7 Autologous Tissue Substitute 8 Zooplastic Tissue C Extraluminal Device D Intraluminal Device J Synthetic Substitute K Nonautologous Tissue Substitute M Cardiac Lead N Intracardiac Pacemaker Q Implantable Heart Assist System Y Other Device	Z No Qualifier
A Heart	0 Open 3 Percutaneous 4 Percutaneous Endoscopic	R Short-term External Heart Assist System	S Biventricular Z No Qualifier
A Heart	X External	2 Monitoring Device 3 Infusion Device D Intraluminal Device M Cardiac Lead	Z No Qualifier
W Thoracic Aorta, Descending	3 Percutaneous	R Short-term External Heart Assist System	Z No Qualifier
Y Great Vessel	0 Open 3 Percutaneous 4 Percutaneous Endoscopic	2 Monitoring Device 3 Infusion Device 7 Autologous Tissue Substitute 8 Zooplastic Tissue C Extraluminal Device D Intraluminal Device J Synthetic Substitute K Nonautologous Tissue Substitute Y Other Device	Z No Qualifier
Y Great Vessel	X External	2 Monitoring Device 3 Infusion Device D Intraluminal Device	Z No Qualifier

Section	0	Medical and Surgical
Body System	2	Heart and Great Vessels
Operation	Q	Repair: Restoring, to the extent possible, a body part to its normal anatomic structure and function

Body Part (4th)	Approach (5th)	Device (6th)	Qualifier (7th)
0 Coronary Artery, One Artery 1 Coronary Artery, Two Arteries 2 Coronary Artery, Three Arteries 3 Coronary Artery, Four or More Arteries 4 Coronary Vein 5 Atrial Septum 6 Atrium, Right 7 Atrium, Left 8 Conduction Mechanism 9 Chordae Tendineae A Heart B Heart, Right C Heart, Left D Papillary Muscle H Pulmonary Valve K Ventricle, Right L Ventricle, Left M Ventricular Septum N Pericardium P Pulmonary Trunk Q Pulmonary Artery, Right R Pulmonary Artery, Left S Pulmonary Vein, Right	0 Open 3 Percutaneous 4 Percutaneous Endoscopic	Z No Device	Z No Qualifier

Medical and Surgical, Heart and Great Vessels Tables

Continued →

137

Section	0	Medical and Surgical
Body System	2	Heart and Great Vessels
Operation	Q	Repair: Restoring, to the extent possible, a body part to its normal anatomic structure and function

02Q Continued

Body Part (4th)	Approach (5th)	Device (6th)	Qualifier (7th)
T Pulmonary Vein, Left V Superior Vena Cava W Thoracic Aorta, Descending X Thoracic Aorta, Ascending/Arch			
F Aortic Valve	0 Open 3 Percutaneous 4 Percutaneous Endoscopic	Z No Device	J Truncal Valve Z No Qualifier
G Mitral Valve	0 Open 3 Percutaneous 4 Percutaneous Endoscopic	Z No Device	E Atrioventricular Valve, Left Z No Qualifier
J Tricuspid Valve	0 Open 3 Percutaneous 4 Percutaneous Endoscopic	Z No Device	G Atrioventricular Valve, Right Z No Qualifier

Section	0	Medical and Surgical
Body System	2	Heart and Great Vessels
Operation	R	Replacement: Putting in or on biological or synthetic material that physically takes the place and/or function of all or a portion of a body part

Body Part (4th)	Approach (5th)	Device (6th)	Qualifier (7th)
5 Atrial Septum 6 Atrium, Right 7 Atrium, Left 9 Chordae Tendineae D Papillary Muscle K Ventricle, Right L Ventricle, Left M Ventricular Septum N Pericardium P Pulmonary Trunk Q Pulmonary Artery, Right R Pulmonary Artery, Left S Pulmonary Vein, Right T Pulmonary Vein, Left V Superior Vena Cava W Thoracic Aorta, Descending X Thoracic Aorta, Ascending/Arch	0 Open 4 Percutaneous Endoscopic	7 Autologous Tissue Substitute 8 Zooplastic Tissue J Synthetic Substitute K Nonautologous Tissue Substitute	Z No Qualifier
A Heart	0 Open	L Biologic with Synthetic Substitute, Autoregulated Electrohydraulic M Synthetic Substitute, Pneumatic	Z No Qualifier
F Aortic Valve	0 Open 4 Percutaneous Endoscopic	7 Autologous Tissue Substitute J Synthetic Substitute K Nonautologous Tissue Substitute	Z No Qualifier
F Aortic Valve	0 Open 4 Percutaneous Endoscopic	8 Zooplastic Tissue	N Rapid Deployment Technique Z No Qualifier
F Aortic Valve	3 Percutaneous	7 Autologous Tissue Substitute J Synthetic Substitute K Nonautologous Tissue Substitute	H Transapical Z No Qualifier
F Aortic Valve	3 Percutaneous	8 Zooplastic Tissue	H Transapical N Rapid Deployment Technique Z No Qualifier

Continued →

Section	0	Medical and Surgical
Body System	2	Heart and Great Vessels
Operation	R	Replacement: Putting in or on biological or synthetic material that physically takes the place and/or function of all or a portion of a body part

02R Continued

Body Part (4th)	Approach (5th)	Device (6th)	Qualifier (7th)
G Mitral Valve J Tricuspid Valve	0 Open 4 Percutaneous Endoscopic	7 Autologous Tissue Substitute 8 Zooplastic Tissue J Synthetic Substitute K Nonautologous Tissue Substitute	Z No Qualifier
G Mitral Valve J Tricuspid Valve	3 Percutaneous	7 Autologous Tissue Substitute 8 Zooplastic Tissue J Synthetic Substitute K Nonautologous Tissue Substitute	H Transapical Z No Qualifier
H Pulmonary Valve	0 Open 4 Percutaneous Endoscopic	7 Autologous Tissue Substitute 8 Zooplastic Tissue J Synthetic Substitute K Nonautologous Tissue Substitute	Z No Qualifier
H Pulmonary Valve	3 Percutaneous	7 Autologous Tissue Substitute J Synthetic Substitute K Nonautologous Tissue Substitute	H Transapical Z No Qualifier
H Pulmonary Valve	3 Percutaneous	8 Zooplastic Tissue	H Transapical L In Exisiting Conduit M Native Site Z No Qualifier

Section	0	Medical and Surgical
Body System	2	Heart and Great Vessels
Operation	S	Reposition: Moving to its normal location, or other suitable location, all or a portion of a body part

Body Part (4th)	Approach (5th)	Device (6th)	Qualifier (7th)
0 Coronary Artery, One Artery 1 Coronary Artery, Two Arteries P Pulmonary Trunk Q Pulmonary Artery, Right R Pulmonary Artery, Left S Pulmonary Vein, Right T Pulmonary Vein, Left V Superior Vena Cava W Thoracic Aorta, Descending X Thoracic Aorta, Ascending/Arch	0 Open	Z No Device	Z No Qualifier

Section	0	Medical and Surgical
Body System	2	Heart and Great Vessels
Operation	T	Resection: Cutting out or off, without replacement, all of a body part

Body Part (4th)	Approach (5th)	Device (6th)	Qualifier (7th)
5 Atrial Septum 8 Conduction Mechanism 9 Chordae Tendineae D Papillary Muscle H Pulmonary Valve M Ventricular Septum N Pericardium	0 Open 3 Percutaneous 4 Percutaneous Endoscopic	Z No Device	Z No Qualifier

Section	0	Medical and Surgical
Body System	2	Heart and Great Vessels
Operation	U	Supplement: Putting in or on biological or synthetic material that physically reinforces and/or augments the function of a portion of a body part

Body Part (4th)	Approach (5th)	Device (6th)	Qualifier (7th)
0 Coronary Artery, One Artery 1 Coronary Artery, Two Arteries 2 Coronary Artery, Three Arteries 3 Coronary Artery, Four or More Arteries 5 Atrial Septum 6 Atrium, Right 7 Atrium, Left 9 Chordae Tendineae A Heart D Papillary Muscle H Pulmonary Valve K Ventricle, Right L Ventricle, Left M Ventricular Septum N Pericardium P Pulmonary Trunk Q Pulmonary Artery, Right R Pulmonary Artery, Left S Pulmonary Vein, Right T Pulmonary Vein, Left V Superior Vena Cava W Thoracic Aorta, Descending X Thoracic Aorta, Ascending/Arch	0 Open 3 Percutaneous 4 Percutaneous Endoscopic	7 Autologous Tissue Substitute 8 Zooplastic Tissue J Synthetic Substitute K Nonautologous Tissue Substitute	Z No Qualifier
F Aortic Valve	0 Open 3 Percutaneous 4 Percutaneous Endoscopic	7 Autologous Tissue Substitute 8 Zooplastic Tissue J Synthetic Substitute K Nonautologous Tissue Substitute	J Truncal Valve Z No Qualifier
G Mitral Valve	0 Open 4 Percutaneous Endoscopic	7 Autologous Tissue Substitute 8 Zooplastic Tissue J Synthetic Substitute K Nonautologous Tissue Substitute	E Atrioventricular Valve, Left Z No Qualifier
G Mitral Valve	3 Percutaneous	7 Autologous Tissue Substitute 8 Zooplastic Tissue K Nonautologous Tissue Substitute	E Atrioventricular Valve, Left Z No Qualifier
G Mitral Valve	3 Percutaneous	J Synthetic Substitute	E Atrioventricular Valve, Left H Transapical Z No Qualifier
J Tricuspid Valve	0 Open 3 Percutaneous 4 Percutaneous Endoscopic	7 Autologous Tissue Substitute 8 Zooplastic Tissue J Synthetic Substitute K Nonautologous Tissue Substitute	G Atrioventricular Valve, Right Z No Qualifier

Section	**0**	**Medical and Surgical**	
Body System	**2**	**Heart and Great Vessels**	
Operation	**V**	**Restriction:** Partially closing an orifice or the lumen of a tubular body part	

Body Part (4th)	Approach (5th)	Device (6th)	Qualifier (7th)
A Heart	0 Open 3 Percutaneous 4 Percutaneous Endoscopic	C Extraluminal Device Z No Device	Z No Qualifier
G Mitral Valve	0 Open 3 Percutaneous 4 Percutaneous Endoscopic	Z No Device	Z No Qualifier
L Ventricle, Left P Pulmonary Trunk Q Pulmonary Artery, Right S Pulmonary Vein, Right T Pulmonary Vein, Left V Superior Vena Cava	0 Open 3 Percutaneous 4 Percutaneous Endoscopic	C Extraluminal Device D Intraluminal Device Z No Device	Z No Qualifier
R Pulmonary Artery, Left	0 Open 3 Percutaneous 4 Percutaneous Endoscopic	C Extraluminal Device D Intraluminal Device Z No Device	T Ductus Arteriosus Z No Qualifier
W Thoracic Aorta, Descending X Thoracic Aorta, Ascending/ Arch	0 Open 3 Percutaneous 4 Percutaneous Endoscopic	C Extraluminal Device D Intraluminal Device E Intraluminal Device, Branched or Fenestrated, One or Two Arteries F Intraluminal Device, Branched or Fenestrated, Three or More Arteries Z No Device	Z No Qualifier

Section	**0**	**Medical and Surgical**	
Body System	**2**	**Heart and Great Vessels**	
Operation	**W**	**Revision:** Correcting, to the extent possible, a portion of a malfunctioning device or the position of a displaced device	

Body Part (4th)	Approach (5th)	Device (6th)	Qualifier (7th)
5 Atrial Septum M Ventricular Septum	0 Open 4 Percutaneous Endoscopic	J Synthetic Substitute	Z No Qualifier
A Heart	0 Open 3 Percutaneous 4 Percutaneous Endoscopic	2 Monitoring Device 3 Infusion Device 7 Autologous Tissue Substitute 8 Zooplastic Tissue C Extraluminal Device D Intraluminal Device J Synthetic Substitute K Nonautologous Tissue Substitute M Cardiac Lead N Intracardiac Pacemaker Q Implantable Heart Assist System Y Other Device	Z No Qualifier
A Heart	0 Open 3 Percutaneous 4 Percutaneous Endoscopic	R Short-term External Heart Assist System	S Biventricular Z No Qualifier

Continued →

Section	0	Medical and Surgical
Body System	2	Heart and Great Vessels
Operation	W	Revision: Correcting, to the extent possible, a portion of a malfunctioning device or the position of a displaced device

02W Continued

Body Part (4th)	Approach (5th)	Device (6th)	Qualifier (7th)
A Heart	X External	2 Monitoring Device 3 Infusion Device 7 Autologous Tissue Substitute 8 Zooplastic Tissue C Extraluminal Device D Intraluminal Device J Synthetic Substitute K Nonautologous Tissue Substitute M Cardiac Lead N Intracardiac Pacemaker Q Implantable Heart Assist System	Z No Qualifier
A Heart	X External	R Short-term External Heart Assist System	S Biventricular Z No Qualifier
F Aortic Valve G Mitral Valve H Pulmonary Valve J Tricuspid Valve	0 Open 3 Percutaneous 4 Percutaneous Endoscopic	7 Autologous Tissue Substitute 8 Zooplastic Tissue J Synthetic Substitute K Nonautologous Tissue Substitute	Z No Qualifier
W Thoracic Aorta, Descending	3 Percutaneous	R Short-term External Heart Assist System	Z No Qualifier
Y Great Vessel	0 Open 3 Percutaneous 4 Percutaneous Endoscopic	2 Monitoring Device 3 Infusion Device 7 Autologous Tissue Substitute 8 Zooplastic Tissue C Extraluminal Device D Intraluminal Device J Synthetic Substitute K Nonautologous Tissue Substitute Y Other Device	Z No Qualifier
Y Great Vessel	X External	2 Monitoring Device 3 Infusion Device 7 Autologous Tissue Substitute 8 Zooplastic Tissue C Extraluminal Device D Intraluminal Device J Synthetic Substitute K Nonautologous Tissue Substitute	Z No Qualifier

Section	0	Medical and Surgical
Body System	2	Heart and Great Vessels
Operation	Y	Transplantation: Putting in or on all or a portion of a living body part taken from another individual or animal to physically take the place and/or function of all or a portion of a similar body part

Body Part (4th)	Approach (5th)	Device (6th)	Qualifier (7th)
A Heart	0 Open	Z No Device	0 Allogeneic 1 Syngeneic 2 Zooplastic

AHA Coding Clinic

0210098 Bypass Coronary Artery, One Artery from Right Internal Mammary with Autologous Venous Tissue, Open Approach—AHA CC: 3Q, 2018, 8-9

021009W Bypass Coronary Artery, One Artery from Aorta with Autologous Venous Tissue, Open Approach—AHA CC: 1Q, 2014, 10-11

02100A3 Bypass Coronary Artery, One Artery from Coronary Artery with Autologous Arterial Tissue, Open Approach—AHA CC: 3Q, 2021, 22-23

02100AW Bypass Coronary Artery, One Artery from Aorta with Autologous Arterial Tissue, Open Approach—AHA CC: 4Q, 2016, 83-84

02100Z9 Bypass Coronary Artery, One Artery from Left Internal Mammary, Open Approach—AHA CC: 3Q, 2014, 8, 20-21; 1Q, 2016, 27-28; 4Q, 2016, 83-84

021109W Bypass Coronary Artery, Two Arteries from Aorta with Autologous VenousTissue, Open Approach—AHA CC: 3Q, 2014, 20-21; 4Q, 2016, 83-84

021209W Bypass Coronary Artery, Three Arteries from Aorta with Autologous Venous Tissue, Open Approach—AHA CC: 1Q, 2016, 27-28

02160JQ Bypass Right Atrium to Right Pulmonary Artery with Synthetic Substitute, Open Approach—AHA CC: 3Q, 2014, 29

02163Z7 Bypass Right Atrium to Left Atrium, Percutaneous Approach—AHA CC: 4Q, 2017, 56

02170ZU Bypass Left Atrium to Pulmonary Vein Confluence, Open Approach—AHA CC: 4Q, 2016, 108-109

02173J6 Bypass Left Atrium to Right Atrium with Synthetic Substitute, Percutaneous Approach—AHA CC: 4Q, 2020, 44-45

021K0JP Bypass Right Ventricle to Pulmonary Trunk with Synthetic Substitute, Open Approach—AHA CC: 1Q, 2017, 19-20; 1Q, 2020, 24-25

021K0JQ Bypass Right Ventricle to Right Pulmonary Artery with Synthetic Substitute, Open Approach—AHA CC: 3Q, 2014, 30

021K0KP Bypass Right Ventricle to Pulmonary Trunk with Nonautologous Tissue Substitute, Open Approach—AHA CC: 3Q, 2015, 16-17; 4Q, 2015. 22-23, 25

021V08S Bypass Superior Vena Cava to Right Pulmonary Vein with Zooplastic Tissue, Open Approach—AHA CC: 4Q, 2016, 145

021V09S Bypass Superior Vena Cava to Right Pulmonary Vein with Autologous Venous Tissue, Open Approach—AHA CC: 4Q, 2016, 144

021W0JQ Bypass Thoracic Aorta, Descending to Right Pulmonary Artery with Synthetic Substitute, Open Approach—AHA CC: 3Q, 2014, 3

021W0JV Bypass Thoracic Aorta, Descending to Lower Extremity Artery with Synthetic Substitute, Open Approach—AHA CC: 4Q, 2018, 46

021X0JA Bypass Thoracic Aorta, Ascending/Arch to Innominate Artery with Synthetic Substitute, Open Approach—AHA CC: 3Q, 2019, 30-31; 4Q, 2019, 23; 1Q, 2020, 37

021X0JD Bypass Thoracic Aorta, Ascending/Arch to Carotid with Synthetic Substitute, Open Approach—AHA CC: 3Q, 2019, 30-31

02570ZK Destruction of Left Atrial Appendage, Open Approach—AHA CC: 3Q, 2014, 20-21

02580ZZ Destruction of Conduction Mechanism, Open Approach—AHA CC: 3Q, 2016, 44

02583ZZ Destruction of Conduction Mechanism, Percutaneous Approach—AHA CC: 3Q, 2014, 19; 4Q, 2014, 47-48; 3Q, 2016, 43-44; 1Q, 2020, 32-33

02584ZZ Destruction of Conduction Mechanism, Percutaneous Endoscopic Approach—AHA CC: 1Q, 2020, 32-33

025M3ZZ Destruction of Ventricular Septum, Percutaneous Approach—AHA CC: 3Q, 2018, 27

025N0ZZ Destruction of Pericardium, Open Approach—AHA CC: 2Q, 2016, 17-18

0270346 Dilation of Coronary Artery, One Artery, Bifurcation, with Drug-eluting Intraluminal Device, Percutaneous Approach—AHA CC: 2Q, 2015, 4-5; 4Q, 2016, 88

027034Z Dilation of Coronary Artery, One Artery with Drug-eluting Intraluminal Device, Percutaneous Approach—AHA CC: 2Q, 2014, 4; 2Q, 2015, 3-4; 4Q, 2015, 13-14; 4Q, 2019, 39-40

027037Z Dilation of Coronary Artery, One Artery with Four or More Drug-eluting Intraluminal Devices, Percutaneous Approach—AHA CC: 4Q, 2016, 85-86

02703DZ Dilation of Coronary Artery, One Artery with Intraluminal Device, Percutaneous Approach—AHA CC: 2Q, 2015, 4

02703EZ Dilation of Coronary Artery, One Artery with Two Intraluminal Devices, Percutaneous Approach—AHA CC: 4Q, 2016, 84-85

02703ZZ Dilation of Coronary Artery, One Artery, Percutaneous Approach—AHA CC: 3Q, 2015, 10; 4Q, 2016, 88, 3Q, 2018, 7-8

027134Z Dilation of Coronary Artery, Two Arteries with Drug-eluting Intraluminal Device, Percutaneous Approach—AHA CC: 2Q, 2015, 5

0271356 Dilation of Coronary Artery, Two Arteries, Bifurcation, with Two Drug-eluting Intraluminal Devices, Percutaneous Approach—AHA CC: 4Q, 2016, 87

027136Z Dilation of Coronary Artery, Two Arteries with Three Drug-eluting Intraluminal Devices, Percutaneous Approach—AHA CC: 4Q, 2016, 84-85

027234Z Dilation of Coronary Artery, Three Arteries with Drug-eluting Intraluminal Device, Percutaneous Approach—AHA CC: 2Q, 2015, 3

027H0ZZ Dilation of Pulmonary Valve, Open Approach—AHA CC: 1Q, 2016, 16-17

027L0ZZ Dilation of Left Ventricle, Open Approach—AHA CC: 4Q, 2017, 33

027Q0DZ Dilation of Right Pulmonary Artery with Intraluminal Device, Open Approach—AHA CC: 3Q, 2015, 16-17

027V3ZZ Dilation of Superior Vena Cava, Percutaneous Approach—AHA CC: 3Q, 2018, 10

02BG0ZZ Excision of Mitral Valve, Open Approach—AHA CC: 2Q, 2015, 23-24

02BK3ZX Excision of Right Ventricle, Percutaneous Approach, Diagnostic—AHA CC: 3Q, 2019, 32

Medical and Surgical, Heart and Great Vessels AHA Coding Clinic

02BN0ZZ Excision of Pericardium, Open Approach—AHA CC: 2Q, 2019, 20-21

02CG0ZZ Extirpation of Matter from Mitral Valve, Open Approach—AHA CC: 2Q, 2016, 24-25

02H13DZ Insertion of Intraluminal Device into Coronary Artery, Two Arteries, Percutaneous Approach—AHA CC: 4Q, 2019, 24

02H633Z Insertion of Infusion Device into Right Atrium, Percutaneous Approach—AHA CC: 2Q, 2016, 15-16; 2Q, 2017, 24-26

02H63KZ Insertion of Cardiac Lead into Right Atrium, Percutaneous Approach—AHA CC: 2Q, 2018, 19

02H73DZ Insertion of Intraluminal Device into Left Atrium, Percutaneous Approach—AHA CC: 4Q, 2017, 104-105

02HA0QZ Insertion of Implantable Heart Assist System into Heart, Open Approach—AHA CC: 1Q, 2019, 24

02HA3RJ Insertion of Short-term External Heart Assist System into Heart, Intraoperative, Percutaneous Approach—AHA CC: 4Q, 2017, 43-44

02HA3RS Insertion of Biventricular Short-term External Heart Assist System into Heart, Percutaneous Approach—AHA CC: 4Q, 2016, 138-139

02HA3RZ Insertion of Short-term External Heart Assist System into Heart, Percutaneous Approach—AHA CC: 1Q, 2017, 11-12; 4Q, 2017, 44-45

02HK3DZ Insertion of Intraluminal Device into Right Ventricle, Percutaneous Approach—AHA CC: 2Q, 2015, 31-32

02HK3JZ Insertion of Pacemaker Lead into Right Ventricle, Percutaneous Approach—AHA CC: 2Q, 2022, 25

02HL0DZ Insertion of Intraluminal Device into Left Ventricle, Open Approach—AHA CC: 3Q, 2019, 19-20

02HL3JZ Insertion of Pacemaker Lead into Left Ventricle, Percutaneous Approach—AHA CC: 3Q, 2019, 23

02HP32Z Insertion of Monitoring Device into Pulmonary Trunk, Percutaneous Approach—AHA CC: 3Q, 2015, 35

02HV33Z Insertion of Infusion Device into Superior Vena Cava, Percutaneous Approach—AHA CC: 3Q, 2013, 18; 2Q, 2015, 33-34; 4Q, 2015, 14-15, 28-32; 4Q, 2017, 63-64

02JA3ZZ Inspection of Heart, Percutaneous Approach—AHA CC: 3Q, 2015, 9

02L70CK Occlusion of Left Atrial Appendage with Extraluminal Device, Open Approach—AHA CC: 3Q, 2014, 20-21

02L73DK Occlusion of Left Atrial Appendage with Intraluminal Device, Percutaneous Approach—AHA CC: 4Q, 2018, 94

02LQ3DZ Occlusion of Right Pulmonary Artery with Intraluminal Device, Percutaneous Approach—AHA CC: 4Q, 2017, 34

02LR0ZT Occlusion of Ductus Arteriosus, Open Approach—AHA CC: 4Q, 2015, 23-24

02LS3DZ Occlusion of Right Pulmonary Vein with Intraluminal Device, Percutaneous Approach—AHA CC: 2Q, 2016, 26; 4Q, 2017, 34

02N00ZZ Release Coronary Artery, One Artery, Open Approach—AHA CC: 2Q, 2019, 13-14

02NK0ZZ Release Right Ventricle, Open Approach—AHA CC: 3Q, 2014, 16-17

02NN0ZZ Release Pericardium, Open Approach—AHA CC: 2Q, 2019, 20-21

02PA0QZ Removal of Implantable Heart Assist System from Heart, Open Approach—AHA CC: 1Q, 2019, 24

02PA0RZ Removal of Short-term External Heart Assist System from Heart, Open Approach—AHA CC: 1Q, 2017, 13-14

02PA3DZ Removal of Intraluminal Device from Heart, Percutaneous Approach—AHA CC: 4Q, 2017, 104-105

02PA3MZ Removal of Cardiac Lead from Heart, Percutaneous Approach—AHA CC: 3Q, 2015, 33; 2Q, 2022, 25

02PA3NZ Removal of Intracardiac Pacemaker from Heart, Percutaneous Approach—AHA CC: 4Q, 2016, 96-97

02PA3RZ Removal of Short-term External Heart Assist System from Heart, Percutaneous Approach—AHA CC: 4Q, 2016, 139; 1Q, 2017, 11-12; 4Q, 2017, 44-45; 4Q, 2018, 54

02PY33Z Removal of Infusion Device from Great Vessel, Percutaneous Approach—AHA CC: 4Q, 2015, 31-32; 2Q, 2016, 15-16; 2Q, 2017, 24-26

02PY3JZ Removal of Synthetic Substitute from Great Vessel, Percutaneous Approach—AHA CC: 4Q, 2018, 85

02PYX3Z Removal of Infusion Device from Great Vessel, External Approach—AHA CC: 3Q, 2016, 19

02Q50ZZ Repair Atrial Septum, Open Approach—AHA CC: 4Q, 2015, 23-24

02Q60ZZ Repair Right Atrium, Open Approach—AHA CC: 3Q, 2021, 26-27

02QA0ZZ Repair Heart, Open Approach—AHA CC: 1Q, 2022, 40-41

02QS0ZZ Repair Right Pulmonary Vein, Open Approach—AHA CC: 1Q, 2017, 18-19

02QT0ZZ Repair Left Pulmonary Vein, Open Approach—AHA CC: 1Q, 2017, 18-19

02QV0ZZ Repair Superior Vena Cava, Open Approach—AHA CC: 3Q, 2021, 26-27

02QW0ZZ Repair Thoracic Aorta, Descending, Open Approach—AHA CC: 3Q, 2015, 16

02RF38Z Replacement of Aortic Valve with Zooplastic Tissue, Percutaneous Approach—AHA CC: 1Q, 2019, 31-32

02RF3JZ Replacement of Aortic Valve with Synthetic Substitute, Percutaneous Approach—AHA CC: 4Q, 2019, 24

02RG08Z Replacement of Mitral Valve with Zooplastic Tissue, Open Approach—AHA CC: 3Q, 2019, 23-24

02RJ3JZ Replacement of Tricuspid Valve with Synthetic Substitute, Percutaneous Approach—AHA CC: 4Q, 2017, 56

02RJ48Z Replacement of Tricuspid Valve with Zooplastic Tissue, Percutaneous Endoscopic Approach—AHA CC: 3Q, 2016, 32

02RK0JZ Replacement of Right Ventricle with Synthetic Substitute, Open Approach—AHA CC: 1Q, 2017, 13-14

02RL0JZ Replacement of Left Ventricle with Synthetic Substitute, Open Approach—AHA CC: 1Q, 2017, 13-14

02RW0KZ Replacement of Thoracic Aorta, Descending with Nonautologous Tissue Substitute, Open Approach—AHA CC: 1Q, 2014, 10-11

02RX0JZ Replacement of Thoracic Aorta, Ascending/Arch with Synthetic Substitute, Open Approach—AHA CC: 3Q, 2019, 24; 1Q, 2020, 25-26

02S10ZZ Reposition Coronary Artery, Two Arteries, Open Approach—AHA CC: 4Q, 2016, 103-104

02SP0ZZ Reposition Pulmonary Trunk, Open Approach—AHA CC: 4Q, 2015, 23-24; 4Q, 2016, 103-104

02SW0ZZ Reposition Thoracic Aorta, Descending, Open Approach—AHA CC: 4Q, 2015, 23-24

02SX0ZZ Reposition Thoracic Aorta, Ascending/Arch, Open Approach—AHA CC: 4Q, 2016, 103-104

02U03JZ Supplement Coronary Artery, One Artery with Synthetic Substitute, Percutaneous Approach—AHA CC: 4Q, 2019, 25-26

02U607Z Supplement Right Atrium with Autologous Tissue Substitute, Open Approach—AHA CC: 3Q, 2017, 7-8

02U707Z Supplement Left Atrium with Autologous Tissue Substitute, Open Approach— AHA CC: 3Q, 2017, 7-8

02U73JZ Supplement Left Atrium with Synthetic Substitute, Percutaneous Approach—AHA CC: 1Q, 2022, 37-38

02UA08Z Supplement Heart with Zooplastic Tissue, Open Approach—AHA CC: 1Q, 2022, 39-40

02UF08Z Supplement Aortic Valve with Zooplastic Tissue, Open Approach—AHA CC: 4Q, 2015, 25

02UG08Z Supplement Mitral Valve with Zooplastic Tissue, Open Approach—AHA CC: 4Q, 2017, 36

02UG0JZ Supplement Mitral Valve with Synthetic Substitute, Open Approach—AHA CC: 2Q, 2015, 23-24

02UG3JH Supplement Mitral Valve with Synthetic Substitute, Transapical, Percutaneous Approach—AHA CC: 4Q, 2020, 52

02UG3JZ Supplement Mitral Valve with Synthetic Substitute, Percutaneous Approach—AHA CC: 3Q, 2021, 28; 2Q, 2023, 21

02UM08Z Supplement Ventricular Septum with Zooplastic Tissue, Open Approach—AHA CC: 4Q, 2015, 25

02UM0JZ Supplement Ventricular Septum with Synthetic Substitute, Open Approach—AHA CC: 3Q, 2014, 16-17; 4Q, 2015, 22-23

02UP07Z Supplement Pulmonary Trunk with Autologous Tissue Substitute, Open Approach—AHA CC: 2Q, 2016, 23-24

02UP08Z Supplement Pulmonary Trunk with Zooplastic Tissue, Open Approach—AHA CC: 1Q, 2020, 24-25

02UQ0KZ Supplement Right Pulmonary Artery with Nonautologous Tissue Substitute, Open Approach—AHA CC: 3Q, 2015, 16-17

02UR07Z Supplement Left Pulmonary Artery with Autologous Tissue Substitute, Open Approach—AHA CC: 2Q, 2016, 23-24

02UR0KZ Supplement Left Pulmonary Artery with Nonautologous Tissue Substitute, Open Approach—AHA CC: 3Q, 2015, 16-17

02UW07Z Supplement Thoracic Aorta, Descending with Autologous Tissue Substitute, Open Approach—AHA CC: 4Q, 2015, 23-24

02UW0JZ Supplement Thoracic Aorta, Descending with Synthetic Substitute, Open Approach—AHA CC: 2Q, 2016, 26-27

02UX0KZ Supplement Thoracic Aorta, Ascending/Arch with Nonautologous Tissue Substitute, Open Approach—AHA CC: 1Q, 2017, 19-20

02VG0ZZ Restriction of Mitral Valve, Open Approach—AHA CC: 4Q, 2017, 36

02VL3DZ Restriction of Left Ventricle with Intraluminal Device, Percutaneous Approach—AHA CC: 4Q, 2021, 44-45

02VW0DZ Restriction of Thoracic Aorta, Descending with Intraluminal Device, Open Approach—AHA CC: 1Q, 2020, 25-26

02VW3DZ Restriction of Thoracic Aorta, Descending with Intraluminal Device, Percutaneous Approach—AHA CC: 4Q, 2016, 92-93

02WA3JZ Revision of Synthetic Substitute in Heart, Percutaneous Approach—AHA CC: 3Q, 2014, 31-32

02WA3MZ Revision of Cardiac Lead in Heart, Percutaneous Approach—AHA CC: 3Q, 2015, 32

02WA3NZ Revision of Intracardiac Pacemaker in Heart, Percutaneous Approach—AHA CC: 4Q, 2016, 96

02WAXRZ Revision of Short-term External Heart Assist System in Heart, External Approach—AHA CC: 1Q, 2018, 17

02WY33Z Revision of Infusion Device in Great Vessel, Percutaneous Approach—AHA CC: 3Q, 2018, 9-10

02YA0Z0 Transplantation of Heart, Allogeneic, Open Approach—AHA CC: 3Q, 2013, 18-19

Upper Arteries

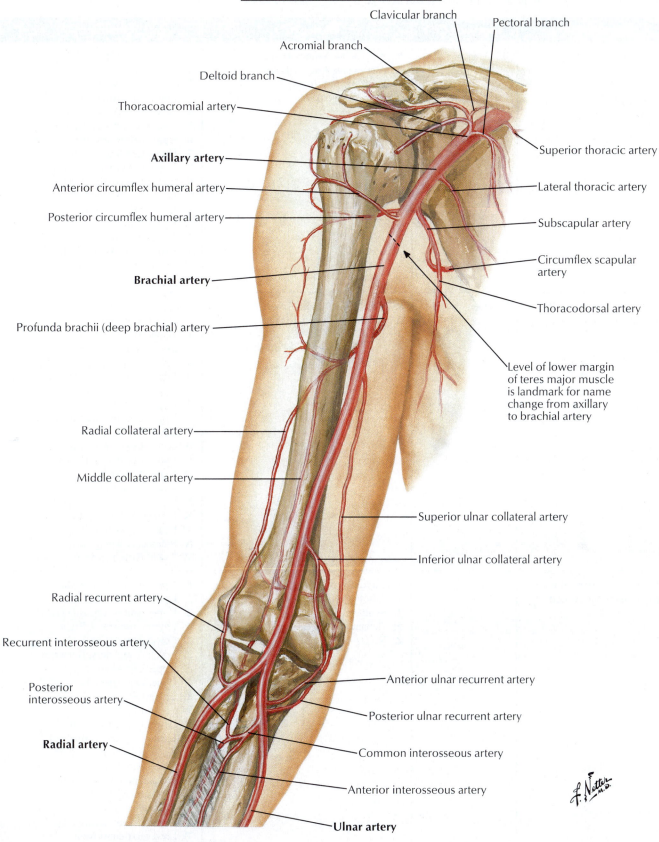

Upper Arteries Tables 031–03W

Section	0	Medical and Surgical
Body System	3	Upper Arteries
Operation	1	**Bypass:** Altering the route of passage of the contents of a tubular body part

Body Part (4th)	Approach (5th)	Device (6th)	Qualifier (7th)
2 Innominate Artery	0 Open	9 Autologous Venous Tissue A Autologous Arterial Tissue J Synthetic Substitute K Nonautologous Tissue Substitute Z No Device	0 Upper Arm Artery, Right 1 Upper Arm Artery, Left 2 Upper Arm Artery, Bilateral 3 Lower Arm Artery, Right 4 Lower Arm Artery, Left 5 Lower Arm Artery, Bilateral 6 Upper Leg Artery, Right 7 Upper Leg Artery, Left 8 Upper Leg Artery, Bilateral 9 Lower Leg Artery, Right B Lower Leg Artery, Left C Lower Leg Artery, Bilateral D Upper Arm Vein F Lower Arm Vein J Extracranial Artery, Right K Extracranial Artery, Left W Lower Extremity Vein
3 Subclavian Artery, Right 4 Subclavian Artery, Left	0 Open	9 Autologous Venous Tissue A Autologous Arterial Tissue J Synthetic Substitute K Nonautologous Tissue Substitute Z No Device	0 Upper Arm Artery, Right 1 Upper Arm Artery, Left 2 Upper Arm Artery, Bilateral 3 Lower Arm Artery, Right 4 Lower Arm Artery, Left 5 Lower Arm Artery, Bilateral 6 Upper Leg Artery, Right 7 Upper Leg Artery, Left 8 Upper Leg Artery, Bilateral 9 Lower Leg Artery, Right B Lower Leg Artery, Left C Lower Leg Artery, Bilateral D Upper Arm Vein F Lower Arm Vein J Extracranial Artery, Right K Extracranial Artery, Left M Pulmonary Artery, Right N Pulmonary Artery, Left W Lower Extremity Vein
5 Axillary Artery, Right 6 Axillary Artery, Left	0 Open	9 Autologous Venous Tissue A Autologous Arterial Tissue J Synthetic Substitute K Nonautologous Tissue Substitute Z No Device	0 Upper Arm Artery, Right 1 Upper Arm Artery, Left 2 Upper Arm Artery, Bilateral 3 Lower Arm Artery, Right 4 Lower Arm Artery, Left 5 Lower Arm Artery, Bilateral 6 Upper Leg Artery, Right 7 Upper Leg Artery, Left 8 Upper Leg Artery, Bilateral 9 Lower Leg Artery, Right B Lower Leg Artery, Left C Lower Leg Artery, Bilateral D Upper Arm Vein F Lower Arm Vein J Extracranial Artery, Right K Extracranial Artery, Left T Abdominal Artery V Superior Vena Cava W Lower Extremity Vein

Continued ➡

Section	0	Medical and Surgical
Body System	3	Upper Arteries
Operation	1	Bypass: Altering the route of passage of the contents of a tubular body part

031 Continued

Body Part (4th)	Approach (5th)	Device (6th)	Qualifier (7th)
7 Brachial Artery, Right	0 Open	9 Autologous Venous Tissue A Autologous Arterial Tissue J Synthetic Substitute K Nonautologous Tissue Substitute Z No Device	0 Upper Arm Artery, Right 3 Lower Arm Artery, Right D Upper Arm Vein F Lower Arm Vein V Superior Vena Cava W Lower Extremity Vein
7 Brachial Artery, Right	3 Percutaneous	Z No Device	F Lower Arm Vein
8 Brachial Artery, Left	0 Open	9 Autologous Venous Tissue A Autologous Arterial Tissue J Synthetic Substitute K Nonautologous Tissue Substitute Z No Device	1 Upper Arm Artery, Left 4 Lower Arm Artery, Left D Upper Arm Vein F Lower Arm Vein V Superior Vena Cava W Lower Extremity Vein
8 Brachial Artery, Left	3 Percutaneous	Z No Device	F Lower Arm Vein
9 Ulnar Artery, Right B Radial Artery, Right	0 Open	9 Autologous Venous Tissue A Autologous Arterial Tissue J Synthetic Substitute K Nonautologous Tissue Substitute Z No Device	3 Lower Arm Artery, Right F Lower Arm Vein
9 Ulnar Artery, Right B Radial Artery, Right	3 Percutaneous	Z No Device	F Lower Arm Vein
A Ulnar Artery, Left C Radial Artery, Left	0 Open	9 Autologous Venous Tissue A Autologous Arterial Tissue J Synthetic Substitute K Nonautologous Tissue Substitute Z No Device	4 Lower Arm Artery, Left F Lower Arm Vein
A Ulnar Artery, Left C Radial Artery, Left	3 Percutaneous	Z No Device	F Lower Arm Vein
G Intracranial Artery S Temporal Artery, Right T Temporal Artery, Left	0 Open	9 Autologous Venous Tissue A Autologous Arterial Tissue J Synthetic Substitute K Nonautologous Tissue Substitute Z No Device	G Intracranial Artery
H Common Carotid Artery, Right J Common Carotid Artery, Left	0 Open	9 Autologous Venous Tissue A Autologous Arterial Tissue J Synthetic Substitute K Nonautologous Tissue Substitute Z No Device	G Intracranial Artery J Extracranial Artery, Right K Extracranial Artery, Left Y Upper Artery
K Internal Carotid Artery, Right L Internal Carotid Artery, Left M External Carotid Artery, Right N External Carotid Artery, Left	0 Open	9 Autologous Venous Tissue A Autologous Arterial Tissue J Synthetic Substitute K Nonautologous Tissue Substitute Z No Device	J Extracranial Artery, Right K Extracranial Artery, Left

Section	0	Medical and Surgical
Body System	3	Upper Arteries
Operation	5	Destruction: Physical eradication of all or a portion of a body part by the direct use of energy, force, or a destructive agent

Body Part (4th)	Approach (5th)	Device (6th)	Qualifier (7th)
0 Internal Mammary Artery, Right	0 Open	Z No Device	Z No Qualifier
1 Internal Mammary Artery, Left	3 Percutaneous		
2 Innominate Artery	4 Percutaneous Endoscopic		
3 Subclavian Artery, Right			
4 Subclavian Artery, Left			
5 Axillary Artery, Right			
6 Axillary Artery, Left			
7 Brachial Artery, Right			
8 Brachial Artery, Left			
9 Ulnar Artery, Right			
A Ulnar Artery, Left			
B Radial Artery, Right			
C Radial Artery, Left			
D Hand Artery, Right			
F Hand Artery, Left			
G Intracranial Artery			
H Common Carotid Artery, Right			
J Common Carotid Artery, Left			
K Internal Carotid Artery, Right			
L Internal Carotid Artery, Left			
M External Carotid Artery, Right			
N External Carotid Artery, Left			
P Vertebral Artery, Right			
Q Vertebral Artery, Left			
R Face Artery			
S Temporal Artery, Right			
T Temporal Artery, Left			
U Thyroid Artery, Right			
V Thyroid Artery, Left			
Y Upper Artery			

Section	0	Medical and Surgical
Body System	3	Upper Arteries
Operation	7	**Dilation:** Expanding an orifice or the lumen of a tubular body part

Body Part (4th)	Approach (5th)	Device (6th)	Qualifier (7th)
0 Internal Mammary Artery, Right 1 Internal Mammary Artery, Left 2 Innominate Artery 3 Subclavian Artery, Right 4 Subclavian Artery, Left 5 Axillary Artery, Right 6 Axillary Artery, Left 7 Brachial Artery, Right 8 Brachial Artery, Left 9 Ulnar Artery, Right A Ulnar Artery, Left B Radial Artery, Right C Radial Artery, Left	0 Open 3 Percutaneous 4 Percutaneous Endoscopic	4 Intraluminal Device, Drug-eluting 5 Intraluminal Device, Drug-eluting, Two 6 Intraluminal Device, Drug-eluting, Three 7 Intraluminal Device, Drug-eluting, Four or More E Intraluminal Devices, Two F Intraluminal Devices, Three G Intraluminal Devices, Four or More	Z No Qualifier
0 Internal Mammary Artery, Right 1 Internal Mammary Artery, Left 2 Innominate Artery 3 Subclavian Artery, Right 4 Subclavian Artery, Left 5 Axillary Artery, Right 6 Axillary Artery, Left 7 Brachial Artery, Right 8 Brachial Artery, Left 9 Ulnar Artery, Right A Ulnar Artery, Left B Radial Artery, Right C Radial Artery, Left	0 Open 3 Percutaneous 4 Percutaneous Endoscopic	D Intraluminal Device Z No Device	1 Drug-Coated Balloon Z No Qualifier
D Hand Artery, Right F Hand Artery, Left G Intracranial Artery H Common Carotid Artery, Right J Common Carotid Artery, Left K Internal Carotid Artery, Right L Internal Carotid Artery, Left M External Carotid Artery, Right N External Carotid Artery, Left P Vertebral Artery, Right Q Vertebral Artery, Left R Face Artery S Temporal Artery, Right T Temporal Artery, Left U Thyroid Artery, Right V Thyroid Artery, Left Y Upper Artery	0 Open 3 Percutaneous 4 Percutaneous Endoscopic	4 Intraluminal Device, Drug-eluting 5 Intraluminal Device, Drug-eluting, Two 6 Intraluminal Device, Drug-eluting, Three 7 Intraluminal Device, Drug-eluting, Four or More D Intraluminal Device E Intraluminal Device, Two F Intraluminal Device, Three G Intraluminal Device, Four or More Z No Device	Z No Qualifier

Section	0	Medical and Surgical
Body System	3	Upper Arteries
Operation	9	Drainage: Taking or letting out fluids and/or gases from a body part

Body Part (4th)	Approach (5th)	Device (6th)	Qualifier (7th)
0 Internal Mammary Artery, Right 1 Internal Mammary Artery, Left 2 Innominate Artery 3 Subclavian Artery, Right 4 Subclavian Artery, Left 5 Axillary Artery, Right 6 Axillary Artery, Left 7 Brachial Artery, Right 8 Brachial Artery, Left 9 Ulnar Artery, Right A Ulnar Artery, Left B Radial Artery, Right C Radial Artery, Left D Hand Artery, Right F Hand Artery, Left G Intracranial Artery H Common Carotid Artery, Right J Common Carotid Artery, Left K Internal Carotid Artery, Right L Internal Carotid Artery, Left M External Carotid Artery, Right N External Carotid Artery, Left P Vertebral Artery, Right Q Vertebral Artery, Left R Face Artery S Temporal Artery, Right T Temporal Artery, Left U Thyroid Artery, Right V Thyroid Artery, Left Y Upper Artery	0 Open 3 Percutaneous 4 Percutaneous Endoscopic	0 Drainage Device	Z No Qualifier
0 Internal Mammary Artery, Right 1 Internal Mammary Artery, Left 2 Innominate Artery 3 Subclavian Artery, Right 4 Subclavian Artery, Left 5 Axillary Artery, Right 6 Axillary Artery, Left 7 Brachial Artery, Right 8 Brachial Artery, Left 9 Ulnar Artery, Right A Ulnar Artery, Left B Radial Artery, Right C Radial Artery, Left D Hand Artery, Right F Hand Artery, Left G Intracranial Artery H Common Carotid Artery, Right J Common Carotid Artery, Left K Internal Carotid Artery, Right L Internal Carotid Artery, Left M External Carotid Artery, Right N External Carotid Artery, Left P Vertebral Artery, Right Q Vertebral Artery, Left R Face Artery S Temporal Artery, Right T Temporal Artery, Left U Thyroid Artery, Right V Thyroid Artery, Left Y Upper Artery	0 Open 3 Percutaneous 4 Percutaneous Endoscopic	Z No Device	X Diagnostic Z No Qualifier

Section	0	Medical and Surgical
Body System	3	Upper Arteries
Operation	B	Excision: Cutting out or off, without replacement, a portion of a body part

Body Part (4th)	Approach (5th)	Device (6th)	Qualifier (7th)
0 Internal Mammary Artery, Right 1 Internal Mammary Artery, Left 2 Innominate Artery 3 Subclavian Artery, Right 4 Subclavian Artery, Left 5 Axillary Artery, Right 6 Axillary Artery, Left 7 Brachial Artery, Right 8 Brachial Artery, Left 9 Ulnar Artery, Right A Ulnar Artery, Left B Radial Artery, Right C Radial Artery, Left D Hand Artery, Right F Hand Artery, Left G Intracranial Artery H Common Carotid Artery, Right J Common Carotid Artery, Left K Internal Carotid Artery, Right L Internal Carotid Artery, Left M External Carotid Artery, Right N External Carotid Artery, Left P Vertebral Artery, Right Q Vertebral Artery, Left R Face Artery S Temporal Artery, Right T Temporal Artery, Left U Thyroid Artery, Right V Thyroid Artery, Left Y Upper Artery	0 Open 3 Percutaneous 4 Percutaneous Endoscopic	Z No Device	X Diagnostic Z No Qualifier

Section	0	Medical and Surgical
Body System	3	Upper Arteries
Operation	C	Extirpation: Taking or cutting out solid matter from a body part

Body Part (4th)	Approach (5th)	Device (6th)	Qualifier (7th)
0 Internal Mammary Artery, Right 1 Internal Mammary Artery, Left 2 Innominate Artery 3 Subclavian Artery, Right 4 Subclavian Artery, Left 5 Axillary Artery, Right 6 Axillary Artery, Left 7 Brachial Artery, Right 8 Brachial Artery, Left 9 Ulnar Artery, Right A Ulnar Artery, Left B Radial Artery, Right C Radial Artery, Left D Hand Artery, Right F Hand Artery, Left R Face Artery S Temporal Artery, Right T Temporal Artery, Left U Thyroid Artery, Right V Thyroid Artery, Left Y Upper Artery	0 Open 3 Percutaneous 4 Percutaneous Endoscopic	Z No Device	Z No Qualifier

Continued →

Section	0	Medical and Surgical
Body System	3	Upper Arteries
Operation	C	Extirpation: Taking or cutting out solid matter from a body part

Body Part (4th)	Approach (5th)	Device (6th)	Qualifier (7th)
G Intracranial Artery H Common Carotid Artery, Right J Common Carotid Artery, Left K Internal Carotid Artery, Right L Internal Carotid Artery, Left M External Carotid Artery, Right N External Carotid Artery, Left P Vertebral Artery, Right Q Vertebral Artery, Left	0 Open 4 Percutaneous Endoscopic	Z No Device	Z No Qualifier
G Intracranial Artery H Common Carotid Artery, Right J Common Carotid Artery, Left K Internal Carotid Artery, Right L Internal Carotid Artery, Left M External Carotid Artery, Right N External Carotid Artery, Left P Vertebral Artery, Right Q Vertebral Artery, Left	3 Percutaneous	Z No Device	7 Stent Retriever Z No Qualifier

Section	0	Medical and Surgical
Body System	3	Upper Arteries
Operation	F	Fragmentation: Breaking solid matter in a body part into pieces

Body Part (4th)	Approach (5th)	Device (6th)	Qualifier (7th)
2 Innominate Artery 3 Subclavian Artery, Right 4 Subclavian Artery, Left 5 Axillary Artery, Right 6 Axillary Artery, Left 7 Brachial Artery, Right 8 Brachial Artery, Left 9 Ulnar Artery, Right A Ulnar Artery, Left B Radial Artery, Right C Radial Artery, Left G Intracranial Artery Y Upper Artery	3 Percutaneous	Z No Device	0 Ultrasonic Z No Qualifier

Section	0	Medical and Surgical
Body System	3	Upper Arteries
Operation	H	Insertion: Putting in a nonbiological appliance that monitors, assists, performs, or prevents a physiological function but does not physically take the place of a body part

Body Part (4th)	Approach (5th)	Device (6th)	Qualifier (7th)
0 Internal Mammary Artery, Right 1 Internal Mammary Artery, Left 2 Innominate Artery 3 Subclavian Artery, Right 4 Subclavian Artery, Left 5 Axillary Artery, Right 6 Axillary Artery, Left 7 Brachial Artery, Right 8 Brachial Artery, Left 9 Ulnar Artery, Right A Ulnar Artery, Left B Radial Artery, Right C Radial Artery, Left D Hand Artery, Right F Hand Artery, Left G Intracranial Artery H Common Carotid Artery, Right J Common Carotid Artery, Left M External Carotid Artery, Right N External Carotid Artery, Left P Vertebral Artery, Right Q Vertebral Artery, Left R Face Artery S Temporal Artery, Right T Temporal Artery, Left U Thyroid Artery, Right V Thyroid Artery, Left	0 Open 3 Percutaneous 4 Percutaneous Endoscopic	3 Infusion Device D Intraluminal Device	Z No Qualifier
K Internal Carotid Artery, Right L Internal Carotid Artery, Left	0 Open 3 Percutaneous 4 Percutaneous Endoscopic	3 Infusion Device D Intraluminal Device M Stimulator Lead	Z No Qualifier
Y Upper Artery	0 Open 3 Percutaneous 4 Percutaneous Endoscopic	2 Monitoring Device 3 Infusion Device D Intraluminal Device Y Other Device	Z No Qualifier

Section	0	Medical and Surgical
Body System	3	Upper Arteries
Operation	J	Inspection: Visually and/or manually exploring a body part

Body Part (4th)	Approach (5th)	Device (6th)	Qualifier (7th)
Y Upper Artery	0 Open 3 Percutaneous 4 Percutaneous Endoscopic X External	Z No Device	Z No Qualifier

Section	0	Medical and Surgical
Body System	3	Upper Arteries
Operation	L	Occlusion: Completely closing an orifice or the lumen of a tubular body part

Body Part (4th)	Approach (5th)	Device (6th)	Qualifier (7th)
0 Internal Mammary Artery, Right 1 Internal Mammary Artery, Left 2 Innominate Artery 3 Subclavian Artery, Right 4 Subclavian Artery, Left 5 Axillary Artery, Right 6 Axillary Artery, Left 7 Brachial Artery, Right 8 Brachial Artery, Left 9 Ulnar Artery, Right A Ulnar Artery, Left B Radial Artery, Right C Radial Artery, Left D Hand Artery, Right F Hand Artery, Left R Face Artery S Temporal Artery, Right T Temporal Artery, Left U Thyroid Artery, Right V Thyroid Artery, Left Y Upper Artery	0 Open 3 Percutaneous 4 Percutaneous Endoscopic	C Extraluminal Device D Intraluminal Device Z No Device	Z No Qualifier
G Intracranial Artery H Common Carotid Artery, Right J Common Carotid Artery, Left K Internal Carotid Artery, Right L Internal Carotid Artery, Left M External Carotid Artery, Right N External Carotid Artery, Left P Vertebral Artery, Right Q Vertebral Artery, Left	0 Open 3 Percutaneous 4 Percutaneous Endoscopic	B Intraluminal Device, Bioactive C Extraluminal Device D Intraluminal Device Z No Device	Z No Qualifier

Section	0	Medical and Surgical
Body System	3	Upper Arteries
Operation	N	Release: Freeing a body part from an abnormal physical constraint by cutting or by the use of force

Body Part (4th)	Approach (5th)	Device (6th)	Qualifier (7th)
0 Internal Mammary Artery, Right 1 Internal Mammary Artery, Left 2 Innominate Artery 3 Subclavian Artery, Right 4 Subclavian Artery, Left 5 Axillary Artery, Right 6 Axillary Artery, Left 7 Brachial Artery, Right 8 Brachial Artery, Left 9 Ulnar Artery, Right A Ulnar Artery, Left B Radial Artery, Right C Radial Artery, Left D Hand Artery, Right F Hand Artery, Left G Intracranial Artery H Common Carotid Artery, Right J Common Carotid Artery, Left K Internal Carotid Artery, Right L Internal Carotid Artery, Left M External Carotid Artery, Right N External Carotid Artery, Left P Vertebral Artery, Right Q Vertebral Artery, Left R Face Artery S Temporal Artery, Right T Temporal Artery, Left U Thyroid Artery, Right V Thyroid Artery, Left Y Upper Artery	0 Open 3 Percutaneous 4 Percutaneous Endoscopic	Z No Device	Z No Qualifier

Section	0	Medical and Surgical
Body System	3	Upper Arteries
Operation	P	Removal: Taking out or off a device from a body part

Body Part (4th)	Approach (5th)	Device (6th)	Qualifier (7th)
Y Upper Artery	0 Open 3 Percutaneous 4 Percutaneous Endoscopic	0 Drainage Device 2 Monitoring Device 3 Infusion Device 7 Autologous Tissue Substitute C Extraluminal Device D Intraluminal Device J Synthetic Substitute K Nonautologous Tissue Substitute M Stimulator Lead Y Other Device	Z No Qualifier
Y Upper Artery	X External	0 Drainage Device 2 Monitoring Device 3 Infusion Device D Intraluminal Device M Stimulator Lead	Z No Qualifier

Section	0	Medical and Surgical
Body System	3	Upper Arteries
Operation	Q	Repair: Restoring, to the extent possible, a body part to its normal anatomic structure and function

Body Part (4th)	Approach (5th)	Device (6th)	Qualifier (7th)
0 Internal Mammary Artery, Right 1 Internal Mammary Artery, Left 2 Innominate Artery 3 Subclavian Artery, Right 4 Subclavian Artery, Left 5 Axillary Artery, Right 6 Axillary Artery, Left 7 Brachial Artery, Right 8 Brachial Artery, Left 9 Ulnar Artery, Right A Ulnar Artery, Left B Radial Artery, Right C Radial Artery, Left D Hand Artery, Right F Hand Artery, Left G Intracranial Artery H Common Carotid Artery, Right J Common Carotid Artery, Left K Internal Carotid Artery, Right L Internal Carotid Artery, Left M External Carotid Artery, Right N External Carotid Artery, Left P Vertebral Artery, Right Q Vertebral Artery, Left R Face Artery S Temporal Artery, Right T Temporal Artery, Left U Thyroid Artery, Right V Thyroid Artery, Left Y Upper Artery	0 Open 3 Percutaneous 4 Percutaneous Endoscopic	Z No Device	Z No Qualifier

03R–03S

Medical and Surgical, Upper Arteries Tables

Section	0	Medical and Surgical
Body System	3	Upper Arteries
Operation	R	**Replacement:** Putting in or on biological or synthetic material that physically takes the place and/or function of all or a portion of a body part

Body Part (4th)	Approach (5th)	Device (6th)	Qualifier (7th)
0 Internal Mammary Artery, Right	**0** Open	**7** Autologous Tissue Substitute	**Z** No Qualifier
1 Internal Mammary Artery, Left	**4** Percutaneous Endoscopic	**J** Synthetic Substitute	
2 Innominate Artery		**K** Nonautologous Tissue Substitute	
3 Subclavian Artery, Right			
4 Subclavian Artery, Left			
5 Axillary Artery, Right			
6 Axillary Artery, Left			
7 Brachial Artery, Right			
8 Brachial Artery, Left			
9 Ulnar Artery, Right			
A Ulnar Artery, Left			
B Radial Artery, Right			
C Radial Artery, Left			
D Hand Artery, Right			
F Hand Artery, Left			
G Intracranial Artery			
H Common Carotid Artery, Right			
J Common Carotid Artery, Left			
K Internal Carotid Artery, Right			
L Internal Carotid Artery, Left			
M External Carotid Artery, Right			
N External Carotid Artery, Left			
P Vertebral Artery, Right			
Q Vertebral Artery, Left			
R Face Artery			
S Temporal Artery, Right			
T Temporal Artery, Left			
U Thyroid Artery, Right			
V Thyroid Artery, Left			
Y Upper Artery			

Section	0	Medical and Surgical
Body System	3	Upper Arteries
Operation	S	**Reposition:** Moving to its normal location, or other suitable location, all or a portion of a body part

Body Part (4th)	Approach (5th)	Device (6th)	Qualifier (7th)
0 Internal Mammary Artery, Right	**0** Open	**Z** No Device	**Z** No Qualifier
1 Internal Mammary Artery, Left	**3** Percutaneous		
2 Innominate Artery	**4** Percutaneous Endoscopic		
3 Subclavian Artery, Right			
4 Subclavian Artery, Left			
5 Axillary Artery, Right			
6 Axillary Artery, Left			
7 Brachial Artery, Right			
8 Brachial Artery, Left			
9 Ulnar Artery, Right			
A Ulnar Artery, Left			
B Radial Artery, Right			
C Radial Artery, Left			
D Hand Artery, Right			
F Hand Artery, Left			
G Intracranial Artery			
H Common Carotid Artery, Right			
J Common Carotid Artery, Left			
K Internal Carotid Artery, Right			
L Internal Carotid Artery, Left			
M External Carotid Artery, Right			
N External Carotid Artery, Left			
P Vertebral Artery, Right			
Q Vertebral Artery, Left			
R Face Artery			
S Temporal Artery, Right			
T Temporal Artery, Left			
U Thyroid Artery, Right			
V Thyroid Artery, Left			
Y Upper Artery			

Section	0	Medical and Surgical
Body System	3	Upper Arteries
Operation	U	**Supplement:** Putting in or on biological or synthetic material that physically reinforces and/or augments the function of a portion of a body part

Body Part (4th)	Approach (5th)	Device (6th)	Qualifier (7th)
0 Internal Mammary Artery, Right	**0** Open	**7** Autologous Tissue Substitute	**Z** No Qualifier
1 Internal Mammary Artery, Left	**3** Percutaneous	**J** Synthetic Substitute	
2 Innominate Artery	**4** Percutaneous Endoscopic	**K** Nonautologous Tissue Substitute	
3 Subclavian Artery, Right			
4 Subclavian Artery, Left			
5 Axillary Artery, Right			
6 Axillary Artery, Left			
7 Brachial Artery, Right			
8 Brachial Artery, Left			
9 Ulnar Artery, Right			
A Ulnar Artery, Left			
B Radial Artery, Right			
C Radial Artery, Left			
D Hand Artery, Right			
F Hand Artery, Left			
G Intracranial Artery			
H Common Carotid Artery, Right			
J Common Carotid Artery, Left			
K Internal Carotid Artery, Right			
L Internal Carotid Artery, Left			
M External Carotid Artery, Right			
N External Carotid Artery, Left			
P Vertebral Artery, Right			
Q Vertebral Artery, Left			
R Face Artery			
S Temporal Artery, Right			
T Temporal Artery, Left			
U Thyroid Artery, Right			
V Thyroid Artery, Left			
Y Upper Artery			

Section   **0**   **Medical and Surgical**
Body System   **3**   **Upper Arteries**
Operation   **V**   **Restriction:** Partially closing an orifice or the lumen of a tubular body part

Body Part (4th)	Approach (5th)	Device (6th)	Qualifier (7th)
0 Internal Mammary Artery, Right 1 Internal Mammary Artery, Left 2 Innominate Artery 3 Subclavian Artery, Right 4 Subclavian Artery, Left 5 Axillary Artery, Right 6 Axillary Artery, Left 7 Brachial Artery, Right 8 Brachial Artery, Left 9 Ulnar Artery, Right A Ulnar Artery, Left B Radial Artery, Right C Radial Artery, Left D Hand Artery, Right F Hand Artery, Left R Face Artery S Temporal Artery, Right T Temporal Artery, Left U Thyroid Artery, Right V Thyroid Artery, Left Y Upper Artery	0 Open 3 Percutaneous 4 Percutaneous Endoscopic	C Extraluminal Device D Intraluminal Device Z No Device	Z No Qualifier
G Intracranial Artery H Common Carotid Artery, Right J Common Carotid Artery, Left K Internal Carotid Artery, Right L Internal Carotid Artery, Left M External Carotid Artery, Right N External Carotid Artery, Left P Vertebral Artery, Right Q Vertebral Artery, Left	0 Open 3 Percutaneous 4 Percutaneous Endoscopic	B Intraluminal Device, Bioactive C Extraluminal Device D Intraluminal Device H Intraluminal Device, Flow Diverter Z No Device	Z No Qualifier

Section   **0**   **Medical and Surgical**
Body System   **3**   **Upper Arteries**
Operation   **W**   **Revision:** Correcting, to the extent possible, a portion of a malfunctioning device or the position of a displaced device

Body Part (4th)	Approach (5th)	Device (6th)	Qualifier (7th)
Y Upper Artery	0 Open 3 Percutaneous 4 Percutaneous Endoscopic	0 Drainage Device 2 Monitoring Device 3 Infusion Device 7 Autologous Tissue Substitute C Extraluminal Device D Intraluminal Device J Synthetic Substitute K Nonautologous Tissue Substitute M Stimulator Lead Y Other Device	Z No Qualifier
Y Upper Artery	X External	0 Drainage Device 2 Monitoring Device 3 Infusion Device 7 Autologous Tissue Substitute C Extraluminal Device D Intraluminal Device J Synthetic Substitute K Nonautologous Tissue Substitute M Neurostimulator Lead	Z No Qualifier

AHA Coding Clinic

03170KF Bypass Right Brachial Artery to Lower Arm Vein with Nonautologous Tissue Substitute, Open Approach—AHA CC: 3Q, 2021, 14-15

03170ZD Bypass Right Brachial Artery to Upper Arm Vein, Open Approach—AHA CC: 4Q, 2013, 125-126

03180JD Bypass Left Brachial Artery to Upper Arm Vein with Synthetic Substitute, Open Approach—AHA CC: 3Q, 2016, 37-38

031C0ZF Bypass Left Radial Artery to Lower Arm Vein, Open Approach—AHA CC: 1Q, 2013, 27-28

031J0JJ Bypass Left Common Carotid Artery to Right Extracranial Artery with Synthetic Substitute, Open Approach—AHA CC: 4Q, 2017, 65

031J0ZK Bypass Left Common Carotid Artery to Left Extracranial Artery, Open Approach—AHA CC: 2Q, 2017, 22

037K3DZ Dilation of Right Internal Carotid Artery with Intraluminal Device, Percutaneous Approach—AHA CC: 3Q, 2019, 29-30

03BN0ZZ Excision of Left External Carotid Artery, Open Approach—AHA CC: 2Q, 2016, 12-14

03C70ZZ Extirpation of Matter from Right Brachial Artery, Open Approach—AHA CC: 3Q, 2020, 38-40

03CG3ZZ Extirpation of Matter from Intracranial Artery, Percutaneous Approach—AHA CC: 1Q, 2022, 43-44

03CK0ZZ Extirpation of Matter from Right Internal Carotid Artery, Open Approach—AHA CC: 2Q, 2016, 11-12

03CL0ZZ Extirpation of Matter from Left Internal Carotid Artery, Open Approach—AHA CC: 2Q, 2021, 13

03CN0ZZ Extirpation of Matter from Left External Carotid Artery, Open Approach—AHA CC: 4Q, 2017, 65

03H40DZ Insertion of Intraluminal Device into Left Subclavian Artery, Open Approach—AHA CC: 1Q, 2020, 25-27

03HY32Z Insertion of Monitoring Device into Upper Artery, Percutaneous Approach—AHA CC: 2Q, 2016, 32-33

03JY0ZZ Inspection of Upper Artery, Open Approach—AHA CC: 1Q, 2015, 29

03JY3ZZ Inspection of Upper Artery, Percutaneous Approach—AHA CC: 1Q, 2021, 16-17

03LG0CZ Occlusion of Intracranial Artery with Extraluminal Device, Open Approach—AHA CC: 2Q, 2016, 30

03LG3DZ Occlusion of Intracranial Artery with Intraluminal Device, Percutaneous Approach—AHA CC: 4Q, 2014, 37

03LL0ZZ Occlusion of Left Internal Carotid Artery, Open Approach—AHA CC: 2Q, 2021, 13

03QH0ZZ Repair Right Common Carotid Artery, Open Approach—AHA CC: 1Q, 2017, 31-32

03SS0ZZ Reposition Right Temporal Artery, Open Approach—AHA CC: 3Q, 2015, 27-28

03UK0JZ Supplement Right Internal Carotid Artery with Synthetic Substitute, Open Approach—AHA CC: 2Q, 2016, 11-12

03VG0CZ Restriction of Intracranial Artery with Extraluminal Device, Open Approach—AHA CC: 1Q, 2019, 22

03VG3DZ Restriction of Intracranial Artery with Intraluminal Device, Percutaneous Approach—AHA CC: 1Q, 2016, 19-20

03VK3DZ Restriction of Right Internal Carotid Artery with Intraluminal Device, Percutaneous Approach—AHA CC: 1Q, 2023, 34-35

03VK3HZ Restriction of Right Internal Carotid Artery with Intraluminal Device, Flow Diverter, Percutaneous Approach—AHA CC: 1Q, 2023, 34-35

03VM3DZ Restriction of Right External Carotid Artery with Intraluminal Device, Percutaneous Approach—AHA CC: 4Q, 2016, 26

03WY0JZ Revision of Synthetic Substitute in Upper Artery, Open Approach—AHA CC: 3Q, 2016, 39-40

03WY3DZ Revision of Intraluminal Device in Upper Artery, Percutaneous Approach—AHA CC: 1Q, 2015, 32-33

Lower Arteries

Arteries

Lower Arteries Tables 041–04W

Section 0 Medical and Surgical
Body System 4 Lower Arteries
Operation 1 Bypass: Altering the route of passage of the contents of a tubular body part

Body Part (4th)	Approach (5th)	Device (6th)	Qualifier (7th)
0 Abdominal Aorta C Common Iliac Artery, Right D Common Iliac Artery, Left	0 Open 4 Percutaneous Endoscopic	9 Autologous Venous Tissue A Autologous Arterial Tissue J Synthetic Substitute K Nonautologous Tissue Substitute Z No Device	0 Abdominal Aorta 1 Celiac Artery 2 Mesenteric Artery 3 Renal Artery, Right 4 Renal Artery, Left 5 Renal Artery, Bilateral 6 Common Iliac Artery, Right 7 Common Iliac Artery, Left 8 Common Iliac Arteries, Bilateral 9 Internal Iliac Artery, Right B Internal Iliac Artery, Left C Internal Iliac Arteries, Bilateral D External Iliac Artery, Right F External Iliac Artery, Left G External Iliac Arteries, Bilateral H Femoral Artery, Right J Femoral Artery, Left K Femoral Arteries, Bilateral Q Lower Extremity Artery R Lower Artery
3 Hepatic Artery 4 Splenic Artery	0 Open 4 Percutaneous Endoscopic	9 Autologous Venous Tissue A Autologous Arterial Tissue J Synthetic Substitute K Nonautologous Tissue Substitute Z No Device	3 Renal Artery, Right 4 Renal Artery, Left 5 Renal Artery, Bilateral
E Internal Iliac Artery, Right F Internal Iliac Artery, Left H External Iliac Artery, Right J External Iliac Artery, Left	0 Open 4 Percutaneous Endoscopic	9 Autologous Venous Tissue A Autologous Arterial Tissue J Synthetic Substitute K Nonautologous Tissue Substitute Z No Device	9 Internal Iliac Artery, Right B Internal Iliac Artery, Left C Internal Iliac Arteries, Bilateral D External Iliac Artery, Right F External Iliac Artery, Left G External Iliac Arteries, Bilateral H Femoral Artery, Right J Femoral Artery, Left K Femoral Arteries, Bilateral P Foot Artery Q Lower Extremity Artery
K Femoral Artery, Right L Femoral Artery, Left	0 Open 4 Percutaneous Endoscopic	9 Autologous Venous Tissue A Autologous Arterial Tissue J Synthetic Substitute K Nonautologous Tissue Substitute Z No Device	H Femoral Artery, Right J Femoral Artery, Left K Femoral Arteries, Bilateral L Popliteal Artery M Peroneal Artery N Posterior Tibial Artery P Foot Artery Q Lower Extremity Artery S Lower Extremity Vein
K Femoral Artery, Right L Femoral Artery, Left	3 Percutaneous	J Synthetic Substitute	Q Lower Extremity Artery S Lower Extremity Vein
M Popliteal Artery, Right N Popliteal Artery, Left	0 Open 4 Percutaneous Endoscopic	9 Autologous Venous Tissue A Autologous Arterial Tissue J Synthetic Substitute K Nonautologous Tissue Substitute Z No Device	L Popliteal Artery M Peroneal Artery P Foot Artery Q Lower Extremity Artery S Lower Extremity Vein

Continued→

Section	0	Medical and Surgical
Body System	4	Lower Arteries
Operation	1	Bypass: Altering the route of passage of the contents of a tubular body part

041 Continued

Body Part (4th)	Approach (5th)	Device (6th)	Qualifier (7th)
M Popliteal Artery, Right N Popliteal Artery, Left	3 Percutaneous	J Synthetic Substitute	Q Lower Extremity Artery S Lower Extremity Vein
P Anterior Tibial Artery, Right Q Anterior Tibial Artery, Left R Posterior Tibial Artery, Right S Posterior Tibial Artery, Left	0 Open 3 Percutaneou 4 Percutaneous Endoscopic	J Synthetic Substitute	Q Lower Extremity Artery S Lower Extremity Vein
T Peroneal Artery, Right U Peroneal Artery, Left V Foot Artery, Right W Foot Artery, Left	0 Open 4 Percutaneous Endoscopic	9 Autologous Venous Tissue A Autologous Arterial Tissue J Synthetic Substitute K Nonautologous Tissue Substitute Z No Device	P Foot Artery Q Lower Extremity Artery S Lower Extremity Vein
T Peroneal Artery, Right U Peroneal Artery, Left V Foot Artery, Right W Foot Artery, Left	3 Percutaneous	J Synthetic Substitute	Q Lower Extremity Artery S Lower Extremity Vein

Section	0	Medical and Surgical
Body System	4	Lower Arteries
Operation	5	Destruction: Physical eradication of all or a portion of a body part by the direct use of energy, force, or a destructive agent

Body Part (4th)	Approach (5th)	Device (6th)	Qualifier (7th)
0 Abdominal Aorta 1 Celiac Artery 2 Gastric Artery 3 Hepatic Artery 4 Splenic Artery 5 Superior Mesenteric Artery 6 Colic Artery, Right 7 Colic Artery, Left 8 Colic Artery, Middle 9 Renal Artery, Right A Renal Artery, Left B Inferior Mesenteric Artery C Common Iliac Artery, Right D Common Iliac Artery, Left E Internal Iliac Artery, Right F Internal Iliac Artery, Left H External Iliac Artery, Right J External Iliac Artery, Left K Femoral Artery, Right L Femoral Artery, Left M Popliteal Artery, Right N Popliteal Artery, Left P Anterior Tibial Artery, Right Q Anterior Tibial Artery, Left R Posterior Tibial Artery, Right S Posterior Tibial Artery, Left T Peroneal Artery, Right U Peroneal Artery, Left V Foot Artery, Right W Foot Artery, Left Y Lower Artery	0 Open 3 Percutaneous 4 Percutaneous Endoscopic	Z No Device	Z No Qualifier

Section	0	Medical and Surgical
Body System	4	Lower Arteries
Operation	7	Dilation: Expanding an orifice or the lumen of a tubular body part

Body Part (4th)	Approach (5th)	Device (6th)	Qualifier (7th)
0 Abdominal Aorta 1 Celiac Artery 2 Gastric Artery 3 Hepatic Artery 4 Splenic Artery 5 Superior Mesenteric Artery 6 Colic Artery, Right 7 Colic Artery, Left 8 Colic Artery, Middle 9 Renal Artery, Right A Renal Artery, Left B Inferior Mesenteric Artery C Common Iliac Artery, Right D Common Iliac Artery, Left E Internal Iliac Artery, Right F Internal Iliac Artery, Left H External Iliac Artery, Right J External Iliac Artery, Left K Femoral Artery, Right L Femoral Artery, Left M Popliteal Artery, Right N Popliteal Artery, Left P Anterior Tibial Artery, Right Q Anterior Tibial Artery, Left R Posterior Tibial Artery, Right S Posterior Tibial Artery, Left T Peroneal Artery, Right U Peroneal Artery, Left V Foot Artery, Right W Foot Artery, Left Y Lower Artery	0 Open 3 Percutaneous 4 Percutaneous Endoscopic	4 Intraluminal Device, Drug-eluting D Intraluminal Device Z No Device	1 Drug-Coated Balloon Z No Qualifier
0 Abdominal Aorta 1 Celiac Artery 2 Gastric Artery 3 Hepatic Artery 4 Splenic Artery 5 Superior Mesenteric Artery 6 Colic Artery, Right 7 Colic Artery, Left 8 Colic Artery, Middle 9 Renal Artery, Right A Renal Artery, Left B Inferior Mesenteric Artery C Common Iliac Artery, Right D Common Iliac Artery, Left E Internal Iliac Artery, Right F Internal Iliac Artery, Left H External Iliac Artery, Right J External Iliac Artery, Left K Femoral Artery, Right L Femoral Artery, Left M Popliteal Artery, Right N Popliteal Artery, Left P Anterior Tibial Artery, Right Q Anterior Tibial Artery, Left R Posterior Tibial Artery, Right S Posterior Tibial Artery, Left T Peroneal Artery, Right U Peroneal Artery, Left V Foot Artery, Right W Foot Artery, Left Y Lower Artery	0 Open 3 Percutaneous 4 Percutaneous Endoscopic	5 Intraluminal Device, Drug-eluting, Two 6 Intraluminal Device, Drug-eluting, Three 7 Intraluminal Device, Drug-eluting, Four or More E Intraluminal Devices, Two F Intraluminal Devices, Three G Intraluminal Devices, Four or More	Z No Qualifier

Section	0	Medical and Surgical
Body System	4	Lower Arteries
Operation	9	Drainage: Taking or letting out fluids and/or gases from a body part

Body Part (4th)	Approach (5th)	Device (6th)	Qualifier (7th)
0 Abdominal Aorta 1 Celiac Artery 2 Gastric Artery 3 Hepatic Artery 4 Splenic Artery 5 Superior Mesenteric Artery 6 Colic Artery, Right 7 Colic Artery, Left 8 Colic Artery, Middle 9 Renal Artery, Right A Renal Artery, Left B Inferior Mesenteric Artery C Common Iliac Artery, Right D Common Iliac Artery, Left E Internal Iliac Artery, Right F Internal Iliac Artery, Left H External Iliac Artery, Right J External Iliac Artery, Left K Femoral Artery, Right L Femoral Artery, Left M Popliteal Artery, Right N Popliteal Artery, Left P Anterior Tibial Artery, Right Q Anterior Tibial Artery, Left R Posterior Tibial Artery, Right S Posterior Tibial Artery, Left T Peroneal Artery, Right U Peroneal Artery, Left V Foot Artery, Right W Foot Artery, Left Y Lower Artery	0 Open 3 Percutaneous 4 Percutaneous Endoscopic	0 Drainage Device	Z No Qualifier
0 Abdominal Aorta 1 Celiac Artery 2 Gastric Artery 3 Hepatic Artery 4 Splenic Artery 5 Superior Mesenteric Artery 6 Colic Artery, Right 7 Colic Artery, Left 8 Colic Artery, Middle 9 Renal Artery, Right A Renal Artery, Left B Inferior Mesenteric Artery C Common Iliac Artery, Right D Common Iliac Artery, Left E Internal Iliac Artery, Right F Internal Iliac Artery, Left H External Iliac Artery, Right J External Iliac Artery, Left K Femoral Artery, Right L Femoral Artery, Left M Popliteal Artery, Right N Popliteal Artery, Left P Anterior Tibial Artery, Right Q Anterior Tibial Artery, Left R Posterior Tibial Artery, Right S Posterior Tibial Artery, Left T Peroneal Artery, Right U Peroneal Artery, Left V Foot Artery, Right W Foot Artery, Left Y Lower Artery	0 Open 3 Percutaneous 4 Percutaneous Endoscopic	Z No Device	X Diagnostic Z No Qualifier

Section	0	Medical and Surgical
Body System	4	Lower Arteries
Operation	B	Excision: Cutting out or off, without replacement, a portion of a body part

Body Part (4th)	Approach (5th)	Device (6th)	Qualifier (7th)
0 Abdominal Aorta	0 Open	Z No Device	X Diagnostic
1 Celiac Artery	3 Percutaneous		Z No Qualifier
2 Gastric Artery	4 Percutaneous Endoscopic		
3 Hepatic Artery			
4 Splenic Artery			
5 Superior Mesenteric Artery			
6 Colic Artery, Right			
7 Colic Artery, Left			
8 Colic Artery, Middle			
9 Renal Artery, Right			
A Renal Artery, Left			
B Inferior Mesenteric Artery			
C Common Iliac Artery, Right			
D Common Iliac Artery, Left			
E Internal Iliac Artery, Right			
F Internal Iliac Artery, Left			
H External Iliac Artery, Right			
J External Iliac Artery, Left			
K Femoral Artery, Right			
L Femoral Artery, Left			
M Popliteal Artery, Right			
N Popliteal Artery, Left			
P Anterior Tibial Artery, Right			
Q Anterior Tibial Artery, Left			
R Posterior Tibial Artery, Right			
S Posterior Tibial Artery, Left			
T Peroneal Artery, Right			
U Peroneal Artery, Left			
V Foot Artery, Right			
W Foot Artery, Left			
Y Lower Artery			

04B

Medical and Surgical, Lower Arteries Tables

Section   **0**   **Medical and Surgical**
Body System   **4**   **Lower Arteries**
Operation   **C**   **Extirpation:** Taking or cutting out solid matter from a body part

Body Part (4th)	Approach (5th)	Device (6th)	Qualifier (7th)
0 Abdominal Aorta	**0** Open	**Z** No Device	**Z** No Qualifier
1 Celiac Artery	**3** Percutaneous		
2 Gastric Artery	**4** Percutaneous		
3 Hepatic Artery	Endoscopic		
4 Splenic Artery			
5 Superior Mesenteric Artery			
6 Colic Artery, Right			
7 Colic Artery, Left			
8 Colic Artery, Middle			
9 Renal Artery, Right			
A Renal Artery, Left			
B Inferior Mesenteric Artery			
C Common Iliac Artery, Right			
D Common Iliac Artery, Left			
E Internal Iliac Artery, Right			
F Internal Iliac Artery, Left			
H External Iliac Artery, Right			
J External Iliac Artery, Left			
K Femoral Artery, Right			
L Femoral Artery, Left			
M Popliteal Artery, Right			
N Popliteal Artery, Left			
P Anterior Tibial Artery, Right			
Q Anterior Tibial Artery, Left			
R Posterior Tibial Artery, Right			
S Posterior Tibial Artery, Left			
T Peroneal Artery, Right			
U Peroneal Artery, Left			
V Foot Artery, Right			
W Foot Artery, Left			
Y Lower Artery			

Section   **0**   **Medical and Surgical**
Body System   **4**   **Lower Arteries**
Operation   **F**   **Fragmentation:** Breaking solid matter in a body part into pieces

Body Part (4th)	Approach (5th)	Device (6th)	Qualifier (7th)
C Common Iliac Artery, Right	**3** Percutaneous	**Z** No Device	**0** Ultrasonic
D Common Iliac Artery, Left			**Z** No Qualifier
E Internal Iliac Artery, Right			
F Internal Iliac Artery, Left			
H External Iliac Artery, Right			
J External Iliac Artery, Left			
K Femoral Artery, Right			
L Femoral Artery, Left			
M Popliteal Artery, Right			
N Popliteal Artery, Left			
P Anterior Tibial Artery, Right			
Q Anterior Tibial Artery, Left			
R Posterior Tibial Artery, Right			
S Posterior Tibial Artery, Left			
T Peroneal Artery, Right			
U Peroneal Artery, Left			
Y Lower Artery			

Section	0	Medical and Surgical
Body System	4	Lower Arteries
Operation	H	Insertion: Putting in a nonbiological appliance that monitors, assists, performs, or prevents a physiological function but does not physically take the place of a body part

Body Part (4th)	Approach (5th)	Device (6th)	Qualifier (7th)
0 Abdominal Aorta	**0** Open **3** Percutaneous **4** Percutaneous Endoscopic	**2** Monitoring Device **3** Infusion Device **D** Intraluminal Device	**Z** No Qualifier
1 Celiac Artery **2** Gastric Artery **3** Hepatic Artery **4** Splenic Artery **5** Superior Mesenteric Artery **6** Colic Artery, Right **7** Colic Artery, Left **8** Colic Artery, Middle **9** Renal Artery, Right **A** Renal Artery, Left **B** Inferior Mesenteric Artery **C** Common Iliac Artery, Right **D** Common Iliac Artery, Left **E** Internal Iliac Artery, Right **F** Internal Iliac Artery, Left **H** External Iliac Artery, Right **J** External Iliac Artery, Left **K** Femoral Artery, Right **L** Femoral Artery, Left **M** Popliteal Artery, Right **N** Popliteal Artery, Left **P** Anterior Tibial Artery, Right **Q** Anterior Tibial Artery, Left **R** Posterior Tibial Artery, Right **S** Posterior Tibial Artery, Left **T** Peroneal Artery, Right **U** Peroneal Artery, Left **V** Foot Artery, Right **W** Foot Artery, Left	**0** Open **3** Percutaneous **4** Percutaneous Endoscopic	**3** Infusion Device **D** Intraluminal Device	**Z** No Qualifier
Y Lower Artery	**0** Open **3** Percutaneous **4** Percutaneous Endoscopic	**2** Monitoring Device **3** Infusion Device **D** Intraluminal Device **Y** Other Device	**Z** No Qualifier

Section	0	Medical and Surgical
Body System	4	Lower Arteries
Operation	J	Inspection: Visually and/or manually exploring a body part

Body Part (4th)	Approach (5th)	Device (6th)	Qualifier (7th)
Y Lower Artery	**0** Open **3** Percutaneous **4** Percutaneous Endoscopic **X** External	**Z** No Device	**Z** No Qualifier

Section	0	Medical and Surgical
Body System	4	Lower Arteries
Operation	L	Occlusion: Completely closing an orifice or the lumen of a tubular body part

Body Part (4th)	Approach (5th)	Device (6th)	Qualifier (7th)
0 Abdominal Aorta	0 Open 3 Percutaneous	C Extraluminal Device Z No Device	Z No Qualifier
0 Abdominal Aorta	0 Open 3 Percutaneous	D Intraluminal Device	J Temporary Z No Qualifier
0 Abdominal Aorta	4 Percutaneous Endoscopic	C Extraluminal Device D Intraluminal Device Z No Device	Z No Qualifier
1 Celiac Artery 2 Gastric Artery 3 Hepatic Artery 4 Splenic Artery 5 Superior Mesenteric Artery 6 Colic Artery, Right 7 Colic Artery, Left 8 Colic Artery, Middle 9 Renal Artery, Right A Renal Artery, Left B Inferior Mesenteric Artery C Common Iliac Artery, Right D Common Iliac Artery, Left H External Iliac Artery, Right J External Iliac Artery, Left K Femoral Artery, Right L Femoral Artery, Left M Popliteal Artery, Right N Popliteal Artery, Left P Anterior Tibial Artery, Right Q Anterior Tibial Artery, Left R Posterior Tibial Artery, Right S Posterior Tibial Artery, Left T Peroneal Artery, Right U Peroneal Artery, Left V Foot Artery, Right W Foot Artery, Left Y Lower Artery	0 Open 3 Percutaneous 4 Percutaneous Endoscopic	C Extraluminal Device D Intraluminal Device Z No Device	Z No Qualifier
E Internal Iliac Artery, Right	0 Open 3 Percutaneous 4 Percutaneous Endoscopic	C Extraluminal Device D Intraluminal Device Z No Device	T Uterine Artery, Right V Prostatic Artery, Right Z No Qualifier
F Internal Iliac Artery, Left	0 Open 3 Percutaneous 4 Percutaneous Endoscopic	C Extraluminal Device D Intraluminal Device Z No Device	U Uterine Artery, Left W Prostatic Artery, Left Z No Qualifier

Section	0	Medical and Surgical
Body System	4	Lower Arteries
Operation	N	Release: Freeing a body part from an abnormal physical constraint by cutting or by the use of force

Body Part (4th)	Approach (5th)	Device (6th)	Qualifier (7th)
0 Abdominal Aorta 1 Celiac Artery 2 Gastric Artery 3 Hepatic Artery 4 Splenic Artery 5 Superior Mesenteric Artery 6 Colic Artery, Right 7 Colic Artery, Left 8 Colic Artery, Middle 9 Renal Artery, Right A Renal Artery, Left B Inferior Mesenteric Artery C Common Iliac Artery, Right D Common Iliac Artery, Left E Internal Iliac Artery, Right F Internal Iliac Artery, Left H External Iliac Artery, Right J External Iliac Artery, Left K Femoral Artery, Right L Femoral Artery, Left M Popliteal Artery, Right N Popliteal Artery, Left P Anterior Tibial Artery, Right Q Anterior Tibial Artery, Left R Posterior Tibial Artery, Right S Posterior Tibial Artery, Left T Peroneal Artery, Right U Peroneal Artery, Left V Foot Artery, Right W Foot Artery, Left Y Lower Artery	0 Open 3 Percutaneous 4 Percutaneous Endoscopic	Z No Device	Z No Qualifier

Section	0	Medical and Surgical
Body System	4	Lower Arteries
Operation	P	Removal: Taking out or off a device from a body part

Body Part (4th)	Approach (5th)	Device (6th)	Qualifier (7th)
Y Lower Artery	0 Open 3 Percutaneous 4 Percutaneous Endoscopic	0 Drainage Device 2 Monitoring Device 3 Infusion Device 7 Autologous Tissue Substitute C Extraluminal Device D Intraluminal Device J Synthetic Substitute K Nonautologous Tissue Substitute Y Other Device	Z No Qualifier
Y Lower Artery	X External	0 Drainage Device 1 Radioactive Element 2 Monitoring Device 3 Infusion Device D Intraluminal Device	Z No Qualifier

Section	0	Medical and Surgical
Body System	4	Lower Arteries
Operation	Q	**Repair:** Restoring, to the extent possible, a body part to its normal anatomic structure and function

Body Part (4th)	Approach (5th)	Device (6th)	Qualifier (7th)
0 Abdominal Aorta	**0** Open	**Z** No Device	**Z** No Qualifier
1 Celiac Artery	**3** Percutaneous		
2 Gastric Artery	**4** Percutaneous		
3 Hepatic Artery	Endoscopic		
4 Splenic Artery			
5 Superior Mesenteric Artery			
6 Colic Artery, Right			
7 Colic Artery, Left			
8 Colic Artery, Middle			
9 Renal Artery, Right			
A Renal Artery, Left			
B Inferior Mesenteric Artery			
C Common Iliac Artery, Right			
D Common Iliac Artery, Left			
E Internal Iliac Artery, Right			
F Internal Iliac Artery, Left			
H External Iliac Artery, Right			
J External Iliac Artery, Left			
K Femoral Artery, Right			
L Femoral Artery, Left			
M Popliteal Artery, Right			
N Popliteal Artery, Left			
P Anterior Tibial Artery, Right			
Q Anterior Tibial Artery, Left			
R Posterior Tibial Artery, Right			
S Posterior Tibial Artery, Left			
T Peroneal Artery, Right			
U Peroneal Artery, Left			
V Foot Artery, Right			
W Foot Artery, Left			
Y Lower Artery			

Section	0	Medical and Surgical
Body System	4	Lower Arteries
Operation	R	Replacement: Putting in or on biological or synthetic material that physically takes the place and/or function of all or a portion of a body part

Body Part (4th)	Approach (5th)	Device (6th)	Qualifier (7th)
0 Abdominal Aorta	0 Open	7 Autologous Tissue Substitute	Z No Qualifier
1 Celiac Artery	4 Percutaneous Endoscopic	J Synthetic Substitute	
2 Gastric Artery		K Nonautologous Tissue Substitute	
3 Hepatic Artery			
4 Splenic Artery			
5 Superior Mesenteric Artery			
6 Colic Artery, Right			
7 Colic Artery, Left			
8 Colic Artery, Middle			
9 Renal Artery, Right			
A Renal Artery, Left			
B Inferior Mesenteric Artery			
C Common Iliac Artery, Right			
D Common Iliac Artery, Left			
E Internal Iliac Artery, Right			
F Internal Iliac Artery, Left			
H External Iliac Artery, Right			
J External Iliac Artery, Left			
K Femoral Artery, Right			
L Femoral Artery, Left			
M Popliteal Artery, Right			
N Popliteal Artery, Left			
P Anterior Tibial Artery, Right			
Q Anterior Tibial Artery, Left			
R Posterior Tibial Artery, Right			
S Posterior Tibial Artery, Left			
T Peroneal Artery, Right			
U Peroneal Artery, Left			
V Foot Artery, Right			
W Foot Artery, Left			
Y Lower Artery			

	Section	0	Medical and Surgical
	Body System	4	Lower Arteries
	Operation	S	Reposition: Moving to its normal location, or other suitable location, all or a portion of a body part

Body Part (4th)	Approach (5th)	Device (6th)	Qualifier (7th)
0 Abdominal Aorta	0 Open	Z No Device	Z No Qualifier
1 Celiac Artery	3 Percutaneous		
2 Gastric Artery	4 Percutaneous Endoscopic		
3 Hepatic Artery			
4 Splenic Artery			
5 Superior Mesenteric Artery			
6 Colic Artery, Right			
7 Colic Artery, Left			
8 Colic Artery, Middle			
9 Renal Artery, Right			
A Renal Artery, Left			
B Inferior Mesenteric Artery			
C Common Iliac Artery, Right			
D Common Iliac Artery, Left			
E Internal Iliac Artery, Right			
F Internal Iliac Artery, Left			
H External Iliac Artery, Right			
J External Iliac Artery, Left			
K Femoral Artery, Right			
L Femoral Artery, Left			
M Popliteal Artery, Right			
N Popliteal Artery, Left			
P Anterior Tibial Artery, Right			
Q Anterior Tibial Artery, Left			
R Posterior Tibial Artery, Right			
S Posterior Tibial Artery, Left			
T Peroneal Artery, Right			
U Peroneal Artery, Left			
V Foot Artery, Right			
W Foot Artery, Left			
Y Lower Artery			

Section	0	**Medical and Surgical**
Body System	4	**Lower Arteries**
Operation	U	**Supplement:** Putting in or on biological or synthetic material that physically reinforces and/or augments the function of a portion of a body part

Body Part (4ᵗʰ)	Approach (5ᵗʰ)	Device (6ᵗʰ)	Qualifier (7ᵗʰ)
0 Abdominal Aorta 1 Celiac Artery 2 Gastric Artery 3 Hepatic Artery 4 Splenic Artery 5 Superior Mesenteric Artery 6 Colic Artery, Right 7 Colic Artery, Left 8 Colic Artery, Middle 9 Renal Artery, Right A Renal Artery, Left B Inferior Mesenteric Artery C Common Iliac Artery, Right D Common Iliac Artery, Left E Internal Iliac Artery, Right F Internal Iliac Artery, Left H External Iliac Artery, Right J External Iliac Artery, Left K Femoral Artery, Right L Femoral Artery, Left M Popliteal Artery, Right N Popliteal Artery, Left P Anterior Tibial Artery, Right Q Anterior Tibial Artery, Left R Posterior Tibial Artery, Right S Posterior Tibial Artery, Left T Peroneal Artery, Right U Peroneal Artery, Left V Foot Artery, Right W Foot Artery, Left Y Lower Artery	0 Open 3 Percutaneous 4 Percutaneous Endoscopic	7 Autologous Tissue Substitute J Synthetic Substitute K Nonautologous Tissue Substitute	Z No Qualifier

Section	0	**Medical and Surgical**
Body System	4	**Lower Arteries**
Operation	V	**Restriction:** Partially closing an orifice or the lumen of a tubular body part

Body Part (4ᵗʰ)	Approach (5ᵗʰ)	Device (6ᵗʰ)	Qualifier (7ᵗʰ)
0 Abdominal Aorta	0 Open 3 Percutaneous 4 Percutaneous Endoscopic	C Extraluminal Device E Intraluminal Device, Branched or Fenestrated, One or Two Arteries F Intraluminal Device, Branched or Fenestrated, Three or More Arteries Z No Device	Z No Qualifier
0 Abdominal Aorta	0 Open 3 Percutaneous 4 Percutaneous Endoscopic	D Intraluminal Device	J Temporary Z No Qualifier

Continued →

Section	0	Medical and Surgical
Body System	4	Lower Arteries
Operation	V	Restriction: Partially closing an orifice or the lumen of a tubular body part

04V Continued

Body Part (4th)	Approach (5th)	Device (6th)	Qualifier (7th)
1 Celiac Artery 2 Gastric Artery 3 Hepatic Artery 4 Splenic Artery 5 Superior Mesenteric Artery 6 Colic Artery, Right 7 Colic Artery, Left 8 Colic Artery, Middle 9 Renal Artery, Right A Renal Artery, Left B Inferior Mesenteric Artery E Internal Iliac Artery, Right F Internal Iliac Artery, Left H External Iliac Artery, Right J External Iliac Artery, Left K Femoral Artery, Right L Femoral Artery, Left M Popliteal Artery, Right N Popliteal Artery, Left P Anterior Tibial Artery, Right Q Anterior Tibial Artery, Left R Posterior Tibial Artery, Right S Posterior Tibial Artery, Left T Peroneal Artery, Right U Peroneal Artery, Left V Foot Artery, Right W Foot Artery, Left Y Lower Artery	0 Open 3 Percutaneous 4 Percutaneous Endoscopic	C Extraluminal Device D Intraluminal Device Z No Device	Z No Qualifier
C Common Iliac Artery, Right D Common Iliac Artery, Left	0 Open 3 Percutaneous 4 Percutaneous Endoscopic	C Extraluminal Device D Intraluminal Device E Intraluminal Device, Branched or Fenestrated, One or Two Arteries Z No Device	Z No Qualifier

Section	0	Medical and Surgical
Body System	4	Lower Arteries
Operation	W	Revision: Correcting, to the extent possible, a portion of a malfunctioning device or the position of a displaced device

Body Part (4th)	Approach (5th)	Device (6th)	Qualifier (7th)
Y Lower Artery	0 Open 3 Percutaneous 4 Percutaneous Endoscopic	0 Drainage Device 2 Monitoring Device 3 Infusion Device 7 Autologous Tissue Substitute C Extraluminal Device D Intraluminal Device J Synthetic Substitute K Nonautologous Tissue Substitute Y Other Device	Z No Qualifier
Y Lower Artery	X External	0 Drainage Device 2 Monitoring Device 3 Infusion Device 7 Autologous Tissue Substitute C Extraluminal Device D Intraluminal Device J Synthetic Substitute K Nonautologus Tissue Substitute	Z No Qualifier

AHA Coding Clinic

04100JH Bypass Abdominal Aorta to Right Femoral Artery with Synthetic Substitute, Open Approach—AHA CC: 3Q, 2022, 5-6

04100Z3 Bypass Abdominal Aorta to Right Renal Artery, Open Approach—AHA CC: 3Q, 2015, 28

04130Z3 Bypass Hepatic Artery to Right Renal Artery, Open Approach—AHA CC: 4Q, 2017, 47

04140Z4 Bypass Splenic Artery to Left Renal Artery, Open Approach—AHA CC: 3Q, 2015, 28; 4Q, 2017, 47

041C0J2 Bypass Right Common Iliac Artery to Mesenteric Artery with Synthetic Substitute, Open Approach—AHA CC: 3Q, 2017, 16

041C0J5 Bypass Right Common Iliac Artery to Bilateral Renal Artery with Synthetic Substitute, Open Approach—AHA CC: 3Q, 2017, 16

041K09N Bypass Right Femoral Artery to Posterior Tibial Artery with Autologous Venous Tissue, Open Approach—AHA CC: 3Q, 2017, 5-6

041K0JL Bypass Right Femoral Artery to Popliteal Artery with Synthetic Substitute, Open Approach—AHA CC: 3Q, 2018, 25

041K0JN Bypass Right Femoral Artery to Posterior Tibial Artery with Synthetic Substitute, Open Approach—AHA CC: 2Q, 2016, 18-19; 3Q, 2017, 5-6

041M09P Bypass Right Popliteal Artery to Foot Artery with Autologous Venous Tissue, Open Approach—AHA CC: 1Q, 2017, 32-33

047H3Z1 Dilation of Right External Iliac Artery using Drug-Coated Balloon, Percutaneous Approach—AHA CC: 4Q, 2020, 50-51

047K3D1 Dilation of Right Femoral Artery with Intraluminal Device, using Drug-Coated Balloon, Percutaneous Approach—AHA CC: 4Q, 2015, 7,15

047K3Z1 Dilation of Right Femoral Artery using Drug-Coated Balloon, Percutaneous Approach—AHA CC: 4Q, 2020, 50-51

047K3Z6 Dilation of Right Femoral Artery, Bifurcation, Percutaneous Approach—AHA CC: 4Q, 2016, 88-89

047L3Z1 Dilation of Left Femoral Artery using Drug-Coated Balloon, Percutaneous Approach—AHA CC: 4Q, 2015, 15

04CH0ZZ Extirpation of Matter from Right External Iliac Artery, Open Approach—AHA CC: 1Q, 2021, 15-16

04CJ0ZZ Extirpation of Matter from Left External Iliac Artery, Open Approach—AHA CC: 1Q, 2016, 31; 1Q, 2021, 15-16

04CK3Z6 Extirpation of Matter from Right Femoral Artery, Bifurcation, Percutaneous Approach—AHA CC: 4Q, 2016, 88-89

04CL3ZZ Extirpation of Matter from Left Femoral Artery, Percutaneous Approach—AHA CC: 1Q, 2015, 36

04FC3ZZ Fragmentation of Right Common Iliac Artery, Percutaneous Approach—AHA CC: 4Q, 2020, 51-52

04FH3ZZ Fragmentation of Right External Iliac Artery, Percutaneous Approach—AHA CC: 4Q, 2020, 50-52

04FK3ZZ Fragmentation of Right Femoral Artery, Percutaneous Approach—AHA CC: 4Q, 2020, 50-51

04H03DZ Insertion of Intraluminal Device into Abdominal Aorta, Percutaneous Approach—AHA CC: 3Q, 2022, 19-20

04H13DZ Insertion of Intraluminal Device into Celiac Artery, Percutaneous Approach—AHA CC: 1Q, 2019, 23

04H53DZ Insertion of Intraluminal Device into Superior Mesenteric Artery, Percutaneous Approach—AHA CC: 1Q, 2019, 23

04H93DZ Insertion of Intraluminal Device into Right Renal Artery, Percutaneous Approach—AHA CC: 1Q, 2019, 23

04HA3DZ Insertion of Intraluminal Device into Left Renal Artery, Percutaneous Approach—AHA CC: 1Q, 2019, 23

04HY32Z Insertion of Monitoring Device into Lower Artery, Percutaneous Approach—AHA CC: 1Q, 2017, 30

04HY33Z Insertion of Infusion Device into Lower Artery, Percutaneous Approach—AHA CC: 3Q, 2019, 20-21

04JY3ZZ Inspection of Lower Artery, Percutaneous Approach—AHA CC: 4Q, 2022, 56

04L24ZZ Occlusion of Gastric Artery, Percutaneous Endoscopic Approach—AHA CC: 3Q, 2020, 43

04L33DZ Occlusion of Hepatic Artery with Intraluminal Device, Percutaneous Approach—AHA CC: 3Q, 2014, 26-27

04L73DZ Occlusion of Left Colic Artery with Intraluminal Device, Percutaneous Approach—AHA CC: 1Q, 2014, 24

04LB3DZ Occlusion of Inferior Mesenteric Artery with Intraluminal Device, Percutaneous Approach—AHA CC: 1Q, 2014, 24

04LE3DT Occlusion of Right Uterine Artery with Intraluminal Device, Percutaneous Approach—AHA CC: 2Q, 2015, 27

04LE3DV Occlusion of Right Prostatic Artery with Intraluminal Device, Percutaneous Approach—AHA CC: 4Q, 2022, 56

04LH0CZ Occlusion of Right External Iliac Artery with Extraluminal Device, Open Approach—AHA CC: 2Q, 2018, 18-19

04LJ0CZ Occlusion of Left External Iliac Artery with Extraluminal Device, Open Approach—AHA CC: 2Q, 2018, 18-19

04N10ZZ Release Celiac Artery, Open Approach—AHA CC: 2Q, 2015, 28

04PY33Z Removal of Infusion Device from Lower Artery, Percutaneous Approach—AHA CC: 3Q, 2019, 20-21

04QK0ZZ Repair Right Femoral Artery, Open Approach—AHA CC: 1Q, 2014, 21-22

04R00JZ Replacement of Abdominal Aorta with Synthetic Substitute, Open Approach—AHA CC: 3Q, 2022, 5-6

04R10JZ Replacement of Celiac Artery with Synthetic Substitute, Open Approach—AHA CC: 2Q, 2015, 28

04RD0JZ Replacement of Left Common Iliac Artery with Synthetic Substitute, Open Approach—AHA CC: 3Q, 2022, 5-6

04UJ0KZ Supplement Left External Iliac Artery with Nonautologous Tissue Substitute, Open Approach—AHA CC: 1Q, 2016, 31

04UK0KZ Supplement Right Femoral Artery with Nonautologous Tissue Substitute, Open Approach—AHA CC: 4Q, 2014, 37-38

04UK3JZ Supplement Right Femoral Artery with Synthetic Substitute, Percutaneous Approach—AHA CC: 1Q, 2014, 22-23

04UR07Z Supplement Right Posterior Tibial Artery with Autologous Tissue Substitute, Open Approach—AHA CC: 2Q, 2016, 18-19

04V00DZ Restriction of Abdominal Aorta with Intraluminal Device, Open Approach—AHA CC: 1Q, 2019, 22

04V03DZ Restriction of Abdominal Aorta with Intraluminal Device, Percutaneous Approach—AHA CC: 1Q, 2014, 9; 3Q, 2016, 39

04V03E6 Restriction of Abdominal Aorta, Bifurcation, with Branched or Fenestrated Intraluminal Device, One or Two Arteries, Percutaneous Approach—AHA CC: 4Q, 2016, 91-92

04V03F6 Restriction of Abdominal Aorta, Bifurcation, with Branched or Fenestrated Intraluminal Device, Three or More Arteries, Percutaneous Approach—AHA CC: 4Q, 2016, 92-94

04V43DZ Restriction of Splenic Artery with Intraluminal Device, Percutaneous Approach—AHA CC: 3Q, 2021, 23

04VC3EZ Restriction of Right Common Iliac Artery with Branched or Fenestrated Intraluminal Device, One or Two Arteries, Percutaneous Approach—AHA CC: 4Q, 2016, 93-94

04VD3EZ Restriction of Left Common Iliac Artery with Branched or Fenestrated Intraluminal Device, One or Two Arteries, Percutaneous Approach—AHA CC: 4Q, 2016, 93-94

04WY07Z Revision of Autologous Tissue Substitute in Lower Artery, Open Approach—AHA CC: 1Q, 2015, 36-37

04WY0JZ Revision of Synthetic Substitute in Lower Artery, Open Approach—AHA CC: 2Q, 2019, 14-15

04WY37Z Revision of Autologous Tissue Substitute in Lower Artery, Percutaneous Approach—AHA CC: 1Q, 2014, 22

04WY3DZ Revision of Intraluminal Device in Lower Artery, Percutaneous Approach—AHA CC: 1Q, 2014, 9-10; 3Q, 2020, 6

Upper Veins

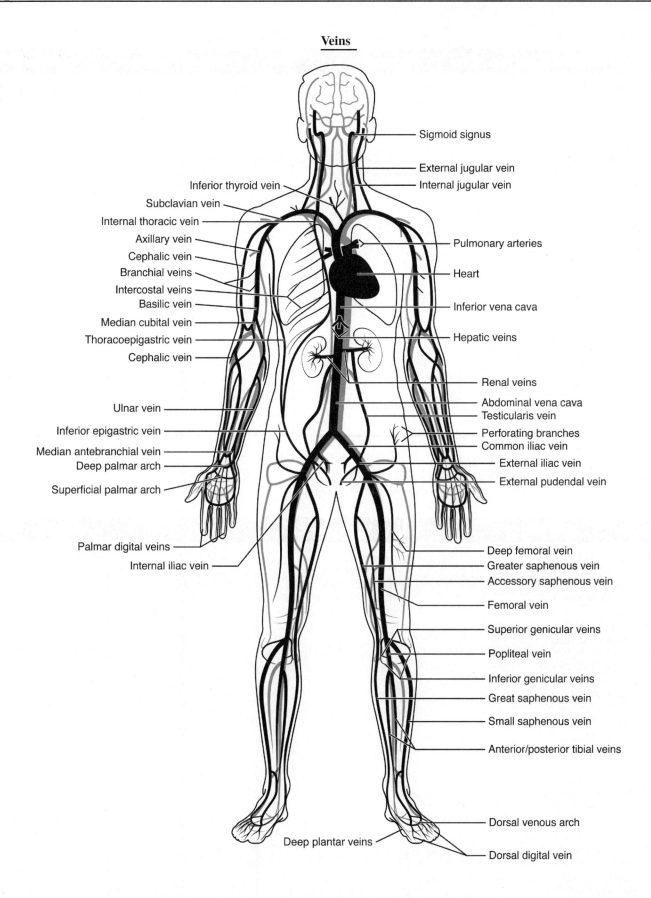

Upper Veins Tables 051–05W

Section	0	Medical and Surgical
Body System	5	Upper Veins
Operation	1	**Bypass:** Altering the route of passage of the contents of a tubular body part

Body Part (4th)	Approach (5th)	Device (6th)	Qualifier (7th)
0 Azygos Vein	0 Open	7 Autologous Tissue Substitute	Y Upper Vein
1 Hemiazygos Vein	4 Percutaneous Endoscopic	9 Autologous Venous Tissue	
3 Innominate Vein, Right		A Autologous Arterial Tissue	
4 Innominate Vein, Left		J Synthetic Substitute	
5 Subclavian Vein, Right		K Nonautologous Tissue Substitute	
6 Subclavian Vein, Left		Z No Device	
7 Axillary Vein, Right			
8 Axillary Vein, Left			
9 Brachial Vein, Right			
A Brachial Vein, Left			
B Basilic Vein, Right			
C Basilic Vein, Left			
D Cephalic Vein, Right			
F Cephalic Vein, Left			
G Hand Vein, Right			
H Hand Vein, Left			
L Intracranial Vein			
M Internal Jugular Vein, Right			
N Internal Jugular Vein, Left			
P External Jugular Vein, Right			
Q External Jugular Vein, Left			
R Vertebral Vein, Right			
S Vertebral Vein, Left			
T Face Vein, Right			
V Face Vein, Left			

Section	0	Medical and Surgical
Body System	5	Upper Veins
Operation	5	**Destruction:** Physical eradication of all or a portion of a body part by the direct use of energy, force, or a destructive agent

Body Part (4th)	Approach (5th)	Device (6th)	Qualifier (7th)
0 Azygos Vein	0 Open	Z No Device	Z No Qualifier
1 Hemiazygos Vein	3 Percutaneous		
3 Innominate Vein, Right	4 Percutaneous Endoscopic		
4 Innominate Vein, Left			
5 Subclavian Vein, Right			
6 Subclavian Vein, Left			
7 Axillary Vein, Right			
8 Axillary Vein, Left			
9 Brachial Vein, Right			
A Brachial Vein, Left			
B Basilic Vein, Right			
C Basilic Vein, Left			
D Cephalic Vein, Right			
F Cephalic Vein, Left			
G Hand Vein, Right			
H Hand Vein, Left			
L Intracranial Vein			
M Internal Jugular Vein, Right			
N Internal Jugular Vein, Left			
P External Jugular Vein, Right			
Q External Jugular Vein, Left			
R Vertebral Vein, Right			
S Vertebral Vein, Left			
T Face Vein, Right			
V Face Vein, Left			
Y Upper Vein			

Section	0	Medical and Surgical
Body System	5	Upper Veins
Operation	7	**Dilation:** Expanding an orifice or the lumen of a tubular body part

Body Part (4th)	Approach (5th)	Device (6th)	Qualifier (7th)
0 Azygos Vein 1 Hemiazygos Vein G Hand Vein, Right H Hand Vein, Left L Intracranial Vein M Internal Jugular Vein, Right N Internal Jugular Vein, Left P External Jugular Vein, Right Q External Jugular Vein, Left R Vertebral Vein, Right S Vertebral Vein, Left T Face Vein, Right V Face Vein, Left Y Upper Vein	0 Open 3 Percutaneous 4 Percutaneous Endoscopic	D Intraluminal Device Z No Device	Z No Qualifier
3 Innominate Vein, Right 4 Innominate Vein, Left 5 Subclavian Vein, Right 6 Subclavian Vein, Left 7 Axillary Vein, Right 8 Axillary Vein, Left 9 Brachial Vein, Right A Brachial Vein, Left B Basilic Vein, Right C Basilic Vein, Left D Cephalic Vein, Right F Cephalic Vein, Left	0 Open 3 Percutaneous 4 Percutaneous Endoscopic	D Intraluminal Device Z No Device	1 Drug-Coated Balloon Z No Qualifier

Section	0	Medical and Surgical
Body System	5	Upper Veins
Operation	9	**Drainage:** Taking or letting out fluids and/or gases from a body part

Body Part (4th)	Approach (5th)	Device (6th)	Qualifier (7th)
0 Azygos Vein 1 Hemiazygos Vein 3 Innominate Vein, Right 4 Innominate Vein, Left 5 Subclavian Vein, Right 6 Subclavian Vein, Left 7 Axillary Vein, Right 8 Axillary Vein, Left 9 Brachial Vein, Right A Brachial Vein, Left B Basilic Vein, Right C Basilic Vein, Left D Cephalic Vein, Right F Cephalic Vein, Left G Hand Vein, Right H Hand Vein, Left L Intracranial Vein M Internal Jugular Vein, Right N Internal Jugular Vein, Left P External Jugular Vein, Right Q External Jugular Vein, Left R Vertebral Vein, Right S Vertebral Vein, Left T Face Vein, Right V Face Vein, Left Y Upper Vein	0 Open 3 Percutaneous 4 Percutaneous Endoscopic	0 Drainage Device	Z No Qualifier

Continued →

059–05B

Medical and Surgical, Upper Veins Tables

Section	0	Medical and Surgical	*059 Continued*
Body System	5	Upper Veins	
Operation	9	Drainage: Taking or letting out fluids and/or gases from a body part	

Body Part (4th)	Approach (5th)	Device (6th)	Qualifier (7th)
0 Azygos Vein	0 Open	Z No Device	X Diagnostic
1 Hemiazygos Vein	3 Percutaneous		Z No Qualifier
3 Innominate Vein, Right	4 Percutaneous Endoscopic		
4 Innominate Vein, Left			
5 Subclavian Vein, Right			
6 Subclavian Vein, Left			
7 Axillary Vein, Right			
8 Axillary Vein, Left			
9 Brachial Vein, Right			
A Brachial Vein, Left			
B Basilic Vein, Right			
C Basilic Vein, Left			
D Cephalic Vein, Right			
F Cephalic Vein, Left			
G Hand Vein, Right			
H Hand Vein, Left			
L Intracranial Vein			
M Internal Jugular Vein, Right			
N Internal Jugular Vein, Left			
P External Jugular Vein, Right			
Q External Jugular Vein, Left			
R Vertebral Vein, Right			
S Vertebral Vein, Left			
T Face Vein, Right			
V Face Vein, Left			
Y Upper Vein			

Section	0	Medical and Surgical
Body System	5	Upper Veins
Operation	B	Excision: Cutting out or off, without replacement, a portion of a body part

Body Part (4th)	Approach (5th)	Device (6th)	Qualifier (7th)
0 Azygos Vein	0 Open	Z No Device	X Diagnostic
1 Hemiazygos Vein	3 Percutaneous		Z No Qualifier
3 Innominate Vein, Right	4 Percutaneous Endoscopic		
4 Innominate Vein, Left			
5 Subclavian Vein, Right			
6 Subclavian Vein, Left			
7 Axillary Vein, Right			
8 Axillary Vein, Left			
9 Brachial Vein, Right			
A Brachial Vein, Left			
B Basilic Vein, Right			
C Basilic Vein, Left			
D Cephalic Vein, Right			
F Cephalic Vein, Left			
G Hand Vein, Right			
H Hand Vein, Left			
L Intracranial Vein			
M Internal Jugular Vein, Right			
N Internal Jugular Vein, Left			
P External Jugular Vein, Right			
Q External Jugular Vein, Left			
R Vertebral Vein, Right			
S Vertebral Vein, Left			
T Face Vein, Right			
V Face Vein, Left			
Y Upper Vein			

Section	0	Medical and Surgical
Body System	5	Upper Veins
Operation	C	Extirpation: Taking or cutting out solid matter from a body part

Body Part (4th)	Approach (5th)	Device (6th)	Qualifier (7th)
0 Azygos Vein	0 Open	Z No Device	Z No Qualifier
1 Hemiazygos Vein	3 Percutaneous		
3 Innominate Vein, Right	4 Percutaneous Endoscopic		
4 Innominate Vein, Left			
5 Subclavian Vein, Right			
6 Subclavian Vein, Left			
7 Axillary Vein, Right			
8 Axillary Vein, Left			
9 Brachial Vein, Right			
A Brachial Vein, Left			
B Basilic Vein, Right			
C Basilic Vein, Left			
D Cephalic Vein, Right			
F Cephalic Vein, Left			
G Hand Vein, Right			
H Hand Vein, Left			
L Intracranial Vein			
M Internal Jugular Vein, Right			
N Internal Jugular Vein, Left			
P External Jugular Vein, Right			
Q External Jugular Vein, Left			
R Vertebral Vein, Right			
S Vertebral Vein, Left			
T Face Vein, Right			
V Face Vein, Left			
Y Upper Vein			

Section	0	Medical and Surgical
Body System	5	Upper Veins
Operation	D	Extraction: Pulling or stripping out or off all or a portion of a body part by the use of force

Body Part (4th)	Approach (5th)	Device (6th)	Qualifier (7th)
9 Brachial Vein, Right	0 Open	Z No Device	Z No Qualifier
A Brachial Vein, Left	3 Percutaneous		
B Basilic Vein, Right			
C Basilic Vein, Left			
D Cephalic Vein, Right			
F Cephalic Vein, Left			
G Hand Vein, Right			
H Hand Vein, Left			
Y Upper Vein			

Section	0	Medical and Surgical
Body System	5	Upper Veins
Operation	F	Fragmentation: Breaking solid matter in a body part into pieces

Body Part (4th)	Approach (5th)	Device (6th)	Qualifier (7th)
3 Innominate Vein, Right	3 Percutaneous	Z No Device	0 Ultrasonic
4 Innominate Vein, Left			Z No Qualifier
5 Subclavian Vein, Right			
6 Subclavian Vein, Left			
7 Axillary Vein, Right			
8 Axillary Vein, Left			
9 Brachial Vein, Right			
A Brachial Vein, Left			
B Basilic Vein, Right			
C Basilic Vein, Left			
D Cephalic Vein, Right			
F Cephalic Vein, Left			
Y Upper Vein			

05H–05J

Section   **0**   **Medical and Surgical**
Body System   **5**   **Upper Veins**
Operation   **H**   **Insertion:** Putting in a nonbiological appliance that monitors, assists, performs, or prevents a physiological function but does not physically take the place of a body part

Body Part (4ᵗʰ)	Approach (5ᵗʰ)	Device (6ᵗʰ)	Qualifier (7ᵗʰ)
0 Azygos Vein	**0** Open **3** Percutaneous **4** Percutaneous Endoscopic	**2** Monitoring Device **3** Infusion Device **D** Intraluminal Device **M** Neurostimulator Lead	**Z** No Qualifier
1 Hemiazygos Vein **5** Subclavian Vein, Right **6** Subclavian Vein, Left **7** Axillary Vein, Right **8** Axillary Vein, Left **9** Brachial Vein, Right **A** Brachial Vein, Left **B** Basilic Vein, Right **C** Basilic Vein, Left **D** Cephalic Vein, Right **F** Cephalic Vein, Left **G** Hand Vein, Right **H** Hand Vein, Left **L** Intracranial Vein **M** Internal Jugular Vein, Right **N** Internal Jugular Vein, Left **P** External Jugular Vein, Right **Q** External Jugular Vein, Left **R** Vertebral Vein, Right **S** Vertebral Vein, Left **T** Face Vein, Right **V** Face Vein, Left	**0** Open **3** Percutaneous **4** Percutaneous Endoscopic	**3** Infusion Device **D** Intraluminal Device	**Z** No Qualifier
3 Innominate Vein, Right **4** Innominate Vein, Left	**0** Open **3** Percutaneous **4** Percutaneous Endoscopic	**3** Infusion Device **D** Intraluminal Device **M** Neurostimulator Lead	**Z** No Qualifier
Y Upper Vein	**0** Open **3** Percutaneous **4** Percutaneous Endoscopic	**2** Monitoring Device **3** Infusion Device **D** Intraluminal Device **Y** Other Device	**Z** No Qualifier

Section   **0**   **Medical and Surgical**
Body System   **5**   **Upper Veins**
Operation   **J**   **Inspection:** Visually and/or manually exploring a body part

Body Part (4ᵗʰ)	Approach (5ᵗʰ)	Device (6ᵗʰ)	Qualifier (7ᵗʰ)
Y Upper Vein	**0** Open **3** Percutaneous **4** Percutaneous Endoscopic **X** External	**Z** No Device	**Z** No Qualifier

Medical and Surgical, Upper Veins Tables

184

Section	0	Medical and Surgical
Body System	5	Upper Veins
Operation	L	Occlusion: Completely closing an orifice or the lumen of a tubular body part

Body Part (4th)	Approach (5th)	Device (6th)	Qualifier (7th)
0 Azygos Vein	0 Open	C Extraluminal Device	Z No Qualifier
1 Hemiazygos Vein	3 Percutaneous	D Intraluminal Device	
3 Innominate Vein, Right	4 Percutaneous Endoscopic	Z No Device	
4 Innominate Vein, Left			
5 Subclavian Vein, Right			
6 Subclavian Vein, Left			
7 Axillary Vein, Right			
8 Axillary Vein, Left			
9 Brachial Vein, Right			
A Brachial Vein, Left			
B Basilic Vein, Right			
C Basilic Vein, Left			
D Cephalic Vein, Right			
F Cephalic Vein, Left			
G Hand Vein, Right			
H Hand Vein, Left			
L Intracranial Vein			
M Internal Jugular Vein, Right			
N Internal Jugular Vein, Left			
P External Jugular Vein, Right			
Q External Jugular Vein, Left			
R Vertebral Vein, Right			
S Vertebral Vein, Left			
T Face Vein, Right			
V Face Vein, Left			
Y Upper Vein			

Section	0	Medical and Surgical
Body System	5	Upper Veins
Operation	N	Release: Freeing a body part from an abnormal physical constraint by cutting or by the use of force

Body Part (4th)	Approach (5th)	Device (6th)	Qualifier (7th)
0 Azygos Vein	0 Open	Z No Device	Z No Qualifier
1 Hemiazygos Vein	3 Percutaneous		
3 Innominate Vein, Right	4 Percutaneous Endoscopic		
4 Innominate Vein, Left			
5 Subclavian Vein, Right			
6 Subclavian Vein, Left			
7 Axillary Vein, Right			
8 Axillary Vein, Left			
9 Brachial Vein, Right			
A Brachial Vein, Left			
B Basilic Vein, Right			
C Basilic Vein, Left			
D Cephalic Vein, Right			
F Cephalic Vein, Left			
G Hand Vein, Right			
H Hand Vein, Left			
L Intracranial Vein			
M Internal Jugular Vein, Right			
N Internal Jugular Vein, Left			
P External Jugular Vein, Right			
Q External Jugular Vein, Left			
R Vertebral Vein, Right			
S Vertebral Vein, Left			
T Face Vein, Right			
V Face Vein, Left			
Y Upper Vein			

05P–05Q

Medical and Surgical, Upper Veins Tables

Section	0	Medical and Surgical
Body System	5	Upper Veins
Operation	P	Removal: Taking out or off a device from a body part

Body Part (4th)	Approach (5th)	Device (6th)	Qualifier (7th)
0 Azygos Vein	0 Open 3 Percutaneous 4 Percutaneous Endoscopic X External	2 Monitoring Device M Neurostimulator Lead	Z No Qualifier
3 Innominate Vein, Right 4 Innominate Vein, Left	0 Open 3 Percutaneous 4 Percutaneous Endoscopic X External	M Neurostimulator Lead	Z No Qualifier
Y Upper Vein	0 Open 3 Percutaneous 4 Percutaneous Endoscopic	0 Drainage Device 2 Monitoring Device 3 Infusion Device 7 Autologous Tissue Substitute C Extraluminal Device D Intraluminal Device J Synthetic Substitute K Nonautologous Tissue Substitute Y Other Device	Z No Qualifier
Y Upper Vein	X External	0 Drainage Device 2 Monitoring Device 3 Infusion Device D Intraluminal Device	Z No Qualifier

Section	0	Medical and Surgical
Body System	5	Upper Veins
Operation	Q	Repair: Restoring, to the extent possible, a body part to its normal anatomic structure and function

Body Part (4th)	Approach (5th)	Device (6th)	Qualifier (7th)
0 Azygos Vein 1 Hemiazygos Vein 3 Innominate Vein, Right 4 Innominate Vein, Left 5 Subclavian Vein, Right 6 Subclavian Vein, Left 7 Axillary Vein, Right 8 Axillary Vein, Left 9 Brachial Vein, Right A Brachial Vein, Left B Basilic Vein, Right C Basilic Vein, Left D Cephalic Vein, Right F Cephalic Vein, Left G Hand Vein, Right H Hand Vein, Left L Intracranial Vein M Internal Jugular Vein, Right N Internal Jugular Vein, Left P External Jugular Vein, Right Q External Jugular Vein, Left R Vertebral Vein, Right S Vertebral Vein, Left T Face Vein, Right V Face Vein, Left Y Upper Vein	0 Open 3 Percutaneous 4 Percutaneous Endoscopic	Z No Device	Z No Qualifier

186

Section	0	Medical and Surgical
Body System	5	Upper Veins
Operation	R	Replacement: Putting in or on biological or synthetic material that physically takes the place and/or function of all or a portion of a body part

Body Part (4th)	Approach (5th)	Device (6th)	Qualifier (7th)
0 Azygos Vein	0 Open	7 Autologous Tissue Substitute	Z No Qualifier
1 Hemiazygos Vein	4 Percutaneous Endoscopic	J Synthetic Substitute	
3 Innominate Vein, Right		K Nonautologous Tissue Substitute	
4 Innominate Vein, Left			
5 Subclavian Vein, Right			
6 Subclavian Vein, Left			
7 Axillary Vein, Right			
8 Axillary Vein, Left			
9 Brachial Vein, Right			
A Brachial Vein, Left			
B Basilic Vein, Right			
C Basilic Vein, Left			
D Cephalic Vein, Right			
F Cephalic Vein, Left			
G Hand Vein, Right			
H Hand Vein, Left			
L Intracranial Vein			
M Internal Jugular Vein, Right			
N Internal Jugular Vein, Left			
P External Jugular Vein, Right			
Q External Jugular Vein, Left			
R Vertebral Vein, Right			
S Vertebral Vein, Left			
T Face Vein, Right			
V Face Vein, Left			
Y Upper Vein			

Section	0	Medical and Surgical
Body System	5	Upper Veins
Operation	S	Reposition: Moving to its normal location, or other suitable location, all or a portion of a body part

Body Part (4th)	Approach (5th)	Device (6th)	Qualifier (7th)
0 Azygos Vein	0 Open	Z No Device	Z No Qualifier
1 Hemiazygos Vein	3 Percutaneous		
3 Innominate Vein, Right	4 Percutaneous Endoscopic		
4 Innominate Vein, Left			
5 Subclavian Vein, Right			
6 Subclavian Vein, Left			
7 Axillary Vein, Right			
8 Axillary Vein, Left			
9 Brachial Vein, Right			
A Brachial Vein, Left			
B Basilic Vein, Right			
C Basilic Vein, Left			
D Cephalic Vein, Right			
F Cephalic Vein, Left			
G Hand Vein, Right			
H Hand Vein, Left			
L Intracranial Vein			
M Internal Jugular Vein, Right			
N Internal Jugular Vein, Left			
P External Jugular Vein, Right			
Q External Jugular Vein, Left			
R Vertebral Vein, Right			
S Vertebral Vein, Left			
T Face Vein, Right			
V Face Vein, Left			
Y Upper Vein			

	Section	0	Medical and Surgical
	Body System	5	Upper Veins
	Operation	U	Supplement: Putting in or on biological or synthetic material that physically reinforces and/or augments the function of a portion of a body part

Body Part (4th)	Approach (5th)	Device (6th)	Qualifier (7th)
0 Azygos Vein	0 Open	7 Autologous Tissue Substitute	Z No Qualifier
1 Hemiazygos Vein	3 Percutaneous	J Synthetic Substitute	
3 Innominate Vein, Right	4 Percutaneous Endoscopic	K Nonautologous Tissue Substitute	
4 Innominate Vein, Left			
5 Subclavian Vein, Right			
6 Subclavian Vein, Left			
7 Axillary Vein, Right			
8 Axillary Vein, Left			
9 Brachial Vein, Right			
A Brachial Vein, Left			
B Basilic Vein, Right			
C Basilic Vein, Left			
D Cephalic Vein, Right			
F Cephalic Vein, Left			
G Hand Vein, Right			
H Hand Vein, Left			
L Intracranial Vein			
M Internal Jugular Vein, Right			
N Internal Jugular Vein, Left			
P External Jugular Vein, Right			
Q External Jugular Vein, Left			
R Vertebral Vein, Right			
S Vertebral Vein, Left			
T Face Vein, Right			
V Face Vein, Left			
Y Upper Vein			

	Section	0	Medical and Surgical
	Body System	5	Upper Veins
	Operation	V	Restriction: Partially closing an orifice or the lumen of a tubular body part

Body Part (4th)	Approach (5th)	Device (6th)	Qualifier (7th)
0 Azygos Vein	0 Open	C Extraluminal Device	Z No Qualifier
1 Hemiazygos Vein	3 Percutaneous	D Intraluminal Device	
3 Innominate Vein, Right	4 Percutaneous Endoscopic	Z No Device	
4 Innominate Vein, Left			
5 Subclavian Vein, Right			
6 Subclavian Vein, Left			
7 Axillary Vein, Right			
8 Axillary Vein, Left			
9 Brachial Vein, Right			
A Brachial Vein, Left			
B Basilic Vein, Right			
C Basilic Vein, Left			
D Cephalic Vein, Right			
F Cephalic Vein, Left			
G Hand Vein, Right			
H Hand Vein, Left			
L Intracranial Vein			
M Internal Jugular Vein, Right			
N Internal Jugular Vein, Left			
P External Jugular Vein, Right			
Q External Jugular Vein, Left			
R Vertebral Vein, Right			
S Vertebral Vein, Left			
T Face Vein, Right			
V Face Vein, Left			
Y Upper Vein			

Section	0	Medical and Surgical
Body System	5	Upper Veins
Operation	W	Revision: Correcting, to the extent possible, a portion of a malfunctioning device or the position of a displaced device

Body Part (4th)	Approach (5th)	Device (6th)	Qualifier (7th)
0 Azygos Vein	0 Open 3 Percutaneous 4 Percutaneous Endoscopic X External	2 Monitoring Device M Neurostimulator Lead	Z No Qualifier
3 Innominate Vein, Right 4 Innominate Vein, Left	0 Open 3 Percutaneous 4 Percutaneous Endoscopic X External	M Neurostimulator Lead	Z No Qualifier
Y Upper Vein	0 Open 3 Percutaneous 4 Percutaneous Endoscopic	0 Drainage Device 2 Monitoring Device 3 Infusion Device 7 Autologous Tissue Substitute C Extraluminal Device D Intraluminal Device J Synthetic Substitute K Nonautologous Tissue Substitute Y Other Device	Z No Qualifier
Y Upper Vein	X External	0 Drainage Device 2 Monitoring Device 3 Infusion Device 7 Autologous Tissue Substitute C Extraluminal Device D Intraluminal Device J Synthetic Substitute K Nonautologus Tissue Substitute	Z No Qualifier

AHA Coding Clinic

051Q49Y Bypass Left External Jugular Vein to Upper Vein with Autologous Venous Tissue, Percutaneous Endoscopic Approach—AHA CC: 1Q, 2020, 28-29

05733DZ Dilation of Right Innominate Vein with Intraluminal Device, Percutaneous Approach—AHA CC: 3Q, 2020, 38-40

059430Z Drainage of Left Innominate Vein with Drainage Device, Percutaneous Approach—AHA CC: 3Q, 2018, 7

05BD0ZZ Excision of Right Cephalic Vein, Open Approach—AHA CC: 3Q, 2020, 40

05BL0ZZ Excision of Intracranial Vein, Open Approach—AHA CC: 1Q, 2020, 24; 2Q, 2021, 15-16

05BN0ZZ Excision of Left Internal Jugular Vein, Open Approach—AHA CC: 2Q, 2016, 12-14

05BQ0ZZ Excision of Left External Jugular Vein, Open Approach—AHA CC: 2Q, 2016, 12-14

05CD0ZZ Extirpation of Matter from Right Cephalic Vein, Open Approach—AHA CC: 3Q, 2020, 37-40

05H032Z Insertion of Monitoring Device into Azygos Vein, Percutaneous Approach—AHA CC: 4Q, 2016, 98-99

05H43MZ Insertion of Neurostimulator Lead into Left Innominate Vein, Percutaneous Approach—AHA CC: 4Q, 2016, 98-99

05Q40ZZ Repair Left Innominate Vein, Open Approach—AHA CC: 3Q, 2017, 15-16

05SD0ZZ Reposition Right Cephalic Vein, Open Approach—AHA CC: 4Q, 2013, 125-126

05VD0ZZ Restriction of Right Cephalic Vein, Open Approach—AHA CC: 3Q, 2020, 37-38

Lower Veins

Lower Veins Tables 061–06W

Section   0   **Medical and Surgical**
Body System   6   **Lower Veins**
Operation   1   **Bypass:** Altering the route of passage of the contents of a tubular body part

Body Part (4th)	Approach (5th)	Device (6th)	Qualifier (7th)
0 Inferior Vena Cava	0 Open 4 Percutaneous Endoscopic	7 Autologous Tissue Substitute 9 Autologous Venous Tissue A Autologous Arterial Tissue J Synthetic Substitute K Nonautologous Tissue Substitute Z No Device	5 Superior Mesenteric Vein 6 Inferior Mesenteric Vein P Pulmonary Trunk Q Pulmonary Artery, Right R Pulmonary Artery, Left Y Lower Vein
1 Splenic Vein	0 Open 4 Percutaneous Endoscopic	7 Autologous Tissue Substitute 9 Autologous Venous Tissue A Autologous Arterial Tissue J Synthetic Substitute K Nonautologous Tissue Substitute Z No Device	9 Renal Vein, Right B Renal Vein, Left Y Lower Vein
2 Gastric Vein 3 Esophageal Vein 4 Hepatic Vein 5 Superior Mesenteric Vein 6 Inferior Mesenteric Vein 7 Colic Vein 9 Renal Vein, Right B Renal Vein, Left C Common Iliac Vein, Right D Common Iliac Vein, Left F External Iliac Vein, Right G External Iliac Vein, Left H Hypogastric Vein, Right J Hypogastric Vein, Left M Femoral Vein, Right N Femoral Vein, Left P Saphenous Vein, Right Q Saphenous Vein, Left T Foot Vein, Right V Foot Vein, Left	0 Open 4 Percutaneous Endoscopic	7 Autologous Tissue Substitute 9 Autologous Venous Tissue A Autologous Arterial Tissue J Synthetic Substitute K Nonautologous Tissue Substitute Z No Device	Y Lower Vein
8 Portal Vein	0 Open	7 Autologous Tissue Substitute 9 Autologous Venous Tissue A Autologous Arterial Tissue J Synthetic Substitute K Nonautologous Tissue Substitute Z No Device	9 Renal Vein, Right B Renal Vein, Left Y Lower Vein
8 Portal Vein	3 Percutaneous	J Synthetic Substitute	4 Hepatic Vein Y Lower Vein
8 Portal Vein	4 Percutaneous Endoscopic	7 Autologous Tissue Substitute 9 Autologous Venous Tissue A Autologous Arterial Tissue K Nonautologous Tissue Substitute Z No Device	9 Renal Vein, Right B Renal Vein, Left Y Lower Vein
8 Portal Vein	4 Percutaneous Endoscopic	J Synthetic Substitute	4 Hepatic Vein 9 Renal Vein, Right B Renal Vein, Left Y Lower Vein

Section	0	Medical and Surgical
Body System	6	Lower Veins
Operation	5	Destruction: Physical eradication of all or a portion of a body part by the direct use of energy, force, or a destructive agent

Body Part (4th)	Approach (5th)	Device (6th)	Qualifier (7th)
0 Inferior Vena Cava 1 Splenic Vein 2 Gastric Vein 3 Esophageal Vein 4 Hepatic Vein 5 Superior Mesenteric Vein 6 Inferior Mesenteric Vein 7 Colic Vein 8 Portal Vein 9 Renal Vein, Right B Renal Vein, Left C Common Iliac Vein, Right D Common Iliac Vein, Left F External Iliac Vein, Right G External Iliac Vein, Left H Hypogastric Vein, Right J Hypogastric Vein, Left M Femoral Vein, Right N Femoral Vein, Left P Saphenous Vein, Right Q Saphenous Vein, Left T Foot Vein, Right V Foot Vein, Left	0 Open 3 Percutaneous 4 Percutaneous Endoscopic	Z No Device	Z No Qualifier
Y Lower Vein	0 Open 3 Percutaneous 4 Percutaneous Endoscopic	Z No Device	C Hemorrhoidal Plexus Z No Qualifier

Section	0	Medical and Surgical
Body System	6	Lower Veins
Operation	7	Dilation: Expanding an orifice or the lumen of a tubular body part

Body Part (4th)	Approach (5th)	Device (6th)	Qualifier (7th)
0 Inferior Vena Cava 1 Splenic Vein 2 Gastric Vein 3 Esophageal Vein 4 Hepatic Vein 5 Superior Mesenteric Vein 6 Inferior Mesenteric Vein 7 Colic Vein 8 Portal Vein 9 Renal Vein, Right B Renal Vein, Left C Common Iliac Vein, Right D Common Iliac Vein, Left F External Iliac Vein, Right G External Iliac Vein, Left H Hypogastric Vein, Right J Hypogastric Vein, Left M Femoral Vein, Right N Femoral Vein, Left P Saphenous Vein, Right Q Saphenous Vein, Left T Foot Vein, Right V Foot Vein, Left Y Lower Vein	0 Open 3 Percutaneous 4 Percutaneous Endoscopic	D Intraluminal Device Z No Device	Z No Qualifier

Section	0	Medical and Surgical
Body System	6	Lower Veins
Operation	9	**Drainage:** Taking or letting out fluids and/or gases from a body part

Body Part (4th)	Approach (5th)	Device (6th)	Qualifier (7th)
0 Inferior Vena Cava	**0** Open	**0** Drainage Device	**Z** No Qualifier
1 Splenic Vein	**3** Percutaneous		
2 Gastric Vein	**4** Percutaneous Endoscopic		
3 Esophageal Vein			
4 Hepatic Vein			
5 Superior Mesenteric Vein			
6 Inferior Mesenteric Vein			
7 Colic Vein			
8 Portal Vein			
9 Renal Vein, Right			
B Renal Vein, Left			
C Common Iliac Vein, Right			
D Common Iliac Vein, Left			
F External Iliac Vein, Right			
G External Iliac Vein, Left			
H Hypogastric Vein, Right			
J Hypogastric Vein, Left			
M Femoral Vein, Right			
N Femoral Vein, Left			
P Saphenous Vein, Right			
Q Saphenous Vein, Left			
T Foot Vein, Right			
V Foot Vein, Left			
Y Lower Vein			
0 Inferior Vena Cava	**0** Open	**Z** No Device	**X** Diagnostic
1 Splenic Vein	**3** Percutaneous		**Z** No Qualifier
2 Gastric Vein	**4** Percutaneous Endoscopic		
3 Esophageal Vein			
4 Hepatic Vein			
5 Superior Mesenteric Vein			
6 Inferior Mesenteric Vein			
7 Colic Vein			
8 Portal Vein			
9 Renal Vein, Right			
B Renal Vein, Left			
C Common Iliac Vein, Right			
D Common Iliac Vein, Left			
F External Iliac Vein, Right			
G External Iliac Vein, Left			
H Hypogastric Vein, Right			
J Hypogastric Vein, Left			
M Femoral Vein, Right			
N Femoral Vein, Left			
P Saphenous Vein, Right			
Q Saphenous Vein, Left			
T Foot Vein, Right			
V Foot Vein, Left			
Y Lower Vein			

06B–06C

Medical and Surgical, Lower Veins Tables

Section	0	Medical and Surgical
Body System	6	Lower Veins
Operation	B	**Excision:** Cutting out or off, without replacement, a portion of a body part

Body Part (4th)	Approach (5th)	Device (6th)	Qualifier (7th)
0 Inferior Vena Cava **1** Splenic Vein **2** Gastric Vein **3** Esophageal Vein **4** Hepatic Vein **5** Superior Mesenteric Vein **6** Inferior Mesenteric Vein **7** Colic Vein **8** Portal Vein **9** Renal Vein, Right **B** Renal Vein, Left **C** Common Iliac Vein, Right **D** Common Iliac Vein, Left **F** External Iliac Vein, Right **G** External Iliac Vein, Left **H** Hypogastric Vein, Right **J** Hypogastric Vein, Left **M** Femoral Vein, Right **N** Femoral Vein, Left **P** Saphenous Vein, Right **Q** Saphenous Vein, Left **T** Foot Vein, Right **V** Foot Vein, Left	**0** Open **3** Percutaneous **4** Percutaneous Endoscopic	**Z** No Device	**X** Diagnostic **Z** No Qualifier
Y Lower Vein	**0** Open **3** Percutaneous **4** Percutaneous Endoscopic	**Z** No Device	**C** Hemorrhoidal Plexus **X** Diagnostic **Z** No Qualifier

Section	0	Medical and Surgical
Body System	6	Lower Veins
Operation	C	**Extirpation:** Taking or cutting out solid matter from a body part

Body Part (4th)	Approach (5th)	Device (6th)	Qualifier (7th)
0 Inferior Vena Cava **1** Splenic Vein **2** Gastric Vein **3** Esophageal Vein **4** Hepatic Vein **5** Superior Mesenteric Vein **6** Inferior Mesenteric Vein **7** Colic Vein **8** Portal Vein **9** Renal Vein, Right **B** Renal Vein, Left **C** Common Iliac Vein, Right **D** Common Iliac Vein, Left **F** External Iliac Vein, Right **G** External Iliac Vein, Left **H** Hypogastric Vein, Right **J** Hypogastric Vein, Left **M** Femoral Vein, Right **N** Femoral Vein, Left **P** Saphenous Vein, Right **Q** Saphenous Vein, Left **T** Foot Vein, Right **V** Foot Vein, Left **Y** Lower Vein	**0** Open **3** Percutaneous **4** Percutaneous Endoscopic	**Z** No Device	**Z** No Qualifier

194

Section	0	Medical and Surgical
Body System	6	Lower Veins
Operation	D	**Extraction:** Pulling or stripping out or off all or a portion of a body part by the use of force

Body Part (4th)	Approach (5th)	Device (6th)	Qualifier (7th)
M Femoral Vein, Right N Femoral Vein, Left P Saphenous Vein, Right Q Saphenous Vein, Left T Foot Vein, Right V Foot Vein, Left Y Lower Vein	0 Open 3 Percutaneous 4 Percutaneous Endoscopic	Z No Device	Z No Qualifier

Section	0	Medical and Surgical
Body System	6	Lower Veins
Operation	F	**Fragmentation:** Breaking solid matter in a body part into pieces

Body Part (4th)	Approach (5th)	Device (6th)	Qualifier (7th)
C Common Iliac Vein, Right D Common Iliac Vein, Left F External Iliac Vein, Right G External Iliac Vein, Left H Hypogastric Vein, Right J Hypogastric Vein, Left M Femoral Vein, Right N Femoral Vein, Left P Saphenous Vein, Right Q Saphenous Vein, Left Y Lower Vein	3 Percutaneous	Z No Device	0 Ultrasonic Z No Qualifier

Section	0	Medical and Surgical
Body System	6	Lower Veins
Operation	H	**Insertion:** Putting in a nonbiological appliance that monitors, assists, performs, or prevents a physiological function but does not physically take the place of a body part

Body Part (4th)	Approach (5th)	Device (6th)	Qualifier (7th)
0 Inferior Vena Cava	0 Open 3 Percutaneous	3 Infusion Device	T Via Umbilical Vein Z No Qualifier
0 Inferior Vena Cava	0 Open 3 Percutaneous	D Intraluminal Device	Z No Qualifier
0 Inferior Vena Cava	4 Percutaneous Endoscopic	3 Infusion Device D Intraluminal Device	Z No Qualifier

Continued →

195

Section	0	Medical and Surgical	*06H Continued*
Body System	6	Lower Veins	
Operation	H	**Insertion:** Putting in a nonbiological appliance that monitors, assists, performs, or prevents a physiological function but does not physically take the place of a body part	

Body Part (4th)	Approach (5th)	Device (6th)	Qualifier (7th)
1 Splenic Vein 2 Gastric Vein 3 Esophageal Vein 4 Hepatic Vein 5 Superior Mesenteric Vein 6 Inferior Mesenteric Vein 7 Colic Vein 8 Portal Vein 9 Renal Vein, Right B Renal Vein, Left C Common Iliac Vein, Right D Common Iliac Vein, Left F External Iliac Vein, Right G External Iliac Vein, Left H Hypogastric Vein, Right J Hypogastric Vein, Left M Femoral Vein, Right N Femoral Vein, Left P Saphenous Vein, Right Q Saphenous Vein, Left T Foot Vein, Right V Foot Vein, Left	0 Open 3 Percutaneous 4 Percutaneous Endoscopic	3 Infusion Device D Intraluminal Device	Z No Qualifier
Y Lower Vein	0 Open 3 Percutaneous 4 Percutaneous Endoscopic	2 Monitoring Device 3 Infusion Device D Intraluminal Device Y Other Device	Z No Qualifier

Section	0	Medical and Surgical
Body System	6	Lower Veins
Operation	J	**Inspection:** Visually and/or manually exploring a body part

Body Part (4th)	Approach (5th)	Device (6th)	Qualifier (7th)
Y Lower Vein	0 Open 3 Percutaneous 4 Percutaneous Endoscopic X External	Z No Device	Z No Qualifier

Section	0	Medical and Surgical
Body System	6	Lower Veins
Operation	L	Occlusion: Completely closing an orifice or the lumen of a tubular body part

Body Part (4th)	Approach (5th)	Device (6th)	Qualifier (7th)
0 Inferior Vena Cava 1 Splenic Vein 4 Hepatic Vein 5 Superior Mesenteric Vein 6 Inferior Mesenteric Vein 7 Colic Vein 8 Portal Vein 9 Renal Vein, Right B Renal Vein, Left C Common Iliac Vein, Right D Common Iliac Vein, Left F External Iliac Vein, Right G External Iliac Vein, Left H Hypogastric Vein, Right J Hypogastric Vein, Left M Femoral Vein, Right N Femoral Vein, Left P Saphenous Vein, Right Q Saphenous Vein, Left T Foot Vein, Right V Foot Vein, Left	0 Open 3 Percutaneous 4 Percutaneous Endoscopic	C Extraluminal Device D Intraluminal Device Z No Device	Z No Qualifier
2 Gastric Vein 3 Esophageal Vein	0 Open 3 Percutaneous 4 Percutaneous Endoscopic 7 Via Natural or Artificial Opening 8 Via Natural or Artificial Opening Endoscopic	C Extraluminal Device D Intraluminal Device Z No Device	Z No Qualifier
Y Lower Vein	0 Open 3 Percutaneous 4 Percutaneous Endoscopic 7 Via Natural or Artificial Opening 8 Via Natural or Artificial Opening Endoscopic	C Extraluminal Device D Intraluminal Device Z No Device	C Hemorrhoidal Plexus Z No Qualifier

Section	0	Medical and Surgical
Body System	6	Lower Veins
Operation	N	Release: Freeing a body part from an abnormal physical constraint by cutting or by the use of force

Body Part (4th)	Approach (5th)	Device (6th)	Qualifier (7th)
0 Inferior Vena Cava 1 Splenic Vein 2 Gastric Vein 3 Esophageal Vein 4 Hepatic Vein 5 Superior Mesenteric Vein 6 Inferior Mesenteric Vein 7 Colic Vein 8 Portal Vein 9 Renal Vein, Right B Renal Vein, Left C Common Iliac Vein, Right D Common Iliac Vein, Left F External Iliac Vein, Right G External Iliac Vein, Left H Hypogastric Vein, Right J Hypogastric Vein, Left M Femoral Vein, Right N Femoral Vein, Left P Saphenous Vein, Right Q Saphenous Vein, Left T Foot Vein, Right V Foot Vein, Left Y Lower Vein	0 Open 3 Percutaneous 4 Percutaneous Endoscopic	Z No Device	Z No Qualifier

06P–06Q

Section	0	Medical and Surgical
Body System	6	Lower Veins
Operation	P	**Removal:** Taking out or off a device from a body part

Body Part (4th)	Approach (5th)	Device (6th)	Qualifier (7th)
Y Lower Vein	0 Open 3 Percutaneous 4 Percutaneous Endoscopic	0 Drainage Device 2 Monitoring Device 3 Infusion Device 7 Autologous Tissue Substitute C Extraluminal Device D Intraluminal Device J Synthetic Substitute K Nonautologous Tissue Substitute Y Other Device	Z No Qualifier
Y Lower Vein	X External	0 Drainage Device 2 Monitoring Device 3 Infusion Device D Intraluminal Device	Z No Qualifier

Section	0	Medical and Surgical
Body System	6	Lower Veins
Operation	Q	**Repair:** Restoring, to the extent possible, a body part to its normal anatomic structure and function

Body Part (4th)	Approach (5th)	Device (6th)	Qualifier (7th)
0 Inferior Vena Cava 1 Splenic Vein 2 Gastric Vein 3 Esophageal Vein 4 Hepatic Vein 5 Superior Mesenteric Vein 6 Inferior Mesenteric Vein 7 Colic Vein 8 Portal Vein 9 Renal Vein, Right B Renal Vein, Left C Common Iliac Vein, Right D Common Iliac Vein, Left F External Iliac Vein, Right G External Iliac Vein, Left H Hypogastric Vein, Right J Hypogastric Vein, Left M Femoral Vein, Right N Femoral Vein, Left P Saphenous Vein, Right Q Saphenous Vein, Left T Foot Vein, Right V Foot Vein, Left Y Lower Vein	0 Open 3 Percutaneous 4 Percutaneous Endoscopic	Z No Device	Z No Qualifier

Medical and Surgical, Lower Veins Tables

Section	0	Medical and Surgical
Body System	6	Lower Veins
Operation	R	Replacement: Putting in or on biological or synthetic material that physically takes the place and/or function of all or a portion of a body part

Body Part (4th)	Approach (5th)	Device (6th)	Qualifier (7th)
0 Inferior Vena Cava	0 Open	7 Autologous Tissue Substitute	Z No Qualifier
1 Splenic Vein	4 Percutaneous Endoscopic	J Synthetic Substitute	
2 Gastric Vein		K Nonautologous Tissue Substitute	
3 Esophageal Vein			
4 Hepatic Vein			
5 Superior Mesenteric Vein			
6 Inferior Mesenteric Vein			
7 Colic Vein			
8 Portal Vein			
9 Renal Vein, Right			
B Renal Vein, Left			
C Common Iliac Vein, Right			
D Common Iliac Vein, Left			
F External Iliac Vein, Right			
G External Iliac Vein, Left			
H Hypogastric Vein, Right			
J Hypogastric Vein, Left			
M Femoral Vein, Right			
N Femoral Vein, Left			
P Saphenous Vein, Right			
Q Saphenous Vein, Left			
T Foot Vein, Right			
V Foot Vein, Left			
Y Lower Vein			

Section	0	Medical and Surgical
Body System	6	Lower Veins
Operation	S	Reposition: Moving to its normal location, or other suitable location, all or a portion of a body part

Body Part (4th)	Approach (5th)	Device (6th)	Qualifier (7th)
0 Inferior Vena Cava	0 Open	Z No Device	Z No Qualifier
1 Splenic Vein	3 Percutaneous		
2 Gastric Vein	4 Percutaneous Endoscopic		
3 Esophageal Vein			
4 Hepatic Vein			
5 Superior Mesenteric Vein			
6 Inferior Mesenteric Vein			
7 Colic Vein			
8 Portal Vein			
9 Renal Vein, Right			
B Renal Vein, Left			
C Common Iliac Vein, Right			
D Common Iliac Vein, Left			
F External Iliac Vein, Right			
G External Iliac Vein, Left			
H Hypogastric Vein, Right			
J Hypogastric Vein, Left			
M Femoral Vein, Right			
N Femoral Vein, Left			
P Saphenous Vein, Right			
Q Saphenous Vein, Left			
T Foot Vein, Right			
V Foot Vein, Left			
Y Lower Vein			

Section	0	Medical and Surgical
Body System	6	Lower Veins
Operation	U	Supplement: Putting in or on biological or synthetic material that physically reinforces and/or augments the function of a portion of a body part

Body Part (4th)	Approach (5th)	Device (6th)	Qualifier (7th)
0 Inferior Vena Cava	0 Open	7 Autologous Tissue Substitute	Z No Qualifier
1 Splenic Vein	3 Percutaneous	J Synthetic Substitute	
2 Gastric Vein	4 Percutaneous Endoscopic	K Nonautologous Tissue Substitute	
3 Esophageal Vein			
4 Hepatic Vein			
5 Superior Mesenteric Vein			
6 Inferior Mesenteric Vein			
7 Colic Vein			
8 Portal Vein			
9 Renal Vein, Right			
B Renal Vein, Left			
C Common Iliac Vein, Right			
D Common Iliac Vein, Left			
F External Iliac Vein, Right			
G External Iliac Vein, Left			
H Hypogastric Vein, Right			
J Hypogastric Vein, Left			
M Femoral Vein, Right			
N Femoral Vein, Left			
P Saphenous Vein, Right			
Q Saphenous Vein, Left			
T Foot Vein, Right			
V Foot Vein, Left			
Y Lower Vein			

Section	0	Medical and Surgical
Body System	6	Lower Veins
Operation	V	Restriction: Partially closing an orifice or the lumen of a tubular body part

Body Part (4th)	Approach (5th)	Device (6th)	Qualifier (7th)
0 Inferior Vena Cava	0 Open	C Extraluminal Device	Z No Qualifier
1 Splenic Vein	3 Percutaneous	D Intraluminal Device	
2 Gastric Vein	4 Percutaneous Endoscopic	Z No Device	
3 Esophageal Vein			
4 Hepatic Vein			
5 Superior Mesenteric Vein			
6 Inferior Mesenteric Vein			
7 Colic Vein			
8 Portal Vein			
9 Renal Vein, Right			
B Renal Vein, Left			
C Common Iliac Vein, Right			
D Common Iliac Vein, Left			
F External Iliac Vein, Right			
G External Iliac Vein, Left			
H Hypogastric Vein, Right			
J Hypogastric Vein, Left			
M Femoral Vein, Right			
N Femoral Vein, Left			
P Saphenous Vein, Right			
Q Saphenous Vein, Left			
T Foot Vein, Right			
V Foot Vein, Left			
Y Lower Vein			

Section	0	Medical and Surgical
Body System	6	Lower Veins
Operation	W	Revision: Correcting, to the extent possible, a portion of a malfunctioning device or the position of a displaced device

Body Part (4th)	Approach (5th)	Device (6th)	Qualifier (7th)
Y Lower Vein	**0** Open **3** Percutaneous **4** Percutaneous Endoscopic **X** External	**0** Drainage Device **2** Monitoring Device **3** Infusion Device **7** Autologous Tissue Substitute **C** Extraluminal Device **D** Intraluminal Device **J** Synthetic Substitute **K** Nonautologous Tissue Substitute **Y** Other Device	**Z** No Qualifier
Y Lower Vein	**X** External	**0** Drainage Device **2** Monitoring Device **3** Infusion Device **7** Autologous Tissue Substitute **C** Extraluminal Device **D** Intraluminal Device **J** Synthetic Substitute **K** Nonautologus Tissue Substitute	**Z** No Qualifier

AHA Coding Clinic

06100JP Bypass Inferior Vena Cava to Pulmonary Trunk with Synthetic Substitute, Open Approach—AHA CC: 4Q, 2017, 37-38

06BP0ZZ Excision of Right Saphenous Vein, Open Approach—AHA CC: 1Q, 2014, 10-11; 2Q, 2016, 18-19; 1Q, 2017, 31-32; 3Q. 2017, 5-6

06BP4ZZ Excision of Right Saphenous Vein, Percutaneous Endoscopic Approach—AHA CC: 3Q, 2014, 20-21

06BQ0ZZ Excision of Left Saphenous Vein, Open Approach—AHA CC: 1Q, 2017, 32-33; 1Q, 2020, 28-29

06BQ4ZZ Excision of Left Saphenous Vein, Percutaneous Endoscopic Approach—AHA CC: 3Q, 2014, 20-21; 1Q, 2016, 27-28

06H033T Insertion of Infusion Device, Via Umbilical Vein, into Inferior Vena Cava, Percutaneous Approach—AHA CC: 1Q, 2017, 31

06H033Z Insertion of Infusion Device into Inferior Vena Cava, Percutaneous Approach—AHA CC: 3Q, 2013, 18-19

06HY33Z Insertion of Infusion Device into Lower Vein, Percutaneous Approach—AHA CC: 1Q, 2017, 31; 3Q, 2021, 18-19

06L34CZ Occlusion of Esophageal Vein with Extraluminal Device, Percutaneous Endoscopic Approach—AHA CC: 4Q, 2013, 112-113

06L38CZ Occlusion of Esophageal Vein with Extraluminal Device, Via Natural or Artificial Opening Endoscopic—AHA CC: 4Q, 2017, 57-58

06L84CZ Occlusion of Portal Vein with Extraluminal Device, Percutaneous Endoscopic Approach—AHA CC: 4Q, 2021, 48-50

06LF0CZ Occlusion of Right External Iliac Vein with Extraluminal Device, Open Approach—AHA CC: 2Q, 2018, 18-19

06LG0CZ Occlusion of Left External Iliac Vein with Extraluminal Device, Open Approach—AHA CC: 2Q, 2018, 18-19

06LY3DZ Occlusion of Lower Vein with Intraluminal Device, Percutaneous Approach—AHA CC: 3Q, 2020, 44-45

06PY33Z Removal of Infusion Device from Lower Vein, Percutaneous Approach—AHA CC: 3Q, 2021, 18-19

06V03DZ Restriction of Inferior Vena Cava with Intraluminal Device, Percutaneous Approach—AHA CC: 3Q, 2018, 11

06WY3DZ Revision of Intraluminal Device in Lower Vein, Percutaneous Approach—AHA CC: 3Q, 2014, 25-26

06WY3JZ Revision of Synthetic Substitute in Lower Vein, Percutaneous Approach—AHA CC: 1Q, 2018, 10; 2Q, 2019, 39

Lymphatic and Hemic System

Lymph Vessels and Nodes of Head and Neck; Lymphatic Drainage of Mouth and Pharynx

*The supraclavicular group of nodes (also known as the lower deep cervical group), especially on the left, are also sometimes referred to as the signal or sentinel lymph nodes of Virchow or Troisier, especially when sufficiently enlarged and palpable. These nodes (or a single node) are so termed because they may be the first recognized presumptive evidence of malignant disease in the viscera.

© 2006 Elsevier Inc. All rights reserved. www.netterimages.com

Lymph Vessels and Nodes of Mammary Gland Lymphatic Drainage

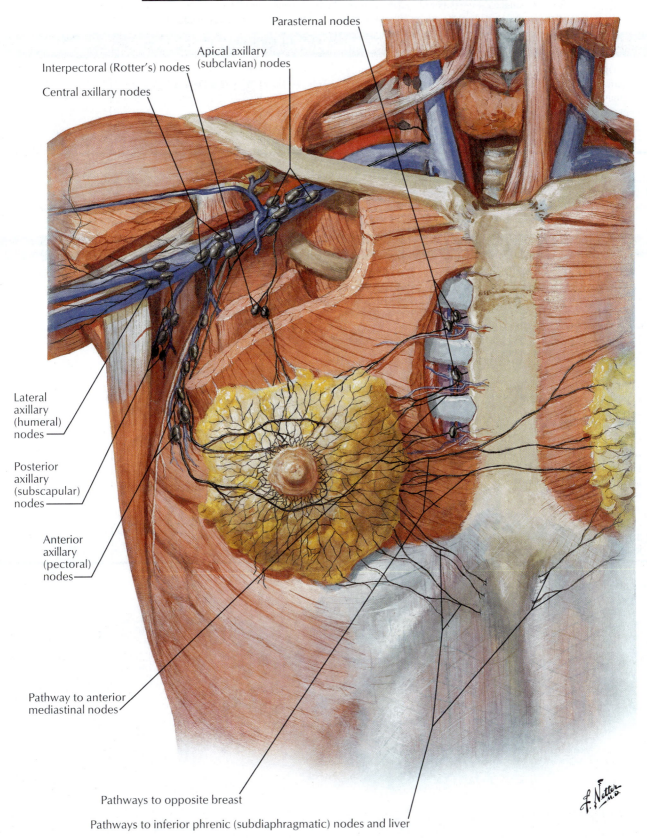

Lymphatic and Hemic Systems Tables 072–07Y

Section	0	Medical and Surgical
Body System	7	Lymphatic and Hemic Systems
Operation	2	**Change:** Taking out or off a device from a body part and putting back an identical or similar device in or on the same body part without cutting or puncturing the skin or a mucous membrane

Body Part (4th)	Approach (5th)	Device (6th)	Qualifier (7th)
K Thoracic Duct L Cisterna Chyli M Thymus N Lymphatic P Spleen T Bone Marrow	X External	0 Drainage Device Y Other Device	Z No Qualifier

Section	0	Medical and Surgical
Body System	7	Lymphatic and Hemic Systems
Operation	5	**Destruction:** Physical eradication of all or a portion of a body part by the direct use of energy, force, or a destructive agent

Body Part (4th)	Approach (5th)	Device (6th)	Qualifier (7th)
0 Lymphatic, Head 1 Lymphatic, Right Neck 2 Lymphatic, Left Neck 3 Lymphatic, Right Upper Extremity 4 Lymphatic, Left Upper Extremity 5 Lymphatic, Right Axillary 6 Lymphatic, Left Axillary 7 Lymphatic, Thorax 8 Lymphatic, Internal Mammary, Right 9 Lymphatic, Internal Mammary, Left B Lymphatic, Mesenteric C Lymphatic, Pelvis D Lymphatic, Aortic F Lymphatic, Right Lower Extremity G Lymphatic, Left Lower Extremity H Lymphatic, Right Inguinal J Lymphatic, Left Inguinal K Thoracic Duct L Cisterna Chyli M Thymus P Spleen	0 Open 3 Percutaneous 4 Percutaneous Endoscopic	Z No Device	Z No Qualifier

Section	0	Medical and Surgical
Body System	7	Lymphatic and Hemic Systems
Operation	9	Drainage: Taking or letting out fluids and/or gases from a body part

Body Part (4th)	Approach (5th)	Device (6th)	Qualifier (7th)
0 Lymphatic, Head 1 Lymphatic, Right Neck 2 Lymphatic, Left Neck 3 Lymphatic, Right Upper Extremity 4 Lymphatic, Left Upper Extremity 5 Lymphatic, Right Axillary 6 Lymphatic, Left Axillary 7 Lymphatic, Thorax 8 Lymphatic, Internal Mammary, Right 9 Lymphatic, Internal Mammary, Left B Lymphatic, Mesenteric C Lymphatic, Pelvis D Lymphatic, Aortic F Lymphatic, Right Lower Extremity G Lymphatic, Left Lower Extremity H Lymphatic, Right Inguinal J Lymphatic, Left Inguinal K Thoracic Duct L Cisterna Chyli	0 Open 3 Percutaneous 4 Percutaneous Endoscopic 8 Via Natural or Artificial Opening Endoscopic	0 Drainage Device	Z No Qualifier
0 Lymphatic, Head 1 Lymphatic, Right Neck 2 Lymphatic, Left Neck 3 Lymphatic, Right Upper Extremity 4 Lymphatic, Left Upper Extremity 5 Lymphatic, Right Axillary 6 Lymphatic, Left Axillary 7 Lymphatic, Thorax 8 Lymphatic, Internal Mammary, Right 9 Lymphatic, Internal Mammary, Left B Lymphatic, Mesenteric C Lymphatic, Pelvis D Lymphatic, Aortic F Lymphatic, Right Lower Extremity G Lymphatic, Left Lower Extremity H Lymphatic, Right Inguinal J Lymphatic, Left Inguinal K Thoracic Duct L Cisterna Chyli	0 Open 3 Percutaneous 4 Percutaneous Endoscopic 8 Via Natural or Artificial Opening Endoscopic	Z No Device	X Diagnostic Z No Qualifier
M Thymus P Spleen T Bone Marrow	0 Open 3 Percutaneous 4 Percutaneous Endoscopic	0 Drainage Device	Z No Qualifier
M Thymus P Spleen T Bone Marrow	0 Open 3 Percutaneous 4 Percutaneous Endoscopic	Z No Device	X No Diagnostic Z No Qualifier

07B–07C

Medical and Surgical, Lymphatic and Hemic System Tables

Section	0	Medical and Surgical
Body System	7	Lymphatic and Hemic Systems
Operation	B	Excision: Cutting out or off, without replacement, a portion of a body part

Body Part (4th)	Approach (5th)	Device (6th)	Qualifier (7th)
0 Lymphatic, Head 1 Lymphatic, Right Neck 2 Lymphatic, Left Neck 3 Lymphatic, Right Upper Extremity 4 Lymphatic, Left Upper Extremity 5 Lymphatic, Right Axillary 6 Lymphatic, Left Axillary 7 Lymphatic, Thorax 8 Lymphatic, Internal Mammary, Right 9 Lymphatic, Internal Mammary, Left B Lymphatic, Mesenteric C Lymphatic, Pelvis D Lymphatic, Aortic F Lymphatic, Right Lower Extremity G Lymphatic, Left Lower Extremity H Lymphatic, Right Inguinal J Lymphatic, Left Inguinal K Thoracic Duct L Cisterna Chyli M Thymus P Spleen	0 Open 3 Percutaneous 4 Percutaneous Endoscopic	Z No Device	X Diagnostic Z No Qualifier

Section	0	Medical and Surgical
Body System	7	Lymphatic and Hemic Systems
Operation	C	Extirpation: Taking or cutting out solid matter from a body part

Body Part (4th)	Approach (5th)	Device (6th)	Qualifier (7th)
0 Lymphatic, Head 1 Lymphatic, Right Neck 2 Lymphatic, Left Neck 3 Lymphatic, Right Upper Extremity 4 Lymphatic, Left Upper Extremity 5 Lymphatic, Right Axillary 6 Lymphatic, Left Axillary 7 Lymphatic, Thorax 8 Lymphatic, Internal Mammary, Right 9 Lymphatic, Internal Mammary, Left B Lymphatic, Mesenteric C Lymphatic, Pelvis D Lymphatic, Aortic F Lymphatic, Right Lower Extremity G Lymphatic, Left Lower Extremity H Lymphatic, Right Inguinal J Lymphatic, Left Inguinal K Thoracic Duct L Cisterna Chyli M Thymus P Spleen	0 Open 3 Percutaneous 4 Percutaneous Endoscopic	Z No Device	Z No Qualifier

Section	0	Medical and Surgical
Body System	7	Lymphatic and Hemic Systems
Operation	D	Extraction: Pulling or stripping out or off all or a portion of a body part by the use of force

Body Part (4th)	Approach (5th)	Device (6th)	Qualifier (7th)
0 Lymphatic, Head 1 Lymphatic, Right Neck 2 Lymphatic, Left Neck 3 Lymphatic, Right Upper Extremity 4 Lymphatic, Left Upper Extremity 5 Lymphatic, Right Axillary 6 Lymphatic, Left Axillary 7 Lymphatic, Thorax 8 Lymphatic, Internal Mammary, Right 9 Lymphatic, Internal Mammary, Left B Lymphatic, Mesenteric C Lymphatic, Pelvis D Lymphatic, Aortic F Lymphatic, Right Lower Extremity G Lymphatic, Left Lower Extremity H Lymphatic, Right Inguinal J Lymphatic, Left Inguinal K Thoracic Duct L Cisterna Chyli	3 Percutaneous 4 Percutaneous Endoscopic 8 Via Natural or Artificial Opening Endoscopic	Z No Device	X Diagnostic
M Thymus P Spleen	3 Percutaneous 4 Percutaneous Endoscopic	Z No Device	X No Diagnostic
Q Bone Marrow, Sternum R Bone Marrow, Iliac S Bone Marrow, Vertebral T Bone Marrow	0 Open 3 Percutaneous	Z No Device	X Diagnostic Z No Qualifier

Section	0	Medical and Surgical
Body System	7	Lymphatic and Hemic Systems
Operation	H	Insertion: Putting in a nonbiological appliance that monitors, assists, performs, or prevents a physiological function but does not physically take the place of a body part

Body Part (4th)	Approach (5th)	Device (6th)	Qualifier (7th)
K Thoracic Duct L Cisterna Chyli M Thymus N Lymphatic P Spleen T Bone Marrow	0 Open 3 Percutaneous 4 Percutaneous Endoscopic	1 Radioactive Element 3 Infusion Device Y Other Device	Z No Qualifier

Section	0	Medical and Surgical
Body System	7	Lymphatic and Hemic Systems
Operation	J	Inspection: Visually and/or manually exploring a body part

Body Part (4th)	Approach (5th)	Device (6th)	Qualifier (7th)
K Thoracic Duct L Cisterna Chyli M Thymus T Bone Marrow	0 Open 3 Percutaneous 4 Percutaneous Endoscopic	Z No Device	Z No Qualifier
N Lymphatic	0 Open 3 Percutaneous 4 Percutaneous Endoscopic 8 Via Natural or Artificial Opening Endoscopic X External	Z No Device	Z No Qualifier
P Spleen	0 Open 3 Percutaneous 4 Percutaneous Endoscopic X External	Z No Device	Z No Qualifier

07L–07N

Medical and Surgical, Lymphatic and Hemic System Tables

Section	0	Medical and Surgical
Body System	7	Lymphatic and Hemic Systems
Operation	L	Occlusion: Completely closing an orifice or the lumen of a tubular body part

Body Part (4th)	Approach (5th)	Device (6th)	Qualifier (7th)
0 Lymphatic, Head 1 Lymphatic, Right Neck 2 Lymphatic, Left Neck 3 Lymphatic, Right Upper Extremity 4 Lymphatic, Left Upper Extremity 5 Lymphatic, Right Axillary 6 Lymphatic, Left Axillary 7 Lymphatic, Thorax 8 Lymphatic, Internal Mammary, Right 9 Lymphatic, Internal Mammary, Left B Lymphatic, Mesenteric C Lymphatic, Pelvis D Lymphatic, Aortic F Lymphatic, Right Lower Extremity G Lymphatic, Left Lower Extremity H Lymphatic, Right Inguinal J Lymphatic, Left Inguinal K Thoracic Duct L Cisterna Chyli	0 Open 3 Percutaneous 4 Percutaneous Endoscopic	C Extraluminal Device D Intraluminal Device Z No Device	Z No Qualifier

Section	0	Medical and Surgical
Body System	7	Lymphatic and Hemic Systems
Operation	N	Release: Freeing a body part from an abnormal physical constraint by cutting or by the use of force

Body Part (4th)	Approach (5th)	Device (6th)	Qualifier (7th)
0 Lymphatic, Head 1 Lymphatic, Right Neck 2 Lymphatic, Left Neck 3 Lymphatic, Right Upper Extremity 4 Lymphatic, Left Upper Extremity 5 Lymphatic, Right Axillary 6 Lymphatic, Left Axillary 7 Lymphatic, Thorax 8 Lymphatic, Internal Mammary, Right 9 Lymphatic, Internal Mammary, Left B Lymphatic, Mesenteric C Lymphatic, Pelvis D Lymphatic, Aortic F Lymphatic, Right Lower Extremity G Lymphatic, Left Lower Extremity H Lymphatic, Right Inguinal J Lymphatic, Left Inguinal K Thoracic Duct L Cisterna Chyli M Thymus P Spleen	0 Open 3 Percutaneous 4 Percutaneous Endoscopic	Z No Device	Z No Qualifier

208

Section	0	Medical and Surgical
Body System	7	Lymphatic and Hemic Systems
Operation	P	Removal: Taking out or off a device from a body part

Body Part (4th)	Approach (5th)	Device (6th)	Qualifier (7th)
K Thoracic Duct L Cisterna Chyli N Lymphatic	0 Open 3 Percutaneous 4 Percutaneous Endoscopic	0 Drainage Device 3 Infusion Device 7 Autologous Tissue Substitute C Extraluminal Device D Intraluminal Device J Synthetic Substitute K Nonautologous Tissue Substitute Y Other Device	Z No Qualifier
K Thoracic Duct L Cisterna Chyli N Lymphatic	X External	0 Drainage Device 3 Infusion Device D Intraluminal Device	Z No Qualifier
M Thymus P Spleen	0 Open 3 Percutaneous 4 Percutaneous Endoscopic	0 Drainage Device 3 Infusion Device Y Other Device	Z No Qualifier
M Thymus P Spleen	X External	0 Drainage Device 3 Infusion Device	Z No Qualifier
T Bone Marrow	0 Open 3 Percutaneous 4 Percutaneous Endoscopic X External	0 Drainage Device	Z No Qualifier

Section	0	Medical and Surgical
Body System	7	Lymphatic and Hemic Systems
Operation	Q	Repair: Restoring, to the extent possible, a body part to its normal anatomic structure and function

Body Part (4th)	Approach (5th)	Device (6th)	Qualifier (7th)
0 Lymphatic, Head 1 Lymphatic, Right Neck 2 Lymphatic, Left Neck 3 Lymphatic, Right Upper Extremity 4 Lymphatic, Left Upper Extremity 5 Lymphatic, Right Axillary 6 Lymphatic, Left Axillary 7 Lymphatic, Thorax 8 Lymphatic, Internal Mammary, Right 9 Lymphatic, Internal Mammary, Left B Lymphatic, Mesenteric C Lymphatic, Pelvis D Lymphatic, Aortic F Lymphatic, Right Lower Extremity G Lymphatic, Left Lower Extremity H Lymphatic, Right Inguinal J Lymphatic, Left Inguinal K Thoracic Duct L Cisterna Chyli	0 Open 3 Percutaneous 4 Percutaneous Endoscopic 8 Via Natural or Artificial Opening Endoscopic	Z No Device	Z No Qualifier
M Thymus P Spleen	0 Open 3 Percutaneous 4 Percutaneous Endoscopic	Z No Device	Z No Qualifier

07S–07U

Medical and Surgical, Lymphatic and Hemic System Tables

Section	0	Medical and Surgical
Body System	7	Lymphatic and Hemic Systems
Operation	S	Reposition: Moving to its normal location, or other suitable location, all or a portion of a body part

Body Part (4th)	Approach (5th)	Device (6th)	Qualifier (7th)
M Thymus P Spleen	0 Open	Z No Device	Z No Qualifier

Section	0	Medical and Surgical
Body System	7	Lymphatic and Hemic Systems
Operation	T	Resection: Cutting out or off, without replacement, all of a body part

Body Part (4th)	Approach (5th)	Device (6th)	Qualifier (7th)
0 Lymphatic, Head 1 Lymphatic, Right Neck 2 Lymphatic, Left Neck 3 Lymphatic, Right Upper Extremity 4 Lymphatic, Left Upper Extremity 5 Lymphatic, Right Axillary 6 Lymphatic, Left Axillary 7 Lymphatic, Thorax 8 Lymphatic, Internal Mammary, Right 9 Lymphatic, Internal Mammary, Left B Lymphatic, Mesenteric C Lymphatic, Pelvis D Lymphatic, Aortic F Lymphatic, Right Lower Extremity G Lymphatic, Left Lower Extremity H Lymphatic, Right Inguinal J Lymphatic, Left Inguinal K Thoracic Duct L Cisterna Chyli M Thymus P Spleen	0 Open 4 Percutaneous Endoscopic	Z No Device	Z No Qualifier

Section	0	Medical and Surgical
Body System	7	Lymphatic and Hemic Systems
Operation	U	Supplement: Putting in or on biological or synthetic material that physically reinforces and/or augments the function of a portion of a body part

Body Part (4th)	Approach (5th)	Device (6th)	Qualifier (7th)
0 Lymphatic, Head 1 Lymphatic, Right Neck 2 Lymphatic, Left Neck 3 Lymphatic, Right Upper Extremity 4 Lymphatic, Left Upper Extremity 5 Lymphatic, Right Axillary 6 Lymphatic, Left Axillary 7 Lymphatic, Thorax 8 Lymphatic, Internal Mammary, Right 9 Lymphatic, Internal Mammary, Left B Lymphatic, Mesenteric C Lymphatic, Pelvis D Lymphatic, Aortic F Lymphatic, Right Lower Extremity G Lymphatic, Left Lower Extremity H Lymphatic, Right Inguinal J Lymphatic, Left Inguinal K Thoracic Duct L Cisterna Chyli	0 Open 4 Percutaneous Endoscopic	7 Autologous Tissue Substitute J Synthetic Substitute K Nonautologous Tissue Substitute	Z No Qualifier

210

Section	0	Medical and Surgical
Body System	7	Lymphatic and Hemic Systems
Operation	V	**Restriction:** Partially closing an orifice or the lumen of a tubular body part

Body Part (4th)	Approach (5th)	Device (6th)	Qualifier (7th)
0 Lymphatic, Head 1 Lymphatic, Right Neck 2 Lymphatic, Left Neck 3 Lymphatic, Right Upper Extremity 4 Lymphatic, Left Upper Extremity 5 Lymphatic, Right Axillary 6 Lymphatic, Left Axillary 7 Lymphatic, Thorax 8 Lymphatic, Internal Mammary, Right 9 Lymphatic, Internal Mammary, Left B Lymphatic, Mesenteric C Lymphatic, Pelvis D Lymphatic, Aortic F Lymphatic, Right Lower Extremity G Lymphatic, Left Lower Extremity H Lymphatic, Right Inguinal J Lymphatic, Left Inguinal K Thoracic Duct L Cisterna Chyli	0 Open 3 Percutaneous 4 Percutaneous Endoscopic	C Extraluminal Device D Intraluminal Device Z No Device	Z No Qualifier

Section	0	Medical and Surgical
Body System	7	Lymphatic and Hemic Systems
Operation	W	**Revision:** Correcting, to the extent possible, a portion of a malfunctioning device or the position of a displaced device

Body Part (4th)	Approach (5th)	Device (6th)	Qualifier (7th)
K Thoracic Duct L Cisterna Chyli N Lymphatic	0 Open 3 Percutaneous 4 Percutaneous Endoscopic	0 Drainage Device 3 Infusion Device 7 Autologous Tissue Substitute C Extraluminal Device D Intraluminal Device J Synthetic Substitute K Nonautologous Tissue Substitute Y Other Device	Z No Qualifier
K Thoracic Duct L Cisterna Chyli N Lymphatic	X External	0 Drainage Device 3 Infusion Device 7 Autologous Tissue Substitute C Extraluminal Device D Intraluminal Device J Synthetic Substitute K Nonautologous Tissue Substitute	Z No Qualifier
M Thymus P Spleen	0 Open 3 Percutaneous 4 Percutaneous Endoscopic	0 Drainage Device 3 Infusion Device Y Other Device	Z No Qualifier
M Thymus P Spleen	X External	0 Drainage Device 3 Infusion Device	Z No Qualifier
T Bone Marrow	0 Open 3 Percutaneous 4 Percutaneous Endoscopic X External	0 Drainage Device	Z No Qualifier

Section	0	Medical and Surgical
Body System	7	Lymphatic and Hemic Systems
Operation	Y	**Transplantation:** Putting in or on all or a portion of a living body part taken from another individual or animal to physically take the place and/or function of all or a portion of a similar body part

Body Part (4ᵗʰ)	Approach (5ᵗʰ)	Device (6ᵗʰ)	Qualifier (7ᵗʰ)
M Thymus P Spleen	0 Open	Z No Device	0 Allogeneic 1 Syngeneic 2 Zooplastic

AHA Coding Clinic

079T3ZX Drainage of Bone Marrow, Percutaneous Approach, Diagnostic—AHA CC: 4Q, 2021, 47-48

07B60ZX Excision of Left Axillary Lymphatic, Percutaneous Approach, Diagnostic—AHA CC: 1Q, 2022, 14-15

07B74ZX Excision of Thorax Lymphatic, Percutaneous Endoscopic Approach, Diagnostic—AHA CC: 1Q, 2014, 20-21, 26; 3Q, 2014, 10-11

07BB0ZZ Excision of Mesenteric Lymphatic, Open Approach—AHA CC: 1Q, 2019, 6-7

07BD0ZZ Excision of Aortic Lymphatic, Open Approach—AHA CC: 1Q, 2019, 6-7

07DT3ZX Extraction of Bone Marrow, Percutaneous Approach, Diagnostic—AHA CC: 4Q, 2021, 47-48

07Q60ZZ Repair Left Axillary Lymphatic, Open Approach—AHA CC: 1Q, 2017, 34

07T10ZZ Resection of Right Neck Lymphatic, Open Approach—AHA CC: 3Q, 2014, 9-10

07T20ZZ Resection of Left Neck Lymphatic, Open Approach—AHA CC: 3Q, 2014, 9-10; 2Q, 2016, 12-14

07T50ZZ Resection of Right Axillary Lymphatic, Open Approach—AHA CC: 1Q, 2016, 30

07TM0ZZ Resection of Thymus, Open Approach—AHA CC: 3Q, 2014, 16-17

07TP0ZZ Resection of Spleen, Open Approach—AHA CC: 4Q, 2015, 13

07YM0Z0 Transplantation of Thymus, Allogeneic, Open Approach—AHA CC: 3Q, 2019, 29

Eye

Anatomy of the Eyeball

Horizontal section

Eyelid

Eye Muscles

Eye Tables 080–08X

Section	0	**Medical and Surgical**
Body System	8	**Eye**
Operation	0	**Alteration:** Modifying the anatomic structure of a body part without affecting the function of the body part

Body Part (4th)	Approach (5th)	Device (6th)	Qualifier (7th)
N Upper Eyelid, Right P Upper Eyelid, Left Q Lower Eyelid, Right R Lower Eyelid, Left	0 Open 3 Percutaneous X External	7 Autologous Tissue Substitute J Synthetic Substitute K Nonautologous Tissue Substitute Z No Device	Z No Qualifier

214

Section	0	Medical and Surgical
Body System	8	Eye
Operation	1	**Bypass:** Altering the route of passage of the contents of a tubular body part

Body Part (4th)	Approach (5th)	Device (6th)	Qualifier (7th)
2 Anterior Chamber, Right 3 Anterior Chamber, Left	3 Percutaneous	J Synthetic Substitute K Nonautologous Tissue Substitute Z No Device	4 Sclera
X Lacrimal Duct, Right Y Lacrimal Duct, Left	0 Open 3 Percutaneous	J Synthetic Substitute K Nonautologous Tissue Substitute Z No Device	3 Nasal Cavity

Section	0	Medical and Surgical
Body System	8	Eye
Operation	2	**Change:** Taking out or off a device from a body part and putting back an identical or similar device in or on the same body part without cutting or puncturing the skin or a mucous membrane

Body Part (4th)	Approach (5th)	Device (6th)	Qualifier (7th)
0 Eye, Right 1 Eye, Left	X External	0 Drainage Device Y Other Device	Z No Qualifier

Section	0	Medical and Surgical
Body System	8	Eye
Operation	5	**Destruction:** Physical eradication of all or a portion of a body part by the direct use of energy, force, or a destructive agent

Body Part (4th)	Approach (5th)	Device (6th)	Qualifier (7th)
0 Eye, Right 1 Eye, Left 6 Sclera, Right 7 Sclera, Left 8 Cornea, Right 9 Cornea, Left S Conjunctiva, Right T Conjunctiva, Left	X External	Z No Device	Z No Qualifier
2 Anterior Chamber, Right 3 Anterior Chamber, Left 4 Vitreous, Right 5 Vitreous, Left C Iris, Right D Iris, Left E Retina, Right F Retina, Left G Retinal Vessel, Right H Retinal Vessel, Left J Lens, Right K Lens, Left	3 Percutaneous	Z No Device	Z No Qualifier
A Choroid, Right B Choroid, Left L Extraocular Muscle, Right M Extraocular Muscle, Left V Lacrimal Gland, Right W Lacrimal Gland, Left	0 Open 3 Percutaneous	Z No Device	Z No Qualifier
N Upper Eyelid, Right P Upper Eyelid, Left Q Lower Eyelid, Right R Lower Eyelid, Left	0 Open 3 Percutaneous X External	Z No Device	Z No Qualifier
X Lacrimal Duct, Right Y Lacrimal Duct, Left	0 Open 3 Percutaneous 7 Via Natural or Artificial Opening 8 Via Natural or Artificial Opening Endoscopic	Z No Device	Z No Qualifier

087–089

Medical and Surgical, Eye Tables

Section	0	Medical and Surgical
Body System	8	Eye
Operation	7	Dilation: Expanding an orifice or the lumen of a tubular body part

Body Part (4th)	Approach (5th)	Device (6th)	Qualifier (7th)
X Lacrimal Duct, Right Y Lacrimal Duct, Left	0 Open 3 Percutaneous 7 Via Natural or Artificial Opening 8 Via Natural or Artificial Opening Endoscopic	D Intraluminal Device Z No Device	Z No Qualifier

Section	0	Medical and Surgical
Body System	8	Eye
Operation	9	Drainage: Taking or letting out fluids and/or gases from a body part

Body Part (4th)	Approach (5th)	Device (6th)	Qualifier (7th)
0 Eye, Right 1 Eye, Left 6 Sclera, Right 7 Sclera, Left 8 Cornea, Right 9 Cornea, Left S Conjunctiva, Right T Conjunctiva, Left	X External	0 Drainage Device	Z No Qualifier
0 Eye, Right 1 Eye, Left 6 Sclera, Right 7 Sclera, Left 8 Cornea, Right 9 Cornea, Left S Conjunctiva, Right T Conjunctiva, Left	X External	Z No Device	X Diagnostic Z No Qualifier
2 Anterior Chamber, Right 3 Anterior Chamber, Left 4 Vitreous, Right 5 Vitreous, Left C Iris, Right D Iris, Left E Retina, Right F Retina, Left G Retinal Vessel, Right H Retinal Vessel, Left J Lens, Right K Lens, Left	3 Percutaneous	0 Drainage Device	Z No Qualifier
2 Anterior Chamber, Right 3 Anterior Chamber, Left 4 Vitreous, Right 5 Vitreous, Left C Iris, Right D Iris, Left E Retina, Right F Retina, Left G Retinal Vessel, Right H Retinal Vessel, Left J Lens, Right K Lens, Left	3 Percutaneous	Z No Device	X Diagnostic Z No Qualifier
A Choroid, Right B Choroid, Left L Extraocular Muscle, Right M Extraocular Muscle, Left V Lacrimal Gland, Right W Lacrimal Gland, Left	0 Open 3 Percutaneous	0 Drainage Device	Z No Qualifier

Continued →

Section	0	Medical and Surgical							*089 Continued*
Body System	8	Eye							
Operation	9	**Drainage:** Taking or letting out fluids and/or gases from a body part							

Body Part (4th)	Approach (5th)	Device (6th)	Qualifier (7th)
A Choroid, Right B Choroid, Left L Extraocular Muscle, Right M Extraocular Muscle, Left V Lacrimal Gland, Right W Lacrimal Gland, Left	0 Open 3 Percutaneous	Z No Device	X Diagnostic Z No Qualifier
N Upper Eyelid, Right P Upper Eyelid, Left Q Lower Eyelid, Right R Lower Eyelid, Left	0 Open 3 Percutaneous X External	0 Drainage Device	Z No Qualifier
N Upper Eyelid, Right P Upper Eyelid, Left Q Lower Eyelid, Right R Lower Eyelid, Left	0 Open 3 Percutaneous X External	Z No Device	X Diagnostic Z No Qualifier
X Lacrimal Duct, Right Y Lacrimal Duct, Left	0 Open 3 Percutaneous 7 Via Natural or Artificial Opening 8 Via Natural or Artificial Opening Endoscopic	0 Drainage Device	Z No Qualifier
X Lacrimal Duct, Right Y Lacrimal Duct, Left	0 Open 3 Percutaneous 7 Via Natural or Artificial Opening 8 Via Natural or Artificial Opening Endoscopic	Z No Device	X Diagnostic Z No Qualifier

Section	0	**Medical and Surgical**						
Body System	8	**Eye**						
Operation	B	**Excision:** Cutting out or off, without replacement, a portion of a body part						

Body Part (4th)	Approach (5th)	Device (6th)	Qualifier (7th)
0 Eye, Right 1 Eye, Left N Upper Eyelid, Right P Upper Eyelid, Left Q Lower Eyelid, Right R Lower Eyelid, Left	0 Open 3 Percutaneous X External	Z No Device	X Diagnostic Z No Qualifier
4 Vitreous, Right 5 Vitreous, Left C Iris, Right D Iris, Left E Retina, Right F Retina, Left J Lens, Right K Lens, Left	3 Percutaneous	Z No Device	X Diagnostic Z No Qualifier
6 Sclera, Right 7 Sclera, Left 8 Cornea, Right 9 Cornea, Left S Conjunctiva, Right T Conjunctiva, Left	X External	Z No Device	X Diagnostic Z No Qualifier

Continued ➡

Section 0 Medical and Surgical
Body System 8 Eye
Operation B Excision: Cutting out or off, without replacement, a portion of a body part

Body Part (4th)	Approach (5th)	Device (6th)	Qualifier (7th)
A Choroid, Right B Choroid, Left L Extraocular Muscle, Right M Extraocular Muscle, Left V Lacrimal Gland, Right W Lacrimal Gland, Left	0 Open 3 Percutaneous	Z No Device	X Diagnostic Z No Qualifier
X Lacrimal Duct, Right Y Lacrimal Duct, Left	0 Open 3 Percutaneous 7 Via Natural or Artificial Opening 8 Via Natural or Artificial Opening Endoscopic	Z No Device	X Diagnostic Z No Qualifier

Section 0 Medical and Surgical
Body System 8 Eye
Operation C Extirpation: Taking or cutting out solid matter from a body part

Body Part (4th)	Approach (5th)	Device (6th)	Qualifier (7th)
0 Eye, Right 1 Eye, Left 6 Sclera, Right 7 Sclera, Left 8 Cornea, Right 9 Cornea, Left S Conjunctiva, Right T Conjunctiva, Left	X External	Z No Device	Z No Qualifier
2 Anterior Chamber, Right 3 Anterior Chamber, Left 4 Vitreous, Right 5 Vitreous, Left C Iris, Right D Iris, Left E Retina, Right F Retina, Left G Retinal Vessel, Right H Retinal Vessel, Left J Lens, Right K Lens, Left	3 Percutaneous X External	Z No Device	Z No Qualifier
A Choroid, Right B Choroid, Left L Extraocular Muscle, Right M Extraocular Muscle, Left N Upper Eyelid, Right P Upper Eyelid, Left Q Lower Eyelid, Right R Lower Eyelid, Left V Lacrimal Gland, Right W Lacrimal Gland, Left	0 Open 3 Percutaneous X External	Z No Device	Z No Qualifier
X Lacrimal Duct, Right Y Lacrimal Duct, Left	0 Open 3 Percutaneous 7 Via Natural or Artificial Opening 8 Via Natural or Artificial Opening Endoscopic	Z No Device	Z No Qualifier

Section	0	Medical and Surgical
Body System	8	Eye
Operation	D	Extraction: Pulling or stripping out or off all or a portion of a body part by the use of force

Body Part (4th)	Approach (5th)	Device (6th)	Qualifier (7th)
8 Cornea, Right 9 Cornea, Left	X External	Z No Device	X Diagnostic Z No Qualifier
J Lens, Right K Lens, Left	3 Percutaneous	Z No Device	Z No Qualifier

Section	0	Medical and Surgical
Body System	8	Eye
Operation	F	Fragmentation: Breaking solid matter in a body part into pieces

Body Part (4th)	Approach (5th)	Device (6th)	Qualifier (7th)
4 Vitreous, Right 5 Vitreous, Left	3 Percutaneous X External	Z No Device	Z No Qualifier

Section	0	Medical and Surgical
Body System	8	Eye
Operation	H	Insertion: Putting in a nonbiological appliance that monitors, assists, performs, or prevents a physiological function but does not physically take the place of a body part

Body Part (4th)	Approach (5th)	Device (6th)	Qualifier (7th)
0 Eye, Right 1 Eye, Left	0 Open	5 Epiretinal Visual Prosthesis Y Other Device	Z No Qualifier
0 Eye, Right 1 Eye, Left	3 Percutaneous	1 Radioactive Element 3 Infusion Device Y Other Device	Z No Qualifier
0 Eye, Right 1 Eye, Left	7 Via Natural or Artificial Opening 8 Via Natural or Artificial Opening Endoscopic	Y Other Device	Z No Qualifier
0 Eye, Right 1 Eye, Left	X External	1 Radioactive Element 3 Infusion Device	Z No Qualifier

Section	0	Medical and Surgical
Body System	8	Eye
Operation	J	Inspection: Visually and/or manually exploring a body part

Body Part (4th)	Approach (5th)	Device (6th)	Qualifier (7th)
0 Eye, Right 1 Eye, Left J Lens, Right K Lens, Left	X External	Z No Device	Z No Qualifier
L Extraocular Muscle, Right M Extraocular Muscle, Left	0 Open X External	Z No Device	Z No Qualifier

08D–08J

Medical and Surgical, Eye Tables

219

Section	0	Medical and Surgical
Body System	8	Eye
Operation	L	Occlusion: Completely closing an orifice or the lumen of a tubular body part

Body Part (4th)	Approach (5th)	Device (6th)	Qualifier (7th)
X Lacrimal Duct, Right Y Lacrimal Duct, Left	0 Open 3 Percutaneous	C Extraluminal Device D Intraluminal Device Z No Device	Z No Qualifier
X Lacrimal Duct, Right Y Lacrimal Duct, Left	7 Via Natural or Artificial Opening 8 Via Natural or Artificial Opening Endoscopic	D Intraluminal Device Z No Device	Z No Qualifier

Section	0	Medical and Surgical
Body System	8	Eye
Operation	M	Reattachment: Putting back in or on all or a portion of a separated body part to its normal location or other suitable location

Body Part (4th)	Approach (5th)	Device (6th)	Qualifier (7th)
N Upper Eyelid, Right P Upper Eyelid, Left Q Lower Eyelid, Right R Lower Eyelid, Left	X External	Z No Device	Z No Qualifier

Section	0	Medical and Surgical
Body System	8	Eye
Operation	N	Release: Freeing a body part from an abnormal physical constraint by cutting or by the use of force

Body Part (4th)	Approach (5th)	Device (6th)	Qualifier (7th)
0 Eye, Right 1 Eye, Left 6 Sclera, Right 7 Sclera, Left 8 Cornea, Right 9 Cornea, Left S Conjunctiva, Right T Conjunctiva, Left	X External	Z No Device	Z No Qualifier
2 Anterior Chamber, Right 3 Anterior Chamber, Left 4 Vitreous, Right 5 Vitreous, Left C Iris, Right D Iris, Left E Retina, Right F Retina, Left G Retinal Vessel, Right H Retinal Vessel, Left J Lens, Right K Lens, Left	3 Percutaneous	Z No Device	Z No Qualifier
A Choroid, Right B Choroid, Left L Extraocular Muscle, Right M Extraocular Muscle, Left V Lacrimal Gland, Right W Lacrimal Gland, Left	0 Open 3 Percutaneous	Z No Device	Z No Qualifier
N Upper Eyelid, Right P Upper Eyelid, Left Q Lower Eyelid, Right R Lower Eyelid, Left	0 Open 3 Percutaneous X External	Z No Device	Z No Qualifier
X Lacrimal Duct, Right Y Lacrimal Duct, Left	0 Open 3 Percutaneous 7 Via Natural or Artificial Opening 8 Via Natural or Artificial Opening Endoscopic	Z No Device	Z No Qualifier

Section	0	Medical and Surgical
Body System	8	Eye
Operation	P	Removal: Taking out or off a device from a body part

Body Part (4th)	Approach (5th)	Device (6th)	Qualifier (7th)
0 Eye, Right 1 Eye, Left	0 Open 3 Percutaneous 7 Via Natural or Artificial Opening 8 Via Natural or Artificial Opening Endoscopic	0 Drainage Device 1 Radioactive Element 3 Infusion Device 7 Autologous Tissue Substitute C Extraluminal Device D Intraluminal Device J Synthetic Substitute K Nonautologous Tissue Substitute Y Other Device	Z No Qualifier
0 Eye, Right 1 Eye, Left	X External	0 Drainage Device 1 Radioactive Element 3 Infusion Device 7 Autologous Tissue Substitute C Extraluminal Device D Intraluminal Device J Synthetic Substitute K Nonautologous Tissue Substitute	Z No Qualifier
J Lens, Right K Lens, Left	3 Percutaneous	J Synthetic Substitute Y Other Device	Z No Qualifier
L Extraocular Muscle, Right M Extraocular Muscle, Left	0 Open 3 Percutaneous	0 Drainage Device 7 Autologous Tissue Substitute J Synthetic Substitute K Nonautologous Tissue Substitute Y Other Device	Z No Qualifier

Section	0	Medical and Surgical
Body System	8	Eye
Operation	Q	Repair: Restoring, to the extent possible, a body part to its normal anatomic structure and function

Body Part (4th)	Approach (5th)	Device (6th)	Qualifier (7th)
0 Eye, Right 1 Eye, Left 6 Sclera, Right 7 Sclera, Left 8 Cornea, Right 9 Cornea, Left S Conjunctiva, Right T Conjunctiva, Left	X External	Z No Device	Z No Qualifier
2 Anterior Chamber, Right 3 Anterior Chamber, Left 4 Vitreous, Right 5 Vitreous, Left C Iris, Right D Iris, Left E Retina, Right F Retina, Left G Retinal Vessel, Right H Retinal Vessel, Left J Lens, Right K Lens, Left	3 Percutaneous	Z No Device	Z No Qualifier

Continued →

08Q–08R

Section   **0**   **Medical and Surgical**
Body System   **8**   **Eye**
Operation   **Q**   **Repair:** Restoring, to the extent possible, a body part to its normal anatomic structure and function

08Q Continued

Body Part (4th)	Approach (5th)	Device (6th)	Qualifier (7th)
A Choroid, Right B Choroid, Left L Extraocular Muscle, Right M Extraocular Muscle, Left V Lacrimal Gland, Right W Lacrimal Gland, Left	0 Open 3 Percutaneous	Z No Device	Z No Qualifier
N Upper Eyelid, Right P Upper Eyelid, Left Q Lower Eyelid, Right R Lower Eyelid, Left	0 Open 3 Percutaneous X External	Z No Device	Z No Qualifier
X Lacrimal Duct, Right Y Lacrimal Duct, Left	0 Open 3 Percutaneous 7 Via Natural or Artificial Opening 8 Via Natural or Artificial Opening Endoscopic	Z No Device	Z No Qualifier

Section   **0**   **Medical and Surgical**
Body System   **8**   **Eye**
Operation   **R**   **Replacement:** Putting in or on biological or synthetic material that physically takes the place and/or function of all or a portion of a body part

Body Part (4th)	Approach (5th)	Device (6th)	Qualifier (7th)
0 Eye, Right 1 Eye, Left A Choroid, Right B Choroid, Left	0 Open 3 Percutaneous	7 Autologous Tissue Substitute J Synthetic Substitute K Nonautologous Tissue Substitute	Z No Qualifier
4 Vitreous, Right 5 Vitreous, Left C Iris, Right D Iris, Left G Retinal Vessel, Right H Retinal Vessel, Left	3 Percutaneous	7 Autologous Tissue Substitute J Synthetic Substitute K Nonautologous Tissue Substitute	Z No Qualifier
6 Sclera, Right 7 Sclera, Left S Conjunctiva, Right T Conjunctiva, Left	X External	7 Autologous Tissue Substitute J Synthetic Substitute K Nonautologous Tissue Substitute	Z No Qualifier
8 Cornea, Right 9 Cornea, Left	3 Percutaneous X External	7 Autologous Tissue Substitute J Synthetic Substitute K Nonautologous Tissue Substitute	Z No Qualifier
J Lens, Right K Lens, Left	3 Percutaneous	0 Synthetic Substitute, Intraocular Telescope 7 Autologous Tissue Substitute J Synthetic Substitute K Nonautologous Tissue Substitute	Z No Qualifier
N Upper Eyelid, Right P Upper Eyelid, Left Q Lower Eyelid, Right R Lower Eyelid, Left	0 Open 3 Percutaneous X External	7 Autologous Tissue Substitute J Synthetic Substitute K Nonautologous Tissue Substitute	Z No Qualifier
X Lacrimal Duct, Right Y Lacrimal Duct, Left	0 Open 3 Percutaneous 7 Via Natural or Artificial Opening 8 Via Natural or Artificial Opening Endoscopic	7 Autologous Tissue Substitute J Synthetic Substitute K Nonautologous Tissue Substitute	Z No Qualifier

Medical and Surgical, Eye Tables

Section	0	Medical and Surgical
Body System	8	Eye
Operation	S	Reposition: Moving to its normal location, or other suitable location, all or a portion of a body part

Body Part (4th)	Approach (5th)	Device (6th)	Qualifier (7th)
C Iris, Right D Iris, Left G Retinal Vessel, Right H Retinal Vessel, Left J Lens, Right K Lens, Left	3 Percutaneous	Z No Device	Z No Qualifier
L Extraocular Muscle, Right M Extraocular Muscle, Left V Lacrimal Gland, Right W Lacrimal Gland, Left	0 Open 3 Percutaneous	Z No Device	Z No Qualifier
N Upper Eyelid, Right P Upper Eyelid, Left Q Lower Eyelid, Right R Lower Eyelid, Left	0 Open 3 Percutaneous X External	Z No Device	Z No Qualifier
X Lacrimal Duct, Right Y Lacrimal Duct, Left	0 Open 3 Percutaneous 7 Via Natural or Artificial Opening 8 Via Natural or Artificial Opening Endoscopic	Z No Device	Z No Qualifier

Section	0	Medical and Surgical
Body System	8	Eye
Operation	T	Resection: Cutting out or off, without replacement, all of a body part

Body Part (4th)	Approach (5th)	Device (6th)	Qualifier (7th)
0 Eye, Right 1 Eye, Left 8 Cornea, Right 9 Cornea, Left	X External	Z No Device	Z No Qualifier
4 Vitreous, Right 5 Vitreous, Left C Iris, Right D Iris, Left J Lens, Right K Lens, Left	3 Percutaneous	Z No Device	Z No Qualifier
L Extraocular Muscle, Right M Extraocular Muscle, Left V Lacrimal Gland, Right W Lacrimal Gland, Left	0 Open 3 Percutaneous	Z No Device	Z No Qualifier
N Upper Eyelid, Right P Upper Eyelid, Left Q Lower Eyelid, Right R Lower Eyelid, Left	0 Open X External	Z No Device	Z No Qualifier
X Lacrimal Duct, Right Y Lacrimal Duct, Left	0 Open 3 Percutaneous 7 Via Natural or Artificial Opening 8 Via Natural or Artificial Opening Endoscopic	Z No Device	Z No Qualifier

Section   **0**   **Medical and Surgical**
Body System   **8**   **Eye**
Operation   **U**   **Supplement:** Putting in or on biological or synthetic material that physically reinforces and/or augments the function of a portion of a body part

Body Part (4th)	Approach (5th)	Device (6th)	Qualifier (7th)
0 Eye, Right **1** Eye, Left **C** Iris, Right **D** Iris, Left **E** Retina, Right **F** Retina, Left **G** Retinal Vessel, Right **H** Retinal Vessel, Left **L** Extraocular Muscle, Right **M** Extraocular Muscle, Left	**0** Open **3** Percutaneous	**7** Autologous Tissue Substitute **J** Synthetic Substitute **K** Nonautologous Tissue Substitute	**Z** No Qualifier
8 Cornea, Right **9** Cornea, Left **N** Upper Eyelid, Right **P** Upper Eyelid, Left **Q** Lower Eyelid, Right **R** Lower Eyelid, Left	**0** Open **3** Percutaneous **X** External	**7** Autologous Tissue Substitute **J** Synthetic Substitute **K** Nonautologous Tissue Substitute	**Z** No Qualifier
X Lacrimal Duct, Right **Y** Lacrimal Duct, Left	**0** Open **3** Percutaneous **7** Via Natural or Artificial Opening **8** Via Natural or Artificial Opening Endoscopic	**7** Autologous Tissue Substitute **J** Synthetic Substitute **K** Nonautologous Tissue Substitute	**Z** No Qualifier

Section   **0**   **Medical and Surgical**
Body System   **8**   **Eye**
Operation   **V**   **Restriction:** Partially closing an orifice or the lumen of a tubular body part

Body Part (4th)	Approach (5th)	Device (6th)	Qualifier (7th)
X Lacrimal Duct, Right **Y** Lacrimal Duct, Left	**0** Open **3** Percutaneous	**C** Extraluminal Device **D** Intraluminal Device **Z** No Device	**Z** No Qualifier
X Lacrimal Duct, Right **Y** Lacrimal Duct, Left	**7** Via Natural or Artificial Opening **8** Via Natural or Artificial Opening Endoscopic	**D** Intraluminal Device **Z** No Device	**Z** No Qualifier

Section   **0**   **Medical and Surgical**
Body System   **8**   **Eye**
Operation   **W**   **Revision:** Correcting, to the extent possible, a portion of a malfunctioning device or the position of a displaced device

Body Part (4th)	Approach (5th)	Device (6th)	Qualifier (7th)
0 Eye, Right **1** Eye, Left	**0** Open **3** Percutaneous **7** Via Natural or Artificial Opening **8** Via Natural or Artificial Opening Endoscopic	**0** Drainage Device **3** Infusion Device **7** Autologous Tissue Substitute **C** Extraluminal Device **D** Intraluminal Device **J** Synthetic Substitute **K** Nonautologous Tissue Substitute **Y** Other Device	**Z** No Qualifier
0 Eye, Right **1** Eye, Left	**X** External	**0** Drainage Device **3** Infusion Device **7** Autologous Tissue Substitute **C** Extraluminal Device **D** Intraluminal Device **J** Synthetic Substitute **K** Nonautologous Tissue Substitute	**Z** No Qualifier

Continued ➡

Section	0	Medical and Surgical
Body System	8	Eye
Operation	W	**Revision:** Correcting, to the extent possible, a portion of a malfunctioning device or the position of a displaced device

08W Continued

Body Part (4ᵗʰ)	Approach (5ᵗʰ)	Device (6ᵗʰ)	Qualifier (7ᵗʰ)
J Lens, Right K Lens, Left	3 Percutaneous	J Synthetic Substitute Y Other Device	Z No Qualifier
J Lens, Right K Lens, Left	X External	J Synthetic Substitute	Z No Qualifier
L Extraocular Muscle, Right M Extraocular Muscle, Left	0 Open 3 Percutaneous	0 Drainage Device 7 Autologous Tissue Substitute J Synthetic Substitute K Nonautologous Tissue Substitute Y Other Device	Z No Qualifier

Section	0	Medical and Surgical
Body System	8	Eye
Operation	X	**Transfer:** Moving, without taking out, all or a portion of a body part to another location to take over the function of all or a portion of a body part

Body Part (4ᵗʰ)	Approach (5ᵗʰ)	Device (6ᵗʰ)	Qualifier (7ᵗʰ)
L Extraocular Muscle, Right M Extraocular Muscle, Left	0 Open 3 Percutaneous	Z No Device	Z No Qualifier

AHA Coding Clinic

08133J4 Bypass Left Anterior Chamber to Sclera with Synthetic Substitute, Percutaneous Approach—AHA CC: 1Q, 2019, 27-28

08923ZZ Drainage of Right Anterior Chamber, Percutaneous Approach—AHA CC: 2Q, 2016, 21-22

08B43ZZ Excision of Right Vitreous, Percutaneous Approach—AHA CC: 4Q, 2014, 36-37

08B53ZZ Excision of Left Vitreous, Percutaneous Approach—AHA CC: 4Q, 2014, 35-36

08J0XZZ Inspection of Right Eye, External Approach—AHA CC: 1Q, 2015, 35-36

08NC3ZZ Release Right Iris, Percutaneous Approach—AHA CC: 2Q, 2015, 24-25

08Q7XZZ Repair Left Sclera, External Approach—AHA CC: 3Q, 2018, 13

08Q9XZZ Repair Left Cornea, External Approach—AHA CC: 3Q, 2018, 13

08R8XKZ Replacement of Right Cornea with Nonautologous Tissue Substitute, External Approach—AHA CC: 2Q, 2015, 24-26

08T1XZZ Resection of Left Eye, External Approach—AHA CC: 2Q, 2015, 12-13

08TM0ZZ Resection of Left Extraocular Muscle, Open Approach—AHA CC: 2Q, 2015, 12-13

08TR0ZZ Resection of Left Lower Eyelid, Open Approach—AHA CC: 2Q, 2015, 12-13

08U9XKZ Supplement Left Cornea with Nonautologous Tissue Substitute, External Approach—AHA CC: 3Q, 2014, 31

Ear, Nose, Sinus

Nose and Sinuses

Frontal view

Coronal section

Anatomy of nasal cavity and sinuses

Sagittal section

Paranasal sinuses

© Elsevier Inc. All rights reserved. www.netterimages.com

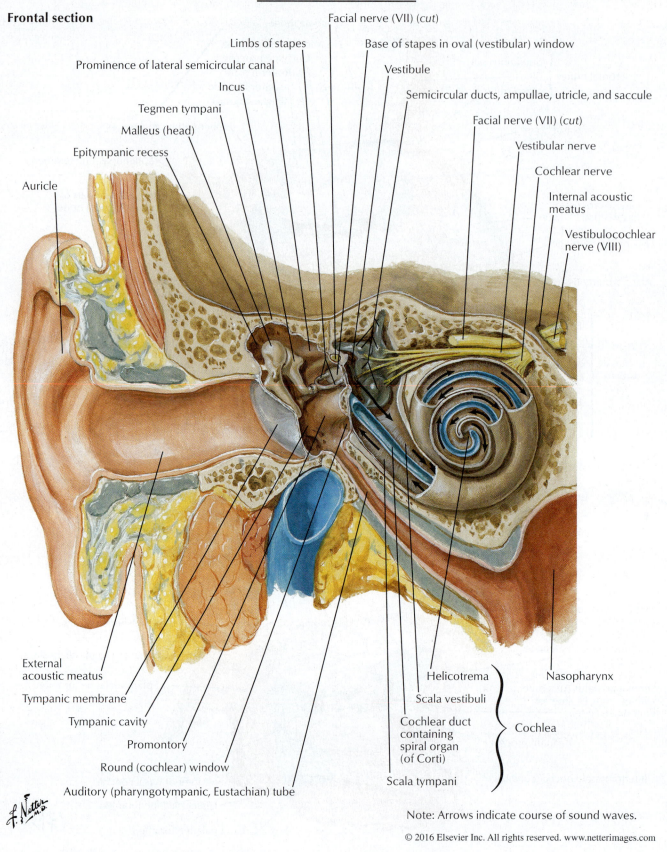

Ear, Nose, Sinus Tables 090–09W

Section	0	Medical and Surgical
Body System	9	Ear, Nose, Sinus
Operation	0	**Alteration:** Modifying the anatomic structure of a body part without affecting the function of the body part

Body Part (4th)	Approach (5th)	Device (6th)	Qualifier (7th)
0 External Ear, Right 1 External Ear, Left 2 External Ear, Bilateral K Nasal Mucosa and Soft Tissue	0 Open 3 Percutaneous 4 Percutaneous Endoscopic X External	7 Autologous Tissue Substitute J Synthetic Substitute K Nonautologous Tissue Substitute Z No Device	Z No Qualifier

Section	0	Medical and Surgical
Body System	9	Ear, Nose, Sinus
Operation	1	**Bypass:** Altering the route of passage of the contents of a tubular body part

Body Part (4th)	Approach (5th)	Device (6th)	Qualifier (7th)
D Inner Ear, Right E Inner Ear, Left	0 Open	7 Autologous Tissue Substitute J Synthetic Substitute K Nonautologous Tissue Substitute Z No Device	0 Endolymphatic

Section	0	Medical and Surgical
Body System	9	Ear, Nose, Sinus
Operation	2	**Change:** Taking out or off a device from a body part and putting back an identical or similar device in or on the same body part without cutting or puncturing the skin or a mucous membrane

Body Part (4th)	Approach (5th)	Device (6th)	Qualifier (7th)
H Ear, Right J Ear, Left K Nasal Mucosa and Soft Tissue Y Sinus	X External	0 Drainage Device Y Other Device	Z No Qualifier

Section	0	Medical and Surgical
Body System	9	Ear, Nose, Sinus
Operation	3	**Control:** Stopping, or attempting to stop, postprocedural or other acute bleeding

Body Part (4th)	Approach (5th)	Device (6th)	Qualifier (7th)
K Nasal Mucosa and Soft Tissue	7 Via Natural or Artificial Opening 8 Via Natural or Artificial Opening Endoscopic	Z No Device	Z No Qualifier

Section	0	Medical and Surgical
Body System	9	Ear, Nose, Sinus
Operation	5	**Destruction:** Physical eradication of all or a portion of a body part by the direct use of energy, force, or a destructive agent

Body Part (4th)	Approach (5th)	Device (6th)	Qualifier (7th)
0 External Ear, Right 1 External Ear, Left	0 Open 3 Percutaneous 4 Percutaneous Endoscopic X External	Z No Device	Z No Qualifier
3 External Auditory Canal, Right 4 External Auditory Canal, Left	0 Open 3 Percutaneous 4 Percutaneous Endoscopic 7 Via Natural or Artificial Opening 8 Via Natural or Artificial Opening Endoscopic X External	Z No Device	Z No Qualifier
5 Middle Ear, Right 6 Middle Ear, Left 9 Auditory Ossicle, Right A Auditory Ossicle, Left D Inner Ear, Right E Inner Ear, Left	0 Open 8 Via Natural or Artificial Opening Endoscopic	Z No Device	Z No Qualifier

Continued →

Section 0 Medical and Surgical
Body System 9 Ear, Nose, Sinus
Operation 5 Destruction: Physical eradication of all or a portion of a body part by the direct use of energy, force, or a destructive agent

Body Part (4th)	Approach (5th)	Device (6th)	Qualifier (7th)
7 Tympanic Membrane, Right 8 Tympanic Membrane, Left F Eustachian Tube, Right G Eustachian Tube, Left L Nasal Turbinate N Nasopharynx	0 Open 3 Percutaneous 4 Percutaneous Endoscopic 7 Via Natural or Artificial Opening 8 Via Natural or Artificial Opening Endoscopic	Z No Device	Z No Qualifier
B Mastoid Sinus, Right C Mastoid Sinus, Left M Nasal Septum P Accessory Sinus Q Maxillary Sinus, Right R Maxillary Sinus, Left S Frontal Sinus, Right T Frontal Sinus, Left U Ethmoid Sinus, Right V Ethmoid Sinus, Left W Sphenoid Sinus, Right X Sphenoid Sinus, Left	0 Open 3 Percutaneous 4 Percutaneous Endoscopic 8 Via Natural or Artificial Opening Endoscopic	Z No Device	Z No Qualifier
K Nasal Mucosa and Soft Tissue	0 Open 3 Percutaneous 4 Percutaneous Endoscopic 8 Via Natural or Artificial Opening Endoscopic X External	Z No Device	Z No Qualifier

Section 0 Medical and Surgical
Body System 9 Ear, Nose, Sinus
Operation 7 Dilation: Expanding an orifice or the lumen of a tubular body part

Body Part (4th)	Approach (5th)	Device (6th)	Qualifier (7th)
F Eustachian Tube, Right G Eustachian Tube, Left	0 Open 7 Via Natural or Artificial Opening 8 Via Natural or Artificial Opening Endoscopic	D Intraluminal Device Z No Device	Z No Qualifier
F Eustachian Tube, Right G Eustachian Tube, Left	3 Percutaneous 4 Percutaneous Endoscopic	Z No Device	Z No Qualifier

Section 0 Medical and Surgical
Body System 9 Ear, Nose, Sinus
Operation 8 Division: Cutting into a body part, without draining fluids and/or gases from the body part, in order to separate or transect a body part

Body Part (4th)	Approach (5th)	Device (6th)	Qualifier (7th)
L Nasal Turbinate	0 Open 3 Percutaneous 4 Percutaneous Endoscopic 7 Via Natural or Artificial Opening 8 Via Natural or Artificial Opening Endoscopic	Z No Device	Z No Qualifier

Section	0	Medical and Surgical
Body System	9	Ear, Nose, Sinus
Operation	9	Drainage: Taking or letting out fluids and/or gases from a body part

Body Part (4th)	Approach (5th)	Device (6th)	Qualifier (7th)
0 External Ear, Right 1 External Ear, Left	0 Open 3 Percutaneous 4 Percutaneous Endoscopic X External	0 Drainage Device	Z No Qualifier
0 External Ear, Right 1 External Ear, Left	0 Open 3 Percutaneous 4 Percutaneous Endoscopic X External	Z No Device	X Diagnostic Z No Qualifier
3 External Auditory Canal, Right 4 External Auditory Canal, Left K Nasal Mucosa and Soft Tissue	0 Open 3 Percutaneous 4 Percutaneous Endoscopic 7 Via Natural or Artificial Opening 8 Via Natural or Artificial Opening Endoscopic X External	0 Drainage Device	Z No Qualifier
3 External Auditory Canal, Right 4 External Auditory Canal, Left K Nasal Mucosa and Soft Tissue	0 Open 3 Percutaneous 4 Percutaneous Endoscopic 7 Via Natural or Artificial Opening 8 Via Natural or Artificial Opening Endoscopic X External	Z No Device	X Diagnostic Z No Qualifier
5 Middle Ear, Right 6 Middle Ear, Left 9 Auditory Ossicle, Right A Auditory Ossicle, Left D Inner Ear, Right E Inner Ear, Left	0 Open 7 Via Natural or Artificial Opening 8 Via Natural or Artificial Opening Endoscopic	0 Drainage Device	Z No Qualifier
5 Middle Ear, Right 6 Middle Ear, Left 9 Auditory Ossicle, Right A Auditory Ossicle, Left D Inner Ear, Right E Inner Ear, Left	0 Open 7 Via Natural or Artificial Opening 8 Via Natural or Artificial Opening Endoscopic	Z No Device	X Diagnostic Z No Qualifier
7 Tympanic Membrane, Right 8 Tympanic Membrane, Left B Mastoid Sinus, Right C Mastoid Sinus, Left F Eustachian Tube, Right G Eustachian Tube, Left L Nasal Turbinate M Nasal Septum N Nasopharynx P Accessory Sinus Q Maxillary Sinus, Right R Maxillary Sinus, Left S Frontal Sinus, Right T Frontal Sinus, Left U Ethmoid Sinus, Right V Ethmoid Sinus, Left W Sphenoid Sinus, Right X Sphenoid Sinus, Left	0 Open 3 Percutaneous 4 Percutaneous Endoscopic 7 Via Natural or Artificial Opening 8 Via Natural or Artificial Opening Endoscopic	0 Drainage Device	Z No Qualifier

Continued ➝

Section	0	Medical and Surgical			099 Continued
Body System	9	Ear, Nose, Sinus			
Operation	9	**Drainage:** Taking or letting out fluids and/or gases from a body part			

Body Part (4th)	Approach (5th)	Device (6th)	Qualifier (7th)
7 Tympanic Membrane, Right 8 Tympanic Membrane, Left B Mastoid Sinus, Right C Mastoid Sinus, Left F Eustachian Tube, Right G Eustachian Tube, Left L Nasal Turbinate M Nasal Septum N Nasopharynx P Accessory Sinus Q Maxillary Sinus, Right R Maxillary Sinus, Left S Frontal Sinus, Right T Frontal Sinus, Left U Ethmoid Sinus, Right V Ethmoid Sinus, Left W Sphenoid Sinus, Right X Sphenoid Sinus, Left	0 Open 3 Percutaneous 4 Percutaneous Endoscopic 7 Via Natural or Artificial Opening 8 Via Natural or Artificial Opening Endoscopic	Z No Device	X Diagnostic Z No Qualifier

Section	0	Medical and Surgical
Body System	9	Ear, Nose, Sinus
Operation	B	**Excision:** Cutting out or off, without replacement, a portion of a body part

Body Part (4th)	Approach (5th)	Device (6th)	Qualifier (7th)
0 External Ear, Right 1 External Ear, Left	0 Open 3 Percutaneous 4 Percutaneous Endoscopic X External	Z No Device	X Diagnostic Z No Qualifier
3 External Auditory Canal, Right 4 External Auditory Canal, Left	0 Open 3 Percutaneous 4 Percutaneous Endoscopic 7 Via Natural or Artificial Opening 8 Via Natural or Artificial Opening Endoscopic X External	Z No Device	X Diagnostic Z No Qualifier
5 Middle Ear, Right 6 Middle Ear, Left 9 Auditory Ossicle, Right A Auditory Ossicle, Left D Inner Ear, Right E Inner Ear, Left	0 Open 8 Via Natural or Artificial Opening Endoscopic	Z No Device	X Diagnostic Z No Qualifier
7 Tympanic Membrane, Right 8 Tympanic Membrane, Left F Eustachian Tube, Right G Eustachian Tube, Left L Nasal Turbinate N Nasopharynx	0 Open 3 Percutaneous 4 Percutaneous Endoscopic 7 Via Natural or Artificial Opening 8 Via Natural or Artificial Opening Endoscopic	Z No Device	X Diagnostic Z No Qualifier
B Mastoid Sinus, Right C Mastoid Sinus, Left M Nasal Septum P Accessory Sinus Q Maxillary Sinus, Right R Maxillary Sinus, Left S Frontal Sinus, Right T Frontal Sinus, Left U Ethmoid Sinus, Right V Ethmoid Sinus, Left W Sphenoid Sinus, Right X Sphenoid Sinus, Left	0 Open 3 Percutaneous 4 Percutaneous Endoscopic 8 Via Natural or Artificial Opening Endoscopic	Z No Device	X Diagnostic Z No Qualifier

Continued ➜

Section	0	Medical and Surgical
Body System	9	Ear, Nose, Sinus
Operation	B	Excision: Cutting out or off, without replacement, a portion of a body part

Body Part (4th)	Approach (5th)	Device (6th)	Qualifier (7th)
K Nasal Mucosa and Soft Tissue	0 Open 3 Percutaneous 4 Percutaneous Endoscopic 8 Via Natural or Artificial Opening Endoscopic X External	Z No Device	X Diagnostic Z No Qualifier

Section	0	Medical and Surgical
Body System	9	Ear, Nose, Sinus
Operation	C	Extirpation: Taking or cutting out solid matter from a body part

Body Part (4th)	Approach (5th)	Device (6th)	Qualifier (7th)
0 External Ear, Right 1 External Ear, Left	0 Open 3 Percutaneous 4 Percutaneous Endoscopic X External	Z No Device	Z No Qualifier
3 External Auditory Canal, Right 4 External Auditory Canal, Left	0 Open 3 Percutaneous 4 Percutaneous Endoscopic 7 Via Natural or Artificial Opening 8 Via Natural or Artificial Opening Endoscopic X External	Z No Device	Z No Qualifier
5 Middle Ear, Right 6 Middle Ear, Left 9 Auditory Ossicle, Right A Auditory Ossicle, Left D Inner Ear, Right E Inner Ear, Left	0 Open 8 Via Natural or Artificial Opening Endoscopic	Z No Device	Z No Qualifier
7 Tympanic Membrane, Right 8 Tympanic Membrane, Left F Eustachian Tube, Right G Eustachian Tube, Left L Nasal Turbinate N Nasopharynx	0 Open 3 Percutaneous 4 Percutaneous Endoscopic 7 Via Natural or Artificial Opening 8 Via Natural or Artificial Opening Endoscopic	Z No Device	Z No Qualifier
B Mastoid Sinus, Right C Mastoid Sinus, Left M Nasal Septum P Accessory Sinus Q Maxillary Sinus, Right R Maxillary Sinus, Left S Frontal Sinus, Right T Frontal Sinus, Left U Ethmoid Sinus, Right V Ethmoid Sinus, Left W Sphenoid Sinus, Right X Sphenoid Sinus, Left	0 Open 3 Percutaneous 4 Percutaneous Endoscopic 8 Via Natural or Artificial Opening Endoscopic	Z No Device	Z No Qualifier
K Nasal Mucosa and Soft Tissue	0 Open 3 Percutaneous 4 Percutaneous Endoscopic 8 Via Natural or Artificial Opening Endoscopic X External	Z No Device	Z No Qualifier

Section	0	Medical and Surgical
Body System	9	Ear, Nose, Sinus
Operation	D	**Extraction:** Pulling or stripping out or off all or a portion of a body part by the use of force

Body Part (4th)	Approach (5th)	Device (6th)	Qualifier (7th)
7 Tympanic Membrane, Right 8 Tympanic Membrane, Left L Nasal Turbinate	0 Open 3 Percutaneous 4 Percutaneous Endoscopic 7 Via Natural or Artificial Opening 8 Via Natural or Artificial Opening Endoscopic	Z No Device	Z No Qualifier
9 Auditory Ossicle, Right A Auditory Ossicle, Left	0 Open	Z No Device	Z No Qualifier
B Mastoid Sinus, Right C Mastoid Sinus, Left M Nasal Septum P Accessory Sinus Q Maxillary Sinus, Right R Maxillary Sinus, Left S Frontal Sinus, Right T Frontal Sinus, Left U Ethmoid Sinus, Right V Ethmoid Sinus, Left W Sphenoid Sinus, Right X Sphenoid Sinus, Left	0 Open 3 Percutaneous 4 Percutaneous Endoscopic	Z No Device	Z No Qualifier

Section	0	Medical and Surgical
Body System	9	Ear, Nose, Sinus
Operation	H	**Insertion:** Putting in a nonbiological appliance that monitors, assists, performs, or prevents a physiological function but does not physically take the place of a body part

Body Part (4th)	Approach (5th)	Device (6th)	Qualifier (7th)
D Inner Ear, Right E Inner Ear, Left	0 Open 3 Percutaneous 4 Percutaneous Endoscopic	1 Radioactive Element 4 Hearing Device, Bone Conduction 5 Hearing Device, Single Channel Cochlear Prosthesis 6 Hearing Device, Multiple Channel Cochlear Prosthesis S Hearing Device	Z No Qualifier
H Ear, Right J Ear, Left K Nasal Mucosa and Soft Tissue Y Sinus	0 Open 3 Percutaneous 4 Percutaneous Endoscopic 7 Via Natural or Artificial Opening 8 Via Natural or Artificial Opening Endoscopic	1 Radioactive Element Y Other Device	Z No Qualifier
N Nasopharynx	7 Via Natural or Artificial Opening 8 Via Natural or Artificial Opening Endoscopic	1 Radioactive Element B Intraluminal Device, Airway	Z No Qualifier

Section	0	Medical and Surgical
Body System	9	Ear, Nose, Sinus
Operation	J	**Inspection:** Visually and/or manually exploring a body part

Body Part (4th)	Approach (5th)	Device (6th)	Qualifier (7th)
7 Tympanic Membrane, Right 8 Tympanic Membrane, Left H Ear, Right J Ear, Left	0 Open 3 Percutaneous 4 Percutaneous Endoscopic 7 Via Natural or Artificial Opening 8 Via Natural or Artificial Opening Endoscopic X External	Z No Device	Z No Qualifier
D Inner Ear, Right E Inner Ear, Left K Nose Y Sinus	0 Open 3 Percutaneous 4 Percutaneous Endoscopic 8 Via Natural or Artificial Opening Endoscopic X External	Z No Device	Z No Qualifier

Section	0	Medical and Surgical
Body System	9	Ear, Nose, Sinus
Operation	M	Reattachment: Putting back in or on all or a portion of a separated body part to its normal location or other suitable location

Body Part (4th)	Approach (5th)	Device (6th)	Qualifier (7th)
0 External Ear, Right 1 External Ear, Left K Nasal Mucosa and Soft Tissue	X External	Z No Device	Z No Qualifier

Section	0	Medical and Surgical
Body System	9	Ear, Nose, Sinus
Operation	N	Release: Freeing a body part from an abnormal physical constraint by cutting or by the use of force

Body Part (4th)	Approach (5th)	Device (6th)	Qualifier (7th)
0 External Ear, Right 1 External Ear, Left	0 Open 3 Percutaneous 4 Percutaneous Endoscopic X External	Z No Device	Z No Qualifier
3 External Auditory Canal, Right 4 External Auditory Canal, Left	0 Open 3 Percutaneous 4 Percutaneous Endoscopic 7 Via Natural or Artificial Opening 8 Via Natural or Artificial Opening Endoscopic X External	Z No Device	Z No Qualifier
5 Middle Ear, Right 6 Middle Ear, Left 9 Auditory Ossicle, Right A Auditory Ossicle, Left D Inner Ear, Right E Inner Ear, Left	0 Open 8 Via Natural or Artificial Opening Endoscopic	Z No Device	Z No Qualifier
7 Tympanic Membrane, Right 8 Tympanic Membrane, Left F Eustachian Tube, Right G Eustachian Tube, Left L Nasal Turbinate N Nasopharynx	0 Open 3 Percutaneous 4 Percutaneous Endoscopic 7 Via Natural or Artificial Opening 8 Via Natural or Artificial Opening Endoscopic	Z No Device	Z No Qualifier
B Mastoid Sinus, Right C Mastoid Sinus, Left M Nasal Septum P Accessory Sinus Q Maxillary Sinus, Right R Maxillary Sinus, Left S Frontal Sinus, Right T Frontal Sinus, Left U Ethmoid Sinus, Right V Ethmoid Sinus, Left W Sphenoid Sinus, Right X Sphenoid Sinus, Left	0 Open 3 Percutaneous 4 Percutaneous Endoscopic 8 Via Natural or Artificial Opening Endoscopic	Z No Device	Z No Qualifier
K Nasal Mucosa and Soft Tissue	0 Open 3 Percutaneous 4 Percutaneous Endoscopic 8 Via Natural or Artificial Opening Endoscopic X External	Z No Device	Z No Qualifier

Section	0	Medical and Surgical
Body System	9	Ear, Nose, Sinus
Operation	P	**Removal:** Taking out or off a device from a body part

Body Part (4th)	Approach (5th)	Device (6th)	Qualifier (7th)
7 Tympanic Membrane, Right 8 Tympanic Membrane, Left	0 Open 7 Via Natural or Artificial Opening 8 Via Natural or Artificial Opening Endoscopic X External	0 Drainage Device	Z No Qualifier
D Inner Ear, Right E Inner Ear, Left	0 Open 7 Via Natural or Artificial Opening 8 Via Natural or Artificial Opening Endoscopic	S Hearing Device	Z No Qualifier
H Ear, Right J Ear, Left K Nasal Mucosa and Soft Tissue	0 Open 3 Percutaneous 4 Percutaneous Endoscopic 7 Via Natural or Artificial Opening 8 Via Natural or Artificial Opening Endoscopic	0 Drainage Device 7 Autologous Tissue Substitute D Intraluminal Device J Synthetic Substitute K Nonautologous Tissue Substitute Y Other Device	Z No Qualifier
H Ear, Right J Ear, Left K Nasal Mucosa and Soft Tissue	X External	0 Drainage Device 7 Autologous Tissue Substitute D Intraluminal Device J Synthetic Substitute K Nonautologous Tissue Substitute	Z No Qualifier
Y Sinus	0 Open 3 Percutaneous 4 Percutaneous Endoscopic	0 Drainage Device Y Other Device	Z No Qualifier
Y Sinus	7 Via Natural or Artificial Opening 8 Via Natural or Artificial Opening Endoscopic	Y Other Device	Z No Qualifier
Y Sinus	X External	0 Drainage Device	Z No Qualifier

Section	0	Medical and Surgical
Body System	9	Ear, Nose, Sinus
Operation	Q	**Repair:** Restoring, to the extent possible, a body part to its normal anatomic structure and function

Body Part (4th)	Approach (5th)	Device (6th)	Qualifier (7th)
0 External Ear, Right 1 External Ear, Left 2 External Ear, Bilateral	0 Open 3 Percutaneous 4 Percutaneous Endoscopic X External	Z No Device	Z No Qualifier
3 External Auditory Canal, Right 4 External Auditory Canal, Left F Eustachian Tube, Right G Eustachian Tube, Left	0 Open 3 Percutaneous 4 Percutaneous Endoscopic 7 Via Natural or Artificial Opening 8 Via Natural or Artificial Opening Endoscopic X External	Z No Device	Z No Qualifier
5 Middle Ear, Right 6 Middle Ear, Left 9 Auditory Ossicle, Right A Auditory Ossicle, Left D Inner Ear, Right E Inner Ear, Left	0 Open 8 Via Natural or Artificial Opening Endoscopic	Z No Device	Z No Qualifier
7 Tympanic Membrane, Right 8 Tympanic Membrane, Left L Nasal Turbinate N Nasopharynx	0 Open 3 Percutaneous 4 Percutaneous Endoscopic 7 Via Natural or Artificial Opening 8 Via Natural or Artificial Opening Endoscopic	Z No Device	Z No Qualifier

Continued

Section	0	Medical and Surgical
Body System	9	Ear, Nose, Sinus
Operation	Q	Repair: Restoring, to the extent possible, a body part to its normal anatomic structure and function

09Q Continued

Body Part (4th)	Approach (5th)	Device (6th)	Qualifier (7th)
B Mastoid Sinus, Right C Mastoid Sinus, Left M Nasal Septum P Accessory Sinus Q Maxillary Sinus, Right R Maxillary Sinus, Left S Frontal Sinus, Right T Frontal Sinus, Left U Ethmoid Sinus, Right V Ethmoid Sinus, Left W Sphenoid Sinus, Right X Sphenoid Sinus, Left	0 Open 3 Percutaneous 4 Percutaneous Endoscopic 8 Via Natural or Artificial Opening Endoscopic	Z No Device	Z No Qualifier
K Nasal Mucosa and Soft Tissue	0 Open 3 Percutaneous 4 Percutaneous Endoscopic 8 Via Natural or Artificial Opening Endoscopic X External	Z No Device	Z No Qualifier

Section	0	Medical and Surgical
Body System	9	Ear, Nose, Sinus
Operation	R	Replacement: Putting in or on biological or synthetic material that physically takes the place and/or function of all or a portion of a body part

Body Part (4th)	Approach (5th)	Device (6th)	Qualifier (7th)
0 External Ear, Right 1 External Ear, Left 2 External Ear, Bilateral K Nasal Mucosa and Soft Tissue	0 Open X External	7 Autologous Tissue Substitute J Synthetic Substitute K Nonautologous Tissue Substitute	Z No Qualifier
5 Middle Ear, Right 6 Middle Ear, Left 9 Auditory Ossicle, Right A Auditory Ossicle, Left D Inner Ear, Right E Inner Ear, Left	0 Open	7 Autologous Tissue Substitute J Synthetic Substitute K Nonautologous Tissue Substitute	Z No Qualifier
7 Tympanic Membrane, Right 8 Tympanic Membrane, Left N Nasopharynx	0 Open 7 Via Natural or Artificial Opening 8 Via Natural or Artificial Opening Endoscopic	7 Autologous Tissue Substitute J Synthetic Substitute K Nonautologous Tissue Substitute	Z No Qualifier
L Nasal Turbinate	0 Open 3 Percutaneous 4 Percutaneous Endoscopic 7 Via Natural or Artificial Opening 8 Via Natural or Artificial Opening Endoscopic	7 Autologous Tissue Substitute J Synthetic Substitute K Nonautologous Tissue Substitute	Z No Qualifier
M Nasal Septum	0 Open 3 Percutaneous 4 Percutaneous Endoscopic	7 Autologous Tissue Substitute J Synthetic Substitute K Nonautologous Tissue Substitute	Z No Qualifier

Section	0	Medical and Surgical
Body System	9	Ear, Nose, Sinus
Operation	S	Reposition: Moving to its normal location, or other suitable location, all or a portion of a body part

Body Part (4th)	Approach (5th)	Device (6th)	Qualifier (7th)
0 External Ear, Right 1 External Ear, Left 2 External Ear, Bilateral K Nasal Mucosa and Soft Tissue	0 Open 4 Percutaneous Endoscopic X External	Z No Device	Z No Qualifier
7 Tympanic Membrane, Right 8 Tympanic Membrane, Left F Eustachian Tube, Right G Eustachian Tube, Left L Nasal Turbinate	0 Open 4 Percutaneous Endoscopic 7 Via Natural or Artificial Opening 8 Via Natural or Artificial Opening Endoscopic	Z No Device	Z No Qualifier
9 Auditory Ossicle, Right A Auditory Ossicle, Left M Nasal Septum	0 Open 4 Percutaneous Endoscopic	Z No Device	Z No Qualifier

Section	0	Medical and Surgical
Body System	9	Ear, Nose, Sinus
Operation	T	Resection: Cutting out or off, without replacement, all of a body part

Body Part (4th)	Approach (5th)	Device (6th)	Qualifier (7th)
0 External Ear, Right 1 External Ear, Left	0 Open 4 Percutaneous Endoscopic X External	Z No Device	Z No Qualifier
5 Middle Ear, Right 6 Middle Ear, Left 9 Auditory Ossicle, Right A Auditory Ossicle, Left D Inner Ear, Right E Inner Ear, Left	0 Open 8 Via Natural or Artificial Opening Endoscopic	Z No Device	Z No Qualifier
7 Tympanic Membrane, Right 8 Tympanic Membrane, Left F Eustachian Tube, Right G Eustachian Tube, Left L Nasal Turbinate N Nasopharynx	0 Open 4 Percutaneous Endoscopic 7 Via Natural or Artificial Opening 8 Via Natural or Artificial Opening Endoscopic	Z No Device	Z No Qualifier
B Mastoid Sinus, Right C Mastoid Sinus, Left M Nasal Septum P Accessory Sinus Q Maxillary Sinus, Right R Maxillary Sinus, Left S Frontal Sinus, Right T Frontal Sinus, Left U Ethmoid Sinus, Right V Ethmoid Sinus, Left W Sphenoid Sinus, Right X Sphenoid Sinus, Left	0 Open 4 Percutaneous Endoscopic 8 Via Natural or Artificial Opening Endoscopic	Z No Device	Z No Qualifier
K Nasal Mucosa and Soft Tissue	0 Open 4 Percutaneous Endoscopic 8 Via Natural or Artificial Opening Endoscopic X External	Z No Device	Z No Qualifier

Section	0	Medical and Surgical
Body System	9	Ear, Nose, Sinus
Operation	U	Supplement: Putting in or on biological or synthetic material that physically reinforces and/or augments the function of a portion of a body part

Body Part (4th)	Approach (5th)	Device (6th)	Qualifier (7th)
0 External Ear, Right 1 External Ear, Left 2 External Ear, Bilateral	0 Open X External	7 Autologous Tissue Substitute J Synthetic Substitute K Nonautologous Tissue Substitute	Z No Qualifier
5 Middle Ear, Right 6 Middle Ear, Left 9 Auditory Ossicle, Right A Auditory Ossicle, Left D Inner Ear, Right E Inner Ear, Left	0 Open 8 Via Natural or Artificial Opening Endoscopic	7 Autologous Tissue Substitute J Synthetic Substitute K Nonautologous Tissue Substitute	Z No Qualifier
7 Tympanic Membrane, Right 8 Tympanic Membrane, Left N Nasopharynx	0 Open 7 Via Natural or Artificial Opening 8 Via Natural or Artificial Opening Endoscopic	7 Autologous Tissue Substitute J Synthetic Substitute K Nonautologous Tissue Substitute	Z No Qualifier
B Mastoid Sinus, Right C Mastoid Sinus, Left L Nasal Turbinate P Accessory Sinus Q Maxillary Sinus, Right R Maxillary Sinus, Left S Frontal Sinus, Right T Frontal Sinus, Left U Ethmoid Sinus, Right V Ethmoid Sinus, Left W Sphenoid Sinus, Right X Sphenoid Sinus, Left	0 Open 3 Percutaneous 4 Percutaneous Endoscopic 7 Via Natural or Artificial Opening 8 Via Natural or Artificial Opening Endoscopic	7 Autologous Tissue Substitute J Synthetic Substitute K Nonautologous Tissue Substitute	Z No Qualifier
K Nasal Mucosa and Soft Tissue	0 Open 8 Via Natural or Artificial Opening Endoscopic X External	7 Autologous Tissue Substitute J Synthetic Substitute K Nonautologous Tissue Substitute	Z No Qualifier
M Nasal Septum	0 Open 3 Percutaneous 4 Percutaneous Endoscopic 8 Via Natural or Artificial Opening Endoscopic	7 Autologous Tissue Substitute J Synthetic Substitute K Nonautologous Tissue Substitute	Z No Qualifier

Section	0	Medical and Surgical
Body System	9	Ear, Nose, Sinus
Operation	W	Revision: Correcting, to the extent possible, a portion of a malfunctioning device or the position of a displaced device

Body Part (4th)	Approach (5th)	Device (6th)	Qualifier (7th)
7 Tympanic Membrane, Right 8 Tympanic Membrane, Left 9 Auditory Ossicle, Right A Auditory Ossicle, Left	0 Open 7 Via Natural or Artificial Opening 8 Via Natural or Artificial Opening Endoscopic	7 Autologous Tissue Substitute J Synthetic Substitute K Nonautologous Tissue Substitute	Z No Qualifier
D Inner Ear, Right E Inner Ear, Left	0 Open 7 Via Natural or Artificial Opening 8 Via Natural or Artificial Opening Endoscopic	S Hearing Device	Z No Qualifier
H Ear, Right J Ear, Left K Nasal Mucosa and Soft Tissue	0 Open 3 Percutaneous 4 Percutaneous Endoscopic 7 Via Natural or Artificial Opening 8 Via Natural or Artificial Opening Endoscopic	0 Drainage Device 7 Autologous Tissue Substitute D Intraluminal Device J Synthetic Substitute K Nonautologous Tissue Substitute Y Other Device	Z No Qualifier

Continued →

Section	0	Medical and Surgical
Body System	9	Ear, Nose, Sinus
Operation	W	**Revision:** Correcting, to the extent possible, a portion of a malfunctioning device or the position of a displaced device

Body Part (4th)	Approach (5th)	Device (6th)	Qualifier (7th)
H Ear, Right **J** Ear, Left **K** Nasal Mucosa and Soft Tissue	**X** External	**0** Drainage Device **7** Autologous Tissue Substitute **D** Intraluminal Device **J** Synthetic Substitute **K** Nonautologous Tissue Substitute	**Z** No Qualifier
Y Sinus	**0** Open **3** Percutaneous **4** Percutaneous Endoscopic	**0** Drainage Device **Y** Other Device	**Z** No Qualifier
Y Sinus	**7** Via Natural or Artificial Opening **8** Via Natural or Artificial Opening Endoscopic	**Y** Other Device	**Z** No Qualifier
Y Sinus	**X** External	**0** Drainage Device	**Z** No Qualifier

AHA Coding Clinic

093K8ZZ Control Bleeding in Nasal Mucosa and Soft Tissue, Via Natural or Artificial Opening Endoscopic—AHA CC: 4Q, 2018, 38

09HK7YZ Insertion of Other Device into Nasal Mucosa and Soft Tissue, Via Natural or Artificial Opening—AHA CC: 2Q, 2022, 18

09QKXZZ Repair Nasal Mucosa and Soft Tissue, External Approach—AHA CC: 4Q, 2014, 20-21

09QT4ZZ Repair Left Frontal Sinus, Percutaneous Endoscopic Approach—AHA CC: 4Q, 2013, 114

09QW0ZZ Repair Right Sphenoid Sinus, Open Approach—AHA CC: 3Q, 2014, 22-23

09QX0ZZ Repair Left Sphenoid Sinus, Open Approach—AHA CC: 3Q, 2014, 22-23

Respiratory System

Topography of Lungs: Anterior View

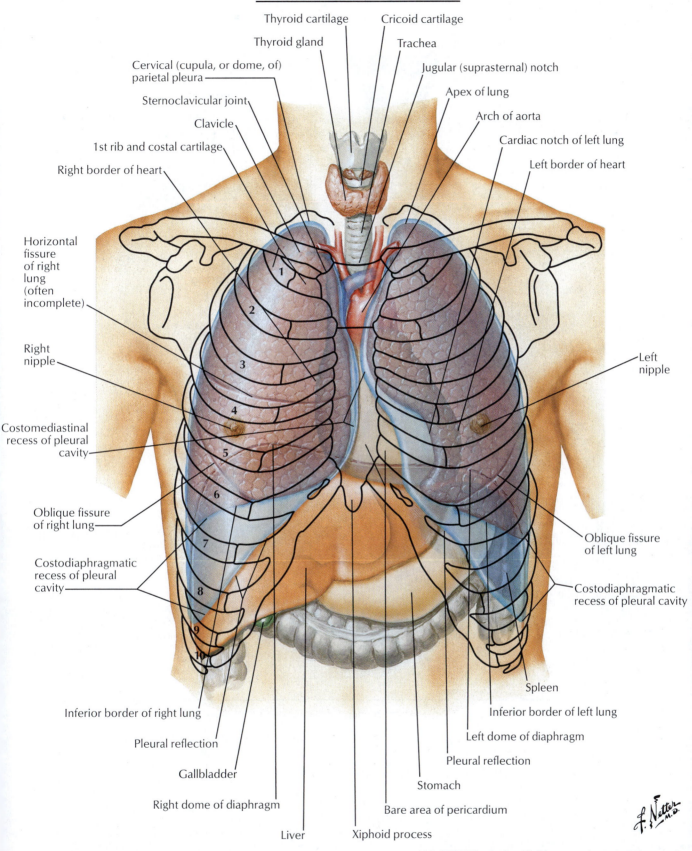

Structure of the Trachea and Major Bronchi

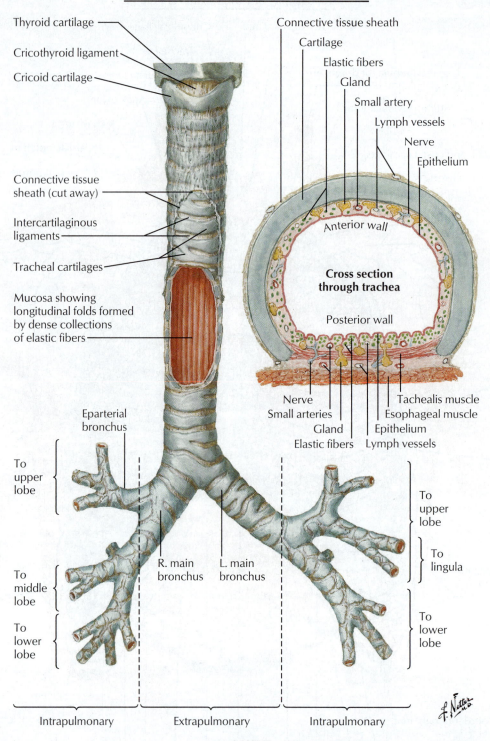

Sublobar Resection and Surgical Lung Biopsy

Segmental resection

Wedge resection or open lung biopsy

Respiratory System Tables 0B1–0BY

Section	0	Medical and Surgical
Body System	B	Respiratory System
Operation	1	Bypass: Altering the route of passage of the contents of a tubular body part

Body Part (4th)	Approach (5th)	Device (6th)	Qualifier (7th)
1 Trachea	0 Open	D Intraluminal Device	6 Esophagus
1 Trachea	0 Open	F Tracheostomy Device Z No Device	4 Cutaneous
1 Trachea	3 Percutaneous 4 Percutaneous Endoscopic	F Tracheostomy Device Z No Device	4 Cutaneous

Section	0	Medical and Surgical
Body System	B	Respiratory System
Operation	2	Change: Taking out or off a device from a body part and putting back an identical or similar device in or on the same body part without cutting or puncturing the skin or a mucous membrane

Body Part (4th)	Approach (5th)	Device (6th)	Qualifier (7th)
0 Tracheobronchial Tree K Lung, Right L Lung, Left Q Pleura T Diaphragm	X External	0 Drainage Device Y Other Device	Z No Qualifier
1 Trachea	X External	0 Drainage Device E Intraluminal Device, Endotracheal Airway F Tracheostomy Device Y Other Device	Z No Qualifier

Section	0	Medical and Surgical
Body System	B	Respiratory System
Operation	5	Destruction: Physical eradication of all or a portion of a body part by the direct use of energy, force, or a destructive agent

Body Part (4th)	Approach (5th)	Device (6th)	Qualifier (7th)
1 Trachea 2 Carina 3 Main Bronchus, Right 4 Upper Lobe Bronchus, Right 5 Middle Lobe Bronchus, Right 6 Lower Lobe Bronchus, Right 7 Main Bronchus, Left 8 Upper Lobe Bronchus, Left 9 Lingula Bronchus B Lower Lobe Bronchus, Left	0 Open 3 Percutaneous 4 Percutaneous Endoscopic 7 Via Natural or Artificial Opening 8 Via Natural or Artificial Opening Endoscopic	Z No Device	Z No Qualifier
C Upper Lung Lobe, Right D Middle Lung Lobe, Right F Lower Lung Lobe, Right G Upper Lung Lobe, Left H Lung Lingula J Lower Lung Lobe, Left K Lung, Right L Lung, Left M Lungs, Bilateral	0 Open 3 Percutaneous 4 Percutaneous Endoscopic	Z No Device	3 Laser Interstitial Thermal Therapy Z No Qualifier
C Upper Lung Lobe, Right D Middle Lung Lobe, Right F Lower Lung Lobe, Right G Upper Lung Lobe, Left H Lung Lingula J Lower Lung Lobe, Left K Lung, Right L Lung, Left M Lungs, Bilateral	7 Via Natural or Artificial Opening 8 Via Natural or Artificial Opening Endoscopic	Z No Device	Z No Qualifier
N Pleura, Right P Pleura, Left T Diaphragm	0 Open 3 Percutaneous 4 Percutaneous Endoscopic	Z No Device	Z No Qualifier

0B7–0B9

Medical and Surgical, Respiratory System Tables

Section	0	Medical and Surgical
Body System	B	Respiratory System
Operation	7	**Dilation:** Expanding an orifice or the lumen of a tubular body part

Body Part (4th)	Approach (5th)	Device (6th)	Qualifier (7th)
1 Trachea 2 Carina 3 Main Bronchus, Right 4 Upper Lobe Bronchus, Right 5 Middle Lobe Bronchus, Right 6 Lower Lobe Bronchus, Right 7 Main Bronchus, Left 8 Upper Lobe Bronchus, Left 9 Lingula Bronchus B Lower Lobe Bronchus, Left	0 Open 3 Percutaneous 4 Percutaneous Endoscopic 7 Via Natural or Artificial Opening 8 Via Natural or Artificial Opening Endoscopic	D Intraluminal Device Z No Device	Z No Qualifier

Section	0	Medical and Surgical
Body System	B	Respiratory System
Operation	9	**Drainage:** Taking or letting out fluids and/or gases from a body part

Body Part (4th)	Approach (5th)	Device (6th)	Qualifier (7th)
1 Trachea 2 Carina 3 Main Bronchus, Right 4 Upper Lobe Bronchus, Right 5 Middle Lobe Bronchus, Right 6 Lower Lobe Bronchus, Right 7 Main Bronchus, Left 8 Upper Lobe Bronchus, Left 9 Lingula Bronchus B Lower Lobe Bronchus, Left C Upper Lung Lobe, Right D Middle Lung Lobe, Right F Lower Lung Lobe, Right G Upper Lung Lobe, Left H Lung Lingula J Lower Lung Lobe, Left K Lung, Right L Lung, Left M Lungs, Bilateral	0 Open 3 Percutaneous 4 Percutaneous Endoscopic 7 Via Natural or Artificial Opening 8 Via Natural or Artificial Opening Endoscopic	0 Drainage Device	Z No Qualifier
1 Trachea 2 Carina 3 Main Bronchus, Right 4 Upper Lobe Bronchus, Right 5 Middle Lobe Bronchus, Right 6 Lower Lobe Bronchus, Right 7 Main Bronchus, Left 8 Upper Lobe Bronchus, Left 9 Lingula Bronchus B Lower Lobe Bronchus, Left C Upper Lung Lobe, Right D Middle Lung Lobe, Right F Lower Lung Lobe, Right G Upper Lung Lobe, Left H Lung Lingula J Lower Lung Lobe, Left K Lung, Right L Lung, Left M Lungs, Bilateral	0 Open 3 Percutaneous 4 Percutaneous Endoscopic 7 Via Natural or Artificial Opening 8 Via Natural or Artificial Opening Endoscopic	Z No Device	X Diagnostic Z No Qualifier
N Pleura, Right P Pleura, Left	0 Open 3 Percutaneous 4 Percutaneous Endoscopic 8 Via Natural or Artificial Opening Endoscopic	0 Drainage Device	Z No Qualifier
N Pleura, Right P Pleura, Left	0 Open 3 Percutaneous 4 Percutaneous Endoscopic 8 Via Natural or Artificial Opening Endoscopic	Z No Device	X Diagnostic Z No Qualifier

Continued →

Section	0	Medical and Surgical
Body System	B	Respiratory System
Operation	9	Drainage: Taking or letting out fluids and/or gases from a body part

0B9 Continued

Body Part (4th)	Approach (5th)	Device (6th)	Qualifier (7th)
T Diaphragm	0 Open 3 Percutaneous 4 Percutaneous Endoscopic	0 Drainage Device	Z No Qualifier
T Diaphragm	0 Open 3 Percutaneous 4 Percutaneous Endoscopic	Z No Device	X Diagnostic Z No Qualifier

Section	0	Medical and Surgical
Body System	B	Respiratory System
Operation	B	Excision: Cutting out or off, without replacement, a portion of a body part

Body Part (4th)	Approach (5th)	Device (6th)	Qualifier (7th)
1 Trachea 2 Carina 3 Main Bronchus, Right 4 Upper Lobe Bronchus, Right 5 Middle Lobe Bronchus, Right 6 Lower Lobe Bronchus, Right 7 Main Bronchus, Left 8 Upper Lobe Bronchus, Left 9 Lingula Bronchus B Lower Lobe Bronchus, Left C Upper Lung Lobe, Right D Middle Lung Lobe, Right F Lower Lung Lobe, Right G Upper Lung Lobe, Left H Lung Lingula J Lower Lung Lobe, Left K Lung, Right L Lung, Left M Lungs, Bilateral	0 Open 3 Percutaneous 4 Percutaneous Endoscopic 7 Via Natural or Artificial Opening 8 Via Natural or Artificial Opening Endoscopic	Z No Device	X Diagnostic Z No Qualifier
N Pleura, Right P Pleura, Left	0 Open 3 Percutaneous 4 Percutaneous Endoscopic 8 Via Natural or Artificial Opening Endoscopic	Z No Device	X Diagnostic Z No Qualifier
T Diaphragm	0 Open 3 Percutaneous 4 Percutaneous Endoscopic	Z No Device	X Diagnostic Z No Qualifier

Section	0	Medical and Surgical
Body System	B	Respiratory System
Operation	C	Extirpation: Taking or cutting out solid matter from a body part

Body Part (4th)	Approach (5th)	Device (6th)	Qualifier (7th)
1 Trachea 2 Carina 3 Main Bronchus, Right 4 Upper Lobe Bronchus, Right 5 Middle Lobe Bronchus, Right 6 Lower Lobe Bronchus, Right 7 Main Bronchus, Left 8 Upper Lobe Bronchus, Left 9 Lingula Bronchus B Lower Lobe Bronchus, Left C Upper Lung Lobe, Right D Middle Lung Lobe, Right F Lower Lung Lobe, Right G Upper Lung Lobe, Left H Lung Lingula J Lower Lung Lobe, Left K Lung, Right L Lung, Left M Lungs, Bilateral	0 Open 3 Percutaneous 4 Percutaneous Endoscopic 7 Via Natural or Artificial Opening 8 Via Natural or Artificial Opening Endoscopic	Z No Device	Z No Qualifier

Continued →

Section	0	Medical and Surgical
Body System	B	Respiratory System
Operation	C	Extirpation: Taking or cutting out solid matter from a body part

Body Part (4th)	Approach (5th)	Device (6th)	Qualifier (7th)
N Pleura, Right P Pleura, Left T Diaphragm	0 Open 3 Percutaneous 4 Percutaneous Endoscopic	Z No Device	Z No Qualifier

Section	0	Medical and Surgical
Body System	B	Respiratory System
Operation	D	Extraction: Pulling or stripping out or off all or a portion of a body part by the use of force

Body Part (4th)	Approach (5th)	Device (6th)	Qualifier (7th)
1 Trachea 2 Carina 3 Main Bronchus, Right 4 Upper Lobe Bronchus, Right 5 Middle Lobe Bronchus, Right 6 Lower Lobe Bronchus, Right 7 Main Bronchus, Left 8 Upper Lobe Bronchus, Left 9 Lingula Bronchus B Lower Lobe Bronchus, Left C Upper Lung Lobe, Right D Middle Lung Lobe, Right F Lower Lung Lobe, Right G Upper Lung Lobe, Left H Lung Lingula J Lower Lung Lobe, Left K Lung, Right L Lung, Left M Lung, Bilateral	4 Percutaneous Endoscopic 8 Via Natural or Artificial Opening Endoscopic	Z No Device	X Diagnostic
N Pleura, Right P Pleura, Left	0 Open 3 Percutaneous 4 Percutaneous Endoscopic	Z No Device	X Diagnostic Z No Qualifier

Section	0	Medical and Surgical
Body System	B	Respiratory System
Operation	F	Fragmentation: Breaking solid matter in a body part into pieces

Body Part (4th)	Approach (5th)	Device (6th)	Qualifier (7th)
1 Trachea 2 Carina 3 Main Bronchus, Right 4 Upper Lobe Bronchus, Right 5 Middle Lobe Bronchus, Right 6 Lower Lobe Bronchus, Right 7 Main Bronchus, Left 8 Upper Lobe Bronchus, Left 9 Lingula Bronchus B Lower Lobe Bronchus, Left	0 Open 3 Percutaneous 4 Percutaneous Endoscopic 7 Via Natural or Artificial Opening 8 Via Natural or Artificial Opening Endoscopic X External	Z No Device	Z No Qualifier

	Section	0	Medical and Surgical
	Body System	B	Respiratory System
	Operation	H	Insertion: Putting in a nonbiological appliance that monitors, assists, performs, or prevents a physiological function but does not physically take the place of a body part

Body Part (4th)	Approach (5th)	Device (6th)	Qualifier (7th)
0 Tracheobronchial Tree	0 Open 3 Percutaneous 4 Percutaneous Endoscopic 7 Via Natural or Artificial Opening 8 Via Natural or Artificial Opening Endoscopic	1 Radioactive Element 2 Monitoring Device 3 Infusion Device D Intraluminal Device Y Other Device	Z No Qualifier
1 Trachea	0 Open	2 Monitoring Device D Intraluminal Device Y Other Device	Z No Qualifier
1 Trachea	3 Percutaneous	D Intraluminal Device E Intraluminal Device, Endotracheal Airway Y Other Device	Z No Qualifier
1 Trachea	4 Percutaneous Endoscopic	D Intraluminal Device Y Other Device	Z No Qualifier
1 Trachea	7 Via Natural or Artificial Opening 8 Via Natural or Artificial Opening Endoscopic	2 Monitoring Device D Intraluminal Device E Intraluminal Device, Endotracheal Airway Y Other Device	Z No Qualifier
3 Main Bronchus, Right 4 Upper Lobe Bronchus, Right 5 Middle Lobe Bronchus, Right 6 Lower Lobe Bronchus, Right 7 Main Bronchus, Left 8 Upper Lobe Bronchus, Left 9 Lingula Bronchus B Lower Lobe Bronchus, Left	0 Open 3 Percutaneous 4 Percutaneous Endoscopic 7 Via Natural or Artificial Opening 8 Via Natural or Artificial Opening Endoscopic	G Intraluminal Device, Endobronchial Valve	Z No Qualifier
K Lung, Right L Lung, Left	0 Open 3 Percutaneous 4 Percutaneous Endoscopic 7 Via Natural or Artificial Opening 8 Via Natural or Artificial Opening Endoscopic	1 Radioactive Element 2 Monitoring Device 3 Infusion Device Y Other Device	Z No Qualifier
Q Pleura	0 Open 3 Percutaneous 4 Percutaneous Endoscopic 7 Via Natural or Artificial Opening 8 Via Natural or Artificial Opening Endoscopic	Y Other Device	Z No Qualifier
T Diaphragm	0 Open 3 Percutaneous 4 Percutaneous Endoscopic	2 Monitoring Device M Diaphragmatic Pacemaker Lead Y Other Device	Z No Qualifier
T Diaphragm	7 Via Natural or Artificial Opening 8 Via Natural or Artificial Opening Endoscopic	Y Other Device	Z No Qualifier

0BJ–0BM

Medical and Surgical, Respiratory System Tables

Section	0	Medical and Surgical
Body System	B	Respiratory System
Operation	J	**Inspection:** Visually and/or manually exploring a body part

Body Part (4th)	Approach (5th)	Device (6th)	Qualifier (7th)
0 Tracheobronchial Tree 1 Trachea K Lung, Right L Lung, Left Q Pleura T Diaphragm	0 Open 3 Percutaneous 4 Percutaneous Endoscopic 7 Via Natural or Artificial Opening 8 Via Natural or Artificial Opening Endoscopic X External	Z No Device	Z No Qualifier

Section	0	Medical and Surgical
Body System	B	Respiratory System
Operation	L	**Occlusion:** Completely closing an orifice or the lumen of a tubular body part

Body Part (4th)	Approach (5th)	Device (6th)	Qualifier (7th)
1 Trachea 2 Carina 3 Main Bronchus, Right 4 Upper Lobe Bronchus, Right 5 Middle Lobe Bronchus, Right 6 Lower Lobe Bronchus, Right 7 Main Bronchus, Left 8 Upper Lobe Bronchus, Left 9 Lingula Bronchus B Lower Lobe Bronchus, Left	0 Open 3 Percutaneous 4 Percutaneous Endoscopic	C Extraluminal Device D Intraluminal Device Z No Device	Z No Qualifier
1 Trachea 2 Carina 3 Main Bronchus, Right 4 Upper Lobe Bronchus, Right 5 Middle Lobe Bronchus, Right 6 Lower Lobe Bronchus, Right 7 Main Bronchus, Left 8 Upper Lobe Bronchus, Left 9 Lingula Bronchus B Lower Lobe Bronchus, Left	7 Via Natural or Artificial Opening 8 Via Natural or Artificial Opening Endoscopic	D Intraluminal Device Z No Device	Z No Qualifier

Section	0	Medical and Surgical
Body System	B	Respiratory System
Operation	M	**Reattachment:** Putting back in or on all or a portion of a separated body part to its normal location or other suitable location

Body Part (4th)	Approach (5th)	Device (6th)	Qualifier (7th)
1 Trachea 2 Carina 3 Main Bronchus, Right 4 Upper Lobe Bronchus, Right 5 Middle Lobe Bronchus, Right 6 Lower Lobe Bronchus, Right 7 Main Bronchus, Left 8 Upper Lobe Bronchus, Left 9 Lingula Bronchus B Lower Lobe Bronchus, Left C Upper Lung Lobe, Right D Middle Lung Lobe, Right F Lower Lung Lobe, Right G Upper Lung Lobe, Left H Lung Lingula J Lower Lung Lobe, Left K Lung, Right L Lung, Left T Diaphragm	0 Open	Z No Device	Z No Qualifier

250

Section	0	Medical and Surgical
Body System	B	Respiratory System
Operation	N	**Release:** Freeing a body part from an abnormal physical constraint by cutting or by the use of force

Body Part (4th)	Approach (5th)	Device (6th)	Qualifier (7th)
1 Trachea 2 Carina 3 Main Bronchus, Right 4 Upper Lobe Bronchus, Right 5 Middle Lobe Bronchus, Right 6 Lower Lobe Bronchus, Right 7 Main Bronchus, Left 8 Upper Lobe Bronchus, Left 9 Lingula Bronchus B Lower Lobe Bronchus, Left C Upper Lung Lobe, Right D Middle Lung Lobe, Right F Lower Lung Lobe, Right G Upper Lung Lobe, Left H Lung Lingula J Lower Lung Lobe, Left K Lung, Right L Lung, Left M Lungs, Bilateral	0 Open 3 Percutaneous 4 Percutaneous Endoscopic 7 Via Natural or Artificial Opening 8 Via Natural or Artificial Opening Endoscopic	Z No Device	Z No Qualifier
N Pleura, Right P Pleura, Left T Diaphragm	0 Open 3 Percutaneous 4 Percutaneous Endoscopic	Z No Device	Z No Qualifier

Section	0	Medical and Surgical
Body System	B	Respiratory System
Operation	P	**Removal:** Taking out or off a device from a body part

Body Part (4th)	Approach (5th)	Device (6th)	Qualifier (7th)
0 Tracheobronchial Tree	0 Open 3 Percutaneous 4 Percutaneous Endoscopic 7 Via Natural or Artificial Opening 8 Via Natural or Artificial Opening Endoscopic	0 Drainage Device 1 Radioactive Element 2 Monitoring Device 3 Infusion Device 7 Autologous Tissue Substitute C Extraluminal Device D Intraluminal Device J Synthetic Substitute K Nonautologous Tissue Substitute Y Other Device	Z No Qualifier
0 Tracheobronchial Tree	X External	0 Drainage Device 1 Radioactive Element 2 Monitoring Device 3 Infusion Device D Intraluminal Device	Z No Qualifier
1 Trachea	0 Open 3 Percutaneous 4 Percutaneous Endoscopic 7 Via Natural or Artificial Opening 8 Via Natural or Artificial Opening Endoscopic	0 Drainage Device 2 Monitoring Device 7 Autologous Tissue Substitute C Extraluminal Device D Intraluminal Device F Tracheostomy Device J Synthetic Substitute K Nonautologous Tissue Substitute	Z No Qualifier
1 Trachea	X External	0 Drainage Device 2 Monitoring Device D Intraluminal Device F Tracheostomy Device	Z No Qualifier

0BP–0BQ

Medical and Surgical, Respiratory System Tables

Section	0	Medical and Surgical			0BP Continued
Body System	B	Respiratory System			
Operation	P	Removal: Taking out or off a device from a body part			

Body Part (4th)	Approach (5th)	Device (6th)	Qualifier (7th)
K Lung, Right L Lung, Left	0 Open 3 Percutaneous 4 Percutaneous Endoscopic 7 Via Natural or Artificial Opening 8 Via Natural or Artificial Opening Endoscopic	0 Drainage Device 1 Radioactive Element 2 Monitoring Device 3 Infusion Device Y Other Device	Z No Qualifier
K Lung, Right L Lung, Left	X External	0 Drainage Device 1 Radioactive Element 2 Monitoring Device 3 Infusion Device	Z No Qualifier
Q Pleura	0 Open 3 Percutaneous 4 Percutaneous Endoscopic 7 Via Natural or Artificial Opening 8 Via Natural or Artificial Opening Endoscopic	0 Drainage Device 1 Radioactive Element 2 Monitoring Device Y Other Device	Z No Qualifier
Q Pleura	X External	0 Drainage Device 1 Radioactive Element 2 Monitoring Device	Z No Qualifier
T Diaphragm	0 Open 3 Percutaneous 4 Percutaneous Endoscopic 7 Via Natural or Artificial Opening 8 Via Natural or Artificial Opening Endoscopic	0 Drainage Device 2 Monitoring Device 7 Autologous Tissue Substitute J Synthetic Substitute K Nonautologous Tissue Substitute M Diaphragmatic Pacemaker Lead Y Other Device	Z No Qualifier
T Diaphragm	X External	0 Drainage Device 2 Monitoring Device M Diaphragmatic Pacemaker Lead	Z No Qualifier

Section	0	Medical and Surgical
Body System	B	Respiratory System
Operation	Q	Repair: Restoring, to the extent possible, a body part to its normal anatomic structure and function

Body Part (4th)	Approach (5th)	Device (6th)	Qualifier (7th)
1 Trachea 2 Carina 3 Main Bronchus, Right 4 Upper Lobe Bronchus, Right 5 Middle Lobe Bronchus, Right 6 Lower Lobe Bronchus, Right 7 Main Bronchus, Left 8 Upper Lobe Bronchus, Left 9 Lingula Bronchus B Lower Lobe Bronchus, Left C Upper Lung Lobe, Right D Middle Lung Lobe, Right F Lower Lung Lobe, Right G Upper Lung Lobe, Left H Lung Lingula J Lower Lung Lobe, Left K Lung, Right L Lung, Left M Lungs, Bilateral	0 Open 3 Percutaneous 4 Percutaneous Endoscopic 7 Via Natural or Artificial Opening 8 Via Natural or Artificial Opening Endoscopic	Z No Device	Z No Qualifier
N Pleura, Right P Pleura, Left T Diaphragm	0 Open 3 Percutaneous 4 Percutaneous Endoscopic	Z No Device	Z No Qualifier

252

Section	0	Medical and Surgical
Body System	B	Respiratory
Operation	R	**Replacement:** Putting in or on biological or synthetic material that physically takes the place and/or function of all or a portion of a body part

Body Part (4th)	Approach (5th)	Device (6th)	Qualifier (7th)
1 Trachea 2 Carina 3 Main Bronchus, Right 4 Upper Lobe Bronchus, Right 5 Middle Lobe Bronchus, Right 6 Lower Lobe Bronchus, Right 7 Main Bronchus, Left 8 Upper Lobe Bronchus, Left 9 Lingula Bronchus B Lower Lobe Bronchus, Left T Diaphragm	0 Open 4 Percutaneous Endoscopic	7 Autologous Tissue Substitute J Synthetic Substitute K Nonautologous Tissue Substitute	Z No Qualifier

Section	0	Medical and Surgical
Body System	B	Respiratory System
Operation	S	**Reposition:** Moving to its normal location, or other suitable location, all or a portion of a body part

Body Part (4th)	Approach (5th)	Device (6th)	Qualifier (7th)
1 Trachea 2 Carina 3 Main Bronchus, Right 4 Upper Lobe Bronchus, Right 5 Middle Lobe Bronchus, Right 6 Lower Lobe Bronchus, Right 7 Main Bronchus, Left 8 Upper Lobe Bronchus, Left 9 Lingula Bronchus B Lower Lobe Bronchus, Left C Upper Lung Lobe, Right D Middle Lung Lobe, Right F Lower Lung Lobe, Right G Upper Lung Lobe, Left H Lung Lingula J Lower Lung Lobe, Left K Lung, Right L Lung, Left T Diaphragm	0 Open	Z No Device	Z No Qualifier

0BT–0BU

Medical and Surgical, Respiratory System Tables

Section	0	Medical and Surgical
Body System	B	Respiratory System
Operation	T	Resection: Cutting out or off, without replacement, all of a body part

Body Part (4th)	Approach (5th)	Device (6th)	Qualifier (7th)
1 Trachea 2 Carina 3 Main Bronchus, Right 4 Upper Lobe Bronchus, Right 5 Middle Lobe Bronchus, Right 6 Lower Lobe Bronchus, Right 7 Main Bronchus, Left 8 Upper Lobe Bronchus, Left 9 Lingula Bronchus B Lower Lobe Bronchus, Left C Upper Lung Lobe, Right D Middle Lung Lobe, Right F Lower Lung Lobe, Right G Upper Lung Lobe, Left H Lung Lingula J Lower Lung Lobe, Left K Lung, Right L Lung, Left M Lungs, Bilateral T Diaphragm	0 Open 4 Percutaneous Endoscopic	Z No Device	Z No Qualifier

Section	0	Medical and Surgical
Body System	B	Respiratory System
Operation	U	Supplement: Putting in or on biological or synthetic material that physically reinforces and/or augments the function of a portion of a body part

Body Part (4th)	Approach (5th)	Device (6th)	Qualifier (7th)
1 Trachea 2 Carina 3 Main Bronchus, Right 4 Upper Lobe Bronchus, Right 5 Middle Lobe Bronchus, Right 6 Lower Lobe Bronchus, Right 7 Main Bronchus, Left 8 Upper Lobe Bronchus, Left 9 Lingula Bronchus B Lower Lobe Bronchus, Left	0 Open 4 Percutaneous Endoscopic 8 Via Natural or Artificial Opening Endoscopic	7 Autologous Tissue Substitute J Synthetic Substitute K Nonautologous Tissue Substitute	Z No Qualifier
T Diaphragm	0 Open 4 Percutaneous Endoscopic	7 Autologous Tissue Substitute J Synthetic Substitute K Nonautologous Tissue Substitute	Z No Qualifier

Section	0	Medical and Surgical
Body System	B	Respiratory System
Operation	V	Restriction: Partially closing an orifice or the lumen of a tubular body part

Body Part (4th)	Approach (5th)	Device (6th)	Qualifier (7th)
1 Trachea 2 Carina 3 Main Bronchus, Right 4 Upper Lobe Bronchus, Right 5 Middle Lobe Bronchus, Right 6 Lower Lobe Bronchus, Right 7 Main Bronchus, Left 8 Upper Lobe Bronchus, Left 9 Lingula Bronchus B Lower Lobe Bronchus, Left	0 Open 3 Percutaneous 4 Percutaneous Endoscopic	C Extraluminal Device D Intraluminal Device Z No Device	Z No Qualifier
1 Trachea 2 Carina 3 Main Bronchus, Right 4 Upper Lobe Bronchus, Right 5 Middle Lobe Bronchus, Right 6 Lower Lobe Bronchus, Right 7 Main Bronchus, Left 8 Upper Lobe Bronchus, Left 9 Lingula Bronchus B Lower Lobe Bronchus, Left	7 Via Natural or Artificial Opening 8 Via Natural or Artificial Opening Endoscopic	D Intraluminal Device Z No Device	Z No Qualifier

Section	0	Medical and Surgical
Body System	B	Respiratory System
Operation	W	Revision: Correcting, to the extent possible, a portion of a malfunctioning device or the position of a displaced device

Body Part (4th)	Approach (5th)	Device (6th)	Qualifier (7th)
0 Tracheobronchial Tree	0 Open 3 Percutaneous 4 Percutaneous Endoscopic 7 Via Natural or Artificial Opening 8 Via Natural or Artificial Opening Endoscopic	0 Drainage Device 2 Monitoring Device 3 Infusion Device 7 Autologous Tissue Substitute C Extraluminal Device D Intraluminal Device J Synthetic Substitute K Nonautologous Tissue Substitute Y Other Device	Z No Qualifier
0 Tracheobronchial Tree	X External	0 Drainage Device 2 Monitoring Device 3 Infusion Device 7 Autologous Tissue Substitute C Extraluminal Device D Intraluminal Device J Synthetic Substitute K Nonautologous Tissue Substitute	Z No Qualifier
1 Trachea	0 Open 3 Percutaneous 4 Percutaneous Endoscopic 7 Via Natural or Artificial Opening 8 Via Natural or Artificial Opening Endoscopic X External	0 Drainage Device 2 Monitoring Device 7 Autologous Tissue Substitute C Extraluminal Device D Intraluminal Device F Tracheostomy Device J Synthetic Substitute K Nonautologous Tissue Substitute	Z No Qualifier

Continued →

0BW–0BY

Section	0	Medical and Surgical
Body System	B	Respiratory System
Operation	W	Revision: Correcting, to the extent possible, a portion of a malfunctioning device or the position of a displaced device

0BW Continued

Body Part (4th)	Approach (5th)	Device (6th)	Qualifier (7th)
K Lung, Right L Lung, Left	0 Open 3 Percutaneous 4 Percutaneous Endoscopic 7 Via Natural or Artificial Opening 8 Via Natural or Artificial Opening Endoscopic	0 Drainage Device 2 Monitoring Device 3 Infusion Device Y Other Device	Z No Qualifier
K Lung, Right L Lung, Left	X External	0 Drainage Device 2 Monitoring Device 3 Infusion Device	Z No Qualifier
Q Pleura	0 Open 3 Percutaneous 4 Percutaneous Endoscopic 7 Via Natural or Artificial Opening 8 Via Natural or Artificial Opening Endoscopic	0 Drainage Device 2 Monitoring Device Y Other Device	Z No Qualifier
Q Pleura	X External	0 Drainage Device 2 Monitoring Device	Z No Qualifier
T Diaphragm	0 Open 3 Percutaneous 4 Percutaneous Endoscopic 7 Via Natural or Artificial Opening 8 Via Natural or Artificial Opening Endoscopic	0 Drainage Device 2 Monitoring Device 7 Autologous Tissue Substitute J Synthetic Substitute K Nonautologous Tissue Substitute M Diaphragmatic Pacemaker Lead Y Other Device	Z No Qualifier
T Diaphragm	X External	0 Drainage Device 2 Monitoring Device 7 Autologous Tissue Substitute J Synthetic Substitute K Nonautologous Tissue Substitute M Diaphragmatic Pacemaker Lead	Z No Qualifier

Section	0	Medical and Surgical
Body System	B	Respiratory System
Operation	Y	Transplantation: Putting in or on all or a portion of a living body part taken from another individual or animal to physically take the place and/or function of all or a portion of a similar body part

Body Part (4th)	Approach (5th)	Device (6th)	Qualifier (7th)
C Upper Lung Lobe, Right D Middle Lung Lobe, Right F Lower Lung Lobe, Right G Upper Lung Lobe, Left H Lung Lingula J Lower Lung Lobe, Left K Lung, Right L Lung, Left M Lungs, Bilateral	0 Open	Z No Device	0 Allogeneic 1 Syngeneic 2 Zooplastic

Medical and Surgical, Respiratory System Tables

AHA Coding Clinic

0B5P0ZZ Destruction of Left Pleura, Open Approach—AHA CC: 2Q, 2016, 17-18

0B948ZX Drainage of Right Upper Lobe Bronchus, Via Natural or Artificial Opening Endoscopic, Diagnostic—AHA CC: 1Q, 2016, 26-27

0B988ZX Drainage of Left Upper Lobe Bronchus, Via Natural or Artificial Opening Endoscopic, Diagnostic—AHA CC: 1Q, 2016, 27

0B9J8ZX Drainage of Left Lower Lung Lobe, Via Natural or Artificial Opening Endoscopic, Diagnostic—AHA CC: 1Q, 2016, 26-27; 1Q, 2017, 51

0B9M8ZZ Drainage of Bilateral Lungs, Via Natural or Artificial Opening Endoscopic—AHA CC: 3Q, 2017, 15

0BB10ZZ Excision of Trachea, Open Approach—AHA CC: 1Q, 2015, 15-16

0BB48ZX Excision of Right Upper Lobe Bronchus, Via Natural or Artificial Opening Endoscopic, Diagnostic—AHA CC: 1Q, 2016, 26-27

0BB88ZX Excision of Left Upper Lobe Bronchus, Via Natural or Artificial Opening Endoscopic, Diagnostic—AHA CC: 1Q, 2016, 27

0BBC8ZX Excision of Right Upper Lung Lobe, Via Natural or Artificial Opening Endoscopic, Diagnostic—AHA CC: 1Q, 2016, 26-27

0BBG8ZX Excision of Left Upper Lung Lobe, Via Natural or Artificial Opening Endoscopic, Diagnostic—AHA CC: 2Q, 2022, 19

0BBK8ZX Excision of Right Lung, Via Natural or Artificial Opening Endoscopic, Diagnostic—AHA CC: 1Q, 2014, 20-21

0BC58ZZ Extirpation of Matter from Right Middle Lobe Bronchus, Via Natural or Artificial Opening Endoscopic—AHA CC: 3Q, 2017, 14-15

0BDC8ZX Extraction of Right Upper Lung Lobe, Via Natural or Artificial Opening Endoscopic, Diagnostic—AHA CC: 3Q, 2020, 40-41

0BDD8ZX Extraction of Right Middle Lung Lobe, Via Natural or Artificial Opening Endoscopic, Diagnostic—AHA CC: 3Q, 2020, 40-41

0BDF8ZX Extraction of Right Lower Lung Lobe, Via Natural or Artificial Opening Endoscopic, Diagnostic—AHA CC: 3Q, 2020, 40-41

0BH17EZ Insertion of Endotracheal Airway into Trachea, Via Natural or Artificial Opening—AHA CC: 4Q, 2014, 3-15; 3Q, 2022, 22-23

0BH18EZ Insertion of Endotracheal Airway into Trachea, Via Natural or Artificial Opening Endoscopic—AHA CC: 4Q, 2014, 3-15

0BHB8GZ Insertion of Endobronchial Valve into Left Lower Lobe Bronchus, Via Natural or Artificial Opening Endoscopic—AHA CC: 3Q, 2019, 33-34

0BJL8ZZ Inspection of Left Lung, Via Natural or Artificial Opening Endoscopic—AHA CC: 1Q, 2014, 20

0BJQ4ZZ Inspection of Pleura, Percutaneous Endoscopic Approach—AHA CC: 2Q, 2015, 31

0BN10ZZ Release Trachea, Open Approach—AHA CC: 3Q, 2015, 15-16

0BNL0ZZ Release Left Lung, Open Approach—AHA CC: 3Q, 2018, 28

0BNN0ZZ Release Right Pleura, Open Approach—AHA CC: 2Q, 2019, 20-21

0BQT4ZZ Repair Diaphragm, Percutaneous Endoscopic Approach—AHA CC: 3Q, 2020, 41-42

0BU18JZ Supplement Trachea with Synthetic Substitute, Via Natural or Artificial Opening Endoscopic—AHA CC: 3Q, 2020, 43-44

0BU307Z Supplement Right Main Bronchus with Autologous Tissue Substitute, Open Approach—AHA CC: 1Q, 2015, 28-29

Mouth and Throat

Glands of the Oral Cavity

Throat

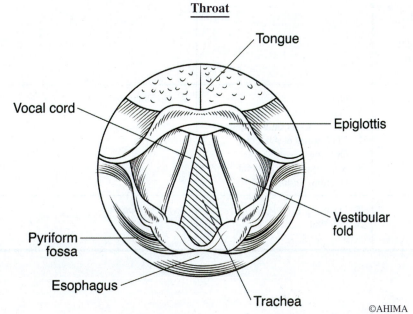

Mouth and Throat Tables 0C0–0CX

Section	0	Medical and Surgical
Body System	C	Mouth and Throat
Operation	0	Alteration: Modifying the anatomic structure of a body part without affecting the function of the body part

Body Part (4th)	Approach (5th)	Device (6th)	Qualifier (7th)
0 Upper Lip 1 Lower Lip	X External	7 Autologous Tissue Substitute J Synthetic Substitute K Nonautologous Tissue Substitute Z No Device	Z No Qualifier

Section	0	Medical and Surgical
Body System	C	Mouth and Throat
Operation	2	Change: Taking out or off a device from a body part and putting back an identical or similar device in or on the same body part without cutting or puncturing the skin or a mucous membrane

Body Part (4th)	Approach (5th)	Device (6th)	Qualifier (7th)
A Salivary Gland S Larynx Y Mouth and Throat	X External	0 Drainage Device Y Other Device	Z No Qualifier

Section	0	Medical and Surgical
Body System	C	Mouth and Throat
Operation	5	Destruction: Physical eradication of all or a portion of a body part by the direct use of energy, force, or a destructive agent

Body Part (4th)	Approach (5th)	Device (6th)	Qualifier (7th)
0 Upper Lip 1 Lower Lip 2 Hard Palate 3 Soft Palate 4 Buccal Mucosa 5 Upper Gingiva 6 Lower Gingiva 7 Tongue N Uvula P Tonsils Q Adenoids	0 Open 3 Percutaneous X External	Z No Device	Z No Qualifier
8 Parotid Gland, Right 9 Parotid Gland, Left B Parotid Duct, Right C Parotid Duct, Left D Sublingual Gland, Right F Sublingual Gland, Left G Submaxillary Gland, Right H Submaxillary Gland, Left J Minor Salivary Gland	0 Open 3 Percutaneous	Z No Device	Z No Qualifier
M Pharynx R Epiglottis S Larynx T Vocal Cord, Right V Vocal Cord, Left	0 Open 3 Percutaneous 4 Percutaneous Endoscopic 7 Via Natural or Artificial Opening 8 Via Natural or Artificial Opening Endoscopic	Z No Device	Z No Qualifier
W Upper Tooth X Lower Tooth	0 Open X External	Z No Device	0 Single 1 Multiple 2 All

Section	0	Medical and Surgical
Body System	C	Mouth and Throat
Operation	7	**Dilation:** Expanding an orifice or the lumen of a tubular body part

Body Part (4th)	Approach (5th)	Device (6th)	Qualifier (7th)
B Parotid Duct, Right C Parotid Duct, Left	0 Open 3 Percutaneous 7 Via Natural or Artificial Opening	D Intraluminal Device Z No Device	Z No Qualifier
M Pharynx	7 Via Natural or Artificial Opening 8 Via Natural or Artificial Opening Endoscopic	D Intraluminal Device Z No Device	Z No Qualifier
S Larynx	0 Open 3 Percutaneous 4 Percutaneous Endoscopic 7 Via Natural or Artificial Opening 8 Via Natural or Artificial Opening Endoscopic	D Intraluminal Device Z No Device	Z No Qualifier

Section	0	Medical and Surgical
Body System	C	Mouth and Throat
Operation	9	**Drainage:** Taking or letting out fluids and/or gases from a body part

Body Part (4th)	Approach (5th)	Device (6th)	Qualifier (7th)
0 Upper Lip 1 Lower Lip 2 Hard Palate 3 Soft Palate 4 Buccal Mucosa 5 Upper Gingiva 6 Lower Gingiva 7 Tongue N Uvula P Tonsils Q Adenoids	0 Open 3 Percutaneous X External	0 Drainage Device	Z No Qualifier
0 Upper Lip 1 Lower Lip 2 Hard Palate 3 Soft Palate 4 Buccal Mucosa 5 Upper Gingiva 6 Lower Gingiva 7 Tongue N Uvula P Tonsils Q Adenoids	0 Open 3 Percutaneous X External	Z No Device	X Diagnostic Z No Qualifier
8 Parotid Gland, Right 9 Parotid Gland, Left B Parotid Duct, Right C Parotid Duct, Left D Sublingual Gland, Right F Sublingual Gland, Left G Submaxillary Gland, Right H Submaxillary Gland, Left J Minor Salivary Gland	0 Open 3 Percutaneous	0 Drainage Device	Z No Qualifier
8 Parotid Gland, Right 9 Parotid Gland, Left B Parotid Duct, Right C Parotid Duct, Left D Sublingual Gland, Right F Sublingual Gland, Left G Submaxillary Gland, Right H Submaxillary Gland, Left J Minor Salivary Gland	0 Open 3 Percutaneous	Z No Device	X Diagnostic Z No Qualifier

Continued →

0C9 Continued

Section	0	Medical and Surgical
Body System	C	Mouth and Throat
Operation	9	Drainage: Taking or letting out fluids and/or gases from a body part

Body Part (4th)	Approach (5th)	Device (6th)	Qualifier (7th)
M Pharynx R Epiglottis S Larynx T Vocal Cord, Right V Vocal Cord, Left	0 Open 3 Percutaneous 4 Percutaneous Endoscopic 7 Via Natural or Artificial Opening 8 Via Natural or Artificial Opening Endoscopic	0 Drainage Device	Z No Qualifier
M Pharynx R Epiglottis S Larynx T Vocal Cord, Right V Vocal Cord, Left	0 Open 3 Percutaneous 4 Percutaneous Endoscopic 7 Via Natural or Artificial Opening 8 Via Natural or Artificial Opening Endoscopic	Z No Device	X Diagnostic Z No Qualifier
W Upper Tooth X Lower Tooth	0 Open X External	0 Drainage Device Z No Device	0 Single 1 Multiple 2 All

Section	0	Medical and Surgical
Body System	C	Mouth and Throat
Operation	B	Excision: Cutting out or off, without replacement, a portion of a body part

Body Part (4th)	Approach (5th)	Device (6th)	Qualifier (7th)
0 Upper Lip 1 Lower Lip 2 Hard Palate 3 Soft Palate 4 Buccal Mucosa 5 Upper Gingiva 6 Lower Gingiva 7 Tongue N Uvula P Tonsils Q Adenoids	0 Open 3 Percutaneous X External	Z No Device	X Diagnostic Z No Qualifier
8 Parotid Gland, Right 9 Parotid Gland, Left B Parotid Duct, Right C Parotid Duct, Left D Sublingual Gland, Right F Sublingual Gland, Left G Submaxillary Gland, Right H Submaxillary Gland, Left J Minor Salivary Gland	0 Open 3 Percutaneous	Z No Device	X Diagnostic Z No Qualifier
M Pharynx R Epiglottis S Larynx T Vocal Cord, Right V Vocal Cord, Left	0 Open 3 Percutaneous 4 Percutaneous Endoscopic 7 Via Natural or Artificial Opening 8 Via Natural or Artificial Opening Endoscopic	Z No Device	X Diagnostic Z No Qualifier
W Upper Tooth X Lower Tooth	0 Open X External	Z No Device	0 Single 1 Multiple 2 All

Section	0	Medical and Surgical
Body System	C	Mouth and Throat
Operation	C	Extirpation: Taking or cutting out solid matter from a body part

Body Part (4th)	Approach (5th)	Device (6th)	Qualifier (7th)
0 Upper Lip 1 Lower Lip 2 Hard Palate 3 Soft Palate 4 Buccal Mucosa 5 Upper Gingiva 6 Lower Gingiva 7 Tongue N Uvula P Tonsils Q Adenoids	0 Open 3 Percutaneous X External	Z No Device	Z No Qualifier
8 Parotid Gland, Right 9 Parotid Gland, Left B Parotid Duct, Right C Parotid Duct, Left D Sublingual Gland, Right F Sublingual Gland, Left G Submaxillary Gland, Right H Submaxillary Gland, Left J Minor Salivary Gland	0 Open 3 Percutaneous	Z No Device	Z No Qualifier
M Pharynx R Epiglottis S Larynx T Vocal Cord, Right V Vocal Cord, Left	0 Open 3 Percutaneous 4 Percutaneous Endoscopic 7 Via Natural or Artificial Opening 8 Via Natural or Artificial Opening Endoscopic	Z No Device	Z No Qualifier
W Upper Tooth X Lower Tooth	0 Open X External	Z No Device	0 Single 1 Multiple 2 All

Section	0	Medical and Surgical
Body System	C	Mouth and Throat
Operation	D	Extraction: Pulling or stripping out or off all or a portion of a body part by the use of force

Body Part (4th)	Approach (5th)	Device (6th)	Qualifier (7th)
T Vocal Cord, Right V Vocal Cord, Left	0 Open 3 Percutaneous 4 Percutaneous Endoscopic 7 Via Natural or Artificial Opening 8 Via Natural or Artificial Opening Endoscopic	Z No Device	Z No Qualifier
W Upper Tooth X Lower Tooth	X External	Z No Device	0 Single 1 Multiple 2 All

Section	0	Medical and Surgical
Body System	C	Mouth and Throat
Operation	F	Fragmentation: Breaking solid matter in a body part into pieces

Body Part (4th)	Approach (5th)	Device (6th)	Qualifier (7th)
B Parotid Duct, Right C Parotid Duct, Left	0 Open 3 Percutaneous 7 Via Natural or Artificial Opening X External	Z No Device	Z No Qualifier

0CH–0CM

Medical and Surgical, Mouth and Throat Tables

Section	0	Medical and Surgical
Body System	C	Mouth and Throat
Operation	H	Insertion: Putting in a nonbiological appliance that monitors, assists, performs, or prevents a physiological function but does not physically take the place of a body part

Body Part (4th)	Approach (5th)	Device (6th)	Qualifier (7th)
7 Tongue	0 Open 3 Percutaneous X External	1 Radioactive Element	Z No Qualifier
A Salivary Gland S Larynx	0 Open 3 Percutaneous 7 Via Natural or Artificial Opening 8 Via Natural or Artificial Opening Endoscopic	1 Radioactive Element Y Other Device	Z No Qualifier
Y Mouth and Throat	0 Open 3 Percutaneous	1 Radioactive Element Y Other Device	Z No Qualifier
Y Mouth and Throat	7 Via Natural or Artificial Opening 8 Via Natural or Artificial Opening Endoscopic	1 Radioactive Element B Intraluminal Device, Airway Y Other Device	Z No Qualifier

Section	0	Medical and Surgical
Body System	C	Mouth and Throat
Operation	J	Inspection: Visually and/or manually exploring a body part

Body Part (4th)	Approach (5th)	Device (6th)	Qualifier (7th)
A SalivaryGland	0 Open 3 Percutaneous X External	Z No Device	Z No Qualifier
S Larynx Y Mouth and Throat	0 Open 3 Percutaneous 4 Percutaneous Endoscopic 7 Via Natural or Artificial Opening 8 Via Natural or Artificial Opening Endoscopic X External	Z No Device	Z No Qualifier

Section	0	Medical and Surgical
Body System	C	Mouth and Throat
Operation	L	Occlusion: Completely closing an orifice or the lumen of a tubular body part

Body Part (4th)	Approach (5th)	Device (6th)	Qualifier (7th)
B Parotid Duct, Right C Parotid Duct, Left	0 Open 3 Percutaneous 4 Percutaneous Endoscopic	C Extraluminal Device D Intraluminal Device Z No Device	Z No Qualifier
B Parotid Duct, Right C Parotid Duct, Left	7 Via Natural or Artificial Opening 8 Via Natural or Artificial Opening Endoscopic	D Intraluminal Device Z No Device	Z No Qualifier

Section	0	Medical and Surgical
Body System	C	Mouth and Throat
Operation	M	Reattachment: Putting back in or on all or a portion of a separated body part to its normal location or other suitable location

Body Part (4th)	Approach (5th)	Device (6th)	Qualifier (7th)
0 Upper Lip 1 Lower Lip 3 Soft Palate 7 Tongue N Uvula	0 Open	Z No Device	Z No Qualifier
W Upper Tooth X Lower Tooth	0 Open X External	Z No Device	0 Single 1 Multiple 2 All

264

Section	0	Medical and Surgical
Body System	C	Mouth and Throat
Operation	N	Release: Freeing a body part from an abnormal physical constraint by cutting or by the use of force

Body Part (4th)	Approach (5th)	Device (6th)	Qualifier (7th)
0 Upper Lip 1 Lower Lip 2 Hard Palate 3 Soft Palate 4 Buccal Mucosa 5 Upper Gingiva 6 Lower Gingiva 7 Tongue N Uvula P Tonsils Q Adenoids	0 Open 3 Percutaneous X External	Z No Device	Z No Qualifier
8 Parotid Gland, Right 9 Parotid Gland, Left B Parotid Duct, Right C Parotid Duct, Left D Sublingual Gland, Right F Sublingual Gland, Left G Submaxillary Gland, Right H Submaxillary Gland, Left J Minor Salivary Gland	0 Open 3 Percutaneous	Z No Device	Z No Qualifier
M Pharynx R Epiglottis S Larynx T Vocal Cord, Right V Vocal Cord, Left	0 Open 3 Percutaneous 4 Percutaneous Endoscopic 7 Via Natural or Artificial Opening 8 Via Natural or Artificial Opening Endoscopic	Z No Device	Z No Qualifier
W Upper Tooth X Lower Tooth	0 Open X External	Z No Device	0 Single 1 Multiple 2 All

Section	0	Medical and Surgical
Body System	C	Mouth and Throat
Operation	P	Removal: Taking out or off a device from a body part

Body Part (4th)	Approach (5th)	Device (6th)	Qualifier (7th)
A Salivary Gland	0 Open 3 Percutaneous	0 Drainage Device C Extraluminal Device Y Other Device	Z No Qualifier
A Salivary Gland	7 Via Natural or Artificial Opening 8 Via Natural or Artificial Opening Endoscopic	Y Other Device	Z No Qualifier
S Larynx	0 Open 3 Percutaneous 7 Via Natural or Artificial Opening 8 Via Natural or Artificial Opening Endoscopic	0 Drainage Device 7 Autologous Tissue Substitute D Intraluminal Device J Synthetic Substitute K Nonautologous Tissue Substitute Y Other Device	Z No Qualifier
S Larynx	X External	0 Drainage Device 7 Autologous Tissue Substitute D Intraluminal Device J Synthetic Substitute K Nonautologous Tissue Substitute	Z No Qualifier

Continued →

0CP–0CQ

Section	0	Medical and Surgical
Body System	C	Mouth and Throat
Operation	P	Removal: Taking out or off a device from a body part

0CP Continued

Body Part (4th)	Approach (5th)	Device (6th)	Qualifier (7th)
Y Mouth and Throat	0 Open 3 Percutaneous 7 Via Natural or Artificial Opening 8 Via Natural or Artificial Opening Endoscopic	0 Drainage Device 1 Radioactive Element 7 Autologous Tissue Substitute D Intraluminal Device J Synthetic Substitute K Nonautologous Tissue Substitute Y Other Device	Z No Qualifier
Y Mouth and Throat	X External	0 Drainage Device 1 Radioactive Element 7 Autologous Tissue Substitute D Intraluminal Device J Synthetic Substitute K Nonautologous Tissue Substitute	Z No Qualifier

Section	0	Medical and Surgical
Body System	C	Mouth and Throat
Operation	Q	Repair: Restoring, to the extent possible, a body part to its normal anatomic structure and function

Body Part (4th)	Approach (5th)	Device (6th)	Qualifier (7th)
0 Upper Lip 1 Lower Lip 2 Hard Palate 3 Soft Palate 4 Buccal Mucosa 5 Upper Gingiva 6 Lower Gingiva 7 Tongue N Uvula P Tonsils Q Adenoids	0 Open 3 Percutaneous X External	Z No Device	Z No Qualifier
8 Parotid Gland, Right 9 Parotid Gland, Left B Parotid Duct, Right C Parotid Duct, Left D Sublingual Gland, Right F Sublingual Gland, Left G Submaxillary Gland, Right H Submaxillary Gland, Left J Minor Salivary Gland	0 Open 3 Percutaneous	Z No Device	Z No Qualifier
M Pharynx R Epiglottis S Larynx T Vocal Cord, Right V Vocal Cord, Left	0 Open 3 Percutaneous 4 Percutaneous Endoscopic 7 Via Natural or Artificial Opening 8 Via Natural or Artificial Opening Endoscopic	Z No Device	Z No Qualifier
W Upper Tooth X Lower Tooth	0 Open X External	Z No Device	0 Single 1 Multiple 2 All

Section	0	Medical and Surgical
Body System	C	Mouth and Throat
Operation	R	Replacement: Putting in or on biological or synthetic material that physically takes the place and/or function of all or a portion of a body part

Body Part (4th)	Approach (5th)	Device (6th)	Qualifier (7th)
0 Upper Lip 1 Lower Lip 2 Hard Palate 3 Soft Palate 4 Buccal Mucosa 5 Upper Gingiva 6 Lower Gingiva 7 Tongue N Uvula	0 Open 3 Percutaneous X External	7 Autologous Tissue Substitute J Synthetic Substitute K Nonautologous Tissue Substitute	Z No Qualifier
B Parotid Duct, Right C Parotid Duct, Left	0 Open 3 Percutaneous	7 Autologous Tissue Substitute J Synthetic Substitute K Nonautologous Tissue Substitute	Z No Qualifier
M Pharynx R Epiglottis S Larynx T Vocal Cord, Right V Vocal Cord, Left	0 Open 7 Via Natural or Artificial Opening 8 Via Natural or Artificial Opening Endoscopic	7 Autologous Tissue Substitute J Synthetic Substitute K Nonautologous Tissue Substitute	Z No Qualifier
W Upper Tooth X Lower Tooth	0 Open X External	7 Autologous Tissue Substitute J Synthetic Substitute K Nonautologous Tissue Substitute	0 Single 1 Multiple 2 All

Section	0	Medical and Surgical
Body System	C	Mouth and Throat
Operation	S	Reposition: Moving to its normal location, or other suitable location, all or a portion of a body part

Body Part (4th)	Approach (5th)	Device (6th)	Qualifier (7th)
0 Upper Lip 1 Lower Lip 2 Hard Palate 3 Soft Palate 7 Tongue N Uvula	0 Open X External	Z No Device	Z No Qualifier
B Parotid Duct, Right C Parotid Duct, Left	0 Open 3 Percutaneous	Z No Device	Z No Qualifier
R Epiglottis S Larynx T Vocal Cord, Right V Vocal Cord, Left	0 Open 7 Via Natural or Artificial Opening 8 Via Natural or Artificial Opening Endoscopic	Z No Device	Z No Qualifier
W Upper Tooth X Lower Tooth	0 Open X External	5 External Fixation Device Z No Device	0 Single 1 Multiple 2 All

Section	0	Medical and Surgical
Body System	C	Mouth and Throat
Operation	T	Resection: Cutting out or off, without replacement, all of a body part

Body Part (4th)	Approach (5th)	Device (6th)	Qualifier (7th)
0 Upper Lip 1 Lower Lip 2 Hard Palate 3 Soft Palate 7 Tongue N Uvula P Tonsils Q Adenoids	0 Open X External	Z No Device	Z No Qualifier
8 Parotid Gland, Right 9 Parotid Gland, Left B Parotid Duct, Right C Parotid Duct, Left D Sublingual Gland, Right F Sublingual Gland, Left G Submaxillary Gland, Right H Submaxillary Gland, Left J Minor Salivary Gland	0 Open	Z No Device	Z No Qualifier
M Pharynx R Epiglottis S Larynx T Vocal Cord, Right V Vocal Cord, Left	0 Open 4 Percutaneous Endoscopic 7 Via Natural or Artificial Opening 8 Via Natural or Artificial Opening Endoscopic	Z No Device	Z No Qualifier
W Upper Tooth X Lower Tooth	0 Open	Z No Device	0 Single 1 Multiple 2 All

Section	0	Medical and Surgical
Body System	C	Mouth and Throat
Operation	U	Supplement: Putting in or on biological or synthetic material that physically reinforces and/or augments the function of a portion of a body part

Body Part (4th)	Approach (5th)	Device (6th)	Qualifier (7th)
0 Upper Lip 1 Lower Lip 2 Hard Palate 3 Soft Palate 4 Buccal Mucosa 5 Upper Gingiva 6 Lower Gingiva 7 Tongue N Uvula	0 Open 3 Percutaneous X External	7 Autologous Tissue Substitute J Synthetic Substitute K Nonautologous Tissue Substitute	Z No Qualifier
M Pharynx R Epiglottis S Larynx T Vocal Cord, Right V Vocal Cord, Left	0 Open 7 Via Natural or Artificial Opening 8 Via Natural or Artificial Opening Endoscopic	7 Autologous Tissue Substitute J Synthetic Substitute K Nonautologous Tissue Substitute	Z No Qualifier

Section	0	Medical and Surgical
Body System	C	Mouth and Throat
Operation	V	Restriction: Partially closing an orifice or the lumen of a tubular body part

Body Part (4th)	Approach (5th)	Device (6th)	Qualifier (7th)
B Parotid Duct, Right **C** Parotid Duct, Left	**0** Open **3** Percutaneous	**C** Extraluminal Device **D** Intraluminal Device **Z** No Device	**Z** No Qualifier
B Parotid Duct, Right **C** Parotid Duct, Left	**7** Via Natural or Artificial Opening **8** Via Natural or Artificial Opening Endoscopic	**D** Intraluminal Device **Z** No Device	**Z** No Qualifier

Section	0	Medical and Surgical
Body System	C	Mouth and Throat
Operation	W	Revision: Correcting, to the extent possible, a portion of a malfunctioning device or the position of a displaced device

Body Part (4th)	Approach (5th)	Device (6th)	Qualifier (7th)
A Salivary Gland	**0** Open **3** Percutaneous	**0** Drainage Device **C** Extraluminal Device **Y** Other Device	**Z** No Qualifier
A Salivary Gland	**7** Via Natural or Artificial Opening **8** Via Natural or Artificial Opening Endoscopic	**Y** Other Device	**Z** No Qualifier
A Salivary Gland	**X** External	**0** Drainage Device **C** Extraluminal Device	**Z** No Qualifier
S Larynx	**0** Open **3** Percutaneous **7** Via Natural or Artificial Opening **8** Via Natural or Artificial Opening Endoscopic	**0** Drainage Device **7** Autologous Tissue Substitute **D** Intraluminal Device **J** Synthetic Substitute **K** Nonautologous Tissue Substitute **Y** Other Device	**Z** No Qualifier
S Larynx	**X** External	**0** Drainage Device **7** Autologous Tissue Substitute **D** Intraluminal Device **J** Synthetic Substitute **K** Nonautologous Tissue Substitute	**Z** No Qualifier
Y Mouth and Throat	**0** Open **3** Percutaneous **7** Via Natural or Artificial Opening **8** Via Natural or Artificial Opening Endoscopic	**0** Drainage Device **1** Radioactive Element **7** Autologous Tissue Substitute **D** Intraluminal Device **J** Synthetic Substitute **K** Nonautologous Tissue Substitute **Y** Other Device	**Z** No Qualifier
Y Mouth and Throat	**X** External	**0** Drainage Device **1** Radioactive Element **7** Autologous Tissue Substitute **D** Intraluminal Device **J** Synthetic Substitute **K** Nonautologous Tissue Substitute	**Z** No Qualifier

Section	0	Medical and Surgical
Body System	C	Mouth and Throat
Operation	X	**Transfer:** Moving, without taking out, all or a portion of a body part to another location to take over the function of all or a portion of a body part

Body Part (4th)	Approach (5th)	Device (6th)	Qualifier (7th)
0 Upper Lip 1 Lower Lip 3 Soft Palate 4 Buccal Mucosa 5 Upper Gingiva 6 Lower Gingiva 7 Tongue	0 Open X External	Z No Device	Z No Qualifier

AHA Coding Clinic

0CB80ZZ Excision of Right Parotid Gland, Open Approach—AHA CC: 3Q, 2014, 21-22

0CBM8ZX Excision of Pharynx, Via Natural or Artificial Opening Endoscopic, Diagnostic—AHA CC: 2Q, 2016, 20

0CBM8ZZ Excision of Pharynx, Via Natural or Artificial Opening Endoscopic—AHA CC: 3Q, 2016, 28-29

0CCH3ZZ Extirpation of Matter from Left Submaxillary Gland, Percutaneous Approach—AHA CC: 2Q, 2016, 20

0CQ50ZZ Repair Upper Gingiva, Open Approach—AHA CC: 1Q, 2017, 20-21

0CR3XJZ Replacement of Soft Palate with Synthetic Substitute, External Approach—AHA CC: 3Q, 2014, 25

0CR4XKZ Replacement of Buccal Mucosa with Nonautologous Tissue Substitute, External Approach—AHA CC: 2Q, 2014, 5-6

0CS20ZZ Reposition Hard Palate, Open Approach—AHA CC: 2Q, 2022, 24-25

0CS30ZZ Reposition Soft Palate, Open Approach—AHA CC: 2Q, 2022, 24-25

0CSR8ZZ Reposition Epiglottis, Via Natural or Artificial Opening Endoscopic—AHA CC: 3Q, 2016, 28-29

0CT90ZZ Resection of Left Parotid Gland, Open Approach—AHA CC: 2Q, 2016, 12-14

0CTW0Z1 Resection of Upper Tooth, Multiple, Open Approach—AHA CC: 3Q, 2014, 23-24

0CTX0Z1 Resection of Lower Tooth, Multiple, Open Approach—AHA CC: 3Q, 2014, 23-24

Gastrointestinal System

Gastrointestinal System: Organization

Stomach, Liver, Gallbladder

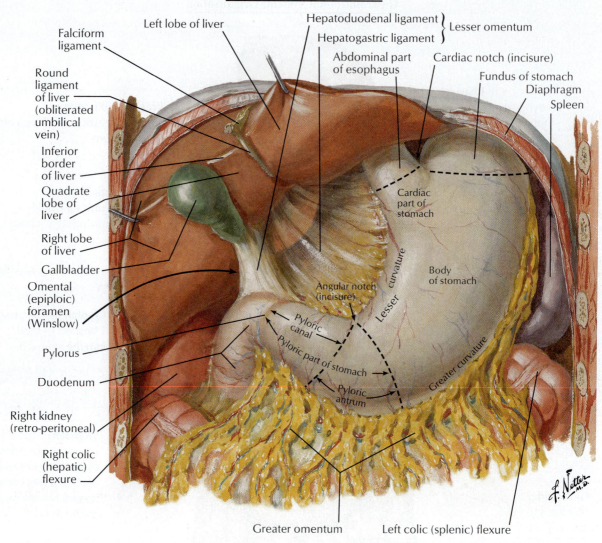

Large Intestine Structure of Colon

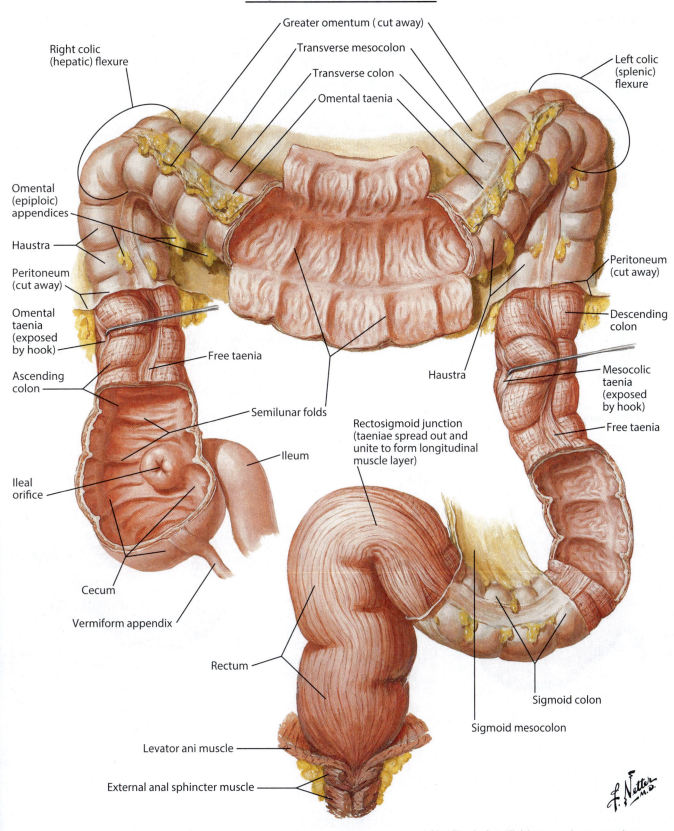

Treatment of Morbid Obesity

Gastric stapling (vertical banded gastroplasty)

Gastric bypass (Roux-en-Y)

Laparoscopic adjustable gastric banding

Sleeve gastrectomy

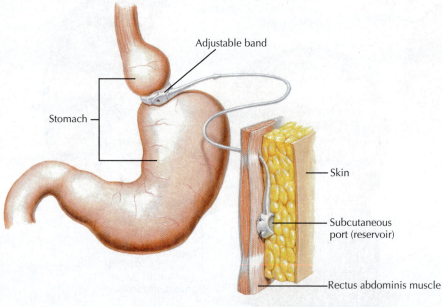

© 2019 Elsevier Inc. All rights reserved. www.netterimages.com

Gastrointestinal System Tables 0D1–0DY

Section	0	Medical and Surgical
Body System	D	Gastrointestinal System
Operation	1	**Bypass:** Altering the route of passage of the contents of a tubular body part

Body Part (4th)	Approach (5th)	Device (6th)	Qualifier (7th)
1 Esophagus, Upper 2 Esophagus, Middle 3 Esophagus, Lower 5 Esophagus	0 Open 4 Percutaneous Endoscopic 8 Via Natural or Artificial Opening Endoscopic	7 Autologous Tissue Substitute J Synthetic Substitute K Nonautologous Tissue Substitute Z No Device	4 Cutaneous 6 Stomach 9 Duodenum A Jejunum B Ileum
1 Esophagus, Upper 2 Esophagus, Middle 3 Esophagus, Lower 5 Esophagus	3 Percutaneous	J Synthetic Substitute	4 Cutaneous
6 Stomach 9 Duodenum	0 Open 4 Percutaneous Endoscopic 8 Via Natural or Artificial Opening Endoscopic	7 Autologous Tissue Substitute J Synthetic Substitute K Nonautologous Tissue Substitute Z No Device	4 Cutaneous 9 Duodenum A Jejunum B Ileum L Transverse Colon
6 Stomach 9 Duodenum	3 Percutaneous	J Synthetic Substitute	4 Cutaneous
8 Small Intestine	0 Open 4 Percutaneous Endoscopic 8 Via Natural or Artificial Opening Endoscopic	7 Autologous Tissue Substitute J Synthetic Substitute K Nonautologous Tissue Z No Device	4 Cutaneous 8 Small Intestine H Cecum K Ascending Colon L Transverse Colon M Descending Colon N Sigmoid Colon P Rectum Q Anus
A Jejunum	0 Open 4 Percutaneous Endoscopic 8 Via Natural or Artificial Opening Endoscopic	7 Autologous Tissue Substitute J Synthetic Substitute K Nonautologous Tissue Substitute Z No Device	4 Cutaneous A Jejunum B Ileum H Cecum K Ascending Colon L Transverse Colon M Descending Colon N Sigmoid Colon P Rectum Q Anus
A Jejunum	3 Percutaneous	J Synthetic Substitute	4 Cutaneous
B Ileum	0 Open 4 Percutaneous Endoscopic 8 Via Natural or Artificial Opening Endoscopic	7 Autologous Tissue Substitute J Synthetic Substitute K Nonautologous Tissue Substitute Z No Device	4 Cutaneous B Ileum H Cecum K Ascending Colon L Transverse Colon M Descending Colon N Sigmoid Colon P Rectum Q Anus
B Ileum	3 Percutaneous	J Synthetic Substitute	4 Cutaneous
E Large Intestine	0 Open 4 Percutaneous Endoscopic 8 Via Natural or Artificial Opening Endoscopic	7 Autologous Tissue Substitute J Synthetic Substitute K Nonautologous Tissue Z No Device	4 Cutaneous E Large Intestine P Rectum

Continued →

Section	0	Medical and Surgical
Body System	D	Gastrointestinal System
Operation	1	**Bypass:** Altering the route of passage of the contents of a tubular body part

0D1 Continued

Body Part (4th)	Approach (5th)	Device (6th)	Qualifier (7th)
H Cecum	0 Open 4 Percutaneous Endoscopic 8 Via Natural or Artificial Opening Endoscopic	7 Autologous Tissue Substitute J Synthetic Substitute K Nonautologous Tissue Substitute Z No Device	4 Cutaneous H Cecum K Ascending Colon L Transverse Colon M Descending Colon N Sigmoid Colon P Rectum
H Cecum	3 Percutaneous	J Synthetic Substitute	4 Cutaneous
K Ascending Colon	0 Open 4 Percutaneous Endoscopic 8 Via Natural or Artificial Opening Endoscopic	7 Autologous Tissue Substitute J Synthetic Substitute K Nonautologous Tissue Substitute Z No Device	4 Cutaneous K Ascending Colon L Transverse Colon M Descending Colon N Sigmoid Colon P Rectum
K Ascending Colon	3 Percutaneous	J Synthetic Substitute	4 Cutaneous
L Transverse Colon	0 Open 4 Percutaneous Endoscopic 8 Via Natural or Artificial Opening Endoscopic	7 Autologous Tissue Substitute J Synthetic Substitute K Nonautologous Tissue Substitute Z No Device	4 Cutaneous L Transverse Colon M Descending Colon N Sigmoid Colon P Rectum
L Transverse Colon	3 Percutaneous	J Synthetic Substitute	4 Cutaneous
M Descending Colon	0 Open 4 Percutaneous Endoscopic 8 Via Natural or Artificial Opening Endoscopic	7 Autologous Tissue Substitute J Synthetic Substitute K Nonautologous Tissue Substitute Z No Device	4 Cutaneous M Descending Colon N Sigmoid Colon P Rectum
M Descending Colon	3 Percutaneous	J Synthetic Substitute	4 Cutaneous
N Sigmoid Colon	0 Open 4 Percutaneous Endoscopic 8 Via Natural or Artificial Opening Endoscopic	7 Autologous Tissue Substitute J Synthetic Substitute K Nonautologous Tissue Substitute Z No Device	4 Cutaneous N Sigmoid Colon P Rectum
N Sigmoid Colon	3 Percutaneous	J Synthetic Substitute	4 Cutaneous

Section	0	Medical and Surgical
Body System	D	Gastrointestinal System
Operation	2	**Change:** Taking out or off a device from a body part and putting back an identical or similar device in or on the same body part without cutting or puncturing the skin or a mucous membrane

Body Part (4th)	Approach (5th)	Device (6th)	Qualifier (7th)
0 Upper Intestinal Tract D Lower Intestinal Tract	X External	0 Drainage Device U Feeding Device Y Other Device	Z No Qualifier
U Omentum V Mesentery W Peritoneum	X External	0 Drainage Device Y Other Device	Z No Qualifier

Section	0	Medical and Surgical
Body System	D	Gastrointestinal System
Operation	5	**Destruction:** Physical eradication of all or a portion of a body part by the direct use of energy, force, or a destructive agent

Body Part (4th)	Approach (5th)	Device (6th)	Qualifier (7th)
1 Esophagus, Upper 2 Esophagus, Middle 3 Esophagus, Lower 4 Esophagogastric Junction 5 Esophagus 6 Stomach 7 Stomach, Pylorus 8 Small Intestine 9 Duodenum A Jejunum B Ileum C Ileocecal Valve E Large Intestine F Large Intestine, Right G Large Intestine, Left H Cecum J Appendix K Ascending Colon L Transverse Colon M Descending Colon N Sigmoid Colon P Rectum	0 Open 3 Percutaneous 4 Percutaneous Endoscopic	Z No Device	3 Laser Interstitial Thermal Therapy Z No Qualifier
1 Esophagus, Upper 2 Esophagus, Middle 3 Esophagus, Lower 4 Esophagogastric Junction 5 Esophagus 6 Stomach 7 Stomack, Pylorus 8 Small Intestine 9 Duodenum A Jejunum B Ileum C Ileocecal Valve E Large Intestine F Large Intestine, Right G Large Intestine, Left H Cecum J Appendix K Ascending Colon L Transverse Colon M Descending Colon N Sigmoid Colon P Rectum	7 Via Natural or Artificial Opening 8 Via Natural or Artificial Opening Endoscopic	Z No Device	Z No Qualifier
Q Anus	0 Open 3 Percutaneous 4 Percutaneous Endoscopic	Z No Device	3 Laser Interstitial Thermal Therapy Z No Qualifier
Q Anus	7 Via Natural or Artificial Opening 8 Via Natural or Artificial Opening Endoscopic X External	Z No Device	Z No Qualifier
R Anal Sphincter U Omentum V Mesentery W Peritoneum	0 Open 3 Percutaneous 4 Percutaneous Endoscopic	Z No Device	Z No Qualifier

Section	0	Medical and Surgical
Body System	D	Gastrointestinal System
Operation	7	Dilation: Expanding an orifice or the lumen of a tubular body part

Body Part (4th)	Approach (5th)	Device (6th)	Qualifier (7th)
1 Esophagus, Upper 2 Esophagus, Middle 3 Esophagus, Lower 4 Esophagogastric Junction 5 Esophagus 6 Stomach 7 Stomach, Pylorus 8 Small Intestine 9 Duodenum A Jejunum B Ileum C Ileocecal Valve E Large Intestine F Large Intestine, Right G Large Intestine, Left H Cecum K Ascending Colon L Transverse Colon M Descending Colon N Sigmoid Colon P Rectum Q Anus	0 Open 3 Percutaneous 4 Percutaneous Endoscopic 7 Via Natural or Artificial Opening 8 Via Natural or Artificial Opening Endoscopic	D Intraluminal Device Z No Device	Z No Qualifier

Section	0	Medical and Surgical
Body System	D	Gastrointestinal System
Operation	8	Division: Cutting into a body part, without draining fluids and/or gases from the body part, in order to separate or transect a body part

Body Part (4th)	Approach (5th)	Device (6th)	Qualifier (7th)
4 Esophagogastric Junction 7 Stomach, Pylorus	0 Open 3 Percutaneous 4 Percutaneous Endoscopic 7 Via Natural or Artificial Opening 8 Via Natural or Artificial Opening Endoscopic	Z No Device	Z No Qualifier
R Anal Sphincter	0 Open 3 Percutaneous	Z No Device	Z No Qualifier

Section   **0**   **Medical and Surgical**
Body System   **D**   **Gastrointestinal System**
Operation   **9**   **Drainage:** Taking or letting out fluids and/or gases from a body part

Body Part (4th)	Approach (5th)	Device (6th)	Qualifier (7th)
1 Esophagus, Upper 2 Esophagus, Middle 3 Esophagus, Lower 4 Esophagogastric Junction 5 Esophagus 6 Stomach 7 Stomach, Pylorus 8 Small Intestine 9 Duodenum A Jejunum B Ileum C Ileocecal Valve E Large Intestine F Large Intestine, Right G Large Intestine, Left H Cecum J Appendix K Ascending Colon L Transverse Colon M Descending Colon N Sigmoid Colon P Rectum	0 Open 3 Percutaneous 4 Percutaneous Endoscopic 7 Via Natural or Artificial Opening 8 Via Natural or Artificial Opening Endoscopic	0 Drainage Device	Z No Qualifier
1 Esophagus, Upper 2 Esophagus, Middle 3 Esophagus, Lower 4 Esophagogastric Junction 5 Esophagus 6 Stomach 7 Stomach, Pylorus 8 Small Intestine 9 Duodenum A Jejunum B Ileum C Ileocecal Valve E Large Intestine F Large Intestine, Right G Large Intestine, Left H Cecum J Appendix K Ascending Colon L Transverse Colon M Descending Colon N Sigmoid Colon P Rectum	0 Open 3 Percutaneous 4 Percutaneous Endoscopic 7 Via Natural or Artificial Opening 8 Via Natural or Artificial Opening Endoscopic	Z No Device	X Diagnostic Z No Qualifier
Q Anus	0 Open 3 Percutaneous 4 Percutaneous Endoscopic 7 Via Natural or Artificial Opening 8 Via Natural or Artificial Opening Endoscopic X External	0 Drainage Device	Z No Qualifier
Q Anus	0 Open 3 Percutaneous 4 Percutaneous Endoscopic 7 Via Natural or Artificial Opening 8 Via Natural or Artificial Opening Endoscopic X External	Z No Device	X Diagnostic Z No Qualifier

Continued →

0D9-0DB

Medical and Surgical, Gastrointestinal System Tables

0D9 Continued

Section	0	Medical and Surgical
Body System	D	Gastrointestinal System
Operation	9	Drainage: Taking or letting out fluids and/or gases from a body part

Body Part (4th)	Approach (5th)	Device (6th)	Qualifier (7th)
R Anal Sphincter U Omentum V Mesentery W Peritoneum	0 Open 3 Percutaneous 4 Percutaneous Endoscopic	0 Drainage Device	Z No Qualifier
R Anal Sphincter U Omentum V Mesentery W Peritoneum	0 Open 3 Percutaneous 4 Percutaneous Endoscopic	Z No Device	X Diagnostic Z No Qualifier

Section	0	Medical and Surgical
Body System	D	Gastrointestinal System
Operation	B	Excision: Cutting out or off, without replacement, a portion of a body part

Body Part (4th)	Approach (5th)	Device (6th)	Qualifier (7th)
1 Esophagus, Upper 2 Esophagus, Middle 3 Esophagus, Lower 4 Esophagogastric Junction 5 Esophagus 7 Stomach, Pylorus 8 Small Intestine 9 Duodenum A Jejunum B Ileum C Ileocecal Valve E Large Intestine F Large Intestine, Right H Cecum J Appendix K Ascending Colon P Rectum	0 Open 3 Percutaneous 4 Percutaneous Endoscopic 7 Via Natural or Artificial Opening 8 Via Natural or Artificial Opening Endoscopic	Z No Device	X Diagnostic Z No Qualifier
6 Stomach	0 Open 3 Percutaneous 4 Percutaneous Endoscopic 7 Via Natural or Artificial Opening 8 Via Natural or Artificial Opening Endoscopic	Z No Device	3 Vertical X Diagnostic Z No Qualifier
G Large Intestine, Left L Transverse Colon M Descending Colon N Sigmoid Colon	0 Open 3 Percutaneous 4 Percutaneous Endoscopic 7 Via Natural or Artificial Opening 8 Via Natural or Artificial Opening Endoscopic	Z No Device	X Diagnostic Z No Qualifier
G Large Intestine, Left L Transverse Colon M Descending Colon N Sigmoid Colon	F Via Natural or Artificial Opening With Percutaneous Endoscopic Assistance	Z No Device	Z No Qualifier
Q Anus	0 Open 3 Percutaneous 4 Percutaneous Endoscopic 7 Via Natural or Artificial Opening 8 Via Natural or Artificial Opening Endoscopic X External	Z No Device	X Diagnostic Z No Qualifier
R Anal Sphincter U Omentum V Mesentery W Peritoneum	0 Open 3 Percutaneous 4 Percutaneous Endoscopic	Z No Device	X Diagnostic Z No Qualifier

280

Section	0	Medical and Surgical
Body System	D	Gastrointestinal System
Operation	C	Extirpation: Taking or cutting out solid matter from a body part

Body Part (4th)	Approach (5th)	Device (6th)	Qualifier (7th)
1 Esophagus, Upper 2 Esophagus, Middle 3 Esophagus, Lower 4 Esophagogastric Junction 5 Esophagus 6 Stomach 7 Stomach, Pylorus 8 Small Intestine 9 Duodenum A Jejunum B Ileum C Ileocecal Valve E Large Intestine F Large Intestine, Right G Large Intestine, Left H Cecum J Appendix K Ascending Colon L Transverse Colon M Descending Colon N Sigmoid Colon P Rectum	0 Open 3 Percutaneous 4 Percutaneous Endoscopic 7 Via Natural or Artificial Opening 8 Via Natural or Artificial Opening Endoscopic	Z No Device	Z No Qualifier
Q Anus	0 Open 3 Percutaneous 4 Percutaneous Endoscopic 7 Via Natural or Artificial Opening 8 Via Natural or Artificial Opening Endoscopic X External	Z No Device	Z No Qualifier
R Anal Sphincter U Omentum V Mesentery W Peritoneum	0 Open 3 Percutaneous 4 Percutaneous Endoscopic	Z No Device	Z No Qualifier

0DD–0DF

Medical and Surgical, Gastrointestinal System Tables

Section	0	Medical and Surgical
Body System	D	Gastrointestinal System
Operation	D	**Extraction:** Pulling or stripping out or off all or a portion of a body part by the use of force

Body Part (4th)	Approach (5th)	Device (6th)	Qualifier (7th)
1 Esophagus, Upper 2 Esophagus, Middle 3 Esophagus, Lower 4 Esophagogastric Junction 5 Esophagus 6 Stomach 7 Stomach, Pylorus 8 Small Intestine 9 Duodenum A Jejunum B Ileum C Ileocecal Valve E Large Intestine F Large Intestine, Right G Large Intestine, Left H Cecum J Appendix K Ascending Colon L Transverse Colon M Descending Colon N Sigmoid Colon P Rectum	3 Percutaneous 4 Percutaneous Endoscopic 8 Via Natural or Artificial Opening Endoscopic	Z No Device	X Diagnostic
Q Anus	3 Percutaneous 4 Percutaneous Endoscopic 8 Via Natural or Artificial Opening Endoscopic X External	Z No Device	X Diagnostic

Section	0	Medical and Surgical
Body System	D	Gastrointestinal System
Operation	F	**Fragmentation:** Breaking solid matter in a body part into pieces

Body Part (4th)	Approach (5th)	Device (6th)	Qualifier (7th)
5 Esophagus 6 Stomach 8 Small Intestine 9 Duodenum A Jejunum B Ileum E Large Intestine F Large Intestine, Right G Large Intestine, Left H Cecum J Appendix K Ascending Colon L Transverse Colon M Descending Colon N Sigmoid Colon P Rectum Q Anus	0 Open 3 Percutaneous 4 Percutaneous Endoscopic 7 Via Natural or Artificial Opening 8 Via Natural or Artificial Opening Endoscopic X External	Z No Device	Z No Qualifier

282

Section	0	Medical and Surgical
Body System	D	Gastrointestinal System
Operation	H	Insertion: Putting in a nonbiological appliance that monitors, assists, performs, or prevents a physiological function but does not physically take the place of a body part

Body Part (4th)	Approach (5th)	Device (6th)	Qualifier (7th)
0 Upper Intestinal Tract D Lower Intestinal Tract	0 Open 3 Percutaneous 4 Percutaneous Endoscopic 7 Via Natural or Artificial Opening 8 Via Natural or Artificial Opening Endoscopic	Y Other Device	Z No Qualifier
1 Esophagus, Upper 2 Esophagus, Middle 3 Esophagus, Lower	7 Via Natural or Artificial Opening	J Magnetic Lengthening Device	Z No Qualifier
5 Esophagus	0 Open 3 Percutaneous 4 Percutaneous Endoscopic	1 Radioactive Element 2 Monitoring Device 3 Infusion Device D Intraluminal Device U Feeding Device Y Other Device	Z No Qualifier
5 Esophagus	7 Via Natural or Artificial Opening 8 Via Natural or Artificial Opening Endoscopic	1 Radioactive Element 2 Monitoring Device 3 Infusion Device B Intraluminal Device, Airway D Intraluminal Device U Feeding Device Y Other Device	Z No Qualifier
6 Stomach	0 Open 3 Percutaneous 4 Percutaneous Endoscopic	1 Radioactive Element 2 Monitoring Device 3 Infusion Device D Intraluminal Device M Stimulator Lead U Feeding Device Y Other Device	Z No Qualifier
6 Stomach	7 Via Natural or Artificial Opening 8 Via Natural or Artificial Opening Endoscopic	1 Radioactive Element 2 Monitoring Device 3 Infusion Device D Intraluminal Device U Feeding Device Y Other Device	Z No Qualifier
8 Small Intestine 9 Duodenum A Jejunum B Ileum	0 Open 3 Percutaneous 4 Percutaneous Endoscopic 7 Via Natural or Artificial Opening 8 Via Natural or Artificial Opening Endoscopic	1 Radioactive Element 2 Monitoring Device 3 Infusion Device D Intraluminal Device U Feeding Device	Z No Qualifier
E Large Intestine P Rectum	0 Open 3 Percutaneous 4 Percutaneous Endoscopic 7 Via Natural or Artificial Opening 8 Via Natural or Artificial Opening Endoscopic	1 Radioactive Element D Intraluminal Device	Z No Qualifier
Q Anus	0 Open 3 Percutaneous 4 Percutaneous Endoscopic	D Intraluminal Device L Artificial Sphincter	Z No Qualifier
Q Anus	7 Via Natural or Artificial Opening 8 Via Natural or Artificial Opening Endoscopic	D Intraluminal Device	Z No Qualifier
R Anal Sphincter	0 Open 3 Percutaneous 4 Percutaneous Endoscopic	M Stimulator Lead	Z No Qualifier

0DH

Medical and Surgical, Gastrointestinal System Tables

283

Section	0	Medical and Surgical
Body System	D	Gastrointestinal System
Operation	J	**Inspection:** Visually and/or manually exploring a body part

Body Part (4th)	Approach (5th)	Device (6th)	Qualifier (7th)
0 Upper Intestinal Tract 6 Stomach D Lower Intestinal Tract	0 Open 3 Percutaneous 4 Percutaneous Endoscopic 7 Via Natural or Artificial Opening 8 Via Natural or Artificial Opening Endoscopic X External	Z No Device	Z No Qualifier
U Omentum V Mesentery W Peritoneum	0 Open 3 Percutaneous 4 Percutaneous Endoscopic X External	Z No Device	Z No Qualifier

Section	0	Medical and Surgical
Body System	D	Gastrointestinal System
Operation	L	**Occlusion:** Completely closing an orifice or the lumen of a tubular body part

Body Part (4th)	Approach (5th)	Device (6th)	Qualifier (7th)
1 Esophagus, Upper 2 Esophagus, Middle 3 Esophagus, Lower 4 Esophagogastric Junction 5 Esophagus 6 Stomach 7 Stomach, Pylorus 8 Small Intestine 9 Duodenum A Jejunum B Ileum C Ileocecal Valve E Large Intestine F Large Intestine, Right G Large Intestine, Left H Cecum K Ascending Colon L Transverse Colon M Descending Colon N Sigmoid Colon P Rectum	0 Open 3 Percutaneous 4 Percutaneous Endoscopic	C Extraluminal Device D Intraluminal Device Z No Device	Z No Qualifier
1 Esophagus, Upper 2 Esophagus, Middle 3 Esophagus, Lower 4 Esophagogastric Junction 5 Esophagus 6 Stomach 7 Stomach, Pylorus 8 Small Intestine 9 Duodenum A Jejunum B Ileum C Ileocecal Valve E Large Intestine F Large Intestine, Right G Large Intestine, Left H Cecum K Ascending Colon L Transverse Colon M Descending Colon N Sigmoid Colon P Rectum	7 Via Natural or Artificial Opening 8 Via Natural or Artificial Opening Endoscopic	D Intraluminal Device Z No Device	Z No Qualifier

Section	0	Medical and Surgical
Body System	D	Gastrointestinal System
Operation	L	Occlusion: Completely closing an orifice or the lumen of a tubular body part

Body Part (4th)	Approach (5th)	Device (6th)	Qualifier (7th)
Q Anus	0 Open 3 Percutaneous 4 Percutaneous Endoscopic X External	C Extraluminal Device D Intraluminal Device Z No Device	Z No Qualifier
Q Anus	7 Via Natural or Artificial Opening 8 Via Natural or Artificial Opening Endoscopic	D Intraluminal Device Z No Device	Z No Qualifier

Section	0	Medical and Surgical
Body System	D	Gastrointestinal System
Operation	M	Reattachment: Putting back in or on all or a portion of a separated body part to its normal location or other suitable location

Body Part (4th)	Approach (5th)	Device (6th)	Qualifier (7th)
5 Esophagus 6 Stomach 8 Small Intestine 9 Duodenum A Jejunum B Ileum E Large Intestine F Large Intestine, Right G Large Intestine, Left H Cecum K Ascending Colon L Transverse Colon M Descending Colon N Sigmoid Colon P Rectum	0 Open 4 Percutaneous Endoscopic	Z No Device	Z No Qualifier

Section	0	Medical and Surgical
Body System	D	Gastrointestinal System
Operation	N	Release: Freeing a body part from an abnormal physical constraint by cutting or by the use of force

Body Part (4th)	Approach (5th)	Device (6th)	Qualifier (7th)
1 Esophagus, Upper 2 Esophagus, Middle 3 Esophagus, Lower 4 Esophagogastric Junction 5 Esophagus 6 Stomach 7 Stomach, Pylorus 8 Small Intestine 9 Duodenum A Jejunum B Ileum C Ileocecal Valve E Large Intestine F Large Intestine, Right G Large Intestine, Left H Cecum J Appendix K Ascending Colon L Transverse Colon M Descending Colon N Sigmoid Colon P Rectum	0 Open 3 Percutaneous 4 Percutaneous Endoscopic 7 Via Natural or Artificial Opening 8 Via Natural or Artificial Opening Endoscopic	Z No Device	Z No Qualifier

0DL Continued

Continued →

0DN Continued

Section	0	Medical and Surgical
Body System	D	Gastrointestinal System
Operation	N	Release: Freeing a body part from an abnormal physical constraint by cutting or by the use of force

Body Part (4th)	Approach (5th)	Device (6th)	Qualifier (7th)
Q Anus	0 Open 3 Percutaneous 4 Percutaneous Endoscopic 7 Via Natural or Artificial Opening 8 Via Natural or Artificial Opening Endoscopic X External	Z No Device	Z No Qualifier
R Anal Sphincter U Omentum V Mesentery W Peritoneum	0 Open 3 Percutaneous 4 Percutaneous Endoscopic	Z No Device	Z No Qualifier

Section	0	Medical and Surgical
Body System	D	Gastrointestinal System
Operation	P	Removal: Taking out or off a device from a body part

Body Part (4th)	Approach (5th)	Device (6th)	Qualifier (7th)
0 Upper Intestinal Tract D Lower Intestinal Tract	0 Open 3 Percutaneous 4 Percutaneous Endoscopic 7 Via Natural or Artificial Opening 8 Via Natural or Artificial Opening Endoscopic	0 Drainage Device 2 Monitoring Device 3 Infusion Device 7 Autologous Tissue Substitute C Extraluminal Device D Intraluminal Device J Synthetic Substitute K Nonautologous Tissue Substitute U Feeding Device Y Other Device	Z No Qualifier
0 Upper Intestinal Tract D Lower Intestinal Tract	X External	0 Drainage Device 2 Monitoring Device 3 Infusion Device D Intraluminal Device U Feeding Device	Z No Qualifier
5 Esophagus	0 Open 3 Percutaneous 4 Percutaneous Endoscopic	1 Radioactive Element 2 Monitoring Device 3 Infusion Device U Feeding Device Y Other Device	Z No Qualifier
5 Esophagus	7 Via Natural or Artificial Opening 8 Via Natural or Artificial Opening Endoscopic	1 Radioactive Element D Intraluminal Device Y Other Device	Z No Qualifier
5 Esophagus	X External	1 Radioactive Element 2 Monitoring Device 3 Infusion Device D Intraluminal Device U Feeding Device	Z No Qualifier

286

Section	0	Medical and Surgical
Body System	D	Gastrointestinal System
Operation	P	Removal: Taking out or off a device from a body part

0DP Continued

Body Part (4th)	Approach (5th)	Device (6th)	Qualifier (7th)
6 Stomach	0 Open 3 Percutaneous 4 Percutaneous Endoscopic	0 Drainage Device 2 Monitoring Device 3 Infusion Device 7 Autologous Tissue Substitute C Extraluminal Device D Intraluminal Device J Synthetic Substitute K Nonautologous Tissue Substitute M Stimulator Lead U Feeding Device Y Other Device	Z No Qualifier
6 Stomach	7 Via Natural or Artificial Opening 8 Via Natural or Artificial Opening Endoscopic	0 Drainage Device 2 Monitoring Device 3 Infusion Device 7 Autologous Tissue Substitute C Extraluminal Device D Intraluminal Device J Synthetic Substitute K Nonautologous Tissue Substitute U Feeding Device Y Other Device	Z No Qualifier
6 Stomach	X External	0 Drainage Device 2 Monitoring Device 3 Infusion Device D Intraluminal Device U Feeding Device	Z No Qualifier
P Rectum	0 Open 3 Percutaneous 4 Percutaneous Endoscopic 7 Via Natural or Artificial Opening 8 Via Natural or Artificial Opening Endoscopic X External	1 Radioactive Element	Z No Qualifier
Q Anus	0 Open 3 Percutaneous 4 Percutaneous Endoscopic 7 Via Natural or Artificial Opening 8 Via Natural or Artificial Opening Endoscopic	L Artificial Sphincter	Z No Qualifier
R Anal Sphincter	0 Open 3 Percutaneous 4 Percutaneous Endoscopic	M Stimulator Lead	Z No Qualifier
U Omentum V Mesentery W Peritoneum	0 Open 3 Percutaneous 4 Percutaneous Endoscopic	0 Drainage Device 1 Radioactive Element 7 Autologous Tissue Substitute J Synthetic Substitute K Nonautologous Tissue Substitute	Z No Qualifier

0DQ–0DR

Medical and Surgical, Gastrointestinal System Tables

Section	0	Medical and Surgical
Body System	D	Gastrointestinal System
Operation	Q	**Repair:** Restoring, to the extent possible, a body part to its normal anatomic structure and function

Body Part (4th)	Approach (5th)	Device (6th)	Qualifier (7th)
1 Esophagus, Upper 2 Esophagus, Middle 3 Esophagus, Lower 4 Esophagogastric Junction 5 Esophagus 6 Stomach 7 Stomach, Pylorus 8 Small Intestine 9 Duodenum A Jejunum B Ileum C Ileocecal Valve E Large Intestine F Large Intestine, Right G Large Intestine, Left H Cecum J Appendix K Ascending Colon L Transverse Colon M Descending Colon N Sigmoid Colon P Rectum	0 Open 3 Percutaneous 4 Percutaneous Endoscopic 7 Via Natural or Artificial Opening 8 Via Natural or Artificial Opening Endoscopic	Z No Device	Z No Qualifier
Q Anus	0 Open 3 Percutaneous 4 Percutaneous Endoscopic 7 Via Natural or Artificial Opening 8 Via Natural or Artificial Opening Endoscopic X External	Z No Device	Z No Qualifier
R Anal Sphincter U Omentum V Mesentery W Peritoneum	0 Open 3 Percutaneous 4 Percutaneous Endoscopic	Z No Device	Z No Qualifier

Section	0	Medical and Surgical
Body System	D	Gastrointestinal System
Operation	R	**Replacement:** Putting in or on biological or synthetic material that physically takes the place and/or function of all or a portion of a body part

Body Part (4th)	Approach (5th)	Device (6th)	Qualifier (7th)
5 Esophagus	0 Open 4 Percutaneous Endoscopic 7 Via Natural or Artificial Opening 8 Via Natural or Artificial Opening Endoscopic	7 Autologous Tissue Substitute J Synthetic Substitute K Nonautologous Tissue Substitute	Z No Qualifier
R Anal Sphincter U Omentum V Mesentery W Peritoneum	0 Open 4 Percutaneous Endoscopic	7 Autologous Tissue Substitute J Synthetic Substitute K Nonautologous Tissue Substitute	Z No Qualifier

Section	0	Medical and Surgical
Body System	D	Gastrointestinal System
Operation	S	Reposition: Moving to its normal location, or other suitable location, all or a portion of a body part

Body Part (4th)	Approach (5th)	Device (6th)	Qualifier (7th)
5 Esophagus 6 Stomach 9 Duodenum A Jejunum B Ileum H Cecum K Ascending Colon L Transverse Colon M Descending Colon N Sigmoid Colon P Rectum Q Anus	0 Open 4 Percutaneous Endoscopic 7 Via Natural or Artificial Opening 8 Via Natural or Artificial Opening Endoscopic X External	Z No Device	Z No Qualifier
8 Small Intestine E Large Intestine	0 Open 4 Percutaneous Endoscopic 7 Via Natural or Artificial Opening 8 Via Natural or Artificial Opening Endoscopic	Z No Device	Z No Qualifier

Section	0	Medical and Surgical
Body System	D	Gastrointestinal System
Operation	T	Resection: Cutting out or off, without replacement, all of a body part

Body Part (4th)	Approach (5th)	Device (6th)	Qualifier (7th)
1 Esophagus, Upper 2 Esophagus, Middle 3 Esophagus, Lower 4 Esophagogastric Junction 5 Esophagus 6 Stomach 7 Stomach, Pylorus 8 Small Intestine 9 Duodenum A Jejunum B Ileum C Ileocecal Valve E Large Intestine F Large Intestine, Right H Cecum J Appendix K Ascending Colon P Rectum Q Anus	0 Open 4 Percutaneous Endoscopic 7 Via Natural or Artificial Opening 8 Via Natural or Artificial Opening Endoscopic	Z No Device	Z No Qualifier
G Large Intestine, Left L Transverse Colon M Descending Colon N Sigmoid Colon	0 Open 4 Percutaneous Endoscopic 7 Via Natural or Artificial Opening 8 Via Natural or Artificial Opening Endoscopic F Via Natural or Artificial Opening With Percutaneous Endoscopic Assistance	Z No Device	Z No Qualifier
R Anal Sphincter U Omentum	0 Open 4 Percutaneous Endoscopic	Z No Device	Z No Qualifier

0DU–0DV

Medical and Surgical, Gastrointestinal System Tables

Section	0	Medical and Surgical
Body System	D	Gastrointestinal System
Operation	U	Supplement: Putting in or on biological or synthetic material that physically reinforces and/or augments the function of a portion of a body part

Body Part (4th)	Approach (5th)	Device (6th)	Qualifier (7th)
1 Esophagus, Upper 2 Esophagus, Middle 3 Esophagus, Lower 4 Esophagogastric Junction 5 Esophagus 6 Stomach 7 Stomach, Pylorus 8 Small Intestine 9 Duodenum A Jejunum B Ileum C Ileocecal Valve E Large Intestine F Large Intestine, Right G Large Intestine, Left H Cecum K Ascending Colon L Transverse Colon M Descending Colon N Sigmoid Colon P Rectum	0 Open 4 Percutaneous Endoscopic 7 Via Natural or Artificial Opening 8 Via Natural or Artificial Opening Endoscopic	7 Autologous Tissue Substitute J Synthetic Substitute K Nonautologous Tissue Substitute	Z No Qualifier
Q Anus	0 Open 4 Percutaneous Endoscopic 7 Via Natural or Artificial Opening 8 Via Natural or Artificial Opening Endoscopic X External	7 Autologous Tissue Substitute J Synthetic Substitute K Nonautologous Tissue Substitute	Z No Qualifier
R Anal Sphincter U Omentum V Mesentery W Peritoneum	0 Open 4 Percutaneous Endoscopic	7 Autologous Tissue Substitute J Synthetic Substitute K Nonautologous Tissue Substitute	Z No Qualifier

Section	0	Medical and Surgical
Body System	D	Gastrointestinal System
Operation	V	Restriction: Partially closing an orifice or the lumen of a tubular body part

Body Part (4th)	Approach (5th)	Device (6th)	Qualifier (7th)
1 Esophagus, Upper 2 Esophagus, Middle 3 Esophagus, Lower 4 Esophagogastric Junction 5 Esophagus 6 Stomach 7 Stomach, Pylorus 8 Small Intestine 9 Duodenum A Jejunum B Ileum C Ileocecal Valve E Large Intestine F Large Intestine, Right G Large Intestine, Left H Cecum K Ascending Colon L Transverse Colon M Descending Colon N Sigmoid Colon P Rectum	0 Open 3 Percutaneous 4 Percutaneous Endoscopic	C Extraluminal Device D Intraluminal Device Z No Device	Z No Qualifier

Continued →

290

0DV Continued

Section	0	Medical and Surgical
Body System	D	Gastrointestinal System
Operation	V	Restriction: Partially closing an orifice or the lumen of a tubular body part

Body Part (4th)	Approach (5th)	Device (6th)	Qualifier (7th)
1 Esophagus, Upper 2 Esophagus, Middle 3 Esophagus, Lower 4 Esophagogastric Junction 5 Esophagus 6 Stomach 7 Stomach, Pylorus 8 Small Intestine 9 Duodenum A Jejunum B Ileum C Ileocecal Valve E Large Intestine F Large Intestine, Right G Large Intestine, Left H Cecum K Ascending Colon L Transverse Colon M Descending Colon N Sigmoid Colon P Rectum	7 Via Natural or Artificial Opening 8 Via Natural or Artificial Opening Endoscopic	D Intraluminal Device Z No Device	Z No Qualifier
Q Anus	0 Open 3 Percutaneous 4 Percutaneous Endoscopic X External	C Extraluminal Device D Intraluminal Device Z No Device	Z No Qualifier
Q Anus	7 Via Natural or Artificial Opening 8 Via Natural or Artificial Opening Endoscopic	D Intraluminal Device Z No Device	Z No Qualifier

Section	0	Medical and Surgical
Body System	D	Gastrointestinal System
Operation	W	Revision: Correcting, to the extent possible, a portion of a malfunctioning device or the position of a displaced device

Body Part (4th)	Approach (5th)	Device (6th)	Qualifier (7th)
0 Upper Intestinal Tract D Lower Intestinal Tract	0 Open 3 Percutaneous 4 Percutaneous Endoscopic 7 Via Natural or Artificial Opening 8 Via Natural or Artificial Opening Endoscopic	0 Drainage Device 2 Monitoring Device 3 Infusion Device 7 Autologous Tissue Substitute C Extraluminal Device D Intraluminal Device J Synthetic Substitute K Nonautologous Tissue Substitute U Feeding Device Y Other Device	Z No Qualifier
0 Upper Intestinal Tract D Lower Intestinal Tract	X External	0 Drainage Device 2 Monitoring Device 3 Infusion Device 7 Autologous Tissue Substitute C Extraluminal Device D Intraluminal Device J Synthetic Substitute K Nonautologous Tissue Substitute U Feeding Device	Z No Qualifier

Continued →

0DV–0DW

Medical and Surgical, Gastrointestinal System Tables

Section	0	Medical and Surgical
Body System	D	Gastrointestinal System
Operation	W	Revision: Correcting, to the extent possible, a portion of a malfunctioning device or the position of a displaced device

0DW Continued

Body Part (4th)	Approach (5th)	Device (6th)	Qualifier (7th)
5 Esophagus	0 Open 3 Percutaneous 4 Percutaneous Endoscopic	Y Other Device	Z No Qualifier
5 Esophagus	7 Via Natural or Artificial Opening 8 Via Natural or Artificial Opening Endoscopic	D Intraluminal Device Y Other Device	Z No Qualifier
5 Esophagus	X External	D Intraluminal Device	Z No Qualifier
6 Stomach	0 Open 3 Percutaneous 4 Percutaneous Endoscopic	0 Drainage Device 2 Monitoring Device 3 Infusion Device 7 Autologous Tissue Substitute C Extraluminal Device D Intraluminal Device J Synthetic Substitute K Nonautologous Tissue Substitute M Stimulator Lead U Feeding Device Y Other Device	Z No Qualifier
6 Stomach	7 Via Natural or Artificial Opening 8 Via Natural or Artificial Opening Endoscopic	0 Drainage Device 2 Monitoring Device 3 Infusion Device 7 Autologous Tissue Substitute C Extraluminal Device D Intraluminal Device J Synthetic Substitute K Nonautologous Tissue Substitute U Feeding Device Y Other Device	Z No Qualifier
6 Stomach	X External	0 Drainage Device 2 Monitoring Device 3 Infusion Device 7 Autologous Tissue Substitute C Extraluminal Device D Intraluminal Device J Synthetic Substitute K Nonautologous Tissue Substitute U Feeding Device	Z No Qualifier
8 Small Intestine E Large Intestine	0 Open 4 Percutaneous Endoscopic 7 Via Natural or Artificial Opening 8 Via Natural or Artificial Opening Endoscopic	7 Autologous Tissue Substitute J Synthetic Substitute K Nonautologous Tissue Substitute	Z No Qualifier
Q Anus	0 Open 3 Percutaneous 4 Percutaneous Endoscopic 7 Via Natural or Artificial Opening 8 Via Natural or Artificial Opening Endoscopic	L Artificial Sphincter	Z No Qualifier
R Anal Sphincter	0 Open 3 Percutaneous 4 Percutaneous Endoscopic	M Stimulator Lead	Z No Qualifier
U Omentum V Mesentery W Peritoneum	0 Open 3 Percutaneous 4 Percutaneous Endoscopic	0 Drainage Device 7 Autologous Tissue Substitute J Synthetic Substitute K Nonautologous Tissue Substitute	Z No Qualifier

Section	0	Medical and Surgical
Body System	D	Gastrointestinal System
Operation	X	**Transfer:** Moving, without taking out, all or a portion of a body part to another location to take over the function of all or a portion of a body part

Body Part (4th)	Approach (5th)	Device (6th)	Qualifier (7th)
6 Stomach	0 Open 4 Percutaneous Endoscopic	Z No Device	5 Esophagus
8 Small Intestine	0 Open 4 Percutaneous Endoscopic	Z No Device	5 Esophagus B Bladder C Ureter, Right D Ureter, Left F Ureters, Bilateral
E Large Intestine	0 Open 4 Percutaneous Endoscopic	Z No Device	5 Esophagus 7 Vagina B Bladder

Section	0	Medical and Surgical
Body System	D	Gastrointestinal System
Operation	Y	**Transplantation:** Putting in or on all or a portion of a living body part taken from another individual or animal to physically take the place and/or function of all or a portion of a similar body part

Body Part (4th)	Approach (5th)	Device (6th)	Qualifier (7th)
5 Esophagus 6 Stomach 8 Small Intestine E Large Intestine	0 Open	Z No Device	0 Allogeneic 1 Syngeneic 2 Zooplastic

AHA Coding Clinic

0D160ZA Bypass Stomach to Jejunum, Open Approach—AHA CC: 2Q, 2017, 17-18

0D194ZB Bypass Duodenum to Ileum, Percutaneous Endoscopic Approach—AHA CC: 2Q, 2016, 31

0D1N0Z4 Bypass Sigmoid Colon to Cutaneous, Open Approach—AHA CC: 4Q, 2014, 41-42

0D20XYZ Change Other Device in Upper Intestinal Tract, External Approach—AHA CC: 1Q, 2022, 45-46

0D2DXUZ Change Feeding Device in Lower Intestinal Tract, External Approach—AHA CC: 1Q, 2019, 26-27

0D5W0ZZ Destruction of Peritoneum, Open Approach—AHA CC: 1Q, 2017, 34-35

0D768ZZ Dilation of Stomach, Via Natural or Artificial Opening Endoscopic—AHA CC: 4Q, 2014, 40

0D7A8ZZ Dilation of Jejunum, Via Natural or Artificial Opening Endoscopic—AHA CC: 4Q, 2014, 40

0D844ZZ Division of Esophagogastric Junction, Percutaneous Endoscopic Approach—AHA CC: 3Q, 2017, 22-23

0D874ZZ Division of Stomach, Pylorus, Percutaneous Endoscopic Approach—AHA CC: 3Q, 2017, 23-24; 2Q, 2019, 15-16

0D9670Z Drainage of Stomach with Drainage Device, Via Natural or Artificial Opening—AHA CC: 2Q, 2015, 29

0DB18ZZ Excision of Upper Esophagus, Via Natural or Artificial Opening Endoscopic—AHA CC: 1Q, 2023, 32-33

0DB28ZX Excision of Middle Esophagus, Via Natural or Artificial Opening Endoscopic, Diagnostic—AHA CC: 1Q, 2016, 24-25

0DB60ZZ Excision of Stomach, Open Approach—AHA CC: 2Q, 2017, 17-18; 1Q, 2019, 4-7

0DB64Z3 Excision of Stomach, Percutaneous Endoscopic Approach, Vertical—AHA CC: 2Q, 2016, 31

0DB80ZZ Excision of Small Intestine, Open Approach—AHA CC: 2Q, 2021, 11-12

0DB90ZZ Excision of Duodenum, Open Approach—AHA CC: 3Q, 2014, 32-33; 1Q, 2019, 4-7

0DBA0ZZ Excision of Jejunum, Open Approach—AHA CC: 1Q, 2019 4-5

0DBA4ZZ Excision of Jejunum, Percutaneous Endoscopic Approach—AHA CC: 2Q, 2019, 15-16

0DBB0ZZ Excision of Ileum, Open Approach—AHA CC: 3Q, 2014, 28-29; 3Q, 2016, 5-6

0DBB4ZZ Excision of Ileum, Percutaneous Endoscopic Approach—AHA CC: 3Q, 2021, 28-29

0DBK8ZZ Excision of Ascending Colon, Via Natural or Artificial Opening Endoscopic—AHA CC: 1Q, 2017, 16

0DBN0ZZ Excision of Sigmoid Colon, Open Approach—AHA CC: 4Q, 2014, 40-41; 1Q, 2019, 27

0DBP0ZZ Excision of Rectum, Open Approach—AHA CC: 1Q, 2019, 27

0DBP7ZZ Excision of Rectum, Via Natural or Artificial Opening—AHA CC: 1Q, 2016, 22

0DBQ0ZZ Excision of Anus, Open Approach—AHA CC: 2Q, 2023, 23-24

0DD68ZX Extraction of Stomach, Via Natural or Artificial Opening Endoscopic, Diagnostic—AHA CC: 4Q, 2017, 42

0DDP8ZX Extraction of Rectum, Via Natural or Artificial Opening Endoscopic, Diagnostic—AHA CC: 1Q, 2021, 20-21

0DH08YZ Insertion of Other Device into Upper Intestinal Tract, Via Natural or Artificial Opening Endoscopic—AHA CC: 1Q, 2022, 44

0DH63UZ Insertion of Feeding Device into Stomach, Percutaneous Approach—AHA CC: 4Q, 2013, 117

0DH67UZ Insertion of Feeding Device into Stomach, Via Natural or Artificial Opening—AHA CC: 3Q, 2016, 26-27

0DH68YZ Insertion of Monitoring Device into Stomach, Via Natural or Artificial Opening Endoscopic—AHA CC: 2Q, 2019, 18

0DHA3UZ Insertion of Feeding Device into Jejunum, Percutaneous Approach—AHA CC: 3Q, 2020, 43

0DJ07ZZ Inspection of Upper Intestinal Tract, Via Natural or Artificial Opening—AHA CC: 2Q, 2016, 20-21

0DJ08ZZ Inspection of Upper Intestinal Tract, Via Natural or Artificial Opening Endoscopic—AHA CC: 3Q, 2015, 24-25

0DJD0ZZ Inspection of Lower Intestinal Tract, Open Approach—AHA CC: 1Q, 2019, 25-26

0DJD8ZZ Inspection of Lower Intestinal Tract, Via Natural or Artificial Opening Endoscopic—AHA CC: 2Q, 2017, 15-16

0DN50ZZ Release Esophagus, Open Approach—AHA CC: 3Q, 2015, 15-16

0DN80ZZ Release Small Intestine, Open Approach—AHA CC: 4Q, 2017, 49-50

0DNW0ZZ Release Peritoneum, Open Approach—AHA CC: 1Q, 2017, 35

0DP68YZ Removal of Other Device from Stomach, Via Natural or Artificial Opening Endoscopic—AHA CC: 2Q, 2019, 18-19

0DQ64ZZ Repair Stomach, Percutaneous Endoscopic Approach—AHA CC: 2Q, 2019, 15-16

0DQ98ZZ Repair Duodenum, Via Natural or Artificial Opening Endoscopic—AHA CC: 4Q, 2014, 20

0DQP0ZZ Repair Rectum, Open Approach—AHA CC: 1Q, 2016, 7-8

0DQR0ZZ Repair Anal Sphincter, Open Approach—AHA CC: 1Q, 2016, 7-8

0DQV4ZZ Repair Mesentery, Percutaneous Endoscopic Approach— AHA CC: 1Q, 2018, 11-12

0DS80ZZ Reposition Small Intestine, Open Approach—AHA CC: 4Q, 2017, 49-50

0DSB7ZZ Reposition Ileum, Via Natural or Artificial Opening—AHA CC: 3Q, 2017, 9-10

0DSE0ZZ Reposition Large Intestine, Open Approach—AHA CC: 4Q, 2017, 49-50

0DSK7ZZ Reposition Ascending Colon, Via Natural or Artificial Opening—AHA CC: 3Q, 2017, 9-10

0DSM4ZZ Reposition Descending Colon, Percutaneous Endoscopic Approach—AHA CC: 3Q, 2016, 5-6

0DSP0ZZ Reposition Rectum, Open Approach—AHA CC: 3Q, 2017, 17-18; 1Q, 2019, 30-31

0DT30ZZ Resection of Lower Esophagus, Open Approach—AHA CC: 1Q, 2019, 14-15

0DT90ZZ Resection of Duodenum, Open Approach—AHA CC: 1Q, 2019, 4-7

0DTF0ZZ Resection of Right Large Intestine, Open Approach—AHA CC: 3Q, 2014, 6-7; 4Q, 2014, 42-43

0DTH0ZZ Resection of Cecum, Open Approach—AHA CC: 3Q, 2014, 6

0DTJ0ZZ Resection of Appendix, Open Approach—AHA CC: 4Q, 2017, 49-50

0DTP0ZZ Resection of Rectum, Open Approach—AHA CC: 4Q, 2014, 40-41

0DTQ0ZZ Resection of Anus, Open Approach—AHA CC: 4Q, 2014, 40-41

0DUE07Z Supplement Large Intestine with Autologous Tissue Substitute, Open Approach—AHA CC: 2Q, 2021, 20-21

0DUP0JZ Supplement Rectum with Synthetic Substitute, Open Approach—AHA CC: 1Q, 2019, 30-31

0DUP47Z Supplement Rectum with Autologous Tissue Substitute, Percutaneous Endoscopic Approach—AHA CC: 1Q, 2021, 22-23

0DV40ZZ Restriction of Esophagogastric Junction, Open Approach—AHA CC: 2Q, 2016, 22-23

0DV44ZZ Restriction of Esophagogastric Junction, Percutaneous Endoscopic Approach—AHA CC: 3Q, 2014, 28; 3Q, 2017, 22-23

0DW63CZ Revision of Extraluminal Device in Stomach, Percutaneous Approach—AHA CC: 1Q, 2018, 20

0DW807Z Revision of Autologous Tissue Substitute in Small Intestine, Open Approach—AHA CC: 1Q, 2021, 19-20

0DX60Z5 Transfer Stomach to Esophagus, Open Approach—AHA CC: 2Q, 2016, 22-23; 2Q, 2017, 18

0DX80ZB Transfer Small Intestine to Bladder, Open Approach—AHA CC: 4Q, 2022, 57

0DXE0Z5 Transfer Large Intestine to Esophagus, Open Approach—AHA CC: 1Q, 2019, 14-15

0DXE0Z7 Transfer Large Intestine to Vagina, Open Approach—AHA CC: 4Q, 2019, 30

Hepatobiliary System and Pancreas

Surfaces and Bed of Liver

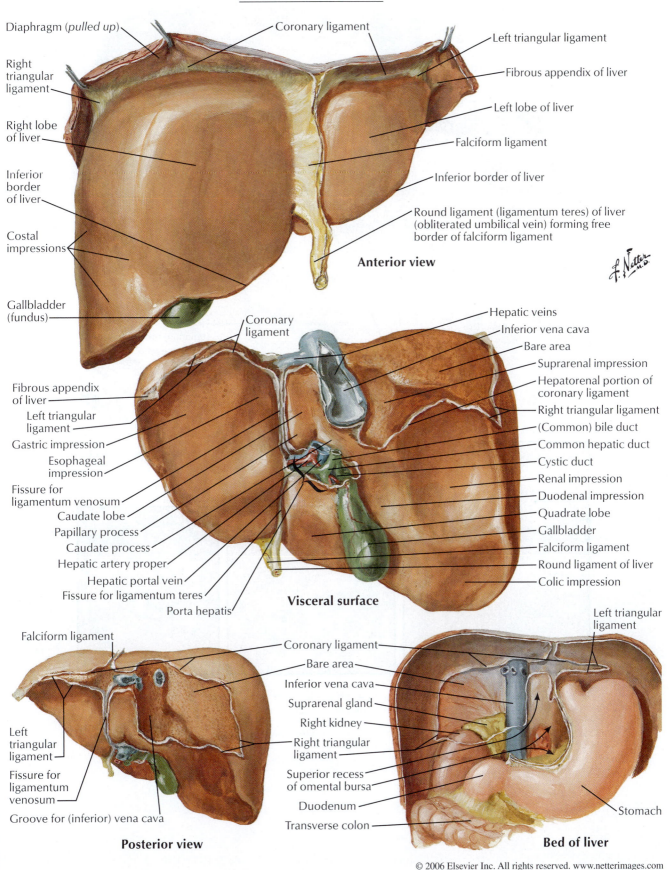

295

Pancreas: Anatomy and Histology

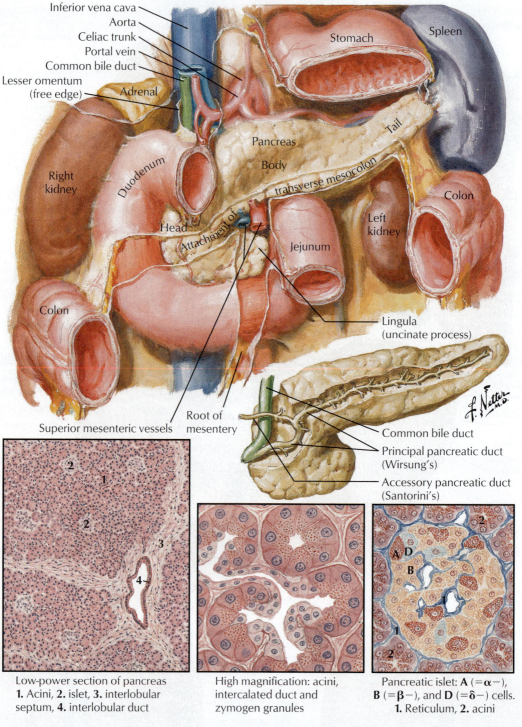

Low-power section of pancreas
1. Acini, **2.** islet, **3.** interlobular septum, **4.** interlobular duct

High magnification: acini, intercalated duct and zymogen granules

Pancreatic islet: **A** (=α−), **B** (=β−), and **D** (=δ−) cells. **1.** Reticulum, **2.** acini

© 2019 Elsevier Inc. All rights reserved. www.netterimages.com

Hepatobiliary System and Pancreas Tables 0F1–0FY

Section	0	Medical and Surgical
Body System	F	Hepatobiliary System and Pancreas
Operation	1	**Bypass:** Altering the route of passage of the contents of a tubular body part

Body Part (4th)	Approach (5th)	Device (6th)	Qualifier (7th)
4 Gallbladder 5 Hepatic Duct, Right 6 Hepatic Duct, Left 7 Hepatic Duct, Common 8 Cystic Duct 9 Common Bile Duct	0 Open 4 Percutaneous Endoscopic	D Intraluminal Device Z No Device	3 Duodenum 4 Stomach 5 Hepatic Duct, Right 6 Hepatic Duct, Left 7 Hepatic Duct, Caudate 8 Cystic Duct 9 Common Bile Duct B Small Intestine
D Pancreatic Duct	0 Open 4 Percutaneous Endoscopic	D Intraluminal Device Z No Device	3 Duodenum 4 Stomach B Small Intestine C Large Intestine
F Pancreatic Duct, Accessory G Pancreas	0 Open 4 Percutaneous Endoscopic	D Intraluminal Device Z No Device	3 Duodenum B Small Intestine C Large Intestine

Section	0	Medical and Surgical
Body System	F	Hepatobiliary System and Pancreas
Operation	2	**Change:** Taking out or off a device from a body part and putting back an identical or similar device in or on the same body part without cutting or puncturing the skin or a mucous membrane

Body Part (4th)	Approach (5th)	Device (6th)	Qualifier (7th)
0 Liver 4 Gallbladder B Hepatobiliary Duct D Pancreatic Duct G Pancreas	X External	0 Drainage Device Y Other Device	Z No Qualifier

Section	0	Medical and Surgical
Body System	F	Hepatobiliary System and Pancreas
Operation	5	**Destruction:** Physical eradication of all or a portion of a body part by the direct use of energy, force, or a destructive agent

Body Part (4th)	Approach (5th)	Device (6th)	Qualifier (7th)
0 Liver 1 Liver, Right Lobe 2 Liver, Left Lobe	0 Open 3 Percutaneous 4 Percutaneous Endoscopic	Z No Device	3 Laser Interstitial Thermal Therapy F Irreversible Electroporation Z No Qualifier
4 Gallbladder	0 Open 3 Percutaneous 4 Percutaneous Endoscopic	Z No Device	3 Laser Interstitial Thermal Therapy Z No Qualifier
4 Gallbladder	8 Via Natural or Artificial Opening Endoscopic	Z No Device	Z No Qualifier
5 Hepatic Duct, Right 6 Hepatic Duct, Left 7 Hepatic Duct, Common 8 Cystic Duct 9 Common Bile Duct C Ampulla of Vater D Pancreatic Duct F Pancreatic Duct, Accessory	0 Open 3 Percutaneous 4 Percutaneous Endoscopic	Z No Device	3 Laser Interstitial Thermal Therapy Z No Qualifier

Continued →

0F5–0F9

Medical and Surgical, Hepatobiliary System and Pancreas Tables

0F5 Continued

Section	0	Medical and Surgical
Body System	F	Hepatobiliary System and Pancreas
Operation	5	Destruction: Physical eradication of all or a portion of a body part by the direct use of energy, force, or a destructive agent

Body Part (4th)	Approach (5th)	Device (6th)	Qualifier (7th)
5 Hepatic Duct, Right 6 Hepatic Duct, Left 7 Hepatic Duct, Common 8 Cystic Duct 9 Common Bile Duct C Ampulla of Vater D Pancreatic Duct F Pancreatic Duct, Accessory	7 Via Natural or Artificial Opening 8 Via Natural or Artificial Opening Endoscopic	Z No Device	Z No Qualifier
G Pancreas	0 Open 3 Percutaneous 4 Percutaneous Endoscopic	Z No Device	3 Laser Interstitial Thermal Therapy F Irreversible Electroporation Z No Qualifier
G Pancreas	8 Via Natural or Artificial Opening Endoscopic	Z No Device	Z No Qualifier

Section	0	Medical and Surgical
Body System	F	Hepatobiliary System and Pancreas
Operation	7	Dilation: Expanding an orifice or the lumen of a tubular body part

Body Part (4th)	Approach (5th)	Device (6th)	Qualifier (7th)
5 Hepatic Duct, Right 6 Hepatic Duct, Left 7 Hepatic Duct, Common 8 Cystic Duct 9 Common Bile Duct C Ampulla of Vater D Pancreatic Duct F Pancreatic Duct, Accessory	0 Open 3 Percutaneous 4 Percutaneous Endoscopic 7 Via Natural or Artificial Opening 8 Via Natural or Artificial Opening Endoscopic	D Intraluminal Device Z No Device	Z No Qualifier

Section	0	Medical and Surgical
Body System	F	Hepatobiliary System and Pancreas
Operation	8	Division: Cutting into a body part, without draining fluids and/or gases from the body part, in order to separate or transect a body part

Body Part (4th)	Approach (5th)	Device (6th)	Qualifier (7th)
0 Liver 1 Liver, Right Lobe 2 Liver, Left Lobe G Pancreas	0 Open 3 Percutaneous 4 Percutaneous Endoscopic	Z No Device	Z No Qualifier

Section	0	Medical and Surgical
Body System	F	Hepatobiliary System and Pancreas
Operation	9	Drainage: Taking or letting out fluids and/or gases from a body part

Body Part (4th)	Approach (5th)	Device (6th)	Qualifier (7th)
0 Liver 1 Liver, Right Lobe 2 Liver, Left Lobe	0 Open 3 Percutaneous 4 Percutaneous Endoscopic	0 Drainage Device	Z No Qualifier

298

Section	0	Medical and Surgical
Body System	F	Hepatobiliary System and Pancreas
Operation	9	Drainage: Taking or letting out fluids and/or gases from a body part

0F9 Continued

Body Part (4th)	Approach (5th)	Device (6th)	Qualifier (7th)
0 Liver 1 Liver, Right Lobe 2 Liver, Left Lobe	0 Open 3 Percutaneous 4 Percutaneous Endoscopic	Z No Device	X Diagnostic Z No Qualifier
4 Gallbladder G Pancreas	0 Open 3 Percutaneous 4 Percutaneous Endoscopic 8 Via Natural or Artificial Opening Endoscopic	0 Drainage Device	Z No Qualifier
4 Gallbladder G Pancreas	0 Open 3 Percutaneous 4 Percutaneous Endoscopic 8 Via Natural or Artificial Opening Endoscopic	Z No Device	X Diagnostic Z No Qualifier
5 Hepatic Duct, Right 6 Hepatic Duct, Left 7 Hepatic Duct, Common 8 Cystic Duct 9 Common Bile Duct C Ampulla of Vater D Pancreatic Duct F Pancreatic Duct, Accessory	0 Open 3 Percutaneous 4 Percutaneous Endoscopic 7 Via Natural or Artificial Opening 8 Via Natural or Artificial Opening Endoscopic	0 Drainage Device	Z No Qualifier
5 Hepatic Duct, Right 6 Hepatic Duct, Left 7 Hepatic Duct, Common 8 Cystic Duct 9 Common Bile Duct C Ampulla of Vater D Pancreatic Duct F Pancreatic Duct, Accessory	0 Open 3 Percutaneous 4 Percutaneous Endoscopic 7 Via Natural or Artificial Opening 8 Via Natural or Artificial Opening Endoscopic	Z No Device	X Diagnostic Z No Qualifier

Section	0	Medical and Surgical
Body System	F	Hepatobiliary System and Pancreas
Operation	B	Excision: Cutting out or off, without replacement, a portion of a body part

Body Part (4th)	Approach (5th)	Device (6th)	Qualifier (7th)
0 Liver 1 Liver, Right Lobe 2 Liver, Left Lobe	0 Open 3 Percutaneous 4 Percutaneous Endoscopic	Z No Device	X Diagnostic Z No Qualifier
4 Gallbladder G Pancreas	0 Open 3 Percutaneous 4 Percutaneous Endoscopic 8 Via Natural or Artificial Opening Endoscopic	Z No Device	X Diagnostic Z No Qualifier
5 Hepatic Duct, Right 6 Hepatic Duct, Left 7 Hepatic Duct, Common 8 Cystic Duct 9 Common Bile Duct C Ampulla of Vater D Pancreatic Duct F Pancreatic Duct, Accessory	0 Open 3 Percutaneous 4 Percutaneous Endoscopic 7 Via Natural or Artificial Opening 8 Via Natural or Artificial Opening Endoscopic	Z No Device	X Diagnostic Z No Qualifier

0F9–0FB

Medical and Surgical, Hepatobiliary System and Pancreas Tables

0FC–0FF

Medical and Surgical, Hepatobiliary System and Pancreas Tables

Section	0	Medical and Surgical
Body System	F	Hepatobiliary System and Pancreas
Operation	C	Extirpation: Taking or cutting out solid matter from a body part

Body Part (4th)	Approach (5th)	Device (6th)	Qualifier (7th)
0 Liver 1 Liver, Right Lobe 2 Liver, Left Lobe	0 Open 3 Percutaneous 4 Percutaneous Endoscopic	Z No Device	Z No Qualifier
4 Gallbladder G Pancreas	0 Open 3 Percutaneous 4 Percutaneous Endoscopic 8 Via Natural or Artificial Opening Endoscopic	Z No Device	Z No Qualifier
5 Hepatic Duct, Right 6 Hepatic Duct, Left 7 Hepatic Duct, Common 8 Cystic Duct 9 Common Bile Duct C Ampulla of Vater D Pancreatic Duct F Pancreatic Duct, Accessory	0 Open 3 Percutaneous 4 Percutaneous Endoscopic 7 Via Natural or Artificial Opening 8 Via Natural or Artificial Opening Endoscopic	Z No Device	Z No Qualifier

Section	0	Medical and Surgical
Body System	F	Hepatobiliary System and Pancreas
Operation	D	Extraction: Pulling or stripping out or off all or a portion of a body part by the use of force

Body Part (4th)	Approach (5th)	Device (6th)	Qualifier (7th)
0 Liver 1 Liver, Right Lobe 2 Liver, Left Lobe	3 Percutaneous 4 Percutaneous Endoscopic	Z No Device	X Diagnostic
4 Gallbladder 5 Hepatic Duct, Right 6 Hepatic Duct, Left 7 Hepatic Duct, Common 8 Cystic Duct 9 Common Bile Duct C Ampulla of Vater D Pancreatic Duct F Pancreatic Duct, Accessory G Pancreas	3 Percutaneous 4 Percutaneous Endoscopic 8 Via Natural or Artificial Opening Endoscopic	Z No Device	X Diagnostic

Section	0	Medical and Surgical
Body System	F	Hepatobiliary System and Pancreas
Operation	F	Fragmentation: Breaking solid matter in a body part into pieces

Body Part (4th)	Approach (5th)	Device (6th)	Qualifier (7th)
4 Gallbladder 5 Hepatic Duct, Right 6 Hepatic Duct, Left 7 Hepatic Duct, Common 8 Cystic Duct 9 Common Bile Duct C Ampulla of Vater D Pancreatic Duct F Pancreatic Duct, Accessory	0 Open 3 Percutaneous 4 Percutaneous Endoscopic 7 Via Natural or Artificial Opening 8 Via Natural or Artificial Opening Endoscopic X External	Z No Device	Z No Qualifier

Section	0	Medical and Surgical
Body System	F	Hepatobiliary System and Pancreas
Operation	H	Insertion: Putting in a nonbiological appliance that monitors, assists, performs, or prevents a physiological function but does not physically take the place of a body part

Body Part (4th)	Approach (5th)	Device (6th)	Qualifier (7th)
0 Liver 4 Gallbladder G Pancreas	0 Open 3 Percutaneous 4 Percutaneous Endoscopic	1 Radioactive Element 2 Monitoring Device 3 Infusion Device Y Other Device	Z No Qualifier
1 Liver, Right Lobe 2 Liver, Left Lobe	0 Open 3 Percutaneous 4 Percutaneous Endoscopic	2 Monitoring Device 3 Infusion Device	Z No Qualifier
B Hepatobiliary Duct D Pancreatic Duct	0 Open 3 Percutaneous 4 Percutaneous Endoscopic 7 Via Natural or Artificial Opening 8 Via Natural or Artificial Opening Endoscopic	1 Radioactive Element 2 Monitoring Device 3 Infusion Device D Intraluminal Device Y Other Device	Z No Qualifier

Section	0	Medical and Surgical
Body System	F	Hepatobiliary System and Pancreas
Operation	J	Inspection: Visually and/or manually exploring a body part

Body Part (4th)	Approach (5th)	Device (6th)	Qualifier (7th)
0 Liver	0 Open 3 Percutaneous 4 Percutaneous Endoscopic X External	Z No Device	Z No Qualifier
4 Gallbladder G Pancreas	0 Open 3 Percutaneous 4 Percutaneous Endoscopic 8 Via Natural or Artificial Opening Endoscopic X External	Z No Device	Z No Qualifier
B Hepatobiliary Duct D Pancreatic Duct	0 Open 3 Percutaneous 4 Percutaneous Endoscopic 7 Via Natural or Artificial Opening 8 Via Natural or Artificial Opening Endoscopic	Z No Device	Z No Qualifier

Section	0	Medical and Surgical
Body System	F	Hepatobiliary System and Pancreas
Operation	L	Occlusion: Completely closing an orifice or the lumen of a tubular body part

Body Part (4th)	Approach (5th)	Device (6th)	Qualifier (7th)
5 Hepatic Duct, Right 6 Hepatic Duct, Left 7 Hepatic Duct, Common 8 Cystic Duct 9 Common Bile Duct C Ampulla of Vater D Pancreatic Duct F Pancreatic Duct, Accessory	0 Open 3 Percutaneous 4 Percutaneous Endoscopic	C Extraluminal Device D Intraluminal Device Z No Device	Z No Qualifier

Continued →

0FL–0FN

Medical and Surgical, Hepatobiliary System and Pancreas Tables

0FL Continued

Section	0	Medical and Surgical
Body System	F	Hepatobiliary System and Pancreas
Operation	L	Occlusion: Completely closing an orifice or the lumen of a tubular body part

Body Part (4th)	Approach (5th)	Device (6th)	Qualifier (7th)
5 Hepatic Duct, Right 6 Hepatic Duct, Left 7 Hepatic Duct, Common 8 Cystic Duct 9 Common Bile Duct C Ampulla of Vater D Pancreatic Duct F Pancreatic Duct, Accessory	7 Via Natural or Artificial Opening 8 Via Natural or Artificial Opening Endoscopic	D Intraluminal Device Z No Device	Z No Qualifier

Section	0	Medical and Surgical
Body System	F	Hepatobiliary System and Pancreas
Operation	M	Reattachment: Putting back in or on all or a portion of a separated body part to its normal location or other suitable location

Body Part (4th)	Approach (5th)	Device (6th)	Qualifier (7th)
0 Liver 1 Liver, Right Lobe 2 Liver, Left Lobe 4 Gallbladder 5 Hepatic Duct, Right 6 Hepatic Duct, Left 7 Hepatic Duct, Common 8 Cystic Duct 9 Common Bile Duct C Ampulla of Vater D Pancreatic Duct F Pancreatic Duct, Accessory G Pancreas	0 Open 4 Percutaneous Endoscopic	Z No Device	Z No Qualifier

Section	0	Medical and Surgical
Body System	F	Hepatobiliary System and Pancreas
Operation	N	Release: Freeing a body part from an abnormal physical constraint by cutting or by the use of force

Body Part (4th)	Approach (5th)	Device (6th)	Qualifier (7th)
0 Liver 1 Liver, Right Lobe 2 Liver, Left Lobe	0 Open 3 Percutaneous 4 Percutaneous Endoscopic	Z No Device	Z No Qualifier
4 Gallbladder G Pancreas	0 Open 3 Percutaneous 4 Percutaneous Endoscopic 8 Via Natural or Artificial Opening Endoscopic	Z No Device	Z No Qualifier
5 Hepatic Duct, Right 6 Hepatic Duct, Left 7 Hepatic Duct, Common 8 Cystic Duct 9 Common Bile Duct C Ampulla of Vater D Pancreatic Duct F Pancreatic Duct, Accessory	0 Open 3 Percutaneous 4 Percutaneous Endoscopic 7 Via Natural or Artificial Opening 8 Via Natural or Artificial Opening Endoscopic	Z No Device	Z No Qualifier

Section	0	Medical and Surgical
Body System	F	Hepatobiliary System and Pancreas
Operation	P	Removal: Taking out or off a device from a body part

Body Part (4th)	Approach (5th)	Device (6th)	Qualifier (7th)
0 Liver	0 Open 3 Percutaneous 4 Percutaneous Endoscopic	0 Drainage Device 2 Monitoring Device 3 Infusion Device Y Other Device	Z No Qualifier
0 Liver	X External	0 Drainage Device 2 Monitoring Device 3 Infusion Device	Z No Qualifier
4 Gallbladder G Pancreas	0 Open 3 Percutaneous 4 Percutaneous Endoscopic X External	0 Drainage Device 2 Monitoring Device 3 Infusion Device D Intraluminal Device Y Other Device	Z No Qualifier
4 Gallbladder G Pancreas	X External	0 Drainage Device 2 Monitoring Device 3 Infusion Device D Intraluminal Device	Z No Qualifier
B Hepatobiliary Duct D Pancreatic Duct	0 Open 3 Percutaneous 4 Percutaneous Endoscopic 7 Via Natural or Artificial Opening 8 Via Natural or Artificial Opening Endoscopic	0 Drainage Device 1 Radioactive Element 2 Monitoring Device 3 Infusion Device 7 Autologous Tissue Substitute C Extraluminal Device D Intraluminal Device J Synthetic Substitute K Nonautologous Tissue Substitute Y Other Device	Z No Qualifier
B Hepatobiliary Duct D Pancreatic Duct	X External	0 Drainage Device 1 Radioactive Element 2 Monitoring Device 3 Infusion Device D Intraluminal Device	Z No Qualifier

Section	0	Medical and Surgical
Body System	F	Hepatobiliary System and Pancreas
Operation	Q	Repair: Restoring, to the extent possible, a body part to its normal anatomic structure and function

Body Part (4th)	Approach (5th)	Device (6th)	Qualifier (7th)
0 Liver 1 Liver, Right Lobe 2 Liver, Left Lobe	0 Open 3 Percutaneous 4 Percutaneous Endoscopic	Z No Device	Z No Qualifier
4 Gallbladder G Pancreas	0 Open 3 Percutaneous 4 Percutaneous Endoscopic 8 Via Natural or Artificial Opening Endoscopic	Z No Device	Z No Qualifier
5 Hepatic Duct, Right 6 Hepatic Duct, Left 7 Hepatic Duct, Common 8 Cystic Duct 9 Common Bile Duct C Ampulla of Vater D Pancreatic Duct F Pancreatic Duct, Accessory	0 Open 3 Percutaneous 4 Percutaneous Endoscopic 7 Via Natural or Artificial Opening 8 Via Natural or Artificial Opening Endoscopic	Z No Device	Z No Qualifier

Section 0 **Medical and Surgical**
Body System F **Hepatobiliary System and Pancreas**
Operation R **Replacement:** Putting in or on biological or synthetic material that physically takes the place and/or function of all or a portion of a body part

Body Part (4th)	Approach (5th)	Device (6th)	Qualifier (7th)
5 Hepatic Duct, Right	0 Open	7 Autologous Tissue Substitute	Z No Qualifier
6 Hepatic Duct, Left	4 Percutaneous Endoscopic	J Synthetic Substitute	
7 Hepatic Duct, Common	8 Via Natural or Artificial	K Nonautologous Tissue Substitute	
8 Cystic Duct	Opening Endoscopic		
9 Common Bile Duct			
C Ampulla of Vater			
D Pancreatic Duct			
F Pancreatic Duct, Accessory			

Section 0 **Medical and Surgical**
Body System F **Hepatobiliary System and Pancreas**
Operation S **Reposition:** Moving to its normal location, or other suitable location, all or a portion of a body part

Body Part (4th)	Approach (5th)	Device (6th)	Qualifier (7th)
0 Liver	0 Open	Z No Device	Z No Qualifier
4 Gallbladder	4 Percutaneous Endoscopic		
5 Hepatic Duct, Right			
6 Hepatic Duct, Left			
7 Hepatic Duct, Common			
8 Cystic Duct			
9 Common Bile Duct			
C Ampulla of Vater			
D Pancreatic Duct			
F Pancreatic Duct, Accessory			
G Pancreas			

Section 0 **Medical and Surgical**
Body System F **Hepatobiliary System and Pancreas**
Operation T **Resection:** Cutting out or off, without replacement, all of a body part

Body Part (4th)	Approach (5th)	Device (6th)	Qualifier (7th)
0 Liver	0 Open	Z No Device	Z No Qualifier
1 Liver, Right Lobe	4 Percutaneous Endoscopic		
2 Liver, Left Lobe			
4 Gallbladder			
G Pancreas			
5 Hepatic Duct, Right	0 Open	Z No Device	Z No Qualifier
6 Hepatic Duct, Left	4 Percutaneous Endoscopic		
7 Hepatic Duct, Common	7 Via Natural or Artificial Opening		
8 Cystic Duct	8 Via Natural or Artificial Opening		
9 Common Bile Duct	Endoscopic		
C Ampulla of Vater			
D Pancreatic Duct			
F Pancreatic Duct, Accessory			

Section	0	Medical and Surgical
Body System	F	Hepatobiliary System and Pancreas
Operation	U	Supplement: Putting in or on biological or synthetic material that physically reinforces and/or augments the function of a portion of a body part

Body Part (4th)	Approach (5th)	Device (6th)	Qualifier (7th)
5 Hepatic Duct, Right 6 Hepatic Duct, Left 7 Hepatic Duct, Common 8 Cystic Duct 9 Common Bile Duct C Ampulla of Vater D Pancreatic Duct F Pancreatic Duct, Accessory	0 Open 3 Percutaneous 4 Percutaneous Endoscopic 8 Via Natural or Artificial Opening Endoscopic	7 Autologous Tissue Substitute J Synthetic Substitute K Nonautologous Tissue Substitute	Z No Qualifier

Section	0	Medical and Surgical
Body System	F	Hepatobiliary System and Pancreas
Operation	V	Restriction: Partially closing an orifice or the lumen of a tubular body part

Body Part (4th)	Approach (5th)	Device (6th)	Qualifier (7th)
5 Hepatic Duct, Right 6 Hepatic Duct, Left 7 Hepatic Duct, Common 8 Cystic Duct 9 Common Bile Duct C Ampulla of Vater D Pancreatic Duct F Pancreatic Duct, Accessory	0 Open 3 Percutaneous 4 Percutaneous Endoscopic	C Extraluminal Device D Intraluminal Device Z No Device	Z No Qualifier
5 Hepatic Duct, Right 6 Hepatic Duct, Left 7 Hepatic Duct, Common 8 Cystic Duct 9 Common Bile Duct C Ampulla of Vater D Pancreatic Duct F Pancreatic Duct, Accessory	7 Via Natural or Artificial Opening 8 Via Natural or Artificial Opening Endoscopic	D Intraluminal Device Z No Device	Z No Qualifier

Section	0	Medical and Surgical
Body System	F	Hepatobiliary System and Pancreas
Operation	W	Revision: Correcting, to the extent possible, a portion of a malfunctioning device or the position of a displaced device

Body Part (4th)	Approach (5th)	Device (6th)	Qualifier (7th)
0 Liver	0 Open 3 Percutaneous 4 Percutaneous Endoscopic	0 Drainage Device 2 Monitoring Device 3 Infusion Device Y Other Device	Z No Qualifier
0 Liver	X External	0 Drainage Device 2 Monitoring Device 3 Infusion Device	Z No Qualifier
4 Gallbladder G Pancreas	0 Open 3 Percutaneous 4 Percutaneous Endoscopic	0 Drainage Device 2 Monitoring Device 3 Infusion Device D Intraluminal Device Y Other Device	Z No Qualifier
4 Gallbladder G Pancreas	X External	0 Drainage Device 2 Monitoring Device 3 Infusion Device D Intraluminal Device	Z No Qualifier

0FW–0FY

Section	0	Medical and Surgical
Body System	F	Hepatobiliary System and Pancreas
Operation	W	Revision: Correcting, to the extent possible, a portion of a malfunctioning device or the position of a displaced device

0FW Continued

Body Part (4ᵗʰ)	Approach (5ᵗʰ)	Device (6ᵗʰ)	Qualifier (7ᵗʰ)
B Hepatobiliary Duct D Pancreatic Duct	0 Open 3 Percutaneous 4 Percutaneous Endoscopic 7 Via Natural or Artificial Opening 8 Via Natural or Artificial Opening Endoscopic	0 Drainage Device 2 Monitoring Device 3 Infusion Device 7 Autologous Tissue Substitute C Extraluminal Device D Intraluminal Device J Synthetic Substitute K Nonautologous Tissue Substitute Y Other Device	Z No Qualifier
B Hepatobiliary Duct D Pancreatic Duct	X External	0 Drainage Device 2 Monitoring Device 3 Infusion Device 7 Autologous Tissue Substitute C Extraluminal Device D Intraluminal Device J Synthetic Substitute K Nonautologous Tissue Substitute	Z No Qualifier

Section	0	Medical and Surgical
Body System	F	Hepatobiliary System and Pancreas
Operation	Y	Transplantation: Putting in or on all or a portion of a living body part taken from another individual or animal to physically take the place and/or function of all or a portion of a similar body part

Body Part (4ᵗʰ)	Approach (5ᵗʰ)	Device (6ᵗʰ)	Qualifier (7ᵗʰ)
0 Liver G Pancreas	0 Open	Z No Device	0 Allogeneic 1 Syngeneic 2 Zooplastic

AHA Coding Clinic

0F1D4Z4 Bypass Pancreatic Duct to Stomach, Percutaneous Endoscopic Approach—AHA CC: 4Q, 2020, 53-54

0F5G4ZF Destruction of Pancreas using Irreversible Electroporation, Percutaneous Endoscopic Approach—AHA CC: 4Q, 2018, 39-40

0F798DZ Dilation of Common Bile Duct with Intraluminal Device, Via Natural or Artificial Opening Endoscopic—AHA CC: 3Q, 2014, 15-16; 1Q, 2016, 25

0F7D8DZ Dilation of Pancreatic Duct with Intraluminal Device, Via Natural or Artificial Opening Endoscopic—AHA CC: 1Q, 2016, 25; 3Q, 2016, 27-28

0F824ZZ Division of Left Lobe Liver, Percutaneous Endoscopic Approach—AHA CC: 4Q, 2021, 48-50

0F9630Z Drainage of Left Hepatic Duct with Drainage Device, Percutaneous Approach—AHA CC: 1Q, 2015, 32

0F9G40Z Drainage of Pancreas with Drainage Device, Percutaneous Endoscopic Approach AHA CC: 3Q, 2014, 15-16

0F9G80Z Drainage of Pancreas with Drainage Device, Via Natural or Artificial Opening Endoscopic—AHA CC: 3Q, 2020 34-35

0FB00ZX Excision of Liver, Open Approach, Diagnostic—AHA CC: 3Q, 2016, 41

0FB90ZZ Excision of Common Bile Duct, Open Approach—AHA CC: 1Q, 2019, 4-7

0FB98ZX Excision of Common Bile Duct, Via Natural or Artificial Opening Endoscopic, Diagnostic—AHA CC: 1Q, 2016, 23-25

0FBD8ZX Excision of Pancreatic Duct, Via Natural or Artificial Opening Endoscopic, Diagnostic—AHA CC: 1Q, 2016, 25

0FBG0ZZ Excision of Pancreas, Open Approach—AHA CC: 3Q, 2014, 32-33; 1Q, 2019, 4-8

0FCG8ZZ Extirpation of Matter from Pancreas, Via Natural or Artificial Opening Endoscopic—AHA CC: 2Q, 2023, 22-23

0FH031Z Insertion of Radioactive Element into Liver, Percutaneous Approach—AHA CC: 2Q, 2022, 26-27

0FQ00ZZ Repair Liver, Open Approach—AHA CC: 4Q, 2013, 109-111

0FQ90ZZ Repair Common Bile Duct, Open Approach—AHA CC: 3Q, 2016, 27

0FT00ZZ Resection of Liver, Open Approach—AHA CC: 4Q, 2012, 99-101

0FT40ZZ Resection of Gallbladder, Open Approach—AHA CC: 1Q, 2019, 4-5

0FT44ZZ Resection of Gallbladder, Percutaneous Endoscopic Approach—AHA CC: 4Q, 2021, 48-50

0FY00Z0 Transplantation of Liver, Allogeneic, Open Approach—AHA CC: 4Q, 2012, 99-101; 3Q, 2014, 13-14

Endocrine System

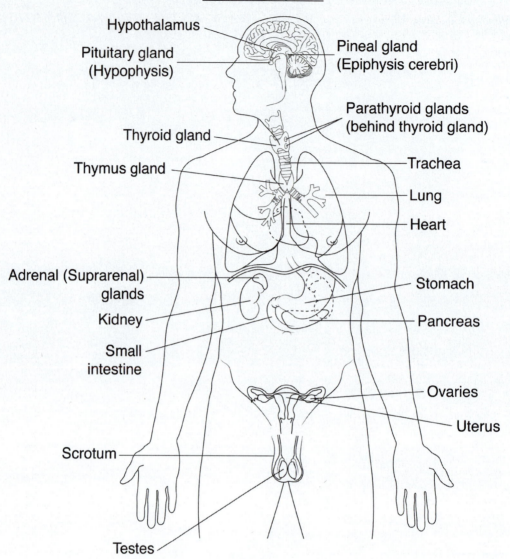

Endocrine System Tables 0G2–0GW

Section	0	Medical and Surgical
Body System	G	Endocrine System
Operation	2	Change: Taking out or off a device from a body part and putting back an identical or similar device in or on the same body part without cutting or puncturing the skin or a mucous membrane

Body Part (4th)	Approach (5th)	Device (6th)	Qualifier (7th)
0 Pituitary Gland 1 Pineal Body 5 Adrenal Gland K Thyroid Gland R Parathyroid Gland S Endocrine Gland	X External	0 Drainage Device Y Other Device	Z No Qualifier

Section	0	Medical and Surgical
Body System	G	Endocrine System
Operation	5	Destruction: Physical eradication of all or a portion of a body part by the direct use of energy, force, or a destructive agent

Body Part (4th)	Approach (5th)	Device (6th)	Qualifier (7th)
0 Pituitary Gland 1 Pineal Body 2 Adrenal Gland, Left 3 Adrenal Gland, Right 4 Adrenal Glands, Bilateral 6 Carotid Body, Left 7 Carotid Body, Right 8 Carotid Bodies, Bilateral 9 Para-aortic Body B Coccygeal Glomus C Glomus Jugulare D Aortic Body F Paraganglion Extremity G Thyroid Gland Lobe, Left H Thyroid Gland Lobe, Right K Thyroid Gland L Superior Parathyroid Gland, Right M Superior Parathyroid Gland, Left N Inferior Parathyroid Gland, Right P Inferior Parathyroid Gland, Left Q Parathyroid Glands, Multiple R Parathyroid Gland	0 Open 3 Percutaneous 4 Percutaneous Endoscopic	Z No Device	3 Laser Interstitial Thermal Therapy Z No Qualifier

Section	0	Medical and Surgical
Body System	G	Endocrine System
Operation	8	Division: Cutting into a body part, without draining fluids and/or gases from the body part, in order to separate or transect a body part

Body Part (4th)	Approach (5th)	Device (6th)	Qualifier (7th)
0 Pituitary Gland J Thyroid Gland Isthmus	0 Open 3 Percutaneous 4 Percutaneous Endoscopic	Z No Device	Z No Qualifier

Section	0	Medical and Surgical
Body System	G	Endocrine System
Operation	9	Drainage: Taking or letting out fluids and/or gases from a body part

Body Part (4th)	Approach (5th)	Device (6th)	Qualifier (7th)
0 Pituitary Gland	0 Open	0 Drainage Device	Z No Qualifier
1 Pineal Body	3 Percutaneous		
2 Adrenal Gland, Left	4 Percutaneous Endoscopic		
3 Adrenal Gland, Right			
4 Adrenal Glands, Bilateral			
6 Carotid Body, Left			
7 Carotid Body, Right			
8 Carotid Bodies, Bilateral			
9 Para-aortic Body			
B Coccygeal Glomus			
C Glomus Jugulare			
D Aortic Body			
F Paraganglion Extremity			
G Thyroid Gland Lobe, Left			
H Thyroid Gland Lobe, Right			
K Thyroid Gland			
L Superior Parathyroid Gland, Right			
M Superior Parathyroid Gland, Left			
N Inferior Parathyroid Gland, Right			
P Inferior Parathyroid Gland, Left			
Q Parathyroid Glands, Multiple			
R Parathyroid Gland			
0 Pituitary Gland	0 Open	Z No Device	X Diagnostic
1 Pineal Body	3 Percutaneous		Z No Qualifier
2 Adrenal Gland, Left	4 Percutaneous Endoscopic		
3 Adrenal Gland, Right			
4 Adrenal Glands, Bilateral			
6 Carotid Body, Left			
7 Carotid Body, Right			
8 Carotid Bodies, Bilateral			
9 Para-aortic Body			
B Coccygeal Glomus			
C Glomus Jugulare			
D Aortic Body			
F Paraganglion Extremity			
G Thyroid Gland Lobe, Left			
H Thyroid Gland Lobe, Right			
K Thyroid Gland			
L Superior Parathyroid Gland, Right			
M Superior Parathyroid Gland, Left			
N Inferior Parathyroid Gland, Right			
P Inferior Parathyroid Gland, Left			
Q Parathyroid Glands, Multiple			
R Parathyroid Gland			

Section	0	Medical and Surgical
Body System	G	Endocrine System
Operation	B	Excision: Cutting out or off, without replacement, a portion of a body part

Body Part (4th)	Approach (5th)	Device (6th)	Qualifier (7th)
0 Pituitary Gland 1 Pineal Body 2 Adrenal Gland, Left 3 Adrenal Gland, Right 4 Adrenal Glands, Bilateral 6 Carotid Body, Left 7 Carotid Body, Right 8 Carotid Bodies, Bilateral 9 Para-aortic Body B Coccygeal Glomus C Glomus Jugulare D Aortic Body F Paraganglion Extremity G Thyroid Gland Lobe, Left H Thyroid Gland Lobe, Right J Thyroid Gland Isthmus L Superior Parathyroid Gland, Right M Superior Parathyroid Gland, Left N Inferior Parathyroid Gland, Right P Inferior Parathyroid Gland, Left Q Parathyroid Glands, Multiple R Parathyroid Gland	0 Open 3 Percutaneous 4 Percutaneous Endoscopic	Z No Device	X Diagnostic Z No Qualifier

Section	0	Medical and Surgical
Body System	G	Endocrine System
Operation	C	Extirpation: Taking or cutting out solid matter from a body part

Body Part (4th)	Approach (5th)	Device (6th)	Qualifier (7th)
0 Pituitary Gland 1 Pineal Body 2 Adrenal Gland, Left 3 Adrenal Gland, Right 4 Adrenal Glands, Bilateral 6 Carotid Body, Left 7 Carotid Body, Right 8 Carotid Bodies, Bilateral 9 Para-aortic Body B Coccygeal Glomus C Glomus Jugulare D Aortic Body F Paraganglion Extremity G Thyroid Gland Lobe, Left H Thyroid Gland Lobe, Right K Thyroid Gland L Superior Parathyroid Gland, Right M Superior Parathyroid Gland, Left N Inferior Parathyroid Gland, Right P Inferior Parathyroid Gland, Left Q Parathyroid Glands, Multiple R Parathyroid Gland	0 Open 3 Percutaneous 4 Percutaneous Endoscopic	Z No Device	Z No Qualifier

Section	0	Medical and Surgical
Body System	G	Endocrine System
Operation	H	Insertion: Putting in a nonbiological appliance that monitors, assists, performs, or prevents a physiological function but does not physically take the place of a body part

Body Part (4th)	Approach (5th)	Device (6th)	Qualifier (7th)
S Endocrine Gland	0 Open 3 Percutaneous 4 Percutaneous Endoscopic	1 Radioactive Element 2 Monitoring Device 3 Infusion Device Y Other Device	Z No Qualifier

0GB–0GH

Medical and Surgical, Endocrine System Tables

0GJ–0GN

Medical and Surgical, Endocrine System Tables

Section	0	Medical and Surgical
Body System	G	Endocrine System
Operation	J	Inspection: Visually and/or manually exploring a body part

Body Part (4th)	Approach (5th)	Device (6th)	Qualifier (7th)
0 Pituitary Gland 1 Pineal Body 5 Adrenal Gland K Thyroid Gland R Parathyroid Gland S Endocrine Gland	0 Open 3 Percutaneous 4 Percutaneous Endoscopic	Z No Device	Z No Qualifier

Section	0	Medical and Surgical
Body System	G	Endocrine System
Operation	M	Reattachment: Putting back in or on all or a portion of a separated body part to its normal location or other suitable location

Body Part (4th)	Approach (5th)	Device (6th)	Qualifier (7th)
2 Adrenal Gland, Left 3 Adrenal Gland, Right G Thyroid Gland Lobe, Left H Thyroid Gland Lobe, Right L Superior Parathyroid Gland, Right M Superior Parathyroid Gland, Left N Inferior Parathyroid Gland, Right P Inferior Parathyroid Gland, Left Q Parathyroid Glands, Multiple R Parathyroid Gland	0 Open 4 Percutaneous Endoscopic	Z No Device	Z No Qualifier

Section	0	Medical and Surgical
Body System	G	Endocrine System
Operation	N	Release: Freeing a body part from an abnormal physical constraint by cutting or by the use of force

Body Part (4th)	Approach (5th)	Device (6th)	Qualifier (7th)
0 Pituitary Gland 1 Pineal Body 2 Adrenal Gland, Left 3 Adrenal Gland, Right 4 Adrenal Glands, Bilateral 6 Carotid Body, Left 7 Carotid Body, Right 8 Carotid Bodies, Bilateral 9 Para-aortic Body B Coccygeal Glomus C Glomus Jugulare D Aortic Body F Paraganglion Extremity G Thyroid Gland Lobe, Left H Thyroid Gland Lobe, Right K Thyroid Gland L Superior Parathyroid Gland, Right M Superior Parathyroid Gland, Left N Inferior Parathyroid Gland, Right P Inferior Parathyroid Gland, Left Q Parathyroid Glands, Multiple R Parathyroid Gland	0 Open 3 Percutaneous 4 Percutaneous Endoscopic	Z No Device	Z No Qualifier

Section	0	Medical and Surgical
Body System	G	Endocrine System
Operation	P	Removal: Taking out or off a device from a body part

Body Part (4th)	Approach (5th)	Device (6th)	Qualifier (7th)
0 Pituitary Gland 1 Pineal Body 5 Adrenal Gland K Thyroid Gland R Parathyroid Gland	0 Open 3 Percutaneous 4 Percutaneous Endoscopic X External	0 Drainage Device	Z No Qualifier
S Endocrine Gland	0 Open 3 Percutaneous 4 Percutaneous Endoscopic	0 Drainage Device 2 Monitoring Device 3 Infusion Device Y Other Device	Z No Qualifier
S Endocrine Gland	X External	0 Drainage Device 2 Monitoring Device 3 Infusion Device	Z No Qualifier

Section	0	Medical and Surgical
Body System	G	Endocrine System
Operation	Q	Repair: Restoring, to the extent possible, a body part to its normal anatomic structure and function

Body Part (4th)	Approach (5th)	Device (6th)	Qualifier (7th)
0 Pituitary Gland 1 Pineal Body 2 Adrenal Gland, Left 3 Adrenal Gland, Right 4 Adrenal Glands, Bilateral 6 Carotid Body, Left 7 Carotid Body, Right 8 Carotid Bodies, Bilateral 9 Para-aortic Body B Coccygeal Glomus C Glomus Jugulare D Aortic Body F Paraganglion Extremity G Thyroid Gland Lobe, Left H Thyroid Gland Lobe, Right J Thyroid Gland Isthmus K Thyroid Gland L Superior Parathyroid Gland, Right M Superior Parathyroid Gland, Left N Inferior Parathyroid Gland, Right P Inferior Parathyroid Gland, Left Q Parathyroid Glands, Multiple R Parathyroid Gland	0 Open 3 Percutaneous 4 Percutaneous Endoscopic	Z No Device	Z No Qualifier

Section	0	Medical and Surgical
Body System	G	Endocrine System
Operation	S	Reposition: Moving to its normal location, or other suitable location, all or a portion of a body part

Body Part (4th)	Approach (5th)	Device (6th)	Qualifier (7th)
2 Adrenal Gland, Left 3 Adrenal Gland, Right G Thyroid Gland Lobe, Left H Thyroid Gland Lobe, Right L Superior Parathyroid Gland, Right M Superior Parathyroid Gland, Left N Inferior Parathyroid Gland, Right P Inferior Parathyroid Gland, Left Q Parathyroid Glands, Multiple R Parathyroid Gland	0 Open 4 Percutaneous Endoscopic	Z No Device	Z No Qualifier

0GT–0GW

Medical and Surgical, Endocrine System Tables and AHA Coding Clinic

Section	0	Medical and Surgical
Body System	G	Endocrine System
Operation	T	**Resection:** Cutting out or off, without replacement, all of a body part

Body Part (4ᵗʰ)	Approach (5ᵗʰ)	Device (6ᵗʰ)	Qualifier (7ᵗʰ)
0 Pituitary Gland	0 Open	Z No Device	Z No Qualifier
1 Pineal Body	4 Percutaneous Endoscopic		
2 Adrenal Gland, Left			
3 Adrenal Gland, Right			
4 Adrenal Glands, Bilateral			
6 Carotid Body, Left			
7 Carotid Body, Right			
8 Carotid Bodies, Bilateral			
9 Para-aortic Body			
B Coccygeal Glomus			
C Glomus Jugulare			
D Aortic Body			
F Paraganglion Extremity			
G Thyroid Gland Lobe, Left			
H Thyroid Gland Lobe, Right			
J Thyroid Gland Isthmus			
K Thyroid Gland			
L Superior Parathyroid Gland, Right			
M Superior Parathyroid Gland, Left			
N Inferior Parathyroid Gland, Right			
P Inferior Parathyroid Gland, Left			
Q Parathyroid Glands, Multiple			
R Parathyroid Gland			

Section	0	Medical and Surgical
Body System	G	Endocrine System
Operation	W	**Revision:** Correcting, to the extent possible, a portion of a malfunctioning device or the position of a displaced device

Body Part (4ᵗʰ)	Approach (5ᵗʰ)	Device (6ᵗʰ)	Qualifier (7ᵗʰ)
0 Pituitary Gland	0 Open	0 Drainage Device	Z No Qualifier
1 Pineal Body	3 Percutaneous		
5 Adrenal Gland	4 Percutaneous Endoscopic		
K Thyroid Gland	X External		
R Parathyroid Gland			
S Endocrine Gland	0 Open	0 Drainage Device	Z No Qualifier
	3 Percutaneous	2 Monitoring Device	
	4 Percutaneous Endoscopic	3 Infusion Device	
		Y Other Device	
S Endocrine Gland	X External	0 Drainage Device	Z No Qualifier
		2 Monitoring Device	
		3 Infusion Device	

AHA Coding Clinic

0GB00ZZ Excision of Pituitary Gland, Open Approach—AHA CC: 3Q, 2014, 22-23

0GB90ZZ Excision of Para-aortic Body, Open Approach—AHA CC: 2Q, 2021, 7

0GBG0ZZ Excision of Left Thyroid Gland Lobe, Open Approach—AHA CC: 2Q, 2017, 20

0GBH0ZZ Excision of Right Thyroid Gland Lobe, Open Approach—AHA CC: 2Q, 2017, 20

Skin and Breast

Cross-Section of the Skin Showing Layers and Types of Infections

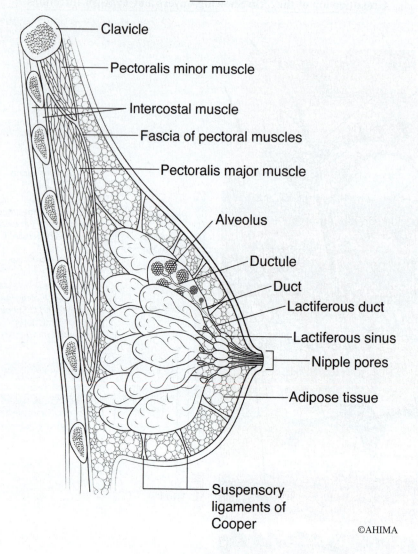

Skin and Breast Tables 0H0–0HX

Section	0	Medical and Surgical
Body System	H	Skin and Breast
Operation	0	Alteration: Modifying the anatomic structure of a body part without affecting the function of the body part

Body Part (4th)	Approach (5th)	Device (6th)	Qualifier (7th)
T Breast, Right U Breast, Left V Breast, Bilateral	0 Open 3 Percutaneous	7 Autologous Tissue Substitute J Synthetic Substitute K Nonautologous Tissue Substitute Z No Device	Z No Qualifier

Section	0	Medical and Surgical
Body System	H	Skin and Breast
Operation	2	Change: Taking out or off a device from a body part and putting back an identical or similar device in or on the same body part without cutting or puncturing the skin or a mucous membrane

Body Part (4th)	Approach (5th)	Device (6th)	Qualifier (7th)
P Skin T Breast, Right U Breast, Left	X External	0 Drainage Device Y Other Device	Z No Qualifier

Section	0	Medical and Surgical
Body System	H	Skin and Breast
Operation	5	Destruction: Physical eradication of all or a portion of a body part by the direct use of energy, force, or a destructive agent

Body Part (4th)	Approach (5th)	Device (6th)	Qualifier (7th)
0 Skin, Scalp 1 Skin, Face 2 Skin, Right Ear 3 Skin, Left Ear 4 Skin, Neck 5 Skin, Chest 6 Skin, Back 7 Skin, Abdomen 8 Skin, Buttock 9 Skin, Perineum A Skin, Inguinal B Skin, Right Upper Arm C Skin, Left Upper Arm D Skin, Right Lower Arm E Skin, Left Lower Arm F Skin, Right Hand G Skin, Left Hand H Skin, Right Upper Leg J Skin, Left Upper Leg K Skin, Right Lower Leg L Skin, Left Lower Leg M Skin, Right Foot N Skin, Left Foot	X External	Z No Device	D Multiple Z No Qualifier
Q Finger Nail R Toe Nail	X External	Z No Device	Z No Device
T Breast, Right U Breast, Left V Breast, Bilateral	0 Open 3 Percutaneous	Z No Device	3 Laser Interstitial Thermal Therapy Z No Qualifier
T Breast, Right U Breast, Left V Breasts, Bilaterial	7 Via Natural or Artificial Opening 8 Via Natural or Artificial Opening Endoscopic	Z No Device	Z No Device

Continued →

Section	0	Medical and Surgical			**0H5 Continued**

Body System   H   Skin and Breast

Operation   5   **Destruction:** Physical eradication of all or a portion of a body part by the direct use of energy, force, or a destructive agent

Body Part (4th)	Approach (5th)	Device (6th)	Qualifier (7th)
W Nipple, Right X Nipple, Left	0 Open 3 Percutaneous 7 Via Natural or Artificial Opening 8 Via Natural or Artificial Opening Endoscopic X External	Z No Device	Z No Qualifier

Section   0   Medical and Surgical

Body System   H   Skin and Breast

Operation   8   **Division:** Cutting into a body part, without draining fluids and/or gases from the body part, in order to separate or transect a body part

Body Part (4th)	Approach (5th)	Device (6th)	Qualifier (7th)
0 Skin, Scalp 1 Skin, Face 2 Skin, Right Ear 3 Skin, Left Ear 4 Skin, Neck 5 Skin, Chest 6 Skin, Back 7 Skin, Abdomen 8 Skin, Buttock 9 Skin, Perineum A Skin, Inguinal B Skin, Right Upper Arm C Skin, Left Upper Arm D Skin, Right Lower Arm E Skin, Left Lower Arm F Skin, Right Hand G Skin, Left Hand H Skin, Right Upper Leg J Skin, Left Upper Leg K Skin, Right Lower Leg L Skin, Left Lower Leg M Skin, Right Foot N Skin, Left Foot	X External	Z No Device	Z No Qualifier

Section	0	Medical and Surgical
Body System	H	Skin and Breast
Operation	9	Drainage: Taking or letting out fluids and/or gases from a body part

Body Part (4th)	Approach (5th)	Device (6th)	Qualifier (7th)
0 Skin, Scalp 1 Skin, Face 2 Skin, Right Ear 3 Skin, Left Ear 4 Skin, Neck 5 Skin, Chest 6 Skin, Back 7 Skin, Abdomen 8 Skin, Buttock 9 Skin, Perineum A Skin, Inguinal B Skin, Right Upper Arm C Skin, Left Upper Arm D Skin, Right Lower Arm E Skin, Left Lower Arm F Skin, Right Hand G Skin, Left Hand H Skin, Right Upper Leg J Skin, Left Upper Leg K Skin, Right Lower Leg L Skin, Left Lower Leg M Skin, Right Foot N Skin, Left Foot Q Finger Nail R Toe Nail	X External	0 Drainage Device	Z No Qualifier
0 Skin, Scalp 1 Skin, Face 2 Skin, Right Ear 3 Skin, Left Ear 4 Skin, Neck 5 Skin, Chest 6 Skin, Back 7 Skin, Abdomen 8 Skin, Buttock 9 Skin, Perineum A Skin, Inguinal B Skin, Right Upper Arm C Skin, Left Upper Arm D Skin, Right Lower Arm E Skin, Left Lower Arm F Skin, Right Hand G Skin, Left Hand H Skin, Right Upper Leg J Skin, Left Upper Leg K Skin, Right Lower Leg L Skin, Left Lower Leg M Skin, Right Foot N Skin, Left Foot Q Finger Nail R Toe Nail	X External	Z No Device	X Diagnostic Z No Qualifier
T Breast, Right U Breast, Left V Breast, Bilateral	0 Open 3 Percutaneous 7 Via Natural or Artificial Opening 8 Via Natural or Artificial Opening Endoscopic	0 Drainage Device	Z No Qualifier
T Breast, Right U Breast, Left V Breast, Bilateral	0 Open 3 Percutaneous 7 Via Natural or Artificial Opening 8 Via Natural or Artificial Opening Endoscopic	Z No Device	X Diagnostic Z No Qualifier

Continued →

0H9–0HB

Medical and Surgical, Skin and Breast Tables

Section	0	Medical and Surgical
Body System	H	Skin and Breast
Operation	9	**Drainage:** Taking or letting out fluids and/or gases from a body part

0H9 Continued

Body Part (4th)	Approach (5th)	Device (6th)	Qualifier (7th)
W Nipple, Right X Nipple, Left	0 Open 3 Percutaneous 7 Via Natural or Artificial Opening 8 Via Natural or Artificial Opening Endoscopic X External	0 Drainage Device	Z No Qualifier
W Nipple, Right X Nipple, Left	0 Open 3 Percutaneous 7 Via Natural or Artificial Opening 8 Via Natural or Artificial Opening Endoscopic X External	Z No Device	X Diagnostic Z No Qualifier

Section	0	Medical and Surgical
Body System	H	Skin and Breast
Operation	B	**Excision:** Cutting out or off, without replacement, a portion of a body part

Body Part (4th)	Approach (5th)	Device (6th)	Qualifier (7th)
0 Skin, Scalp 1 Skin, Face 2 Skin, Right Ear 3 Skin, Left Ear 4 Skin, Neck 5 Skin, Chest 6 Skin, Back 7 Skin, Abdomen 8 Skin, Buttock 9 Skin, Perineum A Skin, Inguinal B Skin, Right Upper Arm C Skin, Left Upper Arm D Skin, Right Lower Arm E Skin, Left Lower Arm F Skin, Right Hand G Skin, Left Hand H Skin, Right Upper Leg J Skin, Left Upper Leg K Skin, Right Lower Leg L Skin, Left Lower Leg M Skin, Right Foot N Skin, Left Foot Q Finger Nail R Toe Nail	X External	Z No Device	X Diagnostic Z No Qualifier
T Breast, Right U Breast, Left V Breast, Bilateral Y Supernumerary Breast	0 Open 3 Percutaneous 7 Via Natural or Artificial Opening 8 Via Natural or Artificial Opening Endoscopic	Z No Device	X Diagnostic Z No Qualifier
W Nipple, Right X Nipple, Left	0 Open 3 Percutaneous 7 Via Natural or Artificial Opening 8 Via Natural or Artificial Opening Endoscopic X External	Z No Device	X Diagnostic Z No Qualifier

Section	0	Medical and Surgical
Body System	H	Skin and Breast
Operation	C	Extirpation: Taking or cutting out solid matter from a body part

Body Part (4th)	Approach (5th)	Device (6th)	Qualifier (7th)
0 Skin, Scalp 1 Skin, Face 2 Skin, Right Ear 3 Skin, Left Ear 4 Skin, Neck 5 Skin, Chest 6 Skin, Back 7 Skin, Abdomen 8 Skin, Buttock 9 Skin, Perineum A Skin, Inguinal B Skin, Right Upper Arm C Skin, Left Upper Arm D Skin, Right Lower Arm E Skin, Left Lower Arm F Skin, Right Hand G Skin, Left Hand H Skin, Right Upper Leg J Skin, Left Upper Leg K Skin, Right Lower Leg L Skin, Left Lower Leg M Skin, Right Foot N Skin, Left Foot Q Finger Nail R Toe Nail	X External	Z No Device	Z No Qualifier
T Breast, Right U Breast, Left V Breast, Bilateral	0 Open 3 Percutaneous 7 Via Natural or Artificial Opening 8 Via Natural or Artificial Opening Endoscopic	Z No Device	Z No Qualifier
W Nipple, Right X Nipple, Left	0 Open 3 Percutaneous 7 Via Natural or Artificial Opening 8 Via Natural or Artificial Opening Endoscopic X External	Z No Device	Z No Qualifier

Section	0	Medical and Surgical
Body System	H	Skin and Breast
Operation	D	**Extraction:** Pulling or stripping out or off all or a portion of a body part by the use of force

Body Part (4th)	Approach (5th)	Device (6th)	Qualifier (7th)
0 Skin, Scalp 1 Skin, Face 2 Skin, Right Ear 3 Skin, Left Ear 4 Skin, Neck 5 Skin, Chest 6 Skin, Back 7 Skin, Abdomen 8 Skin, Buttock 9 Skin, Perineum A Skin, Inguinal B Skin, Right Upper Arm C Skin, Left Upper Arm D Skin, Right Lower Arm E Skin, Left Lower Arm F Skin, Right Hand G Skin, Left Hand H Skin, Right Upper Leg J Skin, Left Upper Leg K Skin, Right Lower Leg L Skin, Left Lower Leg M Skin, Right Foot N Skin, Left Foot Q Finger Nail R Toe Nail S Hair	X External	Z No Device	Z No Qualifier
T Breast, Right U Breast, Left V Breast, Bilateral Y Supernumerary Breast	0 Open	Z No Device	Z No Qualifier

Section	0	Medical and Surgical
Body System	H	Skin and Breast
Operation	H	**Insertion:** Putting in a nonbiological appliance that monitors, assists, performs, or prevents a physiological function but does not physically take the place of a body part

Body Part (4th)	Approach (5th)	Device (6th)	Qualifier (7th)
P Skin	X External	Y Other Device	Z No Qualifier
T Breast, Right U Breast, Left	0 Open 3 Percutaneous 7 Via Natural or Artificial Opening 8 Via Natural or Artificial Opening Endoscopic	1 Radioactive Element N Tissue Expander Y Other Device	Z No Qualifier
V Breast, Bilateral	0 Open 3 Percutaneous 7 Via Natural or Artificial Opening 8 Via Natural or Artificial Opening Endoscopic	1 Radioactive Element N Tissue Expander	Z No Qualifier
W Nipple, Right X Nipple, Left	0 Open 3 Percutaneous 7 Via Natural or Artificial Opening 8 Via Natural or Artificial Opening Endoscopic	1 Radioactive Element N Tissue Expander	Z No Qualifier
W Nipple, Right X Nipple, Left	X External	1 Radioactive Element	Z No Qualifier

Section	0	Medical and Surgical
Body System	H	Skin and Breast
Operation	J	Inspection: Visually and/or manually exploring a body part

Body Part (4th)	Approach (5th)	Device (6th)	Qualifier (7th)
P Skin Q Finger Nail R Toe Nail	X External	Z No Device	Z No Qualifier
T Breast, Right U Breast, Left	0 Open 3 Percutaneous 7 Via Natural or Artificial Opening 8 Via Natural or Artificial Opening Endoscopic	Z No Device	Z No Qualifier

Section	0	Medical and Surgical
Body System	H	Skin and Breast
Operation	M	Reattachment: Putting back in or on all or a portion of a separated body part to its normal location or other suitable location

Body Part (4th)	Approach (5th)	Device (6th)	Qualifier (7th)
0 Skin, Scalp 1 Skin, Face 2 Skin, Right Ear 3 Skin, Left Ear 4 Skin, Neck 5 Skin, Chest 6 Skin, Back 7 Skin, Abdomen 8 Skin, Buttock 9 Skin, Perineum A Skin, Inguinal B Skin, Right Upper Arm C Skin, Left Upper Arm D Skin, Right Lower Arm E Skin, Left Lower Arm F Skin, Right Hand G Skin, Left Hand H Skin, Right Upper Leg J Skin, Left Upper Leg K Skin, Right Lower Leg L Skin, Left Lower Leg M Skin, Right Foot N Skin, Left Foot T Breast, Right U Breast, Left V Breast, Bilateral W Nipple, Right X Nipple, Left	X External	Z No Device	Z No Qualifier

	Section	0	Medical and Surgical
	Body System	H	Skin and Breast
	Operation	N	Release: Freeing a body part from an abnormal physical constraint by cutting or by the use of force

Body Part (4th)	Approach (5th)	Device (6th)	Qualifier (7th)
0 Skin, Scalp 1 Skin, Face 2 Skin, Right Ear 3 Skin, Left Ear 4 Skin, Neck 5 Skin, Chest 6 Skin, Back 7 Skin, Abdomen 8 Skin, Buttock 9 Skin, Perineum A Skin, Inguinal B Skin, Right Upper Arm C Skin, Left Upper Arm D Skin, Right Lower Arm E Skin, Left Lower Arm F Skin, Right Hand G Skin, Left Hand H Skin, Right Upper Leg J Skin, Left Upper Leg K Skin, Right Lower Leg L Skin, Left Lower Leg M Skin, Right Foot N Skin, Left Foot Q Finger Nail R Toe Nail	X External	Z No Device	Z No Qualifier
T Breast, Right U Breast, Left V Breast, Bilateral	0 Open 3 Percutaneous 7 Via Natural or Artificial Opening 8 Via Natural or Artificial Opening Endoscopic	Z No Device	Z No Qualifier
W Nipple, Right X Nipple, Left	0 Open 3 Percutaneous 7 Via Natural or Artificial Opening 8 Via Natural or Artificial Opening Endoscopic X External	Z No Device	Z No Qualifier

0HP–0HQ

Section	0	Medical and Surgical
Body System	H	Skin and Breast
Operation	P	Removal: Taking out or off a device from a body part

Body Part (4th)	Approach (5th)	Device (6th)	Qualifier (7th)
P Skin	X External	0 Drainage Device 7 Autologous Tissue Substitute J Synthetic Substitute K Nonautologous Tissue Substitute Y Other Device	Z No Qualifier
Q Finger Nail R Toe Nail	X External	0 Drainage Device 7 Autologous Tissue Substitute J Synthetic Substitute K Nonautologous Tissue Substitute	Z No Qualifier
S Hair	X External	7 Autologous Tissue Substitute J Synthetic Substitute K Nonautologous Tissue Substitute	Z No Qualifier
T Breast, Right U Breast, Left	0 Open 3 Percutaneous 7 Via Natural or Artificial Opening 8 Via Natural or Artificial Opening Endoscopic	0 Drainage Device 1 Radioactive Element 7 Autologous Tissue Substitute J Synthetic Substitute K Nonautologous Tissue Substitute N Tissue Expander Y Other Device	Z No Qualifier

Section	0	Medical and Surgical
Body System	H	Skin and Breast
Operation	Q	Repair: Restoring, to the extent possible, a body part to its normal anatomic structure and function

Body Part (4th)	Approach (5th)	Device (6th)	Qualifier (7th)
0 Skin, Scalp 1 Skin, Face 2 Skin, Right Ear 3 Skin, Left Ear 4 Skin, Neck 5 Skin, Chest 6 Skin, Back 7 Skin, Abdomen 8 Skin, Buttock 9 Skin, Perineum A Skin, Inguinal B Skin, Right Upper Arm C Skin, Left Upper Arm D Skin, Right Lower Arm E Skin, Left Lower Arm F Skin, Right Hand G Skin, Left Hand H Skin, Right Upper Leg J Skin, Left Upper Leg K Skin, Right Lower Leg L Skin, Left Lower Leg M Skin, Right Foot N Skin, Left Foot Q Finger Nail R Toe Nail	X External	Z No Device	Z No Qualifier
T Breast, Right U Breast, Left V Breast, Bilateral Y Supernumerary Breast	0 Open 3 Percutaneous 7 Via Natural or Artificial Opening 8 Via Natural or Artificial Opening Endoscopic	Z No Device	Z No Qualifier

Continued ➞

Medical and Surgical, Skin and Breast Tables

325

0HQ Continued

Section	0	Medical and Surgical
Body System	H	Skin and Breast
Operation	Q	Repair: Restoring, to the extent possible, a body part to its normal anatomic structure and function

Body Part (4th)	Approach (5th)	Device (6th)	Qualifier (7th)
W Nipple, Right X Nipple, Left	0 Open 3 Percutaneous 7 Via Natural or Artificial Opening 8 Via Natural or Artificial Opening Endoscopic X External	Z No Device	Z No Qualifier

Section	0	Medical and Surgical
Body System	H	Skin and Breast
Operation	R	Replacement: Putting in or on biological or synthetic material that physically takes the place and/or function of all or a portion of a body part

Body Part (4th)	Approach (5th)	Device (6th)	Qualifier (7th)
0 Skin, Scalp 1 Skin, Face 2 Skin, Right Ear 3 Skin, Left Ear 4 Skin, Neck 5 Skin, Chest 6 Skin, Back 7 Skin, Abdomen 8 Skin, Buttock 9 Skin, Perineum A Skin, Inguinal B Skin, Right Upper Arm C Skin, Left Upper Arm D Skin, Right Lower Arm E Skin, Left Lower Arm F Skin, Right Hand G Skin, Left Hand H Skin, Right Upper Leg J Skin, Left Upper Leg K Skin, Right Lower Leg L Skin, Left Lower Leg M Skin, Right Foot N Skin, Left Foot	X External	7 Autologous Tissue Substitute	2 Cell Suspension Technique 3 Full Thickness 4 Partial Thickness
0 Skin, Scalp 1 Skin, Face 2 Skin, Right Ear 3 Skin, Left Ear 4 Skin, Neck 5 Skin, Chest 6 Skin, Back 7 Skin, Abdomen 8 Skin, Buttock 9 Skin, Perineum A Skin, Inguinal B Skin, Right Upper Arm C Skin, Left Upper Arm D Skin, Right Lower Arm E Skin, Left Lower Arm F Skin, Right Hand G Skin, Left Hand H Skin, Right Upper Leg J Skin, Left Upper Leg K Skin, Right Lower Leg L Skin, Left Lower Leg M Skin, Right Foot N Skin, Left Foot	X External	J Synthetic Substitute	3 Full Thickness 4 Partial Thickness Z No Qualifier

Continued →

Section	0	Medical and Surgical
Body System	H	Skin and Breast
Operation	R	**Replacement:** Putting in or on biological or synthetic material that physically takes the place and/or function of all or a portion of a body part

0HR Continued

Body Part (4th)	Approach (5th)	Device (6th)	Qualifier (7th)
0 Skin, Scalp 1 Skin, Face 2 Skin, Right Ear 3 Skin, Left Ear 4 Skin, Neck 5 Skin, Chest 6 Skin, Back 7 Skin, Abdomen 8 Skin, Buttock 9 Skin, Perineum A Skin, Inguinal B Skin, Right Upper Arm C Skin, Left Upper Arm D Skin, Right Lower Arm E Skin, Left Lower Arm F Skin, Right Hand G Skin, Left Hand H Skin, Right Upper Leg J Skin, Left Upper Leg K Skin, Right Lower Leg L Skin, Left Lower Leg M Skin, Right Foot N Skin, Left Foot	X External	K Nonautologous Tissue Substitute	3 Full Thickness 4 Partial Thickness
Q Finger Nail R Toe Nail S Hair	X External	7 Autologous Tissue Substitute J Synthetic Substitute K Nonautologous Tissue Substitute	Z No Qualifier
T Breast, Right U Breast, Left V Breast, Bilateral	0 Open	7 Autologous Tissue Substitute	5 Latissimus Dorsi Myocutaneous Flap 6 Transverse Rectus Abdominis Myocutaneous Flap 7 Deep Inferior Epigastric Artery Perforator Flap 8 Superficial Inferior Epigastric Artery Flap 9 Gluteal Artery Perforator Flap Z No Qualifier
T Breast, Right U Breast, Left V Breast, Bilateral	0 Open	J Synthetic Substitute K Nonautologous Tissue Substitute	Z No Qualifier
T Breast, Right U Breast, Left V Breast, Bilateral	3 Percutaneous	7 Autologous Tissue Substitute J Synthetic Substitute K Nonautologous Tissue Substitute	Z No Qualifier
W Nipple, Right X Nipple, Left	0 Open 3 Percutaneous X External	7 Autologous Tissue Substitute J Synthetic Substitute K Nonautologous Tissue Substitute	Z No Qualifier

0HS–0HU

Medical and Surgical, Skin and Breast Tables

Section	0	Medical and Surgical
Body System	H	Skin and Breast
Operation	S	Reposition: Moving to its normal location, or other suitable location, all or a portion of a body part

Body Part (4th)	Approach (5th)	Device (6th)	Qualifier (7th)
S Hair W Nipple, Right X Nipple, Left	X External	Z No Device	Z No Qualifier
T Breast, Right U Breast, Left V Breast, Bilateral	0 Open	Z No Device	Z No Qualifier

Section	0	Medical and Surgical
Body System	H	Skin and Breast
Operation	T	Resection: Cutting out or off, without replacement, all of a body part

Body Part (4th)	Approach (5th)	Device (6th)	Qualifier (7th)
Q Finger Nail R Toe Nail W Nipple, Right X Nipple, Left	X External	Z No Device	Z No Qualifier
T Breast, Right U Breast, Left V Breast, Bilateral Y Supernumerary Breast	0 Open	Z No Device	Z No Qualifier

Section	0	Medical and Surgical
Body System	H	Skin and Breast
Operation	U	Supplement: Putting in or on biological or synthetic material that physically reinforces and/or augments the function of a portion of a body part

Body Part (4th)	Approach (5th)	Device (6th)	Qualifier (7th)
T Breast, Right U Breast, Left V Breast, Bilateral	0 Open 3 Percutaneous 7 Via Natural or Artificial Opening 8 Via Natural or Artificial Opening Endoscopic	7 Autologous Tissue Substitute J Synthetic Substitute K Nonautologous Tissue Substitute	Z No Qualifier
W Nipple, Right X Nipple, Left	0 Open 3 Percutaneous 7 Via Natural or Artificial Opening 8 Via Natural or Artificial Opening Endoscopic X External	7 Autologous Tissue Substitute J Synthetic Substitute K Nonautologous Tissue Substitute	Z No Qualifier

Section	0	Medical and Surgical
Body System	H	Skin and Breast
Operation	W	Revision: Correcting, to the extent possible, a portion of a malfunctioning device or the position of a displaced device

Body Part (4th)	Approach (5th)	Device (6th)	Qualifier (7th)
P Skin	X External	0 Drainage Device 7 Autologous Tissue Substitute J Synthetic Substitute K Nonautologous Tissue Substitute Y Other Device	Z No Qualifier
Q Finger Nail R Toe Nail	X External	0 Drainage Device 7 Autologous Tissue Substitute J Synthetic Substitute K Nonautologous Tissue Substitute	Z No Qualifier
S Hair	X External	7 Autologous Tissue Substitute J Synthetic Substitute K Nonautologous Tissue Substitute	Z No Qualifier
T Breast, Right U Breast, Left	0 Open 3 Percutaneous 7 Via Natural or Artificial Opening 8 Via Natural or Artificial Opening Endoscopic	0 Drainage Device 7 Autologous Tissue Substitute J Synthetic Substitute K Nonautologous Tissue Substitute N Tissue Expander Y Other Device	Z No Qualifier

Section	0	Medical and Surgical
Body System	H	Skin and Breast
Operation	X	Transfer: Moving, without taking out, all or a portion of a body part to another location to take over the function of all or a portion of a body part

Body Part (4th)	Approach (5th)	Device (6th)	Qualifier (7th)
0 Skin, Scalp 1 Skin, Face 2 Skin, Right Ear 3 Skin, Left Ear 4 Skin, Neck 5 Skin, Chest 6 Skin, Back 7 Skin, Abdomen 8 Skin, Buttock 9 Skin, Perineum A Skin, Inguinal B Skin, Right Upper Arm C Skin, Left Upper Arm D Skin, Right Lower Arm E Skin, Left Lower Arm F Skin, Right Hand G Skin, Left Hand H Skin, Right Upper Leg J Skin, Left Upper Leg K Skin, Right Lower Leg L Skin, Left Lower Leg M Skin, Right Foot N Skin, Left Foot	X External	Z No Device	Z No Qualifier

AHA Coding Clinic

0H0T0ZZ Alteration of Right Breast, Open Approach—AHA CC: 1Q, 2022, 14-16

0HB8XZZ Excision of Buttock Skin, External Approach—AHA CC: 3Q, 2015, 3

0HBHXZZ Excision of Right Upper Leg Skin, External Approach—AHA CC: 1Q, 2020, 31-32

0HBJXZZ Excision of Left Upper Leg Skin, External Approach—AHA CC: 3Q, 2016, 29-30

0HBT0ZZ Excision of Right Breast, Open Approach—AHA CC: 1Q, 2018, 14-15

0HBU0ZZ Excision of Left Breast, Open Approach—AHA CC: 1Q, 2022, 14-15

0HD6XZZ Extraction of Back Skin, External Approach—AHA CC: 3Q, 2015, 5-6

0HDHXZZ Extraction of Right Upper Leg Skin, External Approach—AHA CC: 3Q, 2015, 5

0HHT0NZ Insertion of Tissue Expander into Right Breast, Open Approach—AHA CC: 4Q, 2017, 67

0HHU0YZ Insertion of Other Device into Left Breast, Open Approach—AHA CC: 4Q, 2013, 107

0HHV0NZ Insertion of Tissue Expander into Bilateral Breast, Open Approach—AHA CC: 2Q, 2014, 12

0HPT07Z Removal of Autologous Tissue Substitute from Right Breast, Open Approach—AHA CC: 2Q, 2016, 27

0HPT0NZ Removal of Tissue Expander from Right Breast, Open Approach—AHA CC: 3Q, 2018, 13-14; 3Q, 2022, 20-21

0HPU07Z Removal of Autologous Tissue Substitute from Left Breast, Open Approach—AHA CC: 2Q, 2016, 27

0HPU0NZ Removal of Tissue Expander from Left Breast, Open Approach—AHA CC: 3Q, 2022, 20-21

0HQ9XZZ Repair Perineum Skin, External Approach—AHA CC: 1Q, 2016, 7

0HQEXZZ Repair Left Lower Arm Skin, External Approach—AHA CC: 4Q, 2014, 31-32

0HRMXK3 Replacement of Right Foot Skin with Nonautologous Tissue Substitute, Full Thickness, External Approach—AHA CC: 1Q, 2017, 35-36

0HRNXK3 Replacement of Left Foot Skin with Nonautologous Tissue Substitute, Full Thickness, External Approach—AHA CC: 3Q, 2014, 14-15

0HRU07Z Replacement of Left Breast with Autologous Tissue Substitute, Open Approach—AHA CC: 1Q, 2020, 27-28

0HRV077 Replacement of Bilateral Breast using Deep Inferior Epigastric Artery Perforator Flap, Open Approach—AHA CC: 3Q, 2018, 13-14

0HRX07Z Replacement of Left Nipple with Autologous Tissue Substitute, Open Approach—AHA CC: 1Q, 2022, 15-16

0HTT0ZZ Resection of Right Breast, Open Approach—AHA CC: 4Q, 2014, 34

0HTU0ZZ Resection of Left Breast, Open Approach—AHA CC: 3Q, 2018, 13-14

0HTV0ZZ Resection of Bilateral Breast, Open Approach—AHA CC: 2Q, 2021, 16-17

0HX5XZZ Transfer Chest Skin, External Approach - AHA CC: 2Q, 2023, 30-31

0HX9XZZ Transfer Perineum Skin, External Approach—AHA CC: 3Q, 2022, 13-14; 2Q, 2023, 23-24

Subcutaneous Tissue and Fascia

Subcutaneous Tissue and Fascia Tables 0J0–0JX

Section	0	Medical and Surgical
Body System	J	Subcutaneous Tissue and Fascia
Operation	0	**Alteration:** Modifying the anatomic structure of a body part without affecting the function of the body part

Body Part (4th)	Approach (5th)	Device (6th)	Qualifier (7th)
1 Subcutaneous Tissue and Fascia, Face 4 Subcutaneous Tissue and Fascia, Right Neck 5 Subcutaneous Tissue and Fascia, Left Neck 6 Subcutaneous Tissue and Fascia, Chest 7 Subcutaneous Tissue and Fascia, Back 8 Subcutaneous Tissue and Fascia, Abdomen 9 Subcutaneous Tissue and Fascia, Buttock D Subcutaneous Tissue and Fascia, Right Upper Arm F Subcutaneous Tissue and Fascia, Left Upper Arm G Subcutaneous Tissue and Fascia, Right Lower Arm H Subcutaneous Tissue and Fascia, Left Lower Arm L Subcutaneous Tissue and Fascia, Right Upper Leg M Subcutaneous Tissue and Fascia, Left Upper Leg N Subcutaneous Tissue and Fascia, Right Lower Leg P Subcutaneous Tissue and Fascia, Left Lower Leg	0 Open 3 Percutaneous	Z No Device	Z No Qualifier

Section	0	Medical and Surgical
Body System	J	Subcutaneous Tissue and Fascia
Operation	2	**Change:** Taking out or off a device from a body part and putting back an identical or similar device in or on the same body part without cutting or puncturing the skin or a mucous membrane

Body Part (4th)	Approach (5th)	Device (6th)	Qualifier (7th)
S Subcutaneous Tissue and Fascia, Head and Neck T Subcutaneous Tissue and Fascia, Trunk V Subcutaneous Tissue and Fascia, Upper Extremity W Subcutaneous Tissue and Fascia, Lower Extremity	X External	0 Drainage Device Y Other Device	Z No Qualifier

Section	0	Medical and Surgical
Body System	J	Subcutaneous Tissue and Fascia
Operation	5	**Destruction:** Physical eradication of all or a portion of a body part by the direct use of energy, force, or a destructive agent

Body Part (4th)	Approach (5th)	Device (6th)	Qualifier (7th)
0 Subcutaneous Tissue and Fascia, Scalp 1 Subcutaneous Tissue and Fascia, Face 4 Subcutaneous Tissue and Fascia, Right Neck 5 Subcutaneous Tissue and Fascia, Left Neck 6 Subcutaneous Tissue and Fascia, Chest 7 Subcutaneous Tissue and Fascia, Back 8 Subcutaneous Tissue and Fascia, Abdomen 9 Subcutaneous Tissue and Fascia, Buttock B Subcutaneous Tissue and Fascia, Perineum C Subcutaneous Tissue and Fascia, Pelvic Region D Subcutaneous Tissue and Fascia, Right Upper Arm F Subcutaneous Tissue and Fascia, Left Upper Arm G Subcutaneous Tissue and Fascia, Right Lower Arm H Subcutaneous Tissue and Fascia, Left Lower Arm J Subcutaneous Tissue and Fascia, Right Hand K Subcutaneous Tissue and Fascia, Left Hand L Subcutaneous Tissue and Fascia, Right Upper Leg M Subcutaneous Tissue and Fascia, Left Upper Leg N Subcutaneous Tissue and Fascia, Right Lower Leg P Subcutaneous Tissue and Fascia, Left Lower Leg Q Subcutaneous Tissue and Fascia, Right Foot R Subcutaneous Tissue and Fascia, Left Foot	0 Open 3 Percutaneous	Z No Device	Z No Qualifier

Section	0	Medical and Surgical
Body System	J	Subcutaneous Tissue and Fascia
Operation	8	**Division:** Cutting into a body part, without draining fluids and/or gases from the body part, in order to separate or transect a body part

Body Part (4th)	Approach (5th)	Device (6th)	Qualifier (7th)
0 Subcutaneous Tissue and Fascia, Scalp 1 Subcutaneous Tissue and Fascia, Face 4 Subcutaneous Tissue and Fascia, Right Neck 5 Subcutaneous Tissue and Fascia, Left Neck 6 Subcutaneous Tissue and Fascia, Chest 7 Subcutaneous Tissue and Fascia, Back 8 Subcutaneous Tissue and Fascia, Abdomen 9 Subcutaneous Tissue and Fascia, Buttock B Subcutaneous Tissue and Fascia, Perineum C Subcutaneous Tissue and Fascia, Pelvic Region D Subcutaneous Tissue and Fascia, Right Upper Arm F Subcutaneous Tissue and Fascia, Left Upper Arm G Subcutaneous Tissue and Fascia, Right Lower Arm H Subcutaneous Tissue and Fascia, Left Lower Arm J Subcutaneous Tissue and Fascia, Right Hand K Subcutaneous Tissue and Fascia, Left Hand L Subcutaneous Tissue and Fascia, Right Upper Leg M Subcutaneous Tissue and Fascia, Left Upper Leg N Subcutaneous Tissue and Fascia, Right Lower Leg P Subcutaneous Tissue and Fascia, Left Lower Leg Q Subcutaneous Tissue and Fascia, Right Foot R Subcutaneous Tissue and Fascia, Left Foot S Subcutaneous Tissue and Fascia, Head and Neck T Subcutaneous Tissue and Fascia, Trunk V Subcutaneous Tissue and Fascia, Upper Extremity W Subcutaneous Tissue and Fascia, Lower Extremity	0 Open 3 Percutaneous	Z No Device	Z No Qualifier

Section	0	Medical and Surgical
Body System	J	Subcutaneous Tissue and Fascia
Operation	9	**Drainage:** Taking or letting out fluids and/or gases from a body part

Body Part (4th)	Approach (5th)	Device (6th)	Qualifier (7th)
0 Subcutaneous Tissue and Fascia, Scalp 1 Subcutaneous Tissue and Fascia, Face 4 Subcutaneous Tissue and Fascia, Right Neck 5 Subcutaneous Tissue and Fascia, Left Neck 6 Subcutaneous Tissue and Fascia, Chest 7 Subcutaneous Tissue and Fascia, Back 8 Subcutaneous Tissue and Fascia, Abdomen 9 Subcutaneous Tissue and Fascia, Buttock B Subcutaneous Tissue and Fascia, Perineum C Subcutaneous Tissue and Fascia, Pelvic Region D Subcutaneous Tissue and Fascia, Right Upper Arm F Subcutaneous Tissue and Fascia, Left Upper Arm G Subcutaneous Tissue and Fascia, Right Lower Arm H Subcutaneous Tissue and Fascia, Left Lower Arm J Subcutaneous Tissue and Fascia, Right Hand K Subcutaneous Tissue and Fascia, Left Hand L Subcutaneous Tissue and Fascia, Right Upper Leg M Subcutaneous Tissue and Fascia, Left Upper Leg N Subcutaneous Tissue and Fascia, Right Lower Leg P Subcutaneous Tissue and Fascia, Left Lower Leg Q Subcutaneous Tissue and Fascia, Right Foot R Subcutaneous Tissue and Fascia, Left Foot	0 Open 3 Percutaneous	0 Drainage Device	Z No Qualifier

Continued →

0J9–0JB

Medical and Surgical, Subcutaneous Tissue and Fascia Tables

0J9 Continued

Section	0	Medical and Surgical
Body System	J	Subcutaneous Tissue and Fascia
Operation	9	**Drainage:** Taking or letting out fluids and/or gases from a body part

Body Part (4th)	Approach (5th)	Device (6th)	Qualifier (7th)
0 Subcutaneous Tissue and Fascia, Scalp 1 Subcutaneous Tissue and Fascia, Face 4 Subcutaneous Tissue and Fascia, Right Neck 5 Subcutaneous Tissue and Fascia, Left Neck 6 Subcutaneous Tissue and Fascia, Chest 7 Subcutaneous Tissue and Fascia, Back 8 Subcutaneous Tissue and Fascia, Abdomen 9 Subcutaneous Tissue and Fascia, Buttock B Subcutaneous Tissue and Fascia, Perineum C Subcutaneous Tissue and Fascia, Pelvic Region D Subcutaneous Tissue and Fascia, Right Upper Arm F Subcutaneous Tissue and Fascia, Left Upper Arm G Subcutaneous Tissue and Fascia, Right Lower Arm H Subcutaneous Tissue and Fascia, Left Lower Arm J Subcutaneous Tissue and Fascia, Right Hand K Subcutaneous Tissue and Fascia, Left Hand L Subcutaneous Tissue and Fascia, Right Upper Leg M Subcutaneous Tissue and Fascia, Left Upper Leg N Subcutaneous Tissue and Fascia, Right Lower Leg P Subcutaneous Tissue and Fascia, Left Lower Leg Q Subcutaneous Tissue and Fascia, Right Foot R Subcutaneous Tissue and Fascia, Left Foot	0 Open 3 Percutaneous	Z No Device	X Diagnostic Z No Qualifier

Section	0	Medical and Surgical
Body System	J	Subcutaneous Tissue and Fascia
Operation	B	**Excision:** Cutting out or off, without replacement, a portion of a body part

Body Part (4th)	Approach (5th)	Device (6th)	Qualifier (7th)
0 Subcutaneous Tissue and Fascia, Scalp 1 Subcutaneous Tissue and Fascia, Face 4 Subcutaneous Tissue and Fascia, Right Neck 5 Subcutaneous Tissue and Fascia, Left Neck 6 Subcutaneous Tissue and Fascia, Chest 7 Subcutaneous Tissue and Fascia, Back 8 Subcutaneous Tissue and Fascia, Abdomen 9 Subcutaneous Tissue and Fascia, Buttock B Subcutaneous Tissue and Fascia, Perineum C Subcutaneous Tissue and Fascia, Pelvic Region D Subcutaneous Tissue and Fascia, Right Upper Arm F Subcutaneous Tissue and Fascia, Left Upper Arm G Subcutaneous Tissue and Fascia, Right Lower Arm H Subcutaneous Tissue and Fascia, Left Lower Arm J Subcutaneous Tissue and Fascia, Right Hand K Subcutaneous Tissue and Fascia, Left Hand L Subcutaneous Tissue and Fascia, Right Upper Leg M Subcutaneous Tissue and Fascia, Left Upper Leg N Subcutaneous Tissue and Fascia, Right Lower Leg P Subcutaneous Tissue and Fascia, Left Lower Leg Q Subcutaneous Tissue and Fascia, Right Foot R Subcutaneous Tissue and Fascia, Left Foot	0 Open 3 Percutaneous	Z No Device	X Diagnostic Z No Qualifier

Section	0	Medical and Surgical
Body System	J	Subcutaneous Tissue and Fascia
Operation	C	**Extirpation:** Taking or cutting out solid matter from a body part

Body Part (4th)	Approach (5th)	Device (6th)	Qualifier (7th)
0 Subcutaneous Tissue and Fascia, Scalp 1 Subcutaneous Tissue and Fascia, Face 4 Subcutaneous Tissue and Fascia, Right Neck 5 Subcutaneous Tissue and Fascia, Left Neck 6 Subcutaneous Tissue and Fascia, Chest 7 Subcutaneous Tissue and Fascia, Back 8 Subcutaneous Tissue and Fascia, Abdomen 9 Subcutaneous Tissue and Fascia, Buttock B Subcutaneous Tissue and Fascia, Perineum C Subcutaneous Tissue and Fascia, Pelvic Region D Subcutaneous Tissue and Fascia, Right Upper Arm F Subcutaneous Tissue and Fascia, Left Upper Arm G Subcutaneous Tissue and Fascia, Right Lower Arm H Subcutaneous Tissue and Fascia, Left Lower Arm J Subcutaneous Tissue and Fascia, Right Hand K Subcutaneous Tissue and Fascia, Left Hand L Subcutaneous Tissue and Fascia, Right Upper Leg M Subcutaneous Tissue and Fascia, Left Upper Leg N Subcutaneous Tissue and Fascia, Right Lower Leg P Subcutaneous Tissue and Fascia, Left Lower Leg Q Subcutaneous Tissue and Fascia, Right Foot R Subcutaneous Tissue and Fascia, Left Foot	0 Open 3 Percutaneous	Z No Device	Z No Qualifier

Section	0	Medical and Surgical
Body System	J	Subcutaneous Tissue and Fascia
Operation	D	**Extraction:** Pulling or stripping out or off all or a portion of a body part by the use of force

Body Part (4th)	Approach (5th)	Device (6th)	Qualifier (7th)
0 Subcutaneous Tissue and Fascia, Scalp 1 Subcutaneous Tissue and Fascia, Face 4 Subcutaneous Tissue and Fascia, Right Neck 5 Subcutaneous Tissue and Fascia, Left Neck 6 Subcutaneous Tissue and Fascia, Chest 7 Subcutaneous Tissue and Fascia, Back 8 Subcutaneous Tissue and Fascia, Abdomen 9 Subcutaneous Tissue and Fascia, Buttock B Subcutaneous Tissue and Fascia, Perineum C Subcutaneous Tissue and Fascia, Pelvic Region D Subcutaneous Tissue and Fascia, Right Upper Arm F Subcutaneous Tissue and Fascia, Left Upper Arm G Subcutaneous Tissue and Fascia, Right Lower Arm H Subcutaneous Tissue and Fascia, Left Lower Arm J Subcutaneous Tissue and Fascia, Right Hand K Subcutaneous Tissue and Fascia, Left Hand L Subcutaneous Tissue and Fascia, Right Upper Leg M Subcutaneous Tissue and Fascia, Left Upper Leg N Subcutaneous Tissue and Fascia, Right Lower Leg P Subcutaneous Tissue and Fascia, Left Lower Leg Q Subcutaneous Tissue and Fascia, Right Foot R Subcutaneous Tissue and Fascia, Left Foot	0 Open 3 Percutaneous	Z No Device	Z No Qualifier

Section	0	Medical and Surgical
Body System	J	Subcutaneous Tissue and Fascia
Operation	H	Insertion: Putting in a nonbiological appliance that monitors, assists, performs, or prevents a physiological function but does not physically take the place of a body part

0JH

Body Part (4th)	Approach (5th)	Device (6th)	Qualifier (7th)
0 Subcutaneous Tissue and Fascia, Scalp 1 Subcutaneous Tissue and Fascia, Face 4 Subcutaneous Tissue and Fascia, Right Neck 5 Subcutaneous Tissue and Fascia, Left Neck 9 Subcutaneous Tissue and Fascia, Buttock B Subcutaneous Tissue and Fascia, Perineum C Subcutaneous Tissue and Fascia, Pelvic Region J Subcutaneous Tissue and Fascia, Right Hand K Subcutaneous Tissue and Fascia, Left Hand Q Subcutaneous Tissue and Fascia, Right Foot R Subcutaneous Tissue and Fascia, Left Foot	0 Open 3 Percutaneous	N Tissue Expander	Z No Qualifier
6 Subcutaneous Tissue and Fascia, Chest	0 Open 3 Percutaneous	0 Monitoring Device, Hemodynamic 2 Monitoring Device 4 Pacemaker, Single Chamber 5 Pacemaker, Single Chamber Rate Responsive 6 Pacemaker, Dual Chamber 7 Cardiac Resynchronization Pacemaker Pulse Generator 8 Defibrillator Generator 9 Cardiac Resynchronization Defibrillator Pulse Generator A Contractility Modulation Device B Stimulator Generator, Single Array C Stimulator Generator, Single Array Rechargeable D Stimulator Generator, Multiple Array E Stimulator Generator, Multiple Array Rechargeable F Subcutaneous Defibrillator Lead H Contraceptive Device M Stimulator Generator N Tissue Expander P Cardiac Rhythm Related Device V Infusion Device, Pump W Vascular Access Device, Totally Implantable X Vascular Access Device, Tunneled Y Other Device	Z No Qualifier
7 Subcutaneous Tissue and Fascia, Back	0 Open 3 Percutaneous	B Stimulator Generator, Single Array C Stimulator Generator, Single Array Rechargeable D Stimulator Generator, Multiple Array E Stimulator Generator, Multiple Array Rechargeable M Stimulator Generator N Tissue Expander V Infusion Device, Pump Y Other Device	Z No Qualifier

Continued →

Section	0	Medical and Surgical
Body System	J	Subcutaneous Tissue and Fascia
Operation	H	Insertion: Putting in a nonbiological appliance that monitors, assists, performs, or prevents a physiological function but does not physically take the place of a body part

Body Part (4th)	Approach (5th)	Device (6th)	Qualifier (7th)
8 Subcutaneous Tissue and Fascia, Abdomen	0 Open 3 Percutaneous	0 Monitoring Device, Hemodynamic 2 Monitoring Device 4 Pacemaker, Single Chamber 5 Pacemaker, Single Chamber Rate Responsive 6 Pacemaker, Dual Chamber 7 Cardiac Resynchronization Pacemaker Pulse Generator 8 Defibrillator Generator 9 Cardiac Resynchronization Defibrillator Pulse Generator A Contractility Modulation Device B Stimulator Generator, Single Array C Stimulator Generator, Single Array Rechargeable D Stimulator Generator, Multiple Array E Stimulator Generator, Multiple Array Rechargeable H Contraceptive Device M Stimulator Generator N Tissue Expander P Cardiac Rhythm Related Device V Infusion Device, Pump W Vascular Access Device Totally Implantable X Vascular Access Device, Tunneled Y Other Device	Z No Qualifier
D Subcutaneous Tissue and Fascia, Right Upper Arm F Subcutaneous Tissue and Fascia, Left Upper Arm G Subcutaneous Tissue and Fascia, Right Lower Arm H Subcutaneous Tissue and Fascia, Left Lower Arm L Subcutaneous Tissue and Fascia, Right Upper Leg M Subcutaneous Tissue and Fascia, Left Upper Leg N Subcutaneous Tissue and Fascia, Right Lower Leg P Subcutaneous Tissue and Fascia, Left Lower Leg	0 Open 3 Percutaneous	H Contraceptive Device N Tissue Expander V Infusion Device, Pump W Vascular Access Device, Totally Implantable X Vascular Access Device, Tunneled	Z No Qualifier
S Subcutaneous Tissue and Fascia, Head and Neck V Subcutaneous Tissue and Fascia, Upper Extremity W Subcutaneous Tissue and Fascia, Lower Extremity	0 Open 3 Percutaneous	1 Radioactive Element 3 Infusion Device Y Other Device	Z No Qualifier
T Subcutaneous Tissue and Fascia, Trunk	0 Open 3 Percutaneous	1 Radioactive Element 3 Infusion Device V Infusion Device, Pump Y Other Device	Z No Qualifier

Section	0	Medical and Surgical
Body System	J	Subcutaneous Tissue and Fascia
Operation	J	Inspection: Visually and/or manually exploring a body part

Body Part (4th)	Approach (5th)	Device (6th)	Qualifier (7th)
S Subcutaneous Tissue and Fascia, Head and Neck T Subcutaneous Tissue and Fascia, Trunk V Subcutaneous Tissue and Fascia, Upper Extremity W Subcutaneous Tissue and Fascia, Lower Extremity	0 Open 3 Percutaneous X External	Z No Device	Z No Qualifier

Section   **0**   **Medical and Surgical**
Body System   **J**   **Subcutaneous Tissue and Fascia**
Operation   **N**   **Release:** Freeing a body part from an abnormal physical constraint by cutting or by the use of force

Body Part (4th)	Approach (5th)	Device (6th)	Qualifier (7th)
0 Subcutaneous Tissue and Fascia, Scalp 1 Subcutaneous Tissue and Fascia, Face 4 Subcutaneous Tissue and Fascia, Right Neck 5 Subcutaneous Tissue and Fascia, Left Neck 6 Subcutaneous Tissue and Fascia, Chest 7 Subcutaneous Tissue and Fascia, Back 8 Subcutaneous Tissue and Fascia, Abdomen 9 Subcutaneous Tissue and Fascia, Buttock B Subcutaneous Tissue and Fascia, Perineum C Subcutaneous Tissue and Fascia, Pelvic Region D Subcutaneous Tissue and Fascia, Right Upper Arm F Subcutaneous Tissue and Fascia, Left Upper Arm G Subcutaneous Tissue and Fascia, Right Lower Arm H Subcutaneous Tissue and Fascia, Left Lower Arm J Subcutaneous Tissue and Fascia, Right Hand K Subcutaneous Tissue and Fascia, Left Hand L Subcutaneous Tissue and Fascia, Right Upper Leg M Subcutaneous Tissue and Fascia, Left Upper Leg N Subcutaneous Tissue and Fascia, Right Lower Leg P Subcutaneous Tissue and Fascia, Left Lower Leg Q Subcutaneous Tissue and Fascia, Right Foot R Subcutaneous Tissue and Fascia, Left Foot	0 Open 3 Percutaneous X External	Z No Device	Z No Qualifier

Section   **0**   **Medical and Surgical**
Body System   **J**   **Subcutaneous Tissue and Fascia**
Operation   **P**   **Removal:** Taking out or off a device from a body part

Body Part (4th)	Approach (5th)	Device (6th)	Qualifier (7th)
S Subcutaneous Tissue and Fascia, Head and Neck	0 Open 3 Percutaneous	0 Drainage Device 1 Radioactive Element 3 Infusion Device 7 Autologous Tissue Substitute J Synthetic Substitute K Nonautologous Tissue Substitute N Tissue Expander Y Other Device	Z No Qualifier
S Subcutaneous Tissue and Fascia, Head and Neck	X External	0 Drainage Device 1 Radioactive Element 3 Infusion Device	Z No Qualifier
T Subcutaneous Tissue and Fascia, Trunk	0 Open 3 Percutaneous	0 Drainage Device 1 Radioactive Element 2 Monitoring Device 3 Infusion Device 7 Autologous Tissue Substitute F Subcutaneous Defibrillator Lead H Contraceptive Device J Synthetic Substitute K Nonautologous Tissue Substitute M Stimulator Generator N Tissue Expander P Cardiac Rhythm Related Device V Infusion Device, Pump W Vascular Access Device, Totally Implantable X Vascular Access Device, Tunneled Y Other Device	Z No Qualifier

Continued →

Section	0	Medical and Surgical
Body System	J	Subcutaneous Tissue and Fascia
Operation	P	Removal: Taking out or off a device from a body part

0JP Continued

Body Part (4th)	Approach (5th)	Device (6th)	Qualifier (7th)
T Subcutaneous Tissue and Fascia, Trunk	X External	0 Drainage Device 1 Radioactive Element 2 Monitoring Device 3 Infusion Device H Contraceptive Device V Infusion Device, Pump X Vascular Access Device, Tunneled	Z No Qualifier
V Subcutaneous Tissue and Fascia, Upper Extremity W Subcutaneous Tissue and Fascia, Lower Extremity	0 Open 3 Percutaneous	0 Drainage Device 1 Radioactive Element 3 Infusion Device 7 Autologous Tissue Substitute H Contraceptive Device J Synthetic Substitute K Nonautologous Tissue Substitute N Tissue Expander V Infusion Device, Pump W Vascular Access Device, Totally Implantable X Vascular Access Device, Tunneled Y Other Device	Z No Qualifier
V Subcutaneous Tissue and Fascia, Upper Extremity W Subcutaneous Tissue and Fascia, Lower Extremity	X External	0 Drainage Device 1 Radioactive Element 3 Infusion Device H Contraceptive Device V Infusion Device, Pump X Vascular Access Device, Tunneled	Z No Qualifier

Section	0	Medical and Surgical
Body System	J	Subcutaneous Tissue and Fascia
Operation	Q	Repair: Restoring, to the extent possible, a body part to its normal anatomic structure and function

Body Part (4th)	Approach (5th)	Device (6th)	Qualifier (7th)
0 Subcutaneous Tissue and Fascia, Scalp 1 Subcutaneous Tissue and Fascia, Face 4 Subcutaneous Tissue and Fascia, Right Neck 5 Subcutaneous Tissue and Fascia, Left Neck 6 Subcutaneous Tissue and Fascia, Chest 7 Subcutaneous Tissue and Fascia, Back 8 Subcutaneous Tissue and Fascia, Abdomen 9 Subcutaneous Tissue and Fascia, Buttock B Subcutaneous Tissue and Fascia, Perineum C Subcutaneous Tissue and Fascia, Pelvic Region D Subcutaneous Tissue and Fascia, Right Upper Arm F Subcutaneous Tissue and Fascia, Left Upper Arm G Subcutaneous Tissue and Fascia, Right Lower Arm H Subcutaneous Tissue and Fascia, Left Lower Arm J Subcutaneous Tissue and Fascia, Right Hand K Subcutaneous Tissue and Fascia, Left Hand L Subcutaneous Tissue and Fascia, Right Upper Leg M Subcutaneous Tissue and Fascia, Left Upper Leg N Subcutaneous Tissue and Fascia, Right Lower Leg P Subcutaneous Tissue and Fascia, Left Lower Leg Q Subcutaneous Tissue and Fascia, Right Foot R Subcutaneous Tissue and Fascia, Left Foot	0 Open 3 Percutaneous	Z No Device	Z No Qualifier

0JP–0JQ

Medical and Surgical, Subcutaneous Tissue and Fascia Tables

Section	0	Medical and Surgical
Body System	J	Subcutaneous Tissue and Fascia
Operation	R	**Replacement:** Putting in or on biological or synthetic material that physically takes the place and/or function of all or a portion of a body part

Body Part (4th)	Approach (5th)	Device (6th)	Qualifier (7th)
0 Subcutaneous Tissue and Fascia, Scalp 1 Subcutaneous Tissue and Fascia, Face 4 Subcutaneous Tissue and Fascia, Right Neck 5 Subcutaneous Tissue and Fascia, Left Neck 6 Subcutaneous Tissue and Fascia, Chest 7 Subcutaneous Tissue and Fascia, Back 8 Subcutaneous Tissue and Fascia, Abdomen 9 Subcutaneous Tissue and Fascia, Buttock B Subcutaneous Tissue and Fascia, Perineum C Subcutaneous Tissue and Fascia, Pelvic Region D Subcutaneous Tissue and Fascia, Right Upper Arm F Subcutaneous Tissue and Fascia, Left Upper Arm G Subcutaneous Tissue and Fascia, Right Lower Arm H Subcutaneous Tissue and Fascia, Left Lower Arm J Subcutaneous Tissue and Fascia, Right Hand K Subcutaneous Tissue and Fascia, Left Hand L Subcutaneous Tissue and Fascia, Right Upper Leg M Subcutaneous Tissue and Fascia, Left Upper Leg N Subcutaneous Tissue and Fascia, Right Lower Leg P Subcutaneous Tissue and Fascia, Left Lower Leg Q Subcutaneous Tissue and Fascia, Right Foot R Subcutaneous Tissue and Fascia, Left Foot	0 Open 3 Percutaneous	7 Autologous Tissue Substitute J Synthetic Substitute K Nonautologous Tissue Substitute	Z No Qualifier

Section	0	Medical and Surgical
Body System	J	Subcutaneous Tissue and Fascia
Operation	U	**Supplement:** Putting in or on biological or synthetic material that physically reinforces and/or augments the function of a portion of a body part

Body Part (4th)	Approach (5th)	Device (6th)	Qualifier (7th)
0 Subcutaneous Tissue and Fascia, Scalp 1 Subcutaneous Tissue and Fascia, Face 4 Subcutaneous Tissue and Fascia, Right Neck 5 Subcutaneous Tissue and Fascia, Left Neck 6 Subcutaneous Tissue and Fascia, Chest 7 Subcutaneous Tissue and Fascia, Back 8 Subcutaneous Tissue and Fascia, Abdomen 9 Subcutaneous Tissue and Fascia, Buttock B Subcutaneous Tissue and Fascia, Perineum C Subcutaneous Tissue and Fascia, Pelvic Region D Subcutaneous Tissue and Fascia, Right Upper Arm F Subcutaneous Tissue and Fascia, Left Upper Arm G Subcutaneous Tissue and Fascia, Right Lower Arm H Subcutaneous Tissue and Fascia, Left Lower Arm J Subcutaneous Tissue and Fascia, Right Hand K Subcutaneous Tissue and Fascia, Left Hand L Subcutaneous Tissue and Fascia, Right Upper Leg M Subcutaneous Tissue and Fascia, Left Upper Leg N Subcutaneous Tissue and Fascia, Right Lower Leg P Subcutaneous Tissue and Fascia, Left Lower Leg Q Subcutaneous Tissue and Fascia, Right Foot R Subcutaneous Tissue and Fascia, Left Foot	0 Open 3 Percutaneous	7 Autologous Tissue Substitute J Synthetic Substitute K Nonautologous Tissue Substitute	Z No Qualifier

Section	0	Medical and Surgical
Body System	J	Subcutaneous Tissue and Fascia
Operation	W	Revision: Correcting, to the extent possible, a portion of a malfunctioning device or the position of a displaced device

Body Part (4th)	Approach (5th)	Device (6th)	Qualifier (7th)
S Subcutaneous Tissue and Fascia, Head and Neck	**0** Open **3** Percutaneous	**0** Drainage Device **3** Infusion Device **7** Autologous Tissue Substitute **J** Synthetic Substitute **K** Nonautologous Tissue Substitute **N** Tissue Expander **Y** Other Device	**Z** No Qualifier
S Subcutaneous Tissue and Fascia, Head and Neck	**X** External	**0** Drainage Device **3** Infusion Device **7** Autologous Tissue Substitute **J** Synthetic Substitute **K** Nonautologous Tissue Substitute **N** Tissue Expander	**Z** No Qualifier
T Subcutaneous Tissue and Fascia, Trunk	**0** Open **3** Percutaneous	**0** Drainage Device **2** Monitoring Device **3** Infusion Device **7** Autologous Tissue Substitute **F** Subcutaneous Defibrillator Lead **H** Contraceptive Device **J** Synthetic Substitute **K** Nonautologous Tissue Substitute **M** Stimulator Generator **N** Tissue Expander **P** Cardiac Rhythm Related Device **V** Infusion Device, Pump **W** Vascular Access Device, Totally Implantable **X** Vascular Access Device, Tunneled **Y** Other Device	**Z** No Qualifier
T Subcutaneous Tissue and Fascia, Trunk	**X** External	**0** Drainage Device **2** Monitoring Device **3** Infusion Device **7** Autologous Tissue Substitute **F** Subcutaneous Defibrillator Lead **H** Contraceptive Device **J** Synthetic Substitute **K** Nonautologous Tissue Substitute **M** Stimulator Generator **N** Tissue Expander **P** Cardiac Rhythm Related Device **V** Infusion Device, Pump **W** Vascular Access Device, Totally Implantable **X** Vascular Access Device, Tunneled	**Z** No Qualifier
V Subcutaneous Tissue and Fascia, Upper Extremity **W** Subcutaneous Tissue and Fascia, Lower Extremity	**0** Open **3** Percutaneous	**0** Drainage Device **3** Infusion Device **7** Autologous Tissue Substitute **H** Contraceptive Device **J** Synthetic Substitute **K** Nonautologous Tissue Substitute **N** Tissue Expander **V** Infusion Device, Pump **W** Vascular Access Device, Totally Implantable **X** Vascular Access Device, Tunneled **Y** Other Device	**Z** No Qualifier

Continued ➞

Section	0	Medical and Surgical
Body System	J	Subcutaneous Tissue and Fascia
Operation	W	Revision: Correcting, to the extent possible, a portion of a malfunctioning device or the position of a displaced device

0JW Continued

Body Part (4th)	Approach (5th)	Device (6th)	Qualifier (7th)
V Subcutaneous Tissue and Fascia, Upper Extremity W Subcutaneous Tissue and Fascia, Lower Extremity	X External	0 Drainage Device 3 Infusion Device 7 Autologous Tissue Substitute H Contraceptive Device J Synthetic Substitute K Nonautologous Tissue Substitute N Tissue Expander V Infusion Device, Pump W Vascular Access Device, Totally Implantable X Vascular Access Device, Tunneled	Z No Qualifier

Section	0	Medical and Surgical
Body System	J	Subcutaneous Tissue and Fascia
Operation	X	Transfer: Moving, without taking out, all or a portion of a body part to another location to take over the function of all or a portion of a body part

Body Part (4th)	Approach (5th)	Device (6th)	Qualifier (7th)
0 Subcutaneous Tissue and Fascia, Scalp 1 Subcutaneous Tissue and Fascia, Face 4 Subcutaneous Tissue and Fascia, Right Neck 5 Subcutaneous Tissue and Fascia, Left Neck 6 Subcutaneous Tissue and Fascia, Chest 7 Subcutaneous Tissue and Fascia, Back 8 Subcutaneous Tissue and Fascia, Abdomen 9 Subcutaneous Tissue and Fascia, Buttock B Subcutaneous Tissue and Fascia, Perineum C Subcutaneous Tissue and Fascia, Pelvic Region D Subcutaneous Tissue and Fascia, Right Upper Arm F Subcutaneous Tissue and Fascia, Left Upper Arm G Subcutaneous Tissue and Fascia, Right Lower Arm H Subcutaneous Tissue and Fascia, Left Lower Arm J Subcutaneous Tissue and Fascia, Right Hand K Subcutaneous Tissue and Fascia, Left Hand L Subcutaneous Tissue and Fascia, Right Upper Leg M Subcutaneous Tissue and Fascia, Left Upper Leg N Subcutaneous Tissue and Fascia, Right Lower Leg P Subcutaneous Tissue and Fascia, Left Lower Leg Q Subcutaneous Tissue and Fascia, Right Foot R Subcutaneous Tissue and Fascia, Left Foot	0 Open 3 Percutaneous	Z No Device	B Skin and Subcutaneous Tissue C Skin, Subcutaneous Tissue and Fascia Z No Qualifier

AHA Coding Clinic

0J2TXYZ Change Other Device in Trunk Subcutaneous Tissue and Fascia, External Approach—AHA CC: 2Q, 2017, 26; 3Q, 2018, 10

0J910ZZ Drainage of Face Subcutaneous Tissue and Fascia, Open Approach—AHA CC: 3Q, 2018, 16

0J940ZZ Drainage of Right Neck Subcutaneous Tissue and Fascia, Open Approach—AHA CC: 3Q, 2018, 16-17

0J960ZZ Drainage of Chest Subcutaneous Tissue and Fascia, Open Approach—AHA CC: 3Q, 2015, 23-24

0J9C0ZZ Drainage of Pelvic Region Subcutaneous Tissue and Fascia, Open Approach—AHA CC: 3Q, 2015, 23-24

0J9D0ZZ Drainage of Right Upper Arm Subcutaneous Tissue and Fascia, Open Approach—AHA CC: 3Q, 2015, 23-24

0J9F0ZZ Drainage of Left Upper Arm Subcutaneous Tissue and Fascia, Open Approach—AHA CC: 3Q, 2015, 23-24

0J9L0ZZ Drainage of Right Upper Leg Subcutaneous Tissue and Fascia, Open Approach—AHA CC: 3Q, 2015, 23-24

0J9M0ZZ Drainage of Left Upper Leg Subcutaneous Tissue and Fascia, Open Approach—AHA CC: 3Q, 2015, 23-24

0JB70ZZ Excision of Back Subcutaneous Tissue and Fascia, Open Approach—AHA CC: 1Q, 2018, 7-8; 2Q, 2023, 30

0JB80ZZ Excision of Abdomen Subcutaneous Tissue and Fascia, Open Approach—AHA CC: 3Q, 2014, 22-23; 4Q, 2014, 39-40; 1Q, 2020, 31-32

0JB90ZZ Excision of Buttock Subcutaneous Tissue and Fascia, Open Approach—AHA CC: 3Q, 2015, 6-7

0JB93ZZ Excision of Buttock Subcutaneous Tissue and Fascia, Percutaneous Approach—AHA CC: 3Q, 2019, 25

0JBB0ZZ Excision of Perineum Subcutaneous Tissue and Fascia, Open Approach—AHA CC: 1Q, 2015, 29-30

0JBH0ZZ Excision of Left Lower Arm Subcutaneous Tissue and Fascia, Open Approach—AHA CC: 2Q, 2015, 13

0JBL0ZZ Excision of Right Upper Leg Subcutaneous Tissue and Fascia, Open Approach—AHA CC: 3Q, 2022, 11-13

0JC80ZZ Extirpation of Matter from Abdomen Subcutaneous Tissue and Fascia, Open Approach—AHA CC: 3Q, 2017, 22

0JD70ZZ Extraction of Back Subcutaneous Tissue and Fascia, Open Approach—AHA CC: 3Q, 2016, 21

0JDC0ZZ Extraction of Pelvic Region Subcutaneous Tissue and Fascia, Open Approach—AHA CC: 1Q, 2015, 23

0JDL0ZZ Extraction of Right Upper Leg Subcutaneous Tissue and Fascia, Open Approach—AHA CC: 1Q, 2016, 40

0JDN0ZZ Extraction of Right Lower Leg Subcutaneous Tissue and Fascia, Open Approach—AHA CC: 3Q, 2016, 20-21

0JDR0ZZ Extraction of Left Foot Subcutaneous Tissue and Fascia, Open Approach—AHA CC: 3Q, 2016, 22; 1Q, 2023, 36

0JH608Z Insertion of Defibrillator Generator into Chest Subcutaneous Tissue and Fascia, Open Approach—AHA CC: 4Q, 2012, 104-106

0JH60MZ Insertion of Stimulator Generator into Chest Subcutaneous Tissue and Fascia, Open Approach—AHA CC: 4Q, 2016, 98-99

0JH60PZ Insertion of Cardiac Rhythm Related Device into Chest Subcutaneous Tissue and Fascia, Open Approach—AHA CC: 4Q, 2012, 104-106

0JH60WZ Insertion of Totally Implantable Vascular Access Device into Chest Subcutaneous Tissue and Fascia, Open Approach—AHA CC: 4Q, 2017, 63-64

0JH60XZ Insertion of Tunneled Vascular Access Device into Chest Subcutaneous Tissue and Fascia, Open Approach—AHA CC: 2Q, 2015, 33-34

0JH63VZ Insertion of Infusion Pump into Chest Subcutaneous Tissue and Fascia, Percutaneous Approach—AHA CC: 4Q, 2015, 14-15

0JH63XZ Insertion of Tunneled Vascular Access Device into Chest Subcutaneous Tissue and Fascia, Percutaneous Approach—AHA CC: 4Q, 2015, 30-32; 2Q, 2016, 15-16; 2Q, 2017, 24-26

0JH80VZ Insertion of Infusion Pump into Abdomen Subcutaneous Tissue and Fascia, Open Approach—AHA CC: 3Q, 2014, 19-20

0JH80WZ Insertion of Totally Implantable Vascular Access Device into Abdomen Subcutaneous Tissue and Fascia, Open Approach—AHA CC: 2Q, 2016, 14

0JH80YZ Insertion of Other Device into Abdomen Subcutaneous Tissue and Fascia, Open Approach—AHA CC: 4Q, 2020, 55

0JHS33Z Insertion of Infusion Device into Head and Neck Subcutaneous Tissue and Fascia, Percutaneous Approach—AHA CC: 2Q, 2020, 15-16

0JHT03Z Insertion of Infusion Device into Trunk Subcutaneous Tissue and Fascia, Open Approach—AHA CC: 2Q, 2020, 16-17

0JHT0YZ Insertion of Other Device into Trunk Subcutaneous Tissue and Fascia, Open Approach—AHA CC: 4Q, 2018, 42-43

0JNL0ZZ Release Right Upper Leg Subcutaneous Tissue and Fascia, Open Approach—AHA CC: 3Q, 2017, 11-12

0JNM0ZZ Release Left Upper Leg Subcutaneous Tissue and Fascia, Open Approach—AHA CC: 3Q, 2017, 11-12

0JNN0ZZ Release Right Lower Leg Subcutaneous Tissue and Fascia, Open Approach—AHA CC: 3Q, 2017, 11-12

0JNP0ZZ Release Left Lower Leg Subcutaneous Tissue and Fascia, Open Approach—AHA CC: 3Q, 2017, 11-12

0JNQ0ZZ Release Right Foot Subcutaneous Tissue and Fascia, Open Approach—AHA CC: 3Q, 2017, 11-12

0JNR0ZZ Release Left Foot Subcutaneous Tissue and Fascia, Open Approach—AHA CC: 3Q, 2017, 11-12

0JPT0NZ Removal of Tissue Expander from Trunk Subcutaneous Tissue and Fascia, Open Approach—AHA CC: 4Q, 2013, 109-111

0JPT0PZ Removal of Cardiac Rhythm Related Device from Trunk Subcutaneous Tissue and Fascia, Open Approach—AHA CC: 4Q, 2012, 104-106

0JPT0VZ Removal of Infusion Pump from Trunk Subcutaneous Tissue and Fascia, Open Approach—AHA CC: 3Q, 2014, 19-20

0JPT0XZ Removal of Tunneled Vascular Access Device from Trunk Subcutaneous Tissue and Fascia, Open Approach—AHA CC: 4Q, 2015, 31-32; 2Q, 2016, 15-16

0JPT3JZ Removal of Synthetic Substitute from Trunk Subcutaneous Tissue and Fascia, Percutaneous Approach—AHA CC: 4Q, 2018, 86

0JPT3YZ Removal of Other Device from Trunk Subcutaneous Tissue and Fascia, Percutaneous Approach—AHA CC: 3Q, 2018, 29

0JQ80ZZ Repair Abdomen Subcutaneous Tissue and Fascia, Open Approach—AHA CC: 3Q, 2022, 25

0JQC0ZZ Repair Pelvic Region Subcutaneous Tissue and Fascia, Open Approach—AHA CC: 4Q, 2014, 44-45; 3Q, 2017, 19

0JR107Z Replacement of Face Subcutaneous Tissue and Fascia with Autologous Tissue Substitute, Open Approach—AHA CC: 2Q, 2015, 13

0JU707Z Supplement of Back Subcutaneous Tissue and Fascia with Autologous Tissue Substitute, Open Approach—AHA CC: 1Q, 2018, 7-8

0JUH0KZ Supplement of Left Lower Arm Subcutaneous Tissue and Fascia with Nonautologous Tissue Substitute, Open Approach—AHA CC: 2Q, 2018, 20

0JWS0JZ Revision of Synthetic Substitute in Head and Neck Subcutaneous Tissue and Fascia, Open Approach—AHA CC: 2Q, 2015, 9-10

0JWT0JZ Revision of Synthetic Substitute in Trunk Subcutaneous Tissue and Fascia, Open Approach—AHA CC: 1Q, 2018, 8-9

0JWT03Z Revision of Infusion Device in Trunk Subcutaneous Tissue and Fascia, Open Approach—AHA CC: 3Q, 2022, 25

0JWT0PZ Revision of Cardiac Rhythm Related Device in Trunk Subcutaneous Tissue and Fascia, Open Approach—AHA CC: 4Q, 2012, 104-106

0JWT33Z Revision of Infusion Device in Trunk Subcutaneous Tissue and Fascia, Percutaneous Approach—AHA CC: 4Q, 2015, 33

0JX00ZC Transfer Scalp Subcutaneous Tissue and Fascia with Skin, Subcutaneous Tissue and Fascia, Open Approach—AHA CC: 1Q, 2018, 10

0JX60ZB Transfer Chest Subcutaneous Tissue and Fascia with Skin and Subcutaneous Tissue, Open Approach—AHA CC: 4Q, 2013, 109-111; 2Q, 2021, 16-17

0JX80ZB Transfer Abdomen Subcutaneous Tissue and Fascia with Skin and Subcutaneous Tissue, Open Approach—AHA CC: 4Q, 2013, 109-111

0JXF0ZZ Transfer Left Upper Arm Subcutaneous Tissue and Fascia, Open Approach—AHA CC: 3Q, 2021, 19-20

0JXL0ZZ Transfer Right Upper Leg Subcutaneous Tissue and Fascia, Open Approach—AHA CC: 3Q, 2022, 11-13

0JXN0ZC Transfer Right Lower Leg Subcutaneous Tissue and Fascia with Skin, Subcutaneous Tissue and Fascia, Open Approach—AHA CC: 3Q, 2014, 18-19

Muscles

Muscles

Muscles Tables 0K2–0KX

Section	0	Medical and Surgical
Body System	K	Muscles
Operation	2	**Change:** Taking out or off a device from a body part and putting back an identical or similar device in or on the same body part without cutting or puncturing the skin or a mucous membrane

Body Part (4ᵗʰ)	Approach (5ᵗʰ)	Device (6ᵗʰ)	Qualifier (7ᵗʰ)
X Upper Muscle Y Lower Muscle	X External	0 Drainage Device Y Other Device	Z No Qualifier

Section	0	Medical and Surgical
Body System	K	Muscles
Operation	5	**Destruction:** Physical eradication of all or a portion of a body part by the direct use of energy, force, or a destructive agent

Body Part (4ᵗʰ)	Approach (5ᵗʰ)	Device (6ᵗʰ)	Qualifier (7ᵗʰ)
0 Head Muscle 1 Facial Muscle 2 Neck Muscle, Right 3 Neck Muscle, Left 4 Tongue, Palate, Pharynx Muscle 5 Shoulder Muscle, Right 6 Shoulder Muscle, Left 7 Upper Arm Muscle, Right 8 Upper Arm Muscle, Left 9 Lower Arm and Wrist Muscle, Right B Lower Arm and Wrist Muscle, Left C Hand Muscle, Right D Hand Muscle, Left F Trunk Muscle, Right G Trunk Muscle, Left H Thorax Muscle, Right J Thorax Muscle, Left K Abdomen Muscle, Right L Abdomen Muscle, Left M Perineum Muscle N Hip Muscle, Right P Hip Muscle, Left Q Upper Leg Muscle, Right R Upper Leg Muscle, Left S Lower Leg Muscle, Right T Lower Leg Muscle, Left V Foot Muscle, Right W Foot Muscle, Left	0 Open 3 Percutaneous 4 Percutaneous Endoscopic	Z No Device	Z No Qualifier

Section	0	**Medical and Surgical**	
Body System	K	**Muscles**	
Operation	8	**Division:** Cutting into a body part, without draining fluids and/or gases from the body part, in order to separate or transect a body part	

Body Part (4th)	Approach (5th)	Device (6th)	Qualifier (7th)
0 Head Muscle 1 Facial Muscle 2 Neck Muscle, Right 3 Neck Muscle, Left 5 Shoulder Muscle, Right 6 Shoulder Muscle, Left 7 Upper Arm Muscle, Right 8 Upper Arm Muscle, Left 9 Lower Arm and Wrist Muscle, Right B Lower Arm and Wrist Muscle, Left C Hand Muscle, Right D Hand Muscle, Left F Trunk Muscle, Right G Trunk Muscle, Left H Thorax Muscle, Right J Thorax Muscle, Left K Abdomen Muscle, Right L Abdomen Muscle, Left M Perineum Muscle N Hip Muscle, Right P Hip Muscle, Left Q Upper Leg Muscle, Right R Upper Leg Muscle, Left S Lower Leg Muscle, Right T Lower Leg Muscle, Left V Foot Muscle, Right W Foot Muscle, Left	0 Open 3 Percutaneous 4 Percutaneous Endoscopic	Z No Device	Z No Qualifier
4 Tongue, Palate, Pharynx Muscle	0 Open 3 Percutaneous 4 Percutaneous Endoscopic 7 Via Natural or Artificial Opening 8 Via Natural or Artificial Opening Endoscopic	Z No Device	Z No Qualifier

Section	0	Medical and Surgical
Body System	K	Muscles
Operation	9	**Drainage:** Taking or letting out fluids and/or gases from a body part

Body Part (4th)	Approach (5th)	Device (6th)	Qualifier (7th)
0 Head Muscle 1 Facial Muscle 2 Neck Muscle, Right 3 Neck Muscle, Left 4 Tongue, Palate, Pharynx Muscle 5 Shoulder Muscle, Right 6 Shoulder Muscle, Left 7 Upper Arm Muscle, Right 8 Upper Arm Muscle, Left 9 Lower Arm and Wrist Muscle, Right B Lower Arm and Wrist Muscle, Left C Hand Muscle, Right D Hand Muscle, Left F Trunk Muscle, Right G Trunk Muscle, Left H Thorax Muscle, Right J Thorax Muscle, Left K Abdomen Muscle, Right L Abdomen Muscle, Left M Perineum Muscle N Hip Muscle, Right P Hip Muscle, Left Q Upper Leg Muscle, Right R Upper Leg Muscle, Left S Lower Leg Muscle, Right T Lower Leg Muscle, Left V Foot Muscle, Right W Foot Muscle, Left	0 Open 3 Percutaneous 4 Percutaneous Endoscopic	0 Drainage Device	Z No Qualifier
0 Head Muscle 1 Facial Muscle 2 Neck Muscle, Right 3 Neck Muscle, Left 4 Tongue, Palate, Pharynx Muscle 5 Shoulder Muscle, Right 6 Shoulder Muscle, Left 7 Upper Arm Muscle, Right 8 Upper Arm Muscle, Left 9 Lower Arm and Wrist Muscle, Right B Lower Arm and Wrist Muscle, Left C Hand Muscle, Right D Hand Muscle, Left F Trunk Muscle, Right G Trunk Muscle, Left H Thorax Muscle, Right J Thorax Muscle, Left K Abdomen Muscle, Right L Abdomen Muscle, Left M Perineum Muscle N Hip Muscle, Right P Hip Muscle, Left Q Upper Leg Muscle, Right R Upper Leg Muscle, Left S Lower Leg Muscle, Right T Lower Leg Muscle, Left V Foot Muscle, Right W Foot Muscle, Left	0 Open 3 Percutaneous 4 Percutaneous Endoscopic	Z No Device	X Diagnostic Z No Qualifier

Section	0	Medical and Surgical
Body System	K	Muscles
Operation	B	**Excision:** Cutting out or off, without replacement, a portion of a body part

Body Part (4th)	Approach (5th)	Device (6th)	Qualifier (7th)
0 Head Muscle	0 Open	Z No Device	X Diagnostic
1 Facial Muscle	3 Percutaneous		Z No Qualifier
2 Neck Muscle, Right	4 Percutaneous Endoscopic		
3 Neck Muscle, Left			
4 Tongue, Palate, Pharynx Muscle			
5 Shoulder Muscle, Right			
6 Shoulder Muscle, Left			
7 Upper Arm Muscle, Right			
8 Upper Arm Muscle, Left			
9 Lower Arm and Wrist Muscle, Right			
B Lower Arm and Wrist Muscle, Left			
C Hand Muscle, Right			
D Hand Muscle, Left			
F Trunk Muscle, Right			
G Trunk Muscle, Left			
H Thorax Muscle, Right			
J Thorax Muscle, Left			
K Abdomen Muscle, Right			
L Abdomen Muscle, Left			
M Perineum Muscle			
N Hip Muscle, Right			
P Hip Muscle, Left			
Q Upper Leg Muscle, Right			
R Upper Leg Muscle, Left			
S Lower Leg Muscle, Right			
T Lower Leg Muscle, Left			
V Foot Muscle, Right			
W Foot Muscle, Left			

Section	0	Medical and Surgical
Body System	K	Muscles
Operation	C	**Extirpation:** Taking or cutting out solid matter from a body part

Body Part (4th)	Approach (5th)	Device (6th)	Qualifier (7th)
0 Head Muscle	0 Open	Z No Device	Z No Qualifier
1 Facial Muscle	3 Percutaneous		
2 Neck Muscle, Right	4 Percutaneous Endoscopic		
3 Neck Muscle, Left			
4 Tongue, Palate, Pharynx Muscle			
5 Shoulder Muscle, Right			
6 Shoulder Muscle, Left			
7 Upper Arm Muscle, Right			
8 Upper Arm Muscle, Left			
9 Lower Arm and Wrist Muscle, Right			
B Lower Arm and Wrist Muscle, Left			
C Hand Muscle, Right			
D Hand Muscle, Left			
F Trunk Muscle, Right			
G Trunk Muscle, Left			
H Thorax Muscle, Right			
J Thorax Muscle, Left			
K Abdomen Muscle, Right			
L Abdomen Muscle, Left			
M Perineum Muscle			
N Hip Muscle, Right			
P Hip Muscle, Left			
Q Upper Leg Muscle, Right			
R Upper Leg Muscle, Left			
S Lower Leg Muscle, Right			
T Lower Leg Muscle, Left			
V Foot Muscle, Right			
W Foot Muscle, Left			

Section	0	Medical and Surgical
Body System	K	Muscles
Operation	D	**Extraction:** Pulling or stripping out or off all or a portion of a body part by the use of force

Body Part (4th)	Approach (5th)	Device (6th)	Qualifier (7th)
0 Head Muscle	0 Open	Z No Device	Z No Qualifier
1 Facial Muscle			
2 Neck Muscle, Right			
3 Neck Muscle, Left			
4 Tongue, Palate, Pharynx Muscle			
5 Shoulder Muscle, Right			
6 Shoulder Muscle, Left			
7 Upper Arm Muscle, Right			
8 Upper Arm Muscle, Left			
9 Lower Arm and Wrist Muscle, Right			
B Lower Arm and Wrist Muscle, Left			
C Hand Muscle, Right			
D Hand Muscle, Left			
F Trunk Muscle, Right			
G Trunk Muscle, Left			
H Thorax Muscle, Right			
J Thorax Muscle, Left			
K Abdomen Muscle, Right			
L Abdomen Muscle, Left			
M Perineum			
N Hip Muscle, Right			
P Hip Muscle, Left			
Q Upper Leg Muscle, Right			
R Upper Leg Muscle, Left			
S Lower Leg Muscle, Right			
T Lower Leg Muscle, Left			
V Foot Muscle, Right			
W Foot Muscle, Left			

Section	0	Medical and Surgical
Body System	K	Muscles
Operation	H	**Insertion:** Putting in a nonbiological appliance that monitors, assists, performs, or prevents a physiological function but does not physically take the place of a body part

Body Part (4th)	Approach (5th)	Device (6th)	Qualifier (7th)
X Upper Muscle	0 Open	M Stimulator Lead	Z No Qualifier
Y Lower Muscle	3 Percutaneous	Y Other Device	
	4 Percutaneous Endoscopic		

Section	0	Medical and Surgical
Body System	K	Muscles
Operation	J	**Inspection:** Visually and/or manually exploring a body part

Body Part (4th)	Approach (5th)	Device (6th)	Qualifier (7th)
X Upper Muscle	0 Open	Z No Device	Z No Qualifier
Y Lower Muscle	3 Percutaneous		
	4 Percutaneous Endoscopic		
	X External		

0KM–0KN

Medical and Surgical, Muscles Tables

Section	0	Medical and Surgical
Body System	K	Muscles
Operation	M	Reattachment: Putting back in or on all or a portion of a separated body part to its normal location or other suitable location

Body Part (4th)	Approach (5th)	Device (6th)	Qualifier (7th)
0 Head Muscle	0 Open	Z No Device	Z No Qualifier
1 Facial Muscle	4 Percutaneous Endoscopic		
2 Neck Muscle, Right			
3 Neck Muscle, Left			
4 Tongue, Palate, Pharynx Muscle			
5 Shoulder Muscle, Right			
6 Shoulder Muscle, Left			
7 Upper Arm Muscle, Right			
8 Upper Arm Muscle, Left			
9 Lower Arm and Wrist Muscle, Right			
B Lower Arm and Wrist Muscle, Left			
C Hand Muscle, Right			
D Hand Muscle, Left			
F Trunk Muscle, Right			
G Trunk Muscle, Left			
H Thorax Muscle, Right			
J Thorax Muscle, Left			
K Abdomen Muscle, Right			
L Abdomen Muscle, Left			
M Perineum Muscle			
N Hip Muscle, Right			
P Hip Muscle, Left			
Q Upper Leg Muscle, Right			
R Upper Leg Muscle, Left			
S Lower Leg Muscle, Right			
T Lower Leg Muscle, Left			
V Foot Muscle, Right			
W Foot Muscle, Left			

Section	0	Medical and Surgical
Body System	K	Muscles
Operation	N	Release: Freeing a body part from an abnormal physical constraint by cutting or by the use of force

Body Part (4th)	Approach (5th)	Device (6th)	Qualifier (7th)
0 Head Muscle	0 Open	Z No Device	Z No Qualifier
1 Facial Muscle	3 Percutaneous		
2 Neck Muscle, Right	4 Percutaneous Endoscopic		
3 Neck Muscle, Left	X External		
4 Tongue, Palate, Pharynx Muscle			
5 Shoulder Muscle, Right			
6 Shoulder Muscle, Left			
7 Upper Arm Muscle, Right			
8 Upper Arm Muscle, Left			
9 Lower Arm and Wrist Muscle, Right			
B Lower Arm and Wrist Muscle, Left			
C Hand Muscle, Right			
D Hand Muscle, Left			
F Trunk Muscle, Right			
G Trunk Muscle, Left			
H Thorax Muscle, Right			
J Thorax Muscle, Left			
K Abdomen Muscle, Right			
L Abdomen Muscle, Left			
M Perineum Muscle			
N Hip Muscle, Right			
P Hip Muscle, Left			
Q Upper Leg Muscle, Right			
R Upper Leg Muscle, Left			
S Lower Leg Muscle, Right			
T Lower Leg Muscle, Left			
V Foot Muscle, Right			
W Foot Muscle, Left			

Section	0	Medical and Surgical
Body System	K	Muscles
Operation	P	Removal: Taking out or off a device from a body part

Body Part (4th)	Approach (5th)	Device (6th)	Qualifier (7th)
X Upper Muscle Y Lower Muscle	0 Open 3 Percutaneous 4 Percutaneous Endoscopic	0 Drainage Device 7 Autologous Tissue Substitute J Synthetic Substitute K Nonautologous Tissue Substitute M Stimulator Lead Y Other Device	Z No Qualifier
X Upper Muscle Y Lower Muscle	X External	0 Drainage Device M Stimulator Lead	Z No Qualifier

Section	0	Medical and Surgical
Body System	K	Muscles
Operation	Q	Repair: Restoring, to the extent possible, a body part to its normal anatomic structure and function

Body Part (4th)	Approach (5th)	Device (6th)	Qualifier (7th)
0 Head Muscle 1 Facial Muscle 2 Neck Muscle, Right 3 Neck Muscle, Left 4 Tongue, Palate, Pharynx Muscle 5 Shoulder Muscle, Right 6 Shoulder Muscle, Left 7 Upper Arm Muscle, Right 8 Upper Arm Muscle, Left 9 Lower Arm and Wrist Muscle, Right B Lower Arm and Wrist Muscle, Left C Hand Muscle, Right D Hand Muscle, Left F Trunk Muscle, Right G Trunk Muscle, Left H Thorax Muscle, Right J Thorax Muscle, Left K Abdomen Muscle, Right L Abdomen Muscle, Left M Perineum Muscle N Hip Muscle, Right P Hip Muscle, Left Q Upper Leg Muscle, Right R Upper Leg Muscle, Left S Lower Leg Muscle, Right T Lower Leg Muscle, Left V Foot Muscle, Right W Foot Muscle, Left	0 Open 3 Percutaneous 4 Percutaneous Endoscopic	Z No Device	Z No Qualifier

Section	0	Medical and Surgical
Body System	K	Muscles
Operation	R	Replacement: Putting in or on biological or synthetic material that physically takes the place and/or function of all or a portion of a body part

Body Part (4th)	Approach (5th)	Device (6th)	Qualifier (7th)

0 Head Muscle
1 Facial Muscle
2 Neck Muscle, Right
3 Neck Muscle, Left
4 Tongue, Palate, Pharynx Muscle
5 Shoulder Muscle, Right
6 Shoulder Muscle, Left
7 Upper Arm Muscle, Right
8 Upper Arm Muscle, Left
9 Lower Arm and Wrist Muscle, Right
B Lower Arm and Wrist Muscle, Left
C Hand Muscle, Right
D Hand Muscle, Left
F Trunk Muscle, Right
G Trunk Muscle, Left
H Thorax Muscle, Right
J Thorax Muscle, Left
K Abdomen Muscle, Right
L Abdomen Muscle, Left
M Perineum
N Hip Muscle, Right
P Hip Muscle, Left
Q Upper Leg Muscle, Right
R Upper Leg Muscle, Left
S Lower Leg Muscle, Right
T Lower Leg Muscle, Left
V Foot Muscle, Right
W Foot Muscle, Left
	0 Open
	4 Percutaneous Endoscopic
		7 Autologous Tissue
		  Substitute
		J Synthetic Substitute
		K Nonautologous Tissue
		  Substitute
			Z No Qualifier

Section	0	Medical and Surgical
Body System	K	Muscles
Operation	S	Reposition: Moving to its normal location, or other suitable location, all or a portion of a body part

Body Part (4th)	Approach (5th)	Device (6th)	Qualifier (7th)
0 Head Muscle 1 Facial Muscle 2 Neck Muscle, Right 3 Neck Muscle, Left 4 Tongue, Palate, Pharynx Muscle 5 Shoulder Muscle, Right 6 Shoulder Muscle, Left 7 Upper Arm Muscle, Right 8 Upper Arm Muscle, Left 9 Lower Arm and Wrist Muscle, Right B Lower Arm and Wrist Muscle, Left C Hand Muscle, Right D Hand Muscle, Left F Trunk Muscle, Right G Trunk Muscle, Left H Thorax Muscle, Right J Thorax Muscle, Left K Abdomen Muscle, Right L Abdomen Muscle, Left M Perineum Muscle N Hip Muscle, Right P Hip Muscle, Left Q Upper Leg Muscle, Right R Upper Leg Muscle, Left S Lower Leg Muscle, Right T Lower Leg Muscle, Left V Foot Muscle, Right W Foot Muscle, Left	0 Open 4 Percutaneous Endoscopic	Z No Device	Z No Qualifier

Section	0	Medical and Surgical
Body System	K	Muscles
Operation	T	Resection: Cutting out or off, without replacement, all of a body part

Body Part (4th)	Approach (5th)	Device (6th)	Qualifier (7th)
0 Head Muscle 1 Facial Muscle 2 Neck Muscle, Right 3 Neck Muscle, Left 4 Tongue, Palate, Pharynx Muscle 5 Shoulder Muscle, Right 6 Shoulder Muscle, Left 7 Upper Arm Muscle, Right 8 Upper Arm Muscle, Left 9 Lower Arm and Wrist Muscle, Right B Lower Arm and Wrist Muscle, Left C Hand Muscle, Right D Hand Muscle, Left F Trunk Muscle, Right G Trunk Muscle, Left H Thorax Muscle, Right J Thorax Muscle, Left K Abdomen Muscle, Right L Abdomen Muscle, Left M Perineum Muscle N Hip Muscle, Right P Hip Muscle, Left Q Upper Leg Muscle, Right R Upper Leg Muscle, Left S Lower Leg Muscle, Right T Lower Leg Muscle, Left V Foot Muscle, Right W Foot Muscle, Left	0 Open 4 Percutaneous Endoscopic	Z No Device	Z No Qualifier

Section	0	Medical and Surgical
Body System	K	Muscles
Operation	U	Supplement: Putting in or on biological or synthetic material that physically reinforces and/or augments the function of a portion of a body part

Body Part (4th)	Approach (5th)	Device (6th)	Qualifier (7th)
0 Head Muscle 1 Facial Muscle 2 Neck Muscle, Right 3 Neck Muscle, Left 4 Tongue, Palate, Pharynx Muscle 5 Shoulder Muscle, Right 6 Shoulder Muscle, Left 7 Upper Arm Muscle, Right 8 Upper Arm Muscle, Left 9 Lower Arm and Wrist Muscle, Right B Lower Arm and Wrist Muscle, Left C Hand Muscle, Right D Hand Muscle, Left F Trunk Muscle, Right G Trunk Muscle, Left H Thorax Muscle, Right J Thorax Muscle, Left K Abdomen Muscle, Right L Abdomen Muscle, Left M Perineum Muscle N Hip Muscle, Right P Hip Muscle, Left Q Upper Leg Muscle, Right R Upper Leg Muscle, Left S Lower Leg Muscle, Right T Lower Leg Muscle, Left V Foot Muscle, Right W Foot Muscle, Left	0 Open 4 Percutaneous Endoscopic	7 Autologous Tissue Substitute J Synthetic Substitute K Nonautologous Tissue Substitute	Z No Qualifier

0KT–0KU

Medical and Surgical, Muscles Tables

355

Section   **0**   **Medical and Surgical**
Body System   **K**   **Muscles**
Operation   **W**   **Revision:** Correcting, to the extent possible, a portion of a malfunctioning device or the position of a displaced device

Body Part (4th)	Approach (5th)	Device (6th)	Qualifier (7th)
X Upper Muscle Y Lower Muscle	0 Open 3 Percutaneous 4 Percutaneous Endoscopic	0 Drainage Device 7 Autologous Tissue Substitute J Synthetic Substitute K Nonautologous Tissue Substitute M Stimulator Lead Y Other Device	Z No Qualifier
X Upper Muscle Y Lower Muscle	X External	0 Drainage Device 7 Autologous Tissue Substitute J Synthetic Substitute K Nonautologous Tissue Substitute M Stimulator Lead	Z No Qualifier

Section   **0**   **Medical and Surgical**
Body System   **K**   **Muscles**
Operation   **X**   **Transfer:** Moving, without taking out, all or a portion of a body part to another location to take over the function of all or a portion of a body part

Body Part (4th)	Approach (5th)	Device (6th)	Qualifier (7th)
0 Head Muscle 1 Facial Muscle 2 Neck Muscle, Right 3 Neck Muscle, Left 4 Tongue, Palate, Pharynx Muscle 5 Shoulder Muscle, Right 6 Shoulder Muscle, Left 7 Upper Arm Muscle, Right 8 Upper Arm Muscle, Left 9 Lower Arm and Wrist Muscle, Right B Lower Arm and Wrist Muscle, Left C Hand Muscle, Right D Hand Muscle, Left H Thorax Muscle, Right J Thorax Muscle, Left M Perineum Muscle N Hip Muscle, Right P Hip Muscle, Left Q Upper Leg Muscle, Right R Upper Leg Muscle, Left S Lower Leg Muscle, Right T Lower Leg Muscle, Left V Foot Muscle, Right W Foot Muscle, Left	0 Open 4 Percutaneous Endoscopic	Z No Device	0 Skin 1 Subcutaneous Tissue 2 Skin and Subcutaneous Tissue Z No Qualifier
F Trunk Muscle, Right G Trunk Muscle, Left	0 Open 4 Percutaneous Endoscopic	Z No Device	0 Skin 1 Subcutaneous Tissue 2 Skin and Subcutaneous Tissue 5 Latissimus Dorsi Myocutaneous Flap 7 Deep Inferior Epigastric Artery Perforator Flap 8 Superficial Inferior Epigastric Artery Flap 9 Gluteal Artery Perforator Flap Z No Qualifier
K Abdomen Muscle, Right L Abdomen Muscle, Left	0 Open 4 Percutaneous Endoscopic	Z No Device	0 Skin 1 Subcutaneous Tissue 2 Skin and Subcutaneous Tissue 6 Transverse Rectus Abdominis Myocutaneous Flap Z No Qualifier

AHA Coding Clinic

0K844ZZ Division of Tongue, Palate, Pharynx Muscle, Percutaneous Endoscopic Approach—AHA CC: 2Q, 2020, 25

0KB44ZZ Excision of Tongue, Palate, Pharynx Muscle, Percutaneous Endoscopic Approach—AHA CC: 1Q, 2023, 32-33

0KBN0ZZ Excision of Right Hip Muscle, Open Approach—AHA CC: 3Q, 2016, 20

0KBP0ZZ Excision of Left Hip Muscle, Open Approach—AHA CC: 3Q, 2016, 20; 4Q, 2019, 43-44

0KBR0ZZ Excision of Left Upper Leg Muscle, Open Approach—AHA CC: 1Q, 2020, 27-28

0KDS0ZZ Extraction of Right Lower Leg Muscle, Open Approach—AHA CC: 4Q, 2017, 42

0KHY3YZ Insertion of Other Device into Lower Muscle, Percutaneous Approach—AHA CC: 4Q, 2020, 63-64

0KN84ZZ Release Left Upper Arm Muscle, Percutaneous Endoscopic Approach—AHA CC: 2Q, 2015, 22-23

0KNK0ZZ Release Right Abdomen Muscle, Open Approach—AHA CC: 4Q, 2014, 39-40

0KNL0ZZ Release Left Abdomen Muscle, Open Approach—AHA CC: 4Q, 2014, 39-40

0KNT0ZZ Release Left Lower Leg Muscle, Open Approach—AHA CC: 2Q, 2017, 12-14

0KNV0ZZ Release Right Foot Muscle, Open Approach—AHA CC: 2Q, 2017, 12-14

0KQM0ZZ Repair Perineum Muscle, Open Approach—AHA CC: 4Q, 2013, 120; 1Q, 2016, 7; 2Q, 2016, 34-35; 3Q, 2022, 13-14

0KSQ0ZZ Reposition Right Upper Leg Muscle, Open Approach—AHA CC: 3Q, 2022, 11-13

0KT30ZZ Resection of Left Neck Muscle, Open Approach—AHA CC: 2Q, 2016, 12-14

0KTM0ZZ Resection of Perineum Muscle, Open Approach—AHA CC: 4Q, 2014, 40-41; 1Q, 2015, 38

0KX10Z2 Transfer Facial Muscle with Skin and Subcutaneous Tissue, Open Approach—AHA CC: 3Q, 2015, 33

0KX40Z2 Transfer Tongue, Palate, Pharynx Muscle with Skin and Subcutaneous Tissue, Open Approach—AHA CC: 2Q, 2015, 26

0KXF0Z2 Transfer Right Trunk Muscle with Skin and Subcutaneous Tissue, Open Approach—AHA CC: 2Q, 2014, 12

0KXF0Z5 Transfer Right Trunk Muscle, Latissimus Dorsi Myocutaneous Flap, Open Approach—AHA CC: 4Q, 2017, 67

0KXK0Z6 Transfer Right Abdomen Muscle, Transverse Rectus Abdominis Myocutaneous Flap, Open Approach—AHA CC: 4Q, 2014, 41

0KXL0Z6 Transfer Left Abdomen Muscle, Transverse Rectus Abdominis Myocutaneous Flap, Open Approach—AHA CC: 2Q, 2014, 10-11

0KXQ0ZZ Transfer Right Upper Leg Muscle, Open Approach—AHA CC: 3Q, 2016, 30-31

0KXR0ZZ Transfer Left Upper Leg Muscle, Open Approach—AHA CC: 3Q, 2016, 30-31

Tendons

Shoulder Tendons and Ligaments

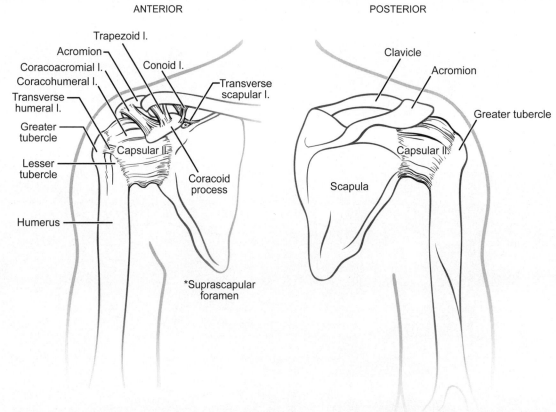

Hip Tendons and Ligaments

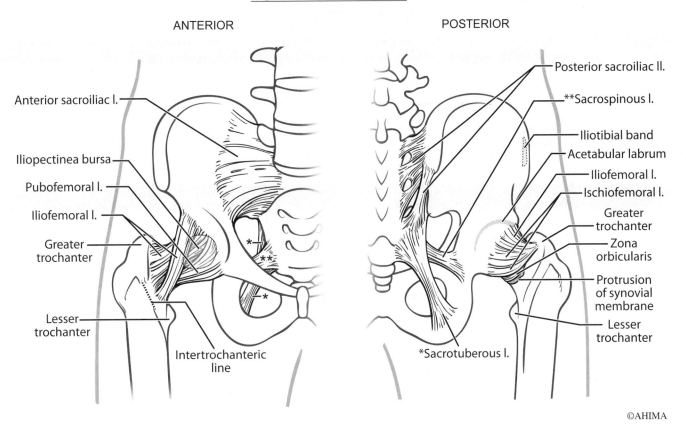

Knee Tendons and Ligaments

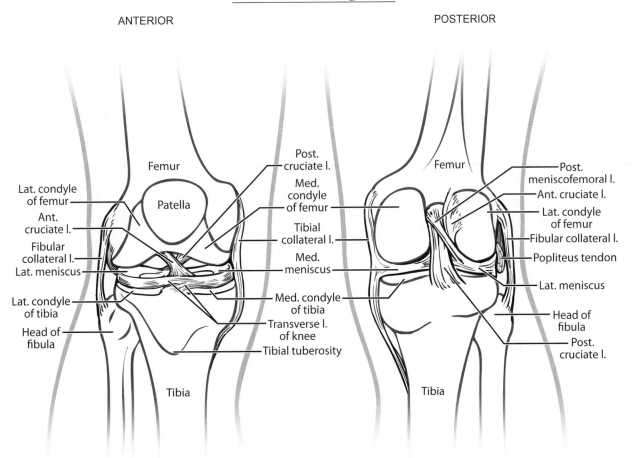

Tendons Tables 0L2–0LX

Section	0	Medical and Surgical
Body System	L	Tendons
Operation	2	**Change:** Taking out or off a device from a body part and putting back an identical or similar device in or on the same body part without cutting or puncturing the skin or a mucous membrane

Body Part (4th)	Approach (5th)	Device (6th)	Qualifier (7th)
X Upper Tendon Y Lower Tendon	X External	0 Drainage Device Y Other Device	Z No Qualifier

Section	0	Medical and Surgical
Body System	L	Tendons
Operation	5	**Destruction:** Physical eradication of all or a portion of a body part by the direct use of energy, force, or a destructive agent

Body Part (4th)	Approach (5th)	Device (6th)	Qualifier (7th)
0 Head and Neck Tendon 1 Shoulder Tendon, Right 2 Shoulder Tendon, Left 3 Upper Arm Tendon, Right 4 Upper Arm Tendon, Left 5 Lower Arm and Wrist Tendon, Right 6 Lower Arm and Wrist Tendon, Left 7 Hand Tendon, Right 8 Hand Tendon, Left 9 Trunk Tendon, Right B Trunk Tendon, Left C Thorax Tendon, Right D Thorax Tendon, Left F Abdomen Tendon, Right G Abdomen Tendon, Left H Perineum Tendon J Hip Tendon, Right K Hip Tendon, Left L Upper Leg Tendon, Right M Upper Leg Tendon, Left N Lower Leg Tendon, Right P Lower Leg Tendon, Left Q Knee Tendon, Right R Knee Tendon, Left S Ankle Tendon, Right T Ankle Tendon, Left V Foot Tendon, Right W Foot Tendon, Left	0 Open 3 Percutaneous 4 Percutaneous Endoscopic	Z No Device	Z No Qualifier

Section	0	Medical and Surgical
Body System	L	Tendons
Operation	8	**Division:** Cutting into a body part, without draining fluids and/or gases from the body part, in order to separate or transect a body part

Body Part (4th)	Approach (5th)	Device (6th)	Qualifier (7th)
0 Head and Neck Tendon	0 Open	Z No Device	Z No Qualifier
1 Shoulder Tendon, Right	3 Percutaneous		
2 Shoulder Tendon, Left	4 Percutaneous Endoscopic		
3 Upper Arm Tendon, Right			
4 Upper Arm Tendon, Left			
5 Lower Arm and Wrist Tendon, Right			
6 Lower Arm and Wrist Tendon, Left			
7 Hand Tendon, Right			
8 Hand Tendon, Left			
9 Trunk Tendon, Right			
B Trunk Tendon, Left			
C Thorax Tendon, Right			
D Thorax Tendon, Left			
F Abdomen Tendon, Right			
G Abdomen Tendon, Left			
H Perineum Tendon			
J Hip Tendon, Right			
K Hip Tendon, Left			
L Upper Leg Tendon, Right			
M Upper Leg Tendon, Left			
N Lower Leg Tendon, Right			
P Lower Leg Tendon, Left			
Q Knee Tendon, Right			
R Knee Tendon, Left			
S Ankle Tendon, Right			
T Ankle Tendon, Left			
V Foot Tendon, Right			
W Foot Tendon, Left			

Section	0	Medical and Surgical
Body System	L	Tendons
Operation	9	**Drainage:** Taking or letting out fluids and/or gases from a body part

Body Part (4th)	Approach (5th)	Device (6th)	Qualifier (7th)
0 Head and Neck Tendon	0 Open	0 Drainage Device	Z No Qualifier
1 Shoulder Tendon, Right	3 Percutaneous		
2 Shoulder Tendon, Left	4 Percutaneous Endoscopic		
3 Upper Arm Tendon, Right			
4 Upper Arm Tendon, Left			
5 Lower Arm and Wrist Tendon, Right			
6 Lower Arm and Wrist Tendon, Left			
7 Hand Tendon, Right			
8 Hand Tendon, Left			
9 Trunk Tendon, Right			
B Trunk Tendon, Left			
C Thorax Tendon, Right			
D Thorax Tendon, Left			
F Abdomen Tendon, Right			
G Abdomen Tendon, Left			
H Perineum Tendon			
J Hip Tendon, Right			
K Hip Tendon, Left			
L Upper Leg Tendon, Right			
M Upper Leg Tendon, Left			
N Lower Leg Tendon, Right			
P Lower Leg Tendon, Left			
Q Knee Tendon, Right			
R Knee Tendon, Left			
S Ankle Tendon, Right			
T Ankle Tendon, Left			
V Foot Tendon, Right			
W Foot Tendon, Left			

Continued →

Section	0	Medical and Surgical
Body System	L	Tendons
Operation	9	Drainage: Taking or letting out fluids and/or gases from a body part

0L9 Continued

Body Part (4th)	Approach (5th)	Device (6th)	Qualifier (7th)
0 Head and Neck Tendon	0 Open	Z No Device	X Diagnostic
1 Shoulder Tendon, Right	3 Percutaneous		Z No Qualifier
2 Shoulder Tendon, Left	4 Percutaneous Endoscopic		
3 Upper Arm Tendon, Right			
4 Upper Arm Tendon, Left			
5 Lower Arm and Wrist Tendon, Right			
6 Lower Arm and Wrist Tendon, Left			
7 Hand Tendon, Right			
8 Hand Tendon, Left			
9 Trunk Tendon, Right			
B Trunk Tendon, Left			
C Thorax Tendon, Right			
D Thorax Tendon, Left			
F Abdomen Tendon, Right			
G Abdomen Tendon, Left			
H Perineum Tendon			
J Hip Tendon, Right			
K Hip Tendon, Left			
L Upper Leg Tendon, Right			
M Upper Leg Tendon, Left			
N Lower Leg Tendon, Right			
P Lower Leg Tendon, Left			
Q Knee Tendon, Right			
R Knee Tendon, Left			
S Ankle Tendon, Right			
T Ankle Tendon, Left			
V Foot Tendon, Right			
W Foot Tendon, Left			

Section	0	Medical and Surgical
Body System	L	Tendons
Operation	B	Excision: Cutting out or off, without replacement, a portion of a body part

Body Part (4th)	Approach (5th)	Device (6th)	Qualifier (7th)
0 Head and Neck Tendon	0 Open	Z No Device	X Diagnostic
1 Shoulder Tendon, Right	3 Percutaneous		Z No Qualifier
2 Shoulder Tendon, Left	4 Percutaneous Endoscopic		
3 Upper Arm Tendon, Right			
4 Upper Arm Tendon, Left			
5 Lower Arm and Wrist Tendon, Right			
6 Lower Arm and Wrist Tendon, Left			
7 Hand Tendon, Right			
8 Hand Tendon, Left			
9 Trunk Tendon, Right			
B Trunk Tendon, Left			
C Thorax Tendon, Right			
D Thorax Tendon, Left			
F Abdomen Tendon, Right			
G Abdomen Tendon, Left			
H Perineum Tendon			
J Hip Tendon, Right			
K Hip Tendon, Left			
L Upper Leg Tendon, Right			
M Upper Leg Tendon, Left			
N Lower Leg Tendon, Right			
P Lower Leg Tendon, Left			
Q Knee Tendon, Right			
R Knee Tendon, Left			
S Ankle Tendon, Right			
T Ankle Tendon, Left			
V Foot Tendon, Right			
W Foot Tendon, Left			

Section	0	Medical and Surgical
Body System	L	Tendons
Operation	C	Extirpation: Taking or cutting out solid matter from a body part

Body Part (4th)	Approach (5th)	Device (6th)	Qualifier (7th)
0 Head and Neck Tendon 1 Shoulder Tendon, Right 2 Shoulder Tendon, Left 3 Upper Arm Tendon, Right 4 Upper Arm Tendon, Left 5 Lower Arm and Wrist Tendon, Right 6 Lower Arm and Wrist Tendon, Left 7 Hand Tendon, Right 8 Hand Tendon, Left 9 Trunk Tendon, Right B Trunk Tendon, Left C Thorax Tendon, Right D Thorax Tendon, Left F Abdomen Tendon, Right G Abdomen Tendon, Left H Perineum Tendon J Hip Tendon, Right K Hip Tendon, Left L Upper Leg Tendon, Right M Upper Leg Tendon, Left N Lower Leg Tendon, Right P Lower Leg Tendon, Left Q Knee Tendon, Right R Knee Tendon, Left S Ankle Tendon, Right T Ankle Tendon, Left V Foot Tendon, Right W Foot Tendon, Left	0 Open 3 Percutaneous 4 Percutaneous Endoscopic	Z No Device	Z No Qualifier

Section	0	Medical and Surgical
Body System	L	Tendons
Operation	D	Extraction: Pulling or stripping out or off all or a portion of a body part by the use of force

Body Part (4th)	Approach (5th)	Device (6th)	Qualifier (7th)
0 Head and Neck Tendon 1 Shoulder Tendon, Right 2 Shoulder Tendon, Left 3 Upper Arm Tendon, Right 4 Upper Arm Tendon, Left 5 Lower Arm and Wrist Tendon, Right 6 Lower Arm and Wrist Tendon, Left 7 Hand Tendon, Right 8 Hand Tendon, Left 9 Trunk Tendon, Right B Trunk Tendon, Left C Thorax Tendon, Right D Thorax Tendon, Left F Abdomen Tendon, Right G Abdomen Tendon, Left H Perineum Tendon J Hip Tendon, Right K Hip Tendon, Left L Upper Leg Tendon, Right M Upper Leg Tendon, Left N Lower Leg Tendon, Right P Lower Leg Tendon, Left Q Knee Tendon, Right R Knee Tendon, Left S Ankle Tendon, Right T Ankle Tendon, Left V Foot Tendon, Right W Foot Tendon, Left	0 Open	Z No Device	Z No Qualifier

Section	0	Medical and Surgical
Body System	L	Tendons
Operation	H	**Inspection:** Putting in a nonbiological appliance that monitors, assists, performs, or prevents a physiological function but does not physically take the place of a body part

Body Part (4th)	Approach (5th)	Device (6th)	Qualifier (7th)
X Upper Tendon Y Lower Tendon	0 Open 3 Percutaneous 4 Percutaneous Endoscopic	Y Other Device	Z No Qualifier

Section	0	Medical and Surgical
Body System	L	Tendons
Operation	J	**Inspection:** Visually and/or manually exploring a body part

Body Part (4th)	Approach (5th)	Device (6th)	Qualifier (7th)
X Upper Tendon Y Lower Tendon	0 Open 3 Percutaneous 4 Percutaneous Endoscopic X External	Z No Device	Z No Qualifier

Section	0	Medical and Surgical
Body System	L	Tendons
Operation	M	**Reattachment:** Putting back in or on all or a portion of a separated body part to its normal location or other suitable location

Body Part (4th)	Approach (5th)	Device (6th)	Qualifier (7th)
0 Head and Neck Tendon 1 Shoulder Tendon, Right 2 Shoulder Tendon, Left 3 Upper Arm Tendon, Right 4 Upper Arm Tendon, Left 5 Lower Arm and Wrist Tendon, Right 6 Lower Arm and Wrist Tendon, Left 7 Hand Tendon, Right 8 Hand Tendon, Left 9 Trunk Tendon, Right B Trunk Tendon, Left C Thorax Tendon, Right D Thorax Tendon, Left F Abdomen Tendon, Right G Abdomen Tendon, Left H Perineum Tendon J Hip Tendon, Right K Hip Tendon, Left L Upper Leg Tendon, Right M Upper Leg Tendon, Left N Lower Leg Tendon, Right P Lower Leg Tendon, Left Q Knee Tendon, Right R Knee Tendon, Left S Ankle Tendon, Right T Ankle Tendon, Left V Foot Tendon, Right W Foot Tendon, Left	0 Open 4 Percutaneous Endoscopic	Z No Device	Z No Qualifier

Section	0	Medical and Surgical
Body System	L	Tendons
Operation	N	**Release:** Freeing a body part from an abnormal physical constraint by cutting or by the use of force

Body Part (4th)	Approach (5th)	Device (6th)	Qualifier (7th)
0 Head and Neck Tendon	0 Open	Z No Device	Z No Qualifier
1 Shoulder Tendon, Right	3 Percutaneous		
2 Shoulder Tendon, Left	4 Percutaneous Endoscopic		
3 Upper Arm Tendon, Right	X External		
4 Upper Arm Tendon, Left			
5 Lower Arm and Wrist Tendon, Right			
6 Lower Arm and Wrist Tendon, Left			
7 Hand Tendon, Right			
8 Hand Tendon, Left			
9 Trunk Tendon, Right			
B Trunk Tendon, Left			
C Thorax Tendon, Right			
D Thorax Tendon, Left			
F Abdomen Tendon, Right			
G Abdomen Tendon, Left			
H Perineum Tendon			
J Hip Tendon, Right			
K Hip Tendon, Left			
L Upper Leg Tendon, Right			
M Upper Leg Tendon, Left			
N Lower Leg Tendon, Right			
P Lower Leg Tendon, Left			
Q Knee Tendon, Right			
R Knee Tendon, Left			
S Ankle Tendon, Right			
T Ankle Tendon, Left			
V Foot Tendon, Right			
W Foot Tendon, Left			

Section	0	Medical and Surgical
Body System	L	Tendons
Operation	P	**Removal:** Taking out or off a device from a body part

Body Part (4th)	Approach (5th)	Device (6th)	Qualifier (7th)
X Upper Tendon Y Lower Tendon	0 Open 3 Percutaneous 4 Percutaneous Endoscopic	0 Drainage Device 7 Autologous Tissue Substitute J Synthetic Substitute K Nonautologous Tissue Substitute Y Other Device	Z No Qualifier
X Upper Tendon Y Lower Tendon	X External	0 Drainage Device	Z No Qualifier

0LQ–0LR

Medical and Surgical, Tendons Tables

Section	0	Medical and Surgical
Body System	L	Tendons
Operation	Q	Repair: Restoring, to the extent possible, a body part to its normal anatomic structure and function

Body Part (4th)	Approach (5th)	Device (6th)	Qualifier (7th)
0 Head and Neck Tendon	0 Open	Z No Device	Z No Qualifier
1 Shoulder Tendon, Right	3 Percutaneous		
2 Shoulder Tendon, Left	4 Percutaneous Endoscopic		
3 Upper Arm Tendon, Right			
4 Upper Arm Tendon, Left			
5 Lower Arm and Wrist Tendon, Right			
6 Lower Arm and Wrist Tendon, Left			
7 Hand Tendon, Right			
8 Hand Tendon, Left			
9 Trunk Tendon, Right			
B Trunk Tendon, Left			
C Thorax Tendon, Right			
D Thorax Tendon, Left			
F Abdomen Tendon, Right			
G Abdomen Tendon, Left			
H Perineum Tendon			
J Hip Tendon, Right			
K Hip Tendon, Left			
L Upper Leg Tendon, Right			
M Upper Leg Tendon, Left			
N Lower Leg Tendon, Right			
P Lower Leg Tendon, Left			
Q Knee Tendon, Right			
R Knee Tendon, Left			
S Ankle Tendon, Right			
T Ankle Tendon, Left			
V Foot Tendon, Right			
W Foot Tendon, Left			

Section	0	Medical and Surgical
Body System	L	Tendons
Operation	R	Replacement: Putting in or on biological or synthetic material that physically takes the place and/or function of all or a portion of a body part

Body Part (4th)	Approach (5th)	Device (6th)	Qualifier (7th)
0 Head and Neck Tendon	0 Open	7 Autologous Tissue Substitute	Z No Qualifier
1 Shoulder Tendon, Right	4 Percutaneous Endoscopic	J Synthetic Substitute	
2 Shoulder Tendon, Left		K Nonautologous Tissue Substitute	
3 Upper Arm Tendon, Right			
4 Upper Arm Tendon, Left			
5 Lower Arm and Wrist Tendon, Right			
6 Lower Arm and Wrist Tendon, Left			
7 Hand Tendon, Right			
8 Hand Tendon, Left			
9 Trunk Tendon, Right			
B Trunk Tendon, Left			
C Thorax Tendon, Right			
D Thorax Tendon, Left			
F Abdomen Tendon, Right			
G Abdomen Tendon, Left			
H Perineum Tendon			
J Hip Tendon, Right			
K Hip Tendon, Left			
L Upper Leg Tendon, Right			
M Upper Leg Tendon, Left			
N Lower Leg Tendon, Right			
P Lower Leg Tendon, Left			
Q Knee Tendon, Right			
R Knee Tendon, Left			
S Ankle Tendon, Right			
T Ankle Tendon, Left			
V Foot Tendon, Right			
W Foot Tendon, Left			

Section	0	Medical and Surgical
Body System	L	Tendons
Operation	S	Reposition: Moving to its normal location, or other suitable location, all or a portion of a body part

Body Part (4th)	Approach (5th)	Device (6th)	Qualifier (7th)
0 Head and Neck Tendon	0 Open	Z No Device	Z No Qualifier
1 Shoulder Tendon, Right	4 Percutaneous Endoscopic		
2 Shoulder Tendon, Left			
3 Upper Arm Tendon, Right			
4 Upper Arm Tendon, Left			
5 Lower Arm and Wrist Tendon, Right			
6 Lower Arm and Wrist Tendon, Left			
7 Hand Tendon, Right			
8 Hand Tendon, Left			
9 Trunk Tendon, Right			
B Trunk Tendon, Left			
C Thorax Tendon, Right			
D Thorax Tendon, Left			
F Abdomen Tendon, Right			
G Abdomen Tendon, Left			
H Perineum Tendon			
J Hip Tendon, Right			
K Hip Tendon, Left			
L Upper Leg Tendon, Right			
M Upper Leg Tendon, Left			
N Lower Leg Tendon, Right			
P Lower Leg Tendon, Left			
Q Knee Tendon, Right			
R Knee Tendon, Left			
S Ankle Tendon, Right			
T Ankle Tendon, Left			
V Foot Tendon, Right			
W Foot Tendon, Left			

Section	0	Medical and Surgical
Body System	L	Tendons
Operation	T	Resection: Cutting out or off, without replacement, all of a body part

Body Part (4th)	Approach (5th)	Device (6th)	Qualifier (7th)
0 Head and Neck Tendon	0 Open	Z No Device	Z No Qualifier
1 Shoulder Tendon, Right	4 Percutaneous Endoscopic		
2 Shoulder Tendon, Left			
3 Upper Arm Tendon, Right			
4 Upper Arm Tendon, Left			
5 Lower Arm and Wrist Tendon, Right			
6 Lower Arm and Wrist Tendon, Left			
7 Hand Tendon, Right			
8 Hand Tendon, Left			
9 Trunk Tendon, Right			
B Trunk Tendon, Left			
C Thorax Tendon, Right			
D Thorax Tendon, Left			
F Abdomen Tendon, Right			
G Abdomen Tendon, Left			
H Perineum Tendon			
J Hip Tendon, Right			
K Hip Tendon, Left			
L Upper Leg Tendon, Right			
M Upper Leg Tendon, Left			
N Lower Leg Tendon, Right			
P Lower Leg Tendon, Left			
Q Knee Tendon, Right			
R Knee Tendon, Left			
S Ankle Tendon, Right			
T Ankle Tendon, Left			
V Foot Tendon, Right			
W Foot Tendon, Left			

0LU–0LW

Section 0 **Medical and Surgical**
Body System L **Tendons**
Operation U **Supplement:** Putting in or on biological or synthetic material that physically reinforces and/or augments the function of a portion of a body part

Body Part (4ᵗʰ)	Approach (5ᵗʰ)	Device (6ᵗʰ)	Qualifier (7ᵗʰ)
0 Head and Neck Tendon	0 Open	7 Autologous Tissue Substitute	Z No Qualifier
1 Shoulder Tendon, Right	4 Percutaneous Endoscopic	J Synthetic Substitute	
2 Shoulder Tendon, Left		K Nonautologous Tissue Substitute	
3 Upper Arm Tendon, Right			
4 Upper Arm Tendon, Left			
5 Lower Arm and Wrist Tendon, Right			
6 Lower Arm and Wrist Tendon, Left			
7 Hand Tendon, Right			
8 Hand Tendon, Left			
9 Trunk Tendon, Right			
B Trunk Tendon, Left			
C Thorax Tendon, Right			
D Thorax Tendon, Left			
F Abdomen Tendon, Right			
G Abdomen Tendon, Left			
H Perineum Tendon			
J Hip Tendon, Right			
K Hip Tendon, Left			
L Upper Leg Tendon, Right			
M Upper Leg Tendon, Left			
N Lower Leg Tendon, Right			
P Lower Leg Tendon, Left			
Q Knee Tendon, Right			
R Knee Tendon, Left			
S Ankle Tendon, Right			
T Ankle Tendon, Left			
V Foot Tendon, Right			
W Foot Tendon, Left			

Section 0 **Medical and Surgical**
Body System L **Tendons**
Operation W **Revision:** Correcting, to the extent possible, a portion of a malfunctioning device or the position of a displaced device

Body Part (4ᵗʰ)	Approach (5ᵗʰ)	Device (6ᵗʰ)	Qualifier (7ᵗʰ)
X Upper Tendon	0 Open	0 Drainage Device	Z No Qualifier
Y Lower Tendon	3 Percutaneous	7 Autologous Tissue Substitute	
	4 Percutaneous Endoscopic	J Synthetic Substitute	
		K Nonautologous Tissue Substitute	
		Y Other Device	
X Upper Tendon	X External	0 Drainage Device	Z No Qualifier
Y Lower Tendon		7 Autologous Tissue Substitute	
		J Synthetic Substitute	
		K Nonautologous Tissue Substitute	

Medical and Surgical, Tendons Tables

Section	0	Medical and Surgical
Body System	L	Tendons
Operation	X	Transfer: Moving, without taking out, all or a portion of a body part to another location to take over the function of all or a portion of a body part

Body Part (4th)	Approach (5th)	Device (6th)	Qualifier (7th)
0 Head and Neck Tendon	0 Open	Z No Device	Z No Qualifier
1 Shoulder Tendon, Right	4 Percutaneous Endoscopic		
2 Shoulder Tendon, Left			
3 Upper Arm Tendon, Right			
4 Upper Arm Tendon, Left			
5 Lower Arm and Wrist Tendon, Right			
6 Lower Arm and Wrist Tendon, Left			
7 Hand Tendon, Right			
8 Hand Tendon, Left			
9 Trunk Tendon, Right			
B Trunk Tendon, Left			
C Thorax Tendon, Right			
D Thorax Tendon, Left			
F Abdomen Tendon, Right			
G Abdomen Tendon, Left			
H Perineum Tendon			
J Hip Tendon, Right			
K Hip Tendon, Left			
L Upper Leg Tendon, Right			
M Upper Leg Tendon, Left			
N Lower Leg Tendon, Right			
P Lower Leg Tendon, Left			
Q Knee Tendon, Right			
R Knee Tendon, Left			
S Ankle Tendon, Right			
T Ankle Tendon, Left			
V Foot Tendon, Right			
W Foot Tendon, Left			

AHA Coding Clinic

0L8J0ZZ Division of Right Hip Tendon, Open Approach—AHA CC: 3Q, 2016, 30-31

0LB60ZZ Excision of Left Lower Arm and Wrist Tendon, Open Approach—AHA CC: 3Q, 2015, 26-27

0LBL0ZZ Excision of Right Upper Leg Tendon, Open Approach—AHA CC: 2Q, 2017, 21-22

0LBP0ZZ Excision of Left Lower Leg Tendon, Open Approach—AHA CC: 3Q, 2014, 18-19

0LBT0ZZ Excision of Left Ankle Tendon, Open Approach—AHA CC: 3Q, 2014, 14-15

0LQ14ZZ Repair Right Shoulder Tendon, Percutaneous Endoscopic Approach—AHA CC: 3Q, 2013, 20-22; 3Q, 2016, 32-33

0LS30ZZ Reposition Right Upper Arm Tendon, Open Approach—AHA CC: 3Q, 2016, 32-33

0LS40ZZ Reposition Left Upper Arm Tendon, Open Approach—AHA CC: 3Q, 2015, 14-15

0LUM0KZ Supplement Left Upper Leg Tendon with Nonautologous Tissue Substitute, Open Approach—AHA CC: 2Q, 2015, 11

0LUQ0KZ Supplement Right Knee Tendon with Nonautologous Tissue Substitute, Open Approach—AHA CC: 2Q, 2015, 11

Bursae and Ligaments

Bursa of the Knee

Ligaments of the Knee

Shoulder Tendons and Ligaments

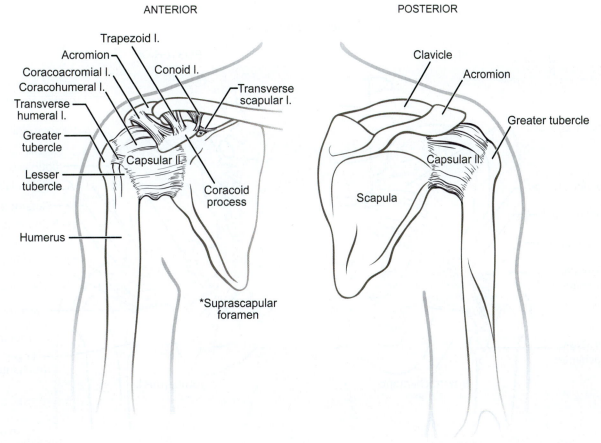

Knee Tendons and Ligaments

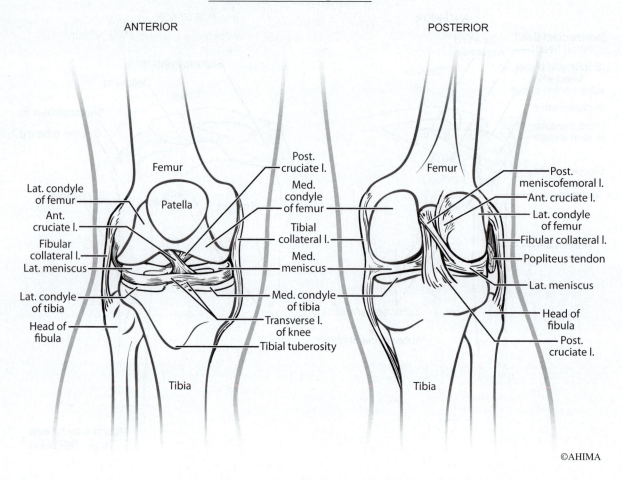

Hip Tendons and Ligaments

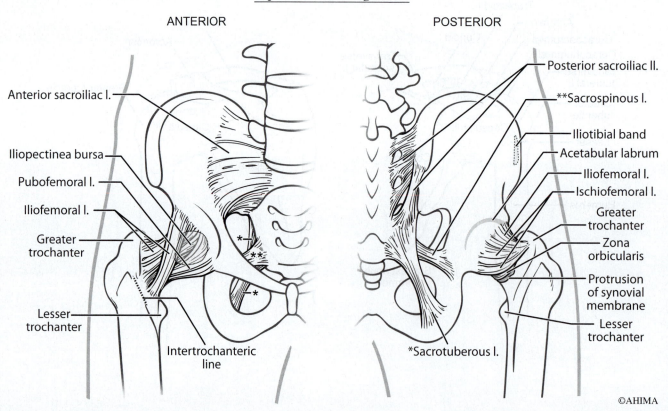

Bursae and Ligaments Tables 0M2–0MX

Section	0	Medical and Surgical
Body System	M	Bursae and Ligaments
Operation	2	**Change:** Taking out or off a device from a body part and putting back an identical or similar device in or on the same body part without cutting or puncturing the skin or a mucous membrane

Body Part (4th)	Approach (5th)	Device (6th)	Qualifier (7th)
X Upper Bursa and Ligament Y Lower Bursa and Ligament	X External	0 Drainage Device Y Other Device	Z No Qualifier

Section	0	Medical and Surgical
Body System	M	Bursae and Ligaments
Operation	5	**Destruction:** Physical eradication of all or a portion of a body part by the direct use of energy, force, or a destructive agent

Body Part (4th)	Approach (5th)	Device (6th)	Qualifier (7th)
0 Head and Neck Bursa and Ligament 1 Shoulder Bursa and Ligament, Right 2 Shoulder Bursa and Ligament, Left 3 Elbow Bursa and Ligament, Right 4 Elbow Bursa and Ligament, Left 5 Wrist Bursa and Ligament, Right 6 Wrist Bursa and Ligament, Left 7 Hand Bursa and Ligament, Right 8 Hand Bursa and Ligament, Left 9 Upper Extremity Bursa and Ligament, Right B Upper Extremity Bursa and Ligament, Left C Upper Spine Bursa and Ligament, Right D Lower Spine Bursa and Ligament, Left F Sternum Bursa and Ligament, Right G Rib(s) Bursa and Ligament, Left H Abdomen Bursa and Ligament, Right J Abdomen Bursa and Ligament, Left K Perineum Bursa and Ligament L Hip Bursa and Ligament, Right M Hip Bursa and Ligament, Left N Knee Bursa and Ligament, Right P Knee Bursa and Ligament, Left Q Ankle Bursa and Ligament, Right R Ankle Bursa and Ligament, Left S Foot Bursa and Ligament, Right T Foot Bursa and Ligament, Left V Lower Extremity Bursa and Ligament, Right W Lower Extremity Bursa and Ligament, Left	0 Open 3 Percutaneous 4 Percutaneous Endoscopic	Z No Device	Z No Qualifier

Section	0	Medical and Surgical
Body System	M	Bursae and Ligaments
Operation	8	**Division:** Cutting into a body part, without draining fluids and/or gases from the body part, in order to separate or transect a body part

Body Part (4th)	Approach (5th)	Device (6th)	Qualifier (7th)
0 Head and Neck Bursa and Ligament	0 Open	Z No Device	Z No Qualifier
1 Shoulder Bursa and Ligament, Right	3 Percutaneous		
2 Shoulder Bursa and Ligament, Left	4 Percutaneous Endoscopic		
3 Elbow Bursa and Ligament, Right			
4 Elbow Bursa and Ligament, Left			
5 Wrist Bursa and Ligament, Right			
6 Wrist Bursa and Ligament, Left			
7 Hand Bursa and Ligament, Right			
8 Hand Bursa and Ligament, Left			
9 Upper Extremity Bursa and Ligament, Right			
B Upper Extremity Bursa and Ligament, Left			
C Upper Spine Bursa and Ligament, Right			
D Lower Spine Bursa and Ligament, Left			
F Sternum Bursa and Ligament, Right			
G Rib(s) Bursa and Ligament, Left			
H Abdomen Bursa and Ligament, Right			
J Abdomen Bursa and Ligament, Left			
K Perineum Bursa and Ligament			
L Hip Bursa and Ligament, Right			
M Hip Bursa and Ligament, Left			
N Knee Bursa and Ligament, Right			
P Knee Bursa and Ligament, Left			
Q Ankle Bursa and Ligament, Right			
R Ankle Bursa and Ligament, Left			
S Foot Bursa and Ligament, Right			
T Foot Bursa and Ligament, Left			
V Lower Extremity Bursa and Ligament, Right			
W Lower Extremity Bursa and Ligament, Left			

Section	0	Medical and Surgical
Body System	M	Bursae and Ligaments
Operation	9	**Drainage:** Taking or letting out fluids and/or gases from a body part

Body Part (4th)	Approach (5th)	Device (6th)	Qualifier (7th)
0 Head and Neck Bursa and Ligament	0 Open	0 Drainage Device	Z No Qualifier
1 Shoulder Bursa and Ligament, Right	3 Percutaneous		
2 Shoulder Bursa and Ligament, Left	4 Percutaneous Endoscopic		
3 Elbow Bursa and Ligament, Right			
4 Elbow Bursa and Ligament, Left			
5 Wrist Bursa and Ligament, Right			
6 Wrist Bursa and Ligament, Left			
7 Hand Bursa and Ligament, Right			
8 Hand Bursa and Ligament, Left			
9 Upper Extremity Bursa and Ligament, Right			
B Upper Extremity Bursa and Ligament, Left			
C Upper Spine Bursa and Ligament, Right			
D Lower Spine Bursa and Ligament, Left			
F Sternum Bursa and Ligament, Right			
G Rib(s) Bursa and Ligament, Left			
H Abdomen Bursa and Ligament, Right			
J Abdomen Bursa and Ligament, Left			
K Perineum Bursa and Ligament			
L Hip Bursa and Ligament, Right			
M Hip Bursa and Ligament, Left			
N Knee Bursa and Ligament, Right			
P Knee Bursa and Ligament, Left			
Q Ankle Bursa and Ligament, Right			
R Ankle Bursa and Ligament, Left			
S Foot Bursa and Ligament, Right			
T Foot Bursa and Ligament, Left			
V Lower Extremity Bursa and Ligament, Right			
W Lower Extremity Bursa and Ligament, Left			

Continued →

Section	0	Medical and Surgical
Body System	M	Bursae and Ligaments
Operation	9	**Drainage:** Taking or letting out fluids and/or gases from a body part

0M9 Continued

Body Part (4ᵗʰ)	Approach (5ᵗʰ)	Device (6ᵗʰ)	Qualifier (7ᵗʰ)
0 Head and Neck Bursa and Ligament 1 Shoulder Bursa and Ligament, Right 2 Shoulder Bursa and Ligament, Left 3 Elbow Bursa and Ligament, Right 4 Elbow Bursa and Ligament, Left 5 Wrist Bursa and Ligament, Right 6 Wrist Bursa and Ligament, Left 7 Hand Bursa and Ligament, Right 8 Hand Bursa and Ligament, Left 9 Upper Extremity Bursa and Ligament, Right B Upper Extremity Bursa and Ligament, Left C Upper Spine Bursa and Ligament, Right D Lower Spine Bursa and Ligament, Left F Sternum Bursa and Ligament, Right G Rib(s) Bursa and Ligament, Left H Abdomen Bursa and Ligament, Right J Abdomen Bursa and Ligament, Left K Perineum Bursa and Ligament L Hip Bursa and Ligament, Right M Hip Bursa and Ligament, Left N Knee Bursa and Ligament, Right P Knee Bursa and Ligament, Left Q Ankle Bursa and Ligament, Right R Ankle Bursa and Ligament, Left S Foot Bursa and Ligament, Right T Foot Bursa and Ligament, Left V Lower Extremity Bursa and Ligament, Right W Lower Extremity Bursa and Ligament, Left	0 Open 3 Percutaneous 4 Percutaneous Endoscopic	Z No Device	X Diagnostic Z No Qualifier

Section	0	Medical and Surgical
Body System	M	Bursae and Ligaments
Operation	B	**Excision:** Cutting out or off, without replacement, a portion of a body part

Body Part (4ᵗʰ)	Approach (5ᵗʰ)	Device (6ᵗʰ)	Qualifier (7ᵗʰ)
0 Head and Neck Bursa and Ligament 1 Shoulder Bursa and Ligament, Right 2 Shoulder Bursa and Ligament, Left 3 Elbow Bursa and Ligament, Right 4 Elbow Bursa and Ligament, Left 5 Wrist Bursa and Ligament, Right 6 Wrist Bursa and Ligament, Left 7 Hand Bursa and Ligament, Right 8 Hand Bursa and Ligament, Left 9 Upper Extremity Bursa and Ligament, Right B Upper Extremity Bursa and Ligament, Left C Upper Spine Bursa and Ligament, Right D Lower Spine Bursa and Ligament, Left F Sternum Bursa and Ligament, Right G Rib(s) Bursa and Ligament, Left H Abdomen Bursa and Ligament, Right J Abdomen Bursa and Ligament, Left K Perineum Bursa and Ligament L Hip Bursa and Ligament, Right M Hip Bursa and Ligament, Left N Knee Bursa and Ligament, Right P Knee Bursa and Ligament, Left Q Ankle Bursa and Ligament, Right R Ankle Bursa and Ligament, Left S Foot Bursa and Ligament, Right T Foot Bursa and Ligament, Left V Lower Extremity Bursa and Ligament, Right W Lower Extremity Bursa and Ligament, Left	0 Open 3 Percutaneous 4 Percutaneous Endoscopic	Z No Device	X Diagnostic Z No Qualifier

Section	0	Medical and Surgical
Body System	M	Bursae and Ligaments
Operation	C	Extirpation: Taking or cutting out solid matter from a body part

Body Part (4th)	Approach (5th)	Device (6th)	Qualifier (7th)
0 Head and Neck Bursa and Ligament 1 Shoulder Bursa and Ligament, Right 2 Shoulder Bursa and Ligament, Left 3 Elbow Bursa and Ligament, Right 4 Elbow Bursa and Ligament, Left 5 Wrist Bursa and Ligament, Right 6 Wrist Bursa and Ligament, Left 7 Hand Bursa and Ligament, Right 8 Hand Bursa and Ligament, Left 9 Upper Extremity Bursa and Ligament, Right B Upper Extremity Bursa and Ligament, Left C Upper Spine Bursa and Ligament, Right D Trunk Bursa and Ligament, Left F Sternum Bursa and Ligament, Right G Rib(s) Bursa and Ligament, Left H Abdomen Bursa and Ligament, Right J Abdomen Bursa and Ligament, Left K Perineum Bursa and Ligament L Hip Bursa and Ligament, Right M Hip Bursa and Ligament, Left N Knee Bursa and Ligament, Right P Knee Bursa and Ligament, Left Q Ankle Bursa and Ligament, Right R Ankle Bursa and Ligament, Left S Foot Bursa and Ligament, Right T Foot Bursa and Ligament, Left V Lower Extremity Bursa and Ligament, Right W Lower Extremity Bursa and Ligament, Left	0 Open 3 Percutaneous 4 Percutaneous Endoscopic	Z No Device	Z No Qualifier

Section	0	Medical and Surgical
Body System	M	Bursae and Ligaments
Operation	D	Extraction: Pulling or stripping out or off all or a portion of a body part by the use of force

Body Part (4th)	Approach (5th)	Device (6th)	Qualifier (7th)
0 Head and Neck Bursa and Ligament 1 Shoulder Bursa and Ligament, Right 2 Shoulder Bursa and Ligament, Left 3 Elbow Bursa and Ligament, Right 4 Elbow Bursa and Ligament, Left 5 Wrist Bursa and Ligament, Right 6 Wrist Bursa and Ligament, Left 7 Hand Bursa and Ligament, Right 8 Hand Bursa and Ligament, Left 9 Upper Extremity Bursa and Ligament, Right B Upper Extremity Bursa and Ligament, Left C Upper Spine Bursa and Ligament, Right D Lower Spine Bursa and Ligament, Left F Sternum Bursa and Ligament, Right G Rib(s) Bursa and Ligament, Left H Abdomen Bursa and Ligament, Right J Abdomen Bursa and Ligament, Left K Perineum Bursa and Ligament L Hip Bursa and Ligament, Right M Hip Bursa and Ligament, Left N Knee Bursa and Ligament, Right P Knee Bursa and Ligament, Left Q Ankle Bursa and Ligament, Right R Ankle Bursa and Ligament, Left S Foot Bursa and Ligament, Right T Foot Bursa and Ligament, Left V Lower Extremity Bursa and Ligament, Right W Lower Extremity Bursa and Ligament, Left	0 Open 3 Percutaneous 4 Percutaneous Endoscopic	Z No Device	Z No Qualifier

Section	0	Medical and Surgical
Body System	M	Bursae and Ligaments
Operation	H	Insertion: Putting in a nonbiological appliance that monitors, assists, performs, or prevents a physiological function but does not physically take the place of a body part

Body Part (4th)	Approach (5th)	Device (6th)	Qualifier (7th)
X Upper Bursa and Ligament Y Lower Bursa and Ligament	0 Open 3 Percutaneous 4 Percutaneous Endoscopic	Y Other Device	Z No Qualifier

Section	0	Medical and Surgical
Body System	M	Bursae and Ligaments
Operation	J	Inspection: Visually and/or manually exploring a body part

Body Part (4th)	Approach (5th)	Device (6th)	Qualifier (7th)
X Upper Bursa and Ligament Y Lower Bursa and Ligament	0 Open 3 Percutaneous 4 Percutaneous Endoscopic X External	Z No Device	Z No Qualifier

Section	0	Medical and Surgical
Body System	M	Bursae and Ligaments
Operation	M	Reattachment: Putting back in or on all or a portion of a separated body part to its normal location or other suitable location

Body Part (4th)	Approach (5th)	Device (6th)	Qualifier (7th)
0 Head and Neck Bursa and Ligament 1 Shoulder Bursa and Ligament, Right 2 Shoulder Bursa and Ligament, Left 3 Elbow Bursa and Ligament, Right 4 Elbow Bursa and Ligament, Left 5 Wrist Bursa and Ligament, Right 6 Wrist Bursa and Ligament, Left 7 Hand Bursa and Ligament, Right 8 Hand Bursa and Ligament, Left 9 Upper Extremity Bursa and Ligament, Right B Upper Extremity Bursa and Ligament, Left C Upper Spine Bursa and Ligament, Right D Lower Spine Bursa and Ligament, Left F Sternum Bursa and Ligament, Right G Rib(s) Bursa and Ligament, Left H Abdomen Bursa and Ligament, Right J Abdomen Bursa and Ligament, Left K Perineum Bursa and Ligament L Hip Bursa and Ligament, Right M Hip Bursa and Ligament, Left N Knee Bursa and Ligament, Right P Knee Bursa and Ligament, Left Q Ankle Bursa and Ligament, Right R Ankle Bursa and Ligament, Left S Foot Bursa and Ligament, Right T Foot Bursa and Ligament, Left V Lower Extremity Bursa and Ligament, Right W Lower Extremity Bursa and Ligament, Left	0 Open 4 Percutaneous Endoscopic	Z No Device	Z No Qualifier

0MN–0MP

Medical and Surgical, Bursae and Ligaments Tables

Section	0	Medical and Surgical
Body System	M	Bursae and Ligaments
Operation	N	**Release:** Freeing a body part from an abnormal physical constraint by cutting or by the use of force

Body Part (4th)	Approach (5th)	Device (6th)	Qualifier (7th)
0 Head and Neck Bursa and Ligament	0 Open	Z No Device	Z No Qualifier
1 Shoulder Bursa and Ligament, Right	3 Percutaneous		
2 Shoulder Bursa and Ligament, Left	4 Percutaneous Endoscopic		
3 Elbow Bursa and Ligament, Right	X External		
4 Elbow Bursa and Ligament, Left			
5 Wrist Bursa and Ligament, Right			
6 Wrist Bursa and Ligament, Left			
7 Hand Bursa and Ligament, Right			
8 Hand Bursa and Ligament, Left			
9 Upper Extremity Bursa and Ligament, Right			
B Upper Extremity Bursa and Ligament, Left			
C Upper Spine Bursa and Ligament, Right			
D Lower Spine Bursa and Ligament, Left			
F Sternum Bursa and Ligament, Right			
G Rib(s) Bursa and Ligament, Left			
H Abdomen Bursa and Ligament, Right			
J Abdomen Bursa and Ligament, Left			
K Perineum Bursa and Ligament			
L Hip Bursa and Ligament, Right			
M Hip Bursa and Ligament, Left			
N Knee Bursa and Ligament, Right			
P Knee Bursa and Ligament, Left			
Q Ankle Bursa and Ligament, Right			
R Ankle Bursa and Ligament, Left			
S Foot Bursa and Ligament, Right			
T Foot Bursa and Ligament, Left			
V Lower Extremity Bursa and Ligament, Right			
W Lower Extremity Bursa and Ligament, Left			

Section	0	Medical and Surgical
Body System	M	Bursae and Ligaments
Operation	P	**Removal:** Taking out or off a device from a body part

Body Part (4th)	Approach (5th)	Device (6th)	Qualifier (7th)
X Upper Bursa and Ligament Y Lower Bursa and Ligament	0 Open 3 Percutaneous 4 Percutaneous Endoscopic	0 Drainage Device 7 Autologous Tissue Substitute J Synthetic Substitute K Nonautologous Tissue Substitute Y Other Device	Z No Qualifier
X Upper Bursa and Ligament Y Lower Bursa and Ligament	X External	0 Drainage Device	Z No Qualifier

378

Section	0	Medical and Surgical
Body System	M	Bursae and Ligaments
Operation	Q	Repair: Restoring, to the extent possible, a body part to its normal anatomic structure and function

Body Part (4th)	Approach (5th)	Device (6th)	Qualifier (7th)
0 Head and Neck Bursa and Ligament	0 Open	Z No Device	Z No Qualifier
1 Shoulder Bursa and Ligament, Right	3 Percutaneous		
2 Shoulder Bursa and Ligament, Left	4 Percutaneous Endoscopic		
3 Elbow Bursa and Ligament, Right			
4 Elbow Bursa and Ligament, Left			
5 Wrist Bursa and Ligament, Right			
6 Wrist Bursa and Ligament, Left			
7 Hand Bursa and Ligament, Right			
8 Hand Bursa and Ligament, Left			
9 Upper Extremity Bursa and Ligament, Right			
B Upper Extremity Bursa and Ligament, Left			
C Upper Spine Bursa and Ligament, Right			
D Lower Spine Bursa and Ligament, Left			
F Sternum Bursa and Ligament, Right			
G Rib(s) Bursa and Ligament, Left			
H Abdomen Bursa and Ligament, Right			
J Abdomen Bursa and Ligament, Left			
K Perineum Bursa and Ligament			
L Hip Bursa and Ligament, Right			
M Hip Bursa and Ligament, Left			
N Knee Bursa and Ligament, Right			
P Knee Bursa and Ligament, Left			
Q Ankle Bursa and Ligament, Right			
R Ankle Bursa and Ligament, Left			
S Foot Bursa and Ligament, Right			
T Foot Bursa and Ligament, Left			
V Lower Extremity Bursa and Ligament, Right			
W Lower Extremity Bursa and Ligament, Left			

Section	0	Medical and Surgical
Body System	M	Bursae and Ligaments
Operation	R	Replacement: Putting in or on biological or synthetic material that physically takes the place and/or function of all or a portion of a body part

Body Part (4th)	Approach (5th)	Device (6th)	Qualifier (7th)
0 Head and Neck Bursa and Ligament	0 Open	7 Autologous Tissue Substitute	Z No Qualifier
1 Shoulder Bursa and Ligament, Right	4 Percutaneous Endoscopic	J Synthetic Substitute	
2 Shoulder Bursa and Ligament, Left		K Nonautologous Tissue Substitute	
3 Elbow Bursa and Ligament, Right			
4 Elbow Bursa and Ligament, Left			
5 Wrist Bursa and Ligament, Right			
6 Wrist Bursa and Ligament, Left			
7 Hand Bursa and Ligament, Right			
8 Hand Bursa and Ligament, Left			
9 Upper Extremity Bursa and Ligament, Right			
B Upper Extremity Bursa and Ligament, Left			
C Upper Spine Bursa and Ligament			
D Lower Spine Bursa and Ligament			
F Sternum Bursa and Ligament			
G Rib(s) Bursa and Ligament			
H Abdomen Bursa and Ligament, Right			
J Abdomen Bursa and Ligament, Left			
K Perineum Bursa and Ligament			
L Hip Bursa and Ligament, Right			
M Hip Bursa and Ligament, Left			
N Knee Bursa and Ligament, Right			
P Knee Bursa and Ligament, Left			
Q Ankle Bursa and Ligament, Right			
R Ankle Bursa and Ligament, Left			
S Foot Bursa and Ligament, Right			
T Foot Bursa and Ligament, Left			
V Lower Extremity Bursa and Ligament, Right			
W Lower Extremity Bursa and Ligament, Left			

0MS–0MT

Section	0	Medical and Surgical
Body System	M	Bursae and Ligaments
Operation	S	Reposition: Moving to its normal location, or other suitable location, all or a portion of a body part

Body Part (4th)	Approach (5th)	Device (6th)	Qualifier (7th)
0 Head and Neck Bursa and Ligament 1 Shoulder Bursa and Ligament, Right 2 Shoulder Bursa and Ligament, Left 3 Elbow Bursa and Ligament, Right 4 Elbow Bursa and Ligament, Left 5 Wrist Bursa and Ligament, Right 6 Wrist Bursa and Ligament, Left 7 Hand Bursa and Ligament, Right 8 Hand Bursa and Ligament, Left 9 Upper Extremity Bursa and Ligament, Right B Upper Extremity Bursa and Ligament, Left C Upper Spine Bursa and Ligament, Right D Lower Spine Bursa and Ligament, Left F Sternum Bursa and Ligament, Right G Rib(s) Bursa and Ligament, Left H Abdomen Bursa and Ligament, Right J Abdomen Bursa and Ligament, Left K Perineum Bursa and Ligament L Hip Bursa and Ligament, Right M Hip Bursa and Ligament, Left N Knee Bursa and Ligament, Right P Knee Bursa and Ligament, Left Q Ankle Bursa and Ligament, Right R Ankle Bursa and Ligament, Left S Foot Bursa and Ligament, Right T Foot Bursa and Ligament, Left V Lower Extremity Bursa and Ligament, Right W Lower Extremity Bursa and Ligament, Left	0 Open 4 Percutaneous Endoscopic	Z No Device	Z No Qualifier

Section	0	Medical and Surgical
Body System	M	Bursae and Ligaments
Operation	T	Resection: Cutting out or off, without replacement, all of a body part

Body Part (4th)	Approach (5th)	Device (6th)	Qualifier (7th)
0 Head and Neck Bursa and Ligament 1 Shoulder Bursa and Ligament, Right 2 Shoulder Bursa and Ligament, Left 3 Elbow Bursa and Ligament, Right 4 Elbow Bursa and Ligament, Left 5 Wrist Bursa and Ligament, Right 6 Wrist Bursa and Ligament, Left 7 Hand Bursa and Ligament, Right 8 Hand Bursa and Ligament, Left 9 Upper Extremity Bursa and Ligament, Right B Upper Extremity Bursa and Ligament, Left C Upper Spine Bursa and Ligament, Right D Lower Spine Bursa and Ligament, Left F Sternum Bursa and Ligament, Right G Rib(s) Bursa and Ligament, Left H Abdomen Bursa and Ligament, Right J Abdomen Bursa and Ligament, Left K Perineum Bursa and Ligament L Hip Bursa and Ligament, Right M Hip Bursa and Ligament, Left N Knee Bursa and Ligament, Right P Knee Bursa and Ligament, Left Q Ankle Bursa and Ligament, Right R Ankle Bursa and Ligament, Left S Foot Bursa and Ligament, Right T Foot Bursa and Ligament, Left V Lower Extremity Bursa and Ligament, Right W Lower Extremity Bursa and Ligament, Left	0 Open 4 Percutaneous Endoscopic	Z No Device	Z No Qualifier

Section	0	Medical and Surgical
Body System	M	Bursae and Ligaments
Operation	U	**Supplement:** Putting in or on biological or synthetic material that physically reinforces and/or augments the function of a portion of a body part

Body Part (4th)	Approach (5th)	Device (6th)	Qualifier (7th)
0 Head and Neck Bursa and Ligament 1 Shoulder Bursa and Ligament, Right 2 Shoulder Bursa and Ligament, Left 3 Elbow Bursa and Ligament, Right 4 Elbow Bursa and Ligament, Left 5 Wrist Bursa and Ligament, Right 6 Wrist Bursa and Ligament, Left 7 Hand Bursa and Ligament, Right 8 Hand Bursa and Ligament, Left 9 Upper Extremity Bursa and Ligament, Right B Upper Extremity Bursa and Ligament, Left C Upper Spine Bursa and Ligament, Right D Lower Spine Bursa and Ligament, Left F Sternum Bursa and Ligament, Right G Rib(s) Bursa and Ligament, Left H Abdomen Bursa and Ligament, Right J Abdomen Bursa and Ligament, Left K Perineum Bursa and Ligament L Hip Bursa and Ligament, Right M Hip Bursa and Ligament, Left N Knee Bursa and Ligament, Right P Knee Bursa and Ligament, Left Q Ankle Bursa and Ligament, Right R Ankle Bursa and Ligament, Left S Foot Bursa and Ligament, Right T Foot Bursa and Ligament, Left V Lower Extremity Bursa and Ligament, Right W Lower Extremity Bursa and Ligament, Left	0 Open 4 Percutaneous Endoscopic	7 Autologous Tissue Substitute J Synthetic Substitute K Nonautologous Tissue Substitute	Z No Qualifier

Section	0	Medical and Surgical
Body System	M	Bursae and Ligaments
Operation	W	**Revision:** Correcting, to the extent possible, a portion of a malfunctioning device or the position of a displaced device

Body Part (4th)	Approach (5th)	Device (6th)	Qualifier (7th)
X Upper Bursa and Ligament Y Lower Bursa and Ligament	0 Open 3 Percutaneous 4 Percutaneous Endoscopic	0 Drainage Device 7 Autologous Tissue Substitute J Synthetic Substitute K Nonautologous Tissue Substitute Y Other Device	Z No Qualifier
X Upper Bursa and Ligament Y Lower Bursa and Ligament	X External	0 Drainage Device 7 Autologous Tissue Substitute J Synthetic Substitute K Nonautologous Tissue Substitute	Z No Qualifier

Section	0	Medical and Surgical
Body System	M	Bursae and Ligaments
Operation	X	**Transfer:** Moving, without taking out, all or a portion of a body part to another location to take over the function of all or a portion of a body part

Body Part (4th)	Approach (5th)	Device (6th)	Qualifier (7th)
0 Head and Neck Bursa and Ligament	0 Open	Z No Device	Z No Qualifier
1 Shoulder Bursa and Ligament, Right	4 Percutaneous Endoscopic		
2 Shoulder Bursa and Ligament, Left			
3 Elbow Bursa and Ligament, Right			
4 Elbow Bursa and Ligament, Left			
5 Wrist Bursa and Ligament, Right			
6 Wrist Bursa and Ligament, Left			
7 Hand Bursa and Ligament, Right			
8 Hand Bursa and Ligament, Left			
9 Upper Extremity Bursa and Ligament, Right			
B Upper Extremity Bursa and Ligament, Left			
C Upper Spine Bursa and Ligament, Right			
D Lower Spine Bursa and Ligament, Left			
F Sternum Bursa and Ligament, Right			
G Rib(s) Bursa and Ligament, Left			
H Abdomen Bursa and Ligament, Right			
J Abdomen Bursa and Ligament, Left			
K Perineum Bursa and Ligament			
L Hip Bursa and Ligament, Right			
M Hip Bursa and Ligament, Left			
N Knee Bursa and Ligament, Right			
P Knee Bursa and Ligament, Left			
Q Ankle Bursa and Ligament, Right			
R Ankle Bursa and Ligament, Left			
S Foot Bursa and Ligament, Right			
T Foot Bursa and Ligament, Left			
V Lower Extremity Bursa and Ligament, Right			
W Lower Extremity Bursa and Ligament, Left			

AHA Coding Clinic

0MM14ZZ Reattachment of Right Shoulder Bursa and Ligament, Percutaneous Endoscopic Approach—AHA CC: 3Q, 2013, 20-22

0MQ00ZZ Repair Head and Neck Bursa and Ligament, Open Approach—AHA CC: 3Q, 2014, 9

0MUN47Z Supplement Right Knee Bursa and Ligament with Autologous Tissue Substitute, Percutaneous Endoscopic Approach— AHA CC: 2Q, 2017, 21-22

Head and Facial Bones

Head and Facial Bones

©AHIMA

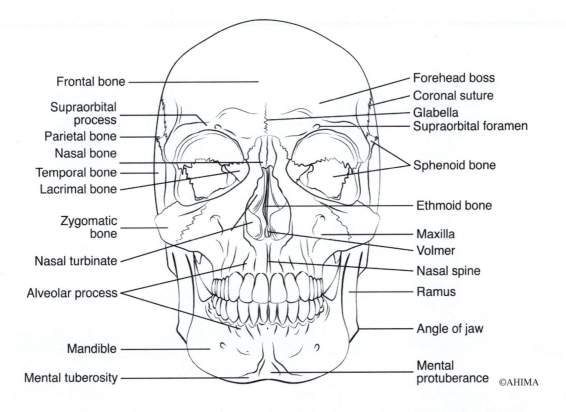

©AHIMA

Head and Facial Bones Tables 0N2–0NW

Section	0	Medical and Surgical
Body System	N	Head and Facial Bones
Operation	2	**Change:** Taking out or off a device from a body part and putting back an identical or similar device in or on the same body part without cutting or puncturing the skin or a mucous membrane

Body Part (4th)	Approach (5th)	Device (6th)	Qualifier (7th)
0 Skull **B** Nasal Bone **W** Facial Bone	**X** External	**0** Drainage Device **Y** Other Device	**Z** No Qualifier

Section	0	Medical and Surgical
Body System	N	Head and Facial Bones
Operation	5	**Destruction:** Physical eradication of all or a portion of a body part by the direct use of energy, force, or a destructive agent

Body Part (4th)	Approach (5th)	Device (6th)	Qualifier (7th)
0 Skull **1** Frontal Bone **3** Parietal Bone, Right **4** Parietal Bone, Left **5** Temporal Bone, Right **6** Temporal Bone, Left **7** Occipital Bone **B** Nasal Bone **C** Sphenoid Bone **F** Ethmoid Bone, Right **G** Ethmoid Bone, Left **H** Lacrimal Bone, Right **J** Lacrimal Bone, Left **K** Palatine Bone, Right **L** Palatine Bone, Left **M** Zygomatic Bone, Right **N** Zygomatic Bone, Left **P** Orbit, Right **Q** Orbit, Left **R** Maxilla **T** Mandible, Right **V** Mandible, Left **X** Hyoid Bone	**0** Open **3** Percutaneous **4** Percutaneous Endoscopic	**Z** No Device	**Z** No Qualifier

Section	0	Medical and Surgical
Body System	N	Head and Facial Bones
Operation	8	**Division:** Cutting into a body part, without draining fluids and/or gases from the body part, in order to separate or transect a body part

Body Part (4th)	Approach (5th)	Device (6th)	Qualifier (7th)
0 Skull	0 Open	Z No Device	Z No Qualifier
1 Frontal Bone	3 Percutaneous		
3 Parietal Bone, Right	4 Percutaneous Endoscopic		
4 Parietal Bone, Left			
5 Temporal Bone, Right			
6 Temporal Bone, Left			
7 Occipital Bone			
B Nasal Bone			
C Sphenoid Bone			
F Ethmoid Bone, Right			
G Ethmoid Bone, Left			
H Lacrimal Bone, Right			
J Lacrimal Bone, Left			
K Palatine Bone, Right			
L Palatine Bone, Left			
M Zygomatic Bone, Right			
N Zygomatic Bone, Left			
P Orbit, Right			
Q Orbit, Left			
R Maxilla			
T Mandible, Right			
V Mandible, Left			
X Hyoid Bone			

Section	0	Medical and Surgical
Body System	N	Head and Facial Bones
Operation	9	**Drainage:** Taking or letting out fluids and/or gases from a body part

Body Part (4th)	Approach (5th)	Device (6th)	Qualifier (7th)
0 Skull	0 Open	0 Drainage Device	Z No Qualifier
1 Frontal Bone	3 Percutaneous		
3 Parietal Bone, Right	4 Percutaneous Endoscopic		
4 Parietal Bone, Left			
5 Temporal Bone, Right			
6 Temporal Bone, Left			
7 Occipital Bone			
B Nasal Bone			
C Sphenoid Bone			
F Ethmoid Bone, Right			
G Ethmoid Bone, Left			
H Lacrimal Bone, Right			
J Lacrimal Bone, Left			
K Palatine Bone, Right			
L Palatine Bone, Left			
M Zygomatic Bone, Right			
N Zygomatic Bone, Left			
P Orbit, Right			
Q Orbit, Left			
R Maxilla			
T Mandible, Right			
V Mandible, Left			
X Hyoid Bone			

Continued →

Section   0   **Medical and Surgical**
Body System   N   **Head and Facial Bones**
Operation   9   **Drainage:** Taking or letting out fluids and/or gases from a body part

Body Part (4ᵗʰ)	Approach (5ᵗʰ)	Device (6ᵗʰ)	Qualifier (7ᵗʰ)
0 Skull	0 Open	Z No Device	X Diagnostic
1 Frontal Bone	3 Percutaneous		Z No Qualifier
3 Parietal Bone, Right	4 Percutaneous Endoscopic		
4 Parietal Bone, Left			
5 Temporal Bone, Right			
6 Temporal Bone, Left			
7 Occipital Bone			
B Nasal Bone			
C Sphenoid Bone			
F Ethmoid Bone, Right			
G Ethmoid Bone, Left			
H Lacrimal Bone, Right			
J Lacrimal Bone, Left			
K Palatine Bone, Right			
L Palatine Bone, Left			
M Zygomatic Bone, Right			
N Zygomatic Bone, Left			
P Orbit, Right			
Q Orbit, Left			
R Maxilla			
T Mandible, Right			
V Mandible, Left			
X Hyoid Bone			

Section   0   **Medical and Surgical**
Body System   N   **Head and Facial Bones**
Operation   B   **Excision:** Cutting out or off, without replacement, a portion of a body part

Body Part (4ᵗʰ)	Approach (5ᵗʰ)	Device (6ᵗʰ)	Qualifier (7ᵗʰ)
0 Skull	0 Open	Z No Device	X Diagnostic
1 Frontal Bone	3 Percutaneous		Z No Qualifier
3 Parietal Bone, Right	4 Percutaneous Endoscopic		
4 Parietal Bone, Left			
5 Temporal Bone, Right			
6 Temporal Bone, Left			
7 Occipital Bone			
B Nasal Bone			
C Sphenoid Bone			
F Ethmoid Bone, Right			
G Ethmoid Bone, Left			
H Lacrimal Bone, Right			
J Lacrimal Bone, Left			
K Palatine Bone, Right			
L Palatine Bone, Left			
M Zygomatic Bone, Right			
N Zygomatic Bone, Left			
P Orbit, Right			
Q Orbit, Left			
R Maxilla			
T Mandible, Right			
V Mandible, Left			
X Hyoid Bone			

Section	0	Medical and Surgical
Body System	N	Head and Facial Bones
Operation	C	Extirpation: Taking or cutting out solid matter from a body part

Body Part (4th)	Approach (5th)	Device (6th)	Qualifier (7th)
1 Frontal Bone 3 Parietal Bone, Right 4 Parietal Bone, Left 5 Temporal Bone, Right 6 Temporal Bone, Left 7 Occipital Bone B Nasal Bone C Sphenoid Bone F Ethmoid Bone, Right G Ethmoid Bone, Left H Lacrimal Bone, Right J Lacrimal Bone, Left K Palatine Bone, Right L Palatine Bone, Left M Zygomatic Bone, Right N Zygomatic Bone, Left P Orbit, Right Q Orbit, Left R Maxilla T Mandible, Right V Mandible, Left X Hyoid Bone	0 Open 3 Percutaneous 4 Percutaneous Endoscopic	Z No Device	Z No Qualifier

Section	0	Medical and Surgical
Body System	N	Head and Facial Bones
Operation	D	Extraction: Pulling or stripping out or off all or a portion of a body part by the use of force

Body Part (4th)	Approach (5th)	Device (6th)	Qualifier (7th)
0 Skull 1 Frontal Bone 3 Parietal Bone, Right 4 Parietal Bone, Left 5 Temporal Bone, Right 6 Temporal Bone, Left 7 Occipital Bone B Nasal Bone C Sphenoid Bone F Ethmoid Bone, Right G Ethmoid Bone, Left H Lacrimal Bone, Right J Lacrimal Bone, Left K Palatine Bone, Right L Palatine Bone, Left M Zygomatic Bone, Right N Zygomatic Bone, Left P Orbit, Right Q Orbit, Left R Maxilla T Mandible, Right V Mandible, Left X Hyoid Bone	0 Open	Z No Device	Z No Qualifier

0NH–0NJ

Medical and Surgical, Head and Facial Bones Tables

Section	**0**	**Medical and Surgical**	
Body System	**N**	**Head and Facial Bones**	
Operation	**H**	**Insertion:** Putting in a nonbiological appliance that monitors, assists, performs, or prevents a physiological function but does not physically take the place of a body part	

Body Part (4th)	Approach (5th)	Device (6th)	Qualifier (7th)
0 Skull	**0** Open	**3** Infusion Device **4** Internal Fixation Device **5** External Fixation Device **M** Bone Growth Stimulator **N** Neurostimulator Generator	**Z** No Qualifier
0 Skull	**3** Percutaneous **4** Percutaneous Endoscopic	**3** Infusion Device **4** Internal Fixation Device **5** External Fixation Device **M** Bone Growth Stimulator	**Z** No Qualifier
1 Frontal Bone **3** Parietal Bone, Right **4** Parietal Bone, Left **7** Occipital Bone **C** Sphenoid Bone **F** Ethmoid Bone, Right **G** Ethmoid Bone, Left **H** Lacrimal Bone, Right **J** Lacrimal Bone, Left **K** Palatine Bone, Right **L** Palatine Bone, Left **M** Zygomatic Bone, Right **N** Zygomatic Bone, Left **P** Orbit, Right **Q** Orbit, Left **X** Hyoid Bone	**0** Open **3** Percutaneous **4** Percutaneous Endoscopic	**4** Internal Fixation Device	**Z** No Qualifier
5 Temporal Bone, Right **6** Temporal Bone, Left	**0** Open **3** Percutaneous **4** Percutaneous Endoscopic	**4** Internal Fixation Device **S** Hearing Device	**Z** No Qualifier
B Nasal Bone	**0** Open **3** Percutaneous **4** Percutaneous Endoscopic	**4** Internal Fixation Device **M** Bone Growth Stimulator	**Z** No Qualifier
R Maxilla **T** Mandible, Right **V** Mandible, Left	**0** Open **3** Percutaneous **4** Percutaneous Endoscopic	**4** Internal Fixation Device **5** External Fixation Device	**Z** No Qualifier
W Facial Bone	**0** Open **3** Percutaneous **4** Percutaneous Endoscopic	**M** Bone Growth Stimulator	**Z** No Qualifier

Section	**0**	**Medical and Surgical**	
Body System	**N**	**Head and Facial Bones**	
Operation	**J**	**Inspection:** Visually and/or manually exploring a body part	

Body Part (4th)	Approach (5th)	Device (6th)	Qualifier (7th)
0 Skull **B** Nasal Bone **W** Facial Bone	**0** Open **3** Percutaneous **4** Percutaneous Endoscopic **X** External	**Z** No Device	**Z** No Qualifier

388

Section	0	Medical and Surgical
Body System	N	Head and Facial Bones
Operation	N	Release: Freeing a body part from an abnormal physical constraint by cutting or by the use of force

Body Part (4th)	Approach (5th)	Device (6th)	Qualifier (7th)
1 Frontal Bone 3 Parietal Bone, Right 4 Parietal Bone, Left 5 Temporal Bone, Right 6 Temporal Bone, Left 7 Occipital Bone B Nasal Bone C Sphenoid Bone F Ethmoid Bone, Right G Ethmoid Bone, Left H Lacrimal Bone, Right J Lacrimal Bone, Left K Palatine Bone, Right L Palatine Bone, Left M Zygomatic Bone, Right N Zygomatic Bone, Left P Orbit, Right Q Orbit, Left R Maxilla T Mandible, Right V Mandible, Left X Hyoid Bone	0 Open 3 Percutaneous 4 Percutaneous Endoscopic	Z No Device	Z No Qualifier

Section	0	Medical and Surgical
Body System	N	Head and Facial Bones
Operation	P	Removal: Taking out or off a device from a body part

Body Part (4th)	Approach (5th)	Device (6th)	Qualifier (7th)
0 Skull	0 Open	0 Drainage Device 3 Infusion Device 4 Internal Fixation Device 5 External Fixation Device 7 Autologous Tissue Substitute J Synthetic Substitute K Nonautologous Tissue Substitute M Bone Growth Stimulator N Neurostimulator Generator S Hearing Device	Z No Qualifier
0 Skull	3 Percutaneous 4 Percutaneous Endoscopic	0 Drainage Device 3 Infusion Device 4 Internal Fixation Device 5 External Fixation Device 7 Autologous Tissue Substitute J Synthetic Substitute K Nonautologous Tissue Substitute M Bone Growth Stimulator S Hearing Device	Z No Qualifier
0 Skull	X External	0 Drainage Device 3 Infusion Device 4 Internal Fixation Device 5 External Fixation Device M Bone Growth Stimulator S Hearing Device	Z No Qualifier
B Nasal Bone W Facial Bone	0 Open 3 Percutaneous 4 Percutaneous Endoscopic	0 Drainage Device 4 Internal Fixation Device 7 Autologous Tissue Substitute J Synthetic Substitute K Nonautologous Tissue Substitute M Bone Growth Stimulator	Z No Qualifier

Continued →

0NP–0NR

Medical and Surgical, Head and Facial Bones Tables

0NP Continued

Section	0	Medical and Surgical
Body System	N	Head and Facial Bones
Operation	P	Removal: Taking out or off a device from a body part

Body Part (4th)	Approach (5th)	Device (6th)	Qualifier (7th)
B Nasal Bone W Facial Bone	X External	0 Drainage Device 4 Internal Fixation Device M Bone Growth Stimulator	Z No Qualifier

Section	0	Medical and Surgical
Body System	N	Head and Facial Bones
Operation	Q	Repair: Restoring, to the extent possible, a body part to its normal anatomic structure and function

Body Part (4th)	Approach (5th)	Device (6th)	Qualifier (7th)
0 Skull 1 Frontal Bone 3 Parietal Bone, Right 4 Parietal Bone, Left 5 Temporal Bone, Right 6 Temporal Bone, Left 7 Occipital Bone B Nasal Bone C Sphenoid Bone F Ethmoid Bone, Right G Ethmoid Bone, Left H Lacrimal Bone, Right J Lacrimal Bone, Left K Palatine Bone, Right L Palatine Bone, Left M Zygomatic Bone, Right N Zygomatic Bone, Left P Orbit, Right Q Orbit, Left R Maxilla T Mandible, Right V Mandible, Left X Hyoid Bone	0 Open 3 Percutaneous 4 Percutaneous Endoscopic X External	Z No Device	Z No Qualifier

Section	0	Medical and Surgical
Body System	N	Head and Facial Bones
Operation	R	Replacement: Putting in or on biological or synthetic material that physically takes the place and/or function of all or a portion of a body part

Body Part (4th)	Approach (5th)	Device (6th)	Qualifier (7th)
0 Skull 1 Frontal Bone 3 Parietal Bone, Right 4 Parietal Bone, Left 5 Temporal Bone, Right 6 Temporal Bone, Left 7 Occipital Bone B Nasal Bone C Sphenoid Bone F Ethmoid Bone, Right G Ethmoid Bone, Left H Lacrimal Bone, Right J Lacrimal Bone, Left K Palatine Bone, Right L Palatine Bone, Left M Zygomatic Bone, Right N Zygomatic Bone, Left P Orbit, Right Q Orbit, Left R Maxilla T Mandible, Right V Mandible, Left X Hyoid Bone	0 Open 3 Percutaneous 4 Percutaneous Endoscopic	7 Autologous Tissue Substitute J Synthetic Substitute K Nonautologous Tissue Substitute	Z No Qualifier

	Section	0	Medical and Surgical
	Body System	N	Head and Facial Bones
	Operation	S	Reposition: Moving to its normal location, or other suitable location, all or a portion of a body part

Body Part (4th)	Approach (5th)	Device (6th)	Qualifier (7th)
0 Skull **R** Maxilla **T** Mandible, Right **V** Mandible, Left	**0** Open **3** Percutaneous **4** Percutaneous Endoscopic	**4** Internal Fixation Device **5** External Fixation Device **Z** No Device	**Z** No Qualifier
0 Skull **R** Maxilla **T** Mandible, Right **V** Mandible, Left	**X** External	**Z** No Device	**Z** No Qualifier
1 Frontal Bone **3** Parietal Bone, Right **4** Parietal Bone, Left **5** Temporal Bone, Right **6** Temporal Bone, Left **7** Occipital Bone **B** Nasal Bone **C** Sphenoid Bone **F** Ethmoid Bone, Right **G** Ethmoid Bone, Left **H** Lacrimal Bone, Right **J** Lacrimal Bone, Left **K** Palatine Bone, Right **L** Palatine Bone, Left **M** Zygomatic Bone, Right **N** Zygomatic Bone, Left **P** Orbit, Right **Q** Orbit, Left **X** Hyoid Bone	**0** Open **3** Percutaneous **4** Percutaneous Endoscopic	**4** Internal Fixation Device **Z** No Device	**Z** No Qualifier
1 Frontal Bone **3** Parietal Bone, Right **4** Parietal Bone, Left **5** Temporal Bone, Right **6** Temporal Bone, Left **7** Occipital Bone **B** Nasal Bone **C** Sphenoid Bone **F** Ethmoid Bone, Right **G** Ethmoid Bone, Left **H** Lacrimal Bone, Right **J** Lacrimal Bone, Left **K** Palatine Bone, Right **L** Palatine Bone, Left **M** Zygomatic Bone, Right **N** Zygomatic Bone, Left **P** Orbit, Right **Q** Orbit, Left **X** Hyoid Bone	**X** External	**Z** No Device	**Z** No Qualifier

0NT-0NU

Medical and Surgical, Head and Facial Bones Tables

Section	0	Medical and Surgical
Body System	N	Head and Facial Bones
Operation	T	Resection: Cutting out or off, without replacement, all of a body part

Body Part (4th)	Approach (5th)	Device (6th)	Qualifier (7th)
1 Frontal Bone 3 Parietal Bone, Right 4 Parietal Bone, Left 5 Temporal Bone, Right 6 Temporal Bone, Left 7 Occipital Bone B Nasal Bone C Sphenoid Bone F Ethmoid Bone, Right G Ethmoid Bone, Left H Lacrimal Bone, Right J Lacrimal Bone, Left K Palatine Bone, Right L Palatine Bone, Left M Zygomatic Bone, Right N Zygomatic Bone, Left P Orbit, Right Q Orbit, Left R Maxilla T Mandible, Right V Mandible, Left X Hyoid Bone	0 Open	Z No Device	Z No Qualifier

Section	0	Medical and Surgical
Body System	N	Head and Facial Bones
Operation	U	Supplement: Putting in or on biological or synthetic material that physically reinforces and/or augments the function of a portion of a body part

Body Part (4th)	Approach (5th)	Device (6th)	Qualifier (7th)
0 Skull 1 Frontal Bone 3 Parietal Bone, Right 4 Parietal Bone, Left 5 Temporal Bone, Right 6 Temporal Bone, Left 7 Occipital Bone B Nasal Bone C Sphenoid Bone F Ethmoid Bone, Right G Ethmoid Bone, Left H Lacrimal Bone, Right J Lacrimal Bone, Left K Palatine Bone, Right L Palatine Bone, Left M Zygomatic Bone, Right N Zygomatic Bone, Left P Orbit, Right Q Orbit, Left R Maxilla T Mandible, Right V Mandible, Left X Hyoid Bone	0 Open 3 Percutaneous 4 Percutaneous Endoscopic	7 Autologous Tissue Substitute J Synthetic Substitute K Nonautologous Tissue Substitute	Z No Qualifier

Section	0	Medical and Surgical
Body System	N	Head and Facial Bones
Operation	W	Revision: Correcting, to the extent possible, a portion of a malfunctioning device or the position of a displaced device

Body Part (4th)	Approach (5th)	Device (6th)	Qualifier (7th)
0 Skull	**0** Open	**0** Drainage Device **3** Infusion Device **4** Internal Fixation Device **5** External Fixation Device **7** Autologous Tissue Substitute **J** Synthetic Substitute **K** Nonautologous Tissue Substitute **M** Bone Growth Stimulator **N** Neurostimulator Generator **S** Hearing Device	**Z** No Qualifier
0 Skull	**3** Percutaneous **4** Percutaneous Endoscopic **X** External	**0** Drainage Device **3** Infusion Device **4** Internal Fixation Device **5** External Fixation Device **7** Autologous Tissue Substitute **J** Synthetic Substitute **K** Nonautologous Tissue Substitute **M** Bone Growth Stimulator **S** Hearing Device	**Z** No Qualifier
B Nasal Bone **W** Facial Bone	**0** Open **3** Percutaneous **4** Percutaneous Endoscopic **X** External	**0** Drainage Device **4** Internal Fixation Device **7** Autologous Tissue Substitute **J** Synthetic Substitute **K** Nonautologous Tissue Substitute **M** Bone Growth Stimulator	**Z** No Qualifier

AHA Coding Clinic

0NBB0ZZ Excision of Nasal Bone, Open Approach—AHA CC: 1Q, 2017, 20-21

0NBQ0ZZ Excision of Left Orbit, Open Approach—AHA CC: 2Q, 2015, 12-13

0NBR0ZZ Excision of Maxilla, Open Approach—AHA CC: 1Q, 2021, 21-22; 2Q, 2022, 18

0NBX0ZZ Excision of Hyoid Bone, Open Approach—AHA CC: 3Q, 2021, 21

0NH004Z Insertion of Internal Fixation Device into Skull, Open Approach—AHA CC: 3Q, 2015, 13-14

0NP004Z Removal of Internal Fixation Device from Skull, Open Approach—AHA CC: 3Q, 2015, 13-14

0NP007Z Removal of Autologous Tissue Substitute from Skull, Open Approach—AHA CC: 1Q, 2023, 31-32

0NR00JZ Replacement of Skull with Synthetic Substitute, Open Approach—AHA CC: 3Q, 2014, 7-8

0NR50JZ Replacement of Right Temporal Bone with Synthetic Substitute, Open Approach—AHA CC: 3Q, 2021, 29-30

0NR70JZ Replacement of Occipital Bone with Synthetic Substitute, Open Approach—AHA CC: 3Q, 2017, 17

0NRR0JZ Replacement of Maxilla with Synthetic Substitute, Open Approach—AHA CC: 1Q, 2021, 21-22

0NRV07Z Replacement of Left Mandible with Autologous Tissue Substitute, Open Approach—AHA CC: 1Q, 2017, 23-24

0NRV0JZ Replacement of Left Mandible with Synthetic Substitute, Open Approach—AHA CC: 1Q, 2017, 23-24

0NS004Z Reposition Skull with Internal Fixation Device, Open Approach—AHA CC: 3Q, 2017, 22

0NS005Z Reposition Skull with External Fixation Device, Open Approach—AHA CC: 3Q, 2013, 24-25

0NS00ZZ Reposition Skull, Open Approach—AHA CC: 3Q, 2015, 17-18; 2Q, 2016, 30

0NS104Z Reposition Frontal Bone with Internal Fixation Device, Open Approach—AHA CC: 3Q, 2013, 25

0NS504Z Reposition Right Temporal Bone with Internal Fixation Device, Open Approach—AHA CC: 3Q, 2015, 27-28

0NSR04Z Reposition Maxilla with Internal Fixation Device, Open Approach—AHA CC: 3Q, 2014, 23-24

0NSR0ZZ Reposition Maxilla, Open Approach—AHA CC: 1Q, 2017, 20-21

0NU00JZ Supplement Skull with Synthetic Substitute, Open Approach—AHA CC: 3Q, 2013, 24-25

0NU50JZ Supplement Right Temporal Bone with Synthetic Substitute, Open Approach—AHA CC: 2Q, 2023, 19-20

0NU50KZ Supplement Right Temporal Bone with Nonautologous Tissue Substitute, Open Approach—AHA CC: 3Q, 2021, 29-30

0NUR07Z Supplement Maxilla with Autologous Tissue Substitute, Open Approach—AHA CC: 3Q, 2016, 29-30

Upper Bones

Bones - Front and Back Views

Cross-section Spine

Hand Bones

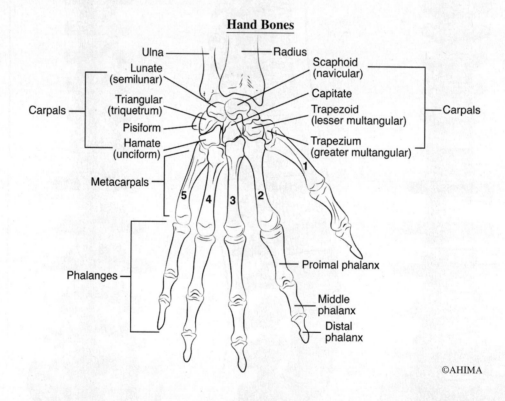

Upper Bones Tables 0P2–0PW

Section	0	Medical and Surgical
Body System	P	Upper Bones
Operation	2	**Change:** Taking out or off a device from a body part and putting back an identical or similar device in or on the same body part without cutting or puncturing the skin or a mucous membrane

Body Part (4th)	Approach (5th)	Device (6th)	Qualifier (7th)
Y Upper Bone	X External	0 Drainage Device Y Other Device	Z No Qualifier

Section	0	Medical and Surgical
Body System	P	Upper Bones
Operation	5	**Destruction:** Physical eradication of all or a portion of a body part by the direct use of energy, force, or a destructive agent

Body Part (4th)	Approach (5th)	Device (6th)	Qualifier (7th)
0 Sternum 1 Ribs, 1 to 2 2 Ribs, 3 or More 5 Scapula, Right 6 Scapula, Left 7 Glenoid Cavity, Right 8 Glenoid Cavity, Left 9 Clavicle, Right B Clavicle, Left C Humeral Head, Right D Humeral Head, Left F Humeral Shaft, Right G Humeral Shaft, Left H Radius, Right J Radius, Left K Ulna, Right L Ulna, Left M Carpal, Right N Carpal, Left P Metacarpal, Right Q Metacarpal, Left R Thumb Phalanx, Right S Thumb Phalanx, Left T Finger Phalanx, Right V Finger Phalanx, Left	0 Open 3 Percutaneous 4 Percutaneous Endoscopic	Z No Device	Z No Qualifier
3 Cervical Vertebra 4 Thoracic Vertebra	0 Open 3 Percutaneous 4 Percutaneous Endoscopic	Z No Device	3 Laser Interstitial Thermal Therapy Z No Qualifier

0P8–0P9

Section	0	Medical and Surgical
Body System	P	Upper Bones
Operation	8	Division: Cutting into a body part, without draining fluids and/or gases from the body part, in order to separate or transect a body part

Body Part (4th)	Approach (5th)	Device (6th)	Qualifier (7th)
0 Sternum	0 Open	Z No Device	Z No Qualifier
1 Ribs, 1 to 2	3 Percutaneous		
2 Ribs, 3 or More	4 Percutaneous Endoscopic		
3 Cervical Vertebra			
4 Thoracic Vertebra			
5 Scapula, Right			
6 Scapula, Left			
7 Glenoid Cavity, Right			
8 Glenoid Cavity, Left			
9 Clavicle, Right			
B Clavicle, Left			
C Humeral Head, Right			
D Humeral Head, Left			
F Humeral Shaft, Right			
G Humeral Shaft, Left			
H Radius, Right			
J Radius, Left			
K Ulna, Right			
L Ulna, Left			
M Carpal, Right			
N Carpal, Left			
P Metacarpal, Right			
Q Metacarpal, Left			
R Thumb Phalanx, Right			
S Thumb Phalanx, Left			
T Finger Phalanx, Right			
V Finger Phalanx, Left			

Section	0	Medical and Surgical
Body System	P	Upper Bones
Operation	9	Drainage: Taking or letting out fluids and/or gases from a body part

Body Part (4th)	Approach (5th)	Device (6th)	Qualifier (7th)
0 Sternum	0 Open	0 Drainage Device	Z No Qualifier
1 Ribs, 1 to 2	3 Percutaneous		
2 Ribs, 3 or More	4 Percutaneous Endoscopic		
3 Cervical Vertebra			
4 Thoracic Vertebra			
5 Scapula, Right			
6 Scapula, Left			
7 Glenoid Cavity, Right			
8 Glenoid Cavity, Left			
9 Clavicle, Right			
B Clavicle, Left			
C Humeral Head, Right			
D Humeral Head, Left			
F Humeral Shaft, Right			
G Humeral Shaft, Left			
H Radius, Right			
J Radius, Left			
K Ulna, Right			
L Ulna, Left			
M Carpal, Right			
N Carpal, Left			
P Metacarpal, Right			
Q Metacarpal, Left			
R Thumb Phalanx, Right			
S Thumb Phalanx, Left			
T Finger Phalanx, Right			
V Finger Phalanx, Left			

Continued →

Section	0	Medical and Surgical
Body System	P	Upper Bones
Operation	9	Drainage: Taking or letting out fluids and/or gases from a body part

0P9 Continued

Body Part (4th)	Approach (5th)	Device (6th)	Qualifier (7th)
0 Sternum 1 Ribs, 1 to 2 2 Ribs, 3 or More 3 Cervical Vertebra 4 Thoracic Vertebra 5 Scapula, Right 6 Scapula, Left 7 Glenoid Cavity, Right 8 Glenoid Cavity, Left 9 Clavicle, Right B Clavicle, Left C Humeral Head, Right D Humeral Head, Left F Humeral Shaft, Right G Humeral Shaft, Left H Radius, Right J Radius, Left K Ulna, Right L Ulna, Left M Carpal, Right N Carpal, Left P Metacarpal, Right Q Metacarpal, Left R Thumb Phalanx, Right S Thumb Phalanx, Left T Finger Phalanx, Right V Finger Phalanx, Left	0 Open 3 Percutaneous 4 Percutaneous Endoscopic	Z No Device	X Diagnostic Z No Qualifier

Section	0	Medical and Surgical
Body System	P	Upper Bones
Operation	B	Excision: Cutting out or off, without replacement, a portion of a body part

Body Part (4th)	Approach (5th)	Device (6th)	Qualifier (7th)
0 Sternum 1 Ribs, 1 to 2 2 Ribs, 3 or More 3 Cervical Vertebra 4 Thoracic Vertebra 5 Scapula, Right 6 Scapula, Left 7 Glenoid Cavity, Right 8 Glenoid Cavity, Left 9 Clavicle, Right B Clavicle, Left C Humeral Head, Right D Humeral Head, Left F Humeral Shaft, Right G Humeral Shaft, Left H Radius, Right J Radius, Left K Ulna, Right L Ulna, Left M Carpal, Right N Carpal, Left P Metacarpal, Right Q Metacarpal, Left R Thumb Phalanx, Right S Thumb Phalanx, Left T Finger Phalanx, Right V Finger Phalanx, Left	0 Open 3 Percutaneous 4 Percutaneous Endoscopic	Z No Device	X Diagnostic Z No Qualifier

Section	0	Medical and Surgical
Body System	P	Upper Bones
Operation	C	**Extirpation:** Taking or cutting out solid matter from a body part

Body Part (4th)	Approach (5th)	Device (6th)	Qualifier (7th)
0 Sternum	0 Open	Z No Device	Z No Qualifier
1 Ribs, 1 to 2	3 Percutaneous		
2 Ribs, 3 or More	4 Percutaneous Endoscopic		
3 Cervical Vertebra			
4 Thoracic Vertebra			
5 Scapula, Right			
6 Scapula, Left			
7 Glenoid Cavity, Right			
8 Glenoid Cavity, Left			
9 Clavicle, Right			
B Clavicle, Left			
C Humeral Head, Right			
D Humeral Head, Left			
F Humeral Shaft, Right			
G Humeral Shaft, Left			
H Radius, Right			
J Radius, Left			
K Ulna, Right			
L Ulna, Left			
M Carpal, Right			
N Carpal, Left			
P Metacarpal, Right			
Q Metacarpal, Left			
R Thumb Phalanx, Right			
S Thumb Phalanx, Left			
T Finger Phalanx, Right			
V Finger Phalanx, Left			

Section	0	Medical and Surgical
Body System	P	Upper Bones
Operation	D	**Extraction:** Pulling or stripping out or off all or a portion of a body part by the use of force

Body Part (4th)	Approach (5th)	Device (6th)	Qualifier (7th)
0 Sternum	0 Open	Z No Device	Z No Qualifier
1 Ribs, 1 to 2			
2 Ribs, 3 or More			
3 Cervical Vertebra			
4 Thoracic Vertebra			
5 Scapula, Right			
6 Scapula, Left			
7 Glenoid Cavity, Right			
8 Glenoid Cavity, Left			
9 Clavical, Right			
B Clavical, Left			
C Humeral Head, Right			
D Humeral Head, Left			
F Humeral Shaft, Right			
G Humeral Shaft, Left			
H Radius, Right			
J Radius, Left			
K Ulna, Right			
L Ulna, Left			
M Carpal, Right			
N Carpal, Left			
P Metacarpal, Right			
Q Metacarpal, Left			
R Thumb Phalanx, Right			
S Thumb Phalanx, Left			
T Finger Phalanx, Right			
V Finger Phalanx, Left			

Section	0	Medical and Surgical
Body System	P	Upper Bones
Operation	H	Insertion: Putting in a nonbiological appliance that monitors, assists, performs, or prevents a physiological function but does not physically take the place of a body part

Body Part (4th)	Approach (5th)	Device (6th)	Qualifier (7th)
0 Sternum	0 Open 3 Percutaneous 4 Percutaneous Endoscopic	0 Internal Fixation Device, Rigid Plate 4 Internal Fixation Device	Z No Qualifier
1 Ribs, 1 to 2 2 Ribs, 3 or More 3 Cervical Vertebra 4 Thoracic Vertebra 5 Scapula, Right 6 Scapula, Left 7 Glenoid Cavity, Right 8 Glenoid Cavity, Left 9 Clavicle, Right B Clavicle, Left	0 Open 3 Percutaneous 4 Percutaneous Endoscopic	4 Internal Fixation Device	Z No Qualifier
C Humeral Head, Right D Humeral Head, Left H Radius, Right J Radius, Left K Ulna, Right L Ulna, Left	0 Open 3 Percutaneous 4 Percutaneous Endoscopic	4 Internal Fixation Device 5 External Fixation Device 6 Internal Fixation Device, Intramedullary 8 External Fixation Device, Limb Lengthening B External Fixation Device, Monoplanar C External Fixation Device, Ring D External Fixation Device, Hybrid	Z No Qualifier
F Humeral Shaft, Right G Humeral Shaft, Left	0 Open 3 Percutaneous 4 Percutaneous Endoscopic	4 Internal Fixation Device 5 External Fixation Device 6 Internal Fixation Device, Intramedullary 7 Internal Fixation Device, Intramedullary Limb Lengthening 8 External Fixation Device, Limb Lengthening B External Fixation Device, Monoplanar C External Fixation Device, Ring D External Fixation Device, Hybrid	Z No Qualifier
M Carpal, Right N Carpal, Left P Metacarpal, Right Q Metacarpal, Left R Thumb Phalanx, Right S Thumb Phalanx, Left T Finger Phalanx, Right V Finger Phalanx, Left	0 Open 3 Percutaneous 4 Percutaneous Endoscopic	4 Internal Fixation Device 5 External Fixation Device	Z No Qualifier
Y Upper Bone	0 Open 3 Percutaneous 4 Percutaneous Endoscopic	M Bone Growth Stimulator	Z No Qualifier

Section	0	Medical and Surgical
Body System	P	Upper Bones
Operation	J	Inspection: Visually and/or manually exploring a body part

Body Part (4th)	Approach (5th)	Device (6th)	Qualifier (7th)
Y Upper Bone	0 Open 3 Percutaneous 4 Percutaneous Endoscopic X External	Z No Device	Z No Qualifier

Section	0	Medical and Surgical
Body System	P	Upper Bones
Operation	N	**Release:** Freeing a body part from an abnormal physical constraint by cutting or by the use of force

Body Part (4th)	Approach (5th)	Device (6th)	Qualifier (7th)
0 Sternum 1 Ribs, 1 to 2 2 Ribs, 3 or More 3 Cervical Vertebra 4 Thoracic Vertebra 5 Scapula, Right 6 Scapula, Left 7 Glenoid Cavity, Right 8 Glenoid Cavity, Left 9 Clavicle, Right B Clavicle, Left C Humeral Head, Right D Humeral Head, Left F Humeral Shaft, Right G Humeral Shaft, Left H Radius, Right J Radius, Left K Ulna, Right L Ulna, Left M Carpal, Right N Carpal, Left P Metacarpal, Right Q Metacarpal, Left R Thumb Phalanx, Right S Thumb Phalanx, Left T Finger Phalanx, Right V Finger Phalanx, Left	0 Open 3 Percutaneous 4 Percutaneous Endoscopic	Z No Device	Z No Qualifier

Section	0	Medical and Surgical
Body System	P	Upper Bones
Operation	P	**Removal:** Taking out or off a device from a body part

Body Part (4th)	Approach (5th)	Device (6th)	Qualifier (7th)
0 Sternum 1 Ribs, 1 to 2 2 Ribs, 3 or More 3 Cervical Vertebra 4 Thoracic Vertebra 5 Scapula, Right 6 Scapula, Left 7 Glenoid Cavity, Right 8 Glenoid Cavity, Left 9 Clavicle, Right B Clavicle, Left	0 Open 3 Percutaneous 4 Percutaneous Endoscopic	4 Internal Fixation Device 7 Autologous Tissue Substitute J Synthetic Substitute K Nonautologous Tissue Substitute	Z No Qualifier
0 Sternum 1 Ribs, 1 to 2 2 Ribs, 3 or More 3 Cervical Vertebra 4 Thoracic Vertebra 5 Scapula, Right 6 Scapula, Left 7 Glenoid Cavity, Right 8 Glenoid Cavity, Left 9 Clavicle, Right B Clavicle, Left	X External	4 Internal Fixation Device	Z No Qualifier

Continued →

Section	0	Medical and Surgical		0PP Continued

Section 0 Medical and Surgical
Body System P Upper Bones
Operation P **Removal:** Taking out or off a device from a body part

Body Part (4ᵗʰ)	Approach (5ᵗʰ)	Device (6ᵗʰ)	Qualifier (7ᵗʰ)
C Humeral Head, Right D Humeral Head, Left F Humeral Shaft, Right G Humeral Shaft, Left H Radius, Right J Radius, Left K Ulna, Right L Ulna, Left M Carpal, Right N Carpal, Left P Metacarpal, Right Q Metacarpal, Left R Thumb Phalanx, Right S Thumb Phalanx, Left T Finger Phalanx, Right V Finger Phalanx, Left	0 Open 3 Percutaneous 4 Percutaneous Endoscopic	4 Internal Fixation Device 5 External Fixation Device 7 Autologous Tissue Substitute J Synthetic Substitute K Nonautologous Tissue Substitute	Z No Qualifier
C Humeral Head, Right D Humeral Head, Left F Humeral Shaft, Right G Humeral Shaft, Left H Radius, Right J Radius, Left K Ulna, Right L Ulna, Left M Carpal, Right N Carpal, Left P Metacarpal, Right Q Metacarpal, Left R Thumb Phalanx, Right S Thumb Phalanx, Left T Finger Phalanx, Right V Finger Phalanx, Left	X External	4 Internal Fixation Device 5 External Fixation Device	Z No Qualifier
Y Upper Bone	0 Open 3 Percutaneous 4 Percutaneous Endoscopic X External	0 Drainage Device M Bone Growth Stimulator	Z No Qualifier

0PQ-0PR

Medical and Surgical, Upper Bones Tables

Section	0	Medical and Surgical
Body System	P	Upper Bones
Operation	Q	**Repair:** Restoring, to the extent possible, a body part to its normal anatomic structure and function

Body Part (4th)	Approach (5th)	Device (6th)	Qualifier (7th)
0 Sternum	0 Open	Z No Device	Z No Qualifier
1 Ribs, 1 to 2	3 Percutaneous		
2 Ribs, 3 or More	4 Percutaneous Endoscopic		
3 Cervical Vertebra	X External		
4 Thoracic Vertebra			
5 Scapula, Right			
6 Scapula, Left			
7 Glenoid Cavity, Right			
8 Glenoid Cavity, Left			
9 Clavicle, Right			
B Clavicle, Left			
C Humeral Head, Right			
D Humeral Head, Left			
F Humeral Shaft, Right			
G Humeral Shaft, Left			
H Radius, Right			
J Radius, Left			
K Ulna, Right			
L Ulna, Left			
M Carpal, Right			
N Carpal, Left			
P Metacarpal, Right			
Q Metacarpal, Left			
R Thumb Phalanx, Right			
S Thumb Phalanx, Left			
T Finger Phalanx, Right			
V Finger Phalanx, Left			

Section	0	Medical and Surgical
Body System	P	Upper Bones
Operation	R	**Replacement:** Putting in or on biological or synthetic material that physically takes the place and/or function of all or a portion of a body part

Body Part (4th)	Approach (5th)	Device (6th)	Qualifier (7th)
0 Sternum	0 Open	7 Autologous Tissue Substitute	Z No Qualifier
1 Ribs, 1 to 2	3 Percutaneous	J Synthetic Substitute	
2 Ribs, 3 or More	4 Percutaneous Endoscopic	K Nonautologous Tissue Substitute	
3 Cervical Vertebra			
4 Thoracic Vertebra			
5 Scapula, Right			
6 Scapula, Left			
7 Glenoid Cavity, Right			
8 Glenoid Cavity, Left			
9 Clavicle, Right			
B Clavicle, Left			
C Humeral Head, Right			
D Humeral Head, Left			
F Humeral Shaft, Right			
G Humeral Shaft, Left			
H Radius, Right			
J Radius, Left			
K Ulna, Right			
L Ulna, Left			
M Carpal, Right			
N Carpal, Left			
P Metacarpal, Right			
Q Metacarpal, Left			
R Thumb Phalanx, Right			
S Thumb Phalanx, Left			
T Finger Phalanx, Right			
V Finger Phalanx, Left			

Section	0	Medical and Surgical
Body System	P	Upper Bones
Operation	S	Reposition: Moving to its normal location, or other suitable location, all or a portion of a body part

Body Part (4th)	Approach (5th)	Device (6th)	Qualifier (7th)
0 Sternum	**0** Open **3** Percutaneous **4** Percutaneous Endoscopic	**0** Internal Fixation Device, Rigid Plate **4** Internal Fixation Device **Z** No Device	**Z** No Qualifier
0 Sternum	**X** External	**Z** No Device	**Z** No Qualifier
1 Ribs, 1 to 2 **2** Ribs, 3 or More **3** Cervical Vertebra **5** Scapula, Right **6** Scapula, Left **7** Glenoid Cavity, Right **8** Glenoid Cavity, Left **9** Clavicle, Right **B** Clavicle, Left	**0** Open **3** Percutaneous **4** Percutaneous Endoscopic	**4** Internal Fixation Device **Z** No Device	**Z** No Qualifier
1 Ribs, 1 to 2 **2** Ribs, 3 or More **3** Cervical Vertebra **5** Scapula, Right **6** Scapula, Left **7** Glenoid Cavity, Right **8** Glenoid Cavity, Left **9** Clavicle, Right **B** Clavicle, Left	**X** External	**Z** No Device	**Z** No Qualifier
4 Thoracic Vertebra	**0** Open **4** Percutaneous Endoscopic	**3** Spinal Stabilization Device, Vertebral Body Tether **4** Internal Fixation Device **Z** No Device	**Z** No Qualifier
4 Thoracic Vertebra	**3** Percutaneous	**4** Internal Fixation Device **Z** No Device	**Z** No Qualifier
4 Thoracic Vertebra	**X** External	**Z** No Device	**Z** No Qualifier
C Humeral Head, Right **D** Humeral Head, Left **F** Humeral Shaft, Right **G** Humeral Shaft, Left **H** Radius, Right **J** Radius, Left **K** Ulna, Right **L** Ulna, Left	**0** Open **3** Percutaneous **4** Percutaneous Endoscopic	**4** Internal Fixation Device **5** External Fixation Device **6** Internal Fixation Device, Intramedullary **B** External Fixation Device, Monoplanar **C** External Fixation Device, Ring **D** External Fixation Device, Hybrid **Z** No Device	**Z** No Qualifier
C Humeral Head, Right **D** Humeral Head, Left **F** Humeral Shaft, Right **G** Humeral Shaft, Left **H** Radius, Right **J** Radius, Left **K** Ulna, Right **L** Ulna, Left	**X** External	**Z** No Device	**Z** No Qualifier
M Carpal, Right **N** Carpal, Left **P** Metacarpal, Right **Q** Metacarpal, Left **R** Thumb Phalanx, Right **S** Thumb Phalanx, Left **T** Finger Phalanx, Right **V** Finger Phalanx, Left	**0** Open **3** Percutaneous **4** Percutaneous Endoscopic	**4** Internal Fixation Device **5** External Fixation Device **Z** No Device	**Z** No Qualifier

Continued →

Section	0	Medical and Surgical			0PS Continued
Body System	P	Upper Bones			
Operation	S	Reposition: Moving to its normal location, or other suitable location, all or a portion of a body part			

Body Part (4th)	Approach (5th)	Device (6th)	Qualifier (7th)
M Carpal, Right N Carpal, Left P Metacarpal, Right Q Metacarpal, Left R Thumb Phalanx, Right S Thumb Phalanx, Left T Finger Phalanx, Right V Finger Phalanx, Left	X External	Z No Device	Z No Qualifier

Section	0	Medical and Surgical
Body System	P	Upper Bones
Operation	T	Resection: Cutting out or off, without replacement, all of a body part

Body Part (4th)	Approach (5th)	Device (6th)	Qualifier (7th)
0 Sternum 1 Ribs, 1 to 2 2 Ribs, 3 or More 5 Scapula, Right 6 Scapula, Left 7 Glenoid Cavity, Right 8 Glenoid Cavity, Left 9 Clavicle, Right B Clavicle, Left C Humeral Head, Right D Humeral Head, Left F Humeral Shaft, Right G Humeral Shaft, Left H Radius, Right J Radius, Left K Ulna, Right L Ulna, Left M Carpal, Right N Carpal, Left P Metacarpal, Right Q Metacarpal, Left R Thumb Phalanx, Right S Thumb Phalanx, Left T Finger Phalanx, Right V Finger Phalanx, Left	0 Open	Z No Device	Z No Qualifier

Section	0	Medical and Surgical
Body System	P	Upper Bones
Operation	U	Supplement: Putting in or on biological or synthetic material that physically reinforces and/or augments the function of a portion of a body part

Body Part (4th)	Approach (5th)	Device (6th)	Qualifier (7th)
0 Sternum	0 Open	7 Autologous Tissue Substitute	Z No Qualifier
1 Ribs, 1 to 2	3 Percutaneous	J Synthetic Substitute	
2 Ribs, 3 or More	4 Percutaneous Endoscopic	K Nonautologous Tissue Substitute	
3 Cervical Vertebra			
4 Thoracic Vertebra			
5 Scapula, Right			
6 Scapula, Left			
7 Glenoid Cavity, Right			
8 Glenoid Cavity, Left			
9 Clavicle, Right			
B Clavicle, Left			
C Humeral Head, Right			
D Humeral Head, Left			
F Humeral Shaft, Right			
G Humeral Shaft, Left			
H Radius, Right			
J Radius, Left			
K Ulna, Right			
L Ulna, Left			
M Carpal, Right			
N Carpal, Left			
P Metacarpal, Right			
Q Metacarpal, Left			
R Thumb Phalanx, Right			
S Thumb Phalanx, Left			
T Finger Phalanx, Right			
V Finger Phalanx, Left			

Section	0	Medical and Surgical
Body System	P	Upper Bones
Operation	W	Revision: Correcting, to the extent possible, a portion of a malfunctioning device or the position of a displaced device

Body Part (4th)	Approach (5th)	Device (6th)	Qualifier (7th)
0 Sternum	0 Open	4 Internal Fixation Device	Z No Qualifier
1 Ribs, 1 to 2	3 Percutaneous	7 Autologous Tissue Substitute	
2 Ribs, 3 or More	4 Percutaneous Endoscopic	J Synthetic Substitute	
3 Cervical Vertebra	X External	K Nonautologous Tissue Substitute	
4 Thoracic Vertebra			
5 Scapula, Right			
6 Scapula, Left			
7 Glenoid Cavity, Right			
8 Glenoid Cavity, Left			
9 Clavicle, Right			
B Clavicle, Left			

Continued →

Section	0	Medical and Surgical			0PW Continued
Body System	P	Upper Bones			
Operation	W	Revision: Correcting, to the extent possible, a portion of a malfunctioning device or the position of a displaced device			

Body Part (4th)	Approach (5th)	Device (6th)	Qualifier (7th)
C Humeral Head, Right **D** Humeral Head, Left **F** Humeral Shaft, Right **G** Humeral Shaft, Left **H** Radius, Right **J** Radius, Left **K** Ulna, Right **L** Ulna, Left **M** Carpal, Right **N** Carpal, Left **P** Metacarpal, Right **Q** Metacarpal, Left **R** Thumb Phalanx, Right **S** Thumb Phalanx, Left **T** Finger Phalanx, Right **V** Finger Phalanx, Left	**0** Open **3** Percutaneous **4** Percutaneous Endoscopic **X** External	**4** Internal Fixation Device **5** External Fixation Device **7** Autologous Tissue Substitute **J** Synthetic Substitute **K** Nonautologous Tissue Substitute	**Z** No Qualifier
Y Upper Bone	**0** Open **3** Percutaneous **4** Percutaneous Endoscopic **X** External	**0** Drainage Device **M** Bone Growth Stimulator	**Z** No Qualifier

AHA Coding Clinic

0PB10ZZ Excision of I to 2 Ribs, Open Approach—AHA CC: 4Q, 2012, 101-102; 4Q, 2013, 109-111

0PB20ZZ Excision of 3 or More Ribs, Open Approach—AHA CC: 4Q, 2013, 109-111

0PB54ZZ Excision of Right Scapula, Percutaneous Endoscopic Approach—AHA CC: 3Q, 2013, 20-22

0PC00ZZ Extirpation of Matter from Sternum, Open Approach—AHA CC: 3Q, 2019, 19

0PCC3ZZ Extirpation of Matter from Right Humeral Head, Percutaneous Approach—AHA CC: 3Q, 2021, 15-16

0PCD3ZZ Extirpation of Matter from Left Humeral Head, Percutaneous Approach—AHA CC: 3Q, 2021, 15-16

0PH000Z Insertion of Rigid Plate Internal Fixation Device into Sternum, Open Approach—AHA CC: 1Q, 2020, 29-30

0PH304Z Insertion of Internal Fixation Device into Cervical Vertebra, Open Approach—AHA CC: 2Q, 2017, 23-24; 2Q, 2019, 40

0PH404Z Insertion of Internal Fixation Device into Thoracic Vertebra, Open Approach—AHA CC: 4Q, 2014, 28-29

0PH504Z Insertion of Internal Fixation Device into Right Scapula, Open Approach—AHA CC: 4Q, 2018, 12-13

0PP404Z Removal of Internal Fixation Device from Thoracic Vertebra, Open Approach—AHA CC: 4Q, 2014, 28-29

0PRH0JZ Replacement of Right Radius with Synthetic Substitute, Open Approach—AHA CC: 4Q, 2018, 92-93

0PS00ZZ Reposition Sternum, Open Approach—AHA CC: 4Q, 2015, 34

0PS204Z Reposition 3 or More Ribs with Internal Fixation Device, Open Approach—AHA CC: 4Q, 2014, 26; 4Q, 2017, 53

0PS3XZZ Reposition Cervical Vertebra, External Approach—AHA CC: 2Q, 2015, 35

0PS404Z Reposition Thoracic Vertebra with Internal Fixation Device, Open Approach—AHA CC: 1Q, 2020, 33-34

0PS444Z Reposition Thoracic Vertebra with Internal Fixation Device, Percutaneous Endoscopic Approach—AHA CC: 3Q, 2018, 26-27

0PS4XZZ Reposition Thoracic Vertebra, External Approach—AHA CC: 1Q, 2016, 21

0PSJ04Z Reposition Left Radius with Internal Fixation Device, Open Approach—AHA CC: 3Q, 2014, 33-34; 4Q, 2014, 32-33

0PSL04Z Reposition Left Ulna with Internal Fixation Device, Open Approach—AHA CC: 4Q, 2014, 32-33

0PTN0ZZ Resection of Left Carpal, Open Approach—AHA CC: 3Q, 2015, 26-27

0PU00JZ Supplement Sternum with Synthetic Substitute, Open Approach—AHA CC: 4Q, 2013, 109-111

0PU30KZ Supplement Cervical Vertebra with Nonautologous Tissue Substitute, Open Approach—AHA CC: 2Q, 2015, 20-21

0PU507Z Supplement Right Scapula with Autologous Tissue Substitute, Open Approach—AHA CC: 4Q, 2018, 12-13

0PU50KZ Supplement Right Scapula with Nonautologous Tissue Substitute, Open Approach—AHA CC: 4Q, 2018, 12-13

0PUC3JZ Supplement Right Humeral Head with Synthetic Substitute, Percutaneous Approach—AHA CC: 3Q, 2021, 15-16

0PUC47Z Supplement Right Humeral Head with Autologous Tissue Substitute, Percutaneous Endoscopic Approach—AHA CC: 2Q, 2023, 24-25

0PUD3JZ Supplement Left Humeral Head with Synthetic Substitute, Percutaneous Approach—AHA CC: 3Q, 2021, 15-16

0PW104Z Revision of Internal Fixation Device in I to 2 Ribs, Open Approach—AHA CC: 4Q, 2014, 26-27

0PW204Z Revision of Internal Fixation Device in 3 or More Ribs, Open Approach—AHA CC: 4Q, 2014, 26-27

0PW404Z Revision of Internal Fixation Device in Thoracic Vertebra, Open Approach—AHA CC: 4Q, 2014, 27-28

Lower Bones

Bones - Front and Back Views

Lower Bones Tables 0Q2–0QW

Section	0	Medical and Surgical
Body System	Q	Lower Bones
Operation	2	**Change:** Taking out or off a device from a body part and putting back an identical or similar device in or on the same body part without cutting or puncturing the skin or a mucous membrane

Body Part (4th)	Approach (5th)	Device (6th)	Qualifier (7th)
Y Lower Bone	**X** External	**0** Drainage Device **Y** Other Device	**Z** No Qualifier

Section	0	Medical and Surgical
Body System	Q	Lower Bones
Operation	5	**Destruction:** Physical eradication of all or a portion of a body part by the direct use of energy, force, or a destructive agent

Body Part (4th)	Approach (5th)	Device (6th)	Qualifier (7th)
0 Lumbar Vertebra **1** Sacrum	**0** Open **3** Percutaneous **4** Percutaneous Endoscopic	**Z** No Device	**3** Laser Interstitial Thermal Therapy **Z** No Qualifier
2 Pelvic Bone, Right **3** Pelvic Bone, Left **4** Acetabulum, Right **5** Acetabulum, Left **6** Upper Femur, Right **7** Upper Femur, Left **8** Femoral Shaft, Right **9** Femoral Shaft, Left **B** Lower Femur, Right **C** Lower Femur, Left **D** Patella, Right **F** Patella, Left **G** Tibia, Right **H** Tibia, Left **J** Fibula, Right **K** Fibula, Left **L** Tarsal, Right **M** Tarsal, Left **N** Metatarsal, Right **P** Metatarsal, Left **Q** Toe Phalanx, Right **R** Toe Phalanx, Left **S** Coccyx	**0** Open **3** Percutaneous **4** Percutaneous Endoscopic	**Z** No Device	**Z** No Qualifier

Section	0	Medical and Surgical
Body System	Q	Lower Bones
Operation	8	**Division:** Cutting into a body part, without draining fluids and/or gases from the body part, in order to separate or transect a body part

Body Part (4th)	Approach (5th)	Device (6th)	Qualifier (7th)
0 Lumbar Vertebra 1 Sacrum 2 Pelvic Bone, Right 3 Pelvic Bone, Left 4 Acetabulum, Right 5 Acetabulum, Left 6 Upper Femur, Right 7 Upper Femur, Left 8 Femoral Shaft, Right 9 Femoral Shaft, Left B Lower Femur, Right C Lower Femur, Left D Patella, Right F Patella, Left G Tibia, Right H Tibia, Left J Fibula, Right K Fibula, Left L Tarsal, Right M Tarsal, Left N Metatarsal, Right P Metatarsal, Left Q Toe Phalanx, Right R Toe Phalanx, Left S Coccyx	0 Open 3 Percutaneous 4 Percutaneous Endoscopic	Z No Device	Z No Qualifier

Section	0	Medical and Surgical
Body System	Q	Lower Bones
Operation	9	**Drainage:** Taking or letting out fluids and/or gases from a body part

Body Part (4th)	Approach (5th)	Device (6th)	Qualifier (7th)
0 Lumbar Vertebra 1 Sacrum 2 Pelvic Bone, Right 3 Pelvic Bone, Left 4 Acetabulum, Right 5 Acetabulum, Left 6 Upper Femur, Right 7 Upper Femur, Left 8 Femoral Shaft, Right 9 Femoral Shaft, Left B Lower Femur, Right C Lower Femur, Left D Patella, Right F Patella, Left G Tibia, Right H Tibia, Left J Fibula, Right K Fibula, Left L Tarsal, Right M Tarsal, Left N Metatarsal, Right P Metatarsal, Left Q Toe Phalanx, Right R Toe Phalanx, Left S Coccyx	0 Open 3 Percutaneous 4 Percutaneous Endoscopic	0 Drainage Device	Z No Qualifier

Continued →

Section	0	Medical and Surgical
Body System	Q	Lower Bones
Operation	9	Drainage: Taking or letting out fluids and/or gases from a body part

Body Part (4th)	Approach (5th)	Device (6th)	Qualifier (7th)
0 Lumbar Vertebra 1 Sacrum 2 Pelvic Bone, Right 3 Pelvic Bone, Left 4 Acetabulum, Right 5 Acetabulum, Left 6 Upper Femur, Right 7 Upper Femur, Left 8 Femoral Shaft, Right 9 Femoral Shaft, Left B Lower Femur, Right C Lower Femur, Left D Patella, Right F Patella, Left G Tibia, Right H Tibia, Left J Fibula, Right K Fibula, Left L Tarsal, Right M Tarsal, Left N Metatarsal, Right P Metatarsal, Left Q Toe Phalanx, Right R Toe Phalanx, Left S Coccyx	0 Open 3 Percutaneous 4 Percutaneous Endoscopic	Z No Device	X Diagnostic Z No Qualifier

Section	0	Medical and Surgical
Body System	Q	Lower Bones
Operation	B	Excision: Cutting out or off, without replacement, a portion of a body part

Body Part (4th)	Approach (5th)	Device (6th)	Qualifier (7th)
0 Lumbar Vertebra 1 Sacrum 2 Pelvic Bone, Right 3 Pelvic Bone, Left 4 Acetabulum, Right 5 Acetabulum, Left 6 Upper Femur, Right 7 Upper Femur, Left 8 Femoral Shaft, Right 9 Femoral Shaft, Left B Lower Femur, Right C Lower Femur, Left D Patella, Right F Patella, Left G Tibia, Right H Tibia, Left J Fibula, Right K Fibula, Left L Tarsal, Right M Tarsal, Left Q Toe Phalanx, Right R Toe Phalanx, Left S Coccyx	0 Open 3 Percutaneous 4 Percutaneous Endoscopic	Z No Device	X Diagnostic Z No Qualifier
N Metatarsal, Right P Metatarsal, Left	0 Open 3 Percutaneous 4 Percutaneous Endoscopic	Z No Device	2 Sesamoid Bone(s) 1st Toe X Diagnostic Z No Qualifier

0QC–0QD

Medical and Surgical, Lower Bones Tables

Section	0	Medical and Surgical
Body System	Q	Lower Bones
Operation	C	**Extirpation:** Taking or cutting out solid matter from a body part

Body Part (4th)	Approach (5th)	Device (6th)	Qualifier (7th)
0 Lumbar Vertebra 1 Sacrum 2 Pelvic Bone, Right 3 Pelvic Bone, Left 4 Acetabulum, Right 5 Acetabulum, Left 6 Upper Femur, Right 7 Upper Femur, Left 8 Femoral Shaft, Right 9 Femoral Shaft, Left B Lower Femur, Right C Lower Femur, Left D Patella, Right F Patella, Left G Tibia, Right H Tibia, Left J Fibula, Right K Fibula, Left L Tarsal, Right M Tarsal, Left N Metatarsal, Right P Metatarsal, Left Q Toe Phalanx, Right R Toe Phalanx, Left S Coccyx	0 Open 3 Percutaneous 4 Percutaneous Endoscopic	Z No Device	Z No Qualifier

Section	0	Medical and Surgical
Body System	Q	Lower Bones
Operation	D	**Extraction:** Pulling or stripping out or off all or a portion of a body part by the use of force

Body Part (4th)	Approach (5th)	Device (6th)	Qualifier (7th)
0 Lumbar Vertebra 1 Sacrum 2 Pelvic Bone, Right 3 Pelvic Bone, Left 4 Acetabulum, Right 5 Acetabulum, Left 6 Upper Femur, Right 7 Upper Femur, Left 8 Femoral Shaft, Right 9 Femoral Shaft, Left B Lower Femur, Right C Lower Femur, Left D Patella, Right F Patella, Left G Tibia, Right H Tibia, Left J Fibula, Right K Fibula, Left L Tarsal, Right M Tarsal, Left N Metatarsal, Right P Metatarsal, Left Q Toe Phalanx, Right R Toe Phalanx, Left S Coccyx	0 Open	Z No Device	Z No Qualifier

Section	0	Medical and Surgical
Body System	Q	Lower Bones
Operation	H	Insertion: Putting in a nonbiological appliance that monitors, assists, performs, or prevents a physiological function but does not physically take the place of a body part

Body Part (4th)	Approach (5th)	Device (6th)	Qualifier (7th)
0 Lumbar Vertebra 1 Sacrum 2 Pelvic Bone, Right 3 Pelvic Bone, Left 4 Acetabulum, Right 5 Acetabulum, Left D Patella, Right F Patella, Left L Tarsal, Right M Tarsal, Left N Metatarsal, Right P Metatarsal, Left Q Toe Phalanx, Right R Toe Phalanx, Left S Coccyx	0 Open 3 Percutaneous 4 Percutaneous Endoscopic	4 Internal Fixation Device 5 External Fixation Device	Z No Qualifier
6 Upper Femur, Right 7 Upper Femur, Left B Lower Femur, Right C Lower Femur, Left J Fibula, Right K Fibula, Left	0 Open 3 Percutaneous 4 Percutaneous Endoscopic	4 Internal Fixation Device 5 External Fixation Device 6 Internal Fixation Device, Intramedullary 8 External Fixation Device, Limb Lengthening B External Fixation Device, Monoplanar C External Fixation Device, Ring D External Fixation Device, Hybrid	Z No Qualifier
8 Femoral Shaft, Right 9 Femoral Shaft, Left G Tibia, Right H Tibia, Left	0 Open 3 Percutaneous 4 Percutaneous Endoscopic	4 Internal Fixation Device 5 External Fixation Device 6 Internal Fixation Device, Intramedullary 7 Internal Fixation Device, Intramedullary Limb Lengthening 8 External Fixation Device, Limb Lengthening B External Fixation Device, Monoplanar C External Fixation Device, Ring D External Fixation Device, Hybrid	Z No Qualifier
Y Lower Bone	0 Open 3 Percutaneous 4 Percutaneous Endoscopic	M Bone Growth Stimulator	Z No Qualifier

Section	0	Medical and Surgical
Body System	Q	Lower Bones
Operation	J	Inspection: Visually and/or manually exploring a body part

Body Part (4th)	Approach (5th)	Device (6th)	Qualifier (7th)
Y Lower Bone	0 Open 3 Percutaneous 4 Percutaneous Endoscopic X External	Z No Device	Z No Qualifier

Section	0	Medical and Surgical
Body System	Q	Lower Bones
Operation	N	**Release:** Freeing a body part from an abnormal physical constraint by cutting or by the use of force

Body Part (4th)	Approach (5th)	Device (6th)	Qualifier (7th)
0 Lumbar Vertebra 1 Sacrum 2 Pelvic Bone, Right 3 Pelvic Bone, Left 4 Acetabulum, Right 5 Acetabulum, Left 6 Upper Femur, Right 7 Upper Femur, Left 8 Femoral Shaft, Right 9 Femoral Shaft, Left B Lower Femur, Right C Lower Femur, Left D Patella, Right F Patella, Left G Tibia, Right H Tibia, Left J Fibula, Right K Fibula, Left L Tarsal, Right M Tarsal, Left N Metatarsal, Right P Metatarsal, Left Q Toe Phalanx, Right R Toe Phalanx, Left S Coccyx	0 Open 3 Percutaneous 4 Percutaneous Endoscopic	Z No Device	Z No Qualifier

Section	0	Medical and Surgical
Body System	Q	Lower Bones
Operation	P	**Removal:** Taking out or off a device from a body part

Body Part (4th)	Approach (5th)	Device (6th)	Qualifier (7th)
0 Lumbar Vertebra 1 Sacrum 2 Pelvic Bone, Right 3 Pelvic Bone, Left 4 Acetabulum, Right 5 Acetabulum, Left 6 Upper Femur, Right 7 Upper Femur, Left 8 Femoral Shaft, Right 9 Femoral Shaft, Left B Lower Femur, Right C Lower Femur, Left D Patella, Right F Patella, Left G Tibia, Right H Tibia, Left J Fibula, Right K Fibula, Left L Tarsal, Right M Tarsal, Left N Metatarsal, Right P Metatarsal, Left Q Toe Phalanx, Right R Toe Phalanx, Left S Coccyx	0 Open 3 Percutaneous 4 Percutaneous Endoscopic	4 Internal Fixation Device 5 External Fixation Device 7 Autologous Tissue Substitute J Synthetic Substitute K Nonautologous Tissue Substitute	Z No Qualifier

Continued →

0QP Continued

Section 0 Medical and Surgical
Body System Q Lower Bones
Operation P Removal: Taking out or off a device from a body part

Body Part (4th)	Approach (5th)	Device (6th)	Qualifier (7th)
0 Lumbar Vertebra 1 Sacrum 2 Pelvic Bone, Right 3 Pelvic Bone, Left 4 Acetabulum, Right 5 Acetabulum, Left 6 Upper Femur, Right 7 Upper Femur, Left 8 Femoral Shaft, Right 9 Femoral Shaft, Left B Lower Femur, Right C Lower Femur, Left D Patella, Right F Patella, Left G Tibia, Right H Tibia, Left J Fibula, Right K Fibula, Left L Tarsal, Right M Tarsal, Left N Metatarsal, Right P Metatarsal, Left Q Toe Phalanx, Right R Toe Phalanx, Left S Coccyx	X External	4 Internal Fixation Device 5 External Fixation Device	Z No Qualifier
Y Lower Bone	0 Open 3 Percutaneous 4 Percutaneous Endoscopic X External	0 Drainage Device M Bone Growth Stimulator	Z No Qualifier

Section 0 Medical and Surgical
Body System Q Lower Bones
Operation Q Repair: Restoring, to the extent possible, a body part to its normal anatomic structure and function

Body Part (4th)	Approach (5th)	Device (6th)	Qualifier (7th)
0 Lumbar Vertebra 1 Sacrum 2 Pelvic Bone, Right 3 Pelvic Bone, Left 4 Acetabulum, Right 5 Acetabulum, Left 6 Upper Femur, Right 7 Upper Femur, Left 8 Femoral Shaft, Right 9 Femoral Shaft, Left B Lower Femur, Right C Lower Femur, Left D Patella, Right F Patella, Left G Tibia, Right H Tibia, Left J Fibula, Right K Fibula, Left L Tarsal, Right M Tarsal, Left N Metatarsal, Right P Metatarsal, Left Q Toe Phalanx, Right R Toe Phalanx, Left S Coccyx	0 Open 3 Percutaneous 4 Percutaneous Endoscopic X External	Z No Device	Z No Qualifier

0QP–0QQ

Medical and Surgical, Lower Bones Tables

Section	0	Medical and Surgical
Body System	Q	Lower Bones
Operation	R	**Replacement:** Putting in or on biological or synthetic material that physically takes the place and/or function of all or a portion of a body part

Body Part (4th)	Approach (5th)	Device (6th)	Qualifier (7th)
0 Lumbar Vertebra 1 Sacrum 2 Pelvic Bone, Right 3 Pelvic Bone, Left 4 Acetabulum, Right 5 Acetabulum, Left 6 Upper Femur, Right 7 Upper Femur, Left 8 Femoral Shaft, Right 9 Femoral Shaft, Left B Lower Femur, Right C Lower Femur, Left D Patella, Right F Patella, Left G Tibia, Right H Tibia, Left J Fibula, Right K Fibula, Left L Tarsal, Right M Tarsal, Left N Metatarsal, Right P Metatarsal, Left Q Toe Phalanx, Right R Toe Phalanx, Left S Coccyx	0 Open 3 Percutaneous 4 Percutaneous Endoscopic	7 Autologous Tissue Substitute J Synthetic Substitute K Nonautologous Tissue Substitute	Z No Qualifier

Section	0	Medical and Surgical
Body System	Q	Lower Bones
Operation	S	**Reposition:** Moving to its normal location, or other suitable location, all or a portion of a body part

Body Part (4th)	Approach (5th)	Device (6th)	Qualifier (7th)
0 Lumbar Vertebra	0 Open 4 Percutaneous Endoscopic	3 Spinal Stabilization Device, Vertebral Body Tether 4 Internal Fixation Device Z No Device	Z No Qualifier
0 Lumbar Vertebra	3 Percutaneous	4 Internal Fixation Device Z No Device	Z No Qualifier
0 Lumbar Vertebra	X External	Z No Device	Z No Qualifier
1 Sacrum 4 Acetabulum, Right 5 Acetabulum, Left S Coccyx	0 Open 3 Percutaneous 4 Percutaneous Endoscopic	4 Internal Fixation Device Z No Device	Z No Qualifier
1 Sacrum 4 Acetabulum, Right 5 Acetabulum, Left S Coccyx	X External	Z No Device	Z No Qualifier
2 Pelvic Bone, Right 3 Pelvic Bone, Left D Patella, Right F Patella, Left L Tarsal, Right M Tarsal, Left Q Toe Phalanx, Right R Toe Phalanx, Left	0 Open 3 Percutaneous 4 Percutaneous Endoscopic	4 Internal Fixation Device 5 External Fixation Device Z No Device	Z No Qualifier

Continued →

0QS Continued

Section	0	Medical and Surgical
Body System	Q	Lower Bones
Operation	S	Reposition: Moving to its normal location, or other suitable location, all or a portion of a body part

Body Part (4th)	Approach (5th)	Device (6th)	Qualifier (7th)
2 Pelvic Bone, Right 3 Pelvic Bone, Left D Patella, Right F Patella, Left L Tarsal, Right M Tarsal, Left Q Toe Phalanx, Right R Toe Phalanx, Left	X External	Z No Device	Z No Qualifier
6 Upper Femur, Right 7 Upper Femur, Left 8 Femoral Shaft, Right 9 Femoral Shaft, Left B Lower Femur, Right C Lower Femur, Left G Tibia, Right H Tibia, Left J Fibula, Right K Fibula, Left	0 Open 3 Percutaneous 4 Percutaneous Endoscopic	4 Internal Fixation Device 5 External Fixation Device 6 Internal Fixation Device, Intramedullary B External Fixation Device, Monoplanar C External Fixation Device, Ring D External Fixation Device, Hybrid Z No Device	Z No Qualifier
6 Upper Femur, Right 7 Upper Femur, Left 8 Femoral Shaft, Right 9 Femoral Shaft, Left B Lower Femur, Right C Lower Femur, Left G Tibia, Right H Tibia, Left J Fibula, Right K Fibula, Left	X External	Z No Device	Z No Qualifier
N Metatarsal, Right P Metatarsal, Left	0 Open 3 Percutaneous 4 Percutaneous Endoscopic	4 Internal Fixation Device 5 External Fixation Device Z No Device	2 Sesamoid Bone(s) 1st Toe Z No Qualifier
N Metatarsal, Right P Metatarsal, Left	X External	Z No Device	2 Sesamoid Bone(s) 1st Toe Z No Qualifier

Section	0	Medical and Surgical
Body System	Q	Lower Bones
Operation	T	Resection: Cutting out or off, without replacement, all of a body part

Body Part (4th)	Approach (5th)	Device (6th)	Qualifier (7th)
2 Pelvic Bone, Right 3 Pelvic Bone, Left 4 Acetabulum, Right 5 Acetabulum, Left 6 Upper Femur, Right 7 Upper Femur, Left 8 Femoral Shaft, Right 9 Femoral Shaft, Left B Lower Femur, Right C Lower Femur, Left D Patella, Right F Patella, Left G Tibia, Right H Tibia, Left J Fibula, Right K Fibula, Left L Tarsal, Right M Tarsal, Left N Metatarsal, Right P Metatarsal, Left Q Toe Phalanx, Right R Toe Phalanx, Left S Coccyx	0 Open	Z No Device	Z No Qualifier

Section 0 **Medical and Surgical**
Body System Q **Lower Bones**
Operation U **Supplement:** Putting in or on biological or synthetic material that physically reinforces and/or augments the function of a portion of a body part

Body Part (4th)	Approach (5th)	Device (6th)	Qualifier (7th)
0 Lumbar Vertebra	0 Open	7 Autologous Tissue Substitute	Z No Qualifier
1 Sacrum	3 Percutaneous	J Synthetic Substitute	
2 Pelvic Bone, Right	4 Percutaneous Endoscopic	K Nonautologous Tissue Substitute	
3 Pelvic Bone, Left			
4 Acetabulum, Right			
5 Acetabulum, Left			
6 Upper Femur, Right			
7 Upper Femur, Left			
8 Femoral Shaft, Right			
9 Femoral Shaft, Left			
B Lower Femur, Right			
C Lower Femur, Left			
D Patella, Right			
F Patella, Left			
G Tibia, Right			
H Tibia, Left			
J Fibula, Right			
K Fibula, Left			
L Tarsal, Right			
M Tarsal, Left			
N Metatarsal, Right			
P Metatarsal, Left			
Q Toe Phalanx, Right			
R Toe Phalanx, Left			
S Coccyx			

Section 0 **Medical and Surgical**
Body System Q **Lower Bones**
Operation W **Revision:** Correcting, to the extent possible, a portion of a malfunctioning device or the position of a displaced device

Body Part (4th)	Approach (5th)	Device (6th)	Qualifier (7th)
0 Lumbar Vertebra	0 Open	4 Internal Fixation Device	Z No Qualifier
1 Sacrum	3 Percutaneous	7 Autologous Tissue Substitute	
4 Acetabulum, Right	4 Percutaneous Endoscopic	J Synthetic Substitute	
5 Acetabulum, Left	X External	K Nonautologous Tissue Substitute	
S Coccyx			
2 Pelvic Bone, Right	0 Open	4 Internal Fixation Device	Z No Qualifier
3 Pelvic Bone, Left	3 Percutaneous	5 External Fixation Device	
6 Upper Femur, Right	4 Percutaneous Endoscopic	7 Autologous Tissue Substitute	
7 Upper Femur, Left	X External	J Synthetic Substitute	
8 Femoral Shaft, Right		K Nonautologous Tissue Substitute	
9 Femoral Shaft, Left			
B Lower Femur, Right			
C Lower Femur, Left			
D Patella, Right			
F Patella, Left			
G Tibia, Right			
H Tibia, Left			
J Fibula, Right			
K Fibula, Left			
L Tarsal, Right			
M Tarsal, Left			
N Metatarsal, Right			
P Metatarsal, Left			
Q Toe Phalanx, Right			
R Toe Phalanx, Left			

Continued →

Section	0	Medical and Surgical				0QW Continued

Section 0 **Medical and Surgical**
Body System Q **Lower Bones**
Operation W **Revision:** Correcting, to the extent possible, a portion of a malfunctioning device or the position of a displaced device

Body Part (4th)	Approach (5th)	Device (6th)	Qualifier (7th)
Y Lower Bone	0 Open 3 Percutaneous 4 Percutaneous Endoscopic X External	0 Drainage Device M Bone Growth Stimulator	Z No Qualifier

AHA Coding Clinic

0Q830ZZ Division of Left Pelvic Bone, Open Approach—AHA CC: 2Q, 2016, 32

0Q923ZX Drainage of Right Pelvic Bone, Percutaneous Approach, Diagnostic—AHA CC: 1Q, 2022, 31-32

0Q933ZX Drainage of Left Pelvic Bone, Percutaneous Approach, Diagnostic—AHA CC: 1Q, 2022, 31-32

0QB10ZZ Excision of Sacrum, Open Approach—AHA CC: 2Q, 2020, 26

0QB20ZZ Excision of Right Pelvic Bone, Open Approach—AHA CC: 2Q, 2014, 6-7; 4Q, 2018, 12-13

0QB30ZZ Excision of Left Pelvic Bone, Open Approach—AHA CC: 2Q, 2019, 19-20

0QB74ZZ Excision of Left Upper Femur, Percutaneous Endoscopic Approach—AHA CC: 4Q, 2014, 25-26

0QBJ0ZZ Excision of Right Fibula, Open Approach—AHA CC: 1Q, 2017, 23-24

0QBK0ZZ Excision of Left Fibula, Open Approach—AHA CC: 2Q, 2013, 39-40

0QBL0ZZ Excision of Right Tarsal, Open Approach—AHA CC: 3Q, 2018, 17-18

0QBN0ZZ Excision of Right Metatarsal, Open Approach—AHA CC: 2Q, 2021, 18-19

0QH204Z Insertion of Internal Fixation Device into Right Pelvic Bone, Open Approach—AHA CC: 1Q, 2017, 21-22

0QH304Z Insertion of Internal Fixation Device into Left Pelvic Bone, Open Approach—AHA CC: 1Q, 2017, 21-22

0QHG04Z Insertion of Internal Fixation Device into Right Tibia, Open Approach—AHA CC: 3Q, 2016, 34-35

0QHH38Z Insertion of Limb Lengthening External Fixation Device into Left Tibia, Percutaneous Approach—AHA CC: 2Q, 2022, 19-21

0QHJ04Z Insertion of Internal Fixation Device into Right Fibula, Open Approach—AHA CC: 3Q, 2016, 34-35

0QHK38Z Insertion of Limb Lengthening External Fixation Device into Left Fibula, Percutaneous Approach—AHA CC: 2Q, 2022, 19-21

0QP004Z Removal of Internal Fixation Device from Lumbar Vertebra, Open Approach—AHA CC: 4Q, 2017, 75

0QP104Z Removal of Internal Fixation Device from Sacrum, Open Approach—AHA CC: 1Q, 2023, 33-34

0QPG04Z Removal of Internal Fixation Device from Right Tibia, Open Approach—AHA CC: 2Q, 2015, 6-7

0QQ10ZZ Repair Sacrum, Open Approach—AHA CC: 3Q, 2014, 24

0QQ20ZZ Repair Right Pelvic Bone, Open Approach—AHA CC: 1Q, 2018, 15

0QQ30ZZ Repair Left Pelvic Bone, Open Approach—AHA CC: 1Q, 2018, 15

0QS004Z Reposition Lumbar Vertebra with Internal Fixation Device, Open Approach—AHA CC: 1Q, 2020, 33-34

0QS504Z Reposition Left Acetabulum with Internal Fixation Device, Open Approach—AHA CC: 2Q, 2016, 32; 1Q, 2018, 25

0QS904Z Reposition Left Femoral Shaft with Internal Fixation Device, Open Approach—AHA CC: 3Q, 2019, 26

0QSC04Z Reposition Left Lower Femur with Internal Fixation Device, Open Approach—AHA CC: 4Q, 2014, 31

0QSF04Z Reposition Left Patella with Internal Fixation Device, Open Approach—AHA CC: 3Q, 2016, 34-35

0QSH04Z Reposition Left Tibia with Internal Fixation Device, Open Approach—AHA CC: 4Q, 2014, 30-31; 3Q, 2016, 34-35

0QSH3CZ Reposition Left Tibia with Ring External Fixation Device, Percutaneous Approach—AHA CC: 2Q, 2022, 19-21

0QSK0ZZ Reposition Left Fibula, Open Approach—AHA CC: 3Q, 2016, 34-35

0QSK3CZ Reposition Left Fibula with Ring External Fixation Device, Percutaneous Approach—AHA CC: 2Q, 2022, 19-21

0QSL04Z Reposition Right Tarsal with Internal Fixation Device, Open Approach—AHA CC: 1Q, 2018, 13

0QSM04Z Reposition Left Tarsal with Internal Fixation Device, Open Approach—AHA CC: 1Q, 2018, 13

0QT60ZZ Resection of Right Upper Femur, Open Approach—AHA CC: 3Q, 2016, 30-31

0QT70ZZ Resection of Left Upper Femur, Open Approach—AHA CC: 3Q, 2015, 26; 3Q, 2016, 30-31

0QTC0ZZ Resection of Left Lower Femur, Open Approach—AHA CC: 4Q, 2014, 30-31

0QU03JZ Supplement Lumbar Vertebra with Synthetic Substitute, Percutaneous Approach—AHA CC: 2Q, 2014, 12-13; 2Q, 2019, 35

0QU20JZ Supplement Right Pelvic Bone with Synthetic Substitute, Open Approach—AHA CC: 2Q, 2013, 35-36

0QU50JZ Supplement Left Acetabulum with Synthetic Substitute, Open Approach—AHA CC: 3Q, 2015, 18-19

0QU90KZ Supplement Left Femoral Shaft with Nonautologous Tissue Substitute, Open Approach—AHA CC: 3Q, 2019, 26

0QUC0KZ Supplement Left Lower Femur with—Nonautologous Tissue Substitute, Open Approach—AHA CC: 4Q, 2014, 31

0QW034Z Revision of Internal Fixation Device in Lumbar Vertebra, Percutaneous Approach—AHA CC: 4Q, 2017, 75

Upper Joints

Intervertebral Joint

Shoulder

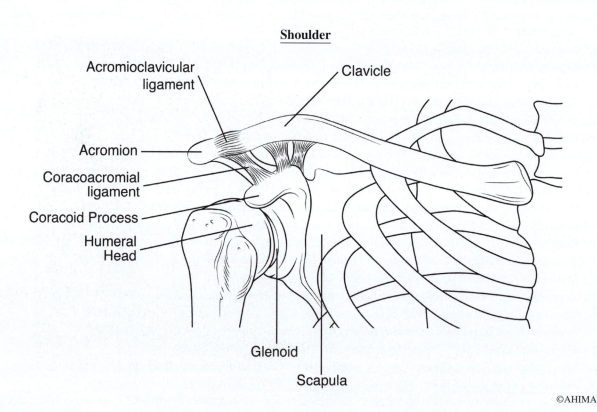

Anterior Interbody Fusion by Dowel Graft

Cervical Spine Injury: Anterior Interbody Fusion by Dowel Graft (Cloward)

Spine exposed by progressive dissection and self-retaining retractors inserted. Disc, osteophytes and bone fragments removed under direct vision

Dowel bone graft obtained from ilium or bone bank is cut 2 mm wider and 2 mm shorter than drill hole. It is impacted after hole is widened with vertebra spreader

Dowel recessed 2 mm below anterior margin of drill hole. When spreader is removed, graft is locked securely in place. Cortical end plates lateral to dowel are perforated and interspace packed with bone dust removed from drill

Follow-up x-ray film. Dowel graft fusion of C5-6 with good union

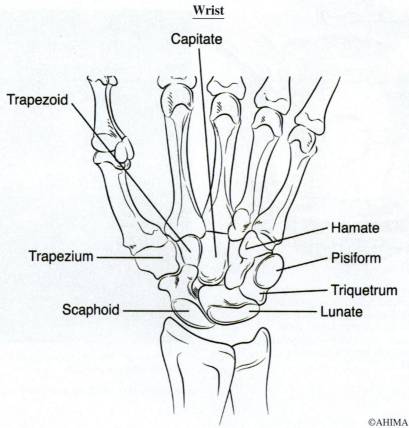

Upper Joints Tables 0R2–0RW

Section	0	Medical and Surgical
Body System	R	Upper Joints
Operation	2	Change: Taking out or off a device from a body part and putting back an identical or similar device in or on the same body part without cutting or puncturing the skin or a mucous membrane

Body Part (4th)	Approach (5th)	Device (6th)	Qualifier (7th)
Y Upper Joint	X External	0 Drainage Device Y Other Device	Z No Qualifier

Section	0	Medical and Surgical
Body System	R	Upper Joints
Operation	5	Destruction: Physical eradication of all or a portion of a body part by the direct use of energy, force, or a destructive agent

Body Part (4th)	Approach (5th)	Device (6th)	Qualifier (7th)
0 Occipital-cervical Joint 1 Cervical Vertebral Joint 3 Cervical Vertebral Disc 4 Cervicothoracic Vertebral Joint 5 Cervicothoracic Vertebral Disc 6 Thoracic Vertebral Joint 9 Thoracic Vertebral Disc A Thoracolumbar Vertebral Joint B Thoracolumbar Vertebral Disc C Temporomandibular Joint, Right D Temporomandibular Joint, Left E Sternoclavicular Joint, Right F Sternoclavicular Joint, Left G Acromioclavicular Joint, Right H Acromioclavicular Joint, Left J Shoulder Joint, Right K Shoulder Joint, Left L Elbow Joint, Right M Elbow Joint, Left N Wrist Joint, Right P Wrist Joint, Left Q Carpal Joint, Right R Carpal Joint, Left S Carpometacarpal Joint, Right T Carpometacarpal Joint, Left U Metacarpophalangeal Joint, Right V Metacarpophalangeal Joint, Left W Finger Phalangeal Joint, Right X Finger Phalangeal Joint, Left	0 Open 3 Percutaneous 4 Percutaneous Endoscopic	Z No Device	Z No Qualifier

Section	0	Medical and Surgical
Body System	R	Upper Joints
Operation	9	Drainage: Taking or letting out fluids and/or gases from a body part

Body Part (4th)	Approach (5th)	Device (6th)	Qualifier (7th)
0 Occipital-cervical Joint 1 Cervical Vertebral Joint 3 Cervical Vertebral Disc 4 Cervicothoracic Vertebral Joint 5 Cervicothoracic Vertebral Disc 6 Thoracic Vertebral Joint 9 Thoracic Vertebral Disc A Thoracolumbar Vertebral Joint B Thoracolumbar Vertebral Disc C Temporomandibular Joint, Right D Temporomandibular Joint, Left E Sternoclavicular Joint, Right F Sternoclavicular Joint, Left G Acromioclavicular Joint, Right H Acromioclavicular Joint, Left J Shoulder Joint, Right K Shoulder Joint, Left L Elbow Joint, Right M Elbow Joint, Left N Wrist Joint, Right P Wrist Joint, Left Q Carpal Joint, Right R Carpal Joint, Left S Carpometacarpal Joint, Right T Carpometacarpal Joint, Left U Metacarpophalangeal Joint, Right V Metacarpophalangeal Joint, Left W Finger Phalangeal Joint, Right X Finger Phalangeal Joint, Left	0 Open 3 Percutaneous 4 Percutaneous Endoscopic	0 Drainage Device	Z No Qualifier
0 Occipital-cervical Joint 1 Cervical Vertebral Joint 3 Cervical Vertebral Disc 4 Cervicothoracic Vertebral Joint 5 Cervicothoracic Vertebral Disc 6 Thoracic Vertebral Joint 9 Thoracic Vertebral Disc A Thoracolumbar Vertebral Joint B Thoracolumbar Vertebral Disc C Temporomandibular Joint, Right D Temporomandibular Joint, Left E Sternoclavicular Joint, Right F Sternoclavicular Joint, Left G Acromioclavicular Joint, Right H Acromioclavicular Joint, Left J Shoulder Joint, Right K Shoulder Joint, Left L Elbow Joint, Right M Elbow Joint, Left N Wrist Joint, Right P Wrist Joint, Left Q Carpal Joint, Right R Carpal Joint, Left S Carpometacarpal Joint, Right T Carpometacarpal Joint, Left U Metacarpophalangeal Joint, Right V Metacarpophalangeal Joint, Left W Finger Phalangeal Joint, Right X Finger Phalangeal Joint, Left	0 Open 3 Percutaneous 4 Percutaneous Endoscopic	Z No Device	X Diagnostic Z No Qualifier

Section	0	Medical and Surgical
Body System	R	Upper Joints
Operation	B	Excision: Cutting out or off, without replacement, a portion of a body part

Body Part (4th)	Approach (5th)	Device (6th)	Qualifier (7th)
0 Occipital-cervical Joint	0 Open	Z No Device	X Diagnostic
1 Cervical Vertebral Joint	3 Percutaneous		Z No Qualifier
3 Cervical Vertebral Disc	4 Percutaneous Endoscopic		
4 Cervicothoracic Vertebral Joint			
5 Cervicothoracic Vertebral Disc			
6 Thoracic Vertebral Joint			
9 Thoracic Vertebral Disc			
A Thoracolumbar Vertebral Joint			
B Thoracolumbar Vertebral Disc			
C Temporomandibular Joint, Right			
D Temporomandibular Joint, Left			
E Sternoclavicular Joint, Right			
F Sternoclavicular Joint, Left			
G Acromioclavicular Joint, Right			
H Acromioclavicular Joint, Left			
J Shoulder Joint, Right			
K Shoulder Joint, Left			
L Elbow Joint, Right			
M Elbow Joint, Left			
N Wrist Joint, Right			
P Wrist Joint, Left			
Q Carpal Joint, Right			
R Carpal Joint, Left			
S Carpometacarpal Joint, Right			
T Carpometacarpal Joint, Left			
U Metacarpophalangeal Joint, Right			
V Metacarpophalangeal Joint, Left			
W Finger Phalangeal Joint, Right			
X Finger Phalangeal Joint, Left			

Section	0	Medical and Surgical
Body System	R	Upper Joints
Operation	C	Extirpation: Taking or cutting out solid matter from a body part

Body Part (4th)	Approach (5th)	Device (6th)	Qualifier (7th)
0 Occipital-cervical Joint 1 Cervical Vertebral Joint 3 Cervical Vertebral Disc 4 Cervicothoracic Vertebral Joint 5 Cervicothoracic Vertebral Disc 6 Thoracic Vertebral Joint 9 Thoracic Vertebral Disc A Thoracolumbar Vertebral Joint B Thoracolumbar Vertebral Disc C Temporomandibular Joint, Right D Temporomandibular Joint, Left E Sternoclavicular Joint, Right F Sternoclavicular Joint, Left G Acromioclavicular Joint, Right H Acromioclavicular Joint, Left J Shoulder Joint, Right K Shoulder Joint, Left L Elbow Joint, Right M Elbow Joint, Left N Wrist Joint, Right P Wrist Joint, Left Q Carpal Joint, Right R Carpal Joint, Left S Carpometacarpal Joint, Right T Carpometacarpal Joint, Left U Metacarpophalangeal Joint, Right V Metacarpophalangeal Joint, Left W Finger Phalangeal Joint, Right X Finger Phalangeal Joint, Left	0 Open 3 Percutaneous 4 Percutaneous Endoscopic	Z No Device	Z No Qualifier

Section	0	Medical and Surgical
Body System	R	Upper Joints
Operation	G	Fusion: Joining together portions of an articular body part rendering the articular body part immobile

Body Part (4th)	Approach (5th)	Device (6th)	Qualifier (7th)
0 Occipital-cervical Joint 1 Cervical Vertebral Joint 2 Cervical Vertebral Joints, 2 or more 4 Cervicothoracic Vertebral Joint 6 Thoracic Vertebral Joint 7 Thoracic Vertebral Joints, 2 to 7 8 Thoracic Vertebral Joints, 8 or more A Thoracolumbar Vertebral Joint	0 Open 3 Percutaneous 4 Percutaneous Endoscopic	7 Autologous Tissue Substitute J Synthetic Substitute K Nonautologous Tissue Substitute	0 Anterior Approach, Anterior Column 1 Posterior Approach, Posterior Column J Posterior Approach, Anterior Column
0 Occipital-cervical Joint 1 Cervical Vertebral Joint 2 Cervical Vertebral Joints, 2 or more 4 Cervicothoracic Vertebral Joint 6 Thoracic Vertebral Joint 7 Thoracic Vertebral Joints, 2 to 7 8 Thoracic Vertebral Joints, 8 or more A Thoracolumbar Vertebral Joint	0 Open 3 Percutaneous 4 Percutaneous Endoscopic	A Interbody Fusion Device	0 Anterior Approach, Anterior Column J Posterior Approach, Anterior Column
C Temporomandibular Joint, Right D Temporomandibular Joint, Left E Sternoclavicular Joint, Right F Sternoclavicular Joint, Left G Acromioclavicular Joint, Right H Acromioclavicular Joint, Left J Shoulder Joint, Right K Shoulder Joint, Left	0 Open 3 Percutaneous 4 Percutaneous Endoscopic	4 Internal Fixation Device 7 Autologous Tissue Substitute J Synthetic Substitute K Nonautologous Tissue Substitute	Z No Qualifier

Continued →

Section	0	Medical and Surgical
Body System	R	Upper Joints
Operation	G	Fusion: Joining together portions of an articular body part rendering the articular body part immobile

0RG Continued

Body Part (4th)	Approach (5th)	Device (6th)	Qualifier (7th)
L Elbow Joint, Right M Elbow Joint, Left N Wrist Joint, Right P Wrist Joint, Left Q Carpal Joint, Right R Carpal Joint, Left S Carpometacarpal Joint, Right T Carpometacarpal Joint, Left U Metacarpophalangeal Joint, Right V Metacarpophalangeal Joint, Left W Finger Phalangeal Joint, Right X Finger Phalangeal Joint, Left	0 Open 3 Percutaneous 4 Percutaneous Endoscopic	3 Internal Fixation Device, Sustained Compression 4 Internal Fixation Device 5 External Fixation Device 7 Autologous Tissue Substitute J Synthetic Substitute K Nonautologous Tissue Substitute	Z No Qualifier

Section	0	Medical and Surgical
Body System	R	Upper Joints
Operation	H	Insertion: Putting in a nonbiological appliance that monitors, assists, performs, or prevents a physiological function but does not physically take the place of a body part

Body Part (4th)	Approach (5th)	Device (6th)	Qualifier (7th)
0 Occipital-cervical Joint 1 Cervical Vertebral Joint 4 Cervicothoracic Vertebral Joint 6 Thoracic Vertebral Joint A Thoracolumbar Vertebral Joint	0 Open 3 Percutaneous 4 Percutaneous Endoscopic	3 Infusion Device 4 Internal Fixation Device 8 Spacer B Spinal Stabilization Device, Interspinous Process C Spinal Stabilization Device, Pedicle-Based D Spinal Stabilization Device, Facet Replacement	Z No Qualifier
3 Cervical Vertebral Disc 5 Cervicothoracic Vertebral Disc 9 Thoracic Vertebral Disc B Thoracolumbar Vertebral Disc	0 Open 3 Percutaneous 4 Percutaneous Endoscopic	3 Infusion Device	Z No Qualifier
C Temporomandibular Joint, Right D Temporomandibular Joint, Left E Sternoclavicular Joint, Right F Sternoclavicular Joint, Left G Acromioclavicular Joint, Right H Acromioclavicular Joint, Left J Shoulder Joint, Right K Shoulder Joint, Left	0 Open 3 Percutaneous 4 Percutaneous Endoscopic	3 Infusion Device 4 Internal Fixation Device 8 Spacer	Z No Qualifier
L Elbow Joint, Right M Elbow Joint, Left N Wrist Joint, Right P Wrist Joint, Left Q Carpal Joint, Right R Carpal Joint, Left S Carpometacarpal Joint, Right T Carpometacarpal Joint, Left U Metacarpophalangeal Joint, Right V Metacarpophalangeal Joint, Left W Finger Phalangeal Joint, Right X Finger Phalangeal Joint, Left	0 Open 3 Percutaneous 4 Percutaneous Endoscopic	3 Infusion Device 4 Internal Fixation Device 5 External Fixation Device 8 Spacer	Z No Qualifier

0RJ-0RN

Section	0	Medical and Surgical
Body System	R	Upper Joints
Operation	J	Inspection: Visually and/or manually exploring a body part

Body Part (4th)	Approach (5th)	Device (6th)	Qualifier (7th)
0 Occipital-cervical Joint 1 Cervical Vertebral Joint 3 Cervical Vertebral Disc 4 Cervicothoracic Vertebral Joint 5 Cervicothoracic Vertebral Disc 6 Thoracic Vertebral Joint 9 Thoracic Vertebral Disc A Thoracolumbar Vertebral Joint B Thoracolumbar Vertebral Disc C Temporomandibular Joint, Right D Temporomandibular Joint, Left E Sternoclavicular Joint, Right F Sternoclavicular Joint, Left G Acromioclavicular Joint, Right H Acromioclavicular Joint, Left J Shoulder Joint, Right K Shoulder Joint, Left L Elbow Joint, Right M Elbow Joint, Left N Wrist Joint, Right P Wrist Joint, Left Q Carpal Joint, Right R Carpal Joint, Left S Carpometacarpal Joint, Right T Carpometacarpal Joint, Left U Metacarpophalangeal Joint, Right V Metacarpophalangeal Joint, Left W Finger Phalangeal Joint, Right X Finger Phalangeal Joint, Left	0 Open 3 Percutaneous 4 Percutaneous Endoscopic X External	Z No Device	Z No Qualifier

Section	0	Medical and Surgical
Body System	R	Upper Joints
Operation	N	Release: Freeing a body part from an abnormal physical constraint by cutting or by the use of force

Body Part (4th)	Approach (5th)	Device (6th)	Qualifier (7th)
0 Occipital-cervical Joint 1 Cervical Vertebral Joint 3 Cervical Vertebral Disc 4 Cervicothoracic Vertebral Joint 5 Cervicothoracic Vertebral Disc 6 Thoracic Vertebral Joint 9 Thoracic Vertebral Disc A Thoracolumbar Vertebral Joint B Thoracolumbar Vertebral Disc C Temporomandibular Joint, Right D Temporomandibular Joint, Left E Sternoclavicular Joint, Right F Sternoclavicular Joint, Left G Acromioclavicular Joint, Right H Acromioclavicular Joint, Left J Shoulder Joint, Right K Shoulder Joint, Left L Elbow Joint, Right M Elbow Joint, Left N Wrist Joint, Right P Wrist Joint, Left Q Carpal Joint, Right R Carpal Joint, Left S Carpometacarpal Joint, Right T Carpometacarpal Joint, Left U Metacarpophalangeal Joint, Right V Metacarpophalangeal Joint, Left W Finger Phalangeal Joint, Right X Finger Phalangeal Joint, Left	0 Open 3 Percutaneous 4 Percutaneous Endoscopic X External	Z No Device	Z No Qualifier

Medical and Surgical, Upper Joints Tables

Section	0	Medical and Surgical
Body System	R	Upper Joints
Operation	P	Removal: Taking out or off a device from a body part

Body Part (4th)	Approach (5th)	Device (6th)	Qualifier (7th)
0 Occipital-cervical Joint 1 Cervical Vertebral Joint 4 Cervicothoracic Vertebral Joint 6 Thoracic Vertebral Joint A Thoracolumbar Vertebral Joint	0 Open 3 Percutaneous 4 Percutaneous Endoscopic	0 Drainage Device 3 Infusion Device 4 Internal Fixation Device 7 Autologous Tissue Substitute 8 Spacer A Interbody Fusion Device J Synthetic Substitute K Nonautologous Tissue Substitute	Z No Qualifier
0 Occipital-cervical Joint 1 Cervical Vertebral Joint 4 Cervicothoracic Vertebral Joint 6 Thoracic Vertebral Joint A Thoracolumbar Vertebral Joint	X External	0 Drainage Device 3 Infusion Device 4 Internal Fixation Device	Z No Qualifier
3 Cervical Vertebral Disc 5 Cervicothoracic Vertebral Disc 9 Thoracic Vertebral Disc B Thoracolumbar Vertebral Disc	0 Open 3 Percutaneous 4 Percutaneous Endoscopic	0 Drainage Device 3 Infusion Device 7 Autologous Tissue Substitute J Synthetic Substitute K Nonautologous Tissue Substitute	Z No Qualifier
3 Cervical Vertebral Disc 5 Cervicothoracic Vertebral Disc 9 Thoracic Vertebral Disc B Thoracolumbar Vertebral Disc	X External	0 Drainage Device 3 Infusion Device	Z No Qualifier
C Temporomandibular Joint, Right D Temporomandibular Joint, Left E Sternoclavicular Joint, Right F Sternoclavicular Joint, Left G Acromioclavicular Joint, Right H Acromioclavicular Joint, Left	0 Open 3 Percutaneous 4 Percutaneous Endoscopic	0 Drainage Device 3 Infusion Device 4 Internal Fixation Device 7 Autologous Tissue Substitute 8 Spacer J Synthetic Substitute K Nonautologous Tissue Substitute	Z No Qualifier
C Temporomandibular Joint, Right D Temporomandibular Joint, Left E Sternoclavicular Joint, Right F Sternoclavicular Joint, Left G Acromioclavicular Joint, Right H Acromioclavicular Joint, Left	X External	0 Drainage Device 3 Infusion Device 4 Internal Fixation Device	Z No Qualifier
J Shoulder Joint, Right K Shoulder Joint, Left	0 Open 3 Percutaneous 4 Percutaneous Endoscopic	0 Drainage Device 3 Infusion Device 4 Internal Fixation Device 7 Autologous Tissue Substitute 8 Spacer K Nonautologous Tissue Substitute	Z No Qualifier
J Shoulder Joint, Right K Shoulder Joint, Left	0 Open 3 Percutaneous 4 Percutaneous Endoscopic	J Synthetic Substitute	6 Humeral Surface 7 Glenoid Surface Z No Device
J Shoulder Joint, Right K Shoulder Joint, Left	X External	0 Drainage Device 3 Infusion Device 4 Internal Fixation Device	Z No Qualifier

Continued →

0RP–0RQ

0RP Continued

Section	0	Medical and Surgical
Body System	R	Upper Joints
Operation	P	Removal: Taking out or off a device from a body part

Body Part (4th)	Approach (5th)	Device (6th)	Qualifier (7th)
L Elbow Joint, Right M Elbow Joint, Left N Wrist Joint, Right P Wrist Joint, Left Q Carpal Joint, Right R Carpal Joint, Left S Carpometacarpal Joint, Right T Carpometacarpal Joint, Left U Metacarpophalangeal Joint, Right V Metacarpophalangeal Joint, Left W Finger Phalangeal Joint, Right X Finger Phalangeal Joint, Left	0 Open 3 Percutaneous 4 Percutaneous Endoscopic	0 Drainage Device 3 Infusion Device 4 Internal Fixation Device 5 External Fixation Device 7 Autologous Tissue Substitute 8 Spacer J Synthetic Substitute K Nonautologous Tissue Substitute	Z No Qualifier
L Elbow Joint, Right M Elbow Joint, Left N Wrist Joint, Right P Wrist Joint, Left Q Carpal Joint, Right R Carpal Joint, Left S Carpometacarpal Joint, Right T Carpometacarpal Joint, Left U Metacarpophalangeal Joint, Right V Metacarpophalangeal Joint, Left W Finger Phalangeal Joint, Right X Finger Phalangeal Joint, Left	X External	0 Drainage Device 3 Infusion Device 4 Internal Fixation Device 5 External Fixation Device	Z No Qualifier

Section	0	Medical and Surgical
Body System	R	Upper Joints
Operation	Q	Repair: Restoring, to the extent possible, a body part to its normal anatomic structure and function

Body Part (4th)	Approach (5th)	Device (6th)	Qualifier (7th)
0 Occipital-cervical Joint 1 Cervical Vertebral Joint 3 Cervical Vertebral Disc 4 Cervicothoracic Vertebral Joint 5 Cervicothoracic Vertebral Disc 6 Thoracic Vertebral Joint 9 Thoracic Vertebral Disc A Thoracolumbar Vertebral Joint B Thoracolumbar Vertebral Disc C Temporomandibular Joint, Right D Temporomandibular Joint, Left E Sternoclavicular Joint, Right F Sternoclavicular Joint, Left G Acromioclavicular Joint, Right H Acromioclavicular Joint, Left J Shoulder Joint, Right K Shoulder Joint, Left L Elbow Joint, Right M Elbow Joint, Left N Wrist Joint, Right P Wrist Joint, Left Q Carpal Joint, Right R Carpal Joint, Left S Carpometacarpal Joint, Right T Carpometacarpal Joint, Left U Metacarpophalangeal Joint, Right V Metacarpophalangeal Joint, Left W Finger Phalangeal Joint, Right X Finger Phalangeal Joint, Left	0 Open 3 Percutaneous 4 Percutaneous Endoscopic X External	Z No Device	Z No Qualifier

Medical and Surgical, Upper Joints Tables

Section	0	**Medical and Surgical**
Body System	R	**Upper Joints**
Operation	R	**Replacement:** Putting in or on biological or synthetic material that physically takes the place and/or function of all or a portion of a body part

Body Part (4th)	Approach (5th)	Device (6th)	Qualifier (7th)
0 Occipital-cervical Joint 1 Cervical Vertebral Joint 3 Cervical Vertebral Disc 4 Cervicothoracic Vertebral Joint 5 Cervicothoracic Vertebral Disc 6 Thoracic Vertebral Joint 9 Thoracic Vertebral Disc A Thoracolumbar Vertebral Joint B Thoracolumbar Vertebral Disc C Temporomandibular Joint, Right D Temporomandibular Joint, Left E Sternoclavicular Joint, Right F Sternoclavicular Joint, Left G Acromioclavicular Joint, Right H Acromioclavicular Joint, Left L Elbow Joint, Right M Elbow Joint, Left N Wrist Joint, Right P Wrist Joint, Left Q Carpal Joint, Right R Carpal Joint, Left S Carpometacarpal Joint, Right T Carpometacarpal Joint, Left U Metacarpophalangeal Joint, Right V Metacarpophalangeal Joint, Left W Finger Phalangeal Joint, Right X Finger Phalangeal Joint, Left	0 Open	7 Autologous Tissue Substitute J Synthetic Substitute K Nonautologous Tissue Substitute	Z No Qualifier
J Shoulder Joint, Right K Shoulder Joint, Left	0 Open	0 Synthetic Substitute, Reverse Ball and Socket 7 Autologous Tissue Substitute K Nonautologous Tissue Substitute	Z No Qualifier
J Shoulder Joint, Right K Shoulder Joint, Left	0 Open	J Synthetic Substitute	6 Humeral Surface 7 Glenoid Surface Z No Qualifier

Section	0	**Medical and Surgical**
Body System	R	**Upper Joints**
Operation	S	**Reposition:** Moving to its normal location, or other suitable location, all or a portion of a body part

Body Part (4th)	Approach (5th)	Device (6th)	Qualifier (7th)
0 Occipital-cervical Joint 1 Cervical Vertebral Joint 4 Cervicothoracic Vertebral Joint 6 Thoracic Vertebral Joint A Thoracolumbar Vertebral Joint C Temporomandibular Joint, Right D Temporomandibular Joint, Left E Sternoclavicular Joint, Right F Sternoclavicular Joint, Left G Acromioclavicular Joint, Right H Acromioclavicular Joint, Left J Shoulder Joint, Right K Shoulder Joint, Left	0 Open 3 Percutaneous 4 Percutaneous Endoscopic X External	4 Internal Fixation Device Z No Device	Z No Qualifier

0RS–0RT

Section 0 Medical and Surgical
Body System R Upper Joints
Operation S Reposition: Moving to its normal location, or other suitable location, all or a portion of a body part

0RS Continued

Body Part (4th)	Approach (5th)	Device (6th)	Qualifier (7th)
L Elbow Joint, Right M Elbow Joint, Left N Wrist Joint, Right P Wrist Joint, Left Q Carpal Joint, Right R Carpal Joint, Left S Carpometacarpal Joint, Right T Carpometacarpal Joint, Left U Metacarpophalangeal Joint, Right V Metacarpophalangeal Joint, Left W Finger Phalangeal Joint, Right X Finger Phalangeal Joint, Left	0 Open 3 Percutaneous 4 Percutaneous Endoscopic X External	4 Internal Fixation Device 5 External Fixation Device Z No Device	Z No Qualifier

Section 0 Medical and Surgical
Body System R Upper Joints
Operation T Resection: Cutting out or off, without replacement, all of a body part

Body Part (4th)	Approach (5th)	Device (6th)	Qualifier (7th)
3 Cervical Vertebral Disc 4 Cervicothoracic Vertebral Joint 5 Cervicothoracic Vertebral Disc 9 Thoracic Vertebral Disc B Thoracolumbar Vertebral Disc C Temporomandibular Joint, Right D Temporomandibular Joint, Left E Sternoclavicular Joint, Right F Sternoclavicular Joint, Left G Acromioclavicular Joint, Right H Acromioclavicular Joint, Left J Shoulder Joint, Right K Shoulder Joint, Left L Elbow Joint, Right M Elbow Joint, Left N Wrist Joint, Right P Wrist Joint, Left Q Carpal Joint, Right R Carpal Joint, Left S Carpometacarpal Joint, Right T Carpometacarpal Joint, Left U Metacarpophalangeal Joint, Right V Metacarpophalangeal Joint, Left W Finger Phalangeal Joint, Right X Finger Phalangeal Joint, Left	0 Open	Z No Device	Z No Qualifier

Medical and Surgical, Upper Joints Tables

434

Section	0	Medical and Surgical
Body System	R	Upper Joints
Operation	U	Supplement: Putting in or on biological or synthetic material that physically reinforces and/or augments the function of a portion of a body part

Body Part (4th)	Approach (5th)	Device (6th)	Qualifier (7th)
0 Occipital-cervical Joint 1 Cervical Vertebral Joint 3 Cervical Vertebral Disc 4 Cervicothoracic Vertebral Joint 5 Cervicothoracic Vertebral Disc 6 Thoracic Vertebral Joint 9 Thoracic Vertebral Disc A Thoracolumbar Vertebral Joint B Thoracolumbar Vertebral Disc C Temporomandibular Joint, Right D Temporomandibular Joint, Left E Sternoclavicular Joint, Right F Sternoclavicular Joint, Left G Acromioclavicular Joint, Right H Acromioclavicular Joint, Left J Shoulder Joint, Right K Shoulder Joint, Left L Elbow Joint, Right M Elbow Joint, Left N Wrist Joint, Right P Wrist Joint, Left Q Carpal Joint, Right R Carpal Joint, Left S Carpometacarpal Joint, Right T Carpometacarpal Joint, Left U Metacarpophalangeal Joint, Right V Metacarpophalangeal Joint, Left W Finger Phalangeal Joint, Right X Finger Phalangeal Joint, Left	0 Open 3 Percutaneous 4 Percutaneous Endoscopic	7 Autologous Tissue Substitute J Synthetic Substitute K Nonautologous Tissue Substitute	Z No Qualifier

Section	0	Medical and Surgical
Body System	R	Upper Joints
Operation	W	Revision: Correcting, to the extent possible, a portion of a malfunctioning device or the position of a displaced device

Body Part (4th)	Approach (5th)	Device (6th)	Qualifier (7th)
0 Occipital-cervical Joint 1 Cervical Vertebral Joint 4 Cervicothoracic Vertebral Joint 6 Thoracic Vertebral Joint A Thoracolumbar Vertebral Joint	0 Open 3 Percutaneous 4 Percutaneous Endoscopic X External	0 Drainage Device 3 Infusion Device 4 Internal Fixation Device 7 Autologous Tissue Substitute 8 Spacer A Interbody Fusion Device J Synthetic Substitute K Nonautologous Tissue Substitute	Z No Qualifier
3 Cervical Vertebral Disc 5 Cervicothoracic Vertebral Disc 9 Thoracic Vertebral Disc B Thoracolumbar Vertebral Disc	0 Open 3 Percutaneous 4 Percutaneous Endoscopic X External	0 Drainage Device 3 Infusion Device 7 Autologous Tissue Substitute J Synthetic Substitute K Nonautologous Tissue Substitute	Z No Qualifier
C Temporomandibular Joint, Right D Temporomandibular Joint, Left E Sternoclavicular Joint, Right F Sternoclavicular Joint, Left G Acromioclavicular Joint, Right H Acromioclavicular Joint, Left	0 Open 3 Percutaneous 4 Percutaneous Endoscopic X External	0 Drainage Device 3 Infusion Device 4 Internal Fixation Device 7 Autologous Tissue Substitute 8 Spacer J Synthetic Substitute K Nonautologous Tissue Substitute	Z No Qualifier

Continued →

Section	0	Medical and Surgical
Body System	R	Upper Joints
Operation	W	Revision: Correcting, to the extent possible, a portion of a malfunctioning device or the position of a displaced device

Body Part (4th)	Approach (5th)	Device (6th)	Qualifier (7th)
J Shoulder Joint, Right K Shoulder Joint, Left	0 Open 3 Percutaneous 4 Percutaneous Endoscopic X External	0 Drainage Device 3 Infusion Device 4 Internal Fixation Device 7 Autologous Tissue Substitute 8 Spacer K Nonautologous Tissue Substitute	Z No Qualifier
J Shoulder Joint, Right K Shoulder Joint, Left	0 Open 3 Percutaneous 4 Percutaneous Endoscopic X External	J Synthetic Substitute	6 Humeral Surface 7 Glenoid Surface Z No Device
L Elbow Joint, Right M Elbow Joint, Left N Wrist Joint, Right P Wrist Joint, Left Q Carpal Joint, Right R Carpal Joint, Left S Carpometacarpal Joint, Right T Carpometacarpal Joint, Left U Metacarpophalangeal Joint, Right V Metacarpophalangeal Joint, Left W Finger Phalangeal Joint, Right X Finger Phalangeal Joint, Left	0 Open 3 Percutaneous 4 Percutaneous Endoscopic X External	0 Drainage Device 3 Infusion Device 4 Internal Fixation Device 5 External Fixation Device 7 Autologous Tissue Substitute 8 Spacer J Synthetic Substitute K Nonautologous Tissue Substitute	Z No Qualifier

AHA Coding Clinic

0RG20A0 Fusion of 2 or more Cervical Vertebral Joints with Interbody Fusion Device, Anterior Approach, Anterior Column, Open Approach—AHA CC: 3Q, 2019, 28

0RG2371 Fusion of 2 or more Cervical Vertebral Joints with Autologous Tissue Substitute, Posterior Approach, Posterior Column, Percutaneous Approach—AHA CC: 2Q, 2019, 19-20

0RG40A0 Fusion of Cervicothoracic Vertebral Joint with Interbody Fusion Device, Anterior Approach, Anterior Column, Open Approach—AHA CC: 1Q, 2013, 29-30; 2Q, 2014, 7-8

0RG7071 Fusion of 2 to 7 Thoracic Vertebral Joints with Autologous Tissue Substitute, Posterior Approach, Posterior Column, Open Approach—AHA CC: 1Q, 2013, 21-23

0RGA071 Fusion of Thoracolumbar Vertebral Joint with Autologous Tissue Substitute, Posterior Approach, Posterior Column, Open Approach—AHA CC: 1Q, 2013, 21-23

0RGW04Z Fusion of Right Finger Phalangeal Joint with Internal Fixation Device, Open Approach—AHA CC: 4Q, 2017, 62

0RHJ04Z Insertion of Internal Fixation Device into Right Shoulder Joint, Open Approach—AHA CC: 3Q, 2016, 32-33

0RNJ4ZZ Release Right Shoulder Joint, Percutaneous Endoscopic Approach—AHA CC: 3Q, 2016, 32-33

0RNK4ZZ Release Left Shoulder Joint, Percutaneous Endoscopic Approach—AHA CC: 2Q, 2015, 22-23

0RQJ4ZZ Repair Right Shoulder Joint, Percutaneous Endoscopic Approach—AHA CC: 1Q, 2016, 30-31

0RRJ00Z Replacement of Right Shoulder Joint with Reverse Ball and Socket Synthetic Substitute, Open Approach—AHA CC: 1Q, 2015, 27

0RRK0J6 Replacement of Left Shoulder Joint with Synthetic Substitute, Humeral Surface, Open Approach—AHA CC: 3Q, 2015, 14-15

0RSH04Z Reposition Left Acromioclavicular Joint with Internal Fixation Device, Open Approach—AHA CC: 3Q, 2019, 26-27

0RSPXZZ Reposition Left Wrist Joint, External Approach—AHA CC: 4Q, 2014, 32-33

0RSR04Z Reposition Left Carpal Joint with Internal Fixation Device, Open Approach—AHA CC: 3Q, 2014, 33-34

0RT50ZZ Resection of Cervicothoracic Vertebral Disc, Open Approach—AHA CC: 2Q, 2014, 7-8

0RUH0KZ Supplement Left Acromioclavicular Joint with Nonautologous Tissue Substitute, Open Approach—AHA CC: 3Q, 2019, 26-27

0RUT07Z Supplement Left Carpometacarpal Joint with Autologous Tissue Substitute, Open Approach—AHA CC: 3Q, 2015, 26-27

Lower Joints

Knee Joint

Ankle

Total Knee Replacement Technique: Steps 1-5

1. Longitudinal 8- to 12-in. skin incision is centered on patella.

2. Capsular incision skirts medial margin of patella and courses distally through periosteum medial to tibial tuberosity.

3. Patella is reflected laterally by raising patellar ligament in continuity with periosteum.

4. If further exposure of the medial knee is needed, a flap can be raised by elevating the deep medial collateral ligament and pes anserinus subperiosteally, aided by external rotation of the tibia.

5. The anterior cruciate ligament and both menisci are excised, and the tibia is subluxated anteriorly.

© 2012 Elsevier Inc. All rights reserved. www.netterimages.com

Total Knee Replacement Technique: Steps 6-9

6. The femoral canal is accessed for placement of guide for distal femoral resections.

7. Femoral size guide is used to determine implant size and rotation.

8. Femoral cutting block is used for anterior, posterior, and chamfer cuts.

9. Tibial cutting block is placed using the aid of an extramedullary alignment rod (pictured, may also use an intramedullary device). The bar can be used to assess slope and alignment of the cut.

© 2012 Elsevier Inc. All rights reserved. www.netterimages.com

Total Knee Replacement Technique: Steps 10-14

10. Tibial cutting block is fixed into place and guide device removed.

11. The proximal tibial articular surface cut is then made with oscillating saw.

12. Trial baseplates are then used to assess the appropriate size of the implant to be used.

13. The trial baseplate is fixed to the tibial surface and a keel punch is used to set rotational alignment and accommodate the stem of the final tibial component

Medial facet   Lateral facet
Articular surface
Transverse section
1 cm

14. Articular surface of patella resected to leave flat surface. Equal amounts to be removed from medial and lateral facets, but at least 1 cm of bone must be left to ensure adequate strength. Using a patella drill template, three holes are drilled into the surface to accommodate the final patellar component, which is cemented in place.

© 2012 Elsevier Inc. All rights reserved. www.netterimages.com

Total Knee Replacement Technique: Steps 15-20

15. Cement is applied to tibial component and cut surfaces of tibia, and component is placed in position. Cement is somewhat less viscous to facilitate penetration into trabecular bone (sagittal section).

16. Extruded cement is removed

18. Extruded cement is removed

17. Cement is applied to posterior limb of femoral component and spread evenly over beveled ends of femur

19. With all components in place, trial polyethylene inserts are used to determine the correct size.

20. Once the final components are in place, the knee is placed through a range of motion and appropriate stress tests. The knee is then irrigated, hemostasis achieved, and the wound is closed.

© 2012 Elsevier Inc. All rights reserved. www.netterimages.com

Lower Joints Tables 0S2–0SW

Section	0	Medical and Surgical
Body System	S	Lower Joints
Operation	2	Change: Taking out or off a device from a body part and putting back an identical or similar device in or on the same body part without cutting or puncturing the skin or a mucous membrane

Body Part (4th)	Approach (5th)	Device (6th)	Qualifier (7th)
Y Lower Joint	X External	0 Drainage Device Y Other Device	Z No Qualifier

Section	0	Medical and Surgical
Body System	S	Lower Joints
Operation	5	Destruction: Physical eradication of all or a portion of a body part by the direct use of energy, force, or a destructive agent

Body Part (4th)	Approach (5th)	Device (6th)	Qualifier (7th)
0 Lumbar Vertebral Joint 2 Lumbar Vertebral Disc 3 Lumbosacral Joint 4 Lumbosacral Disc 5 Sacrococcygeal Joint 6 Coccygeal Joint 7 Sacroiliac Joint, Right 8 Sacroiliac Joint, Left 9 Hip Joint, Right B Hip Joint, Left C Knee Joint, Right D Knee Joint, Left F Ankle Joint, Right G Ankle Joint, Left H Tarsal Joint, Right J Tarsal Joint, Left K Tarsometatarsal Joint, Right L Tarsometatarsal Joint, Left M Metatarsal-Phalangeal Joint, Right N Metatarsal-Phalangeal Joint, Left P Toe Phalangeal Joint, Right Q Toe Phalangeal Joint, Left	0 Open 3 Percutaneous 4 Percutaneous Endoscopic	Z No Device	Z No Qualifier

Section	0	Medical and Surgical
Body System	S	Lower Joints
Operation	9	Drainage: Taking or letting out fluids and/or gases from a body part

Body Part (4th)	Approach (5th)	Device (6th)	Qualifier (7th)
0 Lumbar Vertebral Joint 2 Lumbar Vertebral Disc 3 Lumbosacral Joint 4 Lumbosacral Disc 5 Sacrococcygeal Joint 6 Coccygeal Joint 7 Sacroiliac Joint, Right 8 Sacroiliac Joint, Left 9 Hip Joint, Right B Hip Joint, Left C Knee Joint, Right D Knee Joint, Left F Ankle Joint, Right G Ankle Joint, Left H Tarsal Joint, Right J Tarsal Joint, Left K Tarsometatarsal Joint, Right L Tarsometatarsal Joint, Left M Metatarsal-Phalangeal Joint, Right N Metatarsal-Phalangeal Joint, Left P Toe Phalangeal Joint, Right Q Toe Phalangeal Joint, Left	0 Open 3 Percutaneous 4 Percutaneous Endoscopic	0 Drainage Device	Z No Qualifier
0 Lumbar Vertebral Joint 2 Lumbar Vertebral Disc 3 Lumbosacral Joint 4 Lumbosacral Disc 5 Sacrococcygeal Joint 6 Coccygeal Joint 7 Sacroiliac Joint, Right 8 Sacroiliac Joint, Left 9 Hip Joint, Right B Hip Joint, Left C Knee Joint, Right D Knee Joint, Left F Ankle Joint, Right G Ankle Joint, Left H Tarsal Joint, Right J Tarsal Joint, Left K Tarsometatarsal Joint, Right L Tarsometatarsal Joint, Left M Metatarsal-Phalangeal Joint, Right N Metatarsal-Phalangeal Joint, Left P Toe Phalangeal Joint, Right Q Toe Phalangeal Joint, Left	0 Open 3 Percutaneous 4 Percutaneous Endoscopic	Z No Device	X Diagnostic Z No Qualifier

Section	0	Medical and Surgical
Body System	S	Lower Joints
Operation	B	Excision: Cutting out or off, without replacement, a portion of a body part

Body Part (4th)	Approach (5th)	Device (6th)	Qualifier (7th)
0 Lumbar Vertebral Joint 2 Lumbar Vertebral Disc 3 Lumbosacral Joint 4 Lumbosacral Disc 5 Sacrococcygeal Joint 6 Coccygeal Joint 7 Sacroiliac Joint, Right 8 Sacroiliac Joint, Left 9 Hip Joint, Right B Hip Joint, Left C Knee Joint, Right D Knee Joint, Left F Ankle Joint, Right G Ankle Joint, Left H Tarsal Joint, Right J Tarsal Joint, Left K Tarsometatarsal Joint, Right L Tarsometatarsal Joint, Left M Metatarsal-Phalangeal Joint, Right N Metatarsal-Phalangeal Joint, Left P Toe Phalangeal Joint, Right Q Toe Phalangeal Joint, Left	0 Open 3 Percutaneous 4 Percutaneous Endoscopic	Z No Device	X Diagnostic Z No Qualifier

Section	0	Medical and Surgical
Body System	S	Lower Joints
Operation	C	Extirpation: Taking or cutting out solid matter from a body part

Body Part (4th)	Approach (5th)	Device (6th)	Qualifier (7th)
0 Lumbar Vertebral Joint 2 Lumbar Vertebral Disc 3 Lumbosacral Joint 4 Lumbosacral Disc 5 Sacrococcygeal Joint 6 Coccygeal Joint 7 Sacroiliac Joint, Right 8 Sacroiliac Joint, Left 9 Hip Joint, Right B Hip Joint, Left C Knee Joint, Right D Knee Joint, Left F Ankle Joint, Right G Ankle Joint, Left H Tarsal Joint, Right J Tarsal Joint, Left K Tarsometatarsal Joint, Right L Tarsometatarsal Joint, Left M Metatarsal-Phalangeal Joint, Right N Metatarsal-Phalangeal Joint, Left P Toe Phalangeal Joint, Right Q Toe Phalangeal Joint, Left	0 Open 3 Percutaneous 4 Percutaneous Endoscopic	Z No Device	Z No Qualifier

Section	0	Medical and Surgical
Body System	S	Lower Joints
Operation	G	Fusion: Joining together portions of an articular body part rendering the articular body part immobile

Body Part (4th)	Approach (5th)	Device (6th)	Qualifier (7th)
0 Lumbar Vertebral Joint 1 Lumbar Vertebral Joints, 2 or more 3 Lumbosacral Joint	0 Open 3 Percutaneous 4 Percutaneous Endoscopic	7 Autologous Tissue Substitute J Synthetic Substitute K Nonautologous Tissue Substitute	0 Anterior Approach, Anterior Column 1 Posterior Approach, Posterior Column J Posterior Approach, Anterior Column
0 Lumbar Vertebral Joint 1 Lumbar Vertebral Joints, 2 or more 3 Lumbosacral Joint	0 Open 3 Percutaneous 4 Percutaneous Endoscopic	A Interbody Fusion Device	0 Anterior Approach, Anterior Column J Posterior Approach, Anterior Column
5 Sacrococcygeal Joint 6 Coccygeal Joint 7 Sacroiliac Joint, Right 8 Sacroiliac Joint, Left	0 Open 3 Percutaneous 4 Percutaneous Endoscopic	4 Internal Fixation Device 7 Autologous Tissue Substitute J Synthetic Substitute K Nonautologous Tissue Substitute	Z No Qualifier
9 Hip Joint, Right B Hip Joint, Left C Knee Joint, Right D Knee Joint, Left F Ankle Joint, Right G Ankle Joint, Left H Tarsal Joint, Right J Tarsal Joint, Left K Tarsometatarsal Joint, Right L Tarsometatarsal Joint, Left M Metatarsal-Phalangeal Joint, Right N Metatarsal-Phalangeal Joint, Left P Toe Phalangeal Joint, Right Q Toe Phalangeal Joint, Left	0 Open 3 Percutaneous 4 Percutaneous Endoscopic	3 Internal Fixation Device, Sustained Compression 4 Internal Fixation Device 5 External Fixation Device 7 Autologous Tissue Substitute J Synthetic Substitute K Nonautologous Tissue Substitute	Z No Qualifier

Section	0	Medical and Surgical
Body System	S	Lower Joints
Operation	H	Insertion: Putting in a nonbiological appliance that monitors, assists, performs, or prevents a physiological function but does not physically take the place of a body part

Body Part (4th)	Approach (5th)	Device (6th)	Qualifier (7th)
0 Lumbar Vertebral Joint 3 Lumbosacral Joint	0 Open 3 Percutaneous 4 Percutaneous Endoscopic	3 Infusion Device 4 Internal Fixation Device 8 Spacer B Spinal Stabilization Device, Interspinous Process C Spinal Stabilization Device, Pedicle-Based D Spinal Stabilization Device, Facet Replacement	Z No Qualifier
2 Lumbar Vertebral Disc 4 Lumbosacral Disc	0 Open 3 Percutaneous 4 Percutaneous Endoscopic	3 Infusion Device 8 Spacer	Z No Qualifier
5 Sacrococcygeal Joint 6 Coccygeal Joint 7 Sacroiliac Joint, Right 8 Sacroiliac Joint, Left	0 Open 3 Percutaneous 4 Percutaneous Endoscopic	3 Infusion Device 4 Internal Fixation Device 8 Spacer	Z No Qualifier

Section	0	Medical and Surgical
Body System	S	Lower Joints
Operation	H	Insertion: Putting in a nonbiological appliance that monitors, assists, performs, or prevents a physiological function but does not physically take the place of a body part

Body Part (4th)	Approach (5th)	Device (6th)	Qualifier (7th)
9 Hip Joint, Right B Hip Joint, Left C Knee Joint, Right D Knee Joint, Left F Ankle Joint, Right G Ankle Joint, Left H Tarsal Joint, Right J Tarsal Joint, Left K Tarsometatarsal Joint, Right L Tarsometatarsal Joint, Left M Metatarsal-Phalangeal Joint, Right N Metatarsal-Phalangeal Joint, Left P Toe Phalangeal Joint, Right Q Toe Phalangeal Joint, Left	0 Open 3 Percutaneous 4 Percutaneous Endoscopic	3 Infusion Device 4 Internal Fixation Device 5 External Fixation Device 8 Spacer	Z No Qualifier

Section	0	Medical and Surgical
Body System	S	Lower Joints
Operation	J	Inspection: Visually and/or manually exploring a body part

Body Part (4th)	Approach (5th)	Device (6th)	Qualifier (7th)
0 Lumbar Vertebral Joint 2 Lumbar Vertebral Disc 3 Lumbosacral Joint 4 Lumbosacral Disc 5 Sacrococcygeal Joint 6 Coccygeal Joint 7 Sacroiliac Joint, Right 8 Sacroiliac Joint, Left 9 Hip Joint, Right B Hip Joint, Left C Knee Joint, Right D Knee Joint, Left F Ankle Joint, Right G Ankle Joint, Left H Tarsal Joint, Right J Tarsal Joint, Left K Tarsometatarsal Joint, Right L Tarsometatarsal Joint, Left M Metatarsal-Phalangeal Joint, Right N Metatarsal-Phalangeal Joint, Left P Toe Phalangeal Joint, Right Q Toe Phalangeal Joint, Left	0 Open 3 Percutaneous 4 Percutaneous Endoscopic X External	Z No Device	Z No Qualifier

0SN–0SP

Medical and Surgical, Lower Joints Tables

Section	0	Medical and Surgical
Body System	S	Lower Joints
Operation	N	**Release:** Freeing a body part from an abnormal physical constraint by cutting or by the use of force

Body Part (4th)	Approach (5th)	Device (6th)	Qualifier (7th)
0 Lumbar Vertebral Joint 2 Lumbar Vertebral Disc 3 Lumbosacral Joint 4 Lumbosacral Disc 5 Sacrococcygeal Joint 6 Coccygeal Joint 7 Sacroiliac Joint, Right 8 Sacroiliac Joint, Left 9 Hip Joint, Right B Hip Joint, Left C Knee Joint, Right D Knee Joint, Left F Ankle Joint, Right G Ankle Joint, Left H Tarsal Joint, Right J Tarsal Joint, Left K Tarsometatarsal Joint, Right L Tarsometatarsal Joint, Left M Metatarsal-Phalangeal Joint, Right N Metatarsal-Phalangeal Joint, Left P Toe Phalangeal Joint, Right Q Toe Phalangeal Joint, Left	0 Open 3 Percutaneous 4 Percutaneous Endoscopic X External	Z No Device	Z No Qualifier

Section	0	Medical and Surgical
Body System	S	Lower Joints
Operation	P	**Removal:** Taking out or off a device from a body part

Body Part (4th)	Approach (5th)	Device (6th)	Qualifier (7th)
0 Lumbar Vertebral Joint 3 Lumbosacral Joint	0 Open 3 Percutaneous 4 Percutaneous Endoscopic	0 Drainage Device 3 Infusion Device 4 Internal Fixation Device 7 Autologous Tissue Substitute 8 Spacer A Interbody Fusion Device J Synthetic Substitute K Nonautologous Tissue Substitute	Z No Qualifier
0 Lumbar Vertebral Joint 3 Lumbosacral Joint	X External	0 Drainage Device 3 Infusion Device 4 Internal Fixation Device	Z No Qualifier
2 Lumbar Vertebral Disc 4 Lumbosacral Disc	0 Open 3 Percutaneous 4 Percutaneous Endoscopic	0 Drainage Device 3 Infusion Device 7 Autologous Tissue Substitute J Synthetic Substitute K Nonautologous Tissue Substitute	Z No Qualifier
2 Lumbar Vertebral Disc 4 Lumbosacral Disc	X External	0 Drainage Device 3 Infusion Device	Z No Qualifier
5 Sacrococcygeal Joint 6 Coccygeal Joint 7 Sacroiliac Joint, Right 8 Sacroiliac Joint, Left	0 Open 3 Percutaneous 4 Percutaneous Endoscopic	0 Drainage Device 3 Infusion Device 4 Internal Fixation Device 7 Autologous Tissue Substitute 8 Spacer J Synthetic Substitute K Nonautologous Tissue Substitute	Z No Qualifier

Continued →

448

Section   0   Medical and Surgical
Body System   S   Lower Joints
Operation   P   Removal: Taking out or off a device from a body part

0SP Continued

Body Part (4th)	Approach (5th)	Device (6th)	Qualifier (7th)
5 Sacrococcygeal Joint 6 Coccygeal Joint 7 Sacroiliac Joint, Right 8 Sacroiliac Joint, Left	X External	0 Drainage Device 3 Infusion Device 4 Internal Fixation Device	Z No Qualifier
9 Hip Joint, Right B Hip Joint, Left	0 Open	0 Drainage Device 3 Infusion Device 4 Internal Fixation Device 5 External Fixation Device 7 Autologous Tissue Substitute 8 Spacer 9 Liner B Resurfacing Device E Articulating Spacer J Synthetic Substitute K Nonautologous Tissue Substitute	Z No Qualifier
9 Hip Joint, Right B Hip Joint, Left	3 Percutaneous 4 Percutaneous Endoscopic	0 Drainage Device 3 Infusion Device 4 Internal Fixation Device 5 External Fixation Device 7 Autologous Tissue Substitute 8 Spacer J Synthetic Substitute K Nonautologous Tissue Substitute	Z No Qualifier
9 Hip Joint, Right B Hip Joint, Left	X External	0 Drainage Device 3 Infusion Device 4 Internal Fixation Device 5 External Fixation Device	Z No Qualifier
A Hip Joint, Acetabular Surface, Right E Hip Joint, Acetabular Surface, Left R Hip Joint, Femoral Surface, Right S Hip Joint, Femoral Surface, Left T Knee Joint, Femoral Surface, Right U Knee Joint, Femoral Surface, Left V Knee Joint, Tibial Surface, Right W Knee Joint, Tibial Surface, Left	0 Open 3 Percutaneous 4 Percutaneous Endoscopic	J Synthetic Substitute	Z No Qualifier
C Knee Joint, Right D Knee Joint, Left	0 Open	0 Drainage Device 3 Infusion Device 4 Internal Fixation Device 5 External Fixation Device 7 Autologous Tissue Substitute 8 Spacer 9 Liner E Articulating Spacer K Nonautologous Tissue Substitute L Synthetic Substitute, Unicondylar Medial M Synthetic Substitute, Unicondylar Lateral N Synthetic Substitute, Unicondylar Patellofemoral	Z No Qualifier
C Knee Joint, Right D Knee Joint, Left	0 Open	J Synthetic Substitute	C Patellar Surface Z No Qualifier

Continued →

Section	0	Medical and Surgical		0SP Continued
Body System	S	Lower Joints		
Operation	P	**Removal:** Taking out or off a device from a body part		

Body Part (4th)	Approach (5th)	Device (6th)	Qualifier (7th)
C Knee Joint, Right D Knee Joint, Left	3 Percutaneous 4 Percutaneous Endoscopic	0 Drainage Device 3 Infusion Device 4 Internal Fixation Device 5 External Fixation Device 7 Autologous Tissue Substitute 8 Spacer K Nonautologous Tissue Substitute L Synthetic Substitute, Unicondylar Medial M Synthetic Substitute, Unicondylar Lateral N Synthetic Substitute, Unicondylar Patellofemoral	Z No Qualifier
C Knee Joint, Right D Knee Joint, Left	3 Percutaneous 4 Percutaneous Endoscopic	J Synthetic Substitute	C Patellar Surface Z No Qualifier
C Knee Joint, Right D Knee Joint, Left	X External	0 Drainage Device 3 Infusion Device 4 Internal Fixation Device 5 External Fixation Device	Z No Qualifier
F Ankle Joint, Right G Ankle Joint, Left H Tarsal Joint, Right J Tarsal Joint, Left K Tarsometatarsal Joint, Right L Tarsometatarsal Joint, Left M Metatarsal-Phalangeal Joint, Right N Metatarsal-Phalangeal Joint, Left P Toe Phalangeal Joint, Right Q Toe Phalangeal Joint, Left	0 Open 3 Percutaneous 4 Percutaneous Endoscopic	0 Drainage Device 3 Infusion Device 4 Internal Fixation Device 5 External Fixation Device 7 Autologous Tissue Substitute 8 Spacer J Synthetic Substitute K Nonautologous Tissue Substitute	Z No Qualifier
F Ankle Joint, Right G Ankle Joint, Left H Tarsal Joint, Right J Tarsal Joint, Left K Tarsometatarsal Joint, Right L Tarsometatarsal Joint, Left M Metatarsal-Phalangeal Joint, Right N Metatarsal-Phalangeal Joint, Left P Toe Phalangeal Joint, Right Q Toe Phalangeal Joint, Left	X External	0 Drainage Device 3 Infusion Device 4 Internal Fixation Device 5 External Fixation Device	Z No Qualifier

Section	0	Medical and Surgical
Body System	S	Lower Joints
Operation	Q	**Repair:** Restoring, to the extent possible, a body part to its normal anatomic structure and function

Body Part (4th)	Approach (5th)	Device (6th)	Qualifier (7th)
0 Lumbar Vertebral Joint 2 Lumbar Vertebral Disc 3 Lumbosacral Joint 4 Lumbosacral Disc 5 Sacrococcygeal Joint 6 Coccygeal Joint 7 Sacroiliac Joint, Right 8 Sacroiliac Joint, Left 9 Hip Joint, Right B Hip Joint, Left C Knee Joint, Right D Knee Joint, Left F Ankle Joint, Right G Ankle Joint, Left H Tarsal Joint, Right J Tarsal Joint, Left K Tarsometatarsal Joint, Right L Tarsometatarsal Joint, Left M Metatarsal-Phalangeal Joint, Right N Metatarsal-Phalangeal Joint, Left P Toe Phalangeal Joint, Right Q Toe Phalangeal Joint, Left	0 Open 3 Percutaneous 4 Percutaneous Endoscopic X External	Z No Device	Z No Qualifier

Section	0	Medical and Surgical
Body System	S	Lower Joints
Operation	R	**Replacement:** Putting in or on biological or synthetic material that physically takes the place and/or function of all or a portion of a body part

Body Part (4th)	Approach (5th)	Device (6th)	Qualifier (7th)
0 Lumbar Vertebral Joint 2 Lumbar Vertebral Disc 3 Lumbosacral Joint 4 Lumbosacral Disc 5 Sacrococcygeal Joint 6 Coccygeal Joint 7 Sacroiliac Joint, Right 8 Sacroiliac Joint, Left H Tarsal Joint, Right J Tarsal Joint, Left K Tarsometatarsal Joint, Right L Tarsometatarsal Joint, Left M Metatarsal-Phalangeal Joint, Right N Metatarsal-Phalangeal Joint, Left P Toe Phalangeal Joint, Right Q Toe Phalangeal Joint, Left	0 Open	7 Autologous Tissue Substitute J Synthetic Substitute K Nonautologous Tissue Substitute	Z No Qualifier
9 Hip Joint, Right B Hip Joint, Left	0 Open	1 Synthetic Substitute, Metal 2 Synthetic Substitute, Metal on Polyethylene 3 Synthetic Substitute, Ceramic 4 Synthetic Substitute, Ceramic on Polyethylene 6 Synthetic Substitute, Oxidized Zirconium on Polyethylene J Synthetic Substitute	9 Cemented A Uncemented Z No Qualifier
9 Hip Joint, Right B Hip Joint, Left	0 Open	7 Autologous Tissue Substitute E Articulating Spacer K Nonautologous Tissue Substitute	Z No Qualifier
A Hip Joint, Acetabular Surface, Right E Hip Joint, Acetabular Surface, Left	0 Open	0 Synthetic Substitute, Polyethylene 1 Synthetic Substitute, Metal 3 Synthetic Substitute, Ceramic J Synthetic Substitute	9 Cemented A Uncemented Z No Qualifier

Continued →

Section   **0**   **Medical and Surgical**   *0SR Continued*
Body System   **S**   **Lower Joints**
Operation   **R**   **Replacement:** Putting in or on biological or synthetic material that physically takes the place and/or function of all or a portion of a body part

Body Part (4th)	Approach (5th)	Device (6th)	Qualifier (7th)
A Hip Joint, Acetabular Surface, Right E Hip Joint, Acetabular Surface, Left	0 Open	7 Autologous Tissue Substitute K Nonautologous Tissue Substitute	Z No Qualifier
C Knee Joint, Right D Knee Joint, Left	0 Open	6 Synthetic Substitute, Oxidized Zirconium on Polyethylene J Synthetic Substitute L Synthetic Substitute, Unicondylar Medial M Synthetic Substitute, Unicondylar Lateral N Synthetic Substitute, Unicondylar Patellofemoral	9 Cemented A Uncemented Z No Qualifier
C Knee Joint, Right D Knee Joint, Left	0 Open	7 Autologous Tissue Substitute E Articulating Spacer K Nonautologous Tissue Substitute	Z No Qualifier
F Ankle Joint, Right G Ankle Joint, Left T Knee Joint, Femoral Surface, Right U Knee Joint, Femoral Surface, Left V Knee Joint, Tibial Surface, Right W Knee Joint, Tibial Surface, Left	0 Open	7 Autologous Tissue Substitute K Nonautologous Tissue Substitute	Z No Qualifier
F Ankle Joint, Right G Ankle Joint, Left T Knee Joint, Femoral Surface, Right U Knee Joint, Femoral Surface, Left V Knee Joint, Tibial Surface, Right W Knee Joint, Tibial Surface, Left	0 Open	J Synthetic Substitute	9 Cemented A Uncemented Z No Qualifier
R Hip Joint, Femoral Surface, Right S Hip Joint, Femoral Surface, Left	0 Open	1 Synthetic Substitute, Metal 3 Synthetic Substitute, Ceramic J Synthetic Substitute	9 Cemented A Uncemented Z No Qualifier
R Hip Joint, Femoral Surface, Right S Hip Joint, Femoral Surface, Left	0 Open	7 Autologous Tissue Substitute K Nonautologous Tissue Substitute	Z No Qualifier

Section   **0**   **Medical and Surgical**
Body System   **S**   **Lower Joints**
Operation   **S**   **Reposition:** Moving to its normal location, or other suitable location, all or a portion of a body part

Body Part (4th)	Approach (5th)	Device (6th)	Qualifier (7th)
0 Lumbar Vertebral Joint 3 Lumbosacral Joint 5 Sacrococcygeal Joint 6 Coccygeal Joint 7 Sacroiliac Joint, Right 8 Sacroiliac Joint, Left	0 Open 3 Percutaneous 4 Percutaneous Endoscopic X External	4 Internal Fixation Device Z No Device	Z No Qualifier
9 Hip Joint, Right B Hip Joint, Left C Knee Joint, Right D Knee Joint, Left F Ankle Joint, Right G Ankle Joint, Left H Tarsal Joint, Right J Tarsal Joint, Left K Tarsometatarsal Joint, Right L Tarsometatarsal Joint, Left M Metatarsal-Phalangeal Joint, Right N Metatarsal-Phalangeal Joint, Left P Toe Phalangeal Joint, Right Q Toe Phalangeal Joint, Left	0 Open 3 Percutaneous 4 Percutaneous Endoscopic X External	4 Internal Fixation Device 5 External Fixation Device Z No Device	Z No Qualifier

452

Section	0	Medical and Surgical
Body System	S	Lower Joints
Operation	T	**Resection:** Cutting out or off, without replacement, all of a body part

Body Part (4ᵗʰ)	Approach (5ᵗʰ)	Device (6ᵗʰ)	Qualifier (7ᵗʰ)
2 Lumbar Vertebral Disc 4 Lumbosacral Disc 5 Sacrococcygeal Joint 6 Coccygeal Joint 7 Sacroiliac Joint, Right 8 Sacroiliac Joint, Left 9 Hip Joint, Right B Hip Joint, Left C Knee Joint, Right D Knee Joint, Left F Ankle Joint, Right G Ankle Joint, Left H Tarsal Joint, Right J Tarsal Joint, Left K Tarsometatarsal Joint, Right L Tarsometatarsal Joint, Left M Metatarsal-Phalangeal Joint, Right N Metatarsal-Phalangeal Joint, Left P Toe Phalangeal Joint, Right Q Toe Phalangeal Joint, Left	0 Open	Z No Device	Z No Qualifier

Section	0	Medical and Surgical
Body System	S	Lower Joints
Operation	U	**Supplement:** Putting in or on biological or synthetic material that physically reinforces and/or augments the function of a portion of a body part

Body Part (4ᵗʰ)	Approach (5ᵗʰ)	Device (6ᵗʰ)	Qualifier (7ᵗʰ)
0 Lumbar Vertebral Joint 2 Lumbar Vertebral Disc 3 Lumbosacral Joint 4 Lumbosacral Disc 5 Sacrococcygeal Joint 6 Coccygeal Joint 7 Sacroiliac Joint, Right 8 Sacroiliac Joint, Left F Ankle Joint, Right G Ankle Joint, Left H Tarsal Joint, Right J Tarsal Joint, Left K Tarsometatarsal Joint, Right L Tarsometatarsal Joint, Left M Metatarsal-Phalangeal Joint, Right N Metatarsal-Phalangeal Joint, Left P Toe Phalangeal Joint, Right Q Toe Phalangeal Joint, Left	0 Open 3 Percutaneous 4 Percutaneous Endoscopic	7 Autologous Tissue Substitute J Synthetic Substitute K Nonautologous Tissue Substitute	Z No Qualifier
9 Hip Joint, Right B Hip Joint, Left	0 Open	7 Autologous Tissue Substitute 9 Liner B Resurfacing Device J Synthetic Substitute K Nonautologous Tissue Substitute	Z No Qualifier
9 Hip Joint, Right B Hip Joint, Left	3 Percutaneous 4 Percutaneous Endoscopic	7 Autologous Tissue Substitute J Synthetic Substitute K Nonautologous Tissue Substitute	Z No Qualifier
A Hip Joint, Acetabular Surface, Right E Hip Joint, Acetabular Surface, Left R Hip Joint, Femoral Surface, Right S Hip Joint, Femoral Surface, Left	0 Open	9 Liner B Resurfacing Device	Z No Qualifier

Continued →

Section 0 **Medical and Surgical**
Body System S **Lower Joints**
Operation U **Supplement:** Putting in or on biological or synthetic material that physically reinforces and/or augments the function of a portion of a body part

Body Part (4th)	Approach (5th)	Device (6th)	Qualifier (7th)
C Knee Joint, Right D Knee Joint, Left	0 Open	7 Autologous Tissue Substitute J Synthetic Substitute K Nonautologous Tissue Substitute	Z No Qualifier
C Knee Joint, Right D Knee Joint, Left	0 Open	9 Liner	C Patellar Surface Z No Qualifier
C Knee Joint, Right D Knee Joint, Left	3 Percutaneous 4 Percutaneous Endoscopic	7 Autologous Tissue Substitute J Synthetic Substitute K Nonautologous Tissue Substitute	Z No Qualifier
T Knee Joint, Femoral Surface, Right U Knee Joint, Femoral Surface, Left V Knee Joint, Tibial Surface, Right W Knee Joint, Tibial Surface, Left	0 Open	9 Liner	Z No Qualifier

Section 0 **Medical and Surgical**
Body System S **Lower Joints**
Operation W **Revision:** Correcting, to the extent possible, a portion of a malfunctioning device or the position of a displaced device

Body Part (4th)	Approach (5th)	Device (6th)	Qualifier (7th)
0 Lumbar Vertebral Joint 3 Lumbosacral Joint	0 Open 3 Percutaneous 4 Percutaneous Endoscopic X External	0 Drainage Device 3 Infusion Device 4 Internal Fixation Device 7 Autologous Tissue Substitute 8 Spacer A Interbody Fusion Device J Synthetic Substitute K Nonautologous Tissue Substitute	Z No Qualifier
2 Lumbar Vertebral Disc 4 Lumbosacral Disc	0 Open 3 Percutaneous 4 Percutaneous Endoscopic X External	0 Drainage Device 3 Infusion Device 7 Autologous Tissue Substitute J Synthetic Substitute K Nonautologous Tissue Substitute	Z No Qualifier
5 Sacrococcygeal Joint 6 Coccygeal Joint 7 Sacroiliac Joint, Right 8 Sacroiliac Joint, Left	0 Open 3 Percutaneous 4 Percutaneous Endoscopic X External	0 Drainage Device 3 Infusion Device 4 Internal Fixation Device 7 Autologous Tissue Substitute 8 Spacer J Synthetic Substitute K Nonautologous Tissue Substitute	Z No Qualifier
9 Hip Joint, Right B Hip Joint, Left	0 Open	0 Drainage Device 3 Infusion Device 4 Internal Fixation Device 5 External Fixation Device 7 Autologous Tissue Substitute 8 Spacer 9 Liner B Resurfacing Device J Synthetic Substitute K Nonautologous Tissue Substitute	Z No Qualifier
9 Hip Joint, Right B Hip Joint, Left	3 Percutaneous 4 Percutaneous Endoscopic X External	0 Drainage Device 3 Infusion Device 4 Internal Fixation Device 5 External Fixation Device 7 Autologous Tissue Substitute 8 Spacer J Synthetic Substitute K Nonautologous Tissue Substitute	Z No Qualifier

Continued →

Section	0	Medical and Surgical			0SW Continued
Body System	S	Lower Joints			
Operation	W	Revision: Correcting, to the extent possible, a portion of a malfunctioning device or the position of a displaced device			

Body Part (4th)	Approach (5th)	Device (6th)	Qualifier (7th)
A Hip Joint, Acetabular Surface, Right E Hip Joint, Acetabular Surface, Left R Hip Joint, Femoral Surface, Right S Hip Joint, Femoral Surface, Left T Knee Joint, Femoral Surface, Right U Knee Joint, Femoral Surface, Left V Knee Joint, Tibial Surface, Right W Knee Joint, Tibial Surface, Left	0 Open 3 Percutaneous 4 Percutaneous Endoscopic X External	J Synthetic Substitute	Z No Qualifier
C Knee Joint, Right D Knee Joint, Left	0 Open	0 Drainage Device 3 Infusion Device 4 Internal Fixation Device 5 External Fixation Device 7 Autologous Tissue Substitute 8 Spacer 9 Liner K Nonautologous Tissue Substitute	Z No Qualifier
C Knee Joint, Right D Knee Joint, Left	0 Open	J Synthetic Substitute	C Patellar Surface Z No Qualifier
C Knee Joint, Right D Knee Joint, Left	3 Percutaneous 4 Percutaneous Endoscopic X External	0 Drainage Device 3 Infusion Device 4 Internal Fixation Device 5 External Fixation Device 7 Autologous Tissue Substitute 8 Spacer K Nonautologous Tissue Substitute	Z No Qualifier
C Knee Joint, Right E Knee Joint, Left	3 Percutaneous 4 Percutaneous Endoscopic X External	J Synthetic Substitute	C Patellar Surface Z No Qualifier
F Ankle Joint, Right G Ankle Joint, Left H Tarsal Joint, Right J Tarsal Joint, Left K Tarsometatarsal Joint, Right L Tarsometatarsal Joint, Left M Metatarsal-Phalangeal Joint, Right N Metatarsal-Phalangeal Joint, Left P Toe Phalangeal Joint, Right Q Toe Phalangeal Joint, Left	0 Open 3 Percutaneous 4 Percutaneous Endoscopic X External	0 Drainage Device 3 Infusion Device 4 Internal Fixation Device 5 External Fixation Device 7 Autologous Tissue Substitute 8 Spacer J Synthetic Substitute K Nonautologous Tissue Substitute	Z No Qualifier

AHA Coding Clinic

0S9D4ZZ Drainage of Left Knee Joint, Percutaneous Endoscopic Approach— AHA CC: 2Q, 2018, 17

0SB20ZZ Excision of Lumbar Vertebral Disc, Open Approach—AHA CC: 2Q, 2014, 6-7; 2Q, 2016, 16; 4Q, 2017, 76-77

0SB40ZZ Excision of Lumbosacral Disc, Open Approach—AHA CC: 4Q, 2017, 76-77

0SBD4ZZ Excision of Left Knee Joint, Percutaneous Endoscopic Approach—AHA CC: 1Q, 2015, 34

0SG0071 Fusion of Lumbar Vertebral Joint with Autologous Tissue Substitute, Posterior Approach, Posterior Column, Open Approach—AHA CC: 1Q, 2013, 21-23; 3Q, 2013, 25-26

0SG00AJ Fusion of Lumbar Vertebral Joint with Interbody Fusion Device, Posterior Approach, Anterior Column, Open Approach— AHA CC: 3Q, 2013, 25-26; 3Q, 2022, 21-22

0SG00K1 Fusion of Lumbar Vertebral Joint with Nonautologous Tissue Substitute, Posterior Approach, Posterior Column, Open Approach—AHA CC: 3Q, 2021, 25

0SG107J Fusion of 2 or more Lumbar Vertebral Joints with Autologous Tissue Substitute, Posterior Approach, Anterior Column, Open Approach—AHA CC: 3Q, 2014, 36

0SG10K1 Fusion of 2 or more Lumbar Vertebral Joints with Nonautologous Tissue Substitute, Posterior Approach, Posterior Column, Open Approach—AHA CC: 2Q, 2023, 25-26

0SG834Z Fusion of Left Sacroiliac Joint with Internal Fixation Device, Percutaneous Approach—AHA CC: 2Q, 2022, 23-24

0SGG04Z Fusion of Left Ankle Joint with Internal Fixation Device, Open Approach—AHA CC: 2Q, 2013, 39-40

0SGG07Z Fusion of Left Ankle Joint with Autologous Tissue Substitute, Open Approach—AHA CC: 2Q, 2013, 39-40

0SGJ04Z Fusion of Left Tarsal Joint with Internal Fixation Device, Open Approach—AHA CC: 3Q, 2021, 24

0SGJ07Z Fusion of Left Tarsal Joint with Autologous Tissue Substitute, Open Approach—AHA CC: 3Q, 2021, 24

0SGL04Z Fusion of Left Tarsometatarsal Joint with Internal Fixation Device, Open Approach—AHA CC: 3Q, 2021, 24

0SGL07Z Fusion of Left Tarsometatarsal Joint with Autologous Tissue Substitute, Open Approach—AHA CC: 3Q, 2021, 24

0SH00BZ Insertion of Interspinous Process Spinal Stabilization Device into Lumbar Vertebral Joint, Open Approach—AHA CC: 3Q, 2021, 25

0SH408Z Insertion of Spacer into Lumbosacral Disc, Open Approach—AHA CC: 1Q, 2021, 18-19

0SJG3ZZ Inspection of Left Ankle Joint, Percutaneous Approach—AHA CC: 1Q, 2017, 50

0SNC4ZZ Release Right Knee Joint, Percutaneous Endoscopic Approach—AHA CC: 2Q, 2020, 26-27

0SP909Z Removal of Liner from Right Hip Joint, Open Approach—AHA CC: 2Q, 2015, 19-20; 4Q, 2016, 111-112

0SP90JZ Removal of Synthetic Substitute from Right Hip Joint, Open Approach—AHA CC: 2Q, 2015, 19-20

0SPC0JZ Removal of Synthetic Substitute from Right Knee Joint, Open Approach—AHA CC: 2Q, 2015, 18-19

0SPD0JZ Removal of Synthetic Substitute from Left Knee Joint, Open Approach—AHA CC: 3Q, 2021, 25-26

0SPF0JZ Removal of Synthetic Substitute from Right Ankle Joint, Open Approach—AHA CC: 4Q, 2017, 107-108; 1Q, 2021, 17-18

0SPG04Z Removal of Internal Fixation Device from Left Ankle Joint, Open Approach—AHA CC: 2Q, 2013, 39-40

0SPR0JZ Removal of Synthetic Substitute from Right Hip Joint, Femoral Surface, Open Approach—AHA CC: 4Q, 2016, 111-112

0SPW0JZ Removal of Synthetic Substitute from Left Knee Joint, Tibial Surface, Open Approach—AHA CC: 2Q, 2018, 16-17

0SQB4ZZ Repair Left Hip Joint, Percutaneous Endoscopic Approach—AHA CC: 4Q, 2014, 25-26

0SR9029 Replacement of Right Hip Joint with Metal on Polyethylene Synthetic Substitute, Cemented, Open Approach—AHA CC: 3Q, 2020, 33-34

0SRB02A Replacement of Left Hip Joint with Metal on Polyethylene Synthetic Substitute, Uncemented, Open Approach—AHA CC: 1Q, 2022, 39

0SRB06Z Replacement of Left Hip Joint with Oxidized Zirconium on Polyethylene Synthetic Substitute, Open Approach—AHA CC: 4Q, 2017, 39

0SRB0J9 Replacement of Left Hip Joint with Synthetic Substitute, Cemented, Open Approach—AHA CC: 3Q, 2015, 18-19

0SRC0J9 Replacement of Right Knee Joint with Synthetic Substitute, Cemented, Open Approach—AHA CC: 2Q, 2015, 18-19

0SRD0J9 Replacement of Left Knee Joint with Synthetic Substitute, Cemented, Open Approach—AHA CC: 3Q, 2021, 25-26

0SRD0JZ Replacement of Left Knee Joint with Synthetic Substitute, Open Approach—AHA CC: 4Q, 2016, 109-110

0SRD0LZ Replacement of Left Knee Joint with Unicondylar Synthetic Substitute, Open Approach—AHA CC: 4Q, 2016, 110

0SRF0JA Replacement of Right Ankle Joint with Synthetic Substitute, Uncemented, Open Approach—AHA CC: 4Q, 2017, 107-108

0SRR03A Replacement of Right Hip Joint, Femoral Surface with Ceramic Synthetic Substitute, Uncemented, Open Approach—AHA CC: 2Q, 2015, 19-20

0SRR0J9 Replacement of Right Hip Joint, Femoral Surface with Synthetic Substitute, Cemented, Open Approach—AHA CC: 4Q, 2016, 111-112

0SRW0JZ Replacement of Left Knee Joint, Tibial Surface with Synthetic Substitute, Open Approach—AHA CC: 2Q, 2018, 16-17

0SSB04Z Reposition Left Hip Joint with Internal Fixation Device, Open Approach—AHA CC: 2Q, 2016, 32

0SSG35Z Reposition Left Ankle Joint with External Fixation Device, Percutaneous Approach—AHA CC: 2Q, 2022, 22; 3Q, 2022, 27

0SSJ35Z Reposition Left Tarsal Joint with External Fixation Device, Percutaneous Approach—AHA CC: 3Q, 2022, 27

0STD0ZZ Resection of Left Knee Joint, Open Approach—AHA CC: 4Q, 2014, 30-31

0STM0ZZ Resection of Right Metatarsal-Phalangeal Joint, Open Approach—AHA CC: 1Q, 2016, 20-21

0SUA09Z Supplement Right Hip Joint, Acetabular Surface with Liner, Open Approach—AHA CC: 2Q, 2015, 19-20; 4Q, 2016, 111-112

0SUC07Z Supplement Right Knee Joint with Autologous Tissue Substitute, Open Approach—AHA CC: 1Q, 2022, 47-48

0SUF0JZ Supplement Right Ankle Joint with Synthetic Substitute, Open Approach—AHA CC: 1Q, 2021, 17-18

0SWF0JZ Revision of Synthetic Substitute in Right Ankle Joint, Open Approach—AHA CC: 4Q, 2017, 107-108

0SWW0JZ Revision of Synthetic Substitute in Left Knee Joint, Tibial Surface, Open Approach—AHA CC: 4Q, 2016, 112

Urinary System

Urinary System

Lower Urinary Tract

Renal Revascularization

Bypass to distal extremity of renal artery beyond extensive fibromuscular hyperplasia, employing segment of saphenous vein

Renal artery bypass plus contralateral nephrectomy

Endarterectomy

Patch graft with or without endarterectomy

Renal artery bypass plus patch graft to accessory renal artery

Resection of sacciform aneurysm of renal artery and primary repair

Urinary System Tables 0T1–0TY

Section	0	Medical and Surgical
Body System	T	Urinary System
Operation	1	Bypass: Altering the route of passage of the contents of a tubular body part

Body Part (4th)	Approach (5th)	Device (6th)	Qualifier (7th)
3 Kidney Pelvis, Right 4 Kidney Pelvis, Left	0 Open 4 Percutaneous Endoscopic	7 Autologous Tissue Substitute J Synthetic Substitute K Nonautologous Tissue Substitute Z No Device	3 Kidney Pelvis, Right 4 Kidney Pelvis, Left 6 Ureter, Right 7 Ureter, Left 8 Colon 9 Colocutaneous A Ileum B Bladder C Ileocutaneous D Cutaneous
3 Kidney Pelvis, Right 4 Kidney Pelvis, Left	3 Percutaneous	J Synthetic Substitute	D Cutaneous
6 Ureter, Right 7 Ureter, Left 8 Ureters, Bilateral	0 Open 4 Percutaneous Endoscopic	7 Autologous Tissue Substitute J Synthetic Substitute K Nonautologous Tissue Substitute Z No Device	6 Ureter, Right 7 Ureter, Left 8 Colon 9 Colocutaneous A Ileum B Bladder C Ileocutaneous D Cutaneous
6 Ureter, Right 7 Ureter, Left 8 Ureters, Bilateral	3 Percutaneous	J Synthetic Substitute	D Cutaneous
B Bladder	0 Open 4 Percutaneous Endoscopic	7 Autologous Tissue Substitute J Synthetic Substitute K Nonautologous Tissue Substitute Z No Device	9 Colocutaneous C Ileocutaneous D Cutaneous
B Bladder	3 Percutaneous	J Synthetic Substitute	D Cutaneous

Section	0	Medical and Surgical
Body System	T	Urinary System
Operation	2	Change: Taking out or off a device from a body part and putting back an identical or similar device in or on the same body part without cutting or puncturing the skin or a mucous membrane

Body Part (4th)	Approach (5th)	Device (6th)	Qualifier (7th)
5 Kidney 9 Ureter B Bladder D Urethra	X External	0 Drainage Device Y Other Device	Z No Qualifier

Section	0	Medical and Surgical
Body System	T	Urinary System
Operation	5	Destruction: Physical eradication of all or a portion of a body part by the direct use of energy, force, or a destructive agent

Body Part (4th)	Approach (5th)	Device (6th)	Qualifier (7th)
0 Kidney, Right 1 Kidney, Left 3 Kidney Pelvis, Right 4 Kidney Pelvis, Left 6 Ureter, Right 7 Ureter, Left B Bladder C Bladder Neck	0 Open 3 Percutaneous 4 Percutaneous Endoscopic 7 Via Natural or Artificial Opening 8 Via Natural or Artificial Opening Endoscopic	Z No Device	Z No Qualifier

Continued →

Section	0	Medical and Surgical
Body System	T	Urinary System
Operation	5	Destruction: Physical eradication of all or a portion of a body part by the direct use of energy, force, or a destructive agent

0T5 Continued

Body Part (4th)	Approach (5th)	Device (6th)	Qualifier (7th)
D Urethra	0 Open 3 Percutaneous 4 Percutaneous Endoscopic 7 Via Natural or Artificial Opening 8 Via Natural or Artificial Opening Endoscopic X External	Z No Device	Z No Qualifier

Section	0	Medical and Surgical
Body System	T	Urinary System
Operation	7	Dilation: Expanding an orifice or the lumen of a tubular body part

Body Part (4th)	Approach (5th)	Device (6th)	Qualifier (7th)
3 Kidney Pelvis, Right 4 Kidney Pelvis, Left 6 Ureter, Right 7 Ureter, Left 8 Ureters, Bilateral B Bladder C Bladder Neck D Urethra	0 Open 3 Percutaneous 4 Percutaneous Endoscopic 7 Via Natural or Artificial Opening 8 Via Natural or Artificial Opening Endoscopic	D Intraluminal Device Z No Device	Z No Qualifier

Section	0	Medical and Surgical
Body System	T	Urinary System
Operation	8	Division: Cutting into a body part, without draining fluids and/or gases from the body part, in order to separate or transect a body part

Body Part (4th)	Approach (5th)	Device (6th)	Qualifier (7th)
2 Kidneys, Bilateral C Bladder Neck	0 Open 3 Percutaneous 4 Percutaneous Endoscopic	Z No Device	Z No Qualifier

Section	0	Medical and Surgical
Body System	T	Urinary System
Operation	9	Drainage: Taking or letting out fluids and/or gases from a body part

Body Part (4th)	Approach (5th)	Device (6th)	Qualifier (7th)
0 Kidney, Right 1 Kidney, Left 3 Kidney Pelvis, Right 4 Kidney Pelvis, Left 6 Ureter, Right 7 Ureter, Left 8 Ureters, Bilateral B Bladder C Bladder Neck	0 Open 3 Percutaneous 4 Percutaneous Endoscopic 7 Via Natural or Artificial Opening 8 Via Natural or Artificial Opening Endoscopic	0 Drainage Device	Z No Qualifier
0 Kidney, Right 1 Kidney, Left 3 Kidney Pelvis, Right 4 Kidney Pelvis, Left 6 Ureter, Right 7 Ureter, Left 8 Ureters, Bilateral B Bladder C Bladder Neck	0 Open 3 Percutaneous 4 Percutaneous Endoscopic 7 Via Natural or Artificial Opening 8 Via Natural or Artificial Opening Endoscopic	Z No Device	X Diagnostic Z No Qualifier

Continued →

Section	0	Medical and Surgical
Body System	T	Urinary System
Operation	9	Drainage: Taking or letting out fluids and/or gases from a body part

Body Part (4th)	Approach (5th)	Device (6th)	Qualifier (7th)
D Urethra	**0** Open **3** Percutaneous **4** Percutaneous Endoscopic **7** Via Natural or Artificial Opening **8** Via Natural or Artificial Opening Endoscopic **X** External	**0** Drainage Device	**Z** No Qualifier
D Urethra	**0** Open **3** Percutaneous **4** Percutaneous Endoscopic **7** Via Natural or Artificial Opening **8** Via Natural or Artificial Opening Endoscopic **X** External	**Z** No Device	**X** Diagnostic **Z** No Qualifier

Section	0	Medical and Surgical
Body System	T	Urinary System
Operation	B	Excision: Cutting out or off, without replacement, a portion of a body part

Body Part (4th)	Approach (5th)	Device (6th)	Qualifier (7th)
0 Kidney, Right **1** Kidney, Left **3** Kidney Pelvis, Right **4** Kidney Pelvis, Left **6** Ureter, Right **7** Ureter, Left **B** Bladder **C** Bladder Neck	**0** Open **3** Percutaneous **4** Percutaneous Endoscopic **7** Via Natural or Artificial Opening **8** Via Natural or Artificial Opening Endoscopic	**Z** No Device	**X** Diagnostic **Z** No Qualifier
D Urethra	**0** Open **3** Percutaneous **4** Percutaneous Endoscopic **7** Via Natural or Artificial Opening **8** Via Natural or Artificial Opening Endoscopic **X** External	**Z** No Device	**X** Diagnostic **Z** No Qualifier

Section	0	Medical and Surgical
Body System	T	Urinary System
Operation	C	Extirpation: Taking or cutting out solid matter from a body part

Body Part (4th)	Approach (5th)	Device (6th)	Qualifier (7th)
0 Kidney, Right **1** Kidney, Left **3** Kidney Pelvis, Right **4** Kidney Pelvis, Left **6** Ureter, Right **7** Ureter, Left **B** Bladder **C** Bladder Neck	**0** Open **3** Percutaneous **4** Percutaneous Endoscopic **7** Via Natural or Artificial Opening **8** Via Natural or Artificial Opening Endoscopic	**Z** No Device	**Z** No Qualifier
D Urethra	**0** Open **3** Percutaneous **4** Percutaneous Endoscopic **7** Via Natural or Artificial Opening **8** Via Natural or Artificial Opening Endoscopic **X** External	**Z** No Device	**Z** No Qualifier

0TD-0TH

Medical and Surgical, Urinary System Tables

Section	0	Medical and Surgical
Body System	T	Urinary System
Operation	D	Extraction: Pulling or stripping out or off all or a portion of a body part by the use of force

Body Part (4th)	Approach (5th)	Device (6th)	Qualifier (7th)
0 Kidney, Right 1 Kidney, Left	0 Open 3 Percutaneous 4 Percutaneous Endoscopic	Z No Device	Z No Qualifier

Section	0	Medical and Surgical
Body System	T	Urinary System
Operation	F	Fragmentation: Breaking solid matter in a body part into pieces

Body Part (4th)	Approach (5th)	Device (6th)	Qualifier (7th)
3 Kidney Pelvis, Right 4 Kidney Pelvis, Left 6 Ureter, Right 7 Ureter, Left B Bladder C Bladder Neck D Urethra	0 Open 3 Percutaneous 4 Percutaneous Endoscopic 7 Via Natural or Artificial Opening 8 Via Natural or Artificial Opening Endoscopic X External	Z No Device	Z No Qualifier

Section	0	Medical and Surgical
Body System	T	Urinary System
Operation	H	Insertion: Putting in a nonbiological appliance that monitors, assists, performs, or prevents a physiological function but does not physically take the place of a body part

Body Part (4th)	Approach (5th)	Device (6th)	Qualifier (7th)
5 Kidney	0 Open 3 Percutaneous 4 Percutaneous Endoscopic 7 Via Natural or Artificial Opening 8 Via Natural or Artificial Opening Endoscopic	1 Radioactive Element 2 Monitoring Device 3 Infusion Device Y Other Device	Z No Qualifier
9 Ureter	0 Open 3 Percutaneous 4 Percutaneous Endoscopic 7 Via Natural or Artificial Opening 8 Via Natural or Artificial Opening Endoscopic	1 Radioactive Element 2 Monitoring Device 3 Infusion Device M Stimulator Lead Y Other Device	Z No Qualifier
B Bladder	0 Open 3 Percutaneous 4 Percutaneous Endoscopic 7 Via Natural or Artificial Opening 8 Via Natural or Artificial Opening Endoscopic	1 Radioactive Element 2 Monitoring Device 3 Infusion Device L Artificial Sphincter M Stimulator Lead Y Other Device	Z No Qualifier
C Bladder Neck	0 Open 3 Percutaneous 4 Percutaneous Endoscopic 7 Via Natural or Artificial Opening 8 Via Natural or Artificial Opening Endoscopic	L Artificial Sphincter	Z No Qualifier
D Urethra	0 Open 3 Percutaneous 4 Percutaneous Endoscopic 7 Via Natural or Artificial Opening 8 Via Natural or Artificial Opening Endoscopic	1 Radioactive Element 2 Monitoring Device 3 Infusion Device L Artificial Sphincter Y Other Device	Z No Qualifier
D Urethra	X External	2 Monitoring Device 3 Infusion Device L Artificial Sphincter	Z No Qualifier

464

Section	0	Medical and Surgical
Body System	T	Urinary System
Operation	J	Inspection: Visually and/or manually exploring a body part

Body Part (4th)	Approach (5th)	Device (6th)	Qualifier (7th)
5 Kidney 9 Ureter B Bladder D Urethra	0 Open 3 Percutaneous 4 Percutaneous Endoscopic 7 Via Natural or Artificial Opening 8 Via Natural or Artificial Opening Endoscopic X External	Z No Device	Z No Qualifier

Section	0	Medical and Surgical
Body System	T	Urinary System
Operation	L	Occlusion: Completely closing an orifice or the lumen of a tubular body part

Body Part (4th)	Approach (5th)	Device (6th)	Qualifier (7th)
3 Kidney Pelvis, Right 4 Kidney Pelvis, Left 6 Ureter, Right 7 Ureter, Left B Bladder C Bladder Neck	0 Open 3 Percutaneous 4 Percutaneous Endoscopic	C Extraluminal Device D Intraluminal Device Z No Device	Z No Qualifier
3 Kidney Pelvis, Right 4 Kidney Pelvis, Left 6 Ureter, Right 7 Ureter, Left B Bladder C Bladder Neck	7 Via Natural or Artificial Opening 8 Via Natural or Artificial Opening Endoscopic	D Intraluminal Device Z No Device	Z No Qualifier
D Urethra	0 Open 3 Percutaneous 4 Percutaneous Endoscopic X External	C Extraluminal Device D Intraluminal Device Z No Device	Z No Qualifier
D Urethra	7 Via Natural or Artificial Opening 8 Via Natural or Artificial Opening Endoscopic	D Intraluminal Device Z No Device	Z No Qualifier

Section	0	Medical and Surgical
Body System	T	Urinary System
Operation	M	Reattachment: Putting back in or on all or a portion of a separated body part to its normal location or other suitable location

Body Part (4th)	Approach (5th)	Device (6th)	Qualifier (7th)
0 Kidney, Right 1 Kidney, Left 2 Kidneys, Bilateral 3 Kidney Pelvis, Right 4 Kidney Pelvis, Left 6 Ureter, Right 7 Ureter, Left 8 Ureters, Bilateral B Bladder C Bladder Neck D Urethra	0 Open 4 Percutaneous Endoscopic	Z No Device	Z No Qualifier

0TJ–0TM

Medical and Surgical, Urinary System Tables

465

Section	0	Medical and Surgical
Body System	T	Urinary System
Operation	N	Release: Freeing a body part from an abnormal physical constraint by cutting or by the use of force

Body Part (4th)	Approach (5th)	Device (6th)	Qualifier (7th)
0 Kidney, Right 1 Kidney, Left 3 Kidney Pelvis, Right 4 Kidney Pelvis, Left 6 Ureter, Right 7 Ureter, Left B Bladder C Bladder Neck	0 Open 3 Percutaneous 4 Percutaneous Endoscopic 7 Via Natural or Artificial Opening 8 Via Natural or Artificial Opening Endoscopic	Z No Device	Z No Qualifier
D Urethra	0 Open 3 Percutaneous 4 Percutaneous Endoscopic 7 Via Natural or Artificial Opening 8 Via Natural or Artificial Opening Endoscopic X External	Z No Device	Z No Qualifier

Section	0	Medical and Surgical
Body System	T	Urinary System
Operation	P	Removal: Taking out or off a device from a body part

Body Part (4th)	Approach (5th)	Device (6th)	Qualifier (7th)
5 Kidney	0 Open 3 Percutaneous 4 Percutaneous Endoscopic 7 Via Natural or Artificial Opening 8 Via Natural or Artificial Opening Endoscopic	0 Drainage Device 2 Monitoring Device 3 Infusion Device 7 Autologous Tissue Substitute C Extraluminal Device D Intraluminal Device J Synthetic Substitute K Nonautologous Tissue Substitute Y Other Device	Z No Qualifier
5 Kidney	X External	0 Drainage Device 2 Monitoring Device 3 Infusion Device D Intraluminal Device	Z No Qualifier
9 Ureter	0 Open 3 Percutaneous 4 Percutaneous Endoscopic 7 Via Natural or Artificial Opening 8 Via Natural or Artificial Opening Endoscopic	0 Drainage Device 2 Monitoring Device 3 Infusion Device 7 Autologous Tissue Substitute C Extraluminal Device D Intraluminal Device J Synthetic Substitute K Nonautologous Tissue Substitute M Stimulator Lead Y Other Device	Z No Qualifier
9 Ureter	X External	0 Drainage Device 2 Monitoring Device 3 Infusion Device D Intraluminal Device M Stimulator Lead	Z No Qualifier

Continued →

0TP Continued

Section	0	Medical and Surgical
Body System	T	Urinary System
Operation	P	Removal: Taking out or off a device from a body part

Body Part (4th)	Approach (5th)	Device (6th)	Qualifier (7th)
B Bladder	0 Open 3 Percutaneous 4 Percutaneous Endoscopic 7 Via Natural or Artificial Opening 8 Via Natural or Artificial Opening Endoscopic	0 Drainage Device 2 Monitoring Device 3 Infusion Device 7 Autologous Tissue Substitute C Extraluminal Device D Intraluminal Device J Synthetic Substitute K Nonautologous Tissue Substitute L Artificial Sphincter M Stimulator Lead Y Other Device	Z No Qualifier
B Bladder	X External	0 Drainage Device 2 Monitoring Device 3 Infusion Device D Intraluminal Device L Artificial Sphincter M Stimulator Lead	Z No Qualifier
D Urethra	0 Open 3 Percutaneous 4 Percutaneous Endoscopic 7 Via Natural or Artificial Opening 8 Via Natural or Artificial Opening Endoscopic	0 Drainage Device 2 Monitoring Device 3 Infusion Device 7 Autologous Tissue Substitute C Extraluminal Device D Intraluminal Device J Synthetic Substitute K Nonautologous Tissue Substitute L Artificial Sphincter Y Other Device	Z No Qualifier
D Urethra	X External	0 Drainage Device 2 Monitoring Device 3 Infusion Device D Intraluminal Device L Artificial Sphincter	Z No Qualifier

Section	0	Medical and Surgical
Body System	T	Urinary System
Operation	Q	Repair: Restoring, to the extent possible, a body part to its normal anatomic structure and function

Body Part (4th)	Approach (5th)	Device (6th)	Qualifier (7th)
0 Kidney, Right 1 Kidney, Left 3 Kidney Pelvis, Right 4 Kidney Pelvis, Left 6 Ureter, Right 7 Ureter, Left B Bladder C Bladder Neck	0 Open 3 Percutaneous 4 Percutaneous Endoscopic 7 Via Natural or Artificial Opening 8 Via Natural or Artificial Opening Endoscopic	Z No Device	Z No Qualifier
D Urethra	0 Open 3 Percutaneous 4 Percutaneous Endoscopic 7 Via Natural or Artificial Opening 8 Via Natural or Artificial Opening Endoscopic X External	Z No Device	Z No Qualifier

0TR–0TT

Section 0 **Medical and Surgical**
Body System T **Urinary System**
Operation R **Replacement:** Putting in or on biological or synthetic material that physically takes the place and/or function of all or a portion of a body part

Body Part (4th)	Approach (5th)	Device (6th)	Qualifier (7th)
3 Kidney Pelvis, Right 4 Kidney Pelvis, Left 6 Ureter, Right 7 Ureter, Left B Bladder C Bladder Neck	0 Open 4 Percutaneous Endoscopic 7 Via Natural or Artificial Opening 8 Via Natural or Artificial Opening Endoscopic	7 Autologous Tissue Substitute J Synthetic Substitute K Nonautologous Tissue Substitute	Z No Qualifier
D Urethra	0 Open 4 Percutaneous Endoscopic 7 Via Natural or Artificial Opening 8 Via Natural or Artificial Opening Endoscopic X External	7 Autologous Tissue Substitute J Synthetic Substitute K Nonautologous Tissue Substitute	Z No Qualifier

Section 0 **Medical and Surgical**
Body System T **Urinary System**
Operation S **Reposition:** Moving to its normal location, or other suitable location, all or a portion of a body part

Body Part (4th)	Approach (5th)	Device (6th)	Qualifier (7th)
0 Kidney, Right 1 Kidney, Left 2 Kidneys, Bilateral 3 Kidney Pelvis, Right 4 Kidney Pelvis, Left 6 Ureter, Right 7 Ureter, Left 8 Ureters, Bilateral B Bladder C Bladder Neck D Urethra	0 Open 4 Percutaneous Endoscopic	Z No Device	Z No Qualifier

Section 0 **Medical and Surgical**
Body System T **Urinary System**
Operation T **Resection:** Cutting out or off, without replacement, all of a body part

Body Part (4th)	Approach (5th)	Device (6th)	Qualifier (7th)
0 Kidney, Right 1 Kidney, Left 2 Kidneys, Bilateral	0 Open 4 Percutaneous Endoscopic	Z No Device	Z No Qualifier
3 Kidney Pelvis, Right 4 Kidney Pelvis, Left 6 Ureter, Right 7 Ureter, Left B Bladder C Bladder Neck D Urethra	0 Open 4 Percutaneous Endoscopic 7 Via Natural or Artificial Opening 8 Via Natural or Artificial Opening Endoscopic	Z No Device	Z No Qualifier

Medical and Surgical, Urinary System Tables

Section	0	Medical and Surgical
Body System	T	Urinary System
Operation	U	Supplement: Putting in or on biological or synthetic material that physically reinforces and/or augments the function of a portion of a body part

Body Part (4th)	Approach (5th)	Device (6th)	Qualifier (7th)
3 Kidney Pelvis, Right 4 Kidney Pelvis, Left 6 Ureter, Right 7 Ureter, Left B Bladder C Bladder Neck	0 Open 4 Percutaneous Endoscopic 7 Via Natural or Artificial Opening 8 Via Natural or Artificial Opening Endoscopic	7 Autologous Tissue Substitute J Synthetic Substitute K Nonautologous Tissue Substitute	Z No Qualifier
D Urethra	0 Open 4 Percutaneous Endoscopic 7 Via Natural or Artificial Opening 8 Via Natural or Artificial Opening Endoscopic X External	7 Autologous Tissue Substitute J Synthetic Substitute K Nonautologous Tissue Substitute	Z No Qualifier

Section	0	Medical and Surgical
Body System	T	Urinary System
Operation	V	Restriction: Partially closing an orifice or the lumen of a tubular body part

Body Part (4th)	Approach (5th)	Device (6th)	Qualifier (7th)
3 Kidney Pelvis, Right 4 Kidney Pelvis, Left 6 Ureter, Right 7 Ureter, Left B Bladder C Bladder Neck	0 Open 3 Percutaneous 4 Percutaneous Endoscopic	C Extraluminal Device D Intraluminal Device Z No Device	Z No Qualifier
3 Kidney Pelvis, Right 4 Kidney Pelvis, Left 6 Ureter, Right 7 Ureter, Left B Bladder C Bladder Neck	7 Via Natural or Artificial Opening 8 Via Natural or Artificial Opening Endoscopic	D Intraluminal Device Z No Device	Z No Qualifier
D Urethra	0 Open 3 Percutaneous 4 Percutaneous Endoscopic	C Extraluminal Device D Intraluminal Device Z No Device	Z No Qualifier
D Urethra	7 Via Natural or Artificial Opening 8 Via Natural or Artificial Opening Endoscopic	D Intraluminal Device Z No Device	Z No Qualifier
D Urethra	X External	Z No Device	Z No Qualifier

Section	0	Medical and Surgical
Body System	T	Urinary System
Operation	W	Revision: Correcting, to the extent possible, a portion of a malfunctioning device or the position of a displaced device

Body Part (4th)	Approach (5th)	Device (6th)	Qualifier (7th)
5 Kidney	0 Open 3 Percutaneous 4 Percutaneous Endoscopic 7 Via Natural or Artificial Opening 8 Via Natural or Artificial Opening Endoscopic	0 Drainage Device 2 Monitoring Device 3 Infusion Device 7 Autologous Tissue Substitute C Extraluminal Device D Intraluminal Device J Synthetic Substitute K Nonautologous Tissue Substitute Y Other Device	Z No Qualifier

Continued ➜

Section	0	Medical and Surgical
Body System	T	Urinary System
Operation	W	Revision: Correcting, to the extent possible, a portion of a malfunctioning device or the position of a displaced device

0TW Continued

Body Part (4th)	Approach (5th)	Device (6th)	Qualifier (7th)
5 Kidney	X External	0 Drainage Device 2 Monitoring Device 3 Infusion Device 7 Autologous Tissue Substitute C Extraluminal Device D Intraluminal Device J Synthetic Substitute K Nonautologous Tissue Substitute	Z No Qualifier
9 Ureter	0 Open 3 Percutaneous 4 Percutaneous Endoscopic 7 Via Natural or Artificial Opening 8 Via Natural or Artificial Opening Endoscopic	0 Drainage Device 2 Monitoring Device 3 Infusion Device 7 Autologous Tissue Substitute C Extraluminal Device D Intraluminal Device J Synthetic Substitute K Nonautologous Tissue Substitute M Stimulator Lead Y Other Device	Z No Qualifier
9 Ureter	X External	0 Drainage Device 2 Monitoring Device 3 Infusion Device 7 Autologous Tissue Substitute C Extraluminal Device D Intraluminal Device J Synthetic Substitute K Nonautologous Tissue Substitute M Stimulator Lead	Z No Qualifier
B Bladder	0 Open 3 Percutaneous 4 Percutaneous Endoscopic 7 Via Natural or Artificial Opening 8 Via Natural or Artificial Opening Endoscopic	0 Drainage Device 2 Monitoring Device 3 Infusion Device 7 Autologous Tissue Substitute C Extraluminal Device D Intraluminal Device J Synthetic Substitute K Nonautologous Tissue Substitute L Artificial Sphincter M Stimulator Lead Y Other Device	Z No Qualifier
B Bladder	X External	0 Drainage Device 2 Monitoring Device 3 Infusion Device 7 Autologous Tissue Substitute C Extraluminal Device D Intraluminal Device J Synthetic Substitute K Nonautologous Tissue Substitute L Artificial Sphincter M Stimulator Lead	Z No Qualifier
D Urethra	0 Open 3 Percutaneous 4 Percutaneous Endoscopic 7 Via Natural or Artificial Opening 8 Via Natural or Artificial Opening Endoscopic	0 Drainage Device 2 Monitoring Device 3 Infusion Device 7 Autologous Tissue Substitute C Extraluminal Device D Intraluminal Device J Synthetic Substitute K Nonautologous Tissue Substitute L Artificial Sphincter Y Other Device	Z No Qualifier

Continued →

Section	0	Medical and Surgical	0TW Continued
Body System	T	Urinary System	
Operation	W	Revision: Correcting, to the extent possible, a portion of a malfunctioning device or the position of a displaced device	

Body Part (4th)	Approach (5th)	Device (6th)	Qualifier (7th)
D Urethra	X External	0 Drainage Device 2 Monitoring Device 3 Infusion Device 7 Autologous Tissue Substitute C Extraluminal Device D Intraluminal Device J Synthetic Substitute K Nonautologous Tissue Substitute L Artificial Sphincter	Z No Qualifier

Section	0	Medical and Surgical
Body System	T	Urinary System
Operation	Y	Transplantation: Putting in or on all or a portion of a living body part taken from another individual or animal to physically take the place and/or function of all or a portion of a similar body part

Body Part (4th)	Approach (5th)	Device (6th)	Qualifier (7th)
0 Kidney, Right 1 Kidney, Left	0 Open	Z No Device	0 Allogeneic 1 Syngeneic 2 Zooplastic

AHA Coding Clinic

0T170ZB Bypass Left Ureter to Bladder, Open Approach—AHA CC: 3Q, 2015, 34-35

0T180ZC Bypass Bilateral Ureters to Ileocutaneous, Open Approach—AHA CC: 3Q, 2017, 20-21

0T1B0Z9 Bypass Bladder to Colocutaneous, Open Approach—AHA CC: 3Q, 2017, 21-22

0T768DZ Dilation of Right Ureter with Intraluminal Device, Via Natural or Artificial Opening Endoscopic—AHA CC: 2Q, 2016, 27-28; 4Q, 2017, 111

0T778DZ Dilation of Left Ureter with Intraluminal Device, Via Natural or Artificial Opening Endoscopic—AHA CC: 2Q, 2015, 8-9

0T7D8DZ Dilation of Urethra with Intraluminal Device, Via Natural or Artificial Opening Endoscopic—AHA CC: 4Q, 2013, 123

0T9680Z Drainage of Right Ureter with Drainage Device, Via Natural or Artificial Opening Endoscopic—AHA CC: 3Q, 2017, 19-20

0TBB8ZX Excision of Bladder, Via Natural or Artificial Opening Endoscopic, Diagnostic—AHA CC: 1Q, 2016, 19

0TBB8ZZ Excision of Bladder, Via Natural or Artificial Opening Endoscopic—AHA CC: 2Q, 2014, 8

0TBD8ZZ Excision of Urethra, Via Natural or Artificial Opening Endoscopic—AHA CC: 3Q, 2015, 34

0TC18ZZ Extirpation of Matter from Left Kidney, Via Natural or Artificial Opening Endoscopic—AHA CC: 2Q, 2015, 8-9

0TC48ZZ Extirpation of Matter from Left Kidney Pelvis, Via Natural or Artificial Opening Endoscopic—AHA CC: 2Q, 2015, 7-8

0TC68ZZ Extirpation of Matter from Right Ureter, Via Natural or Artificial Opening Endoscopic—AHA CC: 4Q, 2013, 122-123

0TC78ZZ Extirpation of Matter from Left Ureter, Via Natural or Artificial Opening Endoscopic—AHA CC: 2Q, 2015, 8-9

0TCB8ZZ Extirpation of Matter from Bladder, Via Natural or Artificial Opening Endoscopic—AHA CC: 2Q, 2015, 8-9; 3Q, 2016, 23-24; 3Q, 2019, 4

0TF3XZZ Fragmentation in Right Kidney Pelvis, External Approach—AHA CC: 4Q, 2013, 122

0TP98DZ Removal of Intraluminal Device from Ureter, Via Natural or Artificial Opening Endoscopic—AHA CC: 2Q, 2016, 27-28

0TQD0ZZ Repair Urethra, Open Approach—AHA CC: 1Q, 2017, 37-38

0TRB07Z Replacement of Bladder with Autologous Tissue Substitute, Open Approach—AHA CC: 3Q, 2017, 20-21

0TS60ZZ Reposition Right Ureter, Open Approach—AHA CC: 1Q, 2017, 36-37; 1Q, 2019, 29-30

0TSD0ZZ Reposition Urethra, Open Approach—AHA CC: 1Q, 2016, 15-16

0TT10ZZ Resection of Left Kidney, Open Approach—AHA CC: 3Q, 2014, 16

0TT70ZZ Resection of Left Ureter, Open Approach—AHA CC: 3Q, 2014, 16

0TUB07Z Supplement Bladder with Autologous Tissue Substitute, Open Approach—AHA CC: 3Q, 2017, 21-22

0TUD07Z Supplement Urethra with Autologous Tissue Substitute, Open Approach—AHA CC: 1Q, 2019, 29-30

0TV68ZZ Restriction of Right Ureter, Via Natural or Artificial Opening Endoscopic—AHA CC: 2Q, 2015, 11-12

0TV78ZZ Restriction of Left Ureter, Via Natural or Artificial Opening Endoscopic—AHA CC: 2Q, 2015, 11-12

Female Reproductive System

Cytoreduction Surgery in Ovarian Cancer

Residual tumors >2 cm in diameter after primary surgery associated with decreased survival. Cytoreduction attempts to reduce largest tumor to ≤2 cm in diameter

Extraabdominal involvement and massive involvement of small bowel, porta hepatis, mesenteric root, or aortic nodes preclude successful cytoreduction

Adherent metastatic tumor stripped or obliterated from peritoneal and serosal surfaces. Obstructions or more massive involvement requires more aggressive surgical intervention

Tumor adherent to surfaces rather than invasive of deeper structures can be successfully "peeled off"

© 2023. Netter illustration used with permission of Elsevier Inc. All rights reserved. www.netterimages.com

Female Reproductive System Tables 0U1–0UY

Section	0	Medical and Surgical
Body System	U	Female Reproductive System
Operation	1	Bypass: Altering the route of passage of the contents of a tubular body part

Body Part (4th)	Approach (5th)	Device (6th)	Qualifier (7th)
5 Fallopian Tube, Right 6 Fallopian Tube, Left	0 Open 4 Percutaneous Endoscopic	7 Autologous Tissue Substitute J Synthetic Substitute K Nonautologous Tissue Substitute Z No Device	5 Fallopian Tube, Right 6 Fallopian Tube, Left 9 Uterus

Section	0	Medical and Surgical
Body System	U	Female Reproductive System
Operation	2	Change: Taking out or off a device from a body part and putting back an identical or similar device in or on the same body part without cutting or puncturing the skin or a mucous membrane

Body Part (4th)	Approach (5th)	Device (6th)	Qualifier (7th)
3 Ovary 8 Fallopian Tube M Vulva	X External	0 Drainage Device Y Other Device	Z No Qualifier
D Uterus and Cervix	X External	0 Drainage Device H Contraceptive Device Y Other Device	Z No Qualifier
H Vagina and Cul-de-sac	X External	0 Drainage Device G Intraluminal Device, Pessary Y Other Device	Z No Qualifier

Section	0	Medical and Surgical
Body System	U	Female Reproductive System
Operation	5	Destruction: Physical eradication of all or a portion of a body part by the direct use of energy, force, or a destructive agent

Body Part (4th)	Approach (5th)	Device (6th)	Qualifier (7th)
0 Ovary, Right 1 Ovary, Left 2 Ovaries, Bilateral 4 Uterine Supporting Structure	0 Open 3 Percutaneous 4 Percutaneous Endoscopic 8 Via Natural or Artificial Opening Endoscopic	Z No Device	Z No Qualifier
5 Fallopian Tube, Right 6 Fallopian Tube, Left 7 Fallopian Tubes, Bilateral 9 Uterus B Endometrium C Cervix F Cul-de-sac	0 Open 3 Percutaneous 4 Percutaneous Endoscopic 7 Via Natural or Artificial Opening 8 Via Natural or Artificial Opening Endoscopic	Z No Device	Z No Qualifier
G Vagina K Hymen	0 Open 3 Percutaneous 4 Percutaneous Endoscopic 7 Via Natural or Artificial Opening 8 Via Natural or Artificial Opening Endoscopic X External	Z No Device	Z No Qualifier
J Clitoris L Vestibular Gland M Vulva	0 Open X External	Z No Device	Z No Qualifier

Section 0 **Medical and Surgical**
Body System U **Female Reproductive System**
Operation 7 **Dilation:** Expanding an orifice or the lumen of a tubular body part

Body Part (4th)	Approach (5th)	Device (6th)	Qualifier (7th)
5 Fallopian Tube, Right 6 Fallopian Tube, Left 7 Fallopian Tubes, Bilateral 9 Uterus C Cervix G Vagina	0 Open 3 Percutaneous 4 Percutaneous Endoscopic 7 Via Natural or Artificial Opening 8 Via Natural or Artificial Opening Endoscopic	D Intraluminal Device Z No Device	Z No Qualifier
K Hymen	0 Open 3 Percutaneous 4 Percutaneous Endoscopic 7 Via Natural or Artificial Opening 8 Via Natural or Artificial Opening Endoscopic X External	D Intraluminal Device Z No Device	Z No Qualifier

Section 0 **Medical and Surgical**
Body System U **Female Reproductive System**
Operation 8 **Division:** Cutting into a body part, without draining fluids and/or gases from the body part, in order to separate or transect a body part

Body Part (4th)	Approach (5th)	Device (6th)	Qualifier (7th)
0 Ovary, Right 1 Ovary, Left 2 Ovaries, Bilateral 4 Uterine Supporting Structure	0 Open 3 Percutaneous 4 Percutaneous Endoscopic	Z No Device	Z No Qualifier
K Hymen	7 Via Natural or Artificial Opening 8 Via Natural or Artificial Opening Endoscopic X External	Z No Device	Z No Qualifier

Section 0 **Medical and Surgical**
Body System U **Female Reproductive System**
Operation 9 **Drainage:** Taking or letting out fluids and/or gases from a body part

Body Part (4th)	Approach (5th)	Device (6th)	Qualifier (7th)
0 Ovary, Right 1 Ovary, Left 2 Ovaries, Bilateral	0 Open 3 Percutaneous 4 Percutaneous Endoscopic 8 Via Natural or Artificial Opening Endoscopic	0 Drainage Device	Z No Qualifier
0 Ovary, Right 1 Ovary, Left 2 Ovaries, Bilateral	0 Open 3 Percutaneous 4 Percutaneous Endoscopic 8 Via Natural or Artificial Opening Endoscopic	Z No Device	X Diagnostic Z No Qualifier
0 Ovary, Right 1 Ovary, Left 2 Ovaries, Bilateral	X External	Z No Device	Z No Qualifier
4 Uterine Supporting Structure	0 Open 3 Percutaneous 4 Percutaneous Endoscopic 8 Via Natural or Artificial Opening Endoscopic	0 Drainage Device	Z No Qualifier
4 Uterine Supporting Structure	0 Open 3 Percutaneous 4 Percutaneous Endoscopic 8 Via Natural or Artificial Opening Endoscopic	Z No Device	X Diagnostic Z No Qualifier

Continued ➡

Section	0	Medical and Surgical
Body System	U	Female Reproductive System
Operation	9	Drainage: Taking or letting out fluids and/or gases from a body part

Body Part (4th)	Approach (5th)	Device (6th)	Qualifier (7th)
5 Fallopian Tube, Right 6 Fallopian Tube, Left 7 Fallopian Tubes, Bilateral 9 Uterus C Cervix F Cul-de-sac	0 Open 3 Percutaneous 4 Percutaneous Endoscopic 7 Via Natural or Artificial Opening 8 Via Natural or Artificial Opening Endoscopic	0 Drainage Device	Z No Qualifier
5 Fallopian Tube, Right 6 Fallopian Tube, Left 7 Fallopian Tubes, Bilateral 9 Uterus C Cervix F Cul-de-sac	0 Open 3 Percutaneous 4 Percutaneous Endoscopic 7 Via Natural or Artificial Opening 8 Via Natural or Artificial Opening Endoscopic	Z No Device	X Diagnostic Z No Qualifier
G Vagina K Hymen	0 Open 3 Percutaneous 4 Percutaneous Endoscopic 7 Via Natural or Artificial Opening 8 Via Natural or Artificial Opening Endoscopic X External	0 Drainage Device	Z No Qualifier
G Vagina K Hymen	0 Open 3 Percutaneous 4 Percutaneous Endoscopic 7 Via Natural or Artificial Opening 8 Via Natural or Artificial Opening Endoscopic X External	Z No Device	X Diagnostic Z No Qualifier
J Clitoris L Vestibular Gland M Vulva	0 Open X External	0 Drainage Device	Z No Qualifier
J Clitoris L Vestibular Gland M Vulva	0 Open X External	Z No Device	X Diagnostic Z No Qualifier

Section	0	Medical and Surgical
Body System	U	Female Reproductive System
Operation	B	Excision: Cutting out or off, without replacement, a portion of a body part

Body Part (4th)	Approach (5th)	Device (6th)	Qualifier (7th)
0 Ovary, Right 1 Ovary, Left 2 Ovaries, Bilateral 4 Uterine Supporting Structure 5 Fallopian Tube, Right 6 Fallopian Tube, Left 7 Fallopian Tubes, Bilateral 9 Uterus C Cervix F Cul-de-sac	0 Open 3 Percutaneous 4 Percutaneous Endoscopic 7 Via Natural or Artificial Opening 8 Via Natural or Artificial Opening Endoscopic	Z No Device	X Diagnostic Z No Qualifier

Continued →

0UB–0UD

0UB Continued

Section	0	Medical and Surgical
Body System	U	Female Reproductive System
Operation	B	Excision: Cutting out or off, without replacement, a portion of a body part

Body Part (4th)	Approach (5th)	Device (6th)	Qualifier (7th)
G Vagina K Hymen	0 Open 3 Percutaneous 4 Percutaneous Endoscopic 7 Via Natural or Artificial Opening 8 Via Natural or Artificial Opening Endoscopic X External	Z No Device	X Diagnostic Z No Qualifier
J Clitoris L Vestibular Gland M Vulva	0 Open X External	Z No Device	X Diagnostic Z No Qualifier

Section	0	Medical and Surgical
Body System	U	Female Reproductive System
Operation	C	Extirpation: Taking or cutting out solid matter from a body part

Body Part (4th)	Approach (5th)	Device (6th)	Qualifier (7th)
0 Ovary, Right 1 Ovary, Left 2 Ovaries, Bilateral 4 Uterine Supporting Structure	0 Open 3 Percutaneous 4 Percutaneous Endoscopic 8 Via Natural or Artificial Opening Endoscopic	Z No Device	Z No Qualifier
5 Fallopian Tube, Right 6 Fallopian Tube, Left 7 Fallopian Tubes, Bilateral 9 Uterus B Endometrium C Cervix F Cul-de-sac	0 Open 3 Percutaneous 4 Percutaneous Endoscopic 7 Via Natural or Artificial Opening 8 Via Natural or Artificial Opening Endoscopic	Z No Device	Z No Qualifier
G Vagina K Hymen	0 Open 3 Percutaneous 4 Percutaneous Endoscopic 7 Via Natural or Artificial Opening 8 Via Natural or Artificial Opening Endoscopic X External	Z No Device	Z No Qualifier
J Clitoris L Vestibular Gland M Vulva	0 Open X External	Z No Device	Z No Qualifier

Section	0	Medical and Surgical
Body System	U	Female Reproductive System
Operation	D	Extraction: Pulling or stripping out or off all or a portion of a body part by the use of force

Body Part (4th)	Approach (5th)	Device (6th)	Qualifier (7th)
B Endometrium	7 Via Natural or Artificial Opening 8 Via Natural or Artificial Opening Endoscopic	Z No Device	X Diagnostic Z No Qualifier
N Ova	0 Open 3 Percutaneous 4 Percutaneous Endoscopic	Z No Device	Z No Qualifier

Medical and Surgical, Female Reproductive System Tables

478

Section	0	Medical and Surgical
Body System	U	Female Reproductive System
Operation	F	Fragmentation: Breaking solid matter in a body part into pieces

Body Part (4th)	Approach (5th)	Device (6th)	Qualifier (7th)
5 Fallopian Tube, Right 6 Fallopian Tube, Left 7 Fallopian Tubes, Bilateral 9 Uterus	0 Open 3 Percutaneous 4 Percutaneous Endoscopic 7 Via Natural or Artificial Opening 8 Via Natural or Artificial Opening Endoscopic X External	Z No Device	Z No Qualifier

Section	0	Medical and Surgical
Body System	U	Female Reproductive System
Operation	H	Insertion: Putting in a nonbiological appliance that monitors, assists, performs, or prevents a physiological function but does not physically take the place of a body part

Body Part (4th)	Approach (5th)	Device (6th)	Qualifier (7th)
3 Ovary	0 Open 3 Percutaneous 4 Percutaneous Endoscopic	1 Radioactive Element 3 Infusion Device Y Other Device	Z No Qualifier
3 Ovary	7 Via Natural or Artificial Opening 8 Via Natural or Artificial Opening Endoscopic	1 Radioactive Element Y Other Device	Z No Qualifier
8 Fallopian Tube D Uterus and Cervix H Vagina and Cul-de-sac	0 Open 3 Percutaneous 4 Percutaneous Endoscopic 7 Via Natural or Artificial Opening 8 Via Natural or Artificial Opening Endoscopic	3 Infusion Device Y Other Device	Z No Qualifier
9 Uterus	0 Open 7 Via Natural or Artificial Opening 8 Via Natural or Artificial Opening Endoscopic	1 Radioactive Element H Contraceptive Device	Z No Qualifier
C Cervix	0 Open 3 Percutaneous 4 Percutaneous Endoscopic	1 Radioactive Element	Z No Qualifier
C Cervix	7 Via Natural or Artificial Opening 8 Via Natural or Artificial Opening Endoscopic	1 Radioactive Element H Contraceptive Device	Z No Qualifier
F Cul-de-sac	7 Via Natural or Artificial Opening 8 Via Natural or Artificial Opening Endoscopic	G Intraluminal Device, Pessary	Z No Qualifier
G Vagina	0 Open 3 Percutaneous 4 Percutaneous Endoscopic X External	1 Radioactive Element	Z No Qualifier
G Vagina	7 Via Natural or Artificial Opening 8 Via Natural or Artificial Opening Endoscopic	1 Radioactive Element G Intraluminal Device, Pessary	Z No Qualifier

Section	0	Medical and Surgical
Body System	U	Female Reproductive System
Operation	J	Inspection: Visually and/or manually exploring a body part

Body Part (4th)	Approach (5th)	Device (6th)	Qualifier (7th)
3 Ovary	0 Open 3 Percutaneous 4 Percutaneous Endoscopic 8 Via Natural or Artificial Opening Endoscopic X External	Z No Device	Z No Qualifier

Continued →

0UJ Continued

Section	0	Medical and Surgical
Body System	U	Female Reproductive System
Operation	J	Inspection: Visually and/or manually exploring a body part

Body Part (4th)	Approach (5th)	Device (6th)	Qualifier (7th)
8 Fallopian Tube D Uterus and Cervix H Vagina and Cul-de-sac	0 Open 3 Percutaneous 4 Percutaneous Endoscopic 7 Via Natural or Artificial Opening 8 Via Natural or Artificial Opening Endoscopic X External	Z No Device	Z No Qualifier
M Vulva	0 Open X External	Z No Device	Z No Qualifier

Section	0	Medical and Surgical
Body System	U	Female Reproductive System
Operation	L	Occlusion: Completely closing an orifice or the lumen of a tubular body part

Body Part (4th)	Approach (5th)	Device (6th)	Qualifier (7th)
5 Fallopian Tube, Right 6 Fallopian Tube, Left 7 Fallopian Tubes, Bilateral	0 Open 3 Percutaneous 4 Percutaneous Endoscopic	C Extraluminal Device D Intraluminal Device Z No Device	Z No Qualifier
5 Fallopian Tube, Right 6 Fallopian Tube, Left 7 Fallopian Tubes, Bilateral	7 Via Natural or Artificial Opening 8 Via Natural or Artificial Opening Endoscopic	D Intraluminal Device Z No Device	Z No Qualifier
F Cul-de-sac G Vagina	7 Via Natural or Artificial Opening 8 Via Natural or Artificial Opening Endoscopic	D Intraluminal Device Z No Device	Z No Qualifier

Section	0	Medical and Surgical
Body System	U	Female Reproductive System
Operation	M	Reattachment: Putting back in or on all or a portion of a separated body part to its normal location or other suitable location

Body Part (4th)	Approach (5th)	Device (6th)	Qualifier (7th)
0 Ovary, Right 1 Ovary, Left 2 Ovaries, Bilateral 4 Uterine Supporting Structure 5 Fallopian Tube, Right 6 Fallopian Tube, Left 7 Fallopian Tubes, Bilateral 9 Uterus C Cervix F Cul-de-sac G Vagina	0 Open 4 Percutaneous Endoscopic	Z No Device	Z No Qualifier
J Clitoris M Vulva	X External	Z No Device	Z No Qualifier
K Hymen	0 Open 4 Percutaneous Endoscopic X External	Z No Device	Z No Qualifier

Section	0	Medical and Surgical
Body System	U	Female Reproductive System
Operation	N	Release: Freeing a body part from an abnormal physical constraint by cutting or by the use of force

Body Part (4th)	Approach (5th)	Device (6th)	Qualifier (7th)
0 Ovary, Right 1 Ovary, Left 2 Ovaries, Bilateral 4 Uterine Supporting Structure	0 Open 3 Percutaneous 4 Percutaneous Endoscopic 8 Via Natural or Artificial Opening Endoscopic	Z No Device	Z No Qualifier
5 Fallopian Tube, Right 6 Fallopian Tube, Left 7 Fallopian Tubes, Bilateral 9 Uterus C Cervix F Cul-de-sac	0 Open 3 Percutaneous 4 Percutaneous Endoscopic 7 Via Natural or Artificial Opening 8 Via Natural or Artificial Opening Endoscopic	Z No Device	Z No Qualifier
G Vagina K Hymen	0 Open 3 Percutaneous 4 Percutaneous Endoscopic 7 Via Natural or Artificial Opening 8 Via Natural or Artificial Opening Endoscopic X External	Z No Device	Z No Qualifier
J Clitoris L Vestibular Gland M Vulva	0 Open X External	Z No Device	Z No Qualifier

Section	0	Medical and Surgical
Body System	U	Female Reproductive System
Operation	P	Removal: Taking out or off a device from a body part

Body Part (4th)	Approach (5th)	Device (6th)	Qualifier (7th)
3 Ovary	0 Open 3 Percutaneous 4 Percutaneous Endoscopic	0 Drainage Device 3 Infusion Device Y Other Device	Z No Qualifier
3 Ovary	7 Via Natural or Artificial Opening 8 Via Natural or Artificial Opening Endoscopic	Y Other Device	Z No Qualifier
3 Ovary	X External	0 Drainage Device 3 Infusion Device	Z No Qualifier
8 Fallopian Tube	0 Open 3 Percutaneous 4 Percutaneous Endoscopic 7 Via Natural or Artificial Opening 8 Via Natural or Artificial Opening Endoscopic	0 Drainage Device 3 Infusion Device 7 Autologous Tissue Substitute C Extraluminal Device D Intraluminal Device J Synthetic Substitute K Nonautologous Tissue Substitute Y Other Device	Z No Qualifier
8 Fallopian Tube	X External	0 Drainage Device 3 Infusion Device D Intraluminal Device	Z No Qualifier
D Uterus and Cervix	0 Open 3 Percutaneous 4 Percutaneous Endoscopic 7 Via Natural or Artificial Opening 8 Via Natural or Artificial Opening Endoscopic	0 Drainage Device 1 Radioactive Element 3 Infusion Device 7 Autologous Tissue Substitute C Extraluminal Device D Intraluminal Device H Contraceptive Device J Synthetic Substitute K Nonautologous Tissue Substitute Y Other Device	Z No Qualifier

Continued →

0UP–0UQ

Medical and Surgical, Female Reproductive System Tables

Section	0	Medical and Surgical		*0UP Continued*
Body System	U	Female Reproductive System		
Operation	P	Removal: Taking out or off a device from a body part		

Body Part (4th)	Approach (5th)	Device (6th)	Qualifier (7th)
D Uterus and Cervix	**X** External	**0** Drainage Device **3** Infusion Device **D** Intraluminal Device **H** Contraceptive Device	**Z** No Qualifier
H Vagina and Cul-de-sac	**0** Open **3** Percutaneous **4** Percutaneous Endoscopic **7** Via Natural or Artificial Opening **8** Via Natural or Artificial Opening Endoscopic	**0** Drainage Device **1** Radioactive Element **3** Infusion Device **7** Autologous Tissue Substitute **D** Intraluminal Device **J** Synthetic Substitute **K** Nonautologous Tissue Substitute **Y** Other Device	**Z** No Qualifier
H Vagina and Cul-de-sac	**X** External	**0** Drainage Device **1** Radioactive Element **3** Infusion Device **D** Intraluminal Device	**Z** No Qualifier
M Vulva	**0** Open	**0** Drainage Device **7** Autologous Tissue Substitute **J** Synthetic Substitute **K** Nonautologous Tissue Substitute	**Z** No Qualifier
M Vulva	**X** External	**0** Drainage Device	**Z** No Qualifier

Section	0	Medical and Surgical
Body System	U	Female Reproductive System
Operation	Q	Repair: Restoring, to the extent possible, a body part to its normal anatomic structure and function

Body Part (4th)	Approach (5th)	Device (6th)	Qualifier (7th)
0 Ovary, Right **1** Ovary, Left **2** Ovaries, Bilateral **4** Uterine Supporting Structure	**0** Open **3** Percutaneous **4** Percutaneous Endoscopic **8** Via Natural or Artificial Opening Endoscopic	**Z** No Device	**Z** No Qualifier
5 Fallopian Tube, Right **6** Fallopian Tube, Left **7** Fallopian Tubes, Bilateral **9** Uterus **C** Cervix **F** Cul-de-sac	**0** Open **3** Percutaneous **4** Percutaneous Endoscopic **7** Via Natural or Artificial Opening **8** Via Natural or Artificial Opening Endoscopic	**Z** No Device	**Z** No Qualifier
G Vagina **K** Hymen	**0** Open **3** Percutaneous **4** Percutaneous Endoscopic **7** Via Natural or Artificial Opening **8** Via Natural or Artificial Opening Endoscopic **X** External	**Z** No Device	**Z** No Qualifier
J Clitoris **L** Vestibular Gland **M** Vulva	**0** Open **X** External	**Z** No Device	**Z** No Qualifier

482

Section	0	Medical and Surgical
Body System	U	Female Reproductive System
Operation	S	Reposition: Moving to its normal location, or other suitable location, all or a portion of a body part

Body Part (4th)	Approach (5th)	Device (6th)	Qualifier (7th)
0 Ovary, Right 1 Ovary, Left 2 Ovaries, Bilateral 4 Uterine Supporting Structure 5 Fallopian Tube, Right 6 Fallopian Tube, Left 7 Fallopian Tubes, Bilateral C Cervix F Cul-de-sac	0 Open 4 Percutaneous Endoscopic 8 Via Natural or Artificial Opening Endoscopic	Z No Device	Z No Qualifier
9 Uterus G Vagina	0 Open 4 Percutaneous Endoscopic 7 Via Natural or Artificial Opening 8 Via Natural or Artificial Opening Endoscopic X External	Z No Device	Z No Qualifier

Section	0	Medical and Surgical
Body System	U	Female Reproductive System
Operation	T	Resection: Cutting out or off, without replacement, all of a body part

Body Part (4th)	Approach (5th)	Device (6th)	Qualifier (7th)
0 Ovary, Right 1 Ovary, Left 2 Ovaries, Bilateral 5 Fallopian Tube, Right 6 Fallopian Tube, Left 7 Fallopian Tubes, Bilateral	0 Open 4 Percutaneous Endoscopic 7 Via Natural or Artificial Opening 8 Via Natural or Artificial Opening Endoscopic F Via Natural or Artificial Opening With Percutaneous Endoscopic Assistance	Z No Device	Z No Qualifier
4 Uterine Supporting Structure C Cervix F Cul-de-sac G Vagina	0 Open 4 Percutaneous Endoscopic 7 Via Natural or Artificial Opening 8 Via Natural or Artificial Opening Endoscopic	Z No Device	Z No Qualifier
9 Uterus	0 Open 4 Percutaneous Endoscopic 7 Via Natural or Artificial Opening 8 Via Natural or Artificial Opening Endoscopic F Via Natural or Artificial Opening with Percutaneous Endoscopic Assistance	Z No Device	L Supracervical Z No Qualifier
J Clitoris L Vestibular Gland M Vulva	0 Open X External	Z No Device	Z No Qualifier
K Hymen	0 Open 4 Percutaneous Endoscopic 7 Via Natural or Artificial Opening 8 Via Natural or Artificial Opening Endoscopic X External	Z No Device	Z No Qualifier

0UU–0UW

Medical and Surgical, Female Reproductive System Tables

Section	0	Medical and Surgical
Body System	U	Female Reproductive System
Operation	U	Supplement: Putting in or on biological or synthetic material that physically reinforces and/or augments the function of a portion of a body part

Body Part (4th)	Approach (5th)	Device (6th)	Qualifier (7th)
4 Uterine Supporting Structure	0 Open 4 Percutaneous Endoscopic	7 Autologous Tissue Substitute J Synthetic Substitute K Nonautologous Tissue Substitute	Z No Qualifier
5 Fallopian Tube, Right 6 Fallopian Tube, Left 7 Fallopian Tubes, Bilateral F Cul-de-sac	0 Open 4 Percutaneous Endoscopic 7 Via Natural or Artificial Opening 8 Via Natural or Artificial Opening Endoscopic	7 Autologous Tissue Substitute J Synthetic Substitute K Nonautologous Tissue Substitute	Z No Qualifier
G Vagina K Hymen	0 Open 4 Percutaneous Endoscopic 7 Via Natural or Artificial Opening 8 Via Natural or Artificial Opening Endoscopic X External	7 Autologous Tissue Substitute J Synthetic Substitute K Nonautologous Tissue Substitute	Z No Qualifier
J Clitoris M Vulva	0 Open X External	7 Autologous Tissue Substitute J Synthetic Substitute K Nonautologous Tissue Substitute	Z No Qualifier

Section	0	Medical and Surgical
Body System	U	Female Reproductive System
Operation	V	Restriction: Partially closing an orifice or the lumen of a tubular body part

Body Part (4th)	Approach (5th)	Device (6th)	Qualifier (7th)
C Cervix	0 Open 3 Percutaneous 4 Percutaneous Endoscopic	C Extraluminal Device D Intraluminal Device Z No Device	Z No Qualifier
C Cervix	7 Via Natural or Artificial Opening 8 Via Natural or Artificial Opening Endoscopic	D Intraluminal Device Z No Device	Z No Qualifier

Section	0	Medical and Surgical
Body System	U	Female Reproductive System
Operation	W	Revision: Correcting, to the extent possible, a portion of a malfunctioning device or the position of a displaced device

Body Part (4th)	Approach (5th)	Device (6th)	Qualifier (7th)
3 Ovary	0 Open 3 Percutaneous 4 Percutaneous Endoscopic	0 Drainage Device 3 Infusion Device Y Other Device	Z No Qualifier
3 Ovary	7 Via Natural or Artificial Opening 8 Via Natural or Artificial Opening Endoscopic	Y Other Device	Z No Qualifier
3 Ovary	X External	0 Drainage Device 3 Infusion Device	Z No Qualifier
8 Fallopian Tube	0 Open 3 Percutaneous 4 Percutaneous Endoscopic 7 Via Natural or Artificial Opening 8 Via Natural or Artificial Opening Endoscopic X External	0 Drainage Device 3 Infusion Device 7 Autologous Tissue Substitute C Extraluminal Device D Intraluminal Device J Synthetic Substitute K Nonautologous Tissue Substitute Y Other Device	Z No Qualifier

Continued →

484

Section	0	Medical and Surgical			0UW Continued
Body System	U	Female Reproductive System			
Operation	W	Revision: Correcting, to the extent possible, a portion of a malfunctioning device or the position of a displaced device			

Body Part (4th)	Approach (5th)	Device (6th)	Qualifier (7th)
8 Fallopian Tube	X External	0 Drainage Device 3 Infusion Device 7 Autologous Tissue Substitute C Extraluminal Device D Intraluminal Device J Synthetic Substitute K Nonautologous Tissue Substitute	Z No Qualifier
D Uterus and Cervix	0 Open 3 Percutaneous 4 Percutaneous Endoscopic 7 Via Natural or Artificial Opening 8 Via Natural or Artificial Opening Endoscopic	0 Drainage Device 1 Radioactive Element 3 Infusion Device 7 Autologous Tissue Substitute C Extraluminal Device D Intraluminal Device H Contraceptive Device J Synthetic Substitute K Nonautologous Tissue Substitute Y Other Device	Z No Qualifier
D Uterus and Cervix	X External	0 Drainage Device 3 Infusion Device 7 Autologous Tissue Substitute C Extraluminal Device D Intraluminal Device H Contraceptive Device J Synthetic Substitute K Nonautologous Tissue Substitute	Z No Qualifier
H Vagina and Cul-de-sac	0 Open 3 Percutaneous 4 Percutaneous Endoscopic 7 Via Natural or Artificial Opening 8 Via Natural or Artificial Opening Endoscopic	0 Drainage Device 1 Radioactive Element 3 Infusion Device 7 Autologous Tissue Substitute D Intraluminal Device J Synthetic Substitute K Nonautologous Tissue Substitute Y Other Device	Z No Qualifier
H Vagina and Cul-de-sac	X External	0 Drainage Device 3 Infusion Device 7 Autologous Tissue Substitute D Intraluminal Device J Synthetic Substitute K Nonautologous Tissue Substitute	Z No Qualifier
M Vulva	0 Open X External	0 Drainage Device 7 Autologous Tissue Substitute J Synthetic Substitute K Nonautologous Tissue Substitute	Z No Qualifier

Section	0	Medical and Surgical
Body System	U	Female Reproductive System
Operation	Y	

Transplantation: Putting in or on all or a portion of a living body part taken from another individual or animal to physically take the place and/or function of all or a portion of a similar body part

Body Part (4th)	Approach (5th)	Device (6th)	Qualifier (7th)
0 Ovary, Right 1 Ovary, Left 9 Uterus	0 Open	Z No Device	0 Allogeneic 1 Syngeneic 2 Zooplastic

AHA Coding Clinic

0U7C7ZZ Dilation of Cervix, Via Natural or Artificial Opening—AHA CC: 2Q, 2020, 30

0U9G7ZZ Drainage of Vagina, Via Natural or Artificial Opening—AHA CC: 4Q, 2016, 58-59

0UB64ZZ Excision of Left Fallopian Tube, Percutaneous Endoscopic Approach—AHA CC: 3Q, 2015, 31-32

0UB70ZZ Excision of Bilateral Fallopian Tubes, Open Approach—AHA CC: 3Q, 2015, 31

0UB90ZZ Excision of Uterus, Open Approach—AHA CC: 4Q, 2014, 16

0UBMXZZ Excision of Vulva, External Approach—AHA CC: 3Q, 2014, 12

0UC97ZZ Extirpation of Matter from Uterus, Via Natural or Artificial Opening—AHA CC: 2Q, 2013, 38

0UCC7ZZ Extirpation of Matter from Cervix, Via Natural or Artificial Opening—AHA CC: 3Q, 2015, 30

0UCC8ZZ Extirpation of Matter from Cervix, Via Natural or Artificial Opening Endoscopic—AHA CC: 3Q, 2015, 30-31

0UH97HZ Insertion of Contraceptive Device into Uterus, Via Natural or Artificial Opening—AHA CC: 2Q, 2013, 34

0UHD7YZ Insertion of Other Device into Uterus and Cervix, Via Natural or Artificial Opening—AHA CC: 4Q, 2017, 104; 1Q, 2018, 25

0UJD4ZZ Inspection of Uterus and Cervix, Percutaneous Endoscopic Approach—AHA CC: 1Q, 2015, 33-34

0UPH77Z Removal of Autologous Tissue Substitute from Vagina and Cul-de-sac, Via Natural or Artificial Opening—AHA CC: 3Q, 2022, 13-14

0UQ60ZZ Repair Left Fallopian Tube, Open Approach—AHA CC: 4Q, 2020, 60

0UQJXZZ Repair Clitoris, External Approach—AHA CC: 4Q, 2013, 120-121

0UQMXZZ Repair Vulva, External Approach—AHA CC: 4Q, 2014, 18-19

0US9XZZ Reposition Uterus, External Approach—AHA CC: 1Q, 2016, 9

0UT00ZZ Resection of Right Ovary, Open Approach—AHA CC: 1Q, 2013, 24

0UT20ZZ Resection of Bilateral Ovaries, Open Approach—AHA CC: 1Q, 2015, 33-34

0UT70ZZ Resection of Bilateral Fallopian Tubes, Open Approach—AHA CC: 1Q, 2015, 33-34; 1Q, 2022, 21

0UT90ZZ Resection of Uterus, Open Approach—AHA CC: 3Q, 2013, 28; 1Q, 2015, 33-34; 4Q, 2017, 68; 1Q, 2022, 21

0UT97ZL Resection of Uterus, Supracervical, Via Natural or Artificial Opening—AHA CC: 4Q, 2017, 68

0UTC0ZZ Resection of Cervix, Open Approach—AHA CC: 3Q, 2013, 28; 1Q, 2015, 33-34

0UVC7ZZ Restriction of Cervix, Via Natural or Artificial Opening—AHA CC: 3Q, 2015, 30

Male Reproductive System

Male Reproductive System

Malignant Prostate Surgery I: Laparoscopic and Robotic

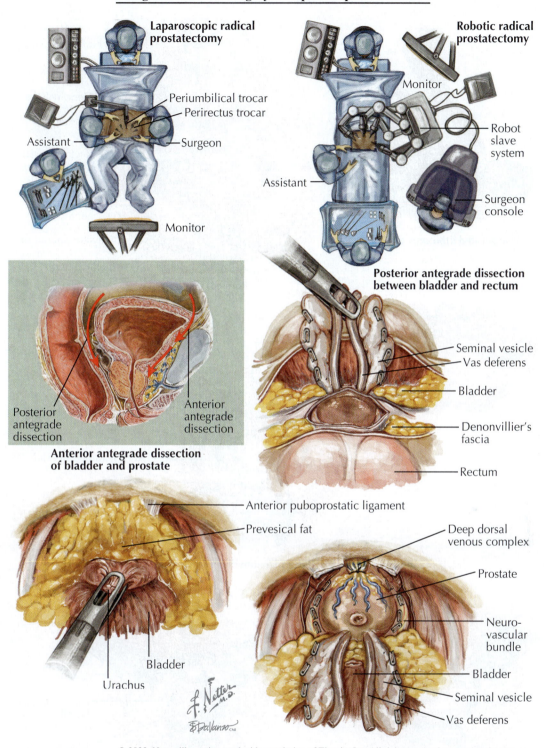

Malignant Prostate Surgery II: Perineal

Male Reproductive System Tables 0V1–0VY

Section	0	Medical and Surgical
Body System	V	Male Reproductive System
Operation	1	Bypass: Altering the route of passage of the contents of a tubular body part

Body Part (4th)	Approach (5th)	Device (6th)	Qualifier (7th)
N Vas Deferens, Right P Vas Deferens, Left Q Vas Deferens, Bilateral	0 Open 4 Percutaneous Endoscopic	7 Autologous Tissue Substitute J Synthetic Substitute K Nonautologous Tissue Substitute Z No Device	J Epididymis, Right K Epididymis, Left N Vas Deferens, Right P Vas Deferens, Left

Section	0	Medical and Surgical
Body System	V	Male Reproductive System
Operation	2	Change: Taking out or off a device from a body part and putting back an identical or similar device in or on the same body part without cutting or puncturing the skin or a mucous membrane

Body Part (4th)	Approach (5th)	Device (6th)	Qualifier (7th)
4 Prostate and Seminal Vesicles 8 Scrotum and Tunica Vaginalis D Testis M Epididymis and Spermatic Cord R Vas Deferens S Penis	X External	0 Drainage Device Y Other Device	Z No Qualifier

Section	0	Medical and Surgical
Body System	V	Male Reproductive System
Operation	5	Destruction: Physical eradication of all or a portion of a body part by the direct use of energy, force, or a destructive agent

Body Part (4th)	Approach (5th)	Device (6th)	Qualifier (7th)
0 Prostate	0 Open 3 Percutaneous 4 Percutaneous Endoscopic	Z No Device	3 Laser Interstitial Thermal Therapy Z No Qualifier
0 Prostate	7 Via Natural or Artificial Opening 8 Via Natural or Artificial Opening Endoscopic	Z No Device	Z No Qualifier
1 Seminal Vesicle, Right 2 Seminal Vesicle, Left 3 Seminal Vesicles, Bilateral 6 Tunica Vaginalis, Right 7 Tunica Vaginalis, Left 9 Testis, Right B Testis, Left C Testes, Bilateral	0 Open 3 Percutaneous 4 Percutaneous Endoscopic	Z No Device	Z No Qualifier
5 Scrotum S Penis T Prepuce	0 Open 3 Percutaneous 4 Percutaneous Endoscopic X External	Z No Device	Z No Qualifier
F Spermatic Cord, Right G Spermatic Cord, Left H Spermatic Cords, Bilateral J Epididymis, Right K Epididymis, Left L Epididymis, Bilateral N Vas Deferens, Right P Vas Deferens, Left Q Vas Deferens, Bilateral	0 Open 3 Percutaneous 4 Percutaneous Endoscopic 8 Via Natural or Artificial Opening Endoscopic	Z No Device	Z No Qualifier

Section	0	Medical and Surgical
Body System	V	Male Reproductive System
Operation	7	Dilation: Expanding an orifice or the lumen of a tubular body part

Body Part (4th)	Approach (5th)	Device (6th)	Qualifier (7th)
N Vas Deferens, Right P Vas Deferens, Left Q Vas Deferens, Bilateral	0 Open 3 Percutaneous 4 Percutaneous Endoscopic	D Intraluminal Device Z No Device	Z No Qualifier

	Section	0	Medical and Surgical
	Body System	V	Male Reproductive System
	Operation	9	Drainage: Taking or letting out fluids and/or gases from a body part

Body Part (4th)	Approach (5th)	Device (6th)	Qualifier (7th)
0 Prostate	**0** Open **3** Percutaneous **4** Percutaneous Endoscopic **7** Via Natural or Artificial Opening **8** Via Natural or Artificial Opening Endoscopic	**0** Drainage Device	**Z** No Qualifier
0 Prostate	**0** Open **3** Percutaneous **4** Percutaneous Endoscopic **7** Via Natural or Artificial Opening **8** Via Natural or Artificial Opening Endoscopic	**Z** No Device	**X** Diagnostic **Z** No Qualifier
1 Seminal Vesicle, Right **2** Seminal Vesicle, Left **3** Seminal Vesicles, Bilateral **6** Tunica Vaginalis, Right **7** Tunica Vaginalis, Left **9** Testis, Right **B** Testis, Left **C** Testes, Bilateral **F** Spermatic Cord, Right **G** Spermatic Cord, Left **H** Spermatic Cords, Bilateral **J** Epididymis, Right **K** Epididymis, Left **L** Epididymis, Bilateral **N** Vas Deferens, Right **P** Vas Deferens, Left **Q** Vas Deferens, Bilateral	**0** Open **3** Percutaneous **4** Percutaneous Endoscopic	**0** Drainage Device	**Z** No Qualifier
1 Seminal Vesicle, Right **2** Seminal Vesicle, Left **3** Seminal Vesicles, Bilateral **6** Tunica Vaginalis, Right **7** Tunica Vaginalis, Left **9** Testis, Right **B** Testis, Left **C** Testes, Bilateral **F** Spermatic Cord, Right **G** Spermatic Cord, Left **H** Spermatic Cords, Bilateral **J** Epididymis, Right **K** Epididymis, Left **L** Epididymis, Bilateral **N** Vas Deferens, Right **P** Vas Deferens, Left **Q** Vas Deferens, Bilateral	**0** Open **3** Percutaneous **4** Percutaneous Endoscopic	**Z** No Device	**X** Diagnostic **Z** No Qualifier
5 Scrotum **S** Penis **T** Prepuce	**0** Open **3** Percutaneous **4** Percutaneous Endoscopic **X** External	**0** Drainage Device	**Z** No Qualifier
5 Scrotum **S** Penis **T** Prepuce	**0** Open **3** Percutaneous **4** Percutaneous Endoscopic **X** External	**Z** No Device	**X** Diagnostic **Z** No Qualifier

Section	0	Medical and Surgical
Body System	V	Male Reproductive System
Operation	B	Excision: Cutting out or off, without replacement, a portion of a body part

Body Part (4th)	Approach (5th)	Device (6th)	Qualifier (7th)
0 Prostate	0 Open 3 Percutaneous 4 Percutaneous Endoscopic 7 Via Natural or Artificial Opening 8 Via Natural or Artificial Opening Endoscopic	Z No Device	X Diagnostic Z No Qualifier
1 Seminal Vesicle, Right 2 Seminal Vesicle, Left 3 Seminal Vesicles, Bilateral 6 Tunica Vaginalis, Right 7 Tunica Vaginalis, Left 9 Testis, Right B Testis, Left C Testes, Bilateral	0 Open 3 Percutaneous 4 Percutaneous Endoscopic	Z No Device	X Diagnostic Z No Qualifier
5 Scrotum S Penis T Prepuce	0 Open 3 Percutaneous 4 Percutaneous Endoscopic X External	Z No Device	X Diagnostic Z No Qualifier
F Spermatic Cord, Right G Spermatic Cord, Left H Spermatic Cords, Bilateral J Epididymis, Right K Epididymis, Left L Epididymis, Bilateral N Vas Deferens, Right P Vas Deferens, Left Q Vas Deferens, Bilateral	0 Open 3 Percutaneous 4 Percutaneous Endoscopic 8 Via Natural or Artificial Opening Endoscopic	Z No Device	X Diagnostic Z No Qualifier

Section	0	Medical and Surgical
Body System	V	Male Reproductive System
Operation	C	Extirpation: Taking or cutting out solid matter from a body part

Body Part (4th)	Approach (5th)	Device (6th)	Qualifier (7th)
0 Prostate	0 Open 3 Percutaneous 4 Percutaneous Endoscopic 7 Via Natural or Artificial Opening 8 Via Natural or Artificial Opening Endoscopic	Z No Device	Z No Qualifier
1 Seminal Vesicle, Right 2 Seminal Vesicle, Left 3 Seminal Vesicles, Bilateral 6 Tunica Vaginalis, Right 7 Tunica Vaginalis, Left 9 Testis, Right B Testis, Left C Testes, Bilateral F Spermatic Cord, Right G Spermatic Cord, Left H Spermatic Cords, Bilateral J Epididymis, Right K Epididymis, Left L Epididymis, Bilateral N Vas Deferens, Right P Vas Deferens, Left Q Vas Deferens, Bilateral	0 Open 3 Percutaneous 4 Percutaneous Endoscopic	Z No Device	Z No Qualifier
5 Scrotum S Penis T Prepuce	0 Open 3 Percutaneous 4 Percutaneous Endoscopic X External	Z No Device	Z No Qualifier

Section 0 **Medical and Surgical**
Body System V **Male Reproductive System**
Operation H **Insertion:** Putting in a nonbiological appliance that monitors, assists, performs, or prevents a physiological function but does not physically take the place of a body part

Body Part (4th)	Approach (5th)	Device (6th)	Qualifier (7th)
0 Prostate	0 Open 3 Percutaneous 4 Percutaneous Endoscopic 7 Via Natural or Artificial Opening 8 Via Natural or Artificial Opening Endoscopic	1 Radioactive Element	Z No Qualifier
4 Prostate and Seminal Vesicles 8 Scrotum and Tunica Vaginalis M Epididymis and Spermatic Cord R Vas Deferens	0 Open 3 Percutaneous 4 Percutaneous Endoscopic 7 Via Natural or Artificial Opening 8 Via Natural or Artificial Opening Endoscopic	3 Infusion Device Y Other Device	Z No Qualifier
D Testis	0 Open 3 Percutaneous 4 Percutaneous Endoscopic 7 Via Natural or Artificial Opening 8 Via Natural or Artificial Opening Endoscopic	1 Radioactive Element 3 Infusion Device Y Other Device	Z No Qualifier
S Penis	0 Open 3 Percutaneous 4 Percutaneous Endoscopic	3 Infusion Device Y Other Device	Z No Qualifier
S Penis	7 Via Natural or Artificial Opening 8 Via Natural or Artificial Opening Endoscopic	Y Other Device	Z No Qualifier
S Penis	X External	3 Infusion Device	Z No Qualifier

Section 0 **Medical and Surgical**
Body System V **Male Reproductive System**
Operation J **Inspection:** Visually and/or manually exploring a body part

Body Part (4th)	Approach (5th)	Device (6th)	Qualifier (7th)
4 Prostate and Seminal Vesicles 8 Scrotum and Tunica Vaginalis D Testis M Epididymis and Spermatic Cord R Vas Deferens S Penis	0 Open 3 Percutaneous 4 Percutaneous Endoscopic X External	Z No Device	Z No Qualifier

Section 0 **Medical and Surgical**
Body System V **Male Reproductive System**
Operation L **Occlusion:** Completely closing an orifice or the lumen of a tubular body part

Body Part (4th)	Approach (5th)	Device (6th)	Qualifier (7th)
F Spermatic Cord, Right G Spermatic Cord, Left H Spermatic Cords, Bilateral N Vas Deferens, Right P Vas Deferens, Left Q Vas Deferens, Bilateral	0 Open 3 Percutaneous 4 Percutaneous Endoscopic 8 Via Natural or Artificial Opening Endoscopic	C Extraluminal Device D Intraluminal Device Z No Device	Z No Qualifier

Section	0	Medical and Surgical
Body System	V	Male Reproductive System
Operation	M	**Reattachment:** Putting back in or on all or a portion of a separated body part to its normal location or other suitable location

Body Part (4th)	Approach (5th)	Device (6th)	Qualifier (7th)
5 Scrotum S Penis	X External	Z No Device	Z No Qualifier
6 Tunica Vaginalis, Right 7 Tunica Vaginalis, Left 9 Testis, Right B Testis, Left C Testes, Bilateral F Spermatic Cord, Right G Spermatic Cord, Left H Spermatic Cords, Bilateral	0 Open 4 Percutaneous Endoscopic	Z No Device	Z No Qualifier

Section	0	Medical and Surgical
Body System	V	Male Reproductive System
Operation	N	**Release:** Freeing a body part from an abnormal physical constraint by cutting or by the use of force

Body Part (4th)	Approach (5th)	Device (6th)	Qualifier (7th)
0 Prostate	0 Open 3 Percutaneous 4 Percutaneous Endoscopic 7 Via Natural or Artificial Opening 8 Via Natural or Artificial Opening Endoscopic	Z No Device	Z No Qualifier
1 Seminal Vesicle, Right 2 Seminal Vesicle, Left 3 Seminal Vesicles, Bilateral 6 Tunica Vaginalis, Right 7 Tunica Vaginalis, Left 9 Testis, Right B Testis, Left C Testes, Bilateral	0 Open 3 Percutaneous 4 Percutaneous Endoscopic	Z No Device	Z No Qualifier
5 Scrotum S Penis T Prepuce	0 Open 3 Percutaneous 4 Percutaneous Endoscopic X External	Z No Device	Z No Qualifier
F Spermatic Cord, Right G Spermatic Cord, Left H Spermatic Cords, Bilateral J Epididymis, Right K Epididymis, Left L Epididymis, Bilateral N Vas Deferens, Right P Vas Deferens, Left Q Vas Deferens, Bilateral	0 Open 3 Percutaneous 4 Percutaneous Endoscopic 8 Via Natural or Artificial Opening Endoscopic	Z No Device	Z No Qualifier

Section	0	Medical and Surgical
Body System	V	Male Reproductive System
Operation	P	**Removal:** Taking out or off a device from a body part

Body Part (4th)	Approach (5th)	Device (6th)	Qualifier (7th)
4 Prostate and Seminal Vesicles	0 Open 3 Percutaneous 4 Percutaneous Endoscopic 7 Via Natural or Artificial Opening 8 Via Natural or Artificial Opening Endoscopic	0 Drainage Device 1 Radioactive Element 3 Infusion Device 7 Autologous Tissue Substitute J Synthetic Substitute K Nonautologous Tissue Substitute Y Other Device	Z No Qualifier

Continued →

495

Section	0	Medical and Surgical
Body System	V	Male Reproductive System
Operation	P	Removal: Taking out or off a device from a body part

0VP Continued

Body Part (4th)	Approach (5th)	Device (6th)	Qualifier (7th)
4 Prostate and Seminal Vesicles	X External	0 Drainage Device 1 Radioactive Element 3 Infusion Device	Z No Qualifier
8 Scrotum and Tunica Vaginalis D Testis S Penis	0 Open 3 Percutaneous 4 Percutaneous Endoscopic 7 Via Natural or Artificial Opening 8 Via Natural or Artificial Opening Endoscopic	0 Drainage Device 3 Infusion Device 7 Autologous Tissue Substitute J Synthetic Substitute K Nonautologous Tissue Substitute Y Other Device	Z No Qualifier
8 Scrotum and Tunica Vaginalis D Testis S Penis	X External	0 Drainage Device 3 Infusion Device	Z No Qualifier
M Epididymis and Spermatic Cord	0 Open 3 Percutaneous 4 Percutaneous Endoscopic 7 Via Natural or Artificial Opening 8 Via Natural or Artificial Opening Endoscopic	0 Drainage Device 3 Infusion Device 7 Autologous Tissue Substitute C Extraluminal Device J Synthetic Substitute K Nonautologous Tissue Substitute Y Other Device	Z No Qualifier
M Epididymis and Spermatic Cord	X External	0 Drainage Device 3 Infusion Device	Z No Qualifier
R Vas Deferens	0 Open 3 Percutaneous 4 Percutaneous Endoscopic 7 Via Natural or Artificial Opening 8 Via Natural or Artificial Opening Endoscopic	0 Drainage Device 3 Infusion Device 7 Autologous Tissue Substitute C Extraluminal Device D Intraluminal Device J Synthetic Substitute K Nonautologous Tissue Substitute Y Other Device	Z No Qualifier
R Vas Deferens	X External	0 Drainage Device 3 Infusion Device D Intraluminal Device	Z No Qualifier

Section	0	Medical and Surgical
Body System	V	Male Reproductive System
Operation	Q	Repair: Restoring, to the extent possible, a body part to its normal anatomic structure and function

Body Part (4th)	Approach (5th)	Device (6th)	Qualifier (7th)
0 Prostate	0 Open 3 Percutaneous 4 Percutaneous Endoscopic 7 Via Natural or Artificial Opening 8 Via Natural or Artificial Opening Endoscopic	Z No Device	Z No Qualifier
1 Seminal Vesicle, Right 2 Seminal Vesicle, Left 3 Seminal Vesicles, Bilateral 6 Tunica Vaginalis, Right 7 Tunica Vaginalis, Left 9 Testis, Right B Testis, Left C Testes, Bilateral	0 Open 3 Percutaneous 4 Percutaneous Endoscopic	Z No Device	Z No Qualifier
5 Scrotum S Penis T Prepuce	0 Open 3 Percutaneous 4 Percutaneous Endoscopic X External	Z No Device	Z No Qualifier

Continued →

496

Section	0	Medical and Surgical
Body System	V	Male Reproductive System
Operation	Q	Repair: Restoring, to the extent possible, a body part to its normal anatomic structure and function

0VQ Continued

Body Part (4th)	Approach (5th)	Device (6th)	Qualifier (7th)
F Spermatic Cord, Right G Spermatic Cord, Left H Spermatic Cords, Bilateral J Epididymis, Right K Epididymis, Left L Epididymis, Bilateral N Vas Deferens, Right P Vas Deferens, Left Q Vas Deferens, Bilateral	0 Open 3 Percutaneous 4 Percutaneous Endoscopic 8 Via Natural or Artificial Opening Endoscopic	Z No Device	Z No Qualifier

Section	0	Medical and Surgical
Body System	V	Male Reproductive System
Operation	R	Replacement: Putting in or on biological or synthetic material that physically takes the place and/or function of all or a portion of a body part

Body Part (4th)	Approach (5th)	Device (6th)	Qualifier (7th)
9 Testis, Right B Testis, Left C Testes, Bilateral	0 Open	J Synthetic Substitute	Z No Qualifier

Section	0	Medical and Surgical
Body System	V	Male Reproductive System
Operation	S	Reposition: Moving to its normal location, or other suitable location, all or a portion of a body part

Body Part (4th)	Approach (5th)	Device (6th)	Qualifier (7th)
9 Testis, Right B Testis, Left C Testes, Bilateral F Spermatic Cord, Right G Spermatic Cord, Left H Spermatic Cords, Bilateral	0 Open 3 Percutaneous 4 Percutaneous Endoscopic 8 Via Natural or Artificial Opening Endoscopic	Z No Device	Z No Qualifier

Section	0	Medical and Surgical
Body System	V	Male Reproductive System
Operation	T	Resection: Cutting out or off, without replacement, all of a body part

Body Part (4th)	Approach (5th)	Device (6th)	Qualifier (7th)
0 Prostate	0 Open 4 Percutaneous Endoscopic 7 Via Natural or Artificial Opening 8 Via Natural or Artificial Opening Endoscopic	Z No Device	Z No Qualifier
1 Seminal Vesicle, Right 2 Seminal Vesicle, Left 3 Seminal Vesicles, Bilateral 6 Tunica Vaginalis, Right 7 Tunica Vaginalis, Left 9 Testis, Right B Testis, Left C Testes, Bilateral F Spermatic Cord, Right G Spermatic Cord, Left H Spermatic Cords, Bilateral J Epididymis, Right K Epididymis, Left L Epididymis, Bilateral N Vas Deferens, Right P Vas Deferens, Left Q Vas Deferens, Bilateral	0 Open 4 Percutaneous Endoscopic	Z No Device	Z No Qualifier

Continued →

Section	0	Medical and Surgical
Body System	V	Male Reproductive System
Operation	T	**Resection:** Cutting out or off, without replacement, all of a body part

Body Part (4th)	Approach (5th)	Device (6th)	Qualifier (7th)
5 Scrotum S Penis T Prepuce	0 Open 4 Percutaneous Endoscopic X External	Z No Device	Z No Qualifier

Section	0	Medical and Surgical
Body System	V	Male Reproductive System
Operation	U	**Supplement:** Putting in or on biological or synthetic material that physically reinforces and/or augments the function of a portion of a body part

Body Part (4th)	Approach (5th)	Device (6th)	Qualifier (7th)
1 Seminal Vesicle, Right 2 Seminal Vesicle, Left 3 Seminal Vesicles, Bilateral 6 Tunica Vaginalis, Right 7 Tunica Vaginalis, Left F Spermatic Cord, Right G Spermatic Cord, Left H Spermatic Cords, Bilateral J Epididymis, Right K Epididymis, Left L Epididymis, Bilateral N Vas Deferens, Right P Vas Deferens, Left Q Vas Deferens, Bilateral	0 Open 4 Percutaneous Endoscopic 8 Via Natural or Artificial Opening Endoscopic	7 Autologous Tissue Substitute J Synthetic Substitute K Nonautologous Tissue Substitute	Z No Qualifier
5 Scrotum S Penis T Prepuce	0 Open 4 Percutaneous Endoscopic X External	7 Autologous Tissue Substitute J Synthetic Substitute K Nonautologous Tissue Substitute	Z No Qualifier
9 Testis, Right B Testis, Left C Testes, Bilateral	0 Open	7 Autologous Tissue Substitute J Synthetic Substitute K Nonautologous Tissue Substitute	Z No Qualifier

Section	0	Medical and Surgical
Body System	V	Male Reproductive System
Operation	W	**Revision:** Correcting, to the extent possible, a portion of a malfunctioning device or the position of a displaced device

Body Part (4th)	Approach (5th)	Device (6th)	Qualifier (7th)
4 Prostate and Seminal Vesicles 8 Scrotum and Tunica Vaginalis D Testis S Penis	0 Open 3 Percutaneous 4 Percutaneous Endoscopic 7 Via Natural or Artificial Opening 8 Via Natural or Artificial Opening Endoscopic	0 Drainage Device 3 Infusion Device 7 Autologous Tissue Substitute J Synthetic Substitute K Nonautologous Tissue Substitute Y Other Device	Z No Qualifier
4 Prostate and Seminal Vesicles 8 Scrotum and Tunica Vaginalis D Testis S Penis	X External	0 Drainage Device 3 Infusion Device 7 Autologous Tissue Substitute J Synthetic Substitute K Nonautologous Tissue Substitute	Z No Qualifier
M Epididymis and Spermatic Cord	0 Open 3 Percutaneous 4 Percutaneous Endoscopic 7 Via Natural or Artificial Opening 8 Via Natural or Artificial Opening Endoscopic	0 Drainage Device 3 Infusion Device 7 Autologous Tissue Substitute C Extraluminal Device J Synthetic Substitute K Nonautologous Tissue Substitute Y Other Device	Z No Qualifier

Section	0	Medical and Surgical
Body System	V	Male Reproductive System
Operation	W	Revision: Correcting, to the extent possible, a portion of a malfunctioning device or the position of a displaced device

0VW Continued

Body Part (4th)	Approach (5th)	Device (6th)	Qualifier (7th)
M Epididymis and Spermatic Cord	X External	0 Drainage Device 3 Infusion Device 7 Autologous Tissue Substitute C Extraluminal Device J Synthetic Substitute K Nonautologous Tissue Substitute	Z No Qualifier
R Vas Deferens	0 Open 3 Percutaneous 4 Percutaneous Endoscopic 7 Via Natural or Artificial Opening 8 Via Natural or Artificial Opening Endoscopic	0 Drainage Device 3 Infusion Device 7 Autologous Tissue Substitute C Extraluminal Device D Intraluminal Device J Synthetic Substitute K Nonautologous Tissue Substitute Y Other Device	Z No Qualifier
R Vas Deferens	X External	0 Drainage Device 3 Infusion Device 7 Autologous Tissue Substitute C Extraluminal Device C Intraluminal Device J Synthetic Substitute K Nonautologous Tissue Substitute	Z No Qualifier

Section	0	Medical and Surgical
Body System	V	Male Reproductive System
Operation	X	Transfer: Moving, without taking out, all or a portion of a body part to another location to take over the function of all or a portion of a body part

Body Part (4th)	Approach (5th)	Device (6th)	Qualifier (7th)
T Prepuce	0 Open X External	Z No Device	D Urethra S Penis

Section	0	Medical and Surgical
Body System	V	Male Reproductive System
Operation	Y	Transplantation: Putting in or on all or a portion of a living body part taken from another individual or animal to physically take the place and/or function of all or a portion of a similar body part

Body Part (4th)	Approach (5th)	Device (6th)	Qualifier (7th)
5 Scrotum 6 Penis	0 Open	Z No Device	0 Allogeneic 1 Syngeneic 2 Zooplastic

AHA Coding Clinic

0VBQ4ZZ Excision of Bilateral Vas Deferens, Percutaneous Endoscopic Approach—AHA CC: 4Q, 2014, 33-34; 1Q, 2016, 23

0VPS0JZ Removal of Synthetic Substitute from Penis, Open Approach—AHA CC: 2Q, 2016, 28-29

0VQS3ZZ Repair Penis, Percutaneous Approach—AHA CC: 3Q, 2018, 12

0VT04ZZ Resection of Prostate, Percutaneous Endoscopic Approach— AHA CC: 4Q, 2014, 33-34

0VT34ZZ Resection of Bilateral Seminal Vesicles, Percutaneous Endoscopic Approach—AHA CC: 4Q, 2014, 33-34

0VUS07Z Supplement Penis with Autologous Tissue Substitute, Open Approach—AHA CC: 1Q, 2020, 31-32

0VUS0JZ Supplement Penis with Synthetic Substitute, Open Approach—AHA CC: 3Q, 2015, 25; 2Q, 2016, 28-29

0VY50Z0 Transplantation of Scrotum, Allogeneic, Open Approach—AHA CC: 4Q, 2020, 58-59

0VYS0Z0 Transplantation of Penis, Allogeneic, Open Approach—AHA CC: 4Q, 2020, 58-59

Anatomical Regions, General

Body Cavities

Body Areas

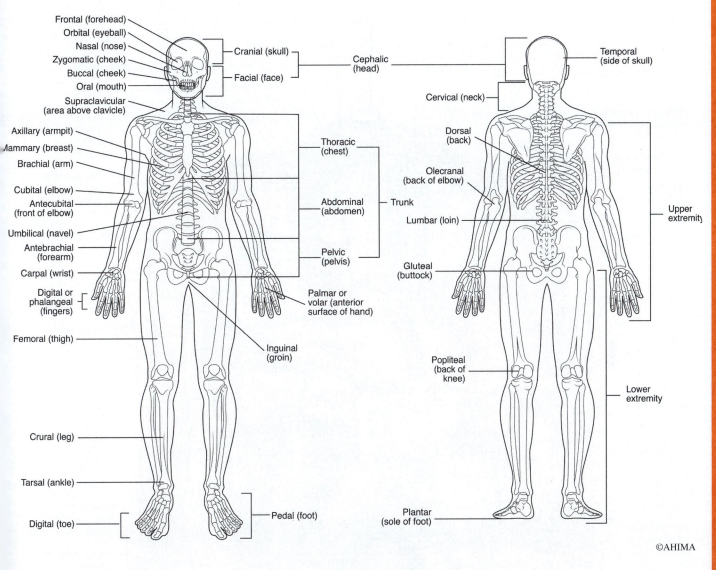

Peritoneum of Posterior Abdominal Wall

Anatomical Regions, General Tables 0W0–0WY

Section	0	Medical and Surgical
Body System	W	Anatomical Regions, General
Operation	0	Alteration: Modifying the anatomic structure of a body part without affecting the function of the body part

Body Part (4th)	Approach (5th)	Device (6th)	Qualifier (7th)
0 Head 2 Face 4 Upper Jaw 5 Lower Jaw 6 Neck 8 Chest Wall F Abdominal Wall K Upper Back L Lower Back M Perineum, Male N Perineum, Female	0 Open 3 Percutaneous 4 Percutaneous Endoscopic	7 Autologous Tissue Substitute J Synthetic Substitute K Nonautologous Tissue Substitute Z No Device	Z No Qualifier

Section	0	Medical and Surgical
Body System	W	Anatomical Regions, General
Operation	1	Bypass: Altering the route of passage of the contents of a tubular body part

Body Part (4th)	Approach (5th)	Device (6th)	Qualifier (7th)
1 Cranial Cavity	0 Open	J Synthetic Substitute	9 Pleural Cavity, Right B Pleural Cavity, Left G Peritoneal Cavity J Pelvic Cavity
9 Pleural Cavity, Right B Pleural Cavity, Left J Pelvic Cavity	0 Open 3 Percutaneous 4 Percutaneous Endoscopic	J Synthetic Substitute	4 Cutaneous 9 Pleural Cavity, Right B Pleural Cavity, Left G Peritoneal Cavity J Pelvic Cavity W Upper Vein Y Lower Vein
G Peritoneal Cavity	0 Open 3 Percutaneous 4 Percutaneous Endoscopic	J Synthetic Substitute	4 Cutaneous 6 Bladder 9 Pleural Cavity, Right B Pleural Cavity, Left G Peritoneal Cavity J Pelvic Cavity W Upper Vein Y Lower Vein

Section	0	Medical and Surgical
Body System	W	Anatomical Regions, General
Operation	2	Change: Taking out or off a device from a body part and putting back an identical or similar device in or on the same body part without cutting or puncturing the skin or a mucous membrane

Body Part (4th)	Approach (5th)	Device (6th)	Qualifier (7th)
0 Head 1 Cranial Cavity 2 Face 4 Upper Jaw 5 Lower Jaw 6 Neck 8 Chest Wall 9 Pleural Cavity, Right B Pleural Cavity, Left C Mediastinum D Pericardial Cavity F Abdominal Wall G Peritoneal Cavity H Retroperitoneum J Pelvic Cavity K Upper Back L Lower Back M Perineum, Male N Perineum, Female	X External	0 Drainage Device Y Other Device	Z No Qualifier

503

0W3–0W8

Medical and Surgical, Anatomical Regions, General Tables

Section	0	Medical and Surgical
Body System	W	Anatomical Regions, General
Operation	3	Control: Stopping, or attempting to stop, postprocedural or other acute bleeding

Body Part (4ᵗʰ)	Approach (5ᵗʰ)	Device (6ᵗʰ)	Qualifier (7ᵗʰ)
0 Head 1 Cranial Cavity 2 Face 4 Upper Jaw 5 Lower Jaw 6 Neck 8 Chest Wall 9 Pleural Cavity, Right B Pleural Cavity, Left C Mediastinum D Pericardial Cavity F Abdominal Wall G Peritoneal Cavity H Retroperitoneum J Pelvic Cavity K Upper Back L Lower Back M Perineum, Male N Perineum, Female	0 Open 3 Percutaneous 4 Percutaneous Endoscopic	Z No Device	Z No Qualifier
3 Oral Cavity and Throat	0 Open 3 Percutaneous 4 Percutaneous Endoscopic 7 Via Natural or Artificial Opening 8 Via Natural or Artificial Opening Endoscopic X External	Z No Device	Z No Qualifier
P Gastrointestinal Tract Q Respiratory Tract R Genitourinary Tract	0 Open 3 Percutaneous 4 Percutaneous Endoscopic 7 Via Natural or Artificial Opening 8 Via Natural or Artificial Opening Endoscopic	Z No Device	Z No Qualifier

Section	0	Medical and Surgical
Body System	W	Anatomical Regions, General
Operation	4	Creation: Putting in or on biological or synthetic material to form a new body part that to the extent possible replicates the anatomic structure or function of an absent body part

Body Part (4ᵗʰ)	Approach (5ᵗʰ)	Device (6ᵗʰ)	Qualifier (7ᵗʰ)
M Perineum, Male	0 Open	7 Autologous Tissue Substitute J Synthetic Substitute K Nonautologous Tissue Substitute	0 Vagina
N Perineum, Female	0 Open	7 Autologous Tissue Substitute J Synthetic Substitute K Nonautologous Tissue Substitute	1 Penis

Section	0	Medical and Surgical
Body System	W	Anatomical Regions, General
Operation	8	Division: Cutting into a body part, without draining fluids and/or gases from the body part, in order to separate or transect a body part

Body Part (4ᵗʰ)	Approach (5ᵗʰ)	Device (6ᵗʰ)	Qualifier (7ᵗʰ)
N Perineum, Female	X External	Z No Device	Z No Qualifier

504

Section	0	Medical and Surgical
Body System	W	Anatomical Regions, General
Operation	9	Drainage: Taking or letting out fluids and/or gases from a body part

Body Part (4th)	Approach (5th)	Device (6th)	Qualifier (7th)
0 Head 1 Cranial Cavity 2 Face 3 Oral Cavity and Throat 4 Upper Jaw 5 Lower Jaw 8 Chest Wall 9 Pleural Cavity, Right B Pleural Cavity, Left C Mediastinum D Pericardial Cavity F Abdominal Wall G Peritoneal Cavity H Retroperitoneum K Upper Back L Lower Back M Perineum, Male N Perineum, Female	0 Open 3 Percutaneous 4 Percutaneous Endoscopic	0 Drainage Device	Z No Qualifier
0 Head 1 Cranial Cavity 2 Face 3 Oral Cavity and Throat 4 Upper Jaw 5 Lower Jaw 8 Chest Wall 9 Pleural Cavity, Right B Pleural Cavity, Left C Mediastinum D Pericardial Cavity F Abdominal Wall G Peritoneal Cavity H Retroperitoneum K Upper Back L Lower Back M Perineum, Male N Perineum, Female	0 Open 3 Percutaneous 4 Percutaneous Endoscopic	Z No Device	X Diagnostic Z No Qualifier
6 Neck J Pelvic Cavity	0 Open 3 Percutaneous 4 Percutaneous Endoscopic 7 Via Natural or Artificial Opening 8 Via Natural or Artificial Opening Endoscopic	0 Drainage Device	Z No Qualifier
6 Neck J Pelvic Cavity	0 Open 3 Percutaneous 4 Percutaneous Endoscopic 7 Via Natural or Artificial Opening 8 Via Natural or Artificial Opening Endoscopic	Z No Device	X Diagnostic Z No Qualifier

Section	0	Medical and Surgical
Body System	W	Anatomical Regions, General
Operation	B	Excision: Cutting out or off, without replacement, a portion of a body part

Body Part (4th)	Approach (5th)	Device (6th)	Qualifier (7th)
0 Head 2 Face 3 Oral Cavity and Throat 4 Upper Jaw 5 Lower Jaw 8 Chest Wall K Upper Back L Lower Back M Perineum, Male N Perineum, Female	0 Open 3 Percutaneous 4 Percutaneous Endoscopic X External	Z No Device	X Diagnostic Z No Qualifier

Continued →

0WB–0WF

Medical and Surgical, Anatomical Regions, General Tables

0WB Continued

Section	0	Medical and Surgical
Body System	W	Anatomical Regions, General
Operation	B	Excision: Cutting out or off, without replacement, a portion of a body part

Body Part (4th)	Approach (5th)	Device (6th)	Qualifier (7th)
6 Neck F Abdominal Wall	0 Open 3 Percutaneous 4 Percutaneous Endoscopic	Z No Device	X Diagnostic Z No Qualifier
6 Neck F Abdominal Wall	X External	Z No Device	2 Stoma X Diagnostic Z No Qualifier
C Mediastinum H Retroperitoneum	0 Open 3 Percutaneous 4 Percutaneous Endoscopic	Z No Device	X Diagnostic Z No Qualifier

Section	0	Medical and Surgical
Body System	W	Anatomical Regions, General
Operation	C	Extirpation: Taking or cutting out solid matter from a body part

Body Part (4th)	Approach (5th)	Device (6th)	Qualifier (7th)
1 Cranial Cavity 3 Oral Cavity and Throat 9 Pleural Cavity, Right B Pleural Cavity, Left C Mediastinum D Pericardial Cavity G Peritoneal Cavity H Retroperitoneum J Pelvic Cavity	0 Open 3 Percutaneous 4 Percutaneous Endoscopic X External	Z No Device	Z No Qualifier
4 Upper Jaw 5 Lower Jaw	0 Open 3 Percutaneous 4 Percutaneous Endoscopic	Z No Device	Z No Qualifier
P Gastrointestinal Tract Q Respiratory Tract R Genitourinary Tract	0 Open 3 Percutaneous 4 Percutaneous Endoscopic 7 Via Natural or Artificial Opening 8 Via Natural or Artificial Opening Endoscopic X External	Z No Device	Z No Qualifier

Section	0	Medical and Surgical
Body System	W	Anatomical Regions, General
Operation	F	Fragmentation: Breaking solid matter in a body part into pieces

Body Part (4th)	Approach (5th)	Device (6th)	Qualifier (7th)
1 Cranial Cavity 3 Oral Cavity and Throat 9 Pleural Cavity, Right B Pleural Cavity, Left C Mediastinum D Pericardial Cavity G Peritoneal Cavity J Pelvic Cavity	0 Open 3 Percutaneous 4 Percutaneous Endoscopic X External	Z No Device	Z No Qualifier
P Gastrointestinal Tract Q Respiratory Tract R Genitourinary Tract	0 Open 3 Percutaneous 4 Percutaneous Endoscopic 7 Via Natural or Artificial Opening 8 Via Natural or Artificial Opening Endoscopic X External	Z No Device	Z No Qualifier

Section	0	Medical and Surgical
Body System	W	Anatomical Regions, General
Operation	H	Insertion: Putting in a nonbiological appliance that monitors, assists, performs, or prevents a physiological function but does not physically take the place of a body part

Body Part (4th)	Approach (5th)	Device (6th)	Qualifier (7th)
0 Head 1 Cranial Cavity 2 Face 3 Oral Cavity and Throat 4 Upper Jaw 5 Lower Jaw 6 Neck 8 Chest Wall 9 Pleural Cavity, Right B Pleural Cavity, Left D Pericardial Cavity F Abdominal Wall G Peritoneal Cavity H Retroperitoneum J Pelvic Cavity K Upper Back L Lower Back M Perineum, Male N Perineum, Female	0 Open 3 Percutaneous 4 Percutaneous Endoscopic	1 Radioactive Element 3 Infusion Device Y Other Device	Z No Qualifier
C Mediastinum	0 Open 3 Percutaneous 4 Percutaneous Endoscopic	1 Radioactive Element 3 Infusion Device G Defibrillator Lead Y Other Device	Z No Qualifier
P Gastrointestinal Tract Q Respiratory Tract R Genitourinary Tract	0 Open 3 Percutaneous 4 Percutaneous Endoscopic 7 Via Natural or Artificial Opening 8 Via Natural or Artificial Opening Endoscopic	1 Radioactive Element 3 Infusion Device Y Other Device	Z No Qualifier

Section	0	Medical and Surgical
Body System	W	Anatomical Regions, General
Operation	J	Inspection: Visually and/or manually exploring a body part

Body Part (4th)	Approach (5th)	Device (6th)	Qualifier (7th)
0 Head 2 Face 3 Oral Cavity and Throat 4 Upper Jaw 5 Lower Jaw 6 Neck 8 Chest Wall F Abdominal Wall K Upper Back L Lower Back M Perineum, Male N Perineum, Female	0 Open 3 Percutaneous 4 Percutaneous Endoscopic X External	Z No Device	Z No Qualifier
1 Cranial Cavity 9 Pleural Cavity, Right B Pleural Cavity, Left C Mediastinum D Pericardial Cavity G Peritoneal Cavity H Retroperitoneum J Pelvic Cavity	0 Open 3 Percutaneous 4 Percutaneous Endoscopic	Z No Device	Z No Qualifier
P Gastrointestinal Tract Q Respiratory Tract R Genitourinary Tract	0 Open 3 Percutaneous 4 Percutaneous Endoscopic 7 Via Natural or Artificial Opening 8 Via Natural or Artificial Opening Endoscopic	Z No Device	Z No Qualifier

Section	0	Medical and Surgical
Body System	W	Anatomical Regions, General
Operation	M	Reattachment: Putting back in or on all or a portion of a separated body part to its normal location or other suitable location

Body Part (4th)	Approach (5th)	Device (6th)	Qualifier (7th)
2 Face 4 Upper Jaw 5 Lower Jaw 6 Neck 8 Chest Wall F Abdominal Wall K Upper Back L Lower Back M Perineum, Male N Perineum, Female	0 Open	Z No Device	Z No Qualifier

Section	0	Medical and Surgical
Body System	W	Anatomical Regions, General
Operation	P	Removal: Taking out or off a device from a body part

Body Part (4th)	Approach (5th)	Device (6th)	Qualifier (7th)
0 Head 2 Face 4 Upper Jaw 5 Lower Jaw 6 Neck 8 Chest Wall F Abdominal Wall K Upper Back L Lower Back M Perineum, Male N Perineum, Female	0 Open 3 Percutaneous 4 Percutaneous Endoscopic X External	0 Drainage Device 1 Radioactive Element 3 Infusion Device 7 Autologous Tissue Substitute J Synthetic Substitute K Nonautologous Tissue Substitute Y Other Device	Z No Qualifier
1 Cranial Cavity 9 Pleural Cavity, Right B Pleural Cavity, Left G Peritoneal Cavity J Pelvic Cavity	0 Open 3 Percutaneous 4 Percutaneous Endoscopic	0 Drainage Device 1 Radioactive Element 3 Infusion Device J Synthetic Substitute Y Other Device	Z No Qualifier
1 Cranial Cavity 9 Pleural Cavity, Right B Pleural Cavity, Left G Peritoneal Cavity J Pelvic Cavity	X External	0 Drainage Device 1 Radioactive Element 3 Infusion Device	Z No Qualifier
C Mediastinum	0 Open 3 Percutaneous 4 Percutaneous Endoscopic X External	0 Drainage Device 1 Radioactive Element 3 Infusion Device 7 Autologous Tissue Substitute G Defibrillator Lead J Synthetic Substitute K Nonautologous Tissue Substitute Y Other Device	Z No Qualifier
D Pericardial Cavity H Retroperitoneum	0 Open 3 Percutaneous 4 Percutaneous Endoscopic	0 Drainage Device 1 Radioactive Element 3 Infusion Device Y Other Device	Z No Qualifier
D Pericardial Cavity H Retroperitoneum	X External	0 Drainage Device 1 Radioactive Element 3 Infusion Device	Z No Qualifier
P Gastrointestinal Tract Q Respiratory Tract R Genitourinary Tract	0 Open 3 Percutaneous 4 Percutaneous Endoscopic 7 Via Natural or Artificial Opening 8 Via Natural or Artificial Opening Endoscopic X External	1 Radioactive Element 3 Infusion Device Y Other Device	Z No Qualifier

Section	0	Medical and Surgical
Body System	W	Anatomical Regions, General
Operation	Q	Repair: Restoring, to the extent possible, a body part to its normal anatomic structure and function

Body Part (4th)	Approach (5th)	Device (6th)	Qualifier (7th)
0 Head 2 Face 3 Oral Cavity and Throat 4 Upper Jaw 5 Lower Jaw 8 Chest Wall K Upper Back L Lower Back M Perineum, Male N Perineum, Female	0 Open 3 Percutaneous 4 Percutaneous Endoscopic X External	Z No Device	Z No Qualifier
6 Neck F Abdominal Wall	0 Open 3 Percutaneous 4 Percutaneous Endoscopic	Z No Device	Z No Qualifier
6 Neck F Abdominal Wall	X External	Z No Device	2 Stoma Z No Qualifier
C Mediastinum	0 Open 3 Percutaneous 4 Percutaneous Endoscopic	Z No Device	Z No Qualifier

Section	0	Medical and Surgical
Body System	W	Anatomical Regions, General
Operation	U	Supplement: Putting in or on biological or synthetic material that physically reinforces and/or augments the function of a portion of a body part

Body Part (4th)	Approach (5th)	Device (6th)	Qualifier (7th)
0 Head 2 Face 4 Upper Jaw 5 Lower Jaw 6 Neck 8 Chest Wall C Mediastinum F Abdominal Wall K Upper Back L Lower Back M Perineum, Male N Perineum, Female	0 Open 4 Percutaneous Endoscopic	7 Autologous Tissue Substitute J Synthetic Substitute K Nonautologous Tissue Substitute	Z No Qualifier

Section	0	Medical and Surgical
Body System	W	Anatomical Regions, General
Operation	W	Revision: Correcting, to the extent possible, a portion of a malfunctioning device or the position of a displaced device

Body Part (4th)	Approach (5th)	Device (6th)	Qualifier (7th)
0 Head 2 Face 4 Upper Jaw 5 Lower Jaw 6 Neck 8 Chest Wall F Abdominal Wall K Upper Back L Lower Back M Perineum, Male N Perineum, Female	0 Open 3 Percutaneous 4 Percutaneous Endoscopic X External	0 Drainage Device 1 Radioactive Element 3 Infusion Device 7 Autologous Tissue Substitute J Synthetic Substitute K Nonautologous Tissue Substitute Y Other Device	Z No Qualifier
1 Cranial Cavity 9 Pleural Cavity, Right B Pleural Cavity, Left G Peritoneal Cavity J Pelvic Cavity	0 Open 3 Percutaneous 4 Percutaneous Endoscopic X External	0 Drainage Device 1 Radioactive Element 3 Infusion Device J Synthetic Substitute Y Other Device	Z No Qualifier
C Mediastinum	0 Open 3 Percutaneous 4 Percutaneous Endoscopic X External	0 Drainage Device 1 Radioactive Element 3 Infusion Device 7 Autologous Tissue Substitute G Defibrillator Lead J Synthetic Substitute K Nonautologous Tissue Substitute Y Other Device	Z No Qualifier

Continued ➔

Section	0	Medical and Surgical			0WW Continued
Body System	W	Anatomical Regions, General			
Operation	W	Revision: Correcting, to the extent possible, a portion of a malfunctioning device or the position of a displaced device			

Body Part (4th)	Approach (5th)	Device (6th)	Qualifier (7th)
D Pericardial Cavity H Retroperitoneum	0 Open 3 Percutaneous 4 Percutaneous Endoscopic X External	0 Drainage Device 1 Radioactive Element 3 Infusion Device Y Other Device	Z No Qualifier
P Gastrointestinal Tract Q Respiratory Tract R Genitourinary Tract	0 Open 3 Percutaneous 4 Percutaneous Endoscopic 7 Via Natural or Artificial Opening 8 Via Natural or Artificial Opening Endoscopic X External	1 Radioactive Element 3 Infusion Device Y Other Device	Z No Qualifier

Section	0	Medical and Surgical
Body System	W	Anatomical Regions, General
Operation	Y	Transplantation: Putting in or on all or a portion of a living body part taken from another individual or animal to physically take the place and/or function of all or a portion of a similar body part

Body Part (4th)	Approach (5th)	Device (6th)	Qualifier (7th)
2 Face	0 Open	Z No Device	0 Allogeneic 1 Syngeneic

AHA Coding Clinic

0W020ZZ Alteration of Face, Open Approach—AHA CC: 1Q, 2015, 31

0W1G3J4 Bypass Peritoneal Cavity to Cutaneous with Synthetic Substitute, Percutaneous Approach—AHA CC: 4Q, 2013, 126-127

0W1G3J6 Bypass Peritoneal Cavity to Bladder with Synthetic Substitute, Percutaneous Approach—AHA CC: 4Q, 2020, 55

0W1G3JW Bypass Peritoneal Cavity to Upper Vein with Synthetic Substitute, Percutaneous Approach—AHA CC: 4Q, 2018, 42-43

0W310ZZ Control Bleeding in Cranial Cavity, Open Approach—AHA CC: 3Q, 2019, 4-5

0W3F0ZZ Control Bleeding in Abdominal Wall, Open Approach—AHA CC: 4Q, 2016, 100-101

0W3P8ZZ Control Bleeding in Gastrointestinal Tract, Via Natural or Artificial Opening Endoscopic—AHA CC: 4Q, 2016, 99-100; 4Q, 2017, 105; 1Q, 2018, 19; 2Q, 2023, 26-27

0W3Q7ZZ Control Bleeding in Respiratory Tract, Via Natural or Artificial Opening—AHA CC: 4Q, 2017, 106

0W3Q8ZZ Control Bleeding in Respiratory Tract, Via Natural or Artificial Opening Endoscopic—AHA CC: 1Q, 2018, 19-20

0W3R7ZZ Control Bleeding in Genitourinary Tract, Via Natural or Artificial Opening—AHA CC: 4Q, 2014, 44

0W930ZZ Drainage of Oral Cavity and Throat, Open Approach—AHA CC: 2Q, 2017, 16-17

0W960ZZ Drainage of Neck, Open Approach—AHA CC: 3Q, 2021, 17-18, 21-22

0W968ZZ Drainage of Neck, Via Natural or Artificial Opening Endoscopic—AHA CC: 4Q, 2022, 60

0W9D0ZZ Drainage of Pericardial Cavity, Open Approach—AHA CC: 3Q, 2021, 26-27

0W9G3ZZ Drainage of Peritoneal Cavity, Percutaneous Approach—AHA CC: 3Q, 2017, 12-13

0WB60ZZ Excision of Neck, Open Approach—AHA CC: 3Q, 2021, 21

0WBF4ZZ Excision of Abdominal Wall, Percutaneous Endoscopic Approach—AHA CC: 1Q, 2016, 21-22

0WBH0ZZ Excision of Retroperitoneum, Open Approach—AHA CC: 1Q, 2019, 27

0WBNXZZ Excision of Female Perineum, External Approach—AHA CC: 4Q, 2013, 119-120

0WC30ZZ Extirpation of Matter from Oral Cavity and Throat, Open Approach—AHA CC: 2Q, 2017, 16

0WCH0ZZ Extirpation of Matter from Retroperitoneum, Open Approach—AHA CC: 1Q, 2022, 42-43

0WCJ0ZZ Extirpation of Matter from Pelvic Cavity, Open Approach—AHA CC: 1Q, 2022, 42-43

0WHG03Z Insertion of Infusion Device into Peritoneal Cavity, Open Approach—AHA CC: 2Q, 2021, 14

0WHG33Z Insertion of Infusion Device into Peritoneal Cavity, Percutaneous Approach—AHA CC: 2Q, 2015, 36; 2Q, 2016, 14

0WHJ01Z Insertion of Radioactive Element into Pelvic Cavity, Open Approach—AHA CC: 4Q, 2019, 43-44

0WJC0ZZ Inspection of Mediastinum, Open Approach—AHA CC: 3Q, 2018, 29

0WJG4ZZ Inspection of Peritoneal Cavity, Percutaneous Endoscopic Approach—AHA CC: 2Q, 2013, 36-37; 1Q, 2019, 4-5, 25; 2Q, 2021, 19-20

0WJJ4ZZ Inspection of Pelvic Cavity, Percutaneous Endoscopic Approach—AHA CC: 4Q, 2016, 58-59

0WQF0ZZ Repair Abdominal Wall, Open Approach—AHA CC: 4Q, 2014, 38-39; 3Q, 2014, 28-29; 3Q, 2016, 6; 3Q, 2017, 8-9

0WU80JZ Supplement Chest Wall with Synthetic Substitute, Open Approach—AHA CC: 4Q, 2012, 101-102

0WUF07Z Supplement Abdominal Wall with Autologous Tissue Substitute, Open Approach—AHA CC: 3Q, 2016, 40-41

0WUF0JZ Supplement Abdominal Wall with Synthetic Substitute, Open Approach—AHA CC: 4Q, 2014, 39-40; 3Q, 2017, 8

0WWG4JZ Revision of Synthetic Substitute in Peritoneal Cavity, Percutaneous Endoscopic Approach—AHA CC: 2Q, 2015, 9-10

Anatomical Regions, Upper Extremities

Anatomical Regions, Upper Extremities Tables 0X0–0XY

Section 0 Medical and Surgical
Body System X Anatomical Regions, Upper Extremities
Operation 0 Alteration: Modifying the anatomic structure of a body part without affecting the function of the body part

Body Part (4ᵗʰ)	Approach (5ᵗʰ)	Device (6ᵗʰ)	Qualifier (7ᵗʰ)
2 Shoulder Region, Right	0 Open	7 Autologous Tissue Substitute	Z No Qualifier
3 Shoulder Region, Left	3 Percutaneous	J Synthetic Substitute	
4 Axilla, Right	4 Percutaneous Endoscopic	K Nonautologous Tissue Substitute	
5 Axilla, Left		Z No Device	
6 Upper Extremity, Right			
7 Upper Extremity, Left			
8 Upper Arm, Right			
9 Upper Arm, Left			
B Elbow Region, Right			
C Elbow Region, Left			
D Lower Arm, Right			
F Lower Arm, Left			
G Wrist Region, Right			
H Wrist Region, Left			

Section 0 Medical and Surgical
Body System X Anatomical Regions, Upper Extremities
Operation 2 Change: Taking out or off a device from a body part and putting back an identical or similar device in or on the same body part without cutting or puncturing the skin or a mucous membrane

Body Part (4ᵗʰ)	Approach (5ᵗʰ)	Device (6ᵗʰ)	Qualifier (7ᵗʰ)
6 Upper Extremity, Right	X External	0 Drainage Device	Z No Qualifier
7 Upper Extremity, Left		Y Other Device	

Section 0 Medical and Surgical
Body System X Anatomical Regions, Upper Extremities
Operation 3 Control: Stopping, or attempting to stop, postprocedural or other acute bleeding

Body Part (4ᵗʰ)	Approach (5ᵗʰ)	Device (6ᵗʰ)	Qualifier (7ᵗʰ)
2 Shoulder Region, Right	0 Open	Z No Device	Z No Qualifier
3 Shoulder Region, Left	3 Percutaneous		
4 Axilla, Right	4 Percutaneous Endoscopic		
5 Axilla, Left			
6 Upper Extremity, Right			
7 Upper Extremity, Left			
8 Upper Arm, Right			
9 Upper Arm, Left			
B Elbow Region, Right			
C Elbow Region, Left			
D Lower Arm, Right			
F Lower Arm, Left			
G Wrist Region, Right			
H Wrist Region, Left			
J Hand, Right			
K Hand, Left			

0X6–0X9

Medical and Surgical, Anatomical Regions, Upper Extremities Tables

Section	0	Medical and Surgical
Body System	X	Anatomical Regions, Upper Extremities
Operation	6	Detachment: Cutting off all or a portion of the upper or lower extremities

Body Part (4th)	Approach (5th)	Device (6th)	Qualifier (7th)
0 Forequarter, Right 1 Forequarter, Left 2 Shoulder Region, Right 3 Shoulder Region, Left B Elbow Region, Right C Elbow Region, Left	0 Open	Z No Device	Z No Qualifier
8 Upper Arm, Right 9 Upper Arm, Left D Lower Arm, Right F Lower Arm, Left	0 Open	Z No Device	1 High 2 Mid 3 Low
J Hand, Right K Hand, Left	0 Open	Z No Device	0 Complete 4 Complete 1st Ray 5 Complete 2nd Ray 6 Complete 3rd Ray 7 Complete 4th Ray 8 Complete 5th Ray 9 Partial 1st Ray B Partial 2nd Ray C Partial 3rd Ray D Partial 4th Ray F Partial 5th Ray
L Thumb, Right M Thumb, Left N Index Finger, Right P Index Finger, Left Q Middle Finger, Right R Middle Finger, Left S Ring Finger, Right T Ring Finger, Left V Little Finger, Right W Little Finger, Left	0 Open	Z No Device	0 Complete 1 High 2 Mid 3 Low

Section	0	Medical and Surgical
Body System	X	Anatomical Regions, Upper Extremities
Operation	9	Drainage: Taking or letting out fluids and/or gases from a body part

Body Part (4th)	Approach (5th)	Device (6th)	Qualifier (7th)
2 Shoulder Region, Right 3 Shoulder Region, Left 4 Axilla, Right 5 Axilla, Left 6 Upper Extremity, Right 7 Upper Extremity, Left 8 Upper Arm, Right 9 Upper Arm, Left B Elbow Region, Right C Elbow Region, Left D Lower Arm, Right F Lower Arm, Left G Wrist Region, Right H Wrist Region, Left J Hand, Right K Hand, Left	0 Open 3 Percutaneous 4 Percutaneous Endoscopic	0 Drainage Device	Z No Qualifier

Continued →

0X9 Continued

Section	0	Medical and Surgical
Body System	X	Anatomical Regions, Upper Extremities
Operation	9	Drainage: Taking or letting out fluids and/or gases from a body part

Body Part (4th)	Approach (5th)	Device (6th)	Qualifier (7th)
2 Shoulder Region, Right 3 Shoulder Region, Left 4 Axilla, Right 5 Axilla, Left 6 Upper Extremity, Right 7 Upper Extremity, Left 8 Upper Arm, Right 9 Upper Arm, Left B Elbow Region, Right C Elbow Region, Left D Lower Arm, Right F Lower Arm, Left G Wrist Region, Right H Wrist Region, Left J Hand, Right K Hand, Left	0 Open 3 Percutaneous 4 Percutaneous Endoscopic	Z No Device	X Diagnostic Z No Qualifier

Section	0	Medical and Surgical
Body System	X	Anatomical Regions, Upper Extremities
Operation	B	Excision: Cutting out or off, without replacement, a portion of a body part

Body Part (4th)	Approach (5th)	Device (6th)	Qualifier (7th)
2 Shoulder Region, Right 3 Shoulder Region, Left 4 Axilla, Right 5 Axilla, Left 6 Upper Extremity, Right 7 Upper Extremity, Left 8 Upper Arm, Right 9 Upper Arm, Left B Elbow Region, Right C Elbow Region, Left D Lower Arm, Right F Lower Arm, Left G Wrist Region, Right H Wrist Region, Left J Hand, Right K Hand, Left	0 Open 3 Percutaneous 4 Percutaneous Endoscopic	Z No Device	X Diagnostic Z No Qualifier

Section	0	Medical and Surgical
Body System	X	Anatomical Regions, Upper Extremities
Operation	H	Insertion: Putting in a nonbiological appliance that monitors, assists, performs, or prevents a physiological function but does not physically take the place of a body part

Body Part (4th)	Approach (5th)	Device (6th)	Qualifier (7th)
2 Shoulder Region, Right 3 Shoulder Region, Left 4 Axilla, Right 5 Axilla, Left 6 Upper Extremity, Right 7 Upper Extremity, Left 8 Upper Arm, Right 9 Upper Arm, Left B Elbow Region, Right C Elbow Region, Left D Lower Arm, Right F Lower Arm, Left G Wrist Region, Right H Wrist Region, Left J Hand, Right K Hand, Left	0 Open 3 Percutaneous 4 Percutaneous Endoscopic	1 Radioactive Element 3 Infusion Device Y Other Device	Z No Qualifier

0XJ–0XP

Medical and Surgical, Anatomical Regions, Upper Extremities Tables

Section	0	Medical and Surgical
Body System	X	Anatomical Regions, Upper Extremities
Operation	J	Inspection: Visually and/or manually exploring a body part

Body Part (4th)	Approach (5th)	Device (6th)	Qualifier (7th)
2 Shoulder Region, Right 3 Shoulder Region, Left 4 Axilla, Right 5 Axilla, Left 6 Upper Extremity, Right 7 Upper Extremity, Left 8 Upper Arm, Right 9 Upper Arm, Left B Elbow Region, Right C Elbow Region, Left D Lower Arm, Right F Lower Arm, Left G Wrist Region, Right H Wrist Region, Left J Hand, Right K Hand, Left	0 Open 3 Percutaneous 4 Percutaneous Endoscopic X External	Z No Device	Z No Qualifier

Section	0	Medical and Surgical
Body System	X	Anatomical Regions, Upper Extremities
Operation	M	Reattachment: Putting back in or on all or a portion of a separated body part to its normal location or other suitable location

Body Part (4th)	Approach (5th)	Device (6th)	Qualifier (7th)
0 Forequarter, Right 1 Forequarter, Left 2 Shoulder Region, Right 3 Shoulder Region, Left 4 Axilla, Right 5 Axilla, Left 6 Upper Extremity, Right 7 Upper Extremity, Left 8 Upper Arm, Right 9 Upper Arm, Left B Elbow Region, Right C Elbow Region, Left D Lower Arm, Right F Lower Arm, Left G Wrist Region, Right H Wrist Region, Left J Hand, Right K Hand, Left L Thumb, Right M Thumb, Left N Index Finger, Right P Index Finger, Left Q Middle Finger, Right R Middle Finger, Left S Ring Finger, Right T Ring Finger, Left V Little Finger, Right W Little Finger, Left	0 Open	Z No Device	Z No Qualifier

Section	0	Medical and Surgical
Body System	X	Anatomical Regions, Upper Extremities
Operation	P	Removal: Taking out or off a device from a body part

Body Part (4th)	Approach (5th)	Device (6th)	Qualifier (7th)
6 Upper Extremity, Right 7 Upper Extremity, Left	0 Open 3 Percutaneous 4 Percutaneous Endoscopic X External	0 Drainage Device 1 Radioactive Element 3 Infusion Device 7 Autologous Tissue Substitute J Synthetic Substitute K Nonautologous Tissue Substitute Y Other Device	Z No Qualifier

Section	0	Medical and Surgical
Body System	X	Anatomical Regions, Upper Extremities
Operation	Q	**Repair:** Restoring, to the extent possible, a body part to its normal anatomic structure and function

Body Part (4th)	Approach (5th)	Device (6th)	Qualifier (7th)
2 Shoulder Region, Right	0 Open	Z No Device	Z No Qualifier
3 Shoulder Region, Left	3 Percutaneous		
4 Axilla, Right	4 Percutaneous Endoscopic		
5 Axilla, Left	X External		
6 Upper Extremity, Right			
7 Upper Extremity, Left			
8 Upper Arm, Right			
9 Upper Arm, Left			
B Elbow Region, Right			
C Elbow Region, Left			
D Lower Arm, Right			
F Lower Arm, Left			
G Wrist Region, Right			
H Wrist Region, Left			
J Hand, Right			
K Hand, Left			
L Thumb, Right			
M Thumb, Left			
N Index Finger, Right			
P Index Finger, Left			
Q Middle Finger, Right			
R Middle Finger, Left			
S Ring Finger, Right			
T Ring Finger, Left			
V Little Finger, Right			
W Little Finger, Left			

Section	0	Medical and Surgical
Body System	X	Anatomical Regions, Upper Extremities
Operation	R	**Replacement:** Putting in or on biological or synthetic material that physically takes the place and/or function of all or a portion of a body part

Body Part (4th)	Approach (5th)	Device (6th)	Qualifier (7th)
L Thumb, Right	0 Open	7 Autologous Tissue Substitute	N Toe, Right
M Thumb, Left	4 Percutaneous Endoscopic		P Toe, Left

Section	0	Medical and Surgical
Body System	X	Anatomical Regions, Upper Extremities
Operation	U	**Supplement:** Putting in or on biological or synthetic material that physically reinforces and/or augments the function of a portion of a body part

Body Part (4th)	Approach (5th)	Device (6th)	Qualifier (7th)
2 Shoulder Region, Right	0 Open	7 Autologous Tissue Substitute	Z No Qualifier
3 Shoulder Region, Left	4 Percutaneous Endoscopic	J Synthetic Substitute	
4 Axilla, Right		K Nonautologous Tissue Substitute	
5 Axilla, Left			
6 Upper Extremity, Right			
7 Upper Extremity, Left			
8 Upper Arm, Right			
9 Upper Arm, Left			
B Elbow Region, Right			
C Elbow Region, Left			
D Lower Arm, Right			
F Lower Arm, Left			
G Wrist Region, Right			
H Wrist Region, Left			
J Hand, Right			
K Hand, Left			
L Thumb, Right			
M Thumb, Left			
N Index Finger, Right			
P Index Finger, Left			
Q Middle Finger, Right			
R Middle Finger, Left			
S Ring Finger, Right			
T Ring Finger, Left			
V Little Finger, Right			
W Little Finger, Left			

Section 0 **Medical and Surgical**
Body System X **Anatomical Regions, Upper Extremities**
Operation W **Revision:** Correcting, to the extent possible, a portion of a malfunctioning device or the position of a displaced device

Body Part (4th)	Approach (5th)	Device (6th)	Qualifier (7th)
6 Upper Extremity, Right 7 Upper Extremity, Left	0 Open 3 Percutaneous 4 Percutaneous Endoscopic X External	0 Drainage Device 3 Infusion Device 7 Autologous Tissue Substitute J Synthetic Substitute K Nonautologous Tissue Substitute Y Other Device	Z No Qualifier

Section 0 **Medical and Surgical**
Body System X **Anatomical Regions, Upper Extremities**
Operation X **Transfer:** Moving, without taking out, all or a portion of a body part to another location to take over the function of all or a portion of a body part

Body Part (4th)	Approach (5th)	Device (6th)	Qualifier (7th)
N Index Finger, Right	0 Open	Z No Device	L Thumb, Right
P Index Finger, Left	0 Open	Z No Device	M Thumb, Left

Section 0 **Medical and Surgical**
Body System X **Anatomical Regions, Upper Extremities**
Operation Y **Transplantation:** Putting in or on all or a portion of a living body part taken from another individual or animal to physically take the place and/or function of all or a portion of a similar body part

Body Part (4th)	Approach (5th)	Device (6th)	Qualifier (7th)
J Hand, Right K Hand, Left	0 Open	Z No Device	0 Allogeneic 1 Syngeneic

AHA Coding Clinic

0X370ZZ Control Bleeding in Left Upper Extremity, Open Approach—AHA CC: 1Q, 2015, 35

0X6M0Z3 Detachment at Left Thumb, Low, Open Approach—AHA CC: 3Q, 2016, 33-34; 1Q, 2017, 52

0X6T0Z3 Detachment at Left Ring Finger, Low, Open Approach—AHA CC: 3Q, 2016, 33-34; 1Q, 2017, 52

0X6V0Z0 Detachment at Right Little Finger, Complete, Open Approach—AHA CC: 2Q, 2017, 18-19

0X6W0Z3 Detachment at Left Little Finger, Low, Open Approach—AHA CC: 3Q, 2016, 33-34; 1Q, 2017, 52

0XH90YZ Insertion of Other Device into Left Upper Arm, Open Approach—AHA CC: 2Q, 2017, 20-21

0XP70YZ Removal of Other Device from Left Upper Extremity, Open Approach—AHA CC: 2Q, 2017, 20-21

Hernia I - Indirect and Direct Inguinal Hernias

Anatomical Regions, Lower Extremities

Anatomical Regions, Lower Extremities 0Y0–0YW

Section	0	Medical and Surgical
Body System	Y	Anatomical Regions, Lower Extremities
Operation	0	Alteration: Modifying the anatomic structure of a body part without affecting the function of the body part

Body Part (4th)	Approach (5th)	Device (6th)	Qualifier (7th)
0 Buttock, Right 1 Buttock, Left 9 Lower Extremity, Right B Lower Extremity, Left C Upper Leg, Right D Upper Leg, Left F Knee Region, Right G Knee Region, Left H Lower Leg, Right J Lower Leg, Left K Ankle Region, Right L Ankle Region, Left	0 Open 3 Percutaneous 4 Percutaneous Endoscopic	7 Autologous Tissue Substitute J Synthetic Substitute K Nonautologous Tissue Substitute Z No Device	Z No Qualifier

Section	0	Medical and Surgical
Body System	Y	Anatomical Regions, Lower Extremities
Operation	2	Change: Taking out or off a device from a body part and putting back an identical or similar device in or on the same body part without cutting or puncturing the skin or a mucous membrane

Body Part (4th)	Approach (5th)	Device (6th)	Qualifier (7th)
9 Lower Extremity, Right B Lower Extremity, Left	X External	0 Drainage Device Y Other Device	Z No Qualifier

Section	0	Medical and Surgical
Body System	Y	Anatomical Regions, Lower Extremities
Operation	3	Control: Stopping, or attempting to stop, postprocedural or other acute bleeding

Body Part (4th)	Approach (5th)	Device (6th)	Qualifier (7th)
0 Buttock, Right 1 Buttock, Left 5 Inguinal Region, Right 6 Inguinal Region, Left 7 Femoral Region, Right 8 Femoral Region, Left 9 Lower Extremity, Right B Lower Extremity, Left C Upper Leg, Right D Upper Leg, Left F Knee Region, Right G Knee Region, Left H Lower Leg, Right J Lower Leg, Left K Ankle Region, Right L Ankle Region, Left M Foot, Right N Foot, Left	0 Open 3 Percutaneous 4 Percutaneous Endoscopic	Z No Device	Z No Qualifier

Section	0	Medical and Surgical
Body System	Y	Anatomical Regions, Lower Extremities
Operation	6	**Detachment:** Cutting off all or a portion of the upper or lower extremities

Body Part (4th)	Approach (5th)	Device (6th)	Qualifier (7th)
2 Hindquarter, Right 3 Hindquarter, Left 4 Hindquarter, Bilateral 7 Femoral Region, Right 8 Femoral Region, Left F Knee Region, Right G Knee Region, Left	0 Open	Z No Device	Z No Qualifier
C Upper Leg, Right D Upper Leg, Left H Lower Leg, Right J Lower Leg, Left	0 Open	Z No Device	1 High 2 Mid 3 Low
M Foot, Right N Foot, Left	0 Open	Z No Device	0 Complete 4 Complete 1st Ray 5 Complete 2nd Ray 6 Complete 3rd Ray 7 Complete 4th Ray 8 Complete 5th Ray 9 Partial 1st Ray B Partial 2nd Ray C Partial 3rd Ray D Partial 4th Ray F Partial 5th Ray
P 1st Toe, Right Q 1st Toe, Left R 2nd Toe, Right S 2nd Toe, Left T 3rd Toe, Right U 3rd Toe, Left V 4th Toe, Right W 4th Toe, Left X 5th Toe, Right Y 5th Toe, Left	0 Open	Z No Device	0 Complete 1 High 2 Mid 3 Low

Section	0	Medical and Surgical
Body System	Y	Anatomical Regions, Lower Extremities
Operation	9	**Drainage:** Taking or letting out fluids and/or gases from a body part

Body Part (4th)	Approach (5th)	Device (6th)	Qualifier (7th)
0 Buttock, Right 1 Buttock, Left 5 Inguinal Region, Right 6 Inguinal Region, Left 7 Femoral Region, Right 8 Femoral Region, Left 9 Lower Extremity, Right B Lower Extremity, Left C Upper Leg, Right D Upper Leg, Left F Knee Region, Right G Knee Region, Left H Lower Leg, Right J Lower Leg, Left K Ankle Region, Right L Ankle Region, Left M Foot, Right N Foot, Left	0 Open 3 Percutaneous 4 Percutaneous Endoscopic	0 Drainage Device	Z No Qualifier

Continued →

0Y9 Continued

Section	0	Medical and Surgical
Body System	Y	Anatomical Regions, Lower Extremities
Operation	9	**Drainage:** Taking or letting out fluids and/or gases from a body part

Body Part (4th)	Approach (5th)	Device (6th)	Qualifier (7th)
0 Buttock, Right 1 Buttock, Left 5 Inguinal Region, Right 6 Inguinal Region, Left 7 Femoral Region, Right 8 Femoral Region, Left 9 Lower Extremity, Right B Lower Extremity, Left C Upper Leg, Right D Upper Leg, Left F Knee Region, Right G Knee Region, Left H Lower Leg, Right J Lower Leg, Left K Ankle Region, Right L Ankle Region, Left M Foot, Right N Foot, Left	0 Open 3 Percutaneous 4 Percutaneous Endoscopic	Z No Device	X Diagnostic Z No Qualifier

Section	0	Medical and Surgical
Body System	Y	Anatomical Regions, Lower Extremities
Operation	B	**Excision:** Cutting out or off, without replacement, a portion of a body part

Body Part (4th)	Approach (5th)	Device (6th)	Qualifier (7th)
0 Buttock, Right 1 Buttock, Left 5 Inguinal Region, Right 6 Inguinal Region, Left 7 Femoral Region, Right 8 Femoral Region, Left 9 Lower Extremity, Right B Lower Extremity, Left C Upper Leg, Right D Upper Leg, Left F Knee Region, Right G Knee Region, Left H Lower Leg, Right J Lower Leg, Left K Ankle Region, Right L Ankle Region, Left M Foot, Right N Foot, Left	0 Open 3 Percutaneous 4 Percutaneous Endoscopic	Z No Device	X Diagnostic Z No Qualifier

Section	0	Medical and Surgical
Body System	Y	Anatomical Regions, Lower Extremities
Operation	H	**Insertion:** Putting in a nonbiological appliance that monitors, assists, performs, or prevents a physiological function but does not physically take the place of a body part

Body Part (4th)	Approach (5th)	Device (6th)	Qualifier (7th)
0 Buttock, Right 1 Buttock, Left 5 Inguinal Region, Right 6 Inguinal Region, Left 7 Femoral Region, Right 8 Femoral Region, Left 9 Lower Extremity, Right B Lower Extremity, Left C Upper Leg, Right D Upper Leg, Left F Knee Region, Right G Knee Region, Left H Lower Leg, Right J Lower Leg, Left K Ankle Region, Right L Ankle Region, Left M Foot, Right N Foot, Left	0 Open 3 Percutaneous 4 Percutaneous Endoscopic	1 Radioactive Element 3 Infusion Device Y Other Device	Z No Qualifier

Section	0	Medical and Surgical
Body System	Y	Anatomical Regions, Lower Extremities
Operation	J	Inspection: Visually and/or manually exploring a body part

Body Part (4th)	Approach (5th)	Device (6th)	Qualifier (7th)
0 Buttock, Right	0 Open	Z No Device	Z No Qualifier
1 Buttock, Left	3 Percutaneous		
5 Inguinal Region, Right	4 Percutaneous Endoscopic		
6 Inguinal Region, Left	X External		
7 Femoral Region, Right			
8 Femoral Region, Left			
9 Lower Extremity, Right			
A Inguinal Region, Bilateral			
B Lower Extremity, Left			
C Upper Leg, Right			
D Upper Leg, Left			
E Femoral Region, Bilateral			
F Knee Region, Right			
G Knee Region, Left			
H Lower Leg, Right			
J Lower Leg, Left			
K Ankle Region, Right			
L Ankle Region, Left			
M Foot, Right			
N Foot, Left			

Section	0	Medical and Surgical
Body System	Y	Anatomical Regions, Lower Extremities
Operation	M	Reattachment: Putting back in or on all or a portion of a separated body part to its normal location or other suitable location

Body Part (4th)	Approach (5th)	Device (6th)	Qualifier (7th)
0 Buttock, Right	0 Open	Z No Device	Z No Qualifier
1 Buttock, Left			
2 Hindquarter, Right			
3 Hindquarter, Left			
4 Hindquarter, Bilateral			
5 Inguinal Region, Right			
6 Inguinal Region, Left			
7 Femoral Region, Right			
8 Femoral Region, Left			
9 Lower Extremity, Right			
B Lower Extremity, Left			
C Upper Leg, Right			
D Upper Leg, Left			
F Knee Region, Right			
G Knee Region, Left			
H Lower Leg, Right			
J Lower Leg, Left			
K Ankle Region, Right			
L Ankle Region, Left			
M Foot, Right			
N Foot, Left			
P 1st Toe, Right			
Q 1st Toe, Left			
R 2nd Toe, Right			
S 2nd Toe, Left			
T 3rd Toe, Right			
U 3rd Toe, Left			
V 4th Toe, Right			
W 4th Toe, Left			
X 5th Toe, Right			
Y 5th Toe, Left			

Section 0 **Medical and Surgical**
Body System Y **Anatomical Regions, Lower Extremities**
Operation P **Removal:** Taking out or off a device from a body part

Body Part (4th)	Approach (5th)	Device (6th)	Qualifier (7th)
9 Lower Extremity, Right B Lower Extremity, Left	0 Open 3 Percutaneous 4 Percutaneous Endoscopic X External	0 Drainage Device 1 Radioactive Element 3 Infusion Device 7 Autologous Tissue Substitute J Synthetic Substitute K Nonautologous Tissue Substitute Y Other Device	Z No Qualifier

Section 0 **Medical and Surgical**
Body System Y **Anatomical Regions, Lower Extremities**
Operation Q **Repair:** Restoring, to the extent possible, a body part to its normal anatomic structure and function

Body Part (4th)	Approach (5th)	Device (6th)	Qualifier (7th)
0 Buttock, Right 1 Buttock, Left 5 Inguinal Region, Right 6 Inguinal Region, Left 7 Femoral Region, Right 8 Femoral Region, Left 9 Lower Extremity, Right A Inguinal Region, Bilateral B Lower Extremity, Left C Upper Leg, Right D Upper Leg, Left E Femoral Region, Bilateral F Knee Region, Right G Knee Region, Left H Lower Leg, Right J Lower Leg, Left K Ankle Region, Right L Ankle Region, Left M Foot, Right N Foot, Left P 1st Toe, Right Q 1st Toe, Left R 2nd Toe, Right S 2nd Toe, Left T 3rd Toe, Right U 3rd Toe, Left V 4th Toe, Right W 4th Toe, Left X 5th Toe, Right Y 5th Toe, Left	0 Open 3 Percutaneous 4 Percutaneous Endoscopic X External	Z No Device	Z No Qualifier

Section	0	Medical and Surgical
Body System	Y	Anatomical Regions, Lower Extremities
Operation	U	Supplement: Putting in or on biological or synthetic material that physically reinforces and/or augments the function of a portion of a body part

Body Part (4th)	Approach (5th)	Device (6th)	Qualifier (7th)
0 Buttock, Right	0 Open	7 Autologous Tissue Substitute	Z No Qualifier
1 Buttock, Left	4 Percutaneous Endoscopic	J Synthetic Substitute	
5 Inguinal Region, Right		K Nonautologous Tissue Substitute	
6 Inguinal Region, Left			
7 Femoral Region, Right			
8 Femoral Region, Left			
9 Lower Extremity, Right			
A Inguinal Region, Bilateral			
B Lower Extremity, Left			
C Upper Leg, Right			
D Upper Leg, Left			
E Femoral Region, Bilateral			
F Knee Region, Right			
G Knee Region, Left			
H Lower Leg, Right			
J Lower Leg, Left			
K Ankle Region, Right			
L Ankle Region, Left			
M Foot, Right			
N Foot, Left			
P 1st Toe, Right			
Q 1st Toe, Left			
R 2nd Toe, Right			
S 2nd Toe, Left			
T 3rd Toe, Right			
U 3rd Toe, Left			
V 4th Toe, Right			
W 4th Toe, Left			
X 5th Toe, Right			
Y 5th Toe, Left			

Section	0	Medical and Surgical
Body System	Y	Anatomical Regions, Lower Extremities
Operation	W	Revision: Correcting, to the extent possible, a portion of a malfunctioning device or the position of a displaced device

Body Part (4th)	Approach (5th)	Device (6th)	Qualifier (7th)
9 Lower Extremity, Right	0 Open	0 Drainage Device	Z No Qualifier
B Lower Extremity, Left	3 Percutaneous	3 Infusion Device	
	4 Percutaneous Endoscopic	7 Autologous Tissue Substitute	
	X External	J Synthetic Substitute	
		K Nonautologous Tissue Substitute	
		Y Other Device	

AHA Coding Clinic

0Y6N0Z0 Detachment at Left Foot, Complete, Open Approach—AHA CC: 1Q, 2015, 28; 1Q, 2017, 22-23

0Y6P0Z3 Detachment at Right 1st Toe, Low, Open Approach—AHA CC: 2Q, 2015, 28-29

0Y6Q0Z3 Detachment at Left 1st Toe, Low, Open Approach—AHA CC: 2Q, 2015, 28-29

0Y950ZZ Drainage of Right Inguinal Region, Open Approach—AHA CC: 1Q, 2015, 23

0Y980ZZ Drainage of Left Femoral Region, Open Approach—AHA CC: 1Q, 2015, 22

0YHC0YZ Insertion of Other Device into Right Upper Leg, Open Approach—AHA CC: 1Q, 2023, 27-30

0YHD0YZ Insertion of Other Device into Left Upper Leg, Open Approach—AHA CC: 1Q, 2023, 27-30

Obstetrics Section (102–10Y)

Within each section of ICD-10-PCS the characters have different meanings. The seven character meanings for the Obstetrics section are illustrated here through the procedure example of *Manually-assisted delivery*.

Section	Body System	Root Operation	Body Part	Approach	Device	Qualifier
Obstetrics	Pregnancy	Delivery	Products of Conception	External	None	None
1	0	E	0	X	Z	Z

Section (Character 1)

All Obstetric procedure codes have a first character value of 1.

Body System (Character 2)

The alphanumeric character for the body system is placed in the second position. The body system applicable to the Obstetrics section is Pregnancy and has a character value of 0.

Root Operations (Character 3)

The alphanumeric character value for root operations is placed in the third position. Listed below are the root operations applicable to the Obstetrics section with their associated meaning.

Character Value	Root Operation	Root Operation Definition
2	Change	Taking out or off a device from a body part and putting back an identical or similar device in or on the same body part without cutting or puncturing the skin or a mucous membrane
9	Drainage	Taking or letting out fluids and/or gases from a body part
A	Abortion	Artificially terminating a pregnancy
D	Extraction	Pulling or stripping out or off all or a portion of a body part by the use of force
E	Delivery	Assisting the passage of the products of conception from the genital canal
H	Insertion	Putting in a nonbiological appliance that monitors, assists, performs, or prevents a physiological function but does not physically take the place of a body part
J	Inspection	Visually and/or manually exploring a body part
P	Removal	Taking out or off a device from a body part, region or orifice
Q	Repair	Restoring, to the extent possible, a body part to its normal anatomic structure and function
S	Reposition	Moving to its normal location, or other suitable location, all or a portion of a body part
T	Resection	Cutting out or off, without replacement, all of a body part
Y	Transplantation	Putting in or on all or a portion of a living body part taken from another individual or animal to physically take the place and/or function of all or a portion of a similar body part

Body Part (Character 4)

For each body system the applicable body part character values will be available for procedure code construction. An example of a body part is Products of Conception.

Approach (Character 5)

The approach is the technique used to reach the procedure site. The following are the approach character values for the Obstetrics section with the associated definitions.

Character Value	Approach	Approach Definition
0	Open	Cutting through the skin or mucous membrane and any other body layers necessary to expose the site of the procedure
3	Percutaneous	Entry, by puncture or minor incision, of instrumentation through the skin or mucous membrane and any other body layers necessary to reach the site of the procedure

Continued →

Character Value	Approach	Approach Definition
4	Percutaneous Endoscopic	Entry, by puncture or minor incision, of instrumentation through the skin or mucous membrane and any other body layers necessary to reach and visualize the site of the procedure
7	Via Natural or Artificial Opening	Entry of instrumentation through a natural or artificial external opening to reach the site of the procedure
8	Via Natural or Artificial Opening Endoscopic	Entry of instrumentation through a natural or artificial external opening to reach and visualize the site of the procedure
X	External	Procedures performed directly on the skin or mucous membrane and procedures performed indirectly by the application of external force through the skin or mucous membrane

Device (Character 6)

Depending on the procedure performed there may or may not be a device used. There are two types of devices included in the Obstetrics section: monitoring electrode and other device. When a device is not utilized during the procedure, the placeholder Z is the character value that should be reported.

Qualifier (Character 7)

The qualifier represents an additional attribute for the procedure when applicable. For example, drainage procedures in this section include several qualifiers including fetal cerebrospinal fluid that is reported with the character value of A. If there is no qualifier for a procedure, the placeholder Z is the character valve that should be reported.

Obstetric Section Guidelines (section 1)

C. Obstetrics Section

Products of Conception
C1. Procedures performed on the products of conception are coded to the Obstetrics section. Procedures performed on the pregnant female other than the products of conception are coded to the appropriate root operation in the Medical and Surgical section.

Example: Amniocentesis is coded to the products of conception body part in the Obstetrics section. Repair of obstetric urethral laceration is coded to the urethra body part in the Medical and Surgical section.

Procedures following delivery or abortion
C2. Procedures performed following a delivery or abortion for curettage of the endometrium or evacuation of retained products of conception are all coded in the Obstetrics section, to the root operation Extraction and the body part Products of Conception, Retained. Diagnostic or therapeutic dilation and curettage performed during times other than the postpartum or post-abortion period are all coded in the Medical and Surgical section, to the root operation Extraction and the body part Endometrium.

Coding Guidelines References

The table below links ICD-10-PCS coding guidelines to Obstetrics section body system tables. The guidelines identified in the table are provided in order to remind users to reference the coding guidelines prior to code reporting. It is imperative to review the ICD-10-PCS coding guidelines to ensure the procedure code being reported is accurate and complete.

Table References

Table	Root Operation	Coding Guideline(s)
102	Change	C1
10D	Extraction	C2

Obstetrics Section Tables

Obstetrics Tables 102–10Y

Section	1	Obstetrics
Body System	0	Pregnancy
Operation	2	**Change:** Taking out or off a device from a body part and putting back an identical or similar device in or on the same body part without cutting or puncturing the skin or a mucous membrane

Body Part (4th)	Approach (5th)	Device (6th)	Qualifier (7th)
0 Products of Conception	7 Via Natural or Artificial Opening	3 Monitoring Electrode Y Other Device	Z No Qualifier

Section	1	Obstetrics
Body System	0	Pregnancy
Operation	9	**Drainage:** Taking or letting out fluids and/or gases from a body part

Body Part (4th)	Approach (5th)	Device (6th)	Qualifier (7th)
0 Products of Conception	0 Open 3 Percutaneous 4 Percutaneous Endoscopic 7 Via Natural or Artificial Opening 8 Via Natural or Artificial Opening Endoscopic	Z No Device	9 Fetal Blood A Fetal Cerebrospinal Fluid B Fetal Fluid, Other C Amniotic Fluid, Therapeutic D Fluid, Other U Amniotic Fluid, Diagnostic

Section	1	Obstetrics
Body System	0	Pregnancy
Operation	A	**Abortion:** Artificially terminating a pregnancy

Body Part (4th)	Approach (5th)	Device (6th)	Qualifier (7th)
0 Products of Conception	0 Open 3 Percutaneous 4 Percutaneous Endoscopic 8 Via Natural or Artificial Opening Endoscopic	Z No Device	Z No Qualifier
0 Products of Conception	7 Via Natural or Artificial Opening	Z No Device	6 Vacuum W Laminaria X Abortifacient Z No Qualifier

Section	1	Obstetrics
Body System	0	Pregnancy
Operation	D	**Extraction:** Pulling or stripping out or off all or a portion of a body part by the use of force

Body Part (4th)	Approach (5th)	Device (6th)	Qualifier (7th)
0 Products of Conception	0 Open	Z No Device	0 High 1 Low 2 Extraperitoneal
0 Products of Conception	7 Via Natural or Artificial Opening	Z No Device	3 Low Forceps 4 Mid Forceps 5 High Forceps 6 Vacuum 7 Internal Version 8 Other

Continued →

Section	1	Obstetrics
Body System	0	Pregnancy
Operation	D	Extraction: Pulling or stripping out or off all or a portion of a body part by the use of force

Body Part (4th)	Approach (5th)	Device (6th)	Qualifier (7th)
1 Products of Conception, Retained	7 Via Natural or Artificial Opening 8 Via Natural or Artificial Opening Endoscopic	Z No Device	9 Manual Z No Qualifier
2 Products of Conception, Ectopic	0 Open 4 Percutaneous Endoscopic 7 Via Natural or Artificial Opening 8 Via Natural or Artificial Opening Endoscopic	Z No Device	Z No Qualifier

Section	1	Obstetrics
Body System	0	Pregnancy
Operation	E	Delivery: Assisting the passage of the products of conception from the genital canal

Body Part (4th)	Approach (5th)	Device (6th)	Qualifier (7th)
0 Products of Conception	X External	Z No Device	Z No Qualifier

Section	1	Obstetrics
Body System	0	Pregnancy
Operation	H	Insertion: Putting in a nonbiological appliance that monitors, assists, performs, or prevents a physiological function but does not physically take the place of a body part

Body Part (4th)	Approach (5th)	Device (6th)	Qualifier (7th)
0 Products of Conception	0 Open 7 Via Natural or Artificial Opening	3 Monitoring Electrode Y Other Device	Z No Qualifier

Section	1	Obstetrics
Body System	0	Pregnancy
Operation	J	Inspection: Visually and/or manually exploring a body part

Body Part (4th)	Approach (5th)	Device (6th)	Qualifier (7th)
0 Products of Conception 1 Products of Conception, Retained 2 Products of Conception, Ectopic	0 Open 3 Percutaneous 4 Percutaneous Endoscopic 7 Via Natural or Artificial Opening 8 Via Natural or Artificial Opening Endoscopic X External	Z No Device	Z No Qualifier

Section	1	Obstetrics
Body System	0	Pregnancy
Operation	P	Removal: Taking out or off a device from a body part, region or orifice

Body Part (4th)	Approach (5th)	Device (6th)	Qualifier (7th)
0 Products of Conception	0 Open 7 Via Natural or Artificial Opening	3 Monitoring Electrode Y Other Device	Z No Qualifier

10Q–10T

Obstetrics Section Tables

Section	1	Obstetrics	
Body System	0	Pregnancy	
Operation	Q	**Repair:** Restoring, to the extent possible, a body part to its normal anatomic structure and function	

Body Part (4th)	Approach (5th)	Device (6th)	Qualifier (7th)
0 Products of Conception	0 Open 3 Percutaneous 4 Percutaneous Endoscopic 7 Via Natural or Artificial Opening 8 Via Natural or Artificial Opening Endoscopic	Y Other Device Z No Device	E Nervous System F Cardiovascular System G Lymphatics and Hemic H Eye J Ear, Nose and Sinus K Respiratory System L Mouth and Throat M Gastrointestinal System N Hepatobiliary and Pancreas P Endocrine System Q Skin R Musculoskeletal System S Urinary System T Female Reproductive System V Male Reproductive System Y Other Body System

Section	1	Obstetrics	
Body System	0	Pregnancy	
Operation	S	**Reposition:** Moving to its normal location, or other suitable location, all or a portion of a body part	

Body Part (4th)	Approach (5th)	Device (6th)	Qualifier (7th)
0 Products of Conception	7 Via Natural or Artificial Opening X External	Z No Device	Z No Qualifier
2 Products of Conception, Ectopic	0 Open 3 Percutaneous 4 Percutaneous Endoscopic 7 Via Natural or Artificial Opening 8 Via Natural or Artificial Opening Endoscopic	Z No Device	Z No Qualifier

Section	1	Obstetrics	
Body System	0	Pregnancy	
Operation	T	**Resection:** Cutting out or off, without replacement, all of a body part	

Body Part (4th)	Approach (5th)	Device (6th)	Qualifier (7th)
2 Products of Conception, Ectopic	0 Open 3 Percutaneous 4 Percutaneous Endoscopic 7 Via Natural or Artificial Opening 8 Via Natural or Artificial Opening Endoscopic	Z No Device	Z No Qualifier

528

Section	1	Obstetrics
Body System	0	Pregnancy
Operation	Y	Transplantation: Putting in or on all or a portion of a living body part taken from another individual or animal to physically take the place and/or function of all or a portion of a similar body part

Body Part (4th)	Approach (5th)	Device (6th)	Qualifier (7th)
0 Products of Conception	3 Percutaneous 4 Percutaneous Endoscopic 7 Via Natural or Artificial Opening	Z No Device	E Nervous System F Cardiovascular System G Lymphatics and Hemic H Eye J Ear, Nose and Sinus K Respiratory System L Mouth and Throat M Gastrointestinal System N Hepatobiliary and Pancreas P Endocrine System Q Skin R Musculoskeletal System S Urinary System T Female Reproductive System V Male Reproductive System Y Other Body System

AHA Coding Clinic

10904ZC Drainage of Amniotic Fluid, Therapeutic from Products of Conception, Percutaneous Endoscopic Approach—AHA CC: 3Q, 2014, 12-13

10907ZC Drainage of Amniotic Fluid, Therapeutic from Products of Conception, Via Natural or Artificial Opening—AHA CC: 2Q, 2014, 9-10

10A07ZZ Abortion of Products of Conception, Via Opening—AHA CC: 1Q, 2022, 41-42

10D00Z0 Extraction of Products of Conception, High, Open Approach— AHA CC: 2Q, 2018, 17-18; 4Q, 2018, 51

10D00Z1 Extraction of Products of Conception, Low, Open Approach—AHA CC: 4Q, 2018, 50-51

10D07Z3 Extraction of Products of Conception, Low Forceps, Via Natural or Artificial Opening—AHA CC: 1Q, 2016, 9-10

10D07Z6 Extraction of Products of Conception, Vacuum, Via Natural or Artificial Opening—AHA CC: 4Q, 2014, 43

10D17ZZ Extraction of Products of Conception, Retained, Via Natural or Artificial Opening—AHA CC: 1Q, 2022, 19

10D20ZZ Extraction of Products of Conception, Ectopic, Open Approach—AHA CC: 1Q, 2021, 52

10D27ZZ Extraction of Products of Conception, Ectopic, Via Natural or Artificial Opening—AHA CC: 4Q, 2020, 60; 1Q, 2021, 52

10E0XZZ Delivery of Products of Conception, External Approach—AHA CC: 2Q, 2014, 9-10; 4Q, 2014, 17-18; 2Q, 2016, 34-35; 3Q, 2017, 5

10H07YZ Insertion of Other Device into Products of Conception, Via Natural or Artificial Opening—AHA CC: 2Q, 2013, 36

10Q00ZK Repair Respiratory System in Products of Conception, Open Approach—AHA CC: 2Q, 2021, 21-22

10Q04ZY Repair Other Body System in Products of Conception, Percutaneous Endoscopic Approach—AHA CC: 3Q, 2014, 12-13

10T24ZZ Resection of Products of Conception, Ectopic, Percutaneous Endoscopic Approach—AHA CC: 3Q, 2015, 32; 3Q, 2020, 47

Placement Section (2W0–2Y5)

Within each section of ICD-10-PCS the characters have different meanings. The seven character meanings for the Placement section are illustrated below through the procedure example of *Placement of pressure dressing on abdominal wall*.

Section	Body System	Root Operation	Body Region	Approach	Device	Qualifier
Placement	Anatomical Regions	Compression	Abdominal Wall	External	Pressure Dressing	None
2	W	1	3	X	6	Z

Section (Character 1)

All Placement procedure codes have a first character value of 2.

Body System (Character 2)

The alphanumeric character for the body system is placed in the second position. There are two character values applicable for the Placement section. The character value of W is reported for anatomical regions. The character value Y is reported for anatomical orifices.

Root Operations (Character 3)

The alphanumeric character value for root operations is placed in the third position. The following are the root operations applicable to the Placement section with their associated meaning.

Character Value	Root Operation	Root Operation Definition
0	Change	Taking out or off a device from a body part and putting back an identical or similar device in or on the same body part without cutting or puncturing the skin or a mucous membrane
1	Compression	Putting pressure on a body region
2	Dressing	Putting material on a body region for protection
3	Immobilization	Limiting or preventing motion of a body region
4	Packing	Putting material in a body region or orifice
5	Removal	Taking out or off a device from a body part
6	Traction	Exerting a pulling force on a body region in a distal direction

Body Region (Character 4)

For each body system the applicable body part character values will be available for procedure code construction. An example of a body region is Chest Wall.

Approach (Character 5)

The only approach technique utilized for the Placement section is External approach and is reported with the character value of X.

Character Value	Approach	Approach Definition
X	External	Procedures performed directly on the skin or mucous membrane and procedures performed indirectly by the application of external force through the skin or mucous membrane

Device (Character 6)

Depending on the procedure performed there may or may not be a device used. There are several types of devices included in the Placement section. Here is a sample list of the devices included in this section:

- Cast
- Packing material
- Pressure dressing
- Traction apparatus

When a device is not utilized during the procedure, the placeholder Z is the character value that should be reported.

Qualifier (Character 7)

The qualifier represents an additional attribute for the procedure when applicable. Currently, there are no qualifiers in the Placement section; therefore, the placeholder character value of Z should be reported.

Coding Guideline References

Before reporting Change and Removal procedures in this section users should review coding guideline B6.1c.

Placement Section Tables

Placement Tables 2W0–2Y5

Section	2	**Placement**
Body System	W	**Anatomical Regions**
Operation	0	**Change:** Taking out or off a device from a body part and putting back an identical or similar device in or on the same body part without cutting or puncturing the skin or a mucous membrane

Body Region (4th)	Approach (5th)	Device (6th)	Qualifier (7th)
0 Head 2 Neck 3 Abdominal Wall 4 Chest Wall 5 Back 6 Inguinal Region, Right 7 Inguinal Region, Left 8 Upper Extremity, Right 9 Upper Extremity, Left A Upper Arm, Right B Upper Arm, Left C Lower Arm, Right D Lower Arm, Left E Hand, Right F Hand, Left G Thumb, Right H Thumb, Left J Finger, Right K Finger, Left L Lower Extremity, Right M Lower Extremity, Left N Upper Leg, Right P Upper Leg, Left Q Lower Leg, Right R Lower Leg, Left S Foot, Right T Foot, Left U Toe, Right V Toe, Left	X External	0 Traction Apparatus 1 Splint 2 Cast 3 Brace 4 Bandage 5 Packing Material 6 Pressure Dressing 7 Intermittent Pressure Device Y Other Device	Z No Qualifier
1 Face	X External	0 Traction Apparatus 1 Splint 2 Cast 3 Brace 4 Bandage 5 Packing Material 6 Pressure Dressing 7 Intermittent Pressure Device 9 Wire Y Other Device	Z No Qualifier

2W1

Section	2	**Placement**
Body System	W	**Anatomical Regions**
Operation	1	**Compression:** Putting pressure on a body region

Body Region (4th)	Approach (5th)	Device (6th)	Qualifier (7th)
0 Head	X External	6 Pressure Dressing	Z No Qualifier
1 Face		7 Intermittent Pressure Device	
2 Neck			
3 Abdominal Wall			
4 Chest Wall			
5 Back			
6 Inguinal Region, Right			
7 Inguinal Region, Left			
8 Upper Extremity, Right			
9 Upper Extremity, Left			
A Upper Arm, Right			
B Upper Arm, Left			
C Lower Arm, Right			
D Lower Arm, Left			
E Hand, Right			
F Hand, Left			
G Thumb, Right			
H Thumb, Left			
J Finger, Right			
K Finger, Left			
L Lower Extremity, Right			
M Lower Extremity, Left			
N Upper Leg, Right			
P Upper Leg, Left			
Q Lower Leg, Right			
R Lower Leg, Left			
S Foot, Right			
T Foot, Left			
U Toe, Right			
V Toe, Left			

Placement Section Tables

Section	2	Placement
Body System	W	Anatomical Regions
Operation	2	**Dressing:** Putting material on a body region for protection

Body Region (4th)	Approach (5th)	Device (6th)	Qualifier (7th)
0 Head	**X** External	**4** Bandage	**Z** No Qualifier
1 Face			
2 Neck			
3 Abdominal Wall			
4 Chest Wall			
5 Back			
6 Inguinal Region, Right			
7 Inguinal Region, Left			
8 Upper Extremity, Right			
9 Upper Extremity, Left			
A Upper Arm, Right			
B Upper Arm, Left			
C Lower Arm, Right			
D Lower Arm, Left			
E Hand, Right			
F Hand, Left			
G Thumb, Right			
H Thumb, Left			
J Finger, Right			
K Finger, Left			
L Lower Extremity, Right			
M Lower Extremity, Left			
N Upper Leg, Right			
P Upper Leg, Left			
Q Lower Leg, Right			
R Lower Leg, Left			
S Foot, Right			
T Foot, Left			
U Toe, Right			
V Toe, Left			

2W3

Section	2	Placement
Body System	W	Anatomical Regions
Operation	3	**Immobilization:** Limiting or preventing motion of a body region

Body Region (4th)	Approach (5th)	Device (6th)	Qualifier (7th)
0 Head 2 Neck 3 Abdominal Wall 4 Chest Wall 5 Back 6 Inguinal Region, Right 7 Inguinal Region, Left 8 Upper Extremity, Right 9 Upper Extremity, Left A Upper Arm, Right B Upper Arm, Left C Lower Arm, Right D Lower Arm, Left E Hand, Right F Hand, Left G Thumb, Right H Thumb, Left J Finger, Right K Finger, Left L Lower Extremity, Right M Lower Extremity, Left N Upper Leg, Right P Upper Leg, Left Q Lower Leg, Right R Lower Leg, Left S Foot, Right T Foot, Left U Toe, Right V Toe, Left	X External	1 Splint 2 Cast 3 Brace Y Other Device	Z No Qualifier
1 Face	X External	1 Splint 2 Cast 3 Brace 9 Wire Y Other Device	Z No Qualifier

Placement Section Tables

Section	2	Placement
Body System	W	Anatomical Regions
Operation	4	Packing: Putting material in a body region or orifice

Body Region (4th)	Approach (5th)	Device (6th)	Qualifier (7th)
0 Head	X External	5 Packing Material	Z No Qualifier
1 Face			
2 Neck			
3 Abdominal Wall			
4 Chest Wall			
5 Back			
6 Inguinal Region, Right			
7 Inguinal Region, Left			
8 Upper Extremity, Right			
9 Upper Extremity, Left			
A Upper Arm, Right			
B Upper Arm, Left			
C Lower Arm, Right			
D Lower Arm, Left			
E Hand, Right			
F Hand, Left			
G Thumb, Right			
H Thumb, Left			
J Finger, Right			
K Finger, Left			
L Lower Extremity, Right			
M Lower Extremity, Left			
N Upper Leg, Right			
P Upper Leg, Left			
Q Lower Leg, Right			
R Lower Leg, Left			
S Foot, Right			
T Foot, Left			
U Toe, Right			
V Toe, Left			

2W5

Section 2 **Placement**
Body System W **Anatomical Regions**
Operation 5 **Removal:** Taking out or off a device from a body part

Body Region (4th)	Approach (5th)	Device (6th)	Qualifier (7th)
0 Head 2 Neck 3 Abdominal Wall 4 Chest Wall 5 Back 6 Inguinal Region, Right 7 Inguinal Region, Left 8 Upper Extremity, Right 9 Upper Extremity, Left A Upper Arm, Right B Upper Arm, Left C Lower Arm, Right D Lower Arm, Left E Hand, Right F Hand, Left G Thumb, Right H Thumb, Left J Finger, Right K Finger, Left L Lower Extremity, Right M Lower Extremity, Left N Upper Leg, Right P Upper Leg, Left Q Lower Leg, Right R Lower Leg, Left S Foot, Right T Foot, Left U Toe, Right V Toe, Left	X External	0 Traction Apparatus 1 Splint 2 Cast 3 Brace 4 Bandage 5 Packing Material 6 Pressure Dressing 7 Intermittent Pressure Device Y Other Device	Z No Qualifier
1 Face	X External	0 Traction Apparatus 1 Splint 2 Cast 3 Brace 4 Bandage 5 Packing Material 6 Pressure Dressing 7 Intermittent Pressure Device 9 Wire Y Other Device	Z No Qualifier

Placement Section Tables

536

Section	2	Placement
Body System	W	Anatomical Regions
Operation	6	Traction: Exerting a pulling force on a body region in a distal direction

Body Region (4th)	Approach (5th)	Device (6th)	Qualifier (7th)
0 Head 1 Face 2 Neck 3 Abdominal Wall 4 Chest Wall 5 Back 6 Inguinal Region, Right 7 Inguinal Region, Left 8 Upper Extremity, Right 9 Upper Extremity, Left A Upper Arm, Right B Upper Arm, Left C Lower Arm, Right D Lower Arm, Left E Hand, Right F Hand, Left G Thumb, Right H Thumb, Left J Finger, Right K Finger, Left L Lower Extremity, Right M Lower Extremity, Left N Upper Leg, Right P Upper Leg, Left Q Lower Leg, Right R Lower Leg, Left S Foot, Right T Foot, Left U Toe, Right V Toe, Left	X External	0 Traction Apparatus Z No Device	Z No Qualifier

Section	2	Placement
Body System	Y	Anatomical Orifices
Operation	0	Change: Taking out or off a device from a body part and putting back an identical or similar device in or on the same body part without cutting or puncturing the skin or a mucous membrane

Body Region (4th)	Approach (5th)	Device (6th)	Qualifier (7th)
0 Mouth and Pharynx 1 Nasal 2 Ear 3 Anorectal 4 Female Genital Tract 5 Urethra	X External	5 Packing Material	Z No Qualifier

Section	2	Placement
Body System	Y	Anatomical Orifices
Operation	4	Packing: Putting material in a body region or orifice

Body Region (4th)	Approach (5th)	Device (6th)	Qualifier (7th)
0 Mouth and Pharynx 1 Nasal 2 Ear 3 Anorectal 4 Female Genital Tract 5 Urethra	X External	5 Packing Material	Z No Qualifier

2Y5

Section	2	Placement
Body System	Y	Anatomical Orifices
Operation	5	Removal: Taking out or off a device from a body part

Body Region (4th)	Approach (5th)	Device (6th)	Qualifier (7th)
0 Mouth and Pharynx **1** Nasal **2** Ear **3** Anorectal **4** Female Genital Tract **5** Urethra	**X** External	**5** Packing Material	**Z** No Qualifier

AHA Coding Clinic

2W60X0Z Traction of Head using Traction Apparatus—AHA CC: 2Q, 2013, 39

2W62X0Z Traction of Neck using Traction Apparatus—AHA CC: 2Q, 2015, 35

2Y41X5Z Packing of Nasal Region using Packing Material—AHA CC: 4Q, 2017, 106; 4Q, 2018, 38

Administration Section (302–3E1)

Within each section of ICD-10-PCS, the characters have different meanings. The seven character meanings for the Administration section are illustrated here through the procedure example of *Nerve block injection to median nerve*.

Section	Body System	Root Operation	Body System/ Region	Approach	Substance	Qualifier
Administration	Physiological System and Anatomical Region	Introduction	Peripheral Nerves and Plexi	Percutaneous	Regional Anesthetic	None
3	E	0	T	3	C	Z

Section (Character 1)

All Administration procedure codes have a first character value of 3.

Body System (Character 2)

The alphanumeric character for the body system is placed in the second position. There are three character values applicable for the Administration section.

Character Value	Character Value Description
0	Circulatory
C	Indwelling Device
E	Physiological System and Anatomical Region

Root Operations (Character 3)

The alphanumeric character value for root operations is placed in the third position. Listed here are the root operations applicable to the Administration section with their associated meaning.

Character Value	Root Operation	Root Operation Definition
0	Introduction	Putting in or on a therapeutic, diagnostic, nutritional, physiological, or prophylactic substance except blood or blood products
1	Irrigation	Putting in or on a cleansing substance
2	Transfusion	Putting in blood or blood products

Body System/Region (Character 4)

For each body system the applicable body part character values will be available for procedure code construction. An example of a body region is upper GI.

Approach (Character 5)

The approach is the technique used to reach the procedure site. Listed here are the approach character values for the Administration with the associated definitions.

Character Value	Approach	Approach Definition
0	Open	Cutting through the skin or mucous membrane and any other body layers necessary to expose the site of the procedure
3	Percutaneous	Entry, by puncture or minor incision, of instrumentation through the skin or mucous membrane and any other body layers necessary to reach the site of the procedure
4	Percutaneous Endoscopic	Entry, by puncture or minor incision, of instrumentation through the skin or mucous membrane and any other body layers necessary to reach and visualize the site of the procedure
7	Via Natural or Artificial Opening	Entry of instrumentation through a natural or artificial external opening to reach the site of the procedure
8	Via Natural or Artificial Opening Endoscopic	Entry of instrumentation through a natural or artificial external opening to reach and visualize the site of the procedure
X	External	Procedures performed directly on the skin or mucous membrane and procedures performed indirectly by the application of external force through the skin or mucous membrane

Substance (Character 6)

In the Administration section a substance is always utilized. The substance is reported in the sixth character position by the type of substance utilized. The following is a sample list of the substances included in this section:

- Anti-inflammatory
- Antineoplastic
- Bone marrow
- Platelet inhibitor
- Whole blood

Qualifier (Character 7)

The qualifier represents an additional attribute for the procedure when applicable. There are several qualifiers included in the Administration section. For example, transfusion procedures in this section include qualifiers including Autologous and Nonautologous that are reported with the character values of 0 and 1, respectively. If there is no qualifier for a procedure, the placeholder Z is the character value that should be reported.

If a coder is unsure of which option to select for the substance qualifier utilized during the procedure, Appendix F can be used to guide the selection. It is important to note that not all substance qualifier categories are provided by CMS in Appendix F. However, for example, the coding scenario indicates that Clolar was introduced percutaneously via the peripheral vein. The coder references Table 3E0 (Introduction in Physiological Systems and Anatomical Regions) under the peripheral vein, percutaneous approach, antineoplastic. Clolar is not a substance qualifier choice. However, the coder can then locate the substance qualifier categories in Appendix F. The category Clofarabine includes Clolar. Therefore, the coder should select P - Clofarabine for the 7th character.

Important Definitions for the Administration Section

Administration Root Operation	Qualifier	Definition
Transfusion (302)	0 - Autologous	Derived or transferred from the same individual's body*
	1 - Nonautologous	Derived or transferred from another individual's body

*Taken from The Free Dictionary by Farlex at www.thefreedictionary.com

Coding Guideline References

Before reporting Transfusion procedures for embryonic stem cells (6th character A), bone marrow (6th character G), cord blood stem cells (6th character X) or hematopoietic stem cells (6th character Y) users should review coding guideline B3.16.

Before reporting Administration codes for all Biliary and Pancreatic Tract (4th character value of J) procedures with a 6th character value of U (Pancreatic Islet Cells), users should review coding guideline B3.16.

Before reporting Irrigation procedures in this section, users should review coding guideline B6.1c.

Administration Section Tables

Administration Tables 302–3E1

Section	3	Administration
Body System	0	Circulatory
Operation	2	**Transfusion:** Putting in blood or blood products

Body System / Region (4th)	Approach (5th)	Substance (6th)	Qualifier (7th)
3 Peripheral Vein 4 Central Vein	3 Percutaneous	A Stem Cells, Embryonic	Z No Qualifier
3 Peripheral Vein 4 Central Vein	3 Percutaneous	C Hematopoietic Stem/Progenitor Cells, Genetically Modified	0 Autologous
3 Peripheral Vein 4 Central Vein	3 Percutaneous	D Pathogen Reduced Cryoprecipitated Fibrinogen Complex	1 Nonautologous
3 Peripheral Vein 4 Central Vein	3 Percutaneous	G Bone Marrow X Stem Cells, Cord Blood Y Stem Cells, Hematopoietic	0 Autologous 2 Allogeneic, Related 3 Allogeneic, Unrelated 4 Allogeneic, Unspecified
3 Peripheral Vein 4 Central Vein	3 Percutaneous	H Whole Blood J Serum Albumin K Frozen Plasma L Fresh Plasma M Plasma Cryoprecipitate N Red Blood Cells P Frozen Red Cells Q White Cells R Platelets S Globulin T Fibrinogen V Antihemophilic Factors W Factor IX	0 Autologous 1 Nonautologous
3 Peripheral Vein 4 Central Vein	3 Percutaneous	U Stem Cells, T-cell Depleted Hematopoietic	2 Allogeneic, Related 3 Allogeneic, Unrelated 4 Allogeneic, Unspecified
7 Products of Conception, Circulatory	3 Percutaneous 7 Via Natural or Artificial Opening	H Whole Blood J Serum Albumin K Frozen Plasma L Fresh Plasma M Plasma Cryoprecipitate N Red Blood Cells P Frozen Red Cells Q White Cells R Platelets S Globulin T Fibrinogen V Antihemophilic Factors W Factor IX	1 Nonautologous
8 Vein	3 Percutaneous	B 4-Factor Prothrombin Complex Concentrate	1 Nonautologous
A Bone Marrow	3 Percutaneous	H Whole Blood J Serum Albumin K Frozen Plasma L Fresh Plasma N Red Blood Cells P Frozen Red Cells R Platelets	0 Autologous 1 Nonautologous

Section	3	Administration
Body System	C	Indwelling Device
Operation	1	**Irrigation:** Putting in or on a cleansing substance

Body System / Region (4th)	Approach (5th)	Substance (6th)	Qualifier (7th)
Z None	X External	8 Irrigating Substance	Z No Qualifier

Section 3 **Administration**
Body System E **Physiological Systems and Anatomical Regions**
Operation 0 **Introduction:** Putting in or on a therapeutic, diagnostic, nutritional, physiological, or prophylactic substance except blood or blood products

Body System / Region (4th)	Approach (5th)	Substance (6th)	Qualifier (7th)
0 Skin and Mucous Membranes	X External	0 Antineoplastic	5 Other Antineoplastic M Monoclonal Antibody
0 Skin and Mucous Membranes	X External	2 Anti-infective	8 Oxazolidinones 9 Other Anti-infective
0 Skin and Mucous Membranes	X External	3 Anti-inflammatory B Anesthetic Agent K Other Diagnostic Substance M Pigment N Analgesics, Hypnotics, Sedatives T Destructive Agent	Z No Qualifier
0 Skin and Mucous Membranes	X External	G Other Therapeutic Substance	C Other Substance
1 Subcutaneous Tissue	0 Open	2 Anti-infective	A Anti-Infective Envelope
1 Subcutaneous Tissue	3 Percutaneous	0 Antineoplastic	5 Other Antineoplastic M Monoclonal Antibody
1 Subcutaneous Tissue	3 Percutaneous	2 Anti-infective	8 Oxazolidinones 9 Other Anti-infective A Anti-Infective Envelope
1 Subcutaneous Tissue	3 Percutaneous	3 Anti-inflammatory 6 Nutritional Substance 7 Electrolytic and Water Balance Substance B Anesthetic Agent H Radioactive Substance K Other Diagnostic Substance N Analgesics, Hypnotics, Sedatives T Destructive Agent	Z No Qualifier
1 Subcutaneous Tissue	3 Percutaneous	4 Serum, Toxoid and Vaccine	0 Influenza Vaccine Z No Qualifier
1 Subcutaneous Tissue	3 Percutaneous	G Other Therapeutic Substance	C Other Substance
1 Subcutaneous Tissue	3 Percutaneous	V Hormone	G Insulin J Other Hormone
2 Muscle	3 Percutaneous	0 Antineoplastic	5 Other Antineoplastic M Monoclonal Antibody
2 Muscle	3 Percutaneous	2 Anti-infective	8 Oxazolidinones 9 Other Anti-infective
2 Muscle	3 Percutaneous	3 Anti-inflammatory 6 Nutritional Substance 7 Electrolytic and Water Balance Substance B Anesthetic Agent H Radioactive Substance K Other Diagnostic Substance N Analgesics, Hypnotics, Sedatives T Destructive Agent	Z No Qualifier
2 Muscle	3 Percutaneous	4 Serum, Toxoid and Vaccine	0 Influenza Vaccine Z No Qualifier
2 Muscle	3 Percutaneous	G Other Therapeutic Substance	C Other Substance

Continued →

Section 3 Administration
Body System E Physiological Systems and Anatomical Regions
Operation 0 Introduction: Putting in or on a therapeutic, diagnostic, nutritional, physiological, or prophylactic substance except blood or blood products

3E0 Continued

Body System / Region (4th)	Approach (5th)	Substance (6th)	Qualifier (7th)
3 Peripheral Vein	0 Open	0 Antineoplastic	2 High-dose Interleukin-2 3 Low-dose Interleukin-2 5 Other Antineoplastic M Monoclonal Antibody P Clofarabine
3 Peripheral Vein	0 Open	1 Thrombolytic	6 Recombinant Human-activated Protein C 7 Other Thrombolytic
3 Peripheral Vein	0 Open	2 Anti-infective	8 Oxazolidinones 9 Other Anti-infective
3 Peripheral Vein	0 Open	3 Anti-inflammatory 4 Serum, Toxoid and Vaccine 6 Nutritional Substance 7 Electrolytic and Water Balance Substance F Intracirculatory Anesthetic H Radioactive Substance K Other Diagnostic Substance N Analgesics, Hypnotics, Sedatives P Platelet Inhibitor R Antiarrhythmic T Destructive Agent X Vasopressor	Z No Qualifier
3 Peripheral Vein	0 Open	G Other Therapeutic Substance	C Other Substance N Blood Brain Barrier Disruption
3 Peripheral Vein	0 Open	U Pancreatic Islet Cells	0 Autologous 1 Nonautologous
3 Peripheral Vein	0 Open	V Hormone	G Insulin H Human B-type Natriuretic Peptide J Other Hormone
3 Peripheral Vein	0 Open	W Immunotherapeutic	K Immunostimulator L Immunosuppressive
3 Peripheral Vein	3 Percutaneous	0 Antineoplastic	2 High-dose Interleukin-2 3 Low-dose Interleukin-2 5 Other Antineoplastic M Monoclonal Antibody P Clofarabine
3 Peripheral Vein	3 Percutaneous	1 Thrombolytic	6 Recombinant Human-activated Protein C 7 Other Thrombolytic
3 Peripheral Vein	3 Percutaneous	2 Anti-infective	8 Oxazolidinones 9 Other Anti-infective
3 Peripheral Vein	3 Percutaneous	3 Anti-inflammatory 4 Serum, Toxoid and Vaccine 6 Nutritional Substance 7 Electrolytic and Water Balance Substance F Intracirculatory Anesthetic H Radioactive Substance K Other Diagnostic Substance N Analgesics, Hypnotics, Sedatives P Platelet Inhibitor R Antiarrhythmic T Destructive Agent X Vasopressor	Z No Qualifier

Continued →

543

Section	**3**	**Administration**	
Body System	**E**	**Physiological Systems and Anatomical Regions**	
Operation	**0**	**Introduction:** Putting in or on a therapeutic, diagnostic, nutritional, physiological, or prophylactic substance except blood or blood products	

3E0 Continued

Body System / Region (4th)	Approach (5th)	Substance (6th)	Qualifier (7th)
3 Peripheral Vein	3 Percutaneous	G Other Therapeutic Substance	C Other Substance N Blood Brain Barrier Disruption Q Glucarpidase R Other Therapeutic Monoclonal Antibody
3 Peripheral Vein	3 Percutaneous	U Pancreatic Islet Cells	0 Autologous 1 Nonautologous
3 Peripheral Vein	3 Percutaneous	V Hormone	G Insulin H Human B-type Natriuretic Peptide J Other Hormone
3 Peripheral Vein	3 Percutaneous	W Immunotherapeutic	K Immunostimulator L Immunosuppressive
4 Central Vein	0 Open	0 Antineoplastic	2 High-dose Interleukin-2 3 Low-dose Interleukin-2 5 Other Antineoplastic M Monoclonal Antibody P Clofarabine
4 Central Vein	0 Open	1 Thrombolytic	6 Recombinant Human-activated Protein C 7 Other Thrombolytic
4 Central Vein	0 Open	2 Anti-infective	8 Oxazolidinones 9 Other Anti-infective
4 Central Vein	0 Open	3 Anti-inflammatory 4 Serum, Toxoid and Vaccine 6 Nutritional Substance 7 Electrolytic and Water Balance Substance F Intracirculatory Anesthetic H Radioactive Substance K Other Diagnostic Substance N Analgesics, Hypnotics, Sedatives P Platelet Inhibitor R Antiarrhythmic T Destructive Agent X Vasopressor	Z No Qualifier
4 Central Vein	0 Open	G Other Therapeutic Substance	C Other Substance N Blood Brain Barrier Disruption
4 Central Vein	0 Open	V Hormone	G Insulin H Human B-type Natriuretic Peptide J Other Hormone
4 Central Vein	0 Open	W Immunotherapeutic	K Immunostimulator L Immunosuppressive
4 Central Vein	3 Percutaneous	0 Antineoplastic	2 High-dose Interleukin-2 3 Low-dose Interleukin-2 5 Other Antineoplastic M Monoclonal Antibody P Clofarabine

Section	3	Administration
Body System	E	Physiological Systems and Anatomical Regions
Operation	0	Introduction: Putting in or on a therapeutic, diagnostic, nutritional, physiological, or prophylactic substance except blood or blood products

3E0 Continued

3E0

Body System / Region (4th)	Approach (5th)	Substance (6th)	Qualifier (7th)
4 Central Vein	3 Percutaneous	1 Thrombolytic	6 Recombinant Human-activated Protein C 7 Other Thrombolytic
4 Central Vein	3 Percutaneous	2 Anti-infective	8 Oxazolidinones 9 Other Anti-infective
4 Central Vein	3 Percutaneous	3 Anti-inflammatory 4 Serum, Toxoid and Vaccine 6 Nutritional Substance 7 Electrolytic and Water Balance Substance F Intracirculatory Anesthetic H Radioactive Substance K Other Diagnostic Substance N Analgesics, Hypnotics, Sedatives P Platelet Inhibitor R Antiarrhythmic T Destructive Agent X Vasopressor	Z No Qualifier
4 Central Vein	3 Percutaneous	G Other Therapeutic Substance	C Other Substance N Blood Brain Barrier Disruption Q Glucarpidase R Other Therapeutic Monoclonal Antibody
4 Central Vein	3 Percutaneous	V Hormone	G Insulin H Human B-type Natriuretic Peptide J Other Hormone
4 Central Vein	3 Percutaneous	W Immunotherapeutic	K Immunostimulator L Immunosuppressive
5 Peripheral Artery 6 Central Artery	0 Open 3 Percutaneous	0 Antineoplastic	2 High-dose Interleukin-2 3 Low-dose Interleukin-2 5 Other Antineoplastic M Monoclonal Antibody P Clofarabine
5 Peripheral Artery 6 Central Artery	0 Open 3 Percutaneous	1 Thrombolytic	6 Recombinant Human-activated Protein C 7 Other Thrombolytic
5 Peripheral Artery 6 Central Artery	0 Open 3 Percutaneous	2 Anti-infective	8 Oxazolidinones 9 Other Anti-infective
5 Peripheral Artery 6 Central Artery	0 Open 3 Percutaneous	3 Anti-inflammatory 4 Serum, Toxoid and Vaccine 6 Nutritional Substance 7 Electrolytic and Water Balance Substance F Intracirculatory Anesthetic H Radioactive Substance K Other Diagnostic Substance N Analgesics, Hypnotics, Sedatives P Platelet Inhibitor R Antiarrhythmic T Destructive Agent X Vasopressor	Z No Qualifier
5 Peripheral Artery 6 Central Artery	0 Open 3 Percutaneous	G Other Therapeutic Substance	C Other Substance N Blood Brain Barrier Disruption

Continued →

Administration Section Tables

545

Section	3	Administration
Body System	E	Physiological Systems and Anatomical Regions
Operation	0	**Introduction:** Putting in or on a therapeutic, diagnostic, nutritional, physiological, or prophylactic substance except blood or blood products

3E0 Continued

Body System / Region (4th)	Approach (5th)	Substance (6th)	Qualifier (7th)
5 Peripheral Artery 6 Central Artery	0 Open 3 Percutaneous	V Hormone	G Insulin H Human B-type Natriuretic Peptide J Other Hormone
5 Peripheral Artery 6 Central Artery	0 Open 3 Percutaneous	W Immunotherapeutic	K Immunostimulator L Immunosuppressive
7 Coronary Artery 8 Heart	0 Open 3 Percutaneous	1 Thrombolytic	6 Recombinant Human-activated Protein C 7 Other Thrombolytic
7 Coronary Artery 8 Heart	0 Open 3 Percutaneous	G Other Therapeutic Substance	C Other Substance
7 Coronary Artery 8 Heart	0 Open 3 Percutaneous	K Other Diagnostic Substance P Platelet Inhibitor	Z No Qualifier
7 Coronary Artery 8 Heart	4 Percutaneous Endoscopic	G Other Therapeutic Substance	C Other Substance
9 Nose	3 Percutaneous 7 Via Natural or Artificial Opening X External	0 Antineoplastic	5 Other Antineoplastic M Monoclonal Antibody
9 Nose	3 Percutaneous 7 Via Natural or Artificial Opening X External	2 Anti-infective	8 Oxazolidinones 9 Other Anti-infective
9 Nose	3 Percutaneous 7 Via Natural or Artificial Opening X External	3 Anti-inflammatory 4 Serum, Toxoid and Vaccine B Anesthetic Agent H Radioactive Substance K Other Diagnostic Substance N Analgesics, Hypnotics, Sedatives T Destructive Agent	Z No Qualifier
9 Nose	3 Percutaneous 7 Via Natural or Artificial Opening X External	G Other Therapeutic Substance	C Other Substance
A Bone Marrow	3 Percutaneous	0 Antineoplastic	5 Other Antineoplastic M Monoclonal Antibody
A Bone Marrow	3 Percutaneous	G Other Therapeutic Substance	C Other Substance
B Ear	3 Percutaneous 7 Via Natural or Artificial Opening X External	0 Antineoplastic	4 Liquid Brachytherapy Radioisotope 5 Other Antineoplastic M Monoclonal Antibody
B Ear	3 Percutaneous 7 Via Natural or Artificial Opening X External	2 Anti-infective	8 Oxazolidinones 9 Other Anti-infective

Continued →

546

Section	3	Administration
Body System	E	Physiological Systems and Anatomical Regions
Operation	0	Introduction: Putting in or on a therapeutic, diagnostic, nutritional, physiological, or prophylactic substance except blood or blood products

3E0 Continued

Body System / Region (4th)	Approach (5th)	Substance (6th)	Qualifier (7th)
B Ear	3 Percutaneous 7 Via Natural or Artificial Opening X External	3 Anti-inflammatory B Anesthetic Agent H Radioactive Substance K Other Diagnostic Substance N Analgesics, Hypnotics, Sedatives T Destructive Agent	Z No Qualifier
B Ear	3 Percutaneous 7 Via Natural or Artificial Opening X External	G Other Therapeutic Substance	C Other Substance
C Eye	3 Percutaneous 7 Via Natural or Artificial Opening X External	0 Antineoplastic	4 Liquid Brachytherapy Radioisotope 5 Other Antineoplastic M Monoclonal Antibody
C Eye	3 Percutaneous 7 Via Natural or Artificial Opening X External	2 Anti-infective	8 Oxazolidinones 9 Other Anti-infective
C Eye	3 Percutaneous 7 Via Natural or Artificial Opening X External	3 Anti-inflammatory B Anesthetic Agent H Radioactive Substance K Other Diagnostic Substance M Pigment N Analgesics, Hypnotics, Sedatives T Destructive Agent	Z No Qualifier
C Eye	3 Percutaneous 7 Via Natural or Artificial Opening X External	G Other Therapeutic Substance	C Other Substance
C Eye	3 Percutaneous 7 Via Natural or Artificial Opening X External	S Gas	F Other Gas
D Mouth and Pharynx	3 Percutaneous 7 Via Natural or Artificial Opening X External	0 Antineoplastic	4 Liquid Brachytherapy Radioisotope 5 Other Antineoplastic M Monoclonal Antibody
D Mouth and Pharynx	3 Percutaneous 7 Via Natural or Artificial Opening X External	2 Anti-infective	8 Oxazolidinones 9 Other Anti-infective
D Mouth and Pharynx	3 Percutaneous 7 Via Natural or Artificial Opening X External	3 Anti-inflammatory 4 Serum, Toxoid and Vaccine 6 Nutritional Substance 7 Electrolytic and Water Balance Substance B Anesthetic Agent H Radioactive Substance K Other Diagnostic Substance N Analgesics, Hypnotics, Sedatives R Antiarrhythmic T Destructive Agent	Z No Qualifier

Administration Section Tables

547

Section	3	Administration
Body System	E	Physiological Systems and Anatomical Regions
Operation	0	Introduction: Putting in or on a therapeutic, diagnostic, nutritional, physiological, or prophylactic substance except blood or blood products

3E0 Continued

Body System / Region (4th)	Approach (5th)	Substance (6th)	Qualifier (7th)
D Mouth and Pharynx	3 Percutaneous 7 Via Natural or Artificial Opening X External	G Other Therapeutic Substance	C Other Substance
E Products of Conception G Upper GI H Lower GI K Genitourinary Tract N Male Reproductive	3 Percutaneous 7 Via Natural or Artificial Opening 8 Via Natural or Artificial Opening Endoscopic	0 Antineoplastic	4 Liquid Brachytherapy Radioisotope 5 Other Antineoplastic M Monoclonal Antibody
E Products of Conception G Upper GI H Lower GI K Genitourinary Tract N Male Reproductive	3 Percutaneous 7 Via Natural or Artificial Opening 8 Via Natural or Artificial Opening Endoscopic	2 Anti-infective	8 Oxazolidinones 9 Other Anti-infective
E Products of Conception G Upper GI H Lower GI K Genitourinary Tract N Male Reproductive	3 Percutaneous 7 Via Natural or Artificial Opening 8 Via Natural or Artificial Opening Endoscopic	3 Anti-inflammatory 6 Nutritional Substance 7 Electrolytic and Water Balance Substance B Anesthetic Agent H Radioactive Substance K Other Diagnostic Substance N Analgesics, Hypnotics, Sedatives T Destructive Agent	Z No Qualifier
E Products of Conception G Upper GI H Lower GI K Genitourinary Tract N Male Reproductive	3 Percutaneous 7 Via Natural or Artificial Opening 8 Via Natural or Artificial Opening Endoscopic	G Other Therapeutic Substance	C Other Substance
E Products of Conception G Upper GI H Lower GI K Genitourinary Tract N Male Reproductive	3 Percutaneous 7 Via Natural or Artificial Opening 8 Via Natural or Artificial Opening Endoscopic	S Gas	F Other Gas
E Products of Conception G Upper GI H Lower GI K Genitourinary Tract N Male Reproductive	4 Percutaneous Endoscopic	G Other Therapeutic Substance	C Other Substance
F Respiratory Tract	3 Percutaneous 7 Via Natural or Artificial Opening 8 Via Natural or Artificial Opening Endoscopic	0 Antineoplastic	4 Liquid Brachytherapy Radioisotope 5 Other Antineoplastic M Monoclonal Antibody
F Respiratory Tract	3 Percutaneous 7 Via Natural or Artificial Opening 8 Via Natural or Artificial Opening Endoscopic	2 Anti-infective	8 Oxazolidinones 9 Other Anti-infective

Section 3 Administration
Body System E Physiological Systems and Anatomical Regions
Operation 0 Introduction: Putting in or on a therapeutic, diagnostic, nutritional, physiological, or prophylactic substance except blood or blood products

3E0 Continued

Body System / Region (4th)	Approach (5th)	Substance (6th)	Qualifier (7th)
F Respiratory Tract	3 Percutaneous 7 Via Natural or Artificial Opening 8 Via Natural or Artificial Opening Endoscopic	3 Anti-inflammatory 6 Nutritional Substance 7 Electrolytic and Water Balance Substance B Anesthetic Agent H Radioactive Substance K Other Diagnostic Substance N Analgesics, Hypnotics, Sedatives T Destructive Agent	Z No Qualifier
F Respiratory Tract	3 Percutaneous 7 Via Natural or Artificial Opening 8 Via Natural or Artificial Opening Endoscopic	G Other Therapeutic Substance	C Other Substance
F Respiratory Tract	3 Percutaneous 7 Via Natural or Artificial Opening 8 Via Natural or Artificial Opening Endoscopic	S Gas	D Nitric Oxide F Other Gas
F Respiratory Tract	4 Percutaneous Endoscopic	G Other Therapeutic Substance	C Other Substance
J Biliary and Pancreatic Tract	3 Percutaneous 7 Via Natural or Artificial Opening 8 Via Natural or Artificial Opening Endoscopic	0 Antineoplastic	4 Liquid Brachytherapy Radioisotope 5 Other Antineoplastic M Monoclonal Antibody
J Biliary and Pancreatic Tract	3 Percutaneous 7 Via Natural or Artificial Opening 8 Via Natural or Artificial Opening Endoscopic	2 Anti-infective	8 Oxazolidinones 9 Other Anti-infective
J Biliary and Pancreatic Tract	3 Percutaneous 7 Via Natural or Artificial Opening 8 Via Natural or Artificial Opening Endoscopic	3 Anti-inflammatory 6 Nutritional Substance 7 Electrolytic and Water Balance Substance B Anesthetic Agent H Radioactive Substance K Other Diagnostic Substance N Analgesics, Hypnotics, Sedatives T Destructive Agent	Z No Qualifier
J Biliary and Pancreatic Tract	3 Percutaneous 7 Via Natural or Artificial Opening 8 Via Natural or Artificial Opening Endoscopic	G Other Therapeutic Substance	C Other Substance
J Biliary and Pancreatic Tract	3 Percutaneous 7 Via Natural or Artificial Opening 8 Via Natural or Artificial Opening Endoscopic	S Gas	F Other Gas

Continued →

Section 3 **Administration**
Body System E **Physiological Systems and Anatomical Regions**
Operation 0 **Introduction:** Putting in or on a therapeutic, diagnostic, nutritional, physiological, or prophylactic substance except blood or blood products

3E0 Continued

Body System / Region (4th)	Approach (5th)	Substance (6th)	Qualifier (7th)
J Biliary and Pancreatic Tract	3 Percutaneous 7 Via Natural or Artificial Opening 8 Via Natural or Artificial Opening Endoscopic	U Pancreatic Islet Cells	0 Autologous 1 Nonautologous
J Biliary and Pancreatic Tract	4 Percutaneous Endoscopic	G Other Therapeutic Substance	C Other Substance
L Pleural Cavity	0 Open	5 Adhesion Barrier	Z No Qualifier
L Pleural Cavity	3 Percutaneous	0 Antineoplastic	4 Liquid Brachytherapy Radioisotope 5 Other Antineoplastic M Monoclonal Antibody
L Pleural Cavity	3 Percutaneous	2 Anti-infective	8 Oxazolidinones 9 Other Anti-infective
L Pleural Cavity	3 Percutaneous	3 Anti-inflammatory 5 Adhesion Barrier 6 Nutritional Substance 7 Electrolytic and Water Balance Substance B Anesthetic Agent H Radioactive Substance K Other Diagnostic Substance N Analgesics, Hypnotics, Sedatives T Destructive Agent	Z No Qualifier
L Pleural Cavity	3 Percutaneous	G Other Therapeutic Substance	C Other Substance
L Pleural Cavity	3 Percutaneous	S Gas	F Other Gas
L Pleural Cavity	4 Percutaneous Endoscopic	5 Adhesion Barrier	Z No Qualifier
L Pleural Cavity	4 Percutaneous Endoscopic	G Other Therapeutic Substance	C Other Substance
L Pleural Cavity	7 Via Natural or Artificial Opening	0 Antineoplastic	4 Liquid Brachytherapy Radioisotope 5 Other Antineoplastic M Monoclonal Antibody
L Pleural Cavity	7 Via Natural or Artificial Opening	S Gas	F Other Gas
M Peritoneal Cavity	0 Open	5 Adhesion Barrier	Z No Qualifier
M Peritoneal Cavity	3 Percutaneous	0 Antineoplastic	4 Liquid Brachytherapy Radioisotope 5 Other Antineoplastic M Monoclonal Antibody Y Hyperthermic
M Peritoneal Cavity	3 Percutaneous	2 Anti-infective	8 Oxazolidinones 9 Other Anti-infective

Continued →

Section	3	Administration
Body System	E	Physiological Systems and Anatomical Regions
Operation	0	Introduction: Putting in or on a therapeutic, diagnostic, nutritional, physiological, or prophylactic substance except blood or blood products

3E0 Continued

Body System / Region (4th)	Approach (5th)	Substance (6th)	Qualifier (7th)
M Peritoneal Cavity	3 Percutaneous	3 Anti-inflammatory 5 Adhesion Barrier 6 Nutritional Substance 7 Electrolytic and Water Balance Substance B Anesthetic Agent H Radioactive Substance K Other Diagnostic Substance N Analgesics, Hypnotics, Sedatives T Destructive Agent	Z No Qualifier
M Peritoneal Cavity	3 Percutaneous	G Other Therapeutic Substance	C Other Substance
M Peritoneal Cavity	3 Percutaneous	S Gas	F Other Gas
M Peritoneal Cavity	4 Percutaneous Endoscopic	5 Adhesion Barrier	Z No Qualifier
M Peritoneal Cavity	4 Percutaneous Endoscopic	G Other Therapeutic Substance	C Other Substance
M Peritoneal Cavity	7 Via Natural or Artificial Opening	0 Antineoplastic	4 Liquid Brachytherapy Radioisotope 5 Other Antineoplastic M Monoclonal Antibody
M Peritoneal Cavity	7 Via Natural or Artificial Opening	S Gas	F Other Gas
P Female Reproductive	0 Open	5 Adhesion Barrier	Z No Qualifier
P Female Reproductive	3 Percutaneous	0 Antineoplastic	4 Liquid Brachytherapy Radioisotope 5 Other Antineoplastic M Monoclonal Antibody
P Female Reproductive	3 Percutaneous	2 Anti-infective	8 Oxazolidinones 9 Other Anti-infective
P Female Reproductive	3 Percutaneous	3 Anti-inflammatory 5 Adhesion Barrier 6 Nutritional Substance 7 Electrolytic and Water Balance Substance B Anesthetic Agent H Radioactive Substance K Other Diagnostic Substance L Sperm N Analgesics, Hypnotics, Sedatives T Destructive Agent V Hormone	Z No Qualifier
P Female Reproductive	3 Percutaneous	G Other Therapeutic Substance	C Other Substance
P Female Reproductive	3 Percutaneous	Q Fertilized Ovum	0 Autologous 1 Nonautologous
P Female Reproductive	3 Percutaneous	S Gas	F Other Gas
P Female Reproductive	4 Percutaneous Endoscopic	5 Adhesion Barrier	Z No Qualifier
P Female Reproductive	4 Percutaneous Endoscopic	G Other Therapeutic Substance	C Other Substance
P Female Reproductive	7 Via Natural or Artificial Opening	0 Antineoplastic	4 Liquid Brachytherapy Radioisotope 5 Other Antineoplastic M Monoclonal Antibody

Continued →

551

Section	3	Administration
Body System	E	Physiological Systems and Anatomical Regions
Operation	0	Introduction: Putting in or on a therapeutic, diagnostic, nutritional, physiological, or prophylactic substance except blood or blood products

3E0 Continued

Body System / Region (4th)	Approach (5th)	Substance (6th)	Qualifier (7th)
P Female Reproductive	7 Via Natural or Artificial Opening	2 Anti-infective	8 Oxazolidinones 9 Other Anti-infective
P Female Reproductive	7 Via Natural or Artificial Opening	5 Adhesion Barrier 6 Nutritional Substance 7 Electrolytic and Water Balance Substance B Anesthetic Agent H Radioactive Substance K Other Diagnostic Substance L Sperm N Analgesics, Hypnotics, Sedatives T Destructive Agent V Hormone	Z No Qualifier
P Female Reproductive	7 Via Natural or Artificial Opening	G Other Therapeutic Substance	C Other Substance
P Female Reproductive	7 Via Natural or Artificial Opening	Q Fertilized Ovum	0 Autologous 1 Nonautologous
P Female Reproductive	7 Via Natural or Artificial Opening	S Gas	F Other Gas
P Female Reproductive	8 Via Natural or Artificial Opening Endoscopic	0 Antineoplastic	4 Liquid Brachytherapy Radioisotope 5 Other Antineoplastic M Monoclonal Antibody
P Female Reproductive	8 Via Natural or Artificial Opening Endoscopic	2 Anti-infective	8 Oxazolidinones 9 Other Anti-infective
P Female Reproductive	8 Via Natural or Artificial Opening Endoscopic	3 Anti-inflammatory 6 Nutritional Substance 7 Electrolytic and Water Balance Substance B Anesthetic Agent H Radioactive Substance K Other Diagnostic Substance N Analgesics, Hypnotics, Sedatives T Destructive Agent	Z No Qualifier
P Female Reproductive	8 Via Natural or Artificial Opening Endoscopic	G Other Therapeutic Substance	C Other Substance
P Female Reproductive	8 Via Natural or Artificial Opening Endoscopic	S Gas	F Other Gas
Q Cranial Cavity and Brain	0 Open 3 Percutaneous	0 Antineoplastic	4 Liquid Brachytherapy Radioisotope 5 Other Antineoplastic M Monoclonal Antibody
Q Cranial Cavity and Brain	0 Open 3 Percutaneous	2 Anti-infective	8 Oxazolidinones 9 Other Anti-infective
Q Cranial Cavity and Brain	0 Open 3 Percutaneous	3 Anti-inflammatory 6 Nutritional Substitute 7 Electrolytic and Water Balance Substitute A Stem Cells, Embryonic B Anesthetic Agent H Radioactive Substance K Other Diagnostic Substance N Analgesics, Hypnotics, Sedatives T Destructive Agent	Z No Qualifier

Continued →

Section 3 Administration
Body System E Physiological Systems and Anatomical Regions
Operation 0 Introduction: Putting in or on a therapeutic, diagnostic, nutritional, physiological, or prophylactic substance except blood or blood products

3E0 Continued

Body System / Region (4th)	Approach (5th)	Substance (6th)	Qualifier (7th)
Q Cranial Cavity and Brain	0 Open 3 Percutaneous	E Stem Cells, Somatic	0 Autologous 1 Nonautologous
Q Cranial Cavity and Brain	0 Open 3 Percutaneous	G Other Therapeutic Substance	C Other Substance
Q Cranial Cavity and Brain	0 Open 3 Percutaneous	S Gas	F Other Gas
Q Cranial Cavity and Brain	7 Via Natural or Artificial Opening	0 Antineoplastic	4 Liquid Brachytherapy Radioisotope 5 Other Antineoplastic M Monoclonal Antibody
Q Cranial Cavity and Brain	7 Via Natural or Artificial Opening	S Gas	F Other Gas
R Spinal Canal	0 Open	A Stem Cells, Embryonic	Z No Qualifier
R Spinal Canal	0 Open	E Stem Cells, Somatic	0 Autologous 1 Nonautologous
R Spinal Canal	3 Percutaneous	0 Antineoplastic	2 High-dose Interleukin-2 3 Low-dose Interleukin-2 4 Liquid Brachytherapy Radioisotope 5 Other Antineoplastic M Monoclonal Antibody
R Spinal Canal	3 Percutaneous	2 Anti-infective	8 Oxazolidinones 9 Other Anti-infective
R Spinal Canal	3 Percutaneous	3 Anti-inflammatory 6 Nutritional Substance 7 Electrolytic and Water Balance Substance A Stem Cells, Embryonic B Anesthetic Agent H Radioactive Substance K Other Diagnostic Substance N Analgesics, Hypnotics, Sedatives T Destructive Agent	Z No Qualifier
R Spinal Canal	3 Percutaneous	E Stem Cells, Somatic	0 Autologous 1 Nonautologous
R Spinal Canal	3 Percutaneous	G Other Therapeutic Substance	C Other Substance
R Spinal Canal	3 Percutaneous	S Gas	F Other Gas
R Spinal Canal	7 Via Natural or Artificial Opening	S Gas	F Other Gas
S Epidural Space	3 Percutaneous	0 Antineoplastic	2 High-dose Interleukin-2 3 Low-dose Interleukin-2 4 Liquid Brachytherapy Radioisotope 5 Other Antineoplastic M Monoclonal Antibody
S Epidural Space	3 Percutaneous	2 Anti-infective	8 Oxazolidinones 9 Other Anti-infective

Continued→

Section 3 Administration
Body System E Physiological Systems and Anatomical Regions
Operation 0 Introduction: Putting in or on a therapeutic, diagnostic, nutritional, physiological, or prophylactic substance except blood or blood products

3E0 Continued

Body System / Region (4th)	Approach (5th)	Substance (6th)	Qualifier (7th)
S Epidural Space	3 Percutaneous	3 Anti-inflammatory 6 Nutritional Substance 7 Electrolytic and Water Balance Substance B Anesthetic Agent H Radioactive Substance K Other Diagnostic Substance N Analgesics, Hypnotics, Sedatives T Destructive Agent	Z No Qualifier
S Epidural Space	3 Percutaneous	G Other Therapeutic Substance	C Other Substance
S Epidural Space	3 Percutaneous	S Gas	F Other Gas
S Epidural Space	7 Via Natural or Artificial Opening	S Gas	F Other Gas
T Peripheral Nerves and Plexi X Cranial Nerves	3 Percutaneous	3 Anti-inflammatory B Anesthetic Agent T Destructive Agent	Z No Qualifier
T Peripheral Nerves and Plexi X Cranial Nerves	3 Percutaneous	G Other Therapeutic Substance	C Other Substance
U Joints	0 Open	2 Anti-infective	8 Oxazolidinones 9 Other Anti-infective
U Joints	0 Open	G Other Therapeutic Substance	B Recombinant Bone Morphogenetic Protein
U Joints	3 Percutaneous	0 Antineoplastic	4 Liquid Brachytherapy Radioisotope 5 Other Antineoplastic M Monoclonal Antibody
U Joints	3 Percutaneous	2 Anti-infective	8 Oxazolidinones 9 Other Anti-infective
U Joints	3 Percutaneous	3 Anti-inflammatory 6 Nutritional Substance 7 Electrolytic and Water Balance Substance B Anesthetic Agent H Radioactive Substance K Other Diagnostic Substance N Analgesics, Hypnotics, Sedatives T Destructive Agent	Z No Qualifier
U Joints	3 Percutaneous	G Other Therapeutic Substance	B Recombinant Bone Morphogenetic Protein C Other Substance
U Joints	3 Percutaneous	S Gas	F Other Gas
U Joints	4 Percutaneous Endoscopic	G Other Therapeutic Substance	C Other Substance
V Bones	0 Open	G Other Therapeutic Substance	B Recombinant Bone Morphogenetic Protein C Other Substance
V Bones	3 Percutaneous	0 Antineoplastic	5 Other Antineoplastic M Monoclonal Antibody
V Bones	3 Percutaneous	2 Anti-infective	8 Oxazolidinones 9 Other Anti-infective

Continued →

Section	3	Administration
Body System	E	Physiological Systems and Anatomical Regions
Operation	0	Introduction: Putting in or on a therapeutic, diagnostic, nutritional, physiological, or prophylactic substance except blood or blood products

3E0 Continued

Body System / Region (4th)	Approach (5th)	Substance (6th)	Qualifier (7th)
V Bones	**3** Percutaneous	**3** Anti-inflammatory **6** Nutritional Substance **7** Electrolytic and Water Balance Substance **B** Anesthetic Agent **H** Radioactive Substance **K** Other Diagnostic Substance **N** Analgesics, Hypnotics, Sedatives **T** Destructive Agent	**Z** No Qualifier
V Bones	**3** Percutaneous	**G** Other Therapeutic Substance	**B** Recombinant Bone Morphogenetic Protein **C** Other Substance
V Bones	**4** Percutaneous Endoscopic	**G** Other Therapeutic Substance	**C** Other Substance
W Lymphatics	**3** Percutaneous	**0** Antineoplastic	**5** Other Antineoplastic **M** Monoclonal Antibody
W Lymphatics	**3** Percutaneous	**2** Anti-infective	**8** Oxazolidinones **9** Other Anti-infective
W Lymphatics	**3** Percutaneous	**3** Anti-inflammatory **6** Nutritional Substance **7** Electrolytic and Water Balance Substance **B** Anesthetic Agent **H** Radioactive Substance **K** Other Diagnostic Substance **N** Analgesics, Hypnotics, Sedatives **T** Destructive Agent	**Z** No Qualifier
W Lymphatics	**3** Percutaneous	**G** Other Therapeutic Substance	**C** Other Substance
Y Pericardial Cavity	**3** Percutaneous	**0** Antineoplastic	**4** Liquid Brachytherapy Radioisotope **5** Other Antineoplastic **M** Monoclonal Antibody
Y Pericardial Cavity	**3** Percutaneous	**2** Anti-infective	**8** Oxazolidinones **9** Other Anti-infective
Y Pericardial Cavity	**3** Percutaneous	**3** Anti-inflammatory **6** Nutritional Substance **7** Electrolytic and Water Balance Substance **B** Anesthetic Agent **H** Radioactive Substance **K** Other Diagnostic Substance **N** Analgesics, Hypnotics, Sedatives **T** Destructive Agent	**Z** No Qualifier
Y Pericardial Cavity	**3** Percutaneous	**G** Other Therapeutic Substance	**C** Other Substance
Y Pericardial Cavity	**3** Percutaneous	**S** Gas	**F** Other Gas
Y Pericardial Cavity	**4** Percutaneous Endoscopic	**G** Other Therapeutic Substance	**C** Other Substance
Y Pericardial Cavity	**7** Via Natural or Artificial Opening	**0** Antineoplastic	**4** Liquid Brachytherapy Radioisotope **5** Other Antineoplastic **M** Monoclonal Antibody
Y Pericardial Cavity	**7** Via Natural or Artificial Opening	**S** Gas	**F** Other Gas

Section	3	Administration
Body System	E	Physiological Systems and Anatomical Regions
Operation	1	Irrigation: Putting in or on a cleansing substance

Body System / Region (4th)	Approach (5th)	Substance (6th)	Qualifier (7th)
0 Skin and Mucous Membranes **C** Eye	**3** Percutaneous **X** External	**8** Irrigating Substance	**X** Diagnostic **Z** No Qualifier
9 Nose **B** Ear **F** Respiratory Tract **G** Upper GI **H** Lower GI **J** Biliary and Pancreatic Tract **K** Genitourinary Tract **N** Male Reproductive **P** Female Reproductive	**3** Percutaneous **7** Via Natural or Artificial Opening **8** Via Natural or Artificial Opening Endoscopic	**8** Irrigating Substance	**X** Diagnostic **Z** No Qualifier
L Pleural Cavity **Q** Cranial Cavity and Brain **R** Spinal Canal **S** Epidural Space **Y** Pericardial Cavity	**3** Percutaneous	**8** Irrigating Substance	**X** Diagnostic **Z** No Qualifier
M Peritoneal Cavity	**3** Percutaneous	**8** Irrigating Substance	**X** Diagnostic **Z** No Qualifier
M Peritoneal Cavity	**3** Percutaneous	**9** Dialysate	**Z** No Qualifier
M Peritoneal Cavity	**4** Percutaneous Endoscopic	**8** Irrigating Substance	**X** Diagnostic **Z** No Qualifier
U Joints	**3** Percutaneous **4** Percutaneous Endoscopic	**8** Irrigating Substance	**X** Diagnostic **Z** No Qualifier

AHA Coding Clinic

302A3H1 Transfusion of Nonautologous Whole Blood into Bone Marrow, Percutaneous Approach—AHA CC: 1Q, 2023, 11

3E013GC Introduction of Other Therapeutic Substance into Subcutaneous Tissue, Percutaneous Approach—AHA CC: 2Q, 2014, 10

3E0234Z Introduction of Serum, Toxoid and Vaccine into Muscle, Percutaneous Approach—AHA CC: 4Q, 2014, 16

3E03317 Introduction of Other Thrombolytic into Peripheral Vein, Percutaneous Approach—AHA CC: 4Q, 2013, 124; 4Q, 2020, 49-50

3E033VJ Introduction of Other Hormone into Peripheral Vein, Percutaneous Approach—AHA CC: 4Q, 2014, 17-18

3E04317 Introduction of Other Thrombolytic into Central Vein, Percutaneous Approach—AHA CC: 4Q, 2020, 49-50

3E043GC Introduction of Other Therapeutic Substance into Central Vein, Percutaneous Approach—AHA CC: 3Q, 2022, 26

3E05305 Introduction of Other Antineoplastic into Peripheral Artery, Percutaneous Approach—AHA CC: 1Q, 2015, 38

3E05317 Introduction of Other Thrombolytic into Peripheral Artery, Percutaneous Approach—AHA CC: 4Q, 2020, 49-50

3E06305 Introduction of Other Antineoplastic into Central Artery, Percutaneous Approach—AHA CC: 3Q, 2014 26-27

3E06317 Introduction of Other Thrombolytic into Central Artery, Percutaneous Approach—AHA CC: 4Q, 2014, 19-20; 4Q, 2020, 49-50

3E073GC Introduction of Other Therapeutic Substance into Coronary Artery, Percutaneous Approach—AHA CC: 3Q, 2018. 7-8

3E0E3KZ Other Diagnostic Substance into Products of Conception, Percutaneous Approach—AHA CC: 2Q, 2023, 33-34

3E0G76Z Introduction of Nutritional Substance into Upper GI, Via Natural or Artificial Opening—AHA CC: 2Q, 2015, 29

3E0G8GC Introduction of Other Therapeutic Substance into Upper GI, via Natural or Artificial Opening Endoscopic—AHA CC: 3Q, 2015, 24-25

3E0G8TZ Introduction of Destructive Agent into Upper GI, Via Natural or Artificial Opening Endoscopic—AHA CC: 1Q, 2013, 27

3E0H3GC Introduction of Other Therapeutic Substance into Lower GI, Percutaneous Approach—AHA CC: 1Q, 2017, 37

3E0L3GC Introduction of Other Therapeutic Substance into Pleural Cavity, Percutaneous Approach—AHA CC: 2Q, 2015, 31; 2Q, 2017, 14-15

3E0M30Y Introduction of Hyperthermic Antineoplastic into Peritoneal Cavity, Percutaneous Approach—AHA CC: 4Q, 2019, 37

3E0M3GC Introduction of Other Therapeutic Substance into Peritoneal Cavity, Percutaneous Approach—AHA CC: 4Q, 2014, 38

3E0P7GC Introduction of Other Therapeutic Substance into Female Reproductive, Via Natural or Artificial Opening—AHA CC: 2Q, 2014, 8-9

3E0Q005 Introduction of Other Antineoplastic into Cranial Cavity and Brain, Open Approach—AHA CC: 4Q, 2016, 114

3E0Q305 Introduction of Other Antineoplastic into Cranial Cavity and Brain, Percutaneous Approach—AHA CC: 4Q, 2014, 34-35

3E0R305 Introduction of Other Antineoplastic into Spinal Canal, Percutaneous Approach—AHA CC: 1Q, 2015, 31

3E0U0GB Introduction of Recombinant Bone Morphogenetic Protein into Joints, Open Approach—AHA CC: 1Q, 2018, 8

3E0V0GB Introduction of Recombinant Bone Morphogenetic Protein into Bones, Open Approach—AHA CC: 3Q, 2016, 29-30

Measurement and Monitoring Section (4A0–4B0)

Within each section of ICD-10-PCS the characters have different meanings. The seven character meanings for the Measurement and Monitoring section are illustrated here through the procedure example of *External electrocardiogram (EKG), single reading*.

Section	Body System	Root Operation	Body System	Approach	Function / Device	Qualifier
Measurement and Monitoring	Physiological Systems	Measurement	Cardiac	External	Electrical Activity	None
4	A	0	2	X	4	Z

Section (Character 1)

All Measurement and Monitoring procedure codes have a first character value of 4.

Body System (Character 2)

The alphanumeric character for the body system is placed in the second position. There are two character values applicable for the Measurement and Monitoring section. The character value of A is reported for physiological systems. The character value B is reported for physiological devices.

Root Operations (Character 3)

The alphanumeric character value for root operations is placed in the third position. Listed here are the root operations applicable to the Measurement and Monitoring section with their associated meaning.

Character Value	Root Operation	Root Operation Definition
0	Measurement	Determining the level of a physiological or physical function at a point in time
1	Monitoring	Determining the level of a physiological or physical function repetitively over a period of time

Body System/Region (Character 4)

For each body system the applicable body part character values will be available for procedure code construction. An example of a body region for this section is Respiratory.

Approach (Character 5)

The approach is the technique used to reach the procedure site. The following are the approach character values for the Measurement and Monitoring section with the associated definitions.

Character Value	Approach	Approach Definition
0	Open	Cutting through the skin or mucous membrane and any other body layers necessary to expose the site of the procedure
3	Percutaneous	Entry, by puncture or minor incision, of instrumentation through the skin or mucous membrane and any other body layers necessary to reach the site of the procedure
4	Percutaneous Endoscopic	Entry, by puncture or minor incision, of instrumentation through the skin or mucous membrane and any other body layers necessary to reach and visualize the site of the procedure
7	Via Natural or Artificial Opening	Entry of instrumentation through a natural or artificial external opening to reach the site of the procedure
8	Via Natural or Artificial Opening Endoscopic	Entry of instrumentation through a natural or artificial external opening to reach and visualize the site of the procedure
X	External	Procedures performed directly on the skin or mucous membrane and procedures performed indirectly by the application of external force through the skin or mucous membrane

Function/Device (Character 6)

In the Measurement and Monitoring section a function or device is always utilized. The function or device is reported in the sixth character position by the type of function monitored or measured or by the device utilized. The following is a sample list of the functions and devices included in this section:

- Conductivity
- Flow
- Metabolism
- Pressure
- Sound

Qualifier (Character 7)

The qualifier represents an additional attribute for the procedure when applicable. There are several qualifiers included in the Measurement and Monitoring section. For example, measurement procedures in this section include several qualifiers including stress that is reported with the character value of 4. If there is no qualifier for a procedure, the placeholder Z is the character valve that should be reported.

Measurement and Monitoring Section Tables

Measurement and Monitoring Tables 4A0–4B0

Section	4	Measurement and Monitoring
Body System	A	Physiological Systems
Operation	0	**Measurement:** Determining the level of a physiological or physical function at a point in time

Body System (4th)	Approach (5th)	Function / Device (6th)	Qualifier (7th)
0 Central Nervous	0 Open	2 Conductivity 4 Electrical Activity B Pressure	Z No Qualifier
0 Central Nervous	3 Percutaneous 7 Via Natural or Artificial Opening 8 Via Natural or Artificial Opening Endoscopic	4 Electrical Activity	Z No Qualifier
0 Central Nervous	3 Percutaneous 7 Via Natural or Artificial Opening 8 Via Natural or Artificial Opening Endoscopic	B Pressure K Temperature R Saturation	D Intracranial
0 Central Nervous	X External	2 Conductivity 4 Electrical Activity	Z No Qualifier
1 Peripheral Nervous	0 Open 3 Percutaneous 7 Via Natural or Artificial Opening 8 Via Natural or Artificial Opening Endoscopic X External	2 Conductivity	9 Sensory B Motor
1 Peripheral Nervous	0 Open 3 Percutaneous 7 Via Natural or Artificial Opening 8 Via Natural or Artificial Opening Endoscopic X External	4 Electrical Activity	Z No Qualifier
2 Cardiac	0 Open 3 Percutaneous 7 Via Natural or Artificial Opening 8 Via Natural or Artificial Opening Endoscopic	4 Electrical Activity 9 Output C Rate F Rhythm H Sound P Action Currents	Z No Qualifier
2 Cardiac	0 Open 3 Percutaneous 7 Via Natural or Artificial Opening 8 Via Natural or Artificial Opening Endoscopic	N Sampling and Pressure	6 Right Heart 7 Left Heart 8 Bilateral
2 Cardiac	X External	4 Electrical Activity	A Guidance Z No Qualifier

Continued →

Section	4	Measurement and Monitoring			4A0 Continued
Body System	A	Physiological Systems			
Operation	0	Measurement: Determining the level of a physiological or physical function at a point in time			

Body System (4th)	Approach (5th)	Function / Device (6th)	Qualifier (7th)
2 Cardiac	X External	9 Output C Rate F Rhythm H Sound P Action Currents	Z No Qualifier
2 Cardiac	X External	M Total Activity	4 Stress
3 Arterial	0 Open 3 Percutaneous	5 Flow J Pulse	1 Peripheral 3 Pulmonary C Coronary
3 Arterial	0 Open 3 Percutaneous	B Pressure	1 Peripheral 3 Pulmonary C Coronary F Other Thoracic
3 Arterial	0 Open 3 Percutaneous	H Sound R Saturation	1 Peripheral
3 Arterial	X External	5 Flow	1 Peripheral D Intracranial
3 Arterial	X External	B Pressure H Sound J Pulse R Saturation	1 Peripheral
4 Venous	0 Open 3 Percutaneous	5 Flow B Pressure J Pulse	0 Central 1 Peripheral 2 Portal 3 Pulmonary
4 Venous	0 Open 3 Percutaneous	R Saturation	1 Peripheral
4 Venous	4 Percutaneous Endoscopic	B Pressure	2 Portal
4 Venous	X External	5 Flow B Pressure J Pulse R Saturation	1 Peripheral
5 Circulatory	X External	L Volume	Z No Qualifier
6 Lymphatic	0 Open 3 Percutaneous 7 Via Natural or Artificial Opening 8 Via Natural or Artificial Opening Endoscopic	5 Flow B Pressure	Z No Qualifier
7 Visual	X External	0 Acuity 7 Mobility B Pressure	Z No Qualifier
8 Olfactory	X External	0 Acuity	Z No Qualifier
9 Respiratory	7 Via Natural or Artificial Opening 8 Via Natural or Artificial Opening Endoscopic X External	1 Capacity 5 Flow C Rate D Resistance L Volume M Total Activity	Z No Qualifier
B Gastrointestinal	7 Via Natural or Artificial Opening 8 Via Natural or Artificial Opening Endoscopic	8 Motility B Pressure G Secretion	Z No Qualifier

Continued →

Section 4 Measurement and Monitoring
Body System A Physiological Systems
Operation 0 Measurement: Determining the level of a physiological or physical function at a point in time

4A0 Continued

Body System (4th)	Approach (5th)	Function / Device (6th)	Qualifier (7th)
C Biliary	3 Percutaneous 4 Percutaneous Endoscopic 7 Via Natural or Artificial Opening 8 Via Natural or Artificial Opening Endoscopic	5 Flow B Pressure	Z No Qualifier
D Urinary	7 Via Natural or Artificial Opening 8 Via Natural or Artificial Opening Endoscopic	3 Contractility 5 Flow B Pressure D Resistance L Volume	Z No Qualifier
F Musculoskeletal	3 Percutaneous	3 Contractility	Z No Qualifier
F Musculoskeletal	3 Percutaneous	B Pressure	E Compartment
F Musculoskeletal	X External	3 Contractility	Z No Qualifier
H Products of Conception, Cardiac	7 Via Natural or Artificial Opening 8 Via Natural or Artificial Opening Endoscopic X External	4 Electrical Activity C Rate F Rhythm H Sound	Z No Qualifier
J Products of Conception, Nervous	7 Via Natural or Artificial Opening 8 Via Natural or Artificial Opening Endoscopic X External	2 Conductivity 4 Electrical Activity B Pressure	Z No Qualifier
Z None	7 Via Natural or Artificial Opening	6 Metabolism K Temperature	Z No Qualifier
Z None	X External	6 Metabolism K Temperature Q Sleep	Z No Qualifier

Section 4 Measurement and Monitoring
Body System A Physiological Systems
Operation 1 Monitoring: Determining the level of a physiological or physical function repetitively over a period of time

Body System (4th)	Approach (5th)	Function / Device (6th)	Qualifier (7th)
0 Central Nervous	0 Open	2 Conductivity B Pressure	Z No Qualifier
0 Central Nervous	0 Open	4 Electrical Activity	G Intraoperative Z No Qualifier
0 Central Nervous	3 Percutaneous 7 Via Natural or Artificial Opening 8 Via Natural or Artificial Opening Endoscopic	4 Electrical Activity	G Intraoperative Z No Qualifier
0 Central Nervous	3 Percutaneous 7 Via Natural or Artificial Opening 8 Via Natural or Artificial Opening Endoscopic	B Pressure K Temperature R Saturation	D Intracranial
0 Central Nervous	X External	2 Conductivity	Z No Qualifier
0 Central Nervous	X External	4 Electrical Activity	G Intraoperative Z No Qualifier
1 Peripheral Nervous	0 Open 3 Percutaneous 7 Via Natural or Artificial Opening 8 Via Natural or Artificial Opening Endoscopic X External	2 Conductivity	9 Sensory B Motor

Section	4	Measurement and Monitoring
Body System	A	Physiological Systems
Operation	1	Monitoring: Determining the level of a physiological or physical function repetitively over a period of time

4A1 Continued

Body System (4th)	Approach (5th)	Function / Device (6th)	Qualifier (7th)
1 Peripheral Nervous	0 Open 3 Percutaneous 7 Via Natural or Artificial Opening 8 Via Natural or Artificial Opening Endoscopic X External	4 Electrical Activity	G Intraoperative Z No Qualifier
2 Cardiac	0 Open 3 Percutaneous 7 Via Natural or Artificial Opening 8 Via Natural or Artificial Opening Endoscopic	4 Electrical Activity 9 Output C Rate F Rhythm H Sound	Z No Qualifier
2 Cardiac	X External	4 Electrical Activity	5 Ambulatory Z No Qualifier
2 Cardiac	X External	9 Output C Rate F Rhythm H Sound	Z No Qualifier
2 Cardiac	X External	M Total Activity	4 Stress
2 Cardiac	X External	S Vascular Perfusion	H Indocyanine Green Dye
3 Arterial	0 Open 3 Percutaneous	5 Flow B Pressure J Pulse	1 Peripheral 3 Pulmonary C Coronary
3 Arterial	0 Open 3 Percutaneous	H Sound R Saturation	1 Peripheral
3 Arterial	X External	5 Flow B Pressure H Sound J Pulse R Saturation	1 Peripheral
4 Venous	0 Open 3 Percutaneous	5 Flow B Pressure J Pulse	0 Central 1 Peripheral 2 Portal 3 Pulmonary
4 Venous	0 Open 3 Percutaneous	R Saturation	0 Central 2 Portal 3 Pulmonary
4 Venous	X External	5 Flow B Pressure J Pulse	1 Peripheral
6 Lymphatic	0 Open 3 Percutaneous 7 Via Natural or Artificial Opening 8 Via Natural or Artificial Opening Endoscopic	5 Flow	H Indocyanine Green Dye Z No Qualifier
6 Lymphatic	0 Open 3 Percutaneous 7 Via Natural or Artificial Opening 8 Via Natural or Artificial Opening Endoscopic	B Pressure	Z No Qualifier
9 Respiratory	7 Via Natural or Artificial Opening X External	1 Capacity 5 Flow C Rate D Resistance L Volume	Z No Qualifier
B Gastrointestinal	7 Via Natural or Artificial Opening 8 Via Natural or Artificial Opening Endoscopic	8 Motility B Pressure G Secretion	Z No Qualifier

Continued →

Section	4	Measurement and Monitoring	**4A1 Continued**
Body System	A	Physiological Systems	
Operation	1	Monitoring: Determining the level of a physiological or physical function repetitively over a period of time	

Body System (4th)	Approach (5th)	Function / Device (6th)	Qualifier (7th)
B Gastrointestinal	**X** External	**S** Vascular Perfusion	**H** Indocyanine Green Dye
D Urinary	**7** Via Natural or Artificial Opening **8** Via Natural or Artificial Opening Endoscopic	**3** Contractility **5** Flow **B** Pressure **D** Resistance **L** Volume	**Z** No Qualifier
G Skin and Breast	**X** External	**S** Vascular Perfusion	**H** Indocyanine Green Dye
H Products of Conception, Cardiac	**7** Via Natural or Artificial Opening **8** Via Natural or Artificial Opening Endoscopic **X** External	**4** Electrical Activity **C** Rate **F** Rhythm **H** Sound	**Z** No Qualifier
J Products of Conception, Nervous	**7** Via Natural or Artificial Opening **8** Via Natural or Artificial Opening Endoscopic **X** External	**2** Conductivity **4** Electrical Activity **B** Pressure	**Z** No Qualifier
Z None	**7** Via Natural or Artificial Opening	**K** Temperature	**Z** No Qualifier
Z None	**X** External	**K** Temperature **Q** Sleep	**Z** No Qualifier

Section	4	Measurement and Monitoring
Body System	B	Physiological Devices
Operation	0	Measurement: Determining the level of a physiological or physical function at a point in time

Body System (4th)	Approach (5th)	Function / Device (6th)	Qualifier (7th)
0 Central Nervous	**X** External	**V** Stimulator	**Z** No Qualifier
0 Central Nervous	**X** External	**W** Cerebrospinal Fluid Shunt	**0** Wireless Sensor
1 Peripheral Nervous **F** Musculoskeletal	**X** External	**V** Stimulator	**Z** No Qualifier
2 Cardiac	**X** External	**S** Pacemaker **T** Defibrillator	**Z** No Qualifier
9 Respiratory	**X** External	**S** Pacemaker	**Z** No Qualifier

AHA Coding Clinic

4A0234Z Measurement of Cardiac Electrical Activity, Percutaneous Approach—AHA CC: 1Q, 2022, 46-47

4A023N6 Measurement of Cardiac Sampling and Pressure, Right Heart, Percutaneous Approach—AHA CC: 3Q, 2019, 32

4A023N8 Measurement of Cardiac Sampling and Pressure, Bilateral, Percutaneous Approach—AHA CC: 1Q, 2018, 12-13

4A02X4Z Measurement of Cardiac Electrical Activity, External Approach—AHA CC: 3Q, 2015, 29

4A033BC Measurement of Arterial Pressure, Coronary, Percutaneous Approach—AHA CC: 3Q, 2016, 37

4A0F3BE Measurement of Musculoskeletal Pressure, Compartment, Percutaneous Approach—AHA CC: 4Q, 2020, 63-64

4A103BD Monitoring of Intracranial Pressure, Percutaneous Approach—AHA CC: 2Q, 2016, 29

4A1134G Monitoring of Peripheral Nervous Electrical Activity, Intraoperative, Percutaneous Approach—AHA CC: 4Q, 2014, 28-29

4A11X4G Monitoring of Peripheral Nervous Electrical Activity, Intraoperative, External Approach—AHA CC: 1Q, 2015, 26; 2Q, 2015, 14

4A1239Z Monitoring of Cardiac Output, Percutaneous Approach—AHA CC: 3Q, 2015, 35

4A133B1 Monitoring of Arterial Pressure, Peripheral, Percutaneous Approach, for Continuous Monitoring of Pressure—AHA CC: 2Q, 2016, 33

4A133B3 Monitoring of Arterial Pressure, Pulmonary, Percutaneous Approach—AHA CC: 3Q, 2015, 35

4A133J1 Monitoring of Arterial Pulse, Peripheral, Percutaneous Approach, for Continuous Monitoring of Pulse—AHA CC: 2Q, 2016, 33

Extracorporeal or Systemic Assistance and Performance Section (5A0–5A2)

Within each section of ICD-10-PCS the characters have different meanings. The seven character meanings for the Extracorporeal or Systemic Assistance and Performance section are illustrated here through the procedure example of *Hyperbaric oxygenation of wound*.

Section	Body System	Root Operation	Body System	Duration	Function	Qualifier
Extracorporeal or Systemic Assistance and Performance	Physiological Systems	Assistance	Circulatory	Intermittent	Oxygenation	Hyperbaric
5	A	0	5	1	2	1

Section (Character 1)

All Extracorporeal or Systemic Assistance and Performance procedure codes have a first character value of 5.

Body System (Character 2)

The alphanumeric character for the body system is placed in the second position. There is one character value applicable for the Extracorporeal or Systemic Assistance and Performance section. The character value of A is reported for physiological systems.

Root Operations (Character 3)

The alphanumeric character value for root operations is placed in the third position. Listed here are the root operations applicable to the Extracorporeal or Systemic Assistance and Performance section with their associated meaning.

Character Value	Root Operation	Root Operation Definition
0	Assistance	Taking over a portion of a physiological function by extracorporeal means
1	Performance	Completely taking over a physiological function by extracorporeal means
2	Restoration	Returning, or attempting to return, a physiological function to its original state by extracorporeal means

Body System (Character 4)

For each body system, the applicable body part character values will be available for procedure code construction. An example of a body region for this section is respiratory.

Duration (Character 5)

The duration represents the length of time or frequency for which the assistance or performance is utilized. Some examples of duration are Intermittent, Continuous, or Less than 24 consecutive hours.

Function (Character 6)

In the Extracorporeal or Systemic Assistance and Performance section a function is always reported. The function is reported in the sixth character position. The following is a sample list of the functions utilized in this section:

- Output
- Oxygenation
- Pacing
- Ventilation

Qualifier (Character 7)

The qualifier represents an additional attribute for the procedure when applicable. There are several qualifiers included in the Extracorporeal or Systemic Assistance and Performance section. For example, assistance procedures in this section include several qualifiers including Balloon Pump, which is reported with the character value of 0. If there is no qualifier for a procedure, the placeholder Z is the character valve that should be reported.

Extracorporeal or Systemic Assistance and Performance Section Tables

Extracorporeal or Systemic Assistance and Performance Tables 5A0–5A2

Section	5	Extracorporeal or Systemic Assistance and Performance
Body System	A	Physiological Systems
Operation	0	Assistance: Taking over a portion of a physiological function by extracorporeal means

Body System (4th)	Duration (5th)	Function (6th)	Qualifier (7th)
2 Cardiac	1 Intermittent	1 Output	0 Balloon Pump 5 Pulsatile Compression 6 Other Pump D Impeller Pump
2 Cardiac	2 Continuous	1 Output	0 Balloon Pump 5 Pulsatile Compression 6 Other Pump D Impeller Pump
2 Cardiac	2 Continuous	2 Oxygenation	C Supersaturated
5 Circulatory	1 Intermittent 2 Continuous	2 Oxygenation	1 Hyperbaric
9 Respiratory	2 Continuous	0 Filtration	Z No Qualifier
9 Respiratory	3 Less than 24 Consecutive Hours 4 24-96 Consecutive Hours 5 Greater than 96 Consecutive Hours	5 Ventilation	7 Continuous Positive Airway Pressure 8 Intermittent Positive Airway Pressure 9 Continuous Negative Airway Pressure A High Nasal Flow/Velocity B Intermittent Negative Airway Pressure Z No Qualifier
9 Respiratory	B Less than 8 Consecutive Hours C 8-24 Consecutive Hours D Greater than 24 Consecutive Hours	5 Ventilation	K Intubated Prone Positioning

Section	5	Extracorporeal or Systemic Assistance and Performance
Body System	A	Physiological Systems
Operation	1	Performance: Completely taking over a physiological function by extracorporeal means

Body System (4th)	Duration (5th)	Function (6th)	Qualifier (7th)
2 Cardiac	0 Single	1 Output	2 Manual
2 Cardiac	1 Intermittent	3 Pacing	Z No Qualifier
2 Cardiac	2 Continuous	1 Output	J Automated Z No Qualifier
2 Cardiac	2 Continuous	3 Pacing	Z No Qualifier
5 Circulatory	2 Continuous A Intraoperative	2 Oxygenation	F Membrane, Central G Membrane, Peripheral Veno-arterial H Membrane, Peripheral Veno-venous
9 Respiratory	0 Single	5 Ventilation	4 Nonmechanical
9 Respiratory	3 Less than 24 Consecutive Hours 4 24-96 Consecutive Hours 5 Greater than 96 Consecutive Hours	5 Ventilation	Z No Qualifier
C Biliary	0 Single 6 Multiple	0 Filtration	Z No Qualifier
D Urinary	7 Intermittent, Less than 6 Hours Per Day 8 Prolonged Intermittent, 6-18 Hours Per Day 9 Continuous, Greater than 18 Hours Per Day	0 Filtration	Z No Qualifier

564

Section	5	**Extracorporeal or Systemic Assistance and Performance**
Body System	A	**Physiological Systems**
Operation	2	**Restoration:** Returning, or attempting to return, a physiological function to its original state by extracorporeal means.

Body System (4ᵗʰ)	Duration (5ᵗʰ)	Function (6ᵗʰ)	Qualifier (7ᵗʰ)
2 Cardiac	**0** Single	**4** Rhythm	**Z** No Qualifier

AHA Coding Clinic

5A02110 Assistance with Cardiac Output using Balloon Pump, Intermittent—AHA CC: 3Q, 2022, 23-24

5A02210 Assistance with Cardiac Output using Balloon Pump, Continuous—AHA CC: 3Q, 2013, 18-19; 2Q, 2018, 4-5; 2Q, 2021, 12

5A0221D Assistance with Cardiac Output using Impeller Pump, Continuous—AHA CC: 3Q, 2014, 19; 4Q, 2016, 138-139; 1Q, 2017, 11-12; 4Q, 2017, 43-45

5A09357 Assistance with Respiratory Ventilation, <24 Hrs, CPAP—AHA CC: 4Q, 2014, 9-10; 1Q, 2020, 10-11

5A09457 Assistance with Respiratory Ventilation, 24-96 Hrs, CPAP—AHA CC: 4Q, 2014, 9-10

5A09557 Assistance with Respiratory Ventilation, >96 Hrs, CPAP—AHA CC: 4Q, 2014, 9-10

5A1221Z Performance of Cardiac Output, Continuous—AHA CC: 3Q, 2013, 18-19; 1Q, 2014, 10-11; 3Q, 2014, 16-17, 20-21; 4Q, 2015, 22-25; 1Q, 2016, 27-28; 1Q, 2017, 19-20; 3Q, 2017, 7-8

ECMO, Extracorporeal Oxygenation, Membrane—AHA CC: 3Q, 2019, 19-23; 4Q, 2019, 39-41

5A1223Z Performance of Cardiac Pacing, Continuous—AHA CC: 3Q, 2013, 18-19; 2Q, 2022, 25

5A1522F Extracorporeal Oxygenation, Membrane, Central—AHA CC: 2Q, 2019, 36

5A1522G Extracorporeal Oxygenation, Membrane, Peripheral Veno-arterial—AHA CC: 4Q, 2018, 53-54

5A1522H Extracorporeal Oxygenation, Membrane, Peripheral Veno-venous—AHA CC: 4Q, 2018. 53-54

5A15A2G Extracorporeal Oxygenation, Membrane, Peripheral Veno-arterial, Intraoperative—AHA CC: 4Q, 2019, 39-40

5A1935Z Respiratory Ventilation, Less than 24 Consecutive Hours—AHA CC: 4Q, 2014, 3-15; 1Q, 2018, 13-14

5A1945Z Respiratory Ventilation, 24-96 Consecutive Hours—AHA CC: 4Q, 2014, 3-15

5A1955Z Respiratory Ventilation, Greater than 96 Consecutive Hours—AHA CC: 4Q, 2014, 3-15

5A1C00Z Performance of Biliary Filtration, Single—AHA CC: 1Q, 2016, 28-29

5A1D60Z Performance of Urinary Filtration, Multiple—AHA CC: 1Q, 2016, 29

5A1D70Z Performance of Urinary Filtration, Intermittent, Less than 6 Hours Per Day—AHA CC: 4Q, 2017, 72-73

5A1D80Z Performance of Urinary Filtration, Prolonged Intermittent, 6-18 hours Per Day—AHA CC: 4Q, 2017, 72

5A1D90Z Performance of Urinary Filtration, Continuous, Greater than 18 hours Per Day—AHA CC: 4Q, 2017, 72-73

5A2204Z Restoration of Cardiac Rhythm, Single—AHA CC: 1Q, 2022, 46-47

Extracorporeal or Systemic Therapies Section (6A0–6AB)

Within each section of ICD-10-PCS the characters have different meanings. The seven character meanings for the Extracorporeal or Systemic Therapies section are illustrated here through the procedure example of *Ultraviolet light phototherapy, series treatment*.

Section	Body System	Root Operation	Body System	Duration	Qualifier	Qualifier
Extracorporeal or Systemic Therapies	Physiological Systems	UV Light Therapy	Skin	Multiple	None	None
6	A	8	0	1	Z	Z

Section (Character 1)

All Extracorporeal or Systemic Therapies procedure codes have a first character value of 6.

Body System (Character 2)

The alphanumeric character for the body system is placed in the second position. There is one character value applicable for the Extracorporeal or Systemic Therapies section. The character value of A is reported for physiological systems.

Root Operations (Character 3)

The alphanumeric character value for root operations is placed in the third position. Listed below are the root operations applicable to the Extracorporeal or Systemic Therapies section with their associated meaning.

Character Value	Root Operation	Root Operation Definition
0	Atmospheric Control	Extracorporeal control of atmospheric pressure and composition
1	Decompression	Extracorporeal elimination of undissolved gas from body fluids
2	Electromagnetic Therapy	Extracorporeal treatment by electromagnetic rays
3	Hyperthermia	Extracorporeal raising of body temperature
4	Hypothermia	Extracorporeal lowering of body temperature
5	Pheresis	Extracorporeal separation of blood products
6	Phototherapy	Extracorporeal treatment by light rays
7	Ultrasound Therapy	Extracorporeal treatment by ultrasound
8	Ultraviolet Light Therapy	Extracorporeal treatment by ultraviolet light
9	Shock Wave Therapy	Extracorporeal treatment by shock waves
B	Perfusion	Extracorporeal treatment by diffusion of therapeutic fluid

Body System (Character 4)

For each body system the applicable body part character values will be available for procedure code construction. An example of a body region for this section is Skin.

Duration (Character 5)

The duration represents the number of therapy sessions performed. Single is reported with character value 0; Multiple is reported with character value 1.

Qualifier (Character 6)

Character 6 is the first of two qualifier characters for the Extracorporeal or Systemic Therapies section. The qualifier represents an additional attribute for the procedure when applicable. There are currently no qualifier values for the sixth character position, so the character value of Z is always reported.

Qualifier (Character 7)

Character 7 is the second of two qualifier characters for the Extracorporeal or Systemic Therapies section. The qualifier represents an additional attribute for the procedure when applicable. There are some qualifiers included in the Extracorporeal or Systemic Therapies section. For example, pheresis procedures in this section include several qualifiers including Plasma that is reported with the character value of 3. If there is no qualifier for a procedure, the placeholder Z is the character valve that should be reported.

Extracorporeal or Systemic Therapies Section Tables

Extracorporeal or Systemic Therapies Tables 6A0–6AB

Section	6	Extracorporeal or Systemic Therapies
Body System	A	Physiological Systems
Operation	0	Atmospheric Control: Extracorporeal control of atmospheric pressure and composition

Body System (4ᵗʰ)	Duration (5ᵗʰ)	Qualifier (6ᵗʰ)	Qualifier (7ᵗʰ)
Z None	0 Single 1 Multiple	Z No Qualifier	Z No Qualifier

Section	6	Extracorporeal or Systemic Therapies
Body System	A	Physiological Systems
Operation	1	Decompression: Extracorporeal elimination of undissolved gas from body fluids

Body System (4ᵗʰ)	Duration (5ᵗʰ)	Qualifier (6ᵗʰ)	Qualifier (7ᵗʰ)
5 Circulatory	0 Single 1 Multiple	Z No Qualifier	Z No Qualifier

Section	6	Extracorporeal or Systemic Therapies
Body System	A	Physiological Systems
Operation	2	Electromagnetic Therapy: Extracorporeal treatment by electromagnetic rays

Body System (4ᵗʰ)	Duration (5ᵗʰ)	Qualifier (6ᵗʰ)	Qualifier (7ᵗʰ)
1 Urinary 2 Central Nervous	0 Single 1 Multiple	Z No Qualifier	Z No Qualifier

Section	6	Extracorporeal or Systemic Therapies
Body System	A	Physiological Systems
Operation	3	Hyperthermia: Extracorporeal raising of body temperature

Body System (4ᵗʰ)	Duration (5ᵗʰ)	Qualifier (6ᵗʰ)	Qualifier (7ᵗʰ)
Z None	0 Single 1 Multiple	Z No Qualifier	Z No Qualifier

Section	6	Extracorporeal or Systemic Therapies
Body System	A	Physiological Systems
Operation	4	Hypothermia: Extracorporeal lowering of body temperature

Body System (4ᵗʰ)	Duration (5ᵗʰ)	Qualifier (6ᵗʰ)	Qualifier (7ᵗʰ)
Z None	0 Single 1 Multiple	Z No Qualifier	Z No Qualifier

Section	6	Extracorporeal or Systemic Therapies
Body System	A	Physiological Systems
Operation	5	Pheresis: Extracorporeal separation of blood products

Body System (4ᵗʰ)	Duration (5ᵗʰ)	Qualifier (6ᵗʰ)	Qualifier (7ᵗʰ)
5 Circulatory	0 Single 1 Multiple	Z No Qualifier	0 Erythrocytes 1 Leukocytes 2 Platelets 3 Plasma T Stem Cells, Cord Blood V Stem Cells, Hematopoietic

Section 6 **Extracorporeal or Systemic Therapies**
Body System A **Physiological Systems**
Operation 6 **Phototherapy:** Extracorporeal treatment by light rays

Body System (4th)	Duration (5th)	Qualifier (6th)	Qualifier (7th)
0 Skin 5 Circulatory	0 Single 1 Multiple	Z No Qualifier	Z No Qualifier

Section 6 **Extracorporeal or Systemic Therapies**
Body System A **Physiological Systems**
Operation 7 **Ultrasound Therapy:** Extracorporeal treatment by ultrasound

Body System (4th)	Duration (5th)	Qualifier (6th)	Qualifier (7th)
5 Circulatory	0 Single 1 Multiple	Z No Qualifier	4 Head and Neck Vessels 5 Heart 6 Peripheral Vessels 7 Other Vessels Z No Qualifier

Section 6 **Extracorporeal or Systemic Therapies**
Body System A **Physiological Systems**
Operation 8 **Ultraviolet Light Therapy:** Extracorporeal treatment by ultraviolet light

Body System (4th)	Duration (5th)	Qualifier (6th)	Qualifier (7th)
0 Skin	0 Single 1 Multiple	Z No Qualifier	Z No Qualifier

Section 6 **Extracorporeal or Systemic Therapies**
Body System A **Physiological Systems**
Operation 9 **Shock Wave Therapy:** Extracorporeal treatment by shock waves

Body System (4th)	Duration (5th)	Qualifier (6th)	Qualifier (7th)
3 Musculoskeletal	0 Single 1 Multiple	Z No Qualifier	Z No Qualifier

Section 6 **Extracorporeal or Systemic Therapies**
Body System A **Physiological Systems**
Operation B **Perfusion:** Extracorporeal treatment by diffusion of therapeutic fluid

Body System (4th)	Duration (5th)	Qualifier (6th)	Qualifier (7th)
5 Circulatory B Respiratory System F Hepatobiliary System and Pancreas T Urinary System	0 Single	B Donor Organ	Z No Qualifier

AHA Coding Clinic

6A4Z0ZZ Hypothermia, Single—AHA CC: 2Q, 2019, 17-18
6A550ZT Pheresis of Cord Blood Stem Cells, Single—AHA CC: 1Q, 2022, 48
6A750Z7 Ultrasound Therapy of Other Vessels, Single—AHA CC: 4Q, 2014, 19-20

Osteopathic Section (7W0)

Within each section of ICD-10-PCS, the characters have different meanings. The seven character meanings for the Osteopathic section are illustrated below through the procedure example of Indirect osteopathic treatment of sacrum.

Section	Body System	Root Operation	Body Region	Approach	Method	Qualifier
Osteopathic	Anatomical Regions	Treatment	Sacrum	External	Indirect	None
7	W	0	4	X	4	Z

Section (Character 1)

All Osteopathic procedure codes have a first character value of 7.

Body System (Character 2)

The alphanumeric character for the body system is placed in the second position. There is one character value applicable for the Osteopathic section. The character value of W is reported for anatomical regions.

Root Operations (Character 3)

The alphanumeric character value for root operations is placed in the third position. Listed here is the root operation applicable to the Osteopathic section with its associated meaning.

Character Value	Root Operation	Root Operation Definition
0	Treatment	Manual treatment to eliminate or alleviate somatic dysfunction and related disorders

Body Region (Character 4)

For each body region the applicable body part character values will be available for procedure code construction. An example of a body region for this section is Head.

Approach (Character 5)

The approach is the technique used to reach the procedure site. The following are the approach character values for the Osteopathic section with the associated definitions.

Character Value	Approach	Approach Definition
X	External	Procedures performed directly on the skin or mucous membrane and procedures performed indirectly by the application of external force through the skin or mucous membrane

Method (Character 6)

The method identifies the treatment method used to complete the osteopathic procedure. The available methods are:

- Articulatory-Raising
- Fascial Release
- General Mobilization
- High Velocity-Low Amplitude
- Indirect
- Low Velocity-High Amplitude
- Lymphatic Pump
- Muscle Energy-Isometric
- Muscle Energy-Isotonic
- Other

Qualifier (Character 7)

The qualifier represents an additional attribute for the procedure when applicable. Currently, there are no qualifiers in the Osteopathic section; therefore, the placeholder character value of Z should be reported.

Osteopathic Section Table

Osteopathic Table 7W0

Section   **7**   **Osteopathic**
Body System   **W**   **Anatomical Regions**
Operation   **0**   **Treatment:** Manual treatment to eliminate or alleviate somatic dysfunction and related disorders

Body Region (4th)	Approach (5th)	Method (6th)	Qualifier (7th)
0 Head	X External	0 Articulatory-Raising	Z None
1 Cervical		1 Fascial Release	
2 Thoracic		2 General Mobilization	
3 Lumbar		3 High Velocity-Low Amplitude	
4 Sacrum		4 Indirect	
5 Pelvis		5 Low Velocity-High Amplitude	
6 Lower Extremities		6 Lymphatic Pump	
7 Upper Extremities		7 Muscle Energy-Isometric	
8 Rib Cage		8 Muscle Energy-Isotonic	
9 Abdomen		9 Other Method	

AHA Coding Clinic

No references have been issued for the Osteopathic Section.

Other Procedures Section (8C0–8E0)

Within each section of ICD-10-PCS the characters have different meanings. The seven character meanings for the Other Procedures section are illustrated here through the procedure example of Yoga therapy.

Section	Body System	Root Operation	Body Region	Approach	Method	Qualifier
Other Procedures	Physiological Systems and Anatomical Regions	Other Procedures	None	External	Other Method	Yoga Therapy
8	E	0	Z	X	Y	4

Section (Character 1)

All Other Procedures codes have a first character value of 8.

Body System (Character 2)

The alphanumeric character for the body system is placed in the second position. There are two character values applicable for the Other Procedures section. The character value of C is reported for indwelling device. The character value of E is reported for physiological system and anatomical regions.

Root Operations (Character 3)

The alphanumeric character value for root operations is placed in the third position. Listed here is the root operation applicable to the Other Procedures section with its associated meaning.

Character Value	Root Operation	Root Operation Definition
0	Other Procedures	Methodologies which attempt to remediate or cure a disorder or disease

Body Region (Character 4)

For each body region the applicable body part character values will be available for procedure code construction. An example of a body region for this section is Lower Extremity.

Approach (Character 5)

The approach is the technique used to reach the procedure site. The following are the approach character values for the Other Procedures section with the associated definitions.

Character Value	Approach	Approach Definition
0	Open	Cutting through the skin or mucous membrane and any other body layers necessary to expose the site of the procedure
3	Percutaneous	Entry, by puncture or minor incision, of instrumentation through the skin or mucous membrane and any other body layers necessary to reach the site of the procedure
4	Percutaneous Endoscopic	Entry, by puncture or minor incision, of instrumentation through the skin or mucous membrane and any other body layers necessary to reach and visualize the site of the procedure
7	Via Natural or Artificial Opening	Entry of instrumentation through a natural or artificial external opening to reach the site of the procedure
8	Via Natural or Artificial Opening Endoscopic	Entry of instrumentation through a natural or artificial external opening to reach and visualize the site of the procedure
X	External	Procedures performed directly on the skin or mucous membrane and procedures performed indirectly by the application of external force through the skin or mucous membrane

Method (Character 6)

The method identifies the treatment method used to complete the other procedure. The available methods are:

- Acupuncture
- Collection
- Computer Assisted Procedure
- Near Infrared Spectroscopy
- Robotic Assisted procedure
- Therapeutic Massage
- Other

Qualifier (Character 7)

The qualifier represents an additional attribute for the procedure when applicable. In the preceding example of Yoga therapy, the qualifier of 4 was used to report that the other procedure was Yoga therapy. If there is no qualifier for a procedure, the placeholder Z is the character valve that should be reported.

Other Procedures Section Tables

Other Procedures Tables 8C0–8E0

Section 8 Other Procedures
Body System C Indwelling Device
Operation 0 Other Procedures: Methodologies which attempt to remediate or cure a disorder or disease

Body Region (4th)	Approach (5th)	Method (6th)	Qualifier (7th)
1 Nervous System	X External	6 Collection	J Cerebrospinal Fluid L Other Fluid
2 Circulatory System	X External	6 Collection	K Blood L Other Fluid

Section 8 Other Procedures
Body System E Physiological Systems and Anatomical Regions
Operation 0 Other Procedures: Methodologies which attempt to remediate or cure a disorder or disease

Body Region (4th)	Approach (5th)	Method (6th)	Qualifier (7th)
1 Nervous System	X External	Y Other Method	7 Examination
2 Circulatory System	3 Percutaneous X External	D Near Infrared Spectroscopy	Z No Qualifier
9 Head and Neck Region	0 Open	C Robotic Assisted Procedure	Z No Qualifier
9 Head and Neck Region	0 Open	E Fluorescence Guided Procedure	M Aminolevulinic Acid Z No Qualifier
9 Head and Neck Region	3 Percutaneous 4 Percutaneous Endoscopic 7 Via Natural or Artificial Opening 8 Via Natural or Artificial Opening Endoscopic	C Robotic Assisted Procedure E Fluorescence Guided Procedure	Z No Qualifier
9 Head and Neck Region	X External	B Computer Assisted Procedure	F With Fluoroscopy G With Computerized Tomography H With Magnetic Resonance Imaging Z No Qualifier
9 Head and Neck Region	X External	C Robotic Assisted Procedure	Z No Qualifier
9 Head and Neck Region	X External	Y Other Method	8 Suture Removal
H Integumentary System and Breast	3 Percutaneous	0 Acupuncture	0 Anesthesia Z No Qualifier
H Integumentary System and Breast	X External	6 Collection	2 Breast Milk

Continued →

Section	8	Other Procedures
Body System	E	Physiological Systems and Anatomical Regions
Operation	0	Other Procedures: Methodologies which attempt to remediate or cure a disorder or disease

8E0 Continued

Body Region (4th)	Approach (5th)	Method (6th)	Qualifier (7th)
H Integumentary System and Breast	**X** External	**Y** Other Method	**9** Piercing
K Musculoskeletal System	**X** External	**1** Therapeutic Massage	**Z** No Qualifier
K Musculoskeletal System	**X** External	**Y** Other Method	**7** Examination
U Female Reproductive System	**0** Open **3** Percutaneous **4** Percutaneous Endoscopic **7** Via Natural or Artificial Opening **8** Via Natural or Artificial Opening Endoscopic	**E** Fluorescence Guided Procedure	**N** Pafolacianine
U Female Reproductive System	**X** External	**Y** Other Method	**7** Examination
V Male Reproductive System	**X** External	**1** Therapeutic Massage	**C** Prostate **D** Rectum
V Male Reproductive System	**X** External	**6** Collection	**3** Sperm
W Trunk Region	**0** Open **3** Percutaneous **4** Percutaneous Endoscopic **7** Via Natural or Artificial Opening **8** Via Natural or Artificial Opening Endoscopic	**C** Robotic Assisted Procedure	**Z** No Qualifier
W Trunk Region	**0** Open **3** Percutaneous **4** Percutaneous Endoscopic **7** Via Natural or Artificial Opening **8** Via Natural or Artificial Opening Endoscopic	**E** Fluorescence Guided Procedure	**N** Pafolacianine **Z** No Qualifier
W Trunk Region	**X** External	**B** Computer Assisted Procedure	**F** With Fluoroscopy **G** With Computerized Tomography **H** With Magnetic Resonance Imaging **Z** No Qualifier
W Trunk Region	**X** External	**C** Robotic Assisted Procedure	**Z** No Qualifier
W Trunk Region	**X** External	**Y** Other Method	**8** Suture Removal
X Upper Extremity **Y** Lower Extremity	**0** Open **3** Percutaneous **4** Percutaneous Endoscopic	**C** Robotic Assisted Procedure **E** Fluorescence Guided Procedure	**Z** No Qualifier
X Upper Extremity **Y** Lower Extremity	**X** External	**B** Computer Assisted Procedure	**F** With Fluoroscopy **G** With Computerized Tomography **H** With Magnetic Resonance Imaging **Z** No Qualifier
X Upper Extremity **Y** Lower Extremity	**X** External	**C** Robotic Assisted Procedure	**Z** No Qualifier
X Upper Extremity **Y** Lower Extremity	**X** External	**Y** Other Method	**8** Suture Removal
Z None	**X** External	**Y** Other Method	**1** In Vitro Fertilization **4** Yoga Therapy **5** Meditation **6** Isolation

AHA Coding Clinic

8E09XBZ Computer Assisted Procedure of Head and Neck Region—AHA CC: 2Q, 2021, 19-20

8E0W3CZ Robotic Assisted Procedure of Trunk Region, Percutaneous Approach—AHA CC: 4Q, 2021, 48-50

8E0W4CZ Robotic Assisted Procedure of Trunk Region, Percutaneous Endoscopic Approach—AHA CC: 4Q, 2014, 33-34; 1Q, 2015, 33-34; 1Q, 2019, 30-31; 4Q, 2020, 53-54

Chiropractic Section (9WB)

Within each section of ICD-10-PCS the characters have different meanings. The seven character meanings for the Chiropractic section are illustrated here through the procedure example of Chiropractic treatment of cervical spine, short lever specific contact.

Section	Body System	Root Operation	Body Region	Approach	Method	Qualifier
Chiropractic	Anatomical Regions	Manipulation	Cervical	External	Short Lever Specific Contact	None
9	W	B	1	X	H	Z

Section (Character 1)

All Chiropractic procedure codes have a first character value of 9.

Body System (Character 2)

The alphanumeric character for the body system is placed in the second position. There is one character value applicable for the Chiropractic section. The character value of W is reported for anatomical regions.

Root Operations (Character 3)

The alphanumeric character value for root operations is placed in the third position. The following is the root operation applicable to the Chiropractic section with its associated meaning.

Character Value	Root Operation	Root Operation Definition
B	Manipulation	Manual procedure that involves a directed thrust to move a joint past the physiological range of motion, without exceeding the anatomical limit

Body Region (Character 4)

For each body region the applicable body part character values will be available for procedure code construction. An example of a body region for this section is Rib Cage.

Approach (Character 5)

The approach is the technique used to reach the procedure site. The following are the approach character values for the Chiropractic section with the associated definitions.

Character Value	Approach	Approach Definition
X	External	Procedures performed directly on the skin or mucous membrane and procedures performed indirectly by the application of external force through the skin or mucous membrane

Method (Character 6)

The method identifies the treatment method used to complete the chiropractic procedure. The available methods are:

- Non-Manual
- Indirect Visceral
- Extra-Articular
- Direct-Visual
- Long Lever Specific Contact
- Short Lever Specific Contact
- Long and Short Lever Specific Contact
- Mechanically Assisted
- Other

Qualifier (Character 7)

The qualifier represents an additional attribute for the procedure when applicable. Currently, there are no qualifiers in the Chiropractic section; therefore, the placeholder character value of Z should be reported.

Chiropractic Section Table

Chiropractic Table 9WB

Section	9	Chiropractic
Body System	W	Anatomical Regions
Operation	B	Manipulation: Manual procedure that involves a directed thrust to move a joint past the physiological range of motion, without exceeding the anatomical limit

Body Region (4th)	Approach (5th)	Method (6th)	Qualifier (7th)
0 Head 1 Cervical 2 Thoracic 3 Lumbar 4 Sacrum 5 Pelvis 6 Lower Extremities 7 Upper Extremities 8 Rib Cage 9 Abdomen	X External	B Non-Manual C Indirect Visceral D Extra-Articular F Direct Visceral G Long Lever Specific Contact H Short Lever Specific Contact J Long and Short Lever Specific Contact K Mechanically Assisted L Other Method	Z None

AHA Coding Clinic

No references have been issued for the Chiropractic Section.

Imaging Section (B00–BY4)

Within each section of ICD-10-PCS the characters have different meanings. The seven character meanings for the Imaging section are illustrated here through the procedure example of X-ray right clavicle, limited study.

Section	Body System	Root Type	Body Part	Contrast	Qualifier	Qualifier
Imaging	Non-Axial Upper Bones	Plain Radiography	Clavicle, right	None	None	None
B	P	0	4	Z	Z	Z

Section (Character 1)
All Imaging procedure codes have a first character value of B.

Body System (Character 2)
The alphanumeric character for the body system is placed in the second position. The following are the body systems applicable to the Imaging section.

Character Value	Character Value Description
0	Central Nervous System
2	Heart
3	Upper Arteries
4	Lower Arteries
5	Veins
7	Lymphatic System
8	Eye
9	Ear, Nose, Mouth and Throat
B	Respiratory System
D	Gastrointestinal System
F	Hepatobiliary System and Pancreas
G	Endocrine System
H	Skin, Subcutaneous Tissue and Breast
L	Connective Tissue
N	Skull and Facial Bones
P	Non-Axial Upper Bones
Q	Non-Axial Lower Bones
R	Axial Skeleton, Except Skull and Facial Bones
T	Urinary System
U	Female Reproductive System
V	Male Reproductive System
W	Anatomical Regions
Y	Fetus and Obstetrical

Root Types (Character 3)
The alphanumeric character value for root types is placed in the third position. Listed here are the root types applicable to the Imaging section with their associated meaning.

Character Value	Root Type	Root Type Definition
0	Plain Radiography	Planar display of an image developed from the capture of external ionizing radiation on photographic or photoconductive plate
1	Fluoroscopy	Single plane or bi-plane real time display of an image developed from the capture of external ionizing radiation on a fluorescent screen. The image may also be stored by either digital or analog means

Continued →

Character Value	Root Type	Root Type Definition
2	Computerized Tomography (CT Scan)	Computer reformatted digital display of multiplanar images developed from the capture of multiple exposures of external ionizing radiation
3	Magnetic Resonance Imaging (MRI)	Computer reformatted digital display of multiplanar images developed from the capture of radiofrequency signals emitted by nuclei in a body site excited within a magnetic field
4	Ultrasonography	Real time display of images of anatomy or flow information developed from the capture of reflected and attenuated high frequency sound waves
5	Other Imaging	Other specified modality for visualizing a body part

Body Part (Character 4)

For each body part the applicable body part character values will be available for procedure code construction. An example of a body part for this section is Spinal Cord.

Contrast (Character 5)

When contrast is utilized during an imaging procedure, the corresponding contrast character value should be reported in the fifth character position. The following are the contrast character values for the Imaging section:

- High Osmolar
- Low Osmolar
- Other Contrast

If contrast is not utilized, the placeholder character value of Z should be reported.

Qualifier (Character 6)

This qualifier character specifies when an image taken without contrast is followed by one with contrast. The character value of 0 is reported for Unenhanced and Enhanced.

Qualifier (Character 7)

The qualifier represents an additional attribute for the procedure when applicable. For example, ultrasonography procedures in this section include the qualifier Densitometry that is reported with the character value of 1 for some body parts. If there is no qualifier for a procedure, the placeholder Z is the character valve that should be reported.

Imaging Section Tables

Imaging Tables B00–BY4

Section	B	Imaging
Body System	0	Central Nervous System
Type	0	**Plain Radiography:** Planar display of an image developed from the capture of external ionizing radiation on photographic or photoconductive plate

Body Part (4th)	Contrast (5th)	Qualifier (6th)	Qualifier (7th)
B Spinal Cord	**0** High Osmolar **1** Low Osmolar **Y** Other Contrast **Z** None	**Z** None	**Z** None

Section	B	Imaging
Body System	0	Central Nervous System
Type	1	**Fluoroscopy:** Single plane or bi-plane real time display of an image developed from the capture of external ionizing radiation on a fluorescent screen. The image may also be stored by either digital or analog means

Body Part (4th)	Contrast (5th)	Qualifier (6th)	Qualifier (7th)
B Spinal Cord	**0** High Osmolar **1** Low Osmolar **Y** Other Contrast **Z** None	**Z** None	**Z** None

B02–B20

Imaging Section Tables

Section	B	Imaging
Body System	0	Central Nervous System
Type	2	**Computerized Tomography (CT Scan):** Computer reformatted digital display of multiplanar images developed from the capture of multiple exposures of external ionizing radiation

Body Part (4th)	Contrast (5th)	Qualifier (6th)	Qualifier (7th)
0 Brain 7 Cisterna 8 Cerebral Ventricle(s) 9 Sella Turcica/Pituitary Gland B Spinal Cord	0 High Osmolar 1 Low Osmolar Y Other Contrast	0 Unenhanced and Enhanced Z None	Z None
0 Brain 7 Cisterna 8 Cerebral Ventricle(s) 9 Sella Turcica/Pituitary Gland B Spinal Cord	Z None	Z None	Z None

Section	B	Imaging
Body System	0	Central Nervous System
Type	3	**Magnetic Resonance Imaging (MRI):** Computer reformatted digital display of multiplanar images developed from the capture of radiofrequency signals emitted by nuclei in a body site excited within a magnetic field

Body Part (4th)	Contrast (5th)	Qualifier (6th)	Qualifier (7th)
0 Brain 9 Sella Turcica/Pituitary Gland B Spinal Cord C Acoustic Nerves	Y Other Contrast	0 Unenhanced and Enhanced Z None	Z None
0 Brain 9 Sella Turcica/Pituitary Gland B Spinal Cord C Acoustic Nerves	Z None	Z None	Z None

Section	B	Imaging
Body System	0	Central Nervous System
Type	4	**Ultrasonography:** Real time display of images of anatomy or flow information developed from the capture of reflected and attenuated high frequency sound waves

Body Part (4th)	Contrast (5th)	Qualifier (6th)	Qualifier (7th)
0 Brain B Spinal Cord	Z None	Z None	Z None

Section	B	Imaging
Body System	2	Heart
Type	0	**Plain Radiography:** Planar display of an image developed from the capture of external ionizing radiation on photographic or photoconductive plate

Body Part (4th)	Contrast (5th)	Qualifier (6th)	Qualifier (7th)
0 Coronary Artery, Single 1 Coronary Arteries, Multiple 2 Coronary Artery Bypass Graft, Single 3 Coronary Artery Bypass Grafts, Multiple 4 Heart, Right 5 Heart, Left 6 Heart, Right and Left 7 Internal Mammary Bypass Graft, Right 8 Internal Mammary Bypass Graft, Left F Bypass Graft, Other	0 High Osmolar 1 Low Osmolar Y Other Contrast	Z None	Z None

578

Section	B	Imaging
Body System	2	Heart
Type	1	**Fluoroscopy:** Single plane or bi-plane real time display of an image developed from the capture of external ionizing radiation on a fluorescent screen. The image may also be stored by either digital or analog means

Body Part (4th)	Contrast (5th)	Qualifier (6th)	Qualifier (7th)
0 Coronary Artery, Single 1 Coronary Arteries, Multiple 2 Coronary Artery Bypass Graft, Single 3 Coronary Artery Bypass Grafts, Multiple	0 High Osmolar 1 Low Osmolar Y Other Contrast	1 Laser	0 Intraoperative
0 Coronary Artery, Single 1 Coronary Arteries, Multiple 2 Coronary Artery Bypass Graft, Single 3 Coronary Artery Bypass Grafts, Multiple	0 High Osmolar 1 Low Osmolar Y Other Contrast	Z None	Z None
4 Heart, Right 5 Heart, Left 6 Heart, Right and Left 7 Internal Mammary Bypass Graft, Right 8 Internal Mammary Bypass Graft, Left F Bypass Graft, Other	0 High Osmolar 1 Low Osmolar Y Other Contrast	Z None	Z None

Section	B	Imaging
Body System	2	Heart
Type	2	**Computerized Tomography (CT Scan):** Computer reformatted digital display of multiplanar images developed from the capture of multiple exposures of external ionizing radiation

Body Part (4th)	Contrast (5th)	Qualifier (6th)	Qualifier (7th)
1 Coronary Arteries, Multiple 3 Coronary Artery Bypass Grafts, Multiple 6 Heart, Right and Left	0 High Osmolar 1 Low Osmolar Y Other Contrast	0 Unenhanced and Enhanced Z None	Z None
1 Coronary Arteries, Multiple 3 Coronary Artery Bypass Grafts, Multiple 6 Heart, Right and Left	Z None	2 Intravascular Optical Coherence Z None	Z None

Section	B	Imaging
Body System	2	Heart
Type	3	**Magnetic Resonance Imaging (MRI):** Computer reformatted digital display of multiplanar images developed from the capture of radiofrequency signals emitted by nuclei in a body site excited within a magnetic field

Body Part (4th)	Contrast (5th)	Qualifier (6th)	Qualifier (7th)
1 Coronary Arteries, Multiple 3 Coronary Artery Bypass Grafts, Multiple 6 Heart, Right and Left	Y Other Contrast	0 Unenhanced and Enhanced Z None	Z None
1 Coronary Arteries, Multiple 3 Coronary Artery Bypass Grafts, Multiple 6 Heart, Right and Left	Z None	Z None	Z None

Section	B	Imaging
Body System	2	Heart
Type	4	**Ultrasonography:** Real time display of images of anatomy or flow information developed from the capture of reflected and attenuated high frequency sound waves

Body Part (4th)	Contrast (5th)	Qualifier (6th)	Qualifier (7th)
0 Coronary Artery, Single **1** Coronary Arteries, Multiple **4** Heart, Right **5** Heart, Left **6** Heart, Right and Left **B** Heart with Aorta **C** Pericardium **D** Pediatric Heart	**Y** Other Contrast	**Z** None	**Z** None
0 Coronary Artery, Single **1** Coronary Arteries, Multiple **4** Heart, Right **5** Heart, Left **6** Heart, Right and Left **B** Heart with Aorta **C** Pericardium **D** Pediatric Heart	**Z** None	**Z** None	**3** Intravascular **4** Transesophageal **Z** None

Section	B	Imaging
Body System	3	Upper Arteries
Type	0	**Plain Radiography:** Planar display of an image developed from the capture of external ionizing radiation on photographic or photoconductive plate

Body Part (4th)	Contrast (5th)	Qualifier (6th)	Qualifier (7th)
0 Thoracic Aorta **1** Brachiocephalic-Subclavian Artery, Right **2** Subclavian Artery, Left **3** Common Carotid Artery, Right **4** Common Carotid Artery, Left **5** Common Carotid Arteries, Bilateral **6** Internal Carotid Artery, Right **7** Internal Carotid Artery, Left **8** Internal Carotid Arteries, Bilateral **9** External Carotid Artery, Right **B** External Carotid Artery, Left **C** External Carotid Arteries, Bilateral **D** Vertebral Artery, Right **F** Vertebral Artery, Left **G** Vertebral Arteries, Bilateral **H** Upper Extremity Arteries, Right **J** Upper Extremity Arteries, Left **K** Upper Extremity Arteries, Bilateral **L** Intercostal and Bronchial Arteries **M** Spinal Arteries **N** Upper Arteries, Other **P** Thoraco-Abdominal Aorta **Q** Cervico-Cerebral Arch **R** Intracranial Arteries **S** Pulmonary Artery, Right **T** Pulmonary Artery, Left	**0** High Osmolar **1** Low Osmolar **Y** Other Contrast **Z** None	**Z** None	**Z** None

Section	B	Imaging
Body System	3	Upper Arteries
Type	1	**Fluoroscopy:** Single plane or bi-plane real time display of an image developed from the capture of external ionizing radiation on a fluorescent screen. The image may also be stored by either digital or analog means

Body Part (4th)	Contrast (5th)	Qualifier (6th)	Qualifier (7th)
0 Thoracic Aorta	0 High Osmolar	1 Laser	0 Intraoperative
1 Brachiocephalic-Subclavian Artery, Right	1 Low Osmolar		
2 Subclavian Artery, Left	Y Other Contrast		
3 Common Carotid Artery, Right			
4 Common Carotid Artery, Left			
5 Common Carotid Arteries, Bilateral			
6 Internal Carotid Artery, Right			
7 Internal Carotid Artery, Left			
8 Internal Carotid Arteries, Bilateral			
9 External Carotid Artery, Right			
B External Carotid Artery, Left			
C External Carotid Arteries, Bilateral			
D Vertebral Artery, Right			
F Vertebral Artery, Left			
G Vertebral Arteries, Bilateral			
H Upper Extremity Arteries, Right			
J Upper Extremity Arteries, Left			
K Upper Extremity Arteries, Bilateral			
L Intercostal and Bronchial Arteries			
M Spinal Arteries			
N Upper Arteries, Other			
P Thoraco-Abdominal Aorta			
Q Cervico-Cerebral Arch			
R Intracranial Arteries			
S Pulmonary Artery, Right			
T Pulmonary Artery, Left			
U Pulmonary Trunk			
0 Thoracic Aorta	0 High Osmolar	Z None	Z None
1 Brachiocephalic-Subclavian Artery, Right	1 Low Osmolar		
2 Subclavian Artery, Left	Y Other Contrast		
3 Common Carotid Artery, Right			
4 Common Carotid Artery, Left			
5 Common Carotid Arteries, Bilateral			
6 Internal Carotid Artery, Right			
7 Internal Carotid Artery, Left			
8 Internal Carotid Arteries, Bilateral			
9 External Carotid Artery, Right			
B External Carotid Artery, Left			
C External Carotid Arteries, Bilateral			
D Vertebral Artery, Right			
F Vertebral Artery, Left			
G Vertebral Arteries, Bilateral			
H Upper Extremity Arteries, Right			
J Upper Extremity Arteries, Left			
K Upper Extremity Arteries, Bilateral			
L Intercostal and Bronchial Arteries			
M Spinal Arteries			
N Upper Arteries, Other			
P Thoraco-Abdominal Aorta			
Q Cervico-Cerebral Arch			
R Intracranial Arteries			
S Pulmonary Artery, Right			
T Pulmonary Artery, Left			
U Pulmonary Trunk			

Continued →

B31–B32

Imaging Section Tables

Section	B	Imaging
Body System	3	Upper Arteries
Type	1	**Fluoroscopy:** Single plane or bi-plane real time display of an image developed from the capture of external ionizing radiation on a fluorescent screen. The image may also be stored by either digital or analog means

B31 Continued

Body Part (4th)	Contrast (5th)	Qualifier (6th)	Qualifier (7th)
0 Thoracic Aorta	Z None	Z None	Z None
1 Brachiocephalic-Subclavian Artery, Right			
2 Subclavian Artery, Left			
3 Common Carotid Artery, Right			
4 Common Carotid Artery, Left			
5 Common Carotid Arteries, Bilateral			
6 Internal Carotid Artery, Right			
7 Internal Carotid Artery, Left			
8 Internal Carotid Arteries, Bilateral			
9 External Carotid Artery, Right			
B External Carotid Artery, Left			
C External Carotid Arteries, Bilateral			
D Vertebral Artery, Right			
F Vertebral Artery, Left			
G Vertebral Arteries, Bilateral			
H Upper Extremity Arteries, Right			
J Upper Extremity Arteries, Left			
K Upper Extremity Arteries, Bilateral			
L Intercostal and Bronchial Arteries			
M Spinal Arteries			
N Upper Arteries, Other			
P Thoraco-Abdominal Aorta			
Q Cervico-Cerebral Arch			
R Intracranial Arteries			
S Pulmonary Artery, Right			
T Pulmonary Artery, Left			
U Pulmonary Trunk			

Section	B	Imaging
Body System	3	Upper Arteries
Type	2	**Computerized Tomography (CT Scan):** Computer reformatted digital display of multiplanar images developed from the capture of multiple exposures of external ionizing radiation

Body Part (4th)	Contrast (5th)	Qualifier (6th)	Qualifier (7th)
0 Thoracic Aorta 5 Common Carotid Arteries, Bilateral 8 Internal Carotid Arteries, Bilateral G Vertebral Arteries, Bilateral R Intracranial Arteries S Pulmonary Artery, Right T Pulmonary Artery, Left	0 High Osmolar 1 Low Osmolar Y Other Contrast	Z None	Z None
0 Thoracic Aorta 5 Common Carotid Arteries, Bilateral 8 Internal Carotid Arteries, Bilateral G Vertebral Arteries, Bilateral R Intracranial Arteries S Pulmonary Artery, Right T Pulmonary Artery, Left	Z None	2 Intravascular Optical Coherence Z None	Z None

582

Section	B	Imaging
Body System	3	Upper Arteries
Type	3	Magnetic Resonance Imaging (MRI): Computer reformatted digital display of multiplanar images developed from the capture of radiofrequency signals emitted by nuclei in a body site excited within a magnetic field

Body Part (4th)	Contrast (5th)	Qualifier (6th)	Qualifier (7th)
0 Thoracic Aorta 5 Common Carotid Arteries, Bilateral 8 Internal Carotid Arteries, Bilateral G Vertebral Arteries, Bilateral H Upper Extremity Arteries, Right J Upper Extremity Arteries, Left K Upper Extremity Arteries, Bilateral M Spinal Arteries Q Cervico-Cerebral Arch R Intracranial Arteries	Y Other Contrast	0 Unenhanced and Enhanced Z None	Z None
0 Thoracic Aorta 5 Common Carotid Arteries, Bilateral 8 Internal Carotid Arteries, Bilateral G Vertebral Arteries, Bilateral H Upper Extremity Arteries, Right J Upper Extremity Arteries, Left K Upper Extremity Arteries, Bilateral M Spinal Arteries Q Cervico-Cerebral Arch R Intracranial Arteries	Z None	Z None	Z None

Section	B	Imaging
Body System	3	Upper Arteries
Type	4	Ultrasonography: Real time display of images of anatomy or flow information developed from the capture of reflected and attenuated high frequency sound waves

Body Part (4th)	Contrast (5th)	Qualifier (6th)	Qualifier (7th)
0 Thoracic Aorta 1 Brachiocephalic-Subclavian Artery, Right 2 Subclavian Artery, Left 3 Common Carotid Artery, Right 4 Common Carotid Artery, Left 5 Common Carotid Arteries, Bilateral 6 Internal Carotid Artery, Right 7 Internal Carotid Artery, Left 8 Internal Carotid Arteries, Bilateral H Upper Extremity Arteries, Right J Upper Extremity Arteries, Left K Upper Extremity Arteries, Bilateral R Intracranial Arteries S Pulmonary Artery, Right T Pulmonary Artery, Left V Ophthalmic Arteries	Z None	Z None	3 Intravascular Z None

B40–B41

Section	B	Imaging
Body System	4	Lower Arteries
Type	0	**Plain Radiography:** Planar display of an image developed from the capture of external ionizing radiation on photographic or photoconductive plate

Body Part (4th)	Contrast (5th)	Qualifier (6th)	Qualifier (7th)
0 Abdominal Aorta 2 Hepatic Artery 3 Splenic Arteries 4 Superior Mesenteric Artery 5 Inferior Mesenteric Artery 6 Renal Artery, Right 7 Renal Artery, Left 8 Renal Arteries, Bilateral 9 Lumbar Arteries B Intra-Abdominal Arteries, Other C Pelvic Arteries D Aorta and Bilateral Lower Extremity Arteries F Lower Extremity Arteries, Right G Lower Extremity Arteries, Left J Lower Arteries, Other M Renal Artery Transplant	0 High Osmolar 1 Low Osmolar Y Other Contrast	Z None	Z None

Section	B	Imaging
Body System	4	Lower Arteries
Type	1	**Fluoroscopy:** Single plane or bi-plane real time display of an image developed from the capture of external ionizing radiation on a fluorescent screen. The image may also be stored by either digital or analog means

Body Part (4th)	Contrast (5th)	Qualifier (6th)	Qualifier (7th)
0 Abdominal Aorta 2 Hepatic Artery 3 Splenic Arteries 4 Superior Mesenteric Artery 5 Inferior Mesenteric Artery 6 Renal Artery, Right 7 Renal Artery, Left 8 Renal Arteries, Bilateral 9 Lumbar Arteries B Intra-Abdominal Arteries, Other C Pelvic Arteries D Aorta and Bilateral Lower Extremity Arteries F Lower Extremity Arteries, Right G Lower Extremity Arteries, Left J Lower Arteries, Other	0 High Osmolar 1 Low Osmolar Y Other Contrast	1 Laser	0 Intraoperative
0 Abdominal Aorta 2 Hepatic Artery 3 Splenic Arteries 4 Superior Mesenteric Artery 5 Inferior Mesenteric Artery 6 Renal Artery, Right 7 Renal Artery, Left 8 Renal Arteries, Bilateral 9 Lumbar Arteries B Intra-Abdominal Arteries, Other C Pelvic Arteries D Aorta and Bilateral Lower Extremity Arteries F Lower Extremity Arteries, Right G Lower Extremity Arteries, Left J Lower Arteries, Other	0 High Osmolar 1 Low Osmolar Y Other Contrast	Z None	Z None

Continued →

Section	B	Imaging
Body System	4	Lower Arteries
Type	1	Fluoroscopy: Single plane or bi-plane real time display of an image developed from the capture of external ionizing radiation on a fluorescent screen. The image may also be stored by either digital or analog means

Body Part (4th)	Contrast (5th)	Qualifier (6th)	Qualifier (7th)
0 Abdominal Aorta 2 Hepatic Artery 3 Splenic Arteries 4 Superior Mesenteric Artery 5 Inferior Mesenteric Artery 6 Renal Artery, Right 7 Renal Artery, Left 8 Renal Arteries, Bilateral 9 Lumbar Arteries B Intra-Abdominal Arteries, Other C Pelvic Arteries D Aorta and Bilateral Lower Extremity Arteries F Lower Extremity Arteries, Right G Lower Extremity Arteries, Left J Lower Arteries, Other	Z None	Z None	Z None

Section	B	Imaging
Body System	4	Lower Arteries
Type	2	Computerized Tomography (CT Scan): Computer reformatted digital display of multiplanar images developed from the capture of multiple exposures of external ionizing radiation

Body Part (4th)	Contrast (5th)	Qualifier (6th)	Qualifier (7th)
0 Abdominal Aorta 1 Celiac Artery 4 Superior Mesenteric Artery 8 Renal Arteries, Bilateral C Pelvic Arteries F Lower Extremity Arteries, Right G Lower Extremity Arteries, Left H Lower Extremity Arteries, Bilateral M Renal Artery Transplant	0 High Osmolar 1 Low Osmolar Y Other Contrast	Z None	Z None
0 Abdominal Aorta 1 Celiac Artery 4 Superior Mesenteric Artery 8 Renal Arteries, Bilateral C Pelvic Arteries F Lower Extremity Arteries, Right G Lower Extremity Arteries, Left H Lower Extremity Arteries, Bilateral M Renal Artery Transplant	Z None	2 Intravascular Optical Coherence Z None	Z None

Section	B	Imaging
Body System	4	Lower Arteries
Type	3	Magnetic Resonance Imaging (MRI): Computer reformatted digital display of multiplanar images developed from the capture of radiofrequency signals emitted by nuclei in a body site excited within a magnetic field

Body Part (4th)	Contrast (5th)	Qualifier (6th)	Qualifier (7th)
0 Abdominal Aorta 1 Celiac Artery 4 Superior Mesenteric Artery 8 Renal Arteries, Bilateral C Pelvic Arteries F Lower Extremity Arteries, Right G Lower Extremity Arteries, Left H Lower Extremity Arteries, Bilateral	Y Other Contrast	0 Unenhanced and Enhanced Z None	Z None

Section	B	Imaging
Body System	4	Lower Arteries
Type	3	**Magnetic Resonance Imaging (MRI):** Computer reformatted digital display of multiplanar images developed from the capture of radiofrequency signals emitted by nuclei in a body site excited within a magnetic field

Body Part (4th)	Contrast (5th)	Qualifier (6th)	Qualifier (7th)
0 Abdominal Aorta 1 Celiac Artery 4 Superior Mesenteric Artery 8 Renal Arteries, Bilateral C Pelvic Arteries F Lower Extremity Arteries, Right G Lower Extremity Arteries, Left H Lower Extremity Arteries, Bilateral	Z None	Z None	Z None

Section	B	Imaging
Body System	4	Lower Arteries
Type	4	**Ultrasonography:** Real time display of images of anatomy or flow information developed from the capture of reflected and attenuated high frequency sound waves

Body Part (4th)	Contrast (5th)	Qualifier (6th)	Qualifier (7th)
0 Abdominal Aorta 4 Superior Mesenteric Artery 5 Inferior Mesenteric Artery 6 Renal Artery, Right 7 Renal Artery, Left 8 Renal Arteries, Bilateral B Intra-Abdominal Arteries, Other F Lower Extremity Arteries, Right G Lower Extremity Arteries, Left H Lower Extremity Arteries, Bilateral K Celiac and Mesenteric Arteries L Femoral Artery N Penile Arteries	Z None	Z None	3 Intravascular Z None

Section	B	Imaging
Body System	5	Veins
Type	0	**Plain Radiography:** Planar display of an image developed from the capture of external ionizing radiation on photographic or photoconductive plate

Body Part (4th)	Contrast (5th)	Qualifier (6th)	Qualifier (7th)
0 Epidural Veins	0 High Osmolar	Z None	Z None
1 Cerebral and Cerebellar Veins	1 Low Osmolar		
2 Intracranial Sinuses	Y Other Contrast		
3 Jugular Veins, Right			
4 Jugular Veins, Left			
5 Jugular Veins, Bilateral			
6 Subclavian Vein, Right			
7 Subclavian Vein, Left			
8 Superior Vena Cava			
9 Inferior Vena Cava			
B Lower Extremity Veins, Right			
C Lower Extremity Veins, Left			
D Lower Extremity Veins, Bilateral			
F Pelvic (Iliac) Veins, Right			
G Pelvic (Iliac) Veins, Left			
H Pelvic (Iliac) Veins, Bilateral			
J Renal Vein, Right			
K Renal Vein, Left			
L Renal Veins, Bilateral			
M Upper Extremity Veins, Right			
N Upper Extremity Veins, Left			
P Upper Extremity Veins, Bilateral			
Q Pulmonary Vein, Right			
R Pulmonary Vein, Left			
S Pulmonary Veins, Bilateral			
T Portal and Splanchnic Veins			
V Veins, Other			
W Dialysis Shunt/Fistula			

Section	B	Imaging
Body System	5	Veins
Type	1	**Fluoroscopy:** Single plane or bi-plane real time display of an image developed from the capture of external ionizing radiation on a fluorescent screen. The image may also be stored by either digital or analog means

Body Part (4th)	Contrast (5th)	Qualifier (6th)	Qualifier (7th)
0 Epidural Veins	0 High Osmolar	Z None	A Guidance
1 Cerebral and Cerebellar Veins	1 Low Osmolar		Z None
2 Intracranial Sinuses	Y Other Contrast		
3 Jugular Veins, Right	Z None		
4 Jugular Veins, Left			
5 Jugular Veins, Bilateral			
6 Subclavian Vein, Right			
7 Subclavian Vein, Left			
8 Superior Vena Cava			
9 Inferior Vena Cava			
B Lower Extremity Veins, Right			
C Lower Extremity Veins, Left			
D Lower Extremity Veins, Bilateral			
F Pelvic (Iliac) Veins, Right			
G Pelvic (Iliac) Veins, Left			
H Pelvic (Iliac) Veins, Bilateral			
J Renal Vein, Right			
K Renal Vein, Left			
L Renal Veins, Bilateral			
M Upper Extremity Veins, Right			
N Upper Extremity Veins, Left			
P Upper Extremity Veins, Bilateral			
Q Pulmonary Vein, Right			
R Pulmonary Vein, Left			
S Pulmonary Veins, Bilateral			
T Portal and Splanchnic Veins			
V Veins, Other			
W Dialysis Shunt/Fistula			

Section	B	Imaging
Body System	5	Veins
Type	2	**Computerized Tomography (CT Scan):** Computer reformatted digital display of multiplanar images developed from the capture of multiple exposures of external ionizing radiation

Body Part (4th)	Contrast (5th)	Qualifier (6th)	Qualifier (7th)
2 Intracranial Sinuses 8 Superior Vena Cava 9 Inferior Vena Cava F Pelvic (Iliac) Veins, Right G Pelvic (Iliac) Veins, Left H Pelvic (Iliac) Veins, Bilateral J Renal Vein, Right K Renal Vein, Left L Renal Veins, Bilateral Q Pulmonary Vein, Right R Pulmonary Vein, Left S Pulmonary Veins, Bilateral T Portal and Splanchnic Veins	0 High Osmolar 1 Low Osmolar Y Other Contrast	0 Unenhanced and Enhanced Z None	Z None
2 Intracranial Sinuses 8 Superior Vena Cava 9 Inferior Vena Cava F Pelvic (Iliac) Veins, Right G Pelvic (Iliac) Veins, Left H Pelvic (Iliac) Veins, Bilateral J Renal Vein, Right K Renal Vein, Left L Renal Veins, Bilateral Q Pulmonary Vein, Right R Pulmonary Vein, Left S Pulmonary Veins, Bilateral T Portal and Splanchnic Veins	Z None	2 Intravascular Optical Coherence Z None	Z None

Section	B	Imaging
Body System	5	Veins
Type	3	**Magnetic Resonance Imaging (MRI):** Computer reformatted digital display of multiplanar images developed from the capture of radiofrequency signals emitted by nuclei in a body site excited within a magnetic field

Body Part (4th)	Contrast (5th)	Qualifier (6th)	Qualifier (7th)
1 Cerebral and Cerebellar Veins 2 Intracranial Sinuses 5 Jugular Veins, Bilateral 8 Superior Vena Cava 9 Inferior Vena Cava B Lower Extremity Veins, Right C Lower Extremity Veins, Left D Lower Extremity Veins, Bilateral H Pelvic (Iliac) Veins, Bilateral L Renal Veins, Bilateral M Upper Extremity Veins, Right N Upper Extremity Veins, Left P Upper Extremity Veins, Bilateral S Pulmonary Veins, Bilateral T Portal and Splanchnic Veins V Veins, Other	Y Other Contrast	0 Unenhanced and Enhanced Z None	Z None

Continued →

Section	B	Imaging			**B53 Continued**
Body System	5	Veins			
Type	3	**Magnetic Resonance Imaging (MRI):** Computer reformatted digital display of multiplanar images developed from the capture of radiofrequency signals emitted by nuclei in a body site excited within a magnetic field			

Body Part (4th)	Contrast (5th)	Qualifier (6th)	Qualifier (7th)
1 Cerebral and Cerebellar Veins 2 Intracranial Sinuses 5 Jugular Veins, Bilateral 8 Superior Vena Cava 9 Inferior Vena Cava B Lower Extremity Veins, Right C Lower Extremity Veins, Left D Lower Extremity Veins, Bilateral H Pelvic (Iliac) Veins, Bilateral L Renal Veins, Bilateral M Upper Extremity Veins, Right N Upper Extremity Veins, Left P Upper Extremity Veins, Bilateral S Pulmonary Veins, Bilateral T Portal and Splanchnic Veins V Veins, Other	Z None	Z None	Z None

Section	B	Imaging
Body System	5	Veins
Type	4	**Ultrasonography:** Real time display of images of anatomy or flow information developed from the capture of reflected and attenuated high frequency sound waves

Body Part (4th)	Contrast (5th)	Qualifier (6th)	Qualifier (7th)
3 Jugular Veins, Right 4 Jugular Veins, Left 6 Subclavian Vein, Right 7 Subclavian Vein, Left 8 Superior Vena Cava 9 Inferior Vena Cava B Lower Extremity Veins, Right C Lower Extremity Veins, Left D Lower Extremity Veins, Bilateral J Renal Vein, Right K Renal Vein, Left L Renal Veins, Bilateral M Upper Extremity Veins, Right N Upper Extremity Veins, Left P Upper Extremity Veins, Bilateral T Portal and Splanchnic Veins	Z None	Z None	3 Intravascular A Guidance Z None

Section	B	Imaging
Body System	7	Lymphatic System
Type	0	**Plain Radiography:** Planar display of an image developed from the capture of external ionizing radiation on photographic or photoconductive plate

Body Part (4th)	Contrast (5th)	Qualifier (6th)	Qualifier (7th)
0 Abdominal/Retroperitoneal Lymphatics, Unilateral 1 Abdominal/Retroperitoneal Lymphatics, Bilateral 4 Lymphatics, Head and Neck 5 Upper Extremity Lymphatics, Right 6 Upper Extremity Lymphatics, Left 7 Upper Extremity Lymphatics, Bilateral 8 Lower Extremity Lymphatics, Right 9 Lower Extremity Lymphatics, Left B Lower Extremity Lymphatics, Bilateral C Lymphatics, Pelvic	0 High Osmolar 1 Low Osmolar Y Other Contrast	Z None	Z None

Section   **B**   **Imaging**
Body System   **8**   **Eye**
Type   **0**   **Plain Radiography:** Planar display of an image developed from the capture of external ionizing radiation on photographic or photoconductive plate

Body Part (4th)	Contrast (5th)	Qualifier (6th)	Qualifier (7th)
0 Lacrimal Duct, Right 1 Lacrimal Duct, Left 2 Lacrimal Ducts, Bilateral	0 High Osmolar 1 Low Osmolar Y Other Contrast	Z None	Z None
3 Optic Foramina, Right 4 Optic Foramina, Left 5 Eye, Right 6 Eye, Left 7 Eyes, Bilateral	Z None	Z None	Z None

Section   **B**   **Imaging**
Body System   **8**   **Eye**
Type   **2**   **Computerized Tomography (CT Scan):** Computer reformatted digital display of multiplanar images developed from the capture of multiple exposures of external ionizing radiation

Body Part (4th)	Contrast (5th)	Qualifier (6th)	Qualifier (7th)
5 Eye, Right 6 Eye, Left 7 Eyes, Bilateral	0 High Osmolar 1 Low Osmolar Y Other Contrast	0 Unenhanced and Enhanced Z None	Z None
5 Eye, Right 6 Eye, Left 7 Eyes, Bilateral	Z None	Z None	Z None

Section   **B**   **Imaging**
Body System   **8**   **Eye**
Type   **3**   **Magnetic Resonance Imaging (MRI):** Computer reformatted digital display of multiplanar images developed from the capture of radiofrequency signals emitted by nuclei in a body site excited within a magnetic field

Body Part (4th)	Contrast (5th)	Qualifier (6th)	Qualifier (7th)
5 Eye, Right 6 Eye, Left 7 Eyes, Bilateral	Y Other Contrast	0 Unenhanced and Enhanced Z None	Z None
5 Eye, Right 6 Eye, Left 7 Eyes, Bilateral	Z None	Z None	Z None

Section   **B**   **Imaging**
Body System   **8**   **Eye**
Type   **4**   **Ultrasonography:** Real time display of images of anatomy or flow information developed from the capture of reflected and attenuated high frequency sound waves

Body Part (4th)	Contrast (5th)	Qualifier (6th)	Qualifier (7th)
5 Eye, Right 6 Eye, Left 7 Eyes, Bilateral	Z None	Z None	Z None

Section	B	Imaging
Body System	9	Ear, Nose, Mouth and Throat
Type	0	**Plain Radiography:** Planar display of an image developed from the capture of external ionizing radiation on photographic or photoconductive plate

Body Part (4th)	Contrast (5th)	Qualifier (6th)	Qualifier (7th)
2 Paranasal Sinuses F Nasopharynx/Oropharynx H Mastoids	Z None	Z None	Z None
4 Parotid Gland, Right 5 Parotid Gland, Left 6 Parotid Glands, Bilateral 7 Submandibular Gland, Right 8 Submandibular Gland, Left 9 Submandibular Glands, Bilateral B Salivary Gland, Right C Salivary Gland, Left D Salivary Glands, Bilateral	0 High Osmolar 1 Low Osmolar Y Other Contrast	Z None	Z None

Section	B	Imaging
Body System	9	Ear, Nose, Mouth and Throat
Type	1	**Fluoroscopy:** Single plane or bi-plane real time display of an image developed from the capture of external ionizing radiation on a fluorescent screen. The image may also be stored by either digital or analog means

Body Part (4th)	Contrast (5th)	Qualifier (6th)	Qualifier (7th)
G Pharynx and Epiglottis J Larynx	Y Other Contrast Z None	Z None	Z None

Section	B	Imaging
Body System	9	Ear, Nose, Mouth and Throat
Type	2	**Computerized Tomography (CT Scan):** Computer reformatted digital display of multiplanar images developed from the capture of multiple exposures of external ionizing radiation

Body Part (4th)	Contrast (5th)	Qualifier (6th)	Qualifier (7th)
0 Ear 2 Paranasal Sinuses 6 Parotid Glands, Bilateral 9 Submandibular Glands, Bilateral D Salivary Glands, Bilateral F Nasopharynx/Oropharynx J Larynx	0 High Osmolar 1 Low Osmolar Y Other Contrast	0 Unenhanced and Enhanced Z None	Z None
0 Ear 2 Paranasal Sinuses 6 Parotid Glands, Bilateral 9 Submandibular Glands, Bilateral D Salivary Glands, Bilateral F Nasopharynx/Oropharynx J Larynx	Z None	Z None	Z None

Section	B	Imaging
Body System	9	Ear, Nose, Mouth and Throat
Type	3	**Magnetic Resonance Imaging (MRI):** Computer reformatted digital display of multiplanar images developed from the capture of radiofrequency signals emitted by nuclei in a body site excited within a magnetic field

Body Part (4th)	Contrast (5th)	Qualifier (6th)	Qualifier (7th)
0 Ear 2 Paranasal Sinuses 6 Parotid Glands, Bilateral 9 Submandibular Glands, Bilateral D Salivary Glands, Bilateral F Nasopharynx/Oropharynx J Larynx	Y Other Contrast	0 Unenhanced and Enhanced Z None	Z None

Continued →

B93–BB2

B93 Continued

Section	B	Imaging
Body System	9	Ear, Nose, Mouth and Throat
Type	3	**Magnetic Resonance Imaging (MRI):** Computer reformatted digital display of multiplanar images developed from the capture of radiofrequency signals emitted by nuclei in a body site excited within a magnetic field

Body Part (4th)	Contrast (5th)	Qualifier (6th)	Qualifier (7th)
0 Ear **2** Paranasal Sinuses **6** Parotid Glands, Bilateral **9** Submandibular Glands, Bilateral **D** Salivary Glands, Bilateral **F** Nasopharynx/Oropharynx **J** Larynx	**Z** None	**Z** None	**Z** None

Section	B	Imaging
Body System	B	Respiratory System
Type	0	**Plain Radiography:** Planar display of an image developed from the capture of external ionizing radiation on photographic or photoconductive plate

Body Part (4th)	Contrast (5th)	Qualifier (6th)	Qualifier (7th)
7 Tracheobronchial Tree, Right **8** Tracheobronchial Tree, Left **9** Tracheobronchial Trees, Bilateral	**Y** Other Contrast	**Z** None	**Z** None
D Upper Airways	**Z** None	**Z** None	**Z** None

Section	B	Imaging
Body System	B	Respiratory System
Type	1	**Fluoroscopy:** Single plane or bi-plane real time display of an image developed from the capture of external ionizing radiation on a fluorescent screen. The image may also be stored by either digital or analog means

Body Part (4th)	Contrast (5th)	Qualifier (6th)	Qualifier (7th)
2 Lung, Right **3** Lung, Left **4** Lungs, Bilateral **6** Diaphragm **C** Mediastinum **D** Upper Airways	**Z** None	**Z** None	**Z** None
7 Tracheobronchial Tree, Right **8** Tracheobronchial Tree, Left **9** Tracheobronchial Trees, Bilateral	**Y** Other Contrast	**Z** None	**Z** None

Section	B	Imaging
Body System	B	Respiratory System
Type	2	**Computerized Tomography (CT Scan):** Computer reformatted digital display of multiplanar images developed from the capture of multiple exposures of external ionizing radiation

Body Part (4th)	Contrast (5th)	Qualifier (6th)	Qualifier (7th)
4 Lungs, Bilateral **7** Tracheobronchial Tree, Right **8** Tracheobronchial Tree, Left **9** Tracheobronchial Trees, Bilateral **F** Trachea/Airways	**0** High Osmolar **1** Low Osmolar **Y** Other Contrast	**0** Unenhanced and Enhanced **Z** None	**Z** None
4 Lungs, Bilateral **7** Tracheobronchial Tree, Right **8** Tracheobronchial Tree, Left **9** Tracheobronchial Trees, Bilateral **F** Trachea/Airways	**Z** None	**Z** None	**Z** None

Imaging Section Tables

592

Section	B	Imaging
Body System	B	Respiratory System
Type	3	**Magnetic Resonance Imaging (MRI):** Computer reformatted digital display of multiplanar images developed from the capture of radiofrequency signals emitted by nuclei in a body site excited within a magnetic field

Body Part (4th)	Contrast (5th)	Qualifier (6th)	Qualifier (7th)
4 Lungs, Bilateral	Z None	3 Hyperpolarized Xenon 129 (Xe-129)	Z None
G Lung Apices	Y Other Contrast	0 Unenhanced and Enhanced Z None	Z None
G Lung Apices	Z None	Z None	Z None

Section	B	Imaging
Body System	B	Respiratory System
Type	4	**Ultrasonography:** Real time display of images of anatomy or flow information developed from the capture of reflected and attenuated high frequency sound waves

Body Part (4th)	Contrast (5th)	Qualifier (6th)	Qualifier (7th)
B Pleura C Mediastinum	Z None	Z None	Z None

Section	B	Imaging
Body System	D	Gastrointestinal System
Type	1	**Fluoroscopy:** Single plane or bi-plane real time display of an image developed from the capture of external ionizing radiation on a fluorescent screen. The image may also be stored by either digital or analog means

Body Part (4th)	Contrast (5th)	Qualifier (6th)	Qualifier (7th)
1 Esophagus 2 Stomach 3 Small Bowel 4 Colon 5 Upper GI 6 Upper GI and Small Bowel 9 Duodenum B Mouth/Oropharynx	Y Other Contrast Z None	Z None	Z None

Section	B	Imaging
Body System	D	Gastrointestinal System
Type	2	**Computerized Tomography (CT Scan):** Computer reformatted digital display of multiplanar images developed from the capture of multiple exposures of external ionizing radiation

Body Part (4th)	Contrast (5th)	Qualifier (6th)	Qualifier (7th)
4 Colon	0 High Osmolar 1 Low Osmolar Y Other Contrast	0 Unenhanced and Enhanced Z None	Z None
4 Colon	Z None	Z None	Z None

Section	B	Imaging
Body System	D	Gastrointestinal System
Type	4	**Ultrasonography:** Real time display of images of anatomy or flow information developed from the capture of reflected and attenuated high frequency sound waves

Body Part (4th)	Contrast (5th)	Qualifier (6th)	Qualifier (7th)
1 Esophagus 2 Stomach 7 Gastrointestinal Tract 8 Appendix 9 Duodenum C Rectum	Z None	Z None	Z None

BF0–BF3

Imaging Section Tables

Section	**B**	**Imaging**	
Body System	**F**	**Hepatobiliary System and Pancreas**	
Type	**0**	**Plain Radiography:** Planar display of an image developed from the capture of external ionizing radiation on photographic or photoconductive plate	

Body Part (4th)	Contrast (5th)	Qualifier (6th)	Qualifier (7th)
0 Bile Ducts **3** Gallbladder and Bile Ducts **C** Hepatobiliary System, All	**0** High Osmolar **1** Low Osmolar **Y** Other Contrast	**Z** None	**Z** None

Section	**B**	**Imaging**	
Body System	**F**	**Hepatobiliary System and Pancreas**	
Type	**1**	**Fluoroscopy:** Single plane or bi-plane real time display of an image developed from the capture of external ionizing radiation on a fluorescent screen. The image may also be stored by either digital or analog means	

Body Part (4th)	Contrast (5th)	Qualifier (6th)	Qualifier (7th)
0 Bile Ducts **1** Biliary and Pancreatic Ducts **2** Gallbladder **3** Gallbladder and Bile Ducts **4** Gallbladder, Bile Ducts and Pancreatic Ducts **8** Pancreatic Ducts	**0** High Osmolar **1** Low Osmolar **Y** Other Contrast	**Z** None	**Z** None
5 Liver	**0** High Osmolar **1** Low Osmolar **Y** Other Contrast	**Z** None	**Z** None
5 Liver	**Z** None	**Z** None	**A** Guidance

Section	**B**	**Imaging**	
Body System	**F**	**Hepatobiliary System and Pancreas**	
Type	**2**	**Computerized Tomography (CT Scan):** Computer reformatted digital display of multiplanar images developed from the capture of multiple exposures of external ionizing radiation	

Body Part (4th)	Contrast (5th)	Qualifier (6th)	Qualifier (7th)
5 Liver **6** Liver and Spleen **7** Pancreas **C** Hepatobiliary System, All	**0** High Osmolar **1** Low Osmolar **Y** Other Contrast	**0** Unenhanced and Enhanced **Z** None	**Z** None
5 Liver **6** Liver and Spleen **7** Pancreas **C** Hepatobiliary System, All	**Z** None	**Z** None	**Z** None

Section	**B**	**Imaging**	
Body System	**F**	**Hepatobiliary System and Pancreas**	
Type	**3**	**Magnetic Resonance Imaging (MRI):** Computer reformatted digital display of multiplanar images developed from the capture of radiofrequency signals emitted by nuclei in a body site excited within a magnetic field	

Body Part (4th)	Contrast (5th)	Qualifier (6th)	Qualifier (7th)
5 Liver **6** Liver and Spleen **7** Pancreas	**Y** Other Contrast	**0** Unenhanced and Enhanced **Z** None	**Z** None
5 Liver **6** Liver and Spleen **7** Pancreas	**Z** None	**Z** None	**Z** None

Section	B	Imaging
Body System	F	Hepatobiliary System and Pancreas
Type	4	Ultrasonography: Real time display of images of anatomy or flow information developed from the capture of reflected and attenuated high frequency sound waves

Body Part (4th)	Contrast (5th)	Qualifier (6th)	Qualifier (7th)
0 Bile Ducts 2 Gallbladder 3 Gallbladder and Bile Ducts 5 Liver 6 Liver and Spleen 7 Pancreas C Hepatobiliary System, All	Z None	Z None	Z None

Section	B	Imaging
Body System	F	Hepatobiliary System and Pancreas
Type	5	Other Imaging: Other specified modality for visualizing a body part

Body Part (4th)	Contrast (5th)	Qualifier (6th)	Qualifier (7th)
0 Bile Ducts 2 Gallbladder 3 Gallbladder and Bile Ducts 5 Liver 6 Liver and Spleen 7 Pancreas C Hepatobiliary System, All	2 Fluorescing Agent	0 Indocyanine Green Dye Z None	0 Intraoperative Z None

Section	B	Imaging
Body System	G	Endocrine System
Type	2	Computerized Tomography (CT Scan): Computer reformatted digital display of multiplanar images developed from the capture of multiple exposures of external ionizing radiation

Body Part (4th)	Contrast (5th)	Qualifier (6th)	Qualifier (7th)
2 Adrenal Glands, Bilateral 3 Parathyroid Glands 4 Thyroid Gland	0 High Osmolar 1 Low Osmolar Y Other Contrast	0 Unenhanced and Enhanced Z None	Z None
2 Adrenal Glands, Bilateral 3 Parathyroid Glands 4 Thyroid Gland	Z None	Z None	Z None

Section	B	Imaging
Body System	G	Endocrine System
Type	3	Magnetic Resonance Imaging (MRI): Computer reformatted digital display of multiplanar images developed from the capture of radiofrequency signals emitted by nuclei in a body site excited within a magnetic field

Body Part (4th)	Contrast (5th)	Qualifier (6th)	Qualifier (7th)
2 Adrenal Glands, Bilateral 3 Parathyroid Glands 4 Thyroid Gland	Y Other Contrast	0 Unenhanced and Enhanced Z None	Z None
2 Adrenal Glands, Bilateral 3 Parathyroid Glands 4 Thyroid Gland	Z None	Z None	Z None

Section   **B**   **Imaging**
Body System   **G**   **Endocrine System**
Type   **4**   **Ultrasonography:** Real time display of images of anatomy or flow information developed from the capture of reflected and attenuated high frequency sound waves

Body Part (4th)	Contrast (5th)	Qualifier (6th)	Qualifier (7th)
0 Adrenal Gland, Right 1 Adrenal Gland, Left 2 Adrenal Glands, Bilateral 3 Parathyroid Glands 4 Thyroid Gland	Z None	Z None	Z None

Section   **B**   **Imaging**
Body System   **H**   **Skin, Subcutaneous Tissue and Breast**
Type   **0**   **Plain Radiography:** Planar display of an image developed from the capture of external ionizing radiation on photographic or photoconductive plate

Body Part (4th)	Contrast (5th)	Qualifier (6th)	Qualifier (7th)
0 Breast, Right 1 Breast, Left 2 Breasts, Bilateral	Z None	Z None	Z None
3 Single Mammary Duct, Right 4 Single Mammary Duct, Left 5 Multiple Mammary Ducts, Right 6 Multiple Mammary Ducts, Left	0 High Osmolar 1 Low Osmolar Y Other Contrast Z None	Z None	Z None

Section   **B**   **Imaging**
Body System   **H**   **Skin, Subcutaneous Tissue and Breast**
Type   **3**   **Magnetic Resonance Imaging (MRI):** Computer reformatted digital display of multiplanar images developed from the capture of radiofrequency signals emitted by nuclei in a body site excited within a magnetic field

Body Part (4th)	Contrast (5th)	Qualifier (6th)	Qualifier (7th)
0 Breast, Right 1 Breast, Left 2 Breasts, Bilateral D Subcutaneous Tissue, Head/Neck F Subcutaneous Tissue, Upper Extremity G Subcutaneous Tissue, Thorax H Subcutaneous Tissue, Abdomen and Pelvis J Subcutaneous Tissue, Lower Extremity	Y Other Contrast	0 Unenhanced and Enhanced Z None	Z None
0 Breast, Right 1 Breast, Left 2 Breasts, Bilateral D Subcutaneous Tissue, Head/Neck F Subcutaneous Tissue, Upper Extremity G Subcutaneous Tissue, Thorax H Subcutaneous Tissue, Abdomen and Pelvis J Subcutaneous Tissue, Lower Extremity	Z None	Z None	Z None

Section   **B**   **Imaging**
Body System   **H**   **Skin, Subcutaneous Tissue and Breast**
Type   **4**   **Ultrasonography:** Real time display of images of anatomy or flow information developed from the capture of reflected and attenuated high frequency sound waves

Body Part (4th)	Contrast (5th)	Qualifier (6th)	Qualifier (7th)
0 Breast, Right 1 Breast, Left 2 Breasts, Bilateral 7 Extremity, Upper 8 Extremity, Lower 9 Abdominal Wall B Chest Wall C Head and Neck	Z None	Z None	Z None

Section	B	Imaging
Body System	L	Connective Tissue
Type	3	**Magnetic Resonance Imaging (MRI):** Computer reformatted digital display of multiplanar images developed from the capture of radiofrequency signals emitted by nuclei in a body site excited within a magnetic field

Body Part (4th)	Contrast (5th)	Qualifier (6th)	Qualifier (7th)
0 Connective Tissue, Upper Extremity **1** Connective Tissue, Lower Extremity **2** Tendons, Upper Extremity **3** Tendons, Lower Extremity	**Y** Other Contrast	**0** Unenhanced and Enhanced **Z** None	**Z** None
0 Connective Tissue, Upper Extremity **1** Connective Tissue, Lower Extremity **2** Tendons, Upper Extremity **3** Tendons, Lower Extremity	**Z** None	**Z** None	**Z** None

Section	B	Imaging
Body System	L	Connective Tissue
Type	4	**Ultrasonography:** Real time display of images of anatomy or flow information developed from the capture of reflected and attenuated high frequency sound waves

Body Part (4th)	Contrast (5th)	Qualifier (6th)	Qualifier (7th)
0 Connective Tissue, Upper Extremity **1** Connective Tissue, Lower Extremity **2** Tendons, Upper Extremity **3** Tendons, Lower Extremity	**Z** None	**Z** None	**Z** None

Section	B	Imaging
Body System	N	Skull and Facial Bones
Type	0	**Plain Radiography:** Planar display of an image developed from the capture of external ionizing radiation on photographic or photoconductive plate

Body Part (4th)	Contrast (5th)	Qualifier (6th)	Qualifier (7th)
0 Skull **1** Orbit, Right **2** Orbit, Left **3** Orbits, Bilateral **4** Nasal Bones **5** Facial Bones **6** Mandible **B** Zygomatic Arch, Right **C** Zygomatic Arch, Left **D** Zygomatic Arches, Bilateral **G** Tooth, Single **H** Teeth, Multiple **J** Teeth, All	**Z** None	**Z** None	**Z** None
7 Temporomandibular Joint, Right **8** Temporomandibular Joint, Left **9** Temporomandibular Joints, Bilateral	**0** High Osmolar **1** Low Osmolar **Y** Other Contrast **Z** None	**Z** None	**Z** None

Section	B	Imaging
Body System	N	Skull and Facial Bones
Type	1	**Fluoroscopy:** Single plane or bi-plane real time display of an image developed from the capture of external ionizing radiation on a fluorescent screen. The image may also be stored by either digital or analog means

Body Part (4th)	Contrast (5th)	Qualifier (6th)	Qualifier (7th)
7 Temporomandibular Joint, Right **8** Temporomandibular Joint, Left **9** Temporomandibular Joints, Bilateral	**0** High Osmolar **1** Low Osmolar **Y** Other Contrast **Z** None	**Z** None	**Z** None

Section   B   Imaging
Body System   N   Skull and Facial Bones
Type   2   **Computerized Tomography (CT Scan):** Computer reformatted digital display of multiplanar images developed from the capture of multiple exposures of external ionizing radiation

Body Part (4ᵗʰ)	Contrast (5ᵗʰ)	Qualifier (6ᵗʰ)	Qualifier (7ᵗʰ)
0 Skull 3 Orbits, Bilateral 5 Facial Bones 6 Mandible 9 Temporomandibular Joints, Bilateral F Temporal Bones	0 High Osmolar 1 Low Osmolar Y Other Contrast Z None	Z None	Z None

Section   B   Imaging
Body System   N   Skull and Facial Bones
Type   3   **Magnetic Resonance Imaging (MRI):** Computer reformatted digital display of multiplanar images developed from the capture of radiofrequency signals emitted by nuclei in a body site excited within a magnetic field

Body Part (4ᵗʰ)	Contrast (5ᵗʰ)	Qualifier (6ᵗʰ)	Qualifier (7ᵗʰ)
9 Temporomandibular Joints, Bilateral	Y Other Contrast Z None	Z None	Z None

Section   B   Imaging
Body System   P   Non-Axial Upper Bones
Type   0   **Plain Radiography:** Planar display of an image developed from the capture of external ionizing radiation on photographic or photoconductive plate

Body Part (4ᵗʰ)	Contrast (5ᵗʰ)	Qualifier (6ᵗʰ)	Qualifier (7ᵗʰ)
0 Sternoclavicular Joint, Right 1 Sternoclavicular Joint, Left 2 Sternoclavicular Joints, Bilateral 3 Acromioclavicular Joints, Bilateral 4 Clavicle, Right 5 Clavicle, Left 6 Scapula, Right 7 Scapula, Left A Humerus, Right B Humerus, Left E Upper Arm, Right F Upper Arm, Left J Forearm, Right K Forearm, Left N Hand, Right P Hand, Left R Finger(s), Right S Finger(s), Left X Ribs, Right Y Ribs, Left	Z None	Z None	Z None
8 Shoulder, Right 9 Shoulder, Left C Hand/Finger Joint, Right D Hand/Finger Joint, Left G Elbow, Right H Elbow, Left L Wrist, Right M Wrist, Left	0 High Osmolar 1 Low Osmolar Y Other Contrast Z None	Z None	Z None

Section	B	Imaging
Body System	P	Non-Axial Upper Bones
Type	1	**Fluoroscopy:** Single plane or bi-plane real time display of an image developed from the capture of external ionizing radiation on a fluorescent screen. The image may also be stored by either digital or analog means

Body Part (4th)	Contrast (5th)	Qualifier (6th)	Qualifier (7th)
0 Sternoclavicular Joint, Right 1 Sternoclavicular Joint, Left 2 Sternoclavicular Joints, Bilateral 3 Acromioclavicular Joints, Bilateral 4 Clavicle, Right 5 Clavicle, Left 6 Scapula, Right 7 Scapula, Left A Humerus, Right B Humerus, Left E Upper Arm, Right F Upper Arm, Left J Forearm, Right K Forearm, Left N Hand, Right P Hand, Left R Finger(s), Right S Finger(s), Left X Ribs, Right Y Ribs, Left	Z None	Z None	Z None
8 Shoulder, Right 9 Shoulder, Left L Wrist, Right M Wrist, Left	0 High Osmolar 1 Low Osmolar Y Other Contrast Z None	Z None	Z None
C Hand/Finger Joint, Right D Hand/Finger Joint, Left G Elbow, Right H Elbow, Left	0 High Osmolar 1 Low Osmolar Y Other Contrast	Z None	Z None

Section	B	Imaging
Body System	P	Non-Axial Upper Bones
Type	2	**Computerized Tomography (CT Scan):** Computer reformatted digital display of multiplanar images developed from the capture of multiple exposures of external ionizing radiation

Body Part (4th)	Contrast (5th)	Qualifier (6th)	Qualifier (7th)
0 Sternoclavicular Joint, Right 1 Sternoclavicular Joint, Left W Thorax	0 High Osmolar 1 Low Osmolar Y Other Contrast	Z None	Z None

Section **B** Imaging
Body System **P** Non-Axial Upper Bones
Type **2** **Computerized Tomography (CT Scan):** Computer reformatted digital display of multiplanar images developed from the capture of multiple exposures of external ionizing radiation

BP2 Continued

Body Part (4th)	Contrast (5th)	Qualifier (6th)	Qualifier (7th)
2 Sternoclavicular Joints, Bilateral 3 Acromioclavicular Joints, Bilateral 4 Clavicle, Right 5 Clavicle, Left 6 Scapula, Right 7 Scapula, Left 8 Shoulder, Right 9 Shoulder, Left A Humerus, Right B Humerus, Left E Upper Arm, Right F Upper Arm, Left G Elbow, Right H Elbow, Left J Forearm, Right K Forearm, Left L Wrist, Right M Wrist, Left N Hand, Right P Hand, Left Q Hands and Wrists, Bilateral R Finger(s), Right S Finger(s), Left T Upper Extremity, Right U Upper Extremity, Left V Upper Extremities, Bilateral X Ribs, Right Y Ribs, Left	0 High Osmolar 1 Low Osmolar Y Other Contrast Z None	Z None	Z None
C Hand/Finger Joint, Right D Hand/Finger Joint, Left	Z None	Z None	Z None

Section **B** Imaging
Body System **P** Non-Axial Upper Bones
Type **3** **Magnetic Resonance Imaging (MRI):** Computer reformatted digital display of multiplanar images developed from the capture of radiofrequency signals emitted by nuclei in a body site excited within a magnetic field

Body Part (4th)	Contrast (5th)	Qualifier (6th)	Qualifier (7th)
8 Shoulder, Right 9 Shoulder, Left C Hand/Finger Joint, Right D Hand/Finger Joint, Left E Upper Arm, Right F Upper Arm, Left G Elbow, Right H Elbow, Left J Forearm, Right K Forearm, Left L Wrist, Right M Wrist, Left	Y Other Contrast	0 Unenhanced and Enhanced Z None	Z None

Continued →

BP3 Continued

Section	B	Imaging
Body System	P	Non-Axial Upper Bones
Type	3	**Magnetic Resonance Imaging (MRI):** Computer reformatted digital display of multiplanar images developed from the capture of radiofrequency signals emitted by nuclei in a body site excited within a magnetic field

Body Part (4th)	Contrast (5th)	Qualifier (6th)	Qualifier (7th)
8 Shoulder, Right 9 Shoulder, Left C Hand/Finger Joint, Right D Hand/Finger Joint, Left E Upper Arm, Right F Upper Arm, Left G Elbow, Right H Elbow, Left J Forearm, Right K Forearm, Left L Wrist, Right M Wrist, Left	Z None	Z None	Z None

Section	B	Imaging
Body System	P	Non-Axial Upper Bones
Type	4	**Ultrasonography:** Real time display of images of anatomy or flow information developed from the capture of reflected and attenuated high frequency sound waves

Body Part (4th)	Contrast (5th)	Qualifier (6th)	Qualifier (7th)
8 Shoulder, Right 9 Shoulder, Left G Elbow, Right H Elbow, Left L Wrist, Right M Wrist, Left N Hand, Right P Hand, Left	Z None	Z None	1 Densitometry Z None

Section	B	Imaging
Body System	Q	Non-Axial Lower Bones
Type	0	**Plain Radiography:** Planar display of an image developed from the capture of external ionizing radiation on photographic or photoconductive plate

Body Part (4th)	Contrast (5th)	Qualifier (6th)	Qualifier (7th)
0 Hip, Right 1 Hip, Left	0 High Osmolar 1 Low Osmolar Y Other Contrast	Z None	Z None
0 Hip, Right 1 Hip, Left	Z None	Z None	1 Densitometry Z None
3 Femur, Right 4 Femur, Left	Z None	Z None	1 Densitometry Z None
7 Knee, Right 8 Knee, Left G Ankle, Right H Ankle, Left	0 High Osmolar 1 Low Osmolar Y Other Contrast Z None	Z None	Z None
D Lower Leg, Right F Lower Leg, Left J Calcaneus, Right K Calcaneus, Left L Foot, Right M Foot, Left P Toe(s), Right Q Toe(s), Left V Patella, Right W Patella, Left	Z None	Z None	Z None

Continued →

BQ0–BQ2

Imaging Section Tables

BQ0 Continued

Section	B	Imaging
Body System	Q	Non-Axial Lower Bones
Type	0	**Plain Radiography:** Planar display of an image developed from the capture of external ionizing radiation on photographic or photoconductive plate

Body Part (4ᵗʰ)	Contrast (5ᵗʰ)	Qualifier (6ᵗʰ)	Qualifier (7ᵗʰ)
X Foot/Toe Joint, Right Y Foot/Toe Joint, Left	0 High Osmolar 1 Low Osmolar Y Other Contrast	Z None	Z None

Section	B	Imaging
Body System	Q	Non-Axial Lower Bones
Type	1	**Fluoroscopy:** Single plane or bi-plane real time display of an image developed from the capture of external ionizing radiation on a fluorescent screen. The image may also be stored by either digital or analog means

Body Part (4ᵗʰ)	Contrast (5ᵗʰ)	Qualifier (6ᵗʰ)	Qualifier (7ᵗʰ)
0 Hip, Right 1 Hip, Left 7 Knee, Right 8 Knee, Left G Ankle, Right H Ankle, Left X Foot/Toe Joint, Right Y Foot/Toe Joint, Left	0 High Osmolar 1 Low Osmolar Y Other Contrast Z None	Z None	Z None
3 Femur, Right 4 Femur, Left D Lower Leg, Right F Lower Leg, Left J Calcaneus, Right K Calcaneus, Left L Foot, Right M Foot, Left P Toe(s), Right Q Toe(s), Left V Patella, Right W Patella, Left	Z None	Z None	Z None

Section	B	Imaging
Body System	Q	Non-Axial Lower Bones
Type	2	**Computerized Tomography (CT Scan):** Computer reformatted digital display of multiplanar images developed from the capture of multiple exposures of external ionizing radiation

Body Part (4ᵗʰ)	Contrast (5ᵗʰ)	Qualifier (6ᵗʰ)	Qualifier (7ᵗʰ)
0 Hip, Right 1 Hip, Left 3 Femur, Right 4 Femur, Left 7 Knee, Right 8 Knee, Left D Lower Leg, Right F Lower Leg, Left G Ankle, Right H Ankle, Left J Calcaneus, Right K Calcaneus, Left L Foot, Right M Foot, Left P Toe(s), Right Q Toe(s), Left R Lower Extremity, Right S Lower Extremity, Left V Patella, Right W Patella, Left X Foot/Toe Joint, Right Y Foot/Toe Joint, Left	0 High Osmolar 1 Low Osmolar Y Other Contrast Z None	Z None	Z None

Continued →

Section	B	Imaging
Body System	Q	Non-Axial Lower Bones
Type	2	**Computerized Tomography (CT Scan):** Computer reformatted digital display of multiplanar images developed from the capture of multiple exposures of external ionizing radiation

Body Part (4th)	Contrast (5th)	Qualifier (6th)	Qualifier (7th)
B Tibia/Fibula, Right **C** Tibia/Fibula, Left	**0** High Osmolar **1** Low Osmolar **Y** Other Contrast	**Z** None	**Z** None

Section	B	Imaging
Body System	Q	Non-Axial Lower Bones
Type	3	**Magnetic Resonance Imaging (MRI):** Computer reformatted digital display of multiplanar images developed from the capture of radiofrequency signals emitted by nuclei in a body site excited within a magnetic field

Body Part (4th)	Contrast (5th)	Qualifier (6th)	Qualifier (7th)
0 Hip, Right **1** Hip, Left **3** Femur, Right **4** Femur, Left **7** Knee, Right **8** Knee, Left **D** Lower Leg, Right **F** Lower Leg, Left **G** Ankle, Right **H** Ankle, Left **J** Calcaneus, Right **K** Calcaneus, Left **L** Foot, Right **M** Foot, Left **P** Toe(s), Right **Q** Toe(s), Left **V** Patella, Right **W** Patella, Left	**Y** Other Contrast	**0** Unenhanced and Enhanced **Z** None	**Z** None
0 Hip, Right **1** Hip, Left **3** Femur, Right **4** Femur, Left **7** Knee, Right **8** Knee, Left **D** Lower Leg, Right **F** Lower Leg, Left **G** Ankle, Right **H** Ankle, Left **J** Calcaneus, Right **K** Calcaneus, Left **L** Foot, Right **M** Foot, Left **P** Toe(s), Right **Q** Toe(s), Left **V** Patella, Right **W** Patella, Left	**Z** None	**Z** None	**Z** None

BQ4–BR1

Imaging Section Tables

Section	B	Imaging
Body System	Q	Non-Axial Lower Bones
Type	4	Ultrasonography: Real time display of images of anatomy or flow information developed from the capture of reflected and attenuated high frequency sound waves

Body Part (4th)	Contrast (5th)	Qualifier (6th)	Qualifier (7th)
0 Hip, Right 1 Hip, Left 2 Hips, Bilateral 7 Knee, Right 8 Knee, Left 9 Knees, Bilateral	Z None	Z None	Z None

Section	B	Imaging
Body System	R	Axial Skeleton, Except Skull and Facial Bones
Type	0	Plain Radiography: Planar display of an image developed from the capture of external ionizing radiation on photographic or photoconductive plate

Body Part (4th)	Contrast (5th)	Qualifier (6th)	Qualifier (7th)
0 Cervical Spine 7 Thoracic Spine 9 Lumbar Spine G Whole Spine	Z None	Z None	1 Densitometry Z None
1 Cervical Disc(s) 2 Thoracic Disc(s) 3 Lumbar Disc(s) 4 Cervical Facet Joint(s) 5 Thoracic Facet Joint(s) 6 Lumbar Facet Joint(s) D Sacroiliac Joints	0 High Osmolar 1 Low Osmolar Y Other Contrast Z None	Z None	Z None
8 Thoracolumbar Joint B Lumbosacral Joint C Pelvis F Sacrum and Coccyx H Sternum	Z None	Z None	Z None

Section	B	Imaging
Body System	R	Axial Skeleton, Except Skull and Facial Bones
Type	1	Fluoroscopy: Single plane or bi-plane real time display of an image developed from the capture of external ionizing radiation on a fluorescent screen. The image may also be stored by either digital or analog means

Body Part (4th)	Contrast (5th)	Qualifier (6th)	Qualifier (7th)
0 Cervical Spine 1 Cervical Disc(s) 2 Thoracic Disc(s) 3 Lumbar Disc(s) 4 Cervical Facet Joint(s) 5 Thoracic Facet Joint(s) 6 Lumbar Facet Joint(s) 7 Thoracic Spine 8 Thoracolumbar Joint 9 Lumbar Spine B Lumbosacral Joint C Pelvis D Sacroiliac Joints F Sacrum and Coccyx G Whole Spine H Sternum	0 High Osmolar 1 Low Osmolar Y Other Contrast Z None	Z None	Z None

Section	B	Imaging
Body System	R	Axial Skeleton, Except Skull and Facial Bones
Type	2	**Computerized Tomography (CT Scan):** Computer reformatted digital display of multiplanar images developed from the capture of multiple exposures of external ionizing radiation

Body Part (4th)	Contrast (5th)	Qualifier (6th)	Qualifier (7th)
0 Cervical Spine **7** Thoracic Spine **9** Lumbar Spine **C** Pelvis **D** Sacroiliac Joints **F** Sacrum and Coccyx	**0** High Osmolar **1** Low Osmolar **Y** Other Contrast **Z** None	**Z** None	**Z** None

Section	B	Imaging
Body System	R	Axial Skeleton, Except Skull and Facial Bones
Type	3	**Magnetic Resonance Imaging (MRI):** Computer reformatted digital display of multiplanar images developed from the capture of radiofrequency signals emitted by nuclei in a body site excited within a magnetic field

Body Part (4th)	Contrast (5th)	Qualifier (6th)	Qualifier (7th)
0 Cervical Spine **1** Cervical Disc(s) **2** Thoracic Disc(s) **3** Lumbar Disc(s) **7** Thoracic Spine **9** Lumbar Spine **C** Pelvis **F** Sacrum and Coccyx	**Y** Other Contrast	**0** Unenhanced and Enhanced **Z** None	**Z** None
0 Cervical Spine **1** Cervical Disc(s) **2** Thoracic Disc(s) **3** Lumbar Disc(s) **7** Thoracic Spine **9** Lumbar Spine **C** Pelvis **F** Sacrum and Coccyx	**Z** None	**Z** None	**Z** None

Section	B	Imaging
Body System	R	Axial Skeleton, Except Skull and Facial Bones
Type	4	**Ultrasonography:** Real time display of images of anatomy or flow information developed from the capture of reflected and attenuated high frequency sound waves

Body Part (4th)	Contrast (5th)	Qualifier (6th)	Qualifier (7th)
0 Cervical Spine **7** Thoracic Spine **9** Lumbar Spine **F** Sacrum and Coccyx	**Z** None	**Z** None	**Z** None

Section	B	Imaging
Body System	T	Urinary System
Type	0	**Plain Radiography:** Planar display of an image developed from the capture of external ionizing radiation on photographic or photoconductive plate

Body Part (4th)	Contrast (5th)	Qualifier (6th)	Qualifier (7th)
0 Bladder **1** Kidney, Right **2** Kidney, Left **3** Kidneys, Bilateral **4** Kidneys, Ureters and Bladder **5** Urethra **6** Ureter, Right **7** Ureter, Left **8** Ureters, Bilateral **B** Bladder and Urethra **C** Ileal Diversion Loop	**0** High Osmolar **1** Low Osmolar **Y** Other Contrast **Z** None	**Z** None	**Z** None

BT1–BT3

Imaging Section Tables

Section	B	Imaging
Body System	T	Urinary System
Type	1	**Fluoroscopy:** Single plane or bi-plane real time display of an image developed from the capture of external ionizing radiation on a fluorescent screen. The image may also be stored by either digital or analog means

Body Part (4ᵗʰ)	Contrast (5ᵗʰ)	Qualifier (6ᵗʰ)	Qualifier (7ᵗʰ)
0 Bladder 1 Kidney, Right 2 Kidney, Left 3 Kidneys, Bilateral 4 Kidneys, Ureters and Bladder 5 Urethra 6 Ureter, Right 7 Ureter, Left B Bladder and Urethra C Ileal Diversion Loop D Kidney, Ureter and Bladder, Right F Kidney, Ureter and Bladder, Left G Ileal Loop, Ureters and Kidneys	0 High Osmolar 1 Low Osmolar Y Other Contrast Z None	Z None	Z None

Section	B	Imaging
Body System	T	Urinary System
Type	2	**Computerized Tomography (CT Scan):** Computer reformatted digital display of multiplanar images developed from the capture of multiple exposures of external ionizing radiation

Body Part (4ᵗʰ)	Contrast (5ᵗʰ)	Qualifier (6ᵗʰ)	Qualifier (7ᵗʰ)
0 Bladder 1 Kidney, Right 2 Kidney, Left 3 Kidneys, Bilateral 9 Kidney Transplant	0 High Osmolar 1 Low Osmolar Y Other Contrast	0 Unenhanced and Enhanced Z None	Z None
0 Bladder 1 Kidney, Right 2 Kidney, Left 3 Kidneys, Bilateral 9 Kidney Transplant	Z None	Z None	Z None

Section	B	Imaging
Body System	T	Urinary System
Type	3	**Magnetic Resonance Imaging (MRI):** Computer reformatted digital display of multiplanar images developed from the capture of radiofrequency signals emitted by nuclei in a body site excited within a magnetic field

Body Part (4ᵗʰ)	Contrast (5ᵗʰ)	Qualifier (6ᵗʰ)	Qualifier (7ᵗʰ)
0 Bladder 1 Kidney, Right 2 Kidney, Left 3 Kidneys, Bilateral 9 Kidney Transplant	Y Other Contrast	0 Unenhanced and Enhanced Z None	Z None
0 Bladder 1 Kidney, Right 2 Kidney, Left 3 Kidneys, Bilateral 9 Kidney Transplant	Z None	Z None	Z None

Section	B	Imaging
Body System	T	Urinary System
Type	4	Ultrasonography: Real time display of images of anatomy or flow information developed from the capture of reflected and attenuated high frequency sound waves

Body Part (4th)	Contrast (5th)	Qualifier (6th)	Qualifier (7th)
0 Bladder 1 Kidney, Right 2 Kidney, Left 3 Kidneys, Bilateral 5 Urethra 6 Ureter, Right 7 Ureter, Left 8 Ureters, Bilateral 9 Kidney Transplant J Kidneys and Bladder	Z None	Z None	Z None

Section	B	Imaging
Body System	U	Female Reproductive System
Type	0	Plain Radiography: Planar display of an image developed from the capture of external ionizing radiation on photographic or photoconductive plate

Body Part (4th)	Contrast (5th)	Qualifier (6th)	Qualifier (7th)
0 Fallopian Tube, Right 1 Fallopian Tube, Left 2 Fallopian Tubes, Bilateral 6 Uterus 8 Uterus and Fallopian Tubes 9 Vagina	0 High Osmolar 1 Low Osmolar Y Other Contrast	Z None	Z None

Section	B	Imaging
Body System	U	Female Reproductive System
Type	1	Fluoroscopy: Single plane or bi-plane real time display of an image developed from the capture of external ionizing radiation on a fluorescent screen. The image may also be stored by either digital or analog means

Body Part (4th)	Contrast (5th)	Qualifier (6th)	Qualifier (7th)
0 Fallopian Tube, Right 1 Fallopian Tube, Left 2 Fallopian Tubes, Bilateral 6 Uterus 8 Uterus and Fallopian Tubes 9 Vagina	0 High Osmolar 1 Low Osmolar Y Other Contrast Z None	Z None	Z None

Section	B	Imaging
Body System	U	Female Reproductive System
Type	3	Magnetic Resonance Imaging (MRI): Computer reformatted digital display of multiplanar images developed from the capture of radiofrequency signals emitted by nuclei in a body site excited within a magnetic field

Body Part (4th)	Contrast (5th)	Qualifier (6th)	Qualifier (7th)
3 Ovary, Right 4 Ovary, Left 5 Ovaries, Bilateral 6 Uterus 9 Vagina B Pregnant Uterus C Uterus and Ovaries	Y Other Contrast	0 Unenhanced and Enhanced Z None	Z None
3 Ovary, Right 4 Ovary, Left 5 Ovaries, Bilateral 6 Uterus 9 Vagina B Pregnant Uterus C Uterus and Ovaries	Z None	Z None	Z None

607

Section	B	Imaging
Body System	U	Female Reproductive System
Type	4	Ultrasonography: Real time display of images of anatomy or flow information developed from the capture of reflected and attenuated high frequency sound waves

Body Part (4th)	Contrast (5th)	Qualifier (6th)	Qualifier (7th)
0 Fallopian Tube, Right 1 Fallopian Tube, Left 2 Fallopian Tubes, Bilateral 3 Ovary, Right 4 Ovary, Left 5 Ovaries, Bilateral 6 Uterus C Uterus and Ovaries	Y Other Contrast Z None	Z None	Z None

Section	B	Imaging
Body System	V	Male Reproductive System
Type	0	Plain Radiography: Planar display of an image developed from the capture of external ionizing radiation on photographic or photoconductive plate

Body Part (4th)	Contrast (5th)	Qualifier (6th)	Qualifier (7th)
0 Corpora Cavernosa 1 Epididymis, Right 2 Epididymis, Left 3 Prostate 5 Testicle, Right 6 Testicle, Left 8 Vasa Vasorum	0 High Osmolar 1 Low Osmolar Y Other Contrast	Z None	Z None

Section	B	Imaging
Body System	V	Male Reproductive System
Type	1	Fluoroscopy: Single plane or bi-plane real time display of an image developed from the capture of external ionizing radiation on a fluorescent screen. The image may also be stored by either digital or analog means

Body Part (4th)	Contrast (5th)	Qualifier (6th)	Qualifier (7th)
0 Corpora Cavernosa 8 Vasa Vasorum	0 High Osmolar 1 Low Osmolar Y Other Contrast Z None	Z None	Z None

Section	B	Imaging
Body System	V	Male Reproductive System
Type	2	Computerized Tomography (CT Scan): Computer reformatted digital display of multiplanar images developed from the capture of multiple exposures of external ionizing radiation

Body Part (4th)	Contrast (5th)	Qualifier (6th)	Qualifier (7th)
3 Prostate	0 High Osmolar 1 Low Osmolar Y Other Contrast	0 Unenhanced and Enhanced Z None	Z None
3 Prostate	Z None	Z None	Z None

Section	B	Imaging
Body System	V	Male Reproductive System
Type	3	**Magnetic Resonance Imaging (MRI):** Computer reformatted digital display of multiplanar images developed from the capture of radiofrequency signals emitted by nuclei in a body site excited within a magnetic field

Body Part (4th)	Contrast (5th)	Qualifier (6th)	Qualifier (7th)
0 Corpora Cavernosa **3** Prostate **4** Scrotum **5** Testicle, Right **6** Testicle, Left **7** Testicles, Bilateral	**Y** Other Contrast	**0** Unenhanced and Enhanced **Z** None	**Z** None
0 Corpora Cavernosa **3** Prostate **4** Scrotum **5** Testicle, Right **6** Testicle, Left **7** Testicles, Bilateral	**Z** None	**Z** None	**Z** None

Section	B	Imaging
Body System	V	Male Reproductive System
Type	4	**Ultrasonography:** Real time display of images of anatomy or flow information developed from the capture of reflected and attenuated high frequency sound waves

Body Part (4th)	Contrast (5th)	Qualifier (6th)	Qualifier (7th)
4 Scrotum **9** Prostate and Seminal Vesicles **B** Penis	**Z** None	**Z** None	**Z** None

Section	B	Imaging
Body System	W	Anatomical Regions
Type	0	**Plain Radiography:** Planar display of an image developed from the capture of external ionizing radiation on photographic or photoconductive plate

Body Part (4th)	Contrast (5th)	Qualifier (6th)	Qualifier (7th)
0 Abdomen **1** Abdomen and Pelvis **3** Chest **B** Long Bones, All **C** Lower Extremity **J** Upper Extremity **K** Whole Body **L** Whole Skeleton **M** Whole Body, Infant	**Z** None	**Z** None	**Z** None

Section	B	Imaging
Body System	W	Anatomical Regions
Type	1	**Fluoroscopy:** Single plane or bi-plane real time display of an image developed from the capture of external ionizing radiation on a fluorescent screen. The image may also be stored by either digital or analog means

Body Part (4th)	Contrast (5th)	Qualifier (6th)	Qualifier (7th)
1 Abdomen and Pelvis **9** Head and Neck **C** Lower Extremity **J** Upper Extremity	**0** High Osmolar **1** Low Osmolar **Y** Other Contrast **Z** None	**Z** None	**Z** None

BW2–BW4

Imaging Section Tables

Section	B	Imaging
Body System	W	Anatomical Regions
Type	2	**Computerized Tomography (CT Scan):** Computer reformatted digital display of multiplanar images developed from the capture of multiple exposures of external ionizing radiation

Body Part (4th)	Contrast (5th)	Qualifier (6th)	Qualifier (7th)
0 Abdomen 1 Abdomen and Pelvis 4 Chest and Abdomen 5 Chest, Abdomen and Pelvis 8 Head 9 Head and Neck F Neck G Pelvic Region	0 High Osmolar 1 Low Osmolar Y Other Contrast	0 Unenhanced and Enhanced Z None	Z None
0 Abdomen 1 Abdomen and Pelvis 4 Chest and Abdomen 5 Chest, Abdomen and Pelvis 8 Head 9 Head and Neck F Neck G Pelvic Region	Z None	Z None	Z None

Section	B	Imaging
Body System	W	Anatomical Regions
Type	3	**Magnetic Resonance Imaging (MRI):** Computer reformatted digital display of multiplanar images developed from the capture of radiofrequency signals emitted by nuclei in a body site excited within a magnetic field

Body Part (4th)	Contrast (5th)	Qualifier (6th)	Qualifier (7th)
0 Abdomen 8 Head F Neck G Pelvic Region H Retroperitoneum P Brachial Plexus	Y Other Contrast	0 Unenhanced and Enhanced Z None	Z None
0 Abdomen 8 Head F Neck G Pelvic Region H Retroperitoneum P Brachial Plexus	Z None	Z None	Z None
3 Chest	Y Other Contrast	0 Unenhanced and Enhanced Z None	Z None

Section	B	Imaging
Body System	W	Anatomical Regions
Type	4	**Ultrasonography:** Real time display of images of anatomy or flow information developed from the capture of reflected and attenuated high frequency sound waves

Body Part (4th)	Contrast (5th)	Qualifier (6th)	Qualifier (7th)
0 Abdomen 1 Abdomen and Pelvis F Neck G Pelvic Region	Z None	Z None	Z None

Section	B	Imaging
Body System	W	Anatomical Regions
Type	5	Other Imaging: Other specified modality for visualizing a body part

Body Part (4th)	Contrast (5th)	Qualifier (6th)	Qualifier (7th)
2 Trunk 9 Head and Neck C Lower Extremity J Upper Extremi	Z None	1 Bacterial Autofluorescence	Z None

Section	B	Imaging
Body System	Y	Fetus and Obstetrical
Type	3	Magnetic Resonance Imaging (MRI): Computer reformatted digital display of multiplanar images developed from the capture of radiofrequency signals emitted by nuclei in a body site excited within a magnetic field

Body Part (4th)	Contrast (5th)	Qualifier (6th)	Qualifier (7th)
0 Fetal Head 1 Fetal Heart 2 Fetal Thorax 3 Fetal Abdomen 4 Fetal Spine 5 Fetal Extremities 6 Whole Fetus	Y Other Contrast	0 Unenhanced and Enhanced Z None	Z None
0 Fetal Head 1 Fetal Heart 2 Fetal Thorax 3 Fetal Abdomen 4 Fetal Spine 5 Fetal Extremities 6 Whole Fetus	Z None	Z None	Z None

Section	B	Imaging
Body System	Y	Fetus and Obstetrical
Type	4	Ultrasonography: Real time display of images of anatomy or flow information developed from the capture of reflected and attenuated high frequency sound waves

Body Part (4th)	Contrast (5th)	Qualifier (6th)	Qualifier (7th)
7 Fetal Umbilical Cord 8 Placenta 9 First Trimester, Single Fetus B First Trimester, Multiple Gestation C Second Trimester, Single Fetus D Second Trimester, Multiple Gestation F Third Trimester, Single Fetus G Third Trimester, Multiple Gestation	Z None	Z None	Z None

AHA Coding Clinic

B2151ZZ Fluoroscopy of Left Heart using Low Osmolar Contrast—AHA CC: 1Q, 2018, 12-13

B518ZZA Fluoroscopy of Superior Vena Cava, Guidance, for Fluoroscopic Guidance used to Place the Renal Dialysis Catheter—AHA CC: 4Q, 2015, 30

BF50200 Other Imaging of Bile Ducts using Fluorescing Agent, Indocyanine Green Dye, Intraoperative—AHA CC: 4Q, 2020, 67-68

Nuclear Medicine Section (C01–CW7)

Within each section of ICD-10-PCS the characters have different meanings. The seven character meanings for the Nuclear Medicine section are illustrated here through the procedure example of *Technetium tomo scan of liver*.

Section	Body System	Root Type	Body Part	Radionuclide	Qualifier	Qualifier
Nuclear Medicine	Hepatobiliary and Pancreas	Tomographic (Tomo)	Liver	Technetium 99m	None	None
C	F	2	5	1	Z	Z

Section (Character 1)
All Nuclear Medicine procedure codes have a first character value of C.

Body System (Character 2)
The alphanumeric character for the body system is placed in the second position. The following are the body systems applicable to the Nuclear Medicine section.

Character Value	Character Value Description
0	Central Nervous System
2	Heart
5	Veins
7	Lymphatic System
8	Eye
9	Ear, Nose, Mouth and Throat
B	Respiratory System
D	Gastrointestinal System
F	Hepatobiliary System and Pancreas
G	Endocrine System
H	Skin, Subcutaneous Tissue and Breast
P	Musculoskeletal
T	Urinary System
V	Male Reproductive System
W	Anatomical Regions

Root Types (Character 3)
The alphanumeric character value for root types is placed in the third position. The following are the root types applicable to the Nuclear Medicine section with their associated meaning.

Character Value	Root Type	Root Type Definition
1	Planar Nuclear Medicine Imaging	Introduction of radioactive materials into the body for single plane display of images developed from the capture of radioactive emissions
2	Tomographic (Tomo) Nuclear Medicine Imaging	Introduction of radioactive materials into the body for three dimensional display of images developed from the capture of radioactive emissions
3	Positron Emission Tomographic (PET) Imaging	Introduction of radioactive materials into the body for three dimensional display of images developed from the simultaneous capture, 180 degrees apart, of radioactive emissions
4	Nonimaging Nuclear Medicine Uptake	Introduction of radioactive materials into the body for measurements of organ function, from the detection of radioactive emissions
5	Nonimaging Nuclear Medicine Probe	Introduction of radioactive materials into the body for the study of distribution and fate of certain substances by the detection of radioactive emissions; or, alternatively, measurement of absorption of radioactive emissions from an external source

Continued →

Character Value	Root Type	Root Type Definition
6	Nonimaging Nuclear Medicine Assay	Introduction of radioactive materials into the body for the study of body fluids and blood elements, by the detection of radioactive emissions
7	Systemic Nuclear Medicine Therapy	Introduction of unsealed radioactive materials into the body for treatment

Body Part (Character 4)

For each body part the applicable body part character values will be available for procedure code construction. An example of a body part is Cerebrospinal Fluid.

Radionuclide (Character 5)

When radionuclide is utilized during a nuclear medicine procedure, the corresponding radionuclide character value should be reported in the fifth character position. The following are examples of the radionuclide character values available for the Nuclear Medicine section.

- Krypton (Kr-81m)
- Technetium 99m (Tc-99m)
- Xenon 127 (Xe-127)
- Xenon 133 (Xe-133)
- Other Radionuclide

If radionuclide is not utilized, the placeholder character value of Z should be reported.

Qualifier (Character 6)

The qualifier represents an additional attribute for the procedure when applicable. Currently, there are no qualifiers in the Nuclear Medicine section; therefore, the placeholder character value of Z should be reported.

Qualifier (Character 7)

The qualifier represents an additional attribute for the procedure when applicable. Currently, there are no qualifiers in the Nuclear Medicine section; therefore, the placeholder character value of Z should be reported.

Nuclear Medicine Section Tables

Nuclear Medicine Tables C01–CW7

Section	C	Nuclear Medicine
Body System	0	Central Nervous System
Type	1	**Planar Nuclear Medicine Imaging:** Introduction of radioactive materials into the body for single plane display of images developed from the capture of radioactive emissions

Body Part (4th)	Radionuclide (5th)	Qualifier (6th)	Qualifier (7th)
0 Brain	1 Technetium 99m (Tc-99m) Y Other Radionuclide	Z None	Z None
5 Cerebrospinal Fluid	D Indium 111 (In-111) Y Other Radionuclide	Z None	Z None
Y Central Nervous System	Y Other Radionuclide	Z None	Z None

Section	C	Nuclear Medicine
Body System	0	Central Nervous System
Type	2	**Tomographic (Tomo) Nuclear Medicine Imaging:** Introduction of radioactive materials into the body for three dimensional display of images developed from the capture of radioactive emissions

Body Part (4th)	Radionuclide (5th)	Qualifier (6th)	Qualifier (7th)
0 Brain	**1** Technetium 99m (Tc-99m) **F** Iodine 123 (I-123) **S** Thallium 201 (Tl-201) **Y** Other Radionuclide	**Z** None	**Z** None
5 Cerebrospinal Fluid	**D** Indium 111 (In-111) **Y** Other Radionuclide	**Z** None	**Z** None
Y Central Nervous System	**Y** Other Radionuclide	**Z** None	**Z** None

Section	C	Nuclear Medicine
Body System	0	Central Nervous System
Type	3	**Positron Emission Tomographic (PET) Imaging:** Introduction of radioactive materials into the body for three dimensional display of images developed from the simultaneous capture, 180 degrees apart, of radioactive emissions

Body Part (4th)	Radionuclide (5th)	Qualifier (6th)	Qualifier (7th)
0 Brain	**B** Carbon 11 (C-11) **K** Fluorine 18 (F-18) **M** Oxygen 15 (O-15) **Y** Other Radionuclide	**Z** None	**Z** None
Y Central Nervous System	**Y** Other Radionuclide	**Z** None	**Z** None

Section	C	Nuclear Medicine
Body System	0	Central Nervous System
Type	5	**Nonimaging Nuclear Medicine Probe:** Introduction of radioactive materials into the body for the study of distribution and fate of certain substances by the detection of radioactive emissions; or, alternatively, measurement of absorption of radioactive emissions from an external source

Body Part (4th)	Radionuclide (5th)	Qualifier (6th)	Qualifier (7th)
0 Brain	**V** Xenon 133 (Xe-133) **Y** Other Radionuclide	**Z** None	**Z** None
Y Central Nervous System	**Y** Other Radionuclide	**Z** None	**Z** None

Section	C	Nuclear Medicine
Body System	2	Heart
Type	1	**Planar Nuclear Medicine Imaging:** Introduction of radioactive materials into the body for single plane display of images developed from the capture of radioactive emissions

Body Part (4th)	Radionuclide (5th)	Qualifier (6th)	Qualifier (7th)
6 Heart, Right and Left	**1** Technetium 99m (Tc-99m) **Y** Other Radionuclide	**Z** None	**Z** None
G Myocardium	**1** Technetium 99m (Tc-99m) **D** Indium 111 (In-111) **S** Thallium 201 (Tl-201) **Y** Other Radionuclide **Z** None	**Z** None	**Z** None
Y Heart	**Y** Other Radionuclide	**Z** None	**Z** None

Section	C	Nuclear Medicine
Body System	2	Heart
Type	2	**Tomographic (Tomo) Nuclear Medicine Imaging:** Introduction of radioactive materials into the body for three dimensional display of images developed from the capture of radioactive emissions

Body Part (4ᵗʰ)	Radionuclide (5ᵗʰ)	Qualifier (6ᵗʰ)	Qualifier (7ᵗʰ)
6 Heart, Right and Left	1 Technetium 99m (Tc-99m) Y Other Radionuclide	Z None	Z None
G Myocardium	1 Technetium 99m (Tc-99m) D Indium 111 (In-111) K Fluorine 18 (F-18) S Thallium 201 (Tl-201) Y Other Radionuclide Z None	Z None	Z None
Y Heart	Y Other Radionuclide	Z None	Z None

Section	C	Nuclear Medicine
Body System	2	Heart
Type	3	**Positron Emission Tomographic (PET) Imaging:** Introduction of radioactive materials into the body for three dimensional display of images developed from the simultaneous capture, 180 degrees apart, of radioactive emissions

Body Part (4ᵗʰ)	Radionuclide (5ᵗʰ)	Qualifier (6ᵗʰ)	Qualifier (7ᵗʰ)
G Myocardium	K Fluorine 18 (F-18) M Oxygen 15 (O-15) Q Rubidium 82 (Rb-82) R Nitrogen 13 (N-13) Y Other Radionuclide	Z None	Z None
Y Heart	Y Other Radionuclide	Z None	Z None

Section	C	Nuclear Medicine
Body System	2	Heart
Type	5	**Nonimaging Nuclear Medicine Probe:** Introduction of radioactive materials into the body for the study of distribution and fate of certain substances by the detection of radioactive emissions; or, alternatively, measurement of absorption of radioactive emissions from an external source

Body Part (4ᵗʰ)	Radionuclide (5ᵗʰ)	Qualifier (6ᵗʰ)	Qualifier (7ᵗʰ)
6 Heart, Right and Left	1 Technetium 99m (Tc-99m) Y Other Radionuclide	Z None	Z None
Y Heart	Y Other Radionuclide	Z None	Z None

Section	C	Nuclear Medicine
Body System	5	Veins
Type	1	**Planar Nuclear Medicine Imaging:** Introduction of radioactive materials into the body for single plane display of images developed from the capture of radioactive emissions

Body Part (4ᵗʰ)	Radionuclide (5ᵗʰ)	Qualifier (6ᵗʰ)	Qualifier (7ᵗʰ)
B Lower Extremity Veins, Right C Lower Extremity Veins, Left D Lower Extremity Veins, Bilateral N Upper Extremity Veins, Right P Upper Extremity Veins, Left Q Upper Extremity Veins, Bilateral R Central Veins	1 Technetium 99m (Tc-99m) Y Other Radionuclide	Z None	Z None
Y Veins	Y Other Radionuclide	Z None	Z None

Section	C	Nuclear Medicine
Body System	7	Lymphatic and Hematologic System
Type	1	**Planar Nuclear Medicine Imaging:** Introduction of radioactive materials into the body for single plane display of images developed from the capture of radioactive emissions

Body Part (4th)	Radionuclide (5th)	Qualifier (6th)	Qualifier (7th)
0 Bone Marrow	1 Technetium 99m (Tc-99m) D Indium 111 (In-111) Y Other Radionuclide	Z None	Z None
2 Spleen 5 Lymphatics, Head and Neck D Lymphatics, Pelvic J Lymphatics, Head K Lymphatics, Neck L Lymphatics, Upper Chest M Lymphatics, Trunk N Lymphatics, Upper Extremity P Lymphatics, Lower Extremity	1 Technetium 99m (Tc-99m) Y Other Radionuclide	Z None	Z None
3 Blood	D Indium 111 (In-111) Y Other Radionuclide	Z None	Z None
Y Lymphatic and Hematologic System	Y Other Radionuclide	Z None	Z None

Section	C	Nuclear Medicine
Body System	7	**Lymphatic and Hematologic System**
Type	2	**Tomographic (Tomo) Nuclear Medicine Imaging:** Introduction of radioactive materials into the body for three dimensional display of images developed from the capture of radioactive emissions

Body Part (4th)	Radionuclide (5th)	Qualifier (6th)	Qualifier (7th)
2 Spleen	1 Technetium 99m (Tc-99m) Y Other Radionuclide	Z None	Z None
Y Lymphatic and Hematologic System	Y Other Radionuclide	Z None	Z None

Section	C	Nuclear Medicine
Body System	7	**Lymphatic and Hematologic System**
Type	5	**Nonimaging Nuclear Medicine Probe:** Introduction of radioactive materials into the body for the study of distribution and fate of certain substances by the detection of radioactive emissions; or, alternatively, measurement of absorption of radioactive emissions from an external source

Body Part (4th)	Radionuclide (5th)	Qualifier (6th)	Qualifier (7th)
5 Lymphatics, Head and Neck D Lymphatics, Pelvic J Lymphatics, Head K Lymphatics, Neck L Lymphatics, Upper Chest M Lymphatics, Trunk N Lymphatics, Upper Extremity P Lymphatics, Lower Extremity	1 Technetium 99m (Tc-99m) Y Other Radionuclide	Z None	Z None
Y Lymphatic and Hematologic System	Y Other Radionuclide	Z None	Z None

Section	C	Nuclear Medicine
Body System	7	Lymphatic and Hematologic System
Type	6	**Nonimaging Nuclear Medicine Assay:** Introduction of radioactive materials into the body for the study of body fluids and blood elements, by the detection of radioactive emissions

Body Part (4th)	Radionuclide (5th)	Qualifier (6th)	Qualifier (7th)
3 Blood	1 Technetium 99m (Tc-99m) 7 Cobalt 58 (Co-58) C Cobalt 57 (Co-57) D Indium 111 (In-111) H Iodine 125 (I-125) W Chromium (Cr-51) Y Other Radionuclide	Z None	Z None
Y Lymphatic and Hematologic System	Y Other Radionuclide	Z None	Z None

Section	C	Nuclear Medicine
Body System	8	Eye
Type	1	**Planar Nuclear Medicine Imaging:** Introduction of radioactive materials into the body for single plane display of images developed from the capture of radioactive emissions

Body Part (4th)	Radionuclide (5th)	Qualifier (6th)	Qualifier (7th)
9 Lacrimal Ducts, Bilateral	1 Technetium 99m (Tc-99m) Y Other Radionuclide	Z None	Z None
Y Eye	Y Other Radionuclide	Z None	Z None

Section	C	Nuclear Medicine
Body System	9	Ear, Nose, Mouth and Throat
Type	1	**Planar Nuclear Medicine Imaging:** Introduction of radioactive materials into the body for single plane display of images developed from the capture of radioactive emissions

Body Part (4th)	Radionuclide (5th)	Qualifier (6th)	Qualifier (7th)
B Salivary Glands, Bilateral	1 Technetium 99m (Tc-99m) Y Other Radionuclide	Z None	Z None
Y Ear, Nose, Mouth and Throat	Y Other Radionuclide	Z None	Z None

Section	C	Nuclear Medicine
Body System	B	Respiratory System
Type	1	**Planar Nuclear Medicine Imaging:** Introduction of radioactive materials into the body for single plane display of images developed from the capture of radioactive emissions

Body Part (4th)	Radionuclide (5th)	Qualifier (6th)	Qualifier (7th)
2 Lungs and Bronchi	1 Technetium 99m (Tc-99m) 9 Krypton (Kr-81m) T Xenon 127 (Xe-127) V Xenon 133 (Xe-133) Y Other Radionuclide	Z None	Z None
Y Respiratory System	Y Other Radionuclide	Z None	Z None

Section	C	Nuclear Medicine
Body System	B	Respiratory System
Type	2	**Tomographic (Tomo) Nuclear Medicine Imaging:** Introduction of radioactive materials into the body for three dimensional display of images developed from the capture of radioactive emissions

Body Part (4th)	Radionuclide (5th)	Qualifier (6th)	Qualifier (7th)
2 Lungs and Bronchi	1 Technetium 99m (Tc-99m) 9 Krypton (Kr-81m) Y Other Radionuclide	Z None	Z None
Y Respiratory System	Y Other Radionuclide	Z None	Z None

Section   **C**   **Nuclear Medicine**
Body System   **B**   **Respiratory System**
Type   **3**   **Positron Emission Tomographic (PET) Imaging:** Introduction of radioactive materials into the body for three dimensional display of images developed from the simultaneous capture, 180 degrees apart, of radioactive emissions

Body Part (4th)	Radionuclide (5th)	Qualifier (6th)	Qualifier (7th)
2 Lungs and Bronchi	K Fluorine 18 (F-18) Y Other Radionuclide	Z None	Z None
Y Respiratory System	Y Other Radionuclide	Z None	Z None

Section   **C**   **Nuclear Medicine**
Body System   **D**   **Gastrointestinal System**
Type   **1**   **Planar Nuclear Medicine Imaging:** Introduction of radioactive materials into the body for single plane display of images developed from the capture of radioactive emissions

Body Part (4th)	Radionuclide (5th)	Qualifier (6th)	Qualifier (7th)
5 Upper Gastrointestinal Tract 7 Gastrointestinal Tract	1 Technetium 99m (Tc-99m) D Indium 111 (In-111) Y Other Radionuclide	Z None	Z None
Y Digestive System	Y Other Radionuclide	Z None	Z None

Section   **C**   **Nuclear Medicine**
Body System   **D**   **Gastrointestinal System**
Type   **2**   **Tomographic (Tomo) Nuclear Medicine Imaging:** Introduction of radioactive materials into the body for three dimensional display of images developed from the capture of radioactive emissions

Body Part (4th)	Radionuclide (5th)	Qualifier (6th)	Qualifier (7th)
7 Gastrointestinal Tract	1 Technetium 99m (Tc-99m) D Indium 111 (In-111) Y Other Radionuclide	Z None	Z None
Y Digestive System	Y Other Radionuclide	Z None	Z None

Section   **C**   **Nuclear Medicine**
Body System   **F**   **Hepatobiliary System and Pancreas**
Type   **1**   **Planar Nuclear Medicine Imaging:** Introduction of radioactive materials into the body for single plane display of images developed from the capture of radioactive emissions

Body Part (4th)	Radionuclide (5th)	Qualifier (6th)	Qualifier (7th)
4 Gallbladder 5 Liver 6 Liver and Spleen C Hepatobiliary System, All	1 Technetium 99m (Tc-99m) Y Other Radionuclide	Z None	Z None
Y Hepatobiliary System and Pancreas	Y Other Radionuclide	Z None	Z None

Section   **C**   **Nuclear Medicine**
Body System   **F**   **Hepatobiliary System and Pancreas**
Type   **2**   **Tomographic (Tomo) Nuclear Medicine Imaging:** Introduction of radioactive materials into the body for three dimensional display of images developed from the capture of radioactive emissions

Body Part (4th)	Radionuclide (5th)	Qualifier (6th)	Qualifier (7th)
4 Gallbladder 5 Liver 6 Liver and Spleen	1 Technetium 99m (Tc-99m) Y Other Radionuclide	Z None	Z None
Y Hepatobiliary System and Pancreas	Y Other Radionuclide	Z None	Z None

Section	C	Nuclear Medicine
Body System	G	Endocrine System
Type	1	**Planar Nuclear Medicine Imaging:** Introduction of radioactive materials into the body for single plane display of images developed from the capture of radioactive emissions

Body Part (4th)	Radionuclide (5th)	Qualifier (6th)	Qualifier (7th)
1 Parathyroid Glands	1 Technetium 99m (Tc-99m) S Thallium 201 (Tl-201) Y Other Radionuclide	Z None	Z None
2 Thyroid Gland	1 Technetium 99m (Tc-99m) F Iodine 123 (I-123) G Iodine 131 (I-131) Y Other Radionuclide	Z None	Z None
4 Adrenal Glands, Bilateral	G Iodine 131 (I-131) Y Other Radionuclide	Z None	Z None
Y Endocrine System	Y Other Radionuclide	Z None	Z None

Section	C	Nuclear Medicine
Body System	G	Endocrine System
Type	2	**Tomographic (Tomo) Nuclear Medicine Imaging:** Introduction of radioactive materials into the body for three dimensional display of images developed from the capture of radioactive emissions

Body Part (4th)	Radionuclide (5th)	Qualifier (6th)	Qualifier (7th)
1 Parathyroid Glands	1 Technetium 99m (Tc-99m) S Thallium 201 (Tl-201) Y Other Radionuclide	Z None	Z None
Y Endocrine System	Y Other Radionuclide	Z None	Z None

Section	C	Nuclear Medicine
Body System	G	Endocrine System
Type	4	**Nonimaging Nuclear Medicine Uptake:** Introduction of radioactive materials into the body for measurements of organ function, from the detection of radioactive emissions

Body Part (4th)	Radionuclide (5th)	Qualifier (6th)	Qualifier (7th)
2 Thyroid Gland	1 Technetium 99m (Tc-99m) F Iodine 123 (I-123) G Iodine 131 (I-131) Y Other Radionuclide	Z None	Z None
Y Endocrine System	Y Other Radionuclide	Z None	Z None

Section	C	Nuclear Medicine
Body System	H	Skin, Subcutaneous Tissue and Breast
Type	1	**Planar Nuclear Medicine Imaging:** Introduction of radioactive materials into the body for single plane display of images developed from the capture of radioactive emissions

Body Part (4th)	Radionuclide (5th)	Qualifier (6th)	Qualifier (7th)
0 Breast, Right 1 Breast, Left 2 Breasts, Bilateral	1 Technetium 99m (Tc-99m) S Thallium 201 (Tl-201) Y Other Radionuclide	Z None	Z None
Y Skin, Subcutaneous Tissue and Breast	Y Other Radionuclide	Z None	Z None

Section	C	Nuclear Medicine
Body System	H	Skin, Subcutaneous Tissue and Breast
Type	2	Tomographic (Tomo) Nuclear Medicine Imaging: Introduction of radioactive materials into the body for three dimensional display of images developed from the capture of radioactive emissions

Body Part (4th)	Radionuclide (5th)	Qualifier (6th)	Qualifier (7th)
0 Breast, Right 1 Breast, Left 2 Breasts, Bilateral	1 Technetium 99m (Tc-99m) S Thallium 201 (Tl-201) Y Other Radionuclide	Z None	Z None
Y Skin, Subcutaneous Tissue and Breast	Y Other Radionuclide	Z None	Z None

Section	C	Nuclear Medicine
Body System	P	Musculoskeletal System
Type	1	Planar Nuclear Medicine Imaging: Introduction of radioactive materials into the body for single plane display of images developed from the capture of radioactive emissions

Body Part (4th)	Radionuclide (5th)	Qualifier (6th)	Qualifier (7th)
1 Skull 4 Thorax 5 Spine 6 Pelvis 7 Spine and Pelvis 8 Upper Extremity, Right 9 Upper Extremity, Left B Upper Extremities, Bilateral C Lower Extremity, Right D Lower Extremity, Left F Lower Extremities, Bilateral Z Musculoskeletal System, All	1 Technetium 99m (Tc-99m) Y Other Radionuclide	Z None	Z None
Y Musculoskeletal System, Other	Y Other Radionuclide	Z None	Z None

Section	C	Nuclear Medicine
Body System	P	Musculoskeletal System
Type	2	Tomographic (Tomo) Nuclear Medicine Imaging: Introduction of radioactive materials into the body for three dimensional display of images developed from the capture of radioactive emissions

Body Part (4th)	Radionuclide (5th)	Qualifier (6th)	Qualifier (7th)
1 Skull 2 Cervical Spine 3 Skull and Cervical Spine 4 Thorax 6 Pelvis 7 Spine and Pelvis 8 Upper Extremity, Right 9 Upper Extremity, Left B Upper Extremities, Bilateral C Lower Extremity, Right D Lower Extremity, Left F Lower Extremities, Bilateral G Thoracic Spine H Lumbar Spine J Thoracolumbar Spine	1 Technetium 99m (Tc-99m) Y Other Radionuclide	Z None	Z None
Y Musculoskeletal System, Other	Y Other Radionuclide	Z None	Z None

Section	C	Nuclear Medicine
Body System	P	Musculoskeletal System
Type	5	**Nonimaging Nuclear Medicine Probe:** Introduction of radioactive materials into the body for the study of distribution and fate of certain substances by the detection of radioactive emissions; or, alternatively, measurement of absorption of radioactive emissions from an external source

Body Part (4th)	Radionuclide (5th)	Qualifier (6th)	Qualifier (7th)
5 Spine **N** Upper Extremities **P** Lower Extremities	**Z** None	**Z** None	**Z** None
Y Musculoskeletal System, Other	**Y** Other Radionuclide	**Z** None	**Z** None

Section	C	Nuclear Medicine
Body System	T	Urinary System
Type	1	**Planar Nuclear Medicine Imaging:** Introduction of radioactive materials into the body for single plane display of images developed from the capture of radioactive emissions

Body Part (4th)	Radionuclide (5th)	Qualifier (6th)	Qualifier (7th)
3 Kidneys, Ureters and Bladder	**1** Technetium 99m (Tc-99m) **F** Iodine 123 (I-123) **G** Iodine 131 (I-131) **Y** Other Radionuclide	**Z** None	**Z** None
H Bladder and Ureters	**1** Technetium 99m (Tc-99m) **Y** Other Radionuclide	**Z** None	**Z** None
Y Urinary System	**Y** Other Radionuclide	**Z** None	**Z** None

Section	C	Nuclear Medicine
Body System	T	Urinary System
Type	2	**Tomographic (Tomo) Nuclear Medicine Imaging:** Introduction of radioactive materials into the body for three dimensional display of images developed from the capture of radioactive emissions

Body Part (4th)	Radionuclide (5th)	Qualifier (6th)	Qualifier (7th)
3 Kidneys, Ureters and Bladder	**1** Technetium 99m (Tc-99m) **Y** Other Radionuclide	**Z** None	**Z** None
Y Urinary System	**Y** Other Radionuclide	**Z** None	**Z** None

Section	C	Nuclear Medicine
Body System	T	Urinary System
Type	6	**Nonimaging Nuclear Medicine Assay:** Introduction of radioactive materials into the body for the study of body fluids and blood elements, by the detection of radioactive emissions

Body Part (4th)	Radionuclide (5th)	Qualifier (6th)	Qualifier (7th)
3 Kidneys, Ureters and Bladder	**1** Technetium 99m (Tc-99m) **F** Iodine 123 (I-123) **G** Iodine 131 (I-131) **H** Iodine 125 (I-125) **Y** Other Radionuclide	**Z** None	**Z** None
Y Urinary System	**Y** Other Radionuclide	**Z** None	**Z** None

Section	C	Nuclear Medicine
Body System	V	Male Reproductive System
Type	1	**Planar Nuclear Medicine Imaging:** Introduction of radioactive materials into the body for single plane display of images developed from the capture of radioactive emissions

Body Part (4th)	Radionuclide (5th)	Qualifier (6th)	Qualifier (7th)
9 Testicles, Bilateral	1 Technetium 99m (Tc-99m) Y Other Radionuclide	Z None	Z None
Y Male Reproductive System	Y Other Radionuclide	Z None	Z None

Section	C	Nuclear Medicine
Body System	W	Anatomical Regions
Type	1	**Planar Nuclear Medicine Imaging:** Introduction of radioactive materials into the body for single plane display of images developed from the capture of radioactive emissions

Body Part (4th)	Radionuclide (5th)	Qualifier (6th)	Qualifier (7th)
0 Abdomen 1 Abdomen and Pelvis 4 Chest and Abdomen 6 Chest and Neck B Head and Neck D Lower Extremity J Pelvic Region M Upper Extremity N Whole Body	1 Technetium 99m (Tc-99m) D Indium 111 (In-111) F Iodine 123 (I-123) G Iodine 131 (I-131) L Gallium 67 (Ga-67) S Thallium 201 (Tl-201) Y Other Radionuclide	Z None	Z None
3 Chest	1 Technetium 99m (Tc-99m) D Indium 111 (In-111) F Iodine 123 (I-123) G Iodine 131 (I-131) K Fluorine 18 (F-18) L Gallium 67 (Ga-67) S Thallium 201 (Tl-201) Y Other Radionuclide	Z None	Z None
Y Anatomical Regions, Multiple	Y Other Radionuclide	Z None	Z None
Z Anatomical Region, Other	Z None	Z None	Z None

Section	C	Nuclear Medicine
Body System	W	Anatomical Regions
Type	2	**Tomographic (Tomo) Nuclear Medicine Imaging:** Introduction of radioactive materials into the body for three dimensional display of images developed from the capture of radioactive emissions

Body Part (4th)	Radionuclide (5th)	Qualifier (6th)	Qualifier (7th)
0 Abdomen 1 Abdomen and Pelvis 3 Chest 4 Chest and Abdomen 6 Chest and Neck B Head and Neck D Lower Extremity J Pelvic Region M Upper Extremity	1 Technetium 99m (Tc-99m) D Indium 111 (In-111) F Iodine 123 (I-123) G Iodine 131 (I-131) K Fluorine 18 (F-18) L Gallium 67 (Ga-67) S Thallium 201 (Tl-201) Y Other Radionuclide	Z None	Z None
Y Anatomical Regions, Multiple	Y Other Radionuclide	Z None	Z None

Section	C	Nuclear Medicine
Body System	W	Anatomical Regions
Type	3	**Positron Emission Tomographic (PET) Imaging:** Introduction of radioactive materials into the body for three dimensional display of images developed from the simultaneous capture, 180 degrees apart, of radioactive emissions

Body Part (4th)	Radionuclide (5th)	Qualifier (6th)	Qualifier (7th)
N Whole Body	Y Other Radionuclide	Z None	Z None

Section	C	Nuclear Medicine
Body System	W	Anatomical Regions
Type	5	**Nonimaging Nuclear Medicine Probe:** Introduction of radioactive materials into the body for the study of distribution and fate of certain substances by the detection of radioactive emissions; or, alternatively, measurement of absorption of radioactive emissions from an external source

Body Part (4th)	Radionuclide (5th)	Qualifier (6th)	Qualifier (7th)
0 Abdomen 1 Abdomen and Pelvis 3 Chest 4 Chest and Abdomen 6 Chest and Neck B Head and Neck D Lower Extremity J Pelvic Region M Upper Extremity	1 Technetium 99m (Tc-99m) D Indium 111 (In-111) Y Other Radionuclide	Z None	Z None

Section	C	Nuclear Medicine
Body System	W	Anatomical Regions
Type	7	**Systemic Nuclear Medicine Therapy:** Introduction of unsealed radioactive materials into the body for treatment

Body Part (4th)	Radionuclide (5th)	Qualifier (6th)	Qualifier (7th)
0 Abdomen 3 Chest	N Phosphorus 32 (P-32) Y Other Radionuclide	Z None	Z None
G Thyroid	G Iodine 131 (I-131) Y Other Radionuclide	Z None	Z None
N Whole Body	8 Samarium 153 (Sm-153) G Iodine 131 (I-131) N Phosphorus 32 (P-32) P Strontium 89 (Sr-89) Y Other Radionuclide	Z None	Z None
Y Anatomical Regions, Multiple	Y Other Radionuclide	Z None	Z None

AHA Coding Clinic

No references have been issued for the Nuclear Medicine section.

Radiation Therapy Section (D00–DWY)

Within each section of ICD-10-PCS the characters have different meanings. The seven character meanings for the Radiation Therapy section are illustrated here through the procedure example of *HDR brachytherapy of prostate using Palladium 103*.

Section	Body System	Modality	Treatment Site	Modality Qualifier	Isotope	Qualifier
Radiation Therapy	Male Reproductive System	Brachytherapy	Prostate	High Dose Rate (HDR)	Palladium 103	None
D	V	1	0	9	B	Z

Section (Character 1)

All Radiation Therapy procedure codes have a first character value of D.

Body System (Character 2)

The alphanumeric character for the body system is placed in the second position. The following are the body systems applicable to the Radiation Therapy section.

Character Value	Character Value Description
0	Central and Peripheral Nervous System
7	Lymphatic and Hematologic System
8	Eye
9	Ear, Nose, Mouth and Throat
B	Respiratory System
D	Gastrointestinal System
F	Hepatobiliary System and Pancreas
G	Endocrine System
H	Skin
M	Breast
P	Musculoskeletal
T	Urinary System
U	Female Reproductive System
V	Male Reproductive System
W	Anatomical Regions

Modality (Character 3)

The alphanumeric character value for root types is placed in the third position. The following are the root types applicable to the Radiation Therapy section with their associated meaning.

Character Value	Modality	Modality Definition
0	Beam Radiation	The external use of high-energy radiation such as x-rays, photons, electrons, or protons
1	Brachytherapy	The use of radioactive sources placed directly into a tumor bearing area to generate local regions of high intensity radiation
2	Stereotactic Radiosurgery	The use of external radiation sources either from a linear accelerator or a special Cobalt-60 irradiator to deliver many beams of radiation directly to an internal structure in a single fraction
Y	Other Radiation	Other types of radiation therapy such as hyperthermia, contact radiation and plaque radiation. *See Modality qualifier, character 5, for specified types of other radiation.*

Source: CSI Navigator for Radiation Oncology, 2010

Treatment Site (Character 4)

For each treatment site the applicable body part character values will be available for procedure code construction. An example of a treatment site for this section is Brain Stem.

Modality Qualifier (Character 5)

The modality qualifier further specifies the treatment modality. The following are examples of the modality qualifier values available for the Radiation Therapy section:

- Photons >10 MeV
- Neutrons
- Electrons
- High Dose Rate
- Hyperthermia

Isotope (Character 6)

When an isotope is utilized during a radiation oncology procedure, the corresponding isotope character value should be reported in the sixth character position. The following are examples of the isotope character values available for the Radiation Therapy section:

- Iridium 192 (Ir-192)
- Iodine 125 (I-125)
- Californium 252 (Cf-252)

Qualifier (Character 7)

The qualifier represents an additional attribute for the procedure when applicable. For example, beam radiation procedures in this section include the qualifier Intraoperative that is reported with the character value of 0 for some body parts. If there is no qualifier for a procedure, the placeholder Z is the character value that should be reported.

Radiation Therapy Section Guidelines (section D)

D. Radiation Therapy Section

Brachytherapy
D1.a

Brachytherapy is coded to the modality Brachytherapy in the Radiation Therapy section. When a radioactive brachytherapy source is left in the body at the end of the procedure, it is coded separately to the root operation Insertion with the device value Radioactive Element.

Example: Brachytherapy with implantation of a low dose rate brachytherapy source left in the body at the end of the procedure is coded to the applicable treatment site in section D, Radiation Therapy, with the modality Brachytherapy, the modality qualifier value, Low Dose Rate, and the applicable isotope value and qualifier value. The implantation of the brachytherapy source is coded separately to the device value Radioactive Element in the appropriate Insertion table of the Medical and Surgical section. The Radiation Therapy section code identifies the specific modality and isotope of the brachytherapy, and the root operation Insertion code identifies the implantation of the brachytherapy source that remain in the body at the end of the procedure.

Exception: Implantation of Cesium-131 brachytherapy seeds embedded in a collagen matrix to the treatment site after resection of brain tumor is coded to the root operation Insertion with the device value Radioactive Element, Cesium-131 Collagen Implant. The procedure is coded to the root operation Insertion only, because the device value identifies both the implantation of the radioactive element and a specific brachytherapy isotope that is not included in the Radiation Therapy section tables.

D1.b

A separate procedure to place a temporary applicator for delivering the brachytherapy is coded to the root operation Insertion and the device value Other Device.

Examples: Intrauterine brachytherapy applicator placed as a separate procedure from the brachytherapy procedure is coded to Insertion of Other Device, and the brachytherapy is coded separately using the modality Brachytherapy in the Radiation Therapy section. Intrauterine brachytherapy applicator placed concomitantly with delivery of the brachytherapy dose is coded with a single code using the modality Brachytherapy in the Radiation Therapy section.

Radiation Therapy Section Tables

Radiation Therapy Tables D00–DWY

Section	D	Radiation Therapy
Body System	0	Central and Peripheral Nervous System
Modality	0	Beam Radiation

Treatment Site (4th)	Modality Qualifier (5th)	Isotope (6th)	Qualifier (7th)
0 Brain 1 Brain Stem 6 Spinal Cord 7 Peripheral Nerve	0 Photons <1 MeV 1 Photons 1 - 10 MeV 2 Photons >10 MeV 4 Heavy Particles (Protons,Ions) 5 Neutrons 6 Neutron Capture	Z None	Z None
0 Brain 1 Brain Stem 6 Spinal Cord 7 Peripheral Nerve	3 Electrons	Z None	0 Intraoperative Z None

Section	D	Radiation Therapy
Body System	0	Central and Peripheral Nervous System
Modality	1	Brachytherapy

Treatment Site (4th)	Modality Qualifier (5th)	Isotope (6th)	Qualifier (7th)
0 Brain 1 Brain Stem 6 Spinal Cord 7 Peripheral Nerve	9 High Dose Rate (HDR)	7 Cesium 137 (Cs-137) 8 Iridium 192 (Ir-192) 9 Iodine 125 (I-125) B Palladium 103 (Pd-103) C Californium 252 (Cf-252) Y Other Isotope	Z None
0 Brain 1 Brain Stem 6 Spinal Cord 7 Peripheral Nerve	B Low Dose Rate (LDR)	6 Cesium 131 (Cs-131) 7 Cesium 137 (Cs-137) 8 Iridium 192 (Ir-192) 9 Iodine 125 (I-125) C Californium 252 (Cf-252) Y Other Isotope	Z None
0 Brain 1 Brain Stem 6 Spinal Cord 7 Peripheral Nerve	B Low Dose Rate (LDR)	B Palladium 103 (Pd-103)	1 Unidirectional Source Z None

Section	D	Radiation Therapy
Body System	0	Central and Peripheral Nervous System
Modality	2	Stereotactic Radiosurgery

Treatment Site (4th)	Modality Qualifier (5th)	Isotope (6th)	Qualifier (7th)
0 Brain 1 Brain Stem 6 Spinal Cord 7 Peripheral Nerve	D Stereotactic Other Photon Radiosurgery H Stereotactic Particulate Radiosurgery J Stereotactic Gamma Beam Radiosurgery	Z None	Z None

Section	D	Radiation Therapy
Body System	0	Central and Peripheral Nervous System
Modality	Y	Other Radiation

Treatment Site (4th)	Modality Qualifier (5th)	Isotope (6th)	Qualifier (7th)
0 Brain 1 Brain Stem 6 Spinal Cord 7 Peripheral Nerve	7 Contact Radiation 8 Hyperthermia C Intraoperative Radiation Therapy (IORT) F Plaque Radiation	Z None	Z None

Section	D	Radiation Therapy
Body System	7	Lymphatic and Hematologic System
Modality	0	Beam Radiation

Treatment Site (4th)	Modality Qualifier (5th)	Isotope (6th)	Qualifier (7th)
0 Bone Marrow 1 Thymus 2 Spleen 3 Lymphatics, Neck 4 Lymphatics, Axillary 5 Lymphatics, Thorax 6 Lymphatics, Abdomen 7 Lymphatics, Pelvis 8 Lymphatics, Inguinal	0 Photons <1 MeV 1 Photons 1 - 10 MeV 2 Photons >10 MeV 4 Heavy Particles (Protons,Ions) 5 Neutrons 6 Neutron Capture	Z None	Z None
0 Bone Marrow 1 Thymus 2 Spleen 3 Lymphatics, Neck 4 Lymphatics, Axillary 5 Lymphatics, Thorax 6 Lymphatics, Abdomen 7 Lymphatics, Pelvis 8 Lymphatics, Inguinal	3 Electrons	Z None	0 Intraoperative Z None

Section	D	Radiation Therapy
Body System	7	Lymphatic and Hematologic System
Modality	1	Brachytherapy

Treatment Site (4th)	Modality Qualifier (5th)	Isotope (6th)	Qualifier (7th)
0 Bone Marrow 1 Thymus 2 Spleen 3 Lymphatics, Neck 4 Lymphatics, Axillary 5 Lymphatics, Thorax 6 Lymphatics, Abdomen 7 Lymphatics, Pelvis 8 Lymphatics, Inguinal	9 High Dose Rate (HDR)	7 Cesium 137 (Cs-137) 8 Iridium 192 (Ir-192) 9 Iodine 125 (I-125) B Palladium 103 (Pd-103) C Californium 252 (Cf-252) Y Other Isotope	Z None
0 Bone Marrow 1 Thymus 2 Spleen 3 Lymphatics, Neck 4 Lymphatics, Axillary 5 Lymphatics, Thorax 6 Lymphatics, Abdomen 7 Lymphatics, Pelvis 8 Lymphatics, Inguinal	B Low Dose Rate (LDR)	6 Cesium 131 (Cs-131) 7 Cesium 137 (Cs-137) 8 Iridium 192 (Ir-192) 9 Iodine 125 (I-125) C Californium 252 (Cf-252) Y Other Isotope	Z None
0 Bone Marrow 1 Thymus 2 Spleen 3 Lymphatics, Neck 4 Lymphatics, Axillary 5 Lymphatics, Thorax 6 Lymphatics, Abdomen 7 Lymphatics, Pelvis 8 Lymphatics, Inguinal	B Low Dose Rate (LDR)	B Palladium 103 (Pd-103)	1 Unidirectional Source Z None

Section	D	Radiation Therapy
Body System	7	Lymphatic and Hematologic System
Modality	2	Stereotactic Radiosurgery

Treatment Site (4th)	Modality Qualifier (5th)	Isotope (6th)	Qualifier (7th)
0 Bone Marrow 1 Thymus 2 Spleen 3 Lymphatics, Neck 4 Lymphatics, Axillary 5 Lymphatics, Thorax 6 Lymphatics, Abdomen 7 Lymphatics, Pelvis 8 Lymphatics, Inguinal	D Stereotactic Other Photon Radiosurgery H Stereotactic Particulate Radiosurgery J Stereotactic Gamma Beam Radiosurgery	Z None	Z None

Section	D	Radiation Therapy
Body System	7	Lymphatic and Hematologic System
Modality	Y	Other Radiation

Treatment Site (4th)	Modality Qualifier (5th)	Isotope (6th)	Qualifier (7th)
0 Bone Marrow 1 Thymus 2 Spleen 3 Lymphatics, Neck 4 Lymphatics, Axillary 5 Lymphatics, Thorax 6 Lymphatics, Abdomen 7 Lymphatics, Pelvis 8 Lymphatics, Inguinal	8 Hyperthermia F Plaque Radiation	Z None	Z None

Section	D	Radiation Therapy
Body System	8	Eye
Modality	0	Beam Radiation

Treatment Site (4th)	Modality Qualifier (5th)	Isotope (6th)	Qualifier (7th)
0 Eye	0 Photons <1 MeV 1 Photons 1 - 10 MeV 2 Photons >10 MeV 4 Heavy Particles (Protons,Ions) 5 Neutrons 6 Neutron Capture	Z None	Z None
0 Eye	3 Electrons	Z None	0 Intraoperative Z None

Section	D	Radiation Therapy
Body System	8	Eye
Modality	1	Brachytherapy

Treatment Site (4th)	Modality Qualifier (5th)	Isotope (6th)	Qualifier (7th)
0 Eye	9 High Dose Rate (HDR)	7 Cesium 137 (Cs-137) 8 Iridium 192 (Ir-192) 9 Iodine 125 (I-125) B Palladium 103 (Pd-103) C Californium 252 (Cf-252) Y Other Isotope	Z None
0 Eye	B Low Dose Rate (LDR)	6 Cesium 131 (Cs-131) 7 Cesium 137 (Cs-137) 8 Iridium 192 (Ir-192) 9 Iodine 125 (I-125) C Californium 252 (Cf-252) Y Other Isotope	Z None

Continued →

Section   **D**   **Radiation Therapy**   *D81 Continued*
Body System   **8**   **Eye**
Modality   **1**   **Brachytherapy**

Treatment Site (4ᵗʰ)	Modality Qualifier (5ᵗʰ)	Isotope (6ᵗʰ)	Qualifier (7ᵗʰ)
0 Eye	**B** Low Dose Rate (LDR)	**B** Palladium 103 (Pd-103)	**1** Unidirectional Source **Z** None

Section   **D**   **Radiation Therapy**
Body System   **8**   **Eye**
Modality   **2**   **Stereotactic Radiosurgery**

Treatment Site (4ᵗʰ)	Modality Qualifier (5ᵗʰ)	Isotope (6ᵗʰ)	Qualifier (7ᵗʰ)
0 Eye	**D** Stereotactic Other Photon Radiosurgery **H** Stereotactic Particulate Radiosurgery **J** Stereotactic Gamma Beam Radiosurgery	**Z** None	**Z** None

Section   **D**   **Radiation Therapy**
Body System   **8**   **Eye**
Modality   **Y**   **Other Radiation**

Treatment Site (4ᵗʰ)	Modality Qualifier (5ᵗʰ)	Isotope (6ᵗʰ)	Qualifier (7ᵗʰ)
0 Eye	**7** Contact Radiation **8** Hyperthermia **F** Plaque Radiation	**Z** None	**Z** None

Section   **D**   **Radiation Therapy**
Body System   **9**   **Ear, Nose, Mouth and Throat**
Modality   **0**   **Beam Radiation**

Treatment Site (4ᵗʰ)	Modality Qualifier (5ᵗʰ)	Isotope (6ᵗʰ)	Qualifier (7ᵗʰ)
0 Ear **1** Nose **3** Hypopharynx **4** Mouth **5** Tongue **6** Salivary Glands **7** Sinuses **8** Hard Palate **9** Soft Palate **B** Larynx **D** Nasopharynx **F** Oropharynx	**0** Photons <1 MeV **1** Photons 1 - 10 MeV **2** Photons >10 MeV **4** Heavy Particles (Protons,Ions) **5** Neutrons **6** Neutron Capture	**Z** None	**Z** None
0 Ear **1** Nose **3** Hypopharynx **4** Mouth **5** Tongue **6** Salivary Glands **7** Sinuses **8** Hard Palate **9** Soft Palate **B** Larynx **D** Nasopharynx **F** Oropharynx	**3** Electrons	**Z** None	**0** Intraoperative **Z** None

Section   **D**   **Radiation Therapy**
Body System   **9**   **Ear, Nose, Mouth and Throat**
Modality   **1**   **Brachytherapy**

Treatment Site (4th)	Modality Qualifier (5th)	Isotope (6th)	Qualifier (7th)
0 Ear 1 Nose 3 Hypopharynx 4 Mouth 5 Tongue 6 Salivary Glands 7 Sinuses 8 Hard Palate 9 Soft Palate B Larynx D Nasopharynx F Oropharynx	9 High Dose Rate (HDR)	7 Cesium 137 (Cs-137) 8 Iridium 192 (Ir-192) 9 Iodine 125 (I-125) B Palladium 103 (Pd-103) C Californium 252 (Cf-252) Y Other Isotope	Z None
0 Ear 1 Nose 3 Hypopharynx 4 Mouth 5 Tongue 6 Salivary Glands 7 Sinuses 8 Hard Palate 9 Soft Palate B Larynx D Nasopharynx F Oropharynx	B Low Dose Rate (LDR)	6 Cesium 131 (Cs-131) 7 Cesium 137 (Cs-137) 8 Iridium 192 (Ir-192) 9 Iodine 125 (I-125) C Californium 252 (Cf-252) Y Other Isotope	Z None
0 Ear 1 Nose 3 Hypopharynx 4 Mouth 5 Tongue 6 Salivary Glands 7 Sinuses 8 Hard Palate 9 Soft Palate B Larynx D Nasopharynx F Oropharynx	B Low Dose Rate (LDR)	B Palladium 103 (Pd-103)	1 Unidirectional Source Z None

Section   **D**   **Radiation Therapy**
Body System   **9**   **Ear, Nose, Mouth and Throat**
Modality   **2**   **Stereotactic Radiosurgery**

Treatment Site (4th)	Modality Qualifier (5th)	Isotope (6th)	Qualifier (7th)
0 Ear 1 Nose 4 Mouth 5 Tongue 6 Salivary Glands 7 Sinuses 8 Hard Palate 9 Soft Palate B Larynx C Pharynx D Nasopharynx	D Stereotactic Other Photon Radiosurgery H Stereotactic Particulate Radiosurgery J Stereotactic Gamma Beam Radiosurgery	Z None	Z None

Section	D	Radiation Therapy
Body System	9	Ear, Nose, Mouth and Throat
Modality	Y	Other Radiation

Treatment Site (4th)	Modality Qualifier (5th)	Isotope (6th)	Qualifier (7th)
0 Ear 1 Nose 5 Tongue 6 Salivary Glands 7 Sinuses 8 Hard Palate 9 Soft Palate	7 Contact Radiation 8 Hyperthermia F Plaque Radiation	Z None	Z None
3 Hypopharynx F Oropharynx	7 Contact Radiation 8 Hyperthermia	Z None	Z None
4 Mouth B Larynx D Nasopharynx	7 Contact Radiation 8 Hyperthermia C Intraoperative Radiation Therapy (IORT) F Plaque Radiation	Z None	Z None
C Pharynx	C Intraoperative Radiation Therapy (IORT) F Plaque Radiation	Z None	Z None

Section	D	Radiation Therapy
Body System	B	Respiratory System
Modality	0	Beam Radiation

Treatment Site (4th)	Modality Qualifier (5th)	Isotope (6th)	Qualifier (7th)
0 Trachea 1 Bronchus 2 Lung 5 Pleura 6 Mediastinum 7 Chest Wall 8 Diaphragm	0 Photons <1 MeV 1 Photons 1 - 10 MeV 2 Photons >10 MeV 4 Heavy Particles (Protons,Ions) 5 Neutrons 6 Neutron Capture	Z None	Z None
0 Trachea 1 Bronchus 2 Lung 5 Pleura 6 Mediastinum 7 Chest Wall 8 Diaphragm	3 Electrons	Z None	0 Intraoperative Z None

Section	D	Radiation Therapy
Body System	B	Respiratory System
Modality	1	Brachytherapy

Treatment Site (4th)	Modality Qualifier (5th)	Isotope (6th)	Qualifier (7th)
0 Trachea 1 Bronchus 2 Lung 5 Pleura 6 Mediastinum 7 Chest Wall 8 Diaphragm	9 High Dose Rate (HDR)	7 Cesium 137 (Cs-137) 8 Iridium 192 (Ir-192) 9 Iodine 125 (I-125) B Palladium 103 (Pd-103) C Californium 252 (Cf-252) Y Other Isotope	Z None

Continued →

DB1 Continued

Section	D	Radiation Therapy
Body System	B	Respiratory System
Modality	1	Brachytherapy

Treatment Site (4th)	Modality Qualifier (5th)	Isotope (6th)	Qualifier (7th)
0 Trachea 1 Bronchus 2 Lung 5 Pleura 6 Mediastinum 7 Chest Wall 8 Diaphragm	B Low Dose Rate (LDR)	6 Cesium 131 (Cs-131) 7 Cesium 137 (Cs-137) 8 Iridium 192 (Ir-192) 9 Iodine 125 (I-125) C Californium 252 (Cf-252) Y Other Isotope	Z None
0 Trachea 1 Bronchus 2 Lung 5 Pleura 6 Mediastinum 7 Chest Wall 8 Diaphragm	B Low Dose Rate (LDR)	B Palladium 103 (Pd-103)	1 Unidirectional Source Z None

Section	D	Radiation Therapy
Body System	B	Respiratory System
Modality	2	Stereotactic Radiosurgery

Treatment Site (4th)	Modality Qualifier (5th)	Isotope (6th)	Qualifier (7th)
0 Trachea 1 Bronchus 2 Lung 5 Pleura 6 Mediastinum 7 Chest Wall 8 Diaphragm	D Stereotactic Other Photon Radiosurgery H Stereotactic Particulate Radiosurgery J Stereotactic Gamma Beam Radiosurgery	Z None	Z None

Section	D	Radiation Therapy
Body System	B	Respiratory System
Modality	Y	Other Radiation

Treatment Site (4th)	Modality Qualifier (5th)	Isotope (6th)	Qualifier (7th)
0 Trachea 1 Bronchus 2 Lung 5 Pleura 6 Mediastinum 7 Chest Wall 8 Diaphragm	7 Contact Radiation 8 Hyperthermia F Plaque Radiation	Z None	Z None

Section	D	Radiation Therapy
Body System	D	Gastrointestinal System
Modality	0	Beam Radiation

Treatment Site (4th)	Modality Qualifier (5th)	Isotope (6th)	Qualifier (7th)
0 Esophagus 1 Stomach 2 Duodenum 3 Jejunum 4 Ileum 5 Colon 7 Rectum	0 Photons <1 MeV 1 Photons 1 - 10 MeV 2 Photons >10 MeV 4 Heavy Particles (Protons,Ions) 5 Neutrons 6 Neutron Capture	Z None	Z None

Continued →

632

Section   D   Radiation Therapy
Body System   D   Gastrointestinal System
Modality   0   Beam Radiation

Treatment Site (4th)	Modality Qualifier (5th)	Isotope (6th)	Qualifier (7th)
0 Esophagus 1 Stomach 2 Duodenum 3 Jejunum 4 Ileum 5 Colon 7 Rectum	3 Electrons	Z None	0 Intraoperative Z None

Section   D   Radiation Therapy
Body System   D   Gastrointestinal System
Modality   1   Brachytherapy

Treatment Site (4th)	Modality Qualifier (5th)	Isotope (6th)	Qualifier (7th)
0 Esophagus 1 Stomach 2 Duodenum 3 Jejunum 4 Ileum 5 Colon 7 Rectum	9 High Dose Rate (HDR)	7 Cesium 137 (Cs-137) 8 Iridium 192 (Ir-192) 9 Iodine 125 (I-125) B Palladium 103 (Pd-103) C Californium 252 (Cf-252) Y Other Isotope	Z None
0 Esophagus 1 Stomach 2 Duodenum 3 Jejunum 4 Ileum 5 Colon 7 Rectum	B Low Dose Rate (LDR)	6 Cesium 131 (Cs-131) 7 Cesium 137 (Cs-137) 8 Iridium 192 (Ir-192) 9 Iodine 125 (I-125) C Californium 252 (Cf-252) Y Other Isotope	Z None
0 Esophagus 1 Stomach 2 Duodenum 3 Jejunum 4 Ileum 5 Colon 7 Rectum	B Low Dose Rate (LDR)	B Palladium 103 (Pd-103)	1 Unidirectional Source Z None

Section   D   Radiation Therapy
Body System   D   Gastrointestinal System
Modality   2   Stereotactic Radiosurgery

Treatment Site (4th)	Modality Qualifier (5th)	Isotope (6th)	Qualifier (7th)
0 Esophagus 1 Stomach 2 Duodenum 3 Jejunum 4 Ileum 5 Colon 7 Rectum	D Stereotactic Other Photon Radiosurgery H Stereotactic Particulate Radiosurgery J Stereotactic Gamma Beam Radiosurgery	Z None	Z None

Section   D   Radiation Therapy
Body System   D   Gastrointestinal System
Modality   Y   Other Radiation

Treatment Site (4th)	Modality Qualifier (5th)	Isotope (6th)	Qualifier (7th)
0 Esophagus	7 Contact Radiation 8 Hyperthermia F Plaque Radiation	Z None	Z None

DDY–DF1

Section	D	Radiation Therapy
Body System	D	Gastrointestinal System
Modality	Y	Other Radiation

DDY Continued

Treatment Site (4th)	Modality Qualifier (5th)	Isotope (6th)	Qualifier (7th)
1 Stomach 2 Duodenum 3 Jejunum 4 Ileum 5 Colon 7 Rectum	7 Contact Radiation 8 Hyperthermia C Intraoperative Radiation Therapy (IORT) F Plaque Radiation	Z None	Z None
8 Anus	C Intraoperative Radiation Therapy (IORT) F Plaque Radiation	Z None	Z None

Section	D	Radiation Therapy
Body System	F	Hepatobiliary System and Pancreas
Modality	0	Beam Radiation

Treatment Site (4th)	Modality Qualifier (5th)	Isotope (6th)	Qualifier (7th)
0 Liver 1 Gallbladder 2 Bile Ducts 3 Pancreas	0 Photons <1 MeV 1 Photons 1 - 10 MeV 2 Photons >10 MeV 4 Heavy Particles (Protons,Ions) 5 Neutrons 6 Neutron Capture	Z None	Z None
0 Liver 1 Gallbladder 2 Bile Ducts 3 Pancreas	3 Electrons	Z None	0 Intraoperative Z None

Section	D	Radiation Therapy
Body System	F	Hepatobiliary System and Pancreas
Modality	1	Brachytherapy

Treatment Site (4th)	Modality Qualifier (5th)	Isotope (6th)	Qualifier (7th)
0 Liver 1 Gallbladder 2 Bile Ducts 3 Pancreas	9 High Dose Rate (HDR)	7 Cesium 137 (Cs-137) 8 Iridium 192 (Ir-192) 9 Iodine 125 (I-125) B Palladium 103 (Pd-103) C Californium 252 (Cf-252) Y Other Isotope	Z None
0 Liver 1 Gallbladder 2 Bile Ducts 3 Pancreas	B Low Dose Rate (LDR)	6 Cesium 131 (Cs-131) 7 Cesium 137 (Cs-137) 8 Iridium 192 (Ir-192) 9 Iodine 125 (I-125) C Californium 252 (Cf-252) Y Other Isotope	Z None
0 Liver 1 Gallbladder 2 Bile Ducts 3 Pancreas	B Low Dose Rate (LDR)	B Palladium 103 (Pd-103)	1 Unidirectional Source Z None

Radiation Therapy Section Tables

Section	D	Radiation Therapy
Body System	F	Hepatobiliary System and Pancreas
Modality	2	Stereotactic Radiosurgery

Treatment Site (4th)	Modality Qualifier (5th)	Isotope (6th)	Qualifier (7th)
0 Liver **1** Gallbladder **2** Bile Ducts **3** Pancreas	**D** Stereotactic Other Photon Radiosurgery **H** Stereotactic Particulate Radiosurgery **J** Stereotactic Gamma Beam Radiosurgery	**Z** None	**Z** None

Section	D	Radiation Therapy
Body System	F	Hepatobiliary System and Pancreas
Modality	Y	Other Radiation

Treatment Site (4th)	Modality Qualifier (5th)	Isotope (6th)	Qualifier (7th)
0 Liver **1** Gallbladder **2** Bile Ducts **3** Pancreas	**7** Contact Radiation **8** Hyperthermia **C** Intraoperative Radiation Therapy (IORT) **F** Plaque Radiation	**Z** None	**Z** None

Section	D	Radiation Therapy
Body System	G	Endocrine System
Modality	0	Beam Radiation

Treatment Site (4th)	Modality Qualifier (5th)	Isotope (6th)	Qualifier (7th)
0 Pituitary Gland **1** Pineal Body **2** Adrenal Glands **4** Parathyroid Glands **5** Thyroid	**0** Photons <1 MeV **1** Photons 1 - 10 MeV **2** Photons >10 MeV **5** Neutrons **6** Neutron Capture	**Z** None	**Z** None
0 Pituitary Gland **1** Pineal Body **2** Adrenal Glands **4** Parathyroid Glands **5** Thyroid	**3** Electrons	**Z** None	**0** Intraoperative **Z** None

Section	D	Radiation Therapy
Body System	G	Endocrine System
Modality	1	Brachytherapy

Treatment Site (4th)	Modality Qualifier (5th)	Isotope (6th)	Qualifier (7th)
0 Pituitary Gland **1** Pineal Body **2** Adrenal Glands **4** Parathyroid Glands **5** Thyroid	**9** High Dose Rate (HDR)	**7** Cesium 137 (Cs-137) **8** Iridium 192 (Ir-192) **9** Iodine 125 (I-125) **B** Palladium 103 (Pd-103) **C** Californium 252 (Cf-252) **Y** Other Isotope	**Z** None
0 Pituitary Gland **1** Pineal Body **2** Adrenal Glands **4** Parathyroid Glands **5** Thyroid	**B** Low Dose Rate (LDR)	**6** Cesium 131 (Cs-131) **7** Cesium 137 (Cs-137) **8** Iridium 192 (Ir-192) **9** Iodine 125 (I-125) **C** Californium 252 (Cf-252) **Y** Other Isotope	**Z** None
0 Pituitary Gland **1** Pineal Body **2** Adrenal Glands **4** Parathyroid Glands **5** Thyroid	**B** Low Dose Rate (LDR)	**B** Palladium 103 (Pd-103)	**1** Unidirectional Source **Z** None

Section	D	Radiation Therapy
Body System	G	Endocrine System
Modality	2	Stereotactic Radiosurgery

Treatment Site (4th)	Modality Qualifier (5th)	Isotope (6th)	Qualifier (7th)
0 Pituitary Gland 1 Pineal Body 2 Adrenal Glands 4 Parathyroid Glands 5 Thyroid	D Stereotactic Other Photon Radiosurgery H Stereotactic Particulate Radiosurgery J Stereotactic Gamma Beam Radiosurgery	Z None	Z None

Section	D	Radiation Therapy
Body System	G	Endocrine System
Modality	Y	Other Radiation

Treatment Site (4th)	Modality Qualifier (5th)	Isotope (6th)	Qualifier (7th)
0 Pituitary Gland 1 Pineal Body 2 Adrenal Glands 4 Parathyroid Glands 5 Thyroid	7 Contact Radiation 8 Hyperthermia F Plaque Radiation	Z None	Z None

Section	D	Radiation Therapy
Body System	H	Skin
Modality	0	Beam Radiation

Treatment Site (4th)	Modality Qualifier (5th)	Isotope (6th)	Qualifier (7th)
2 Skin, Face 3 Skin, Neck 4 Skin, Arm 6 Skin, Chest 7 Skin, Back 8 Skin, Abdomen 9 Skin, Buttock B Skin, Leg	0 Photons <1 MeV 1 Photons 1 - 10 MeV 2 Photons >10 MeV 4 Heavy Particles (Protons,Ions) 5 Neutrons 6 Neutron Capture	Z None	Z None
2 Skin, Face 3 Skin, Neck 4 Skin, Arm 6 Skin, Chest 7 Skin, Back 8 Skin, Abdomen 9 Skin, Buttock B Skin, Leg	3 Electrons	Z None	0 Intraoperative Z None

Section	D	Radiation Therapy
Body System	H	Skin
Modality	Y	Other Radiation

Treatment Site (4th)	Modality Qualifier (5th)	Isotope (6th)	Qualifier (7th)
2 Skin, Face 3 Skin, Neck 4 Skin, Arm 6 Skin, Chest 7 Skin, Back 8 Skin, Abdomen 9 Skin, Buttock B Skin, Leg	7 Contact Radiation 8 Hyperthermia F Plaque Radiation	Z None	Z None
5 Skin, Hand C Skin, Foot	F Plaque Radiation	Z None	Z None

Section	D	Radiation Therapy
Body System	M	Breast
Modality	0	Beam Radiation

Treatment Site (4th)	Modality Qualifier (5th)	Isotope (6th)	Qualifier (7th)
0 Breast, Left 1 Breast, Right	0 Photons <1 MeV 1 Photons 1 - 10 MeV 2 Photons >10 MeV 4 Heavy Particles (Protons,Ions) 5 Neutrons 6 Neutron Capture	Z None	Z None
0 Breast, Left 1 Breast, Right	3 Electrons	Z None	0 Intraoperative Z None

Section	D	Radiation Therapy
Body System	M	Breast
Modality	1	Brachytherapy

Treatment Site (4th)	Modality Qualifier (5th)	Isotope (6th)	Qualifier (7th)
0 Breast, Left 1 Breast, Right	9 High Dose Rate (HDR)	7 Cesium 137 (Cs-137) 8 Iridium 192 (Ir-192) 9 Iodine 125 (I-125) B Palladium 103 (Pd-103) C Californium 252 (Cf-252) Y Other Isotope	Z None
0 Breast, Left 1 Breast, Right	B Low Dose Rate (LDR)	6 Cesium 131 (Cs-131) 7 Cesium 137 (Cs-137) 8 Iridium 192 (Ir-192) 9 Iodine 125 (I-125) C Californium 252 (Cf-252) Y Other Isotope	Z None
0 Breast, Left 1 Breast, Right	B Low Dose Rate (LDR)	B Palladium 103 (Pd-103)	1 Unidirectional Source Z None

Section	D	Radiation Therapy
Body System	M	Breast
Modality	2	Stereotactic Radiosurgery

Treatment Site (4th)	Modality Qualifier (5th)	Isotope (6th)	Qualifier (7th)
0 Breast, Left 1 Breast, Right	D Stereotactic Other Photon Radiosurgery H Stereotactic Particulate Radiosurgery J Stereotactic Gamma Beam Radiosurgery	Z None	Z None

Section	D	Radiation Therapy
Body System	M	Breast
Modality	Y	Other Radiation

Treatment Site (4th)	Modality Qualifier (5th)	Isotope (6th)	Qualifier (7th)
0 Breast, Left 1 Breast, Right	7 Contact Radiation 8 Hyperthermia F Plaque Radiation	Z None	Z None

Section   **D**   **Radiation Therapy**
Body System   **P**   **Musculoskeletal System**
Modality   **0**   **Beam Radiation**

Treatment Site (4th)	Modality Qualifier (5th)	Isotope (6th)	Qualifier (7th)
0 Skull 2 Maxilla 3 Mandible 4 Sternum 5 Rib(s) 6 Humerus 7 Radius/Ulna 8 Pelvic Bones 9 Femur B Tibia/Fibula C Other Bone	0 Photons <1 MeV 1 Photons 1 - 10 MeV 2 Photons >10 MeV 4 Heavy Particles (Protons,Ions) 5 Neutrons 6 Neutron Capture	Z None	Z None
0 Skull 2 Maxilla 3 Mandible 4 Sternum 5 Rib(s) 6 Humerus 7 Radius/Ulna 8 Pelvic Bones 9 Femur B Tibia/Fibula C Other Bone	3 Electrons	Z None	0 Intraoperative Z None

Section   **D**   **Radiation Therapy**
Body System   **P**   **Musculoskeletal System**
Modality   **Y**   **Other Radiation**

Treatment Site (4th)	Modality Qualifier (5th)	Isotope (6th)	Qualifier (7th)
0 Skull 2 Maxilla 3 Mandible 4 Sternum 5 Rib(s) 6 Humerus 7 Radius/Ulna 8 Pelvic Bones 9 Femur B Tibia/Fibula C Other Bone	7 Contact Radiation 8 Hyperthermia F Plaque Radiation	Z None	Z None

Section   **D**   **Radiation Therapy**
Body System   **T**   **Urinary System**
Modality   **0**   **Beam Radiation**

Treatment Site (4th)	Modality Qualifier (5th)	Isotope (6th)	Qualifier (7th)
0 Kidney 1 Ureter 2 Bladder 3 Urethra	0 Photons <1 MeV 1 Photons 1 - 10 MeV 2 Photons >10 MeV 4 Heavy Particles (Protons,Ions) 5 Neutrons 6 Neutron Capture	Z None	Z None
0 Kidney 1 Ureter 2 Bladder 3 Urethra	3 Electrons	Z None	0 Intraoperative Z None

Section	D	Radiation Therapy
Body System	T	Urinary System
Modality	1	Brachytherapy

Treatment Site (4th)	Modality Qualifier (5th)	Isotope (6th)	Qualifier (7th)
0 Kidney 1 Ureter 2 Bladder 3 Urethra	9 High Dose Rate (HDR)	7 Cesium 137 (Cs-137) 8 Iridium 192 (Ir-192) 9 Iodine 125 (I-125) B Palladium 103 (Pd-103) C Californium 252 (Cf-252) Y Other Isotope	Z None
0 Kidney 1 Ureter 2 Bladder 3 Urethra	B Low Dose Rate (LDR)	6 Cesium 131 (Cs-131) 7 Cesium 137 (Cs-137) 8 Iridium 192 (Ir-192) 9 Iodine 125 (I-125) C Californium 252 (Cf-252) Y Other Isotope	Z None
0 Kidney 1 Ureter 2 Bladder 3 Urethra	B Low Dose Rate (LDR)	B Palladium 103 (Pd-103)	1 Unidirectional Source Z None

Section	D	Radiation Therapy
Body System	T	Urinary System
Modality	2	Stereotactic Radiosurgery

Treatment Site (4th)	Modality Qualifier (5th)	Isotope (6th)	Qualifier (7th)
0 Kidney 1 Ureter 2 Bladder 3 Urethra	D Stereotactic Other Photon Radiosurgery H Stereotactic Particulate Radiosurgery J Stereotactic Gamma Beam Radiosurgery	Z None	Z None

Section	D	Radiation Therapy
Body System	T	Urinary System
Modality	Y	Other Radiation

Treatment Site (4th)	Modality Qualifier (5th)	Isotope (6th)	Qualifier (7th)
0 Kidney 1 Ureter 2 Bladder 3 Urethra	7 Contact Radiation 8 Hyperthermia C Intraoperative Radiation Therapy (IORT) F Plaque Radiation	Z None	Z None

Section	D	Radiation Therapy
Body System	U	Female Reproductive System
Modality	0	Beam Radiation

Treatment Site (4th)	Modality Qualifier (5th)	Isotope (6th)	Qualifier (7th)
0 Ovary 1 Cervix 2 Uterus	0 Photons <1 MeV 1 Photons 1 - 10 MeV 2 Photons >10 MeV 4 Heavy Particles (Protons,Ions) 5 Neutrons 6 Neutron Capture	Z None	Z None
0 Ovary 1 Cervix 2 Uterus	3 Electrons	Z None	0 Intraoperative Z None

DU1–DV0

Radiation Therapy Section Tables

Section   **D**   **Radiation Therapy**
Body System **U**   **Female Reproductive System**
Modality   **1**   **Brachytherapy**

Treatment Site (4th)	Modality Qualifier (5th)	Isotope (6th)	Qualifier (7th)
0 Ovary **1** Cervix **2** Uterus	**9** High Dose Rate (HDR)	**7** Cesium 137 (Cs-137) **8** Iridium 192 (Ir-192) **9** Iodine 125 (I-125) **B** Palladium 103 (Pd-103) **C** Californium 252 (Cf-252) **Y** Other Isotope	**Z** None
0 Ovary **1** Cervix **2** Uterus	**B** Low Dose Rate (LDR)	**6** Cesium 131 (Cs-131) **7** Cesium 137 (Cs-137) **8** Iridium 192 (Ir-192) **9** Iodine 125 (I-125) **C** Californium 252 (Cf-252) **Y** Other Isotope	**Z** None
0 Ovary **1** Cervix **2** Uterus	**B** Low Dose Rate (LDR)	**B** Palladium 103 (Pd-103)	**1** Unidirectional Source **Z** None

Section   **D**   **Radiation Therapy**
Body System **U**   **Female Reproductive System**
Modality   **2**   **Stereotactic Radiosurgery**

Treatment Site (4th)	Modality Qualifier (5th)	Isotope (6th)	Qualifier (7th)
0 Ovary **1** Cervix **2** Uterus	**D** Stereotactic Other Photon Radiosurgery **H** Stereotactic Particulate Radiosurgery **J** Stereotactic Gamma Beam Radiosurgery	**Z** None	**Z** None

Section   **D**   **Radiation Therapy**
Body System **U**   **Female Reproductive System**
Modality   **Y**   **Other Radiation**

Treatment Site (4th)	Modality Qualifier (5th)	Isotope (6th)	Qualifier (7th)
0 Ovary **1** Cervix **2** Uterus	**7** Contact Radiation **8** Hyperthermia **C** Intraoperative Radiation Therapy (IORT) **F** Plaque Radiation	**Z** None	**Z** None

Section   **D**   **Radiation Therapy**
Body System **V**   **Male Reproductive System**
Modality   **0**   **Beam Radiation**

Treatment Site (4th)	Modality Qualifier (5th)	Isotope (6th)	Qualifier (7th)
0 Prostate **1** Testis	**0** Photons <1 MeV **1** Photons 1 - 10 MeV **2** Photons >10 MeV **4** Heavy Particles (Protons,Ions) **5** Neutrons **6** Neutron Capture	**Z** None	**Z** None
0 Prostate **1** Testis	**3** Electrons	**Z** None	**0** Intraoperative **Z** None

Section	D	Radiation Therapy
Body System	V	Male Reproductive System
Modality	1	Brachytherapy

Treatment Site (4th)	Modality Qualifier (5th)	Isotope (6th)	Qualifier (7th)
0 Prostate 1 Testis	9 High Dose Rate (HDR)	7 Cesium 137 (Cs-137) 8 Iridium 192 (Ir-192) 9 Iodine 125 (I-125) B Palladium 103 (Pd-103) C Californium 252 (Cf-252) Y Other Isotope	Z None
0 Prostate 1 Testis	B Low Dose Rate (LDR)	6 Cesium 131 (Cs-131) 7 Cesium 137 (Cs-137) 8 Iridium 192 (Ir-192) 9 Iodine 125 (I-125) C Californium 252 (Cf-252) Y Other Isotope	Z None
0 Prostate 1 Testis	B Low Dose Rate (LDR)	B Palladium 103 (Pd-103)	1 Unidirectional Source Z None

Section	D	Radiation Therapy
Body System	V	Male Reproductive System
Modality	2	Stereotactic Radiosurgery

Treatment Site (4th)	Modality Qualifier (5th)	Isotope (6th)	Qualifier (7th)
0 Prostate 1 Testis	D Stereotactic Other Photon Radiosurgery H Stereotactic Particulate Radiosurgery J Stereotactic Gamma Beam Radiosurgery	Z None	Z None

Section	D	Radiation Therapy
Body System	V	Male Reproductive System
Modality	Y	Other Radiation

Treatment Site (4th)	Modality Qualifier (5th)	Isotope (6th)	Qualifier (7th)
0 Prostate	7 Contact Radiation 8 Hyperthermia C Intraoperative Radiation Therapy (IORT) F Plaque Radiation	Z None	Z None
1 Testis	7 Contact Radiation 8 Hyperthermia F Plaque Radiation	Z None	Z None

Section	D	Radiation Therapy
Body System	W	Anatomical Regions
Modality	0	Beam Radiation

Treatment Site (4th)	Modality Qualifier (5th)	Isotope (6th)	Qualifier (7th)
1 Head and Neck 2 Chest 3 Abdomen 4 Hemibody 5 Whole Body 6 Pelvic Region	0 Photons <1 MeV 1 Photons 1 - 10 MeV 2 Photons >10 MeV 4 Heavy Particles (Protons,Ions) 5 Neutrons 6 Neutron Capture	Z None	Z None
1 Head and Neck 2 Chest 3 Abdomen 4 Hemibody 5 Whole Body 6 Pelvic Region	3 Electrons	Z None	0 Intraoperative Z None

DW1–DWY

Section	D	Radiation Therapy
Body System	W	Anatomical Regions
Modality	1	Brachytherapy

Treatment Site (4th)	Modality Qualifier (5th)	Isotope (6th)	Qualifier (7th)
0 Cranial Cavity **K** Upper Back **L** Lower Back **P** Gastrointestinal Track **Q** Respiratory Track **R** Genitourinary Track **X** Upper Extremity **Y** Lower Extremity	**B** Low Dose Rate (LDR)	**B** Palladium 103 (Pd-103)	**1** Unidirectional Source **Z** None
1 Head and Neck **2** Chest **3** Abdomen **6** Pelvic Region	**9** High Dose Rate (HDR)	**7** Cesium 137 (Cs-137) **8** Iridium 192 (Ir-192) **9** Iodine 125 (I-125) **B** Palladium 103 (Pd-103) **C** Californium 252 (Cf-252) **Y** Other Isotope	**Z** None
1 Head and Neck **2** Chest **3** Abdomen **6** Pelvic Region	**B** Low Dose Rate (LDR)	**6** Cesium 131 (Cs-131) **7** Cesium 137 (Cs-137) **8** Iridium 192 (Ir-192) **9** Iodine 125 (I-125) **C** Californium 252 (Cf-252) **Y** Other Isotope	**Z** None
1 Head and Neck **2** Chest **3** Abdomen **6** Pelvic Region	**B** Low Dose Rate (LDR)	**B** Palladium 103 (Pd-103)	**1** Unidirectional Source **Z** None

Section	D	Radiation Therapy
Body System	W	Anatomical Regions
Modality	2	Stereotactic Radiosurgery

Treatment Site (4th)	Modality Qualifier (5th)	Isotope (6th)	Qualifier (7th)
1 Head and Neck **2** Chest **3** Abdomen **6** Pelvic Region	**D** Stereotactic Other Photon Radiosurgery **H** Stereotactic Particulate Radiosurgery **J** Stereotactic Gamma Beam Radiosurgery	**Z** None	**Z** None

Section	D	Radiation Therapy
Body System	W	Anatomical Regions
Modality	Y	Other Radiation

Treatment Site (4th)	Modality Qualifier (5th)	Isotope (6th)	Qualifier (7th)
1 Head and Neck **2** Chest **3** Abdomen **4** Hemibody **6** Pelvic Region	**7** Contact Radiation **8** Hyperthermia **F** Plaque Radiation	**Z** None	**Z** None
5 Whole Body	**7** Contact Radiation **8** Hyperthermia **F** Plaque Radiation	**Z** None	**Z** None
5 Whole Body	**G** Isotope Administration	**D** Iodine 131 (I-131) **F** Phosphorus 32 (P-32) **G** Strontium 89 (Sr-89) **H** Strontium 90 (Sr-90) **Y** Other Isotope	**Z** None

AHA Coding Clinic

DF10BYZ Low Dose Rate (LDR) Brachytherapy of Liver using Other Isotope—AHA CC: 2Q, 2022, 26-27

DU11B7Z Low Dose Rate (LDR) Brachytherapy of Cervix using Cesium 137 (Cs-137)—AHA CC: 4Q, 2017, 104

DW16BB1 Low Dose Rate (LDR) Brachytherapy of Pelvic Region using Palladium 103 (Pd-103), Unidirectional Source—AHA CC: 4Q, 2019, 43-44

DWY38ZZ Hyperthermia of Abdomen—AHA CC: 4Q, 2019, 37

Radiation Therapy Section Tables and AHA Coding Clinic

Physical Rehabilitation and Diagnostic Audiology Section (F00–F15)

Within each section of ICD-10-PCS the characters have different meanings. The seven character meanings for the Physical Rehabilitation and Diagnostic Audiology section are illustrated below through the procedure example of *Individual fitting of moveable brace, right knee*.

Section	Section Qualifier	Root Type	Body System/ Region	Type Qualifier	Equipment	Qualifier
Physical Rehabilitation and Diagnostic Audiology	Rehabilitation	Device Fitting	None	Dynamic Orthosis	Orthosis	None
F	0	D	Z	6	E	Z

Section (Character 1)

All Physical Rehabilitation and Diagnostic Audiology procedure codes have a first character value of F.

Section Qualifier (Character 2)

The alphanumeric character in the second character position identifies if the procedure is a physical rehabilitation procedure or a diagnostic audiology procedure. Physical rehabilitation is reported with character value 0, and diagnostic audiology is reported with character value 1.

Root Type (Character 3)

The alphanumeric character value for root types is placed in the third position. The following are the root types applicable to the Physical Rehabilitation and Diagnostic Audiology section with their associated meaning.

Character Value	Root Type	Root Type Definition
0	Speech Assessment	Measurement of speech and related functions
1	Motor and/or Nerve Function Assessment	Measurement of motor, nerve, and related functions
2	Activities of Daily Living Assessment	Measurement of functional level for activities of daily living
3	Hearing Assessment	Measurement of hearing and related functions
4	Hearing Aid Assessment	Measurement of the appropriateness and/or effectiveness of a hearing device
5	Vestibular Assessment	Measurement of the vestibular system and related functions
6	Speech Treatment	Application of techniques to improve, augment, or compensate for speech and related functional impairment
7	Motor Treatment	Exercise or activities to increase or facilitate motor function
8	Activities of Daily Living Treatment	Exercise or activities to facilitate functional competence for activities of daily living
9	Hearing Treatment	Application of techniques to improve, augment, or compensate for hearing and related functional impairment
B	Cochlear Implant Treatment	Application of techniques to improve the communication abilities of individuals with cochlear implant
C	Vestibular Treatment	Application of techniques to improve, augment, or compensate for vestibular and related functional impairment
D	Device Fitting	Fitting of a device designed to facilitate or support achievement of a higher level of function
F	Caregiver Training	Training in activities to support patient's optimal level of function

Body System/Region (Character 4)

For each body system/region the applicable body part character values will be available for procedure code construction. An example of a body region for this section is Musculoskeletal System—Lower Back/Lower Extremity.

Type Qualifier (Character 5)

Type qualifier further specifies the root type procedure. For example, the type qualifier of Gait Training/Functional Ambulation is used with Motor Treatment (character value 7) when applicable.

Equipment (Character 6)

If equipment is utilized during the procedure character six is used to report the type. Some examples of equipment are

- Aerobic Endurance and Conditioning
- Electrotherapeutic
- Mechanical
- Orthosis
- Prosthesis

If equipment is not utilized, the placeholder character value of Z should be reported.

Qualifier (Character 7)

The qualifier represents an additional attribute for the procedure when applicable. Currently, there are no qualifiers in the Physical Rehabilitation and Diagnostic Audiology section; therefore, the placeholder character value of Z should be reported.

Physical Rehabilitation and Diagnostic Audiology Section Tables

Physical Rehabilitation and Diagnostic Audiology Tables F00–F15

Section   F   Physical Rehabilitation and Diagnostic Audiology
Section Qualifier 0   Rehabilitation
Type   0   **Speech Assessment:** Measurement of speech and related functions

Body System / Region (4th)	Type Qualifier (5th)	Equipment (6th)	Qualifier (7th)
3 Neurological System - Whole Body	G Communicative/Cognitive Integration Skills	K Audiovisual M Augmentative / Alternative Communication P Computer Y Other Equipment Z None	Z None
Z None	0 Filtered Speech 3 Staggered Spondaic Word Q Performance Intensity Phonetically Balanced Speech Discrimination R Brief Tone Stimuli S Distorted Speech T Dichotic Stimuli V Temporal Ordering of Stimuli W Masking Patterns	1 Audiometer 2 Sound Field / Booth K Audiovisual Z None	Z None
Z None	1 Speech Threshold 2 Speech/Word Recognition	1 Audiometer 2 Sound Field / Booth 9 Cochlear Implant K Audiovisual Z None	Z None
Z None	4 Sensorineural Acuity Level	1 Audiometer 2 Sound Field / Booth Z None	Z None
Z None	5 Synthetic Sentence Identification	1 Audiometer 2 Sound Field / Booth 9 Cochlear Implant K Audiovisual	Z None
Z None	6 Speech and/or Language Screening 7 Nonspoken Language 8 Receptive/Expressive Language C Aphasia G Communicative/Cognitive Integration Skills L Augmentative/Alternative Communication System	K Audiovisual M Augmentative / Alternative Communication P Computer Y Other Equipment Z None	Z None

Continued

Section	F	Physical Rehabilitation and Diagnostic Audiology	*F00 Continued*
Section Qualifier	0	Rehabilitation	
Type	0	Speech Assessment: Measurement of speech and related functions	

Body System / Region (4th)	Type Qualifier (5th)	Equipment (6th)	Qualifier (7th)
Z None	9 Articulation/Phonology	K Audiovisual P Computer Q Speech Analysis Y Other Equipment Z None	Z None
Z None	B Motor Speech	K Audiovisual N Biosensory Feedback P Computer Q Speech Analysis T Aerodynamic Function Y Other Equipment Z None	Z None
Z None	D Fluency	K Audiovisual N Biosensory Feedback P Computer Q Speech Analysis S Voice Analysis T Aerodynamic Function Y Other Equipment Z None	Z None
Z None	F Voice	K Audiovisual N Biosensory Feedback P Computer S Voice Analysis T Aerodynamic Function Y Other Equipment Z None	Z None
Z None	H Bedside Swallowing and Oral Function P Oral Peripheral Mechanism	Y Other Equipment Z None	Z None
Z None	J Instrumental Swallowing and Oral Function	T Aerodynamic Function W Swallowing Y Other Equipment	Z None
Z None	K Orofacial Myofunctional	K Audiovisual P Computer Y Other Equipment Z None	Z None
Z None	M Voice Prosthetic	K Audiovisual P Computer S Voice Analysis V Speech Prosthesis Y Other Equipment Z None	Z None
Z None	N Non-invasive Instrumental Status	N Biosensory Feedback P Computer Q Speech Analysis S Voice Analysis T Aerodynamic Function Y Other Equipment	Z None
Z None	X Other Specified Central Auditory Processing	Z None	Z None

Section   F   **Physical Rehabilitation and Diagnostic Audiology**
Section Qualifier   0   **Rehabilitation**
Type   1   **Motor and/or Nerve Function Assessment:** Measurement of motor, nerve, and related functions

Body System / Region (4th)	Type Qualifier (5th)	Equipment (6th)	Qualifier (7th)
0 Neurological System - Head and Neck 1 Neurological System - Upper Back / Upper Extremity 2 Neurological System - Lower Back / Lower Extremity 3 Neurological System - Whole Body	0 Muscle Performance	E Orthosis F Assistive, Adaptive, Supportive or Protective U Prosthesis Y Other Equipment Z None	Z None
0 Neurological System - Head and Neck 1 Neurological System - Upper Back / Upper Extremity 2 Neurological System - Lower Back / Lower Extremity 3 Neurological System - Whole Body	1 Integumentary Integrity 3 Coordination/Dexterity 4 Motor Function G Reflex Integrity	Z None	Z None
0 Neurological System - Head and Neck 1 Neurological System - Upper Back / Upper Extremity 2 Neurological System - Lower Back / Lower Extremity 3 Neurological System - Whole Body	5 Range of Motion and Joint Integrity 6 Sensory Awareness/Processing/Integrity	Y Other Equipment Z None	Z None
D Integumentary System - Head and Neck F Integumentary System - Upper Back / Upper Extremity G Integumentary System - Lower Back / Lower Extremity H Integumentary System - Whole Body J Musculoskeletal System - Head and Neck K Musculoskeletal System - Upper Back / Upper Extremity L Musculoskeletal System - Lower Back / Lower Extremity M Musculoskeletal System - Whole Body	0 Muscle Performance	E Orthosis F Assistive, Adaptive, Supportive or Protective U Prosthesis Y Other Equipment Z None	Z None
D Integumentary System - Head and Neck F Integumentary System - Upper Back / Upper Extremity G Integumentary System - Lower Back / Lower Extremity H Integumentary System - Whole Body J Musculoskeletal System - Head and Neck K Musculoskeletal System - Upper Back / Upper Extremity L Musculoskeletal System - Lower Back / Lower Extremity M Musculoskeletal System - Whole Body	1 Integumentary Integrity	Z None	Z None
D Integumentary System - Head and Neck F Integumentary System - Upper Back / Upper Extremity G Integumentary System - Lower Back / Lower Extremity H Integumentary System - Whole Body J Musculoskeletal System - Head and Neck K Musculoskeletal System - Upper Back / Upper Extremity L Musculoskeletal System - Lower Back / Lower Extremity M Musculoskeletal System - Whole Body	5 Range of Motion and Joint Integrity 6 Sensory Awareness/Processing/Integrity	Y Other Equipment Z None	Z None

Continued →

Section	F	Physical Rehabilitation and Diagnostic Audiology		*F01 Continued*
Section Qualifier	0	Rehabilitation		
Type	1	Motor and/or Nerve Function Assessment: Measurement of motor, nerve, and related functions		

Body System / Region (4th)	Type Qualifier (5th)	Equipment (6th)	Qualifier (7th)
N Genitourinary System	0 Muscle Performance	E Orthosis F Assistive, Adaptive, Supportive or Protective U Prosthesis Y Other Equipment Z None	Z None
Z None	2 Visual Motor Integration	K Audiovisual M Augmentative / Alternative Communication N Biosensory Feedback P Computer Q Speech Analysis S Voice Analysis Y Other Equipment Z None	Z None
Z None	7 Facial Nerve Function	7 Electrophysiologic	Z None
Z None	9 Somatosensory Evoked Potentials	J Somatosensory	Z None
Z None	B Bed Mobility C Transfer F Wheelchair Mobility	E Orthosis F Assistive, Adaptive, Supportive or Protective U Prosthesis Z None	Z None
Z None	D Gait and/or Balance	E Orthosis F Assistive, Adaptive, Supportive or Protective U Prosthesis Y Other Equipment Z None	Z None

Section	F	Physical Rehabilitation and Diagnostic Audiology
Section Qualifier	0	Rehabilitation
Type	2	Activities of Daily Living Assessment: Measurement of functional level for activities of daily living

Body System / Region (4th)	Type Qualifier (5th)	Equipment (6th)	Qualifier (7th)
0 Neurological System - Head and Neck	9 Cranial Nerve Integrity D Neuromotor Development	Y Other Equipment Z None	Z None
1 Neurological System - Upper Back / Upper Extremity 2 Neurological System - Lower Back / Lower Extremity 3 Neurological System - Whole Body	D Neuromotor Development	Y Other Equipment Z None	Z None
4 Circulatory System - Head and Neck 5 Circulatory System - Upper Back / Upper Extremity 6 Circulatory System - Lower Back / Lower Extremity 8 Respiratory System - Head and Neck 9 Respiratory System - Upper Back / Upper Extremity B Respiratory System - Lower Back / Lower Extremity	G Ventilation, Respiration and Circulation	C Mechanical G Aerobic Endurance and Conditioning Y Other Equipment Z None	Z None

Section	F	Physical Rehabilitation and Diagnostic Audiology	*F02 Continued*
Section Qualifier	0	Rehabilitation	
Type	2	**Activities of Daily Living Assessment:** Measurement of functional level for activities of daily living	

Body System / Region (4th)	Type Qualifier (5th)	Equipment (6th)	Qualifier (7th)
7 Circulatory System - Whole Body C Respiratory System - Whole Body	7 Aerobic Capacity and Endurance	E Orthosis G Aerobic Endurance and Conditioning U Prosthesis Y Other Equipment Z None	Z None
7 Circulatory System - Whole Body C Respiratory System - Whole Body	G Ventilation, Respiration and Circulation	C Mechanical G Aerobic Endurance and Conditioning Y Other Equipment Z None	Z None
Z None	0 Bathing/Showering 1 Dressing 3 Grooming/Personal Hygiene 4 Home Management	E Orthosis F Assistive, Adaptive, Supportive or Protective U Prosthesis Z None	Z None
Z None	2 Feeding/Eating 8 Anthropometric Characteristics F Pain	Y Other Equipment Z None	Z None
Z None	5 Perceptual Processing	K Audiovisual M Augmentative / Alternative Communication N Biosensory Feedback P Computer Q Speech Analysis S Voice Analysis Y Other Equipment Z None	Z None
Z None	6 Psychosocial Skills	Z None	Z None
Z None	B Environmental, Home and Work Barriers C Ergonomics and Body Mechanics	E Orthosis F Assistive, Adaptive, Supportive or Protective U Prosthesis Y Other Equipment Z None	Z None
Z None	H Vocational Activities and Functional Community or Work Reintegration Skills	E Orthosis F Assistive, Adaptive, Supportive or Protective G Aerobic Endurance and Conditioning U Prosthesis Y Other Equipment Z None	Z None

Section	F	Physical Rehabilitation and Diagnostic Audiology
Section Qualifier	0	Rehabilitation
Type	6	**Speech Treatment:** Application of techniques to improve, augment, or compensate for speech and related functional impairment

Body System / Region (4th)	Type Qualifier (5th)	Equipment (6th)	Qualifier (7th)
3 Neurological System - Whole Body	6 Communicative/Cognitive Integration Skills	K Audiovisual M Augmentative / Alternative Communication P Computer Y Other Equipment Z None	Z None

Continued →

Section　　　　　　F　Physical Rehabilitation and Diagnostic Audiology　　　　　　　　　　　　　　*F06 Continued*
Section Qualifier　0　Rehabilitation
Type　　　　　　　6　**Speech Treatment:** Application of techniques to improve, augment, or compensate for speech and related functional impairment

Body System / Region (4th)	Type Qualifier (5th)	Equipment (6th)	Qualifier (7th)
Z None	0 Nonspoken Language 3 Aphasia 6 Communicative/Cognitive Integration Skills	K Audiovisual M Augmentative / Alternative Communication P Computer Y Other Equipment Z None	Z None
Z None	1 Speech-Language Pathology and Related Disorders Counseling 2 Speech-Language Pathology and Related Disorders Prevention	K Audiovisual Z None	Z None
Z None	4 Articulation/Phonology	K Audiovisual P Computer Q Speech Analysis T Aerodynamic Function Y Other Equipment Z None	Z None
Z None	5 Aural Rehabilitation	K Audiovisual L Assistive Listening M Augmentative / Alternative Communication N Biosensory Feedback P Computer Q Speech Analysis S Voice Analysis Y Other Equipment Z None	Z None
Z None	7 Fluency	4 Electroacoustic Immitance / Acoustic Reflex K Audiovisual N Biosensory Feedback Q Speech Analysis S Voice Analysis T Aerodynamic Function Y Other Equipment Z None	Z None
Z None	8 Motor Speech	K Audiovisual N Biosensory Feedback P Computer Q Speech Analysis S Voice Analysis T Aerodynamic Function Y Other Equipment Z None	Z None
Z None	9 Orofacial Myofunctional	K Audiovisual P Computer Y Other Equipment Z None	Z None
Z None	B Receptive/Expressive Language	K Audiovisual L Assistive Listening M Augmentative / Alternative Communication P Computer Y Other Equipment Z None	Z None

Section	F	Physical Rehabilitation and Diagnostic Audiology		**F06 Continued**
Section Qualifier	0	Rehabilitation		
Type	6	**Speech Treatment:** Application of techniques to improve, augment, or compensate for speech and related functional impairment		

Body System / Region (4th)	Type Qualifier (5th)	Equipment (6th)	Qualifier (7th)
Z None	C Voice	K Audiovisual N Biosensory Feedback P Computer S Voice Analysis T Aerodynamic Function V Speech Prosthesis Y Other Equipment Z None	Z None
Z None	D Swallowing Dysfunction	M Augmentative / Alternative Communication T Aerodynamic Function V Speech Prosthesis Y Other Equipment Z None	Z None

Section	F	Physical Rehabilitation and Diagnostic Audiology
Section Qualifier	0	Rehabilitation
Type	7	**Motor Treatment:** Exercise or activities to increase or facilitate motor function

Body System / Region (4th)	Type Qualifier (5th)	Equipment (6th)	Qualifier (7th)
0 Neurological System - Head and Neck 1 Neurological System - Upper Back / Upper Extremity 2 Neurological System - Lower Back / Lower Extremity 3 Neurological System - Whole Body D Integumentary System - Head and Neck F Integumentary System - Upper Back / Upper Extremity G Integumentary System - Lower Back / Lower Extremity H Integumentary System - Whole Body J Musculoskeletal System - Head and Neck K Musculoskeletal System - Upper Back / Upper Extremity L Musculoskeletal System - Lower Back / Lower Extremity M Musculoskeletal System - Whole Body	0 Range of Motion and Joint Mobility 1 Muscle Performance 2 Coordination/Dexterity 3 Motor Function	E Orthosis F Assistive, Adaptive, Supportive or Protective U Prosthesis Y Other Equipment Z None	Z None
0 Neurological System - Head and Neck 1 Neurological System - Upper Back / Upper Extremity 2 Neurological System - Lower Back / Lower Extremity 3 Neurological System - Whole Body D Integumentary System - Head and Neck F Integumentary System - Upper Back / Upper Extremity G Integumentary System - Lower Back / Lower Extremity H Integumentary System - Whole Body J Musculoskeletal System - Head and Neck K Musculoskeletal System - Upper Back / Upper Extremity L Musculoskeletal System - Lower Back / Lower Extremity M Musculoskeletal System - Whole Body	6 Therapeutic Exercise	B Physical Agents C Mechanical D Electrotherapeutic E Orthosis F Assistive, Adaptive, Supportive or Protective G Aerobic Endurance and Conditioning H Mechanical or Electromechanical U Prosthesis Y Other Equipment Z None	Z None

Continued →

Section	F	Physical Rehabilitation and Diagnostic Audiology
Section Qualifier	0	Rehabilitation
Type	7	**Motor Treatment:** Exercise or activities to increase or facilitate motor function

F07 Continued

Body System / Region (4th)	Type Qualifier (5th)	Equipment (6th)	Qualifier (7th)
0 Neurological System - Head and Neck 1 Neurological System - Upper Back / Upper Extremity 2 Neurological System - Lower Back / Lower Extremity 3 Neurological System - Whole Body D Integumentary System - Head and Neck F Integumentary System - Upper Back / Upper Extremity G Integumentary System - Lower Back / Lower Extremity H Integumentary System - Whole Body J Musculoskeletal System - Head and Neck K Musculoskeletal System - Upper Back / Upper Extremity L Musculoskeletal System - Lower Back / Lower Extremity M Musculoskeletal System - Whole Body	7 Manual Therapy Techniques	Z None	Z None
4 Circulatory System - Head and Neck 5 Circulatory System - Upper Back / Upper Extremity 6 Circulatory System - Lower Back / Lower Extremity 7 Circulatory System - Whole Body 8 Respiratory System - Head and Neck 9 Respiratory System - Upper Back / Upper Extremity B Respiratory System - Lower Back / Lower Extremity C Respiratory System - Whole Body	6 Therapeutic Exercise	B Physical Agents C Mechanical D Electrotherapeutic E Orthosis F Assistive, Adaptive, Supportive or Protective G Aerobic Endurance and Conditioning H Mechanical or Electromechanical U Prosthesis Y Other Equipment Z None	Z None
N Genitourinary System	1 Muscle Performance	E Orthosis F Assistive, Adaptive, Supportive or Protective U Prosthesis Y Other Equipment Z None	Z None
N Genitourinary System	6 Therapeutic Exercise	B Physical Agents C Mechanical D Electrotherapeutic E Orthosis F Assistive, Adaptive, Supportive or Protective G Aerobic Endurance and Conditioning H Mechanical or Electromechanical U Prosthesis Y Other Equipment Z None	Z None
Z None	4 Wheelchair Mobility	D Electrotherapeutic E Orthosis F Assistive, Adaptive, Supportive or Protective U Prosthesis Y Other Equipment Z None	Z None
Z None	5 Bed Mobility	C Mechanical E Orthosis F Assistive, Adaptive, Supportive or Protective U Prosthesis Y Other Equipment Z None	Z None

Continued →

651

Section	F	Physical Rehabilitation and Diagnostic Audiology
Section Qualifier	0	Rehabilitation
Type	7	Motor Treatment: Exercise or activities to increase or facilitate motor function

Body System / Region (4th)	Type Qualifier (5th)	Equipment (6th)	Qualifier (7th)
Z None	8 Transfer Training	C Mechanical D Electrotherapeutic E Orthosis F Assistive, Adaptive, Supportive or Protective U Prosthesis Y Other Equipment Z None	Z None
Z None	9 Gait Training/ Functional Ambulation	C Mechanical D Electrotherapeutic E Orthosis F Assistive, Adaptive, Supportive or Protective G Aerobic Endurance and Conditioning U Prosthesis Y Other Equipment Z None	Z None

Section	F	Physical Rehabilitation and Diagnostic Audiology
Section Qualifier	0	Rehabilitation
Type	8	Activities of Daily Living Treatment: Exercise or activities to facilitate functional competence for activities of daily living

Body System / Region (4th)	Type Qualifier (5th)	Equipment (6th)	Qualifier (7th)
D Integumentary System - Head and Neck F Integumentary System - Upper Back / Upper Extremity G Integumentary System - Lower Back / Lower Extremity H Integumentary System - Whole Body J Musculoskeletal System - Head and Neck K Musculoskeletal System - Upper Back / Upper Extremity L Musculoskeletal System - Lower Back / Lower Extremity M Musculoskeletal System - Whole Body	5 Wound Management	B Physical Agents C Mechanical D Electrotherapeutic E Orthosis F Assistive, Adaptive, Supportive or Protective U Prosthesis Y Other Equipment Z None	Z None
Z None	0 Bathing/Showering Techniques 1 Dressing Techniques 2 Grooming/Personal Hygiene	E Orthosis F Assistive, Adaptive, Supportive or Protective U Prosthesis Y Other Equipment Z None	Z None
Z None	3 Feeding/Eating	C Mechanical D Electrotherapeutic E Orthosis F Assistive, Adaptive, Supportive or Protective U Prosthesis Y Other Equipment Z None	Z None
Z None	4 Home Management	D Electrotherapeutic E Orthosis F Assistive, Adaptive, Supportive or Protective U Prosthesis Y Other Equipment Z None	Z None

Section	F	Physical Rehabilitation and Diagnostic Audiology	*F08 Continued*
Section Qualifier	0	Rehabilitation	
Type	8	**Activities of Daily Living Treatment:** Exercise or activities to facilitate functional competence for activities of daily living	

Body System / Region (4th)	Type Qualifier (5th)	Equipment (6th)	Qualifier (7th)
Z None	6 Psychosocial Skills	Z None	Z None
Z None	7 Vocational Activities and Functional Community or Work Reintegration Skills	B Physical Agents C Mechanical D Electrotherapeutic E Orthosis F Assistive, Adaptive, Supportive or Protective G Aerobic Endurance and Conditioning U Prosthesis Y Other Equipment Z None	Z None

Section	F	Physical Rehabilitation and Diagnostic Audiology
Section Qualifier	0	Rehabilitation
Type	9	**Hearing Treatment:** Application of techniques to improve, augment, or compensate for hearing and related functional impairment

Body System / Region (4th)	Type Qualifier (5th)	Equipment (6th)	Qualifier (7th)
Z None	0 Hearing and Related Disorders Counseling 1 Hearing and Related Disorders Prevention	K Audiovisual Z None	Z None
Z None	2 Auditory Processing	K Audiovisual L Assistive Listening P Computer Y Other Equipment Z None	Z None
Z None	3 Cerumen Management	X Cerumen Management Z None	Z None

Section	F	Physical Rehabilitation and Diagnostic Audiology
Section Qualifier	0	Rehabilitation
Type	B	**Cochlear Implant Treatment:** Application of techniques to improve the communication abilities of individuals with cochlear implant

Body System / Region (4th)	Type Qualifier (5th)	Equipment (6th)	Qualifier (7th)
Z None	0 Cochlear Implant Rehabilitation	1 Audiometer 2 Sound Field / Booth 9 Cochlear Implant K Audiovisual P Computer Y Other Equipment	Z None

Section	F	Physical Rehabilitation and Diagnostic Audiology
Section Qualifier	0	Rehabilitation
Type	C	**Vestibular Treatment:** Application of techniques to improve, augment, or compensate for vestibular and related functional impairment

Body System / Region (4th)	Type Qualifier (5th)	Equipment (6th)	Qualifier (7th)
3 Neurological System - Whole Body H Integumentary System - Whole Body M Musculoskeletal System - Whole Body	3 Postural Control	E Orthosis F Assistive, Adaptive, Supportive or Protective U Prosthesis Y Other Equipment Z None	Z None
Z None	0 Vestibular	8 Vestibular / Balance Z None	Z None
Z None	1 Perceptual Processing 2 Visual Motor Integration	K Audiovisual L Assistive Listening N Biosensory Feedback P Computer Q Speech Analysis S Voice Analysis T Aerodynamic Function Y Other Equipment Z None	Z None

Section	F	Physical Rehabilitation and Diagnostic Audiology
Section Qualifier	0	Rehabilitation
Type	D	**Device Fitting:** Fitting of a device designed to facilitate or support achievement of a higher level of function

Body System / Region (4th)	Type Qualifier (5th)	Equipment (6th)	Qualifier (7th)
Z None	0 Tinnitus Masker	5 Hearing Aid Selection / Fitting / Test Z None	Z None
Z None	1 Monaural Hearing Aid 2 Binaural Hearing Aid 5 Assistive Listening Device	1 Audiometer 2 Sound Field / Booth 5 Hearing Aid Selection / Fitting / Test K Audiovisual L Assistive Listening Z None	Z None
Z None	3 Augmentative/Alternative Communication System	M Augmentative / Alternative Communication	Z None
Z None	4 Voice Prosthetic	S Voice Analysis V Speech Prosthesis	Z None
Z None	6 Dynamic Orthosis 7 Static Orthosis 8 Prosthesis 9 Assistive, Adaptive, Supportive or Protective Devices	E Orthosis F Assistive, Adaptive, Supportive or Protective U Prosthesis Z None	Z None

Section	F	Physical Rehabilitation and Diagnostic Audiology
Section Qualifier	0	Rehabilitation
Type	F	**Caregiver Training:** Training in activities to support patient's optimal level of function

Body System / Region (4th)	Type Qualifier (5th)	Equipment (6th)	Qualifier (7th)
Z None	**0** Bathing/Showering Technique **1** Dressing **2** Feeding and Eating **3** Grooming/Personal Hygiene **4** Bed Mobility **5** Transfer **6** Wheelchair Mobility **7** Therapeutic Exercise **8** Airway Clearance Techniques **9** Wound Management **B** Vocational Activities and Functional Community or Work Reintegration Skills **C** Gait Training/Functional Ambulation **D** Application, Proper Use and Care of Devices **F** Application, Proper Use and Care of Orthoses **G** Application, Proper Use and Care of Prosthesis **H** Home Management	**E** Orthosis **F** Assistive, Adaptive, Supportive or Protective **U** Prosthesis **Z** None	**Z** None
Z None	**J** Communication Skills	**K** Audiovisual **L** Assistive Listening **M** Augmentative / Alternative Communication **P** Computer **Z** None	**Z** None

Section	F	Physical Rehabilitation and Diagnostic Audiology
Section Qualifier	1	Diagnostic Audiology
Type	3	**Hearing Assessment:** Measurement of hearing and related functions

Body System / Region (4th)	Type Qualifier (5th)	Equipment (6th)	Qualifier (7th)
Z None	**0** Hearing Screening	**0** Occupational Hearing **1** Audiometer **2** Sound Field / Booth **3** Tympanometer **8** Vestibular / Balance **9** Cochlear Implant **Z** None	**Z** None
Z None	**1** Pure Tone Audiometry, Air **2** Pure Tone Audiometry, Air and Bone	**0** Occupational Hearing **1** Audiometer **2** Sound Field / Booth **Z** None	**Z** None
Z None	**3** Bekesy Audiometry **6** Visual Reinforcement Audiometry **9** Short Increment Sensitivity Index **B** Stenger **C** Pure Tone Stenger	**1** Audiometer **2** Sound Field / Booth **Z** None	**Z** None
Z None	**4** Conditioned Play Audiometry **5** Select Picture Audiometry	**1** Audiometer **2** Sound Field / Booth **K** Audiovisual **Z** None	**Z** None
Z None	**7** Alternate Binaural or Monaural Loudness Balance	**1** Audiometer **K** Audiovisual **Z** None	**Z** None

Continued ➡

Section   F   Physical Rehabilitation and Diagnostic Audiology
Section Qualifier 1   Diagnostic Audiology
Type   3   Hearing Assessment: Measurement of hearing and related functions

Body System / Region (4th)	Type Qualifier (5th)	Equipment (6th)	Qualifier (7th)
Z None	8 Tone Decay D Tympanometry F Eustachian Tube Function G Acoustic Reflex Patterns H Acoustic Reflex Threshold J Acoustic Reflex Decay	3 Tympanometer 4 Electroacoustic Immitance / Acoustic Reflex Z None	Z None
Z None	K Electrocochleography L Auditory Evoked Potentials	7 Electrophysiologic Z None	Z None
Z None	M Evoked Otoacoustic Emissions, Screening N Evoked Otoacoustic Emissions, Diagnostic	6 Otoacoustic Emission (OAE) Z None	Z None
Z None	P Aural Rehabilitation Status	1 Audiometer 2 Sound Field / Booth 4 Electroacoustic Immitance / Acoustic Reflex 9 Cochlear Implant K Audiovisual L Assistive Listening P Computer Z None	Z None
Z None	Q Auditory Processing	K Audiovisual P Computer Y Other Equipment Z None	Z None

Section   F   Physical Rehabilitation and Diagnostic Audiology
Section Qualifier 1   Diagnostic Audiology
Type   4   Hearing Aid Assessment: Measurement of the appropriateness and/or effectiveness of a hearing device

Body System / Region (4th)	Type Qualifier (5th)	Equipment (6th)	Qualifier (7th)
Z None	0 Cochlear Implant	1 Audiometer 2 Sound Field / Booth 3 Tympanometer 4 Electroacoustic Immitance / Acoustic Reflex 5 Hearing Aid Selection / Fitting / Test 7 Electrophysiologic 9 Cochlear Implant K Audiovisual L Assistive Listening P Computer Y Other Equipment Z None	Z None
Z None	1 Ear Canal Probe Microphone 6 Binaural Electroacoustic Hearing Aid Check 8 Monaural Electroacoustic Hearing Aid Check	5 Hearing Aid Selection / Fitting / Test Z None	Z None

Section	F	Physical Rehabilitation and Diagnostic Audiology		
Section Qualifier	1	Diagnostic Audiology		
Type	4	Hearing Aid Assessment: Measurement of the appropriateness and/or effectiveness of a hearing device		

F14 Continued

Body System / Region (4th)	Type Qualifier (5th)	Equipment (6th)	Qualifier (7th)
Z None	2 Monaural Hearing Aid 3 Binaural Hearing Aid	1 Audiometer 2 Sound Field / Booth 3 Tympanometer 4 Electroacoustic Immitance / Acoustic Reflex 5 Hearing Aid Selection / Fitting / Test K Audiovisual L Assistive Listening P Computer Z None	Z None
Z None	4 Assistive Listening System/ Device Selection	1 Audiometer 2 Sound Field / Booth 3 Tympanometer 4 Electroacoustic Immitance / Acoustic Reflex K Audiovisual L Assistive Listening Z None	Z None
Z None	5 Sensory Aids	1 Audiometer 2 Sound Field / Booth 3 Tympanometer 4 Electroacoustic Immitance / Acoustic Reflex 5 Hearing Aid Selection / Fitting / Test K Audiovisual L Assistive Listening Z None	Z None
Z None	7 Ear Protector Attentuation	0 Occupational Hearing Z None	Z None

Section	F	Physical Rehabilitation and Diagnostic Audiology		
Section Qualifier	1	Diagnostic Audiology		
Type	5	Vestibular Assessment: Measurement of the vestibular system and related functions		

Body System / Region (4th)	Type Qualifier (5th)	Equipment (6th)	Qualifier (7th)
Z None	0 Bithermal, Binaural Caloric Irrigation 1 Bithermal, Monaural Caloric Irrigation 2 Unithermal Binaural Screen 3 Oscillating Tracking 4 Sinusoidal Vertical Axis Rotational 5 Dix-Hallpike Dynamic 6 Computerized Dynamic Posturography	8 Vestibular / Balance Z None	Z None
Z None	7 Tinnitus Masker	5 Hearing Aid Selection / Fitting / Test Z None	Z None

AHA Coding Clinic

No references have been issued for the Physical Rehabilitation and Diagnostic Audiology section.

Mental Health Section (GZ1–GZJ)

Within each section of ICD-10-PCS the characters have different meanings. The seven character meanings for the Mental Health section are illustrated here through the procedure example of *Crisis intervention*.

Section	Body System	Root Type	Qualifier	Qualifier	Qualifier	Qualifier
Mental Health	None	Crisis Intervention	None	None	None	None
G	Z	2	Z	Z	Z	Z

Section (Character 1)

All Mental Health procedure codes have a first character value of G.

Body System (Character 2)

The body system is not specified for mental health; therefore, the placeholder character value of Z is reported in the second character position.

Root Type (Character 3)

The alphanumeric character value for root types is placed in the third position. Listed below are the root types applicable to the Mental Health section with their associated meaning.

Character Value	Root Type	Root Type Definition
1	Psychological Tests	The administration and interpretation of standardized psychological tests and measurement instruments for the assessment of psychological function
2	Crisis Intervention	Treatment of a traumatized, acutely disturbed or distressed individual for the purpose of short-term stabilization
3	Medication Management	Monitoring and adjusting the use of medications for the treatment of a mental health disorder
5	Individual Psychotherapy	Treatment of an individual with a mental health disorder by behavioral, cognitive, psychoanalytic, psychodynamic or psychophysiological means to improve functioning or well-being
6	Counseling	The application of psychological methods to treat an individual with normal developmental issues and psychological problems in order to increase function, improve well-being, alleviate distress, maladjustment or resolve crises
7	Family Psychotherapy	Treatment that includes one or more family members of an individual with a mental health disorder by behavioral, cognitive, psychoanalytic, psychodynamic or psychophysiological means to improve functioning or well-being
B	Electroconvulsive Therapy	The application of controlled electrical voltages to treat a mental health disorder
C	Biofeedback	Provision of information from the monitoring and regulating of physiological processes in conjunction with cognitive-behavioral techniques to improve patient functioning or well-being
F	Hypnosis	Induction of a state of heightened suggestibility by auditory, visual and tactile techniques to elicit an emotional or behavioral response
G	Narcosynthesis	Administration of intravenous barbiturates in order to release suppressed or repressed thoughts
H	Group Psychotherapy	Treatment of two or more individuals with a mental health disorder by behavioral, cognitive, psychoanalytic, psychodynamic or psychophysiological means to improve functioning or well-being
J	Light Therapy	Application of specialized light treatments to improve functioning or well-being

Qualifier (Character 4)

This qualifier further specifies the root type procedure. For example, the qualifier of Development further specifies the type of Psychological Tests.

Qualifier (Character 5)

The qualifier represents an additional attribute for the procedure when applicable. Currently, there are no qualifiers in the Mental Health section; therefore, the placeholder character value of Z should be reported.

Qualifier (Character 6)

The qualifier represents an additional attribute for the procedure when applicable. Currently, there are no qualifiers in the Mental Health section; therefore, the placeholder character value of Z should be reported.

Qualifier (Character 7)

The qualifier represents an additional attribute for the procedure when applicable. Currently, there are no qualifiers in the Mental Health section; therefore, the placeholder character value of Z should be reported.

Mental Health Section Tables

Mental Health Tables GZ1–GZJ

Section	G	Mental Health
Body System	Z	None
Type	1	**Psychological Tests:** The administration and interpretation of standardized psychological tests and measurement instruments for the assessment of psychological function

Qualifier (4th)	Qualifier (5th)	Qualifier (6th)	Qualifier (7th)
0 Developmental 1 Personality and Behavioral 2 Intellectual and Psychoeducational 3 Neuropsychological 4 Neurobehavioral and Cognitive Status	Z None	Z None	Z None

Section	G	Mental Health
Body System	Z	None
Type	2	**Crisis Intervention:** Treatment of a traumatized, acutely disturbed or distressed individual for the purpose of short-term stabilization

Qualifier (4th)	Qualifier (5th)	Qualifier (6th)	Qualifier (7th)
Z None	Z None	Z None	Z None

Section	G	Mental Health
Body System	Z	None
Type	3	**Medication Management:** Monitoring and adjusting the use of medications for the treatment of a mental health disorder

Qualifier (4th)	Qualifier (5th)	Qualifier (6th)	Qualifier (7th)
Z None	Z None	Z None	Z None

Section	G	Mental Health
Body System	Z	None
Type	5	**Individual Psychotherapy:** Treatment of an individual with a mental health disorder by behavioral, cognitive, psychoanalytic, psychodynamic or psychophysiological means to improve functioning or well-being

Qualifier (4th)	Qualifier (5th)	Qualifier (6th)	Qualifier (7th)
0 Interactive 1 Behavioral 2 Cognitive 3 Interpersonal 4 Psychoanalysis 5 Psychodynamic 6 Supportive 8 Cognitive-Behavioral 9 Psychophysiological	Z None	Z None	Z None

Section	G	Mental Health
Body System	Z	None
Type	6	**Counseling:** The application of psychological methods to treat an individual with normal developmental issues and psychological problems in order to increase function, improve well-being, alleviate distress, maladjustment or resolve crises

Qualifier (4th)	Qualifier (5th)	Qualifier (6th)	Qualifier (7th)
0 Educational 1 Vocational 3 Other Counseling	Z None	Z None	Z None

Section	G	Mental Health
Body System	Z	None
Type	7	**Family Psychotherapy:** Treatment that includes one or more family members of an individual with a mental health disorder by behavioral, cognitive, psychoanalytic, psychodynamic or psychophysiological means to improve functioning or well-being

Qualifier (4th)	Qualifier (5th)	Qualifier (6th)	Qualifier (7th)
2 Other Family Psychotherapy	Z None	Z None	Z None

Section	G	Mental Health
Body System	Z	None
Type	B	**Electroconvulsive Therapy:** The application of controlled electrical voltages to treat a mental health disorder

Qualifier (4th)	Qualifier (5th)	Qualifier (6th)	Qualifier (7th)
0 Unilateral-Single Seizure 1 Unilateral-Multiple Seizure 2 Bilateral-Single Seizure 3 Bilateral-Multiple Seizure 4 Other Electroconvulsive Therapy	Z None	Z None	Z None

Section	G	Mental Health
Body System	Z	None
Type	C	**Biofeedback:** Provision of information from the monitoring and regulating of physiological processes in conjunction with cognitive-behavioral techniques to improve patient functioning or well-being

Qualifier (4th)	Qualifier (5th)	Qualifier (6th)	Qualifier (7th)
9 Other Biofeedback	Z None	Z None	Z None

Section	G	Mental Health
Body System	Z	None
Type	F	**Hypnosis:** Induction of a state of heightened suggestibility by auditory, visual and tactile techniques to elicit an emotional or behavioral response

Qualifier (4th)	Qualifier (5th)	Qualifier (6th)	Qualifier (7th)
Z None	Z None	Z None	Z None

Section	G	Mental Health
Body System	Z	None
Type	G	**Narcosynthesis:** Administration of intravenous barbiturates in order to release suppressed or repressed thoughts

Qualifier (4th)	Qualifier (5th)	Qualifier (6th)	Qualifier (7th)
Z None	Z None	Z None	Z None

Section	G	Mental Health
Body System	Z	None
Type	H	Group Psychotherapy: Treatment of two or more individuals with a mental health disorder by behavioral, cognitive, psychoanalytic, psychodynamic or psychophysiological means to improve functioning or well-being

Qualifier (4th)	Qualifier (5th)	Qualifier (6th)	Qualifier (7th)
Z None	Z None	Z None	Z None

Section	G	Mental Health
Body System	Z	None
Type	J	Light Therapy: Application of specialized light treatments to improve functioning or well-being

Qualifier (4th)	Qualifier (5th)	Qualifier (6th)	Qualifier (7th)
Z None	Z None	Z None	Z None

AHA Coding Clinic

No references have been issued for the Mental Health section.

Substance Abuse Treatment Section (HZ2–HZ9)

Within each section of ICD-10-PCS the characters have different meanings. The seven character meanings for the Substance Abuse Treatment section are illustrated below through the procedure example of *Substance abuse family counseling*.

Section	Body System	Root Type	Qualifier	Qualifier	Qualifier	Qualifier
Substance Abuse	None	Family Counseling	Other Family Counseling	None	None	None
H	Z	6	3	Z	Z	Z

Section (Character 1)

All Substance Abuse Treatment procedure codes have a first character value of H.

Body System (Character 2)

The body system is not specified for substance abuse treatment; therefore, the placeholder character value of Z is reported in the second character position.

Root Type (Character 3)

The alphanumeric character value for root types is placed in the third position. The following are the root types applicable to the Substance Abuse Treatment section with their associated meaning.

Character Value	Root Type	Root Type Definition
2	Detoxification Services	Detoxification from alcohol and/or drugs
3	Individual Counseling	The application of psychological methods to treat an individual with addictive behavior
4	Group Counseling	The application of psychological methods to treat two or more individuals with addictive behavior
5	Individual Psychotherapy	Treatment of an individual with addictive behavior by behavioral, cognitive, psychoanalytic, psychodynamic or psychophysiological means
6	Family Counseling	The application of psychological methods that includes one or more family members to treat an individual with addictive behavior
8	Medication Management	Monitoring and adjusting the use of replacement medications for the treatment of addiction
9	Pharmacotherapy	The use of replacement medications for the treatment of addiction

Qualifier (Character 4)

This qualifier further specifies the root type procedure. For example, the qualifier of Cognitive further specifies the type of Individual counseling.

Qualifier (Character 5)

The qualifier represents an additional attribute for the procedure when applicable. Currently, there are no qualifiers in the Substance Abuse Treatment section; therefore, the placeholder character value of Z should be reported.

Qualifier (Character 6)

The qualifier represents an additional attribute for the procedure when applicable. Currently, there are no qualifiers in the Substance Abuse Treatment section; therefore, the placeholder character value of Z should be reported.

Qualifier (Character 7)

The qualifier represents an additional attribute for the procedure when applicable. Currently, there are no qualifiers in the Substance Abuse Treatment section; therefore, the placeholder character value of Z should be reported.

Substance Abuse Treatment Section Tables

Substance Abuse Treatment Tables HZ2–HZ9

Section	H	Substance Abuse Treatment
Body System	Z	None
Type	2	**Detoxification Services:** Detoxification from alcohol and/or drugs

Qualifier (4ᵗʰ)	Qualifier (5ᵗʰ)	Qualifier (6ᵗʰ)	Qualifier (7ᵗʰ)
Z None	**Z** None	**Z** None	**Z** None

Section	H	Substance Abuse Treatment
Body System	Z	None
Type	3	**Individual Counseling:** The application of psychological methods to treat an individual with addictive behavior

Qualifier (4ᵗʰ)	Qualifier (5ᵗʰ)	Qualifier (6ᵗʰ)	Qualifier (7ᵗʰ)
0 Cognitive **1** Behavioral **2** Cognitive-Behavioral **3** 12-Step **4** Interpersonal **5** Vocational **6** Psychoeducation **7** Motivational Enhancement **8** Confrontational **9** Continuing Care **B** Spiritual **C** Pre/Post-Test Infectious Disease	**Z** None	**Z** None	**Z** None

Section	H	Substance Abuse Treatment
Body System	Z	None
Type	4	**Group Counseling:** The application of psychological methods to treat two or more individuals with addictive behavior

Qualifier (4ᵗʰ)	Qualifier (5ᵗʰ)	Qualifier (6ᵗʰ)	Qualifier (7ᵗʰ)
0 Cognitive **1** Behavioral **2** Cognitive-Behavioral **3** 12-Step **4** Interpersonal **5** Vocational **6** Psychoeducation **7** Motivational Enhancement **8** Confrontational **9** Continuing Care **B** Spiritual **C** Pre/Post-Test Infectious Disease	**Z** None	**Z** None	**Z** None

Section	H	Substance Abuse Treatment
Body System	Z	None
Type	5	**Individual Psychotherapy:** Treatment of an individual with addictive behavior by behavioral, cognitive, psychoanalytic, psychodynamic or psychophysiological means

Qualifier (4th)	Qualifier (5th)	Qualifier (6th)	Qualifier (7th)
0 Cognitive 1 Behavioral 2 Cognitive-Behavioral 3 12-Step 4 Interpersonal 5 Interactive 6 Psychoeducation 7 Motivational Enhancement 8 Confrontational 9 Supportive B Psychoanalysis C Psychodynamic D Psychophysiological	Z None	Z None	Z None

Section	H	Substance Abuse Treatment
Body System	Z	None
Type	6	**Family Counseling:** The application of psychological methods that includes one or more family members to treat an individual with addictive behavior

Qualifier (4th)	Qualifier (5th)	Qualifier (6th)	Qualifier (7th)
3 Other Family Counseling	Z None	Z None	Z None

Section	H	Substance Abuse Treatment
Body System	Z	None
Type	8	**Medication Management:** Monitoring and adjusting the use of replacement medications for the treatment of addiction

Qualifier (4th)	Qualifier (5th)	Qualifier (6th)	Qualifier (7th)
0 Nicotine Replacement 1 Methadone Maintenance 2 Levo-alpha-acetyl-methadol (LAAM) 3 Antabuse 4 Naltrexone 5 Naloxone 6 Clonidine 7 Bupropion 8 Psychiatric Medication 9 Other Replacement Medication	Z None	Z None	Z None

Section	H	Substance Abuse Treatment
Body System	Z	None
Type	9	**Pharmacotherapy:** The use of replacement medications for the treatment of addiction

Qualifier (4th)	Qualifier (5th)	Qualifier (6th)	Qualifier (7th)
0 Nicotine Replacement 1 Methadone Maintenance 2 Levo-alpha-acetyl-methadol (LAAM) 3 Antabuse 4 Naltrexone 5 Naloxone 6 Clonidine 7 Bupropion 8 Psychiatric Medication 9 Other Replacement Medication	Z None	Z None	Z None

AHA Coding Clinic

HZ2ZZZZ Detoxification Services for Substance Abuse Treatment—AHA CC: 1Q, 2020, 21-22

HZ98ZZZ Pharmacotherapy for Substance Abuse Treatment, Psychiatric Medication—AHA CC: 1Q, 2020, 21-22

New Technology (X05–XY0)

Within each section of ICD-10-PCS the characters have different meanings. The seven character meanings for the New Technology section are illustrated below through the procedure example of *Introduction of ceftazidime-avibactam anti-infective into peripheral vein, percutaneous approach.*

Section	Body System	Root Operation	Body Part	Approach	Device / Substance / Technology	Qualifier
New Technology	Anatomical Regions	Introduction	Peripheral Vein	Percutaneous	Ceftazidime-Avibactam Anti-infective	New Technology Group 1
X	W	0	3	3	2	1

Section (Character 1)

All New Technology procedure codes have a first character value of X.

Body System (Character 2)

For each body system the applicable body part character values will be available for procedure code construction.

Root Operations (Character 3)

The alphanumeric character value for root operations is placed in the third position. Listed below are the root operations applicable to the New Technology section with their associated meaning.

Character Value	Root Operation	Root Operation Definition
A	Assistance	Taking over a portion of a physiological function by extracorporeal means
C	Extirpation	Taking or cutting out solid matter from a body part
E	Measurement	Determining a level of a physiological or physical function at a point in time
G	Fusion	Joining together portions of an articular body part rendering the articular body part immobile
H	Insertion	Putting in a nonbiological appliance that monitors, assists, performs, or prevents a physiological function bust does not physically take the place of a body part.
J	Inspection	Visually and/or manually exploring a body part
K	Bypass	Altering the route of passage of the contents of a tubular body part
P	Irrigation	Putting in or on a cleansing substance
R	Replacement	Putting in or on biological or synthetic material that physically takes the place and/or function of all or a portion of a body part
S	Reposition	Moving to its normal location, or other suitable location, all or a portion of a body part
U	Supplement	Putting in or on biological or synthetic material that physically reinforces and/or augments the function of a portion of a body part
V	Restriction	Partially closing an orifice or the lumen of a tubular body part
Z	Other Procedures	Methodologies which attempt to remediate or cure a disorder or disease
0	Introduction	Putting in or on a therapeutic, diagnostic, nutritional, physiological, or prophylactic substance except blood or blood products
1	Transfusion In Anatomical Regions	Putting in blood or blood products
2	Monitoring In Joints & Urinary System	Determining the level of a physiological or physical function repetitively
5	Destruction	Physical eradication of all or a portion of a body part by the direct use of energy, force, or a destructive agent
7	Dilation	Expanding an orifice or the lumen of a tubular body part

Body Part (Character 4)

For each body system the applicable body part character values will be available for procedure code construction.

Approach (Character 5)

The approach is the technique used to reach the procedure site. Listed below are the approach character values for the New Technology section with the associated definitions.

Character Value	Approach	Approach Definition
0	Open	Cutting through the skin or mucous membrane and any other body layers necessary to expose the site of the procedure
3	Percutaneous	Entry, by puncture or minor incision, of instrumentation through the skin or mucous membrane and any other body layers necessary to reach the site of the procedure
4	Percutaneous Endoscopic	Entry, by puncture or minor incision, of instrumentation through the skin or mucous membrane and any other body layers necessary to reach and visualize the site of the procedure
7	Via Natural or Artificial Opening	Entry of instrumentation through a natural or artificial external opening to reach the site of the procedure
8	Via Natural or Artificial Opening Endoscopic	Entry of instrumentation through a natural or artificial external opening to reach and visualize the site of the procedure
X	External	Procedures performed directly on the skin or mucous membrane and procedures performed indirectly by the application of external force through the skin or mucous membrane

Device/Substance/Technology (Character 6)

The New Technology section created a place within ICD-10-PCS to include procedure codes for new services that utilize a specific new device, substance, or technology. Procedures in this section may be part of the Inpatient Prospective Payment System (IPPS) new technology add-on payment mechanism. Depending on the procedure performed there is either a device, substance, or new technology utilized.

Qualifier (Character 7)

The qualifier represents the category year in which the new device, substance, or technology was added to the coding system. In federal fiscal year 2016 (October 1, 2015) the first group of device, substance, and technology was added and therefore are labeled as New Technology Group 1.

New Technology Section Guidelines (section X)

E. New Technology Section

General Guidelines

E1.a Section X codes fully represent the specific procedure described in the code title, and do not require any additional codes from other sections of ICD-10-PCS. When section X contains a code title which describes a specific new technology procedure, and it is the only procedure performed, only the X code is reported for the procedure. There is no need to report an additional code in another section of ICD-10-PCS.

Example: XW043A6 Introduction of Cefiderocol Anti-infective into Central Vein, Percutaneous Approach, New Technology Group 6 can be coded to indicate that Cefiderocol Anti-infective was administered via a central vein. A separate code from table 3E0 in the Administration section of ICD-10-PCS is not coded in addition to this code.

E1.b When multiple procedures are performed, New Technology section X codes are coded following the multiple procedures guideline.

Examples: Dual filter cerebral embolic filtration used during transcatheter aortic valve replacement (TAVR), X2A5312 Cerebral Embolic Filtration, Dual Filter in Innominate Artery and Left Common Carotid Artery, Percutaneous Approach, New Technology Group 2, is coded for the cerebral embolic filtration, along with an ICD-10-PCS code for the TAVR procedure. An extracorporeal flow reversal circuit for embolic neuroprotection placed during a transcarotid arterial revascularization procedure, a code from table X2A, Assistance of the Cardiovascular System is coded for the use of the extracoporeal flow reversal circuit, along with an ICD-10-PCS code for the transcarotid arterial revascularization procedure.

New Technology Section Tables

New Technology Tables X05–XY0

Section	X	New Technology
Body System	0	Nervous System
Operation	5	Destruction: Physical eradication of all or a portion of a body part by the direct use of energy, force, or a destructive agent

Body Part (4th)	Approach (5th)	Device/Substance/Technology (6th)	Qualifier (7th)
1 Renal Sympathetic Nerve(s)	3 Percutaneous	2 Ultrasound Ablation	9 New Technology Group 9

Section	X	New Technology
Body System	0	Nervous System
Operation	H	Insertion: Putting in a nonbiological appliance that monitors, assists, performs, or prevents a physiological function but does not physically take the place of a body part

Body Part (4th)	Approach (5th)	Device/Substance/Technology (6th)	Qualifier (7th)
K Sphenopalatine Ganglion	3 Percutaneous	Q Neurostimulator Lead	8 New Technology Group 8
Q Vagus Nerve	3 Percutaneous	R Neurostimulator Lead with Paired Stimulation System	8 New Technology Group 8

Section	X	New Technology
Body System	0	Nervous System
Operation	Z	Other Procedures: Methodologies which attempt to remediate or cure a disorder or disease

Body Part (4th)	Approach (5th)	Device/Substance/Technology (6th)	Qualifier (7th)
0 Prefrontal Cortex	X External	1 Computer-assisted Transcranial Magnetic Stimulation	8 New Technology Group 8

Section	X	New Technology
Body System	2	Cardiovascular
Operation	7	Dilation: Expanding an orifice or the lumen of a tubular body part

Body Part (4th)	Approach (5th)	Device/Substance/Technology (6th)	Qualifier (7th)
H Femoral Artery, Right J Femoral Artery, Left K Popliteal Artery, Proximal Right L Popliteal Artery, Proximal Left M Popliteal Artery, Distal Right N Popliteal Artery, Distal Left P Anterior Tibial Artery, Right Q Anterior Tibial Artery, Left R Posterior Tibial Artery, Right S Posterior Tibial Artery, Left T Peroneal Tibial Artery, Right U Peroneal Tibial Artery, Left	3 Percutaneous	8 Intraluminal Device, Sustained Release Drug-eluting 9 Intraluminal Device, Sustained Release Drug-eluting, Two B Intraluminal Device, Sustained Release Drug-eluting, Three C Intraluminal Device, Sustained Release Drug-eluting, Four or More	5 New Technology Group 5

Section	X	New Technology
Body System	2	Cardiovascular System
Operation	A	Assistance: Taking over a portion of a physiological function by extracorporeal means

Body Part (4th)	Approach (5th)	Device/Substance/Technology (6th)	Qualifier (7th)
5 Innominate Artery and Left Common Carotid Artery	3 Percutaneous	1 Cerebral Embolic Filtration, Dual Filter	2 New Technology Group 2
6 Aortic Arch	3 Percutaneous	2 Cerebral Embolic Filtration, Single Deflection Filter	5 New Technology Group 5
7 Coronary Sinus	3 Percutaneous	5 Intermittent Coronary Sinus Occlusion	8 New Technology Group 8
H Common Carotid Artery, Right J Common Carotid Artery, Left	3 Percutaneous	3 Cerebral Embolic Filtration, Extracorporeal Flow Reversal Circuit	6 New Technology Group 6

Section	X	New Technology
Body System	2	Cardiovascular System
Operation	C	Extirpation: Taking or cutting out solid matter from a body part

Body Part (4th)	Approach (5th)	Device/Substance/Technology (6th)	Qualifier (7th)
P Abdominal Aorta Q Upper Extremity Vein, Right R Upper Extremity Vein, Left S Lower Extremity Artery, Right T Lower Extremity Artery, Left U Lower Extremity Vein, Right V Lower Extremity Vein, Left Y Great Vessel	3 Percutaneous	T Computer-aided Mechanical Aspiration	7 New Technology Group 7

Section	X	New Technology
Body System	2	Cardiovascular System
Operation	H	Insertion: Putting in a nonbiological appliance that monitors, assists, performs, or prevents a physiological function but does not physically take the place of a body part

Body Part (4th)	Approach (5th)	Device/Substance/Technology (6th)	Qualifier (7th)
0 Inferior Vena Cava 1 Superior Vena Cava	3 Percutaneous	R Intraluminal Device, Bioprosthetic Valve	9 New Technology Group 9
2 Femoral Vein, Right 3 Femoral Vein, Left	0 Open	R Intraluminal Device, Bioprosthetic Valve	9 New Technology Group 9
6 Atrium, Right K Ventricle, Right	3 Percutaneous	V Intracardiac Pacemaker, Dual-Chamber	9 New Technology Group 9
L Axillary Artery, Right M Axillary Artery, Left X Thoracic Aorta, Ascending	0 Open	F Conduit to Short-term External Heart Assist System	9 New Technology Group 9

Section	X	New Technology
Body System	2	Cardiovascular System
Operation	J	Inspection: Visually and/or manually exploring a body part

Body Part (4th)	Approach (5th)	Device/Substance/Technology (6th)	Qualifier (7th)
A Heart	X External	4 Transthoracic Echocardiography Computer-aided Guidance	7 New Technology Group 7

Section	X	New Technology
Body System	2	Cardiovascular System
Operation	K	**Bypass:** Altering the route of passage of the contents of a tubular body part

Body Part (4th)	Approach (5th)	Device/Substance/Technology (6th)	Qualifier (7th)
B Radial Artery, Right **C** Radial Artery, Left	**3** Percutaneous	**1** Thermal Resistance Energy	**7** New Technology Group 7
H Femoral Artery, Right **J** Femoral Artery, Left	**3** Percutaneous	**D** Conduit through Femoral Vein to Superficial Femoral Artery **E** Conduit through Femoral Vein to Popliteal Artery	**9** New Technology Group 9

Section	X	New Technology
Body System	2	Cardiovascular System
Operation	R	**Replacement:** Putting in or on biological or synthetic material that physically takes the place and/or function of all or a portion of a body part

Body Part (4th)	Approach (5th)	Device/Substance/Technology (6th)	Qualifier (7th)
X Thoracic Aorta, Arch	**0** Open	**N** Branched Synthetic Substitute with Intraluminal Device	**7** New Technology Group 7

Section	X	New Technology
Body System	2	Cardiovascular System
Operation	U	**Supplement:** Putting in or on biological or synthetic material that physically reinforces and/or augments the function of a portion of a body part

Body Part (4th)	Approach (5th)	Device/Substance/Technology (6th)	Qualifier (7th)
4 Coronary Artery/Arteries	**0** Open	**7** Vein Graft Extraluminal Support Device(s)	**9** New Technology Group 9
Q Upper Extremity Vein, Right **R** Upper Extremity Vein, Left	**0** Open	**P** Synthetic Substitute, Extraluminal Support Device	**9** New Technology Group 9

Section	X	New Technology
Body System	2	Cardiovascular System
Operation	V	**Restriction:** Partially closing an orifice or the lumen of a tubular body part

Body Part (4th)	Approach (5th)	Device/Substance/Technology (6th)	Qualifier (7th)
7 Coronary Sinus	**3** Percutaneous	**Q** Reduction Device	**7** New Technology Group 7
W Thoracic Aorta, Descending	**0** Open	**N** Branched Synthetic Substitute with Intraluminal Device	**7** New Technology Group 7

Section	X	New Technology
Body System	D	Gastrointestinal System
Operation	2	**Monitoring:** Determining the level of a physiological or physical function repetitively over a period of time

Body Part (4th)	Approach (5th)	Device/Substance/Technology (6th)	Qualifier (7th)
G Upper GI **H** Lower GI	**4** Percutaneous Endoscopic **8** Via Natural or Artificial Opening Endoscopic	**V** Oxygen Saturation	**7** New Technology Group 7

XDP-XKU

New Technology Section Tables

Section	X	New Technology
Body System	D	Gastrointestinal System
Operation	P	Irrigation: Putting in or on a cleansing substance

Body Part (4th)	Approach (5th)	Device/Substance/Technology (6th)	Qualifier (7th)
H Lower GI	8 Via Natural or Artificial Opening Endoscopic	K Intraoperative Single-use Oversleeve	7 New Technology Group 7

Section	X	New Technology
Body System	F	Hepatobiliary System and Pancreas
Operation	5	Destruction: Physical eradication of all or a portion of a body part by the direct use of energy, force, or a destructive agent

Body Part (4th)	Approach (5th)	Device/Substance/Technology (6th)	Qualifier (7th)
0 Liver 1 Liver, Right Lobe 2 Liver, Left Lobe	X External	0 Ultrasound-guided Cavitation	8 New Technology Group 8

Section	X	New Technology
Body System	F	Hepatobiliary System and Pancreas
Operation	J	Inspection: Visually and/or manually exploring a body part

Body Part (4th)	Approach (5th)	Device/Substance/Technology (6th)	Qualifier (7th)
B Hepatobiliary Duct D Pancreatic Duct	8 Via Natural or Artificial Opening Endoscopic	A Single-use Duodenoscope	7 New Technology Group 7

Section	X	New Technology
Body System	H	Skin, Subcutaneous Tissue, Fascia and Breast
Operation	R	Replacement: Putting in or on biological or synthetic material that physically takes the place and/or function of all or a portion of a body part

Body Part (4th)	Approach (5th)	Device/Substance/Technology (6th)	Qualifier (7th)
P Skin	X External	F Bioengineered Allogeneic Construct	7 New Technology Group 7

Section	X	New Technology
Body System	K	Muscles, Tendons, Bursae and Ligaments
Operation	U	Supplement: Putting in or on biological or synthetic material that physically reinforces and/or augments the function of a portion of a body part

Body Part (4th)	Approach (5th)	Device/Substance/Technology (6th)	Qualifier (7th)
C Upper Spine Bursa and Ligament D Lower Spine Bursa and Ligament	0 Open	6 Posterior Vertebral Tether	8 New Technology Group 8

Section	X	New Technology
Body System	N	Bones
Operation	H	Insertion: Putting in a nonbiological appliance that monitors, assists, performs, or prevents a physiological function but does not physically take the place of a body part

Body Part (4th)	Approach (5th)	Device/Substance/Technology (6th)	Qualifier (7th)
6 Pelvic Bone, Right 7 Pelvic Bone, Left	0 Open 3 Percutaneous	5 Internal Fixation Device with Tulip Connector	8 New Technology Group 8
G Tibia, Right H Tibia, Left	0 Open	F Tibial Extension with Motion Sensors	9 New Technology Group 9

Section	X	New Technology
Body System	N	Bones
Operation	R	Replacement: Putting in or on biological or synthetic material that physically takes the place and/or function of all or a portion of a body part

Body Part (4th)	Approach (5th)	Device/Substance/Technology (6th)	Qualifier (7th)
8 Skull	0 Open	D Synthetic Substitute, Ultrasound Penetrable	9 New Technology Group 9
L Tarsal, Right M Tarsal, Left	0 Open	9 Synthetic Substitute, Talar Prosthesis	9 New Technology Group 9

Section	X	New Technology
Body System	N	Bones
Operation	S	Reposition: Moving to its normal location, or other suitable location, all or a portion of a body part

Body Part (4th)	Approach (5th)	Device/Substance/Technology (6th)	Qualifier (7th)
0 Lumbar Vertebra	0 Open	3 Magnetically Controlled Growth Rod(s)	2 New Technology Group 2
0 Lumbar Vertebra	0 Open	C Posterior (Dynamic) Distraction Device	7 New Technology Group 7
0 Lumbar Vertebra	3 Percutaneous	3 Magnetically Controlled Growth Rod(s)	2 New Technology Group 2
0 Lumbar Vertebra	3 Percutaneous	C Posterior (Dynamic) Distraction Device	7 New Technology Group
3 Cervical Vertebra	0 Open 3 Percutaneous	3 Magnetically Controlled Growth Rod(s)	2 New Technology Group 2
4 Thoracic Vertebra	0 Open	3 Magnetically Controlled Growth Rod(s)	2 New Technology Group 2
4 Thoracic Vertebra	0 Open	C Posterior (Dynamic) Distraction Device	7 New Technology Group 7
4 Thoracic Vertebra	3 Percutaneous	3 Magnetically Controlled Growth Rod(s)	2 New Technology Group 2
4 Thoracic Vertebra	3 Percutaneous	C Posterior (Dynamic) Distraction Device	7 New Technology Group 7

Section	X	New Technology
Body System	N	Bones
Operation	U	Supplement: Putting in or on biological or synthetic material that physically reinforces and/or augments the function of a portion of a body part

Body Part (4th)	Approach (5th)	Device/Substance/Technology (6th)	Qualifier (7th)
0 Lumbar Vertebra 4 Thoracic Vertebra	3 Percutaneous	5 Synthetic Substitute, Mechanically Expandable (Paired)	6 New Technology Group 6

XRG–XWO

New Technology Section Tables

Section	X	New Technology
Body System	R	Joints
Operation	G	Fusion: Joining together portions of an articular body part rendering the articular body part immobile

Body Part (4th)	Approach (5th)	Device/Substance/Technology (6th)	Qualifier (7th)
A Thoracolumbar Vertebral Joint **B** Lumbar Vertebral Joint **C** Lumbar Vertebral Joints, 2 or more **D** Lumbosacral Joint	**0** Open **3** Percutaneous **4** Percutaneous Endoscopic	**R** Interbody Fusion Device, Custom-Made Anatomically Designed	**7** New Technology Group 7
E Sacroiliac Joint, Right **F** Sacroiliac Joint, Left	**0** Open **3** Percutaneous	**5** Internal Fixation Device with Tulip Connector	**8** New Technology Group 8
J Ankle Joint, Right **K** Ankle Joint, Left **L** Tarsal Joint, Right **M** Tarsal Joint, Left	**0** Open	**B** Internal Fixation Device, Open-truss Design	**9** New Technology Group 9

Section	X	New Technology
Body System	R	Joints
Operation	H	Insertion: Putting in a nonbiological appliance that monitors, assists, performs, or prevents a physiological function but does not physically take the place of a body part

Body Part (4th)	Approach (5th)	Device/Substance/Technology (6th)	Qualifier (7th)
B Lumbar Vertebral Joint **D** Lumbosacral Joint	**0** Open	**1** Posterior Spinal Motion Preservation Device	**8** New Technology Group 8

Section	X	New Technology
Body System	R	Joints
Operation	R	Replacement: Putting in or on biological or synthetic material that physically takes the place and/or function of all or a portion of a body part

Body Part (4th)	Approach (5th)	Device/Substance/Technology (6th)	Qualifier (7th)
G Knee Joint, Right **H** Knee Joint, Left	**0** Open	**L** Synthetic Substitute, Lateral Meniscus **M** Synthetic Substitute, Medial Meniscus	**8** New Technology Group 8

Section	X	New Technology
Body System	T	Urinary System
Operation	2	Monitoring: Determining the level of a physiological or physical function repetitively over a period of time

Body Part (4th)	Approach (5th)	Device/Substance/Technology (6th)	Qualifier (7th)
5 Kidney	**X** External	**E** Fluorescent Pyrazine	**5** New Technology Group 5

Section	X	New Technology
Body System	W	Anatomical Regions
Operation	0	Introduction: Putting in or on a therapeutic, diagnostic, nutritional, physiological, or prophylactic substance except blood or blood products

Body Part (4th)	Approach (5th)	Device/Substance/Technology (6th)	Qualifier (7th)
0 Skin	**X** External	**2** Anacaulase-bcdb	**7** New Technology Group 7
1 Subcutaneous Tissue	**3** Percutaneous	**1** Daratumumab and Hyaluronidase-fihj **4** Teclistamab Antineoplastic	**8** New Technology Group 8
1 Subcutaneous Tissue	**3** Percutaneous	**9** Satrailzumab-mwge	**7** New Technology Group 7

672

Section	X	New Technology
Body System	W	Anatomical Regions
Operation	0	**Introduction:** Putting in or on a therapeutic, diagnostic, nutritional, physiological, or prophylactic substance except blood or blood products

XW0 Continued

Body Part (4th)	Approach (5th)	Device/Substance/Technology (6th)	Qualifier (7th)
1 Subcutaneous Tissue	3 Percutaneous	F Other New Technology Therapeutic Substance	5 New Technology Group 5
1 Subcutaneous Tissue	3 Percutaneous	G REGN-COV2 Monoclonal Antibody H Other New Technology Monoclonal Antibody K Leronlimab Monoclonal Antibody	6 New Technology Group 6
1 Subcutaneous Tissue	3 Percutaneous	L Elranatamab Antineoplastic	9 New Technology Group 9
1 Subcutaneous Tissue	3 Percutaneous	S COVID-19 Vaccine Dose 1	6 New Technology Group 6
1 Subcutaneous Tissue	3 Percutaneous	S Epcoritamab Monoclonal Antibody	9 New Technology Group 9
1 Subcutaneous Tissue	3 Percutaneous	T COVID-19 Vaccine Dose 2 U COVID-19 Vaccine	6 New Technology Group 6
1 Subcutaneous Tissue	3 Percutaneous	V COVID-19 Vaccine Dose 3	7 New Technology Group 7
1 Subcutaneous Tissue	3 Percutaneous	W Caplacizumab	5 New Technology Group 5
1 Subcutaneous Tissue	3 Percutaneous	W COVID-19 Vaccine Booster	7 New Technology Group 7
1 Subcutaneous Tissue	X External	2 Anacaulase-bcdb	7 New Technology Group 7
2 Muscle	0 Open	D Engineered Allogeneic Thymus Tissue	8 New Technology Group 8
2 Muscle	3 Percutaneous	S COVID-19 Vaccine Dose 1 T COVID-19 Vaccine Dose 2 U COVID-19 Vaccine	6 New Technology Group 6
2 Muscle	3 Percutaneous	V COVID-19 Vaccine Dose 3 W COVID-19 Vaccine Booster X Tixagevimab and Cilgavimab Monoclonal Antibody Y Other New Technology Monoclonal Antibody	7 New Technology Group 7
3 Peripheral Vein	3 Percutaneous	0 Brexanolone	6 New Technology Group 6
3 Peripheral Vein	3 Percutaneous	0 Spesolimab Monoclonal Antibody	8 New Technology Group 8
3 Peripheral Vein	3 Percutaneous	2 Nerinitide 3 Durvalumab Antineoplastic	6 New Technology Group 6
3 Peripheral Vein	3 Percutaneous	5 Narsoplimab Monoclonal Antibody	7 New Technology Group 7
3 Peripheral Vein	3 Percutaneous	5 Mosunetuzumab Antineoplastic	8 New Technology Group 8
3 Peripheral Vein	3 Percutaneous	6 Lefamulin Anti-infective	6 New Technology Group 6
3 Peripheral Vein	3 Percutaneous	6 Terlipressin	7 New Technology Group 7
3 Peripheral Vein	3 Percutaneous	6 Afamitresgene Autoleucel Immunotherapy	8 New Technology Group 8
3 Peripheral Vein	3 Percutaneous	7 Coagulation Factor Xa, Inactivated	2 New Technology Group 2
3 Peripheral Vein	3 Percutaneous	7 Trilaciclib	7 New Technology Group 7

Continued →

Section	X	New Technology		XW0 Continued
Body System	W	Anatomical Regions		
Operation	0	**Introduction:** Putting in or on a therapeutic, diagnostic, nutritional, physiological, or prophylactic substance except blood or blood products		

Body Part (4th)	Approach (5th)	Device/Substance/Technology (6th)	Qualifier (7th)
3 Peripheral Vein	3 Percutaneous	7 Tabelecleucel Immunotherapy	8 New Technology Group 8
3 Peripheral Vein	3 Percutaneous	8 Lurbinectedin	7 New Technology Group 7
3 Peripheral Vein	3 Percutaneous	8 Treosulfan	8 New Technology Group 8
3 Peripheral Vein	3 Percutaneous	9 Ceftolozane/Tazobactam Anti-infective	6 New Technology Group 6
3 Peripheral Vein	3 Percutaneous	9 Inebilizumab-cdon	8 New Technology Group 8
3 Peripheral Vein	3 Percutaneous	A Cefiderocol Anti-infective	6 New Technology Group 6
3 Peripheral Vein	3 Percutaneous	A Ciltacabtagene Autoleucel	7 New Technology Group 7
3 Peripheral Vein	3 Percutaneous	B Cytarabine and Daunorubicin Liposome Antineoplastic	3 New Technology Group 3
3 Peripheral Vein	3 Percutaneous	B Omadacycline Anti-infective	6 New Technology Group 6
3 Peripheral Vein	3 Percutaneous	B Amivantamab Monoclonal Antibody	7 New Technology Group 7
3 Peripheral Vein	3 Percutaneous	C Eculizumab	6 New Technology Group 6
3 Peripheral Vein	3 Percutaneous	C Engineered Chimeric Antigen Receptor T-cell Immunotherapy, Autologous	7 New Technology Group 7
3 Peripheral Vein	3 Percutaneous	D Atezolizumab Antineoplastic	6 New Technology Group 6
3 Peripheral Vein	3 Percutaneous	E Remdesivir Anti-infective	5 New Technology Group 5
3 Peripheral Vein	3 Percutaneous	E Etesevimab Monoclonal Antibody	6 New Technology Group 6
3 Peripheral Vein	3 Percutaneous	F Other New Technology Therapeutic Substance	3 New Technology Group 3
3 Peripheral Vein	3 Percutaneous	F Other New Technology Therapeutic Substance	5 New Technology Group 5
3 Peripheral Vein	3 Percutaneous	F Bamlanivimab Monoclonal Antibody	6 New Technology Group 6
3 Peripheral Vein	3 Percutaneous	G Plazomicin Anti-infective	4 New Technology Group 4
3 Peripheral Vein	3 Percutaneous	G Sarilumab	5 New Technology Group 5
3 Peripheral Vein	3 Percutaneous	G REGN-COV2 Monoclonal Antibody	6 New Technology Group 6
3 Peripheral Vein	3 Percutaneous	G Engineered Chimeric Antigen Receptor T-cell Immunotherapy, Allogeneic	7 New Technology Group 7
3 Peripheral Vein	3 Percutaneous	H Synthetic Human Angiotensin II	4 New Technology Group 4
3 Peripheral Vein	3 Percutaneous	H Tocilizumab	5 New Technology Group 5
3 Peripheral Vein	3 Percutaneous	H Other New Technology Monoclonal Antibody	6 New Technology Group 6
3 Peripheral Vein	3 Percutaneous	H Axicabtagene Ciloleucel Immunotherapy J Tisagenlecleucel Immunotherapy	7 New Technology Group 7

Continued →

Section	X	New Technology					XW0 Continued
Body System	W	Anatomical Regions					
Operation	0	Introduction: Putting in or on a therapeutic, diagnostic, nutritional, physiological, or prophylactic substance except blood or blood products					

3	Peripheral Vein	3	Percutaneous	K	Fosfomycin Anti-Infective	5	New Technology Group 5
3	Peripheral Vein	3	Percutaneous	K	Idecabtagene Vicleucel Immunotherapy	7	New Technology Group 7
3	Peripheral Vein	3	Percutaneous	K	Sulbactam-Durlobactam	9	New Technology Group 9
3	Peripheral Vein	3	Percutaneous	L	CD24Fc Immunomodulator	6	New Technology Group 6
3	Peripheral Vein	3	Percutaneous	L Lifileucel Immunotherapy M Brexucabtagene Autoleucel Immunotherapy		7	New Technology Group 7
3	Peripheral Vein	3	Percutaneous	N	Meropenem-vaborbactam Anti-infective	5	New Technology Group 5
3	Peripheral Vein	3	Percutaneous	N	Lisocabtagene Maraleucel Immunotherapy	7	New Technology Group 7
3	Peripheral Vein	3	Percutaneous	P	Glofitamab Antineoplastic	9	New Technology Group 9
3	Peripheral Vein	3	Percutaneous	Q	Tagraxofusp-erzs Antineoplastic	5	New Technology Group 5
3	Peripheral Vein	3	Percutaneous	Q Posoleucel R Rezafungin		9	New Technology Group 9
3	Peripheral Vein	3	Percutaneous	S Iobenguane I-131 Antineoplastic U Imipenem-cilastatin-relebactam Anti-infective W Caplacizumab		5	New Technology Group 5
4	Central Vein	3	Percutaneous	0	Brexanolone	6	New Technology Group 6
4	Central Vein	3	Percutaneous	0	Spesolimab Monoclonal Antibody	8	New Technology Group 8
4	Central Vein	3	Percutaneous	2 Nerinitide 3 Durvalumab antineoplastic		6	New Technology Group 6
4	Central Vein	3	Percutaneous	5	Narsoplimab Monoclonal Antibody	7	New Technology Group 7
4	Central Vein	3	Percutaneous	5	Mosunetuzumab Antineoplastic	8	New Technology Group 8
4	Central Vein	3	Percutaneous	6	Lefamulin Anti-infective	6	New Technology Group 6
4	Central Vein	3	Percutaneous	6	Terlipressin	7	New Technology Group 7
4	Central Vein	3	Percutaneous	6	Afamitresgene Autoleucel Immunotherapy	8	New Technology Group 8
4	Central Vein	3	Percutaneous	7	Coagulation Factor Xa, Inactivated	2	New Technology Group 2
4	Central Vein	3	Percutaneous	7	Trilaciclib	7	New Technology Group 7
4	Central Vein	3	Percutaneous	7	Tabelecleucel Immunotherapy	8	New Technology Group 8
4	Central Vein	3	Percutaneous	8	Lurbinectedin	7	New Technology Group 7
4	Central Vein	3	Percutaneous	8	Treosulfan	8	New Technology Group 8
4	Central Vein	3	Percutaneous	9	Ceftolozane/Tazobactam Anti-infective	6	New Technology Group 6
4	Central Vein	3	Percutaneous	9	Inebilizumab-cdon	8	New Technology Group 8
4	Central Vein	3	Percutaneous	A	Bezlotoxumab Monoclonal Antibody	3	New Technology Group 3
4	Central Vein	3	Percutaneous	A	Cefiderocol Anti-infective	6	New Technology Group 6

Section	X	New Technology
Body System	W	Anatomical Regions
Operation	0	**Introduction:** Putting in or on a therapeutic, diagnostic, nutritional, physiological, or prophylactic substance except blood or blood products

XW0 Continued

Body Part	Approach	Device / Substance / Technology	Qualifier
4 Central Vein	3 Percutaneous	A Ciltacabtagene Autoleucel	7 New Technology Group 7
4 Central Vein	3 Percutaneous	B Cytarabine and Daunorubicin Liposome Antineoplastic	3 New Technology Group 3
4 Central Vein	3 Percutaneous	B Omadacycline Anti-infective	6 New Technology Group 6
4 Central Vein	3 Percutaneous	B Amivantamab Monoclonal Antibody	7 New Technology Group 7
4 Central Vein	3 Percutaneous	C Eculizumab	6 New Technology Group 6
4 Central Vein	3 Percutaneous	C Engineered Chimeric Antigen Receptor T-cell Immunotherapy, Autologous	7 New Technology Group 7
4 Central Vein	3 Percutaneous	D Atezolizumab Antineoplastic	6 New Technology Group 6
4 Central Vein	3 Percutaneous	E Remdesivir Anti-infective	5 New Technology Group 5
4 Central Vein	3 Percutaneous	E Etesevimab Monoclonal Antibody	6 New Technology Group 6
4 Central Vein	3 Percutaneous	F Other New Technology Therapeutic Substance	3 New Technology Group 3
4 Central Vein	3 Percutaneous	F Other New Technology Therapeutic Substance	5 New Technology Group 5
4 Central Vein	3 Percutaneous	F Bamlanivimab Monoclonal Antibody	6 New Technology Group 6
4 Central Vein	3 Percutaneous	G Plazomicin Anti-infective	4 New Technology Group 4
4 Central Vein	3 Percutaneous	G Sarilumab	5 New Technology Group 5
4 Central Vein	3 Percutaneous	G REGN-COV2 Monoclonal Antibody	6 New Technology Group 6
4 Central Vein	3 Percutaneous	G Engineered Chimeric Antigen Receptor T-cell Immunotherapy, Allogeneic	7 New Technology Group 7
4 Central Vein	3 Percutaneous	H Synthetic Human Angiotensin II	4 New Technology Group 4
4 Central Vein	3 Percutaneous	H Tocilizumab	5 New Technology Group 5
4 Central Vein	3 Percutaneous	H Other New Technology Monoclonal Antibody	6 New Technology Group 6
4 Central Vein	3 Percutaneous	H Axicabtagene Ciloleucel Immunotherapy J Tisagenlecleucel Immunotherapy	7 New Technology Group 7
4 Central Vein	3 Percutaneous	K Fosfomycin Anti-Infective	5 New Technology Group 5
4 Central Vein	3 Percutaneous	K Idecabtagene Vicleucel Immunotherapy	7 New Technology Group 7
4 Central Vein	3 Percutaneous	K Sulbactam-Durlobactam	9 New Technology Group 9
4 Central Vein	3 Percutaneous	L CD24Fc Immunomodulator	6 New Technology Group 6
4 Central Vein	3 Percutaneous	L Lifileucel Immunotherapy M Brexucabtagene Autoleucel Immunotherapy	7 New Technology Group 7
4 Central Vein	3 Percutaneous	N Meropenem-vaborbactam Anti-infective	5 New Technology Group 5
4 Central Vein	3 Percutaneous	N Lisocabtagene Maraleucel Immunotherapy	7 New Technology Group 7
4 Central Vein	3 Percutaneous	P Glofitamab Antineoplastic	9 New Technology Group 9

Continued →

Section	X	New Technology
Body System	W	Anatomical Regions
Operation	0	**Introduction:** Putting in or on a therapeutic, diagnostic, nutritional, physiological, or prophylactic substance except blood or blood products

XW0 Continued

4	Central Vein	3	Percutaneous	Q	Tagraxofusp-erzs Antineoplastic	5	New Technology Group 5
4	Central Vein	3	Percutaneous	Q R	Posoleucel Rezafungin	9	New Technology Group 9
4	Central Vein	3	Percutaneous	S U W	Iobenguane I-131 Antineoplastic Imipenem-cilastatin-relebactam Anti-infective Caplacizumab	5	New Technology Group 5
5	Peripheral Artery	3	Percutaneous	T	Melphalan Hydrochloride Antineoplastic	9	New Technology Group 9
9	Nose	7	Via Natural or Artificial Opening	M	Esketamine Hydrochloride	5	New Technology Group 5
D	Mouth and Pharynx	X	External	3	Maribavir Anti-Infective	8	New Technology Group 8
D	Mouth and Pharynx	X	External	6	Lefamulin Anti-infective	6	New Technology Group 6
D	Mouth and Pharynx	X	External	8	Uridine Triacetate	2	New Technology Group 2
D	Mouth and Pharynx	X	External	F J	Other New Technology Therapeutic Substance Apalutamide Antienoplastic	5	New Technology Group 5
D	Mouth and Pharynx	X	External	J	Quizartinib Antineoplastic	9	New Technology Group 9
D	Mouth and Pharynx	X	External	K	Sabizabulin	8	New Technology Group 8
D	Mouth and Pharynx	X	External	L	Erdafitinib Antineoplastic	5	New Technology Group 5
D	Mouth and Pharynx	X	External	M	Baricitinib	6	New Technology Group 6
D	Mouth and Pharynx	X	External	N	SER-109	9	New Technology Group 9
D	Mouth and Pharynx	X	External	R	Venetoclax Antineoplastic	5	New Technology Group 5
D	Mouth and Pharynx	X	External	R	Fostamatinib	7	New Technology Group 7
D	Mouth and Pharynx	X	External	T V	Ruxolitinib Gilteritinib Antineoplastic	5	New Technology Group 5
G	Upper GI	7	Via Natural or Artificial Opening	3 K	Maribavir Anti-Infective Sabizabulin	8	New Technology Group 8
G	Upper GI	7	Via Natural or Artificial Opening	M	Baricitinib	6	New Technology Group 6
G	Upper GI	7	Via Natural or Artificial Opening	R	Fostamatinib	7	New Technology Group 7
G	Upper GI	8	Via Natural or Artificial Opening Endoscopic	8	Mineral-based Topical Hemostatic Agent	6	New Technology Group 6
H	Lower GI	7	Via Natural or Artificial Opening	3 K	Maribavir Anti-Infective Sabizabulin	8	New Technology Group 8

Continued →

677

Section	X	New Technology		
Body System	W	Anatomical Regions		
Operation	0	Introduction: Putting in or on a therapeutic, diagnostic, nutritional, physiological, or prophylactic substance except blood or blood products		

Body Part (4th)		Approach (5th)		Device/Substance/Technology (6th)		Qualifier (7th)	
H	Lower GI	7	Via Natural or Artificial Opening	M	Baricitinib	6	New Technology Group 6
H	Lower GI	7	Via Natural or Artificial Opening	R	Fostamatinib	7	New Technology Group 7
H	Lower GI	7	Via Natural or Artificial Opening	X	Broad Consortium Microbiota-based Live Biotherapeutic Suspension	8	New Technology Group 8
H	Lower GI	8	Via Natural or Artificial Opening Endoscopic	8	Mineral-based topical Hemostatic Agent	6	New Technology Group 6
Q	Cranial Cavity and Brain	3	Percutaneous	1	Eladocagene exuparvovec	6	New Technology Group 6
V	Bones	0	Open	P	Antibiotic-eluting Bone Void Filler	7	New Technology Group 7

Section	X	New Technology		
Body System	W	Anatomical Regions		
Operation	1	Transfusion: Putting in blood or blood products		

Body Part (4th)		Approach (5th)		Device/Substance/Technology (6th)		Qualifier (7th)	
3	Peripheral Vein	3	Percutaneous	2	Plasma, Convalescent (Nonautologous)	5	New Technology Group 5
3	Peripheral Vein	3	Percutaneous	B C	Betibeglogene Autotemcel Omidubicel	8	New Technology Group 8
3	Peripheral Vein	3	Percutaneous	D E	High-Dose Intravenous Immune Globulin Hyperimmune Globulin	7	New Technology Group 7
3	Peripheral Vein	3	Percutaneous	F G	OTL-103 OTL-200	8	New Technology Group 8
3	Peripheral Vein	3	Percutaneous	H	Lovotibeglogene Autotemcel	9	New Technology Group 9
3	Peripheral Vein	3	Percutaneous	J	Exagamglogene Autotemcel	8	New Technology Group 8
4	Central Vein	3	Percutaneous	2	Plasma, Convalescent (Nonautologous)	5	New Technology Group 5
4	Central Vein	3	Percutaneous	B C	Betibeglogene Autotemcel Omidubicel	8	New Technology Group 8
4	Central Vein	3	Percutaneous	D E	High-Dose Intravenous Immune Globulin Hyperimmune Globulin	7	New Technology Group 7
4	Central Vein	3	Percutaneous	F G	OTL-103 OTL-200	8	New Technology Group 8
4	Central Vein	3	Percutaneous	H	Lovotibeglogene Autotemcel	9	New Technology Group 9
4	Central Vein	3	Percutaneous	J	Exagamglogene Autotemcel	8	New Technology Group 8

Section	X	New Technology
Body System	W	Anatomical Regions
Operation	H	Insertion: Putting in a nonbiological appliance that monitors, assists, performs, or prevents a physiological function but does not physically take the place of a body part

Body Part (4th)	Approach (5th)	Device/Substance/Technology (6th)	Qualifier (7th)
D Mouth and Pharynx	**7** Via Natural or Artificial Opening	**Q** Neurostimulator Lead	**7** New Technology Group 7

Section	X	New Technology
Body System	X	Physiological Systems
Operation	2	Monitoring: Determining the level of a physiological or physical function repetitively over a period of time

Body Part (4th)	Approach (5th)	Device/Substance/Technology (6th)	Qualifier (7th)
0 Central Nervous	**X** External	**8** Brain Electrical Activity, Computer-aided Detection and Notification	**9** New Technology Group 9
F Musculoskeletal	**3** Percutaneous	**W** Muscle Compartment Pressure, Micro-Electro-Mechanical System	**9** New Technology Group 9

Section	X	New Technology
Body System	X	Physiological Systems
Operation	E	Measurement: Determining the level of a physiological or physical function at a point in time

Body Part (4th)	Approach (5th)	Device/Substance/Technology (6th)	Qualifier (7th)
0 Central Nervous	**X** External	**0** Intracranial Vascular Activity, Computer-aided Assessment	**7** New Technology Group 7
0 Central Nervous	**X** External	**4** Brain Electrical Activity, Computer-aided Semiologic Analysis	**8** New Technology Group 8
2 Cardiac	**X** External	**1** Output, Computer-aided Assessment	**9** New Technology Group 9
3 Arterial	**X** External	**2** Pulmonary Artery Flow, Computer-aided Triage and Notification	**7** New Technology Group 7
3 Arterial	**X** External	**5** Coronary Artery Flow, Quantitative Flow Ratio Analysis **6** Coronary Artery Flow, Computer-aided Valve Modeling and Notification	**8** New Technology Group 8
5 Circulatory	**X** External	**3** Infection, Whole Blood Reverse Transcription and Quantitative Real-time Polymerase Chain Reaction	**8** New Technology Group 8
5 Circulatory	**X** External	**M** Infection, Whole Blood Nucleic Acid-base Microbial Detection	**5** New Technology Group 5
5 Circulatory	**X** External	**N** Infection, Positive Blood Culture Fluorescence Hybridization for Organism Identification, Concentration and Susceptibility	**6** New Technology Group 6
5 Circulatory	**X** External	**R** Infection, Mechanical Initial Specimen Diversion Technique Using Active Negative Pressure **T** Intracranial Arterial Flow, Whole Blood mRNA **V** Infection, Serum/Plasma Nanoparticle Fluorescence SARS-CoV-2 Antibody Detection	**7** New Technology Group 7
5 Circulatory	**X** External	**Y** Infection, Other Positive Blood/Isolated Colonies Bimodal Phenotypic Susceptibility Technology	**9** New Technology Group 9
9 Nose	**7** Via Natural or Artificial Opening	**U** Infection, Nasopharyngeal Fluid SARS-CoV-2 Polymerase Chain Reaction	**7** New Technology Group 7
B Respiratory	**X** External	**Q** Infection, Lower Respiratory Fluid Nucleic Acid-base Microbial Detection	**6** New Technology Group 6

Section   **X**   **New Technology**
Body System   **Y**   **Extracorporeal**
Operation   **0**   **Introduction:** Putting in or on a therapeutic, diagnostic, nutritional, physiological, or prophylactic substance except blood or blood products

Body Part (4th)	Approach (5th)	Device/Substance/Technology (6th)	Qualifier (7th)
V Vein Graft	**X** External	**8** Endothelial Damage Inhibitor	**3** New Technology Group 3
Y Extracorporeal	**X** External	**2** Taurolidine Anti-infective and Heparin Anticoagulant	**8** New Technology Group 8
Y Extracorporeal	**X** External	**3** Nafamostat Anticoagulant	**7** New Technology Group 7

AHA Coding Clinic

X0HK3Q8 Insertion of Neurostimulator Lead into Sphenopalatine Ganglion, Percutaneous Approach, New Technology Group 8—AHA CC: 4Q, 2022, 63-64

X2A5312 Cerebral Embolic Filtration, Dual Filter in Innominate Artery and Left Common Carotid Artery, Percutaneous Approach, New Technology Group 2—AHA CC: 1Q, 2021, 16-17

X2C0361 Extirpation of Matter from Coronary Artery, One Site Using Orbital Atherectomy Technology, Percutaneous Approach, New Technology Group 1—AHA CC: 4Q, 2015, 13-14

X2RX0N7 Replacement of thoracic aorta, arch using branched synthetic substitute with intraluminal device, open approach, new technology group 7 - AHA CC: 4Q, 2021, 61

X2VW0N7 Restriction of thoracic aorta, descending using branched synthetic substitute with intraluminal device, open approach, new technology group 7 - AHA CC: 4Q, 2021, 61

XNS0032 Reposition of Lumbar Vertebra using Magnetically Controlled Growth Rod(s), Open Approach, New Technology Group 2—AHA CC: 4Q, 2017, 75

XRGB0F3 Fusion of Lumbar Vertebral Joint using Radiolucent Porous Interbody Fusion Device, Open Approach, New Technology Group 3—AHA CC: 4Q, 2017, 76-77

XRGD0F3 Fusion of Lumbosacral Joint using Radiolucent Porous Interbody Fusion Device, Open Approach, New Technology Group 3—AHA CC: 4Q, 2017, 76-77

XV508A4 Destruction of Prostate using Robotic Waterjet Ablation, Via Natural or Artificial Opening Endoscopic, New Technology Group 4—AHA CC: 4Q, 2018, 55

XW013F5 Introduction of Other New Technology Therapeutic Substance into Subcutaneous Tissue, Percutaneous Approach, New Technology Group 5—AHA CC: 3Q, 2020, 19-20; 1Q, 2021, 49-51; 4Q, 2021, 110-111

XW013V7 Introduction of COVID-19 Vaccine Dose 3 into Subcutaneous Tissue, Percutaneous Approach, New Technology Group 7—AHA CC: 1Q, 2022, 5-7

XW013W7 Introduction of COVID-19 Vaccine Booster into Subcutaneous Tissue, Percutaneous Approach, New Technology Group 7—AHA CC: 1Q, 2022, 5-7

XW023V7 Introduction of COVID-19 Vaccine Dose 3 into Muscle, Percutaneous Approach, New Technology Group 7—AHA CC: 1Q, 2022, 5-7

XW023W7 Introduction of COVID-19 Vaccine Booster into Muscle, Percutaneous Approach, New Technology Group 7—AHA CC: 1Q, 2022, 5-7

XW023X7 Introduction of tixagevimab and cilgavimab monoclonal antibody into muscle, percutaneous approach, new technology group 7 - 1Q, 2022, 8

XW023Y7 Introduction of other new technology monoclonal antibody into muscle, percutaneous approach, new technology group 7 - 1Q, 2022, 8

XW033E5 Introduction of Remdesivir Anti-infective into Peripheral Vein, Percutaneous Approach, New Technology Group 5—AHA CC: 3Q, 2020, 18-19

XW033F5 Introduction of Other New Technology Therapeutic Substance into Peripheral Vein, Percutaneous Approach, New Technology Group 5—AHA CC: 3Q, 2020, 19-20; 1Q, 2021, 49-51; 4Q, 2021, 110-111

XW033G5 Introduction of Sarilumab into Peripheral Vein, Percutaneous Approach, New Technology Group 5—AHA CC: 3Q, 2020, 18-19

XW033H5 Introduction of Tocilizumab into Peripheral Vein, Percutaneous Approach, New Technology Group 5—AHA CC: 3Q, 2020, 18-19

XW04331 Introduction of Idarucizumab, Dabigatran Reversal Agent into Central Vein, Percutaneous Approach, New Technology Group 1—AHA CC: 4Q, 2015, 13

XW04351 Introduction of Blinatumomab Antineoplastic into Central Vein, Percutaneous Approach, New Technology Group 1—AHA CC: 4Q, 2015, 14-15

XW043E5 Introduction of Remdesivir Anti-infective into Central Vein, Percutaneous Approach, New Technology Group 5—AHA CC: 3Q, 2020, 18-19

XW043F5 Introduction of Other New Technology Therapeutic Substance into Central Vein, Percutaneous Approach, New Technology Group 5—AHA CC: 3Q, 2020, 19-20; 1Q, 2021, 49-51; 4Q, 2021, 110-111

XW043G5 Introduction of Sarilumab into Central Vein, Percutaneous Approach, New Technology Group 5—AHA CC: 3Q, 2020, 18-19

XW043H5 Introduction of Tocilizumab into Central Vein, Percutaneous Approach, New Technology Group 5—AHA CC: 3Q, 2020, 18-19

XW0DXF5 Introduction of Other New Technology Therapeutic Substance into Mouth and Pharynx, External Approach, New Technology Group 5—AHA CC: 3Q, 2020, 19-20; 1Q, 2021, 49-51; 4Q, 2021, 110-111

XW0DXR7 Introduction of fostamatinib into mouth and pharynx, external approach, new technology group 7 - 1Q, 2022, 7

XW0G7R7 Introduction of fostamatinib into upper GI, via natural or artificial opening, new technology group 7 - 1Q, 2022, 7

XW0G886 Introduction of Mineral-based Topical Hemostatic Agent into Upper GI, Via Natural or Artificial Opening Endoscopic, New Technology Group 6—AHA CC: 2Q, 2023, 26-27

XW0H7R7 Introduction of fostamatinib into lower GI, via natural or artificial opening, new technology group 7 - 1Q, 2022, 7

XW0Q316 Introduction of Eladocagene exuparvovec into Cranial Cavity and Brain, Percutaneous Approach, New Technology Group 6—AHA CC: 4Q, 2020, 73

XW13325 Transfusion of Convalescent Plasma (Nonautologous) into Peripheral Vein, Percutaneous Approach, New Technology Group 5—AHA CC: 3Q, 2020, 19

XW14325 Transfusion of Convalescent Plasma (Nonautologous) into Central Vein, Percutaneous Approach, New Technology Group 5—AHA CC: 3Q, 2020, 19

XXE5XT7 Measurement of Intracranial Arterial Flow, Whole Blood mRNA, New Technology Group 7—AHA CC: 4Q, 2021, 79-80

XXE5XV7 Measurement of Infection, Serum/Plasma Nanoparticle Fluorescence SARS-CoV-2 Antibody Detection, New Technology Group 7—AHA CC: 4Q, 2021, 79-80

XXE97U7 Measurement of Infection, Nasopharyngeal Fluid SARS-CoV-2 Polymerase Chain Reaction, New Technology Group 7—AHA CC: 4Q, 2021, 79-80

Appendix A: Root Operations Definitions

Section 0 - Medical and Surgical — Character 3 - Root Operation	
Alteration (0)	**Definition:** Modifying the anatomic structure of a body part without affecting the function of the body part **Explanation:** Principal purpose is to improve appearance **Includes/Examples:** Face lift, breast augmentation
Bypass (1)	**Definition:** Altering the route of passage of the contents of a tubular body part **Explanation:** Rerouting contents of a body part to a downstream area of the normal route, to a similar route and body part, or to an abnormal route and dissimilar body part. Includes one or more anastomoses, with or without the use of a device **Includes/Examples:** Coronary artery bypass, colostomy formation
Change (2)	**Definition:** Taking out or off a device from a body part and putting back an identical or similar device in or on the same body part without cutting or puncturing the skin or a mucous membrane **Explanation:** All CHANGE procedures are coded using the approach EXTERNAL **Includes/Examples:** Urinary catheter change, gastrostomy tube change
Control (3)	**Definition:** Stopping, or attempting to stop, postprocedural or other acute bleeding **Includes/Examples:** Control of post-prostatectomy hemorrhage, control of intracranial subdural hemorrhage, control of bleeding duodenal ulcer, control of retroperitoneal hemorrhage
Creation (4)	**Definition:** Putting in or on biological or synthetic material to form a new body part that to the extent possible replicates the anatomic structure or function of an absent body part **Explanation:** Used for gender reassignment surgery and corrective procedures in individuals with congenital anomalies **Includes/Examples:** Creation of vagina in a male, creation of right and left atrioventricular valve from common atrioventricular valve
Destruction (5)	**Definition:** Physical eradication of all or a portion of a body part by the direct use of energy, force, or a destructive agent **Explanation:** None of the body part is physically taken out **Includes/Examples:** Fulguration of rectal polyp, cautery of skin lesion
Detachment (6)	**Definition:** Cutting off all or a portion of the upper or lower extremities **Explanation:** The body part value is the site of the detachment, with a qualifier if applicable to further specify the level where the extremity was detached **Includes/Examples:** Below knee amputation, disarticulation of shoulder
Dilation (7)	**Definition:** Expanding an orifice or the lumen of a tubular body part **Explanation:** The orifice can be a natural orifice or an artificially created orifice. Accomplished by stretching a tubular body part using intraluminal pressure or by cutting part of the orifice or wall of the tubular body part **Includes/Examples:** Percutaneous transluminal angioplasty, internal urethrotomy
Division (8)	**Definition:** Cutting into a body part, without draining fluids and/or gases from the body part, in order to separate or transect a body part **Explanation:** All or a portion of the body part is separated into two or more portions **Includes/Examples:** Spinal cordotomy, osteotomy
Drainage (9)	**Definition:** Taking or letting out fluids and/or gases from a body part **Explanation:** The qualifier DIAGNOSTIC is used to identify drainage procedures that are biopsies **Includes/Examples:** Thoracentesis, incision and drainage
Excision (B)	**Definition:** Cutting out or off, without replacement, a portion of a body part **Explanation:** The qualifier DIAGNOSTIC is used to identify excision procedures that are biopsies **Includes/Examples:** Partial nephrectomy, liver biopsy
Extirpation (C)	**Definition:** Taking or cutting out solid matter from a body part **Explanation:** The solid matter may be an abnormal byproduct of a biological function or a foreign body; it may be imbedded in a body part or in the lumen of a tubular body part. The solid matter may or may not have been previously broken into pieces **Includes/Examples:** Thrombectomy, choledocholithotomy
Extraction (D)	**Definition:** Pulling or stripping out or off all or a portion of a body part by the use of force **Explanation:** The qualifier DIAGNOSTIC is used to identify extraction procedures that are biopsies **Includes/Examples:** Dilation and curettage, vein stripping
Fragmentation (F)	**Definition:** Breaking solid matter in a body part into pieces **Explanation:** Physical force (e.g., manual, ultrasonic) applied directly or indirectly is used to break the solid matter into pieces. The solid matter may be an abnormal byproduct of a biological function or a foreign body. The pieces of solid matter are not taken out **Includes/Examples:** Extracorporeal shockwave lithotripsy, transurethral lithotripsy
Fusion (G)	**Definition:** Joining together portions of an articular body part rendering the articular body part immobile **Explanation:** The body part is joined together by fixation device, bone graft, or other means **Includes/Examples:** Spinal fusion, ankle arthrodesis
Insertion (H)	**Definition:** Putting in a nonbiological appliance that monitors, assists, performs, or prevents a physiological function but does not physically take the place of a body part **Includes/Examples:** Insertion of radioactive implant, insertion of central venous catheter

Continued →

Section 0 - Medical and Surgical — Character 3 - Root Operation

Inspection (J)	**Definition:** Visually and/or manually exploring a body part **Explanation:** Visual exploration may be performed with or without optical instrumentation. Manual exploration may be performed directly or through intervening body layers **Includes/Examples:** Diagnostic arthroscopy, exploratory laparotomy
Map (K)	**Definition:** Locating the route of passage of electrical impulses and/or locating functional areas in a body part **Explanation:** Applicable only to the cardiac conduction mechanism and the central nervous system **Includes/Examples:** Cardiac mapping, cortical mapping
Occlusion (L)	**Definition:** Completely closing an orifice or the lumen of a tubular body part **Explanation:** The orifice can be a natural orifice or an artificially created orifice **Includes/Examples:** Fallopian tube ligation, ligation of inferior vena cava
Reattachment (M)	**Definition:** Putting back in or on all or a portion of a separated body part to its normal location or other suitable location **Explanation:** Vascular circulation and nervous pathways may or may not be reestablished **Includes/Examples:** Reattachment of hand, reattachment of avulsed kidney
Release (N)	**Definition:** Freeing a body part from an abnormal physical constraint by cutting or by the use of force **Explanation:** Some of the restraining tissue may be taken out but none of the body part is taken out **Includes/Examples:** Adhesiolysis, carpal tunnel release
Removal (P)	**Definition:** Taking out or off a device from a body part **Explanation:** If a device is taken out and a similar device put in without cutting or puncturing the skin or mucous membrane, the procedure is coded to the root operation CHANGE. Otherwise, the procedure for taking out a device is coded to the root operation REMOVAL **Includes/Examples:** Drainage tube removal, cardiac pacemaker removal
Repair (Q)	**Definition:** Restoring, to the extent possible, a body part to its normal anatomic structure and function **Explanation:** Used only when the method to accomplish the repair is not one of the other root operations **Includes/Examples:** Colostomy takedown, suture of laceration
Replacement (R)	**Definition:** Putting in or on biological or synthetic material that physically takes the place and/or function of all or a portion of a body part **Explanation:** The body part may have been taken out or replaced, or may be taken out, physically eradicated, or rendered nonfunctional during the Replacement procedure. A Removal procedure is coded for taking out the device used in a previous replacement procedure **Includes/Examples:** Total hip replacement, bone graft, free skin graft
Reposition (S)	**Definition:** Moving to its normal location, or other suitable location, all or a portion of a body part **Explanation:** The body part is moved to a new location from an abnormal location, or from a normal location where it is not functioning correctly. The body part may or may not be cut out or off to be moved to the new location **Includes/Examples:** Reposition of undescended testicle, fracture reduction
Resection (T)	**Definition:** Cutting out or off, without replacement, all of a body part **Includes/Examples:** Total nephrectomy, total lobectomy of lung
Restriction (V)	**Definition:** Partially closing an orifice or the lumen of a tubular body part **Explanation:** The orifice can be a natural orifice or an artificially created orifice **Includes/Examples:** Esophagogastric fundoplication, cervical cerclage
Revision (W)	**Definition:** Correcting, to the extent possible, a portion of a malfunctioning device or the position of a displaced device **Explanation:** Revision can include correcting a malfunctioning or displaced device by taking out or putting in components of the device such as a screw or pin **Includes/Examples:** Adjustment of position of pacemaker lead, recementing of hip prosthesis
Supplement (U)	**Definition:** Putting in or on biological or synthetic material that physically reinforces and/or augments the function of a portion of a body part **Explanation:** The biological material is non-living, or is living and from the same individual. The body part may have been previously replaced, and the Supplement procedure is performed to physically reinforce and/or augment the function of the replaced body part **Includes/Examples:** Herniorrhaphy using mesh, mitral valve ring annuloplasty, put a new acetabular liner in a previous hip replacement
Transfer (X)	**Definition:** Moving, without taking out, all or a portion of a body part to another location to take over the function of all or a portion of a body part **Explanation:** The body part transferred remains connected to its vascular and nervous supply **Includes/Examples:** Tendon transfer, skin pedicle flap transfer
Transplantation (Y)	**Definition:** Putting in or on all or a portion of a living body part taken from another individual or animal to physically take the place and/or function of all or a portion of a similar body part **Explanation:** The native body part may or may not be taken out, and the transplanted body part may take over all or a portion of its function **Includes/Examples:** Kidney transplant, heart transplant

Section 1 - Obstetrics — Character 3 - Root Operations Unique to Obstetrics

Abortion (A)	**Definition:** Artificially terminating a pregnancy **Explanation:** Subdivided according to whether an additional device such as a laminaria or abortifacient is used, or whether the abortion was performed by mechanical means **Includes/Example:** Transvaginal abortion using vacuum aspiration technique
Delivery (E)	**Definition:** Assisting the passage of the products of conception from the genital canal **Explanation:** Applies only to manually-assisted, vaginal delivery **Includes/Example:** Manually-assisted delivery

Section 2 - Placement — Character 3 - Root Operation

Change (0)	**Definition:** Taking out or off a device from a body part and putting back an identical or similar device in or on the same body part without cutting or puncturing the skin or a mucous membrane **Includes/Example:** Change of vaginal packing
Compression (1)	**Definition:** Putting pressure on a body region **Includes/Example:** Placement of pressure dressing on abdominal wall
Dressing (2)	**Definition:** Putting material on a body region for protection **Includes/Example:** Application of sterile dressing to head wound
Immobilization (3)	**Definition:** Limiting or preventing motion of a body region **Includes/Example:** Placement of splint on left finger
Packing (4)	**Definition:** Putting material in a body region or orifice **Includes/Example:** Placement of nasal packing
Removal (5)	**Definition:** Taking out or off a device from a body part **Includes/Example:** Removal of cast from right lower leg
Traction (6)	**Definition:** Exerting a pulling force on a body region in a distal direction **Includes/Example:** Lumbar traction using motorized split-traction table

Section 3 - Administration — Character 3 - Root Operation

Introduction (0)	**Definition:** Putting in or on a therapeutic, diagnostic, nutritional, physiological, or prophylactic substance except blood or blood products **Includes/Example:** Nerve block injection to median nerve
Irrigation (1)	**Definition:** Putting in or on a cleansing substance **Includes/Example:** Flushing of eye
Transfusion (2)	**Definition:** Putting in blood or blood products **Includes/Example:** Transfusion of cell saver red cells into central venous line

Section 4 - Measurement and Monitoring — Character 3 - Root Operation

Measurement (0)	**Definition:** Determining the level of a physiological or physical function at a point in time **Includes/Example:** External electrocardiogram (EKG), single reading
Monitoring (1)	**Definition:** Determining the level of a physiological or physical function repetitively over a period of time **Includes/Example:** Urinary pressure monitoring

Section 5 - Extracorporeal Assistance and Performance — Character 3 - Root Operation

Assistance (0)	**Definition:** Taking over a portion of a physiological function by extracorporeal means **Includes/Example:** Hyperbaric oxygenation of wound
Performance (1)	**Definition:** Completely taking over a physiological function by extracorporeal means **Includes/Example:** Cardiopulmonary bypass in conjunction with CABG
Restoration (2)	**Definition:** Returning, or attempting to return, a physiological function to its original state by extracorporeal means. **Includes/Example:** Attempted cardiac defibrillation, unsuccessful

Section 6 - Extracorporeal Therapies — Character 3 - Root Operation

Atmospheric Control (0)	**Definition:** Extracorporeal control of atmospheric pressure and composition **Includes/Example:** Atmospheric control, single treatment
Decompression (1)	**Definition:** Extracorporeal elimination of undissolved gas from body fluids **Includes/Example:** Hyperbaric decompression treatment, single
Electromagnetic Therapy (2)	**Definition:** Extracorporeal treatment by electromagnetic rays **Includes/Example:** Electromagnetic therapy, central nervous, multiple treatments
Hyperthermia (3)	**Definition:** Extracorporeal raising of body temperature **Includes/Example:** Hyperthermia, single treatment
Hypothermia (4)	**Definition:** Extracorporeal lowering of body temperature **Includes/Example:** Whole body hypothermia treatment for temperature imbalances, series treatment
Perfusion (B)	**Definition:** Extracorporeal treatment by diffusion of therapeutic fluid
Pheresis (5)	**Definition:** Extracorporeal separation of blood products **Includes/Example:** Therapeutic leukopheresis, single treatment
Phototherapy (6)	**Definition:** Extracorporeal treatment by light rays **Includes/Example:** Phototherapy of circulatory system, series treatment

Continued →

Section 6 - Extracorporeal Therapies — Character 3 - Root Operation

Shock Wave Therapy (7)	**Definition:** Extracorporeal treatment by shock waves **Includes/Example:** Shock wave therapy, musculoskeletal, single treatment
Ultrasound Therapy (8)	**Definition:** Extracorporeal treatment by ultrasound **Includes/Example:** Ultrasound therapy of the heart, single treatment
Ultraviolet Light Therapy (9)	**Definition:** Extracorporeal treatment by ultraviolet light **Includes/Example:** Ultraviolet light phototherapy, series treatment

Section 7 - Osteopathic — Character 3 - Root Operation

Treatment (0)	**Definition:** Manual treatment to eliminate or alleviate somatic dysfunction and related disorders **Includes/Example:** Fascial release of abdomen, osteopathic treatment

Section 8 - Other Procedures — Character 3 - Root Operation

Other Procedures (0)	**Definition:** Methodologies which attempt to remediate or cure a disorder or disease **Includes/Example:** Acupuncture

Section 9 - Chiropractic — Character 3 - Root Operation

Manipulation (B)	**Definition:** Manual procedure that involves a directed thrust to move a joint past the physiological range of motion, without exceeding the anatomical limit **Includes/Example:** Chiropractic treatment of cervical spine, short lever specific contact

Section X - New Technology — Character 3 - Root Operation

Assistance (A)	**Definition:** Taking over a portion of a physiological function by extracorporeal means
Bypass (K)	**Definition:** Altering the route of passage of the contents of a tubular body part
Destruction (5)	**Definition:** Physical eradication of all or a portion of a body part by the direct use of energy, force, or a destructive agent **Explanation:** None of the body part is physically taken out **Includes/Examples:** Fulguration of rectal polyp, cautery of skin lesion
Dilation (7)	**Definition:** Expanding an orifice or the lumen of a tubular body part **Explanation:** The orifice can be a natural orifice or an artificially created orifice. Accomplished by stretching a tubular body part using intraluminal pressure or by cutting part of the orifice or wall of the tubular body part
Extirpation (C)	**Definition:** Taking or cutting out solid matter from a body part **Explanation:** The solid matter may be an abnormal by product of a biological function or a foreign body; it may be imbedded in a body part or in the lumen of a tubular body part. The solid matter may or may not have been previously broken into pieces **Includes/Example:** Thrombectomy, choledocholithotomy
Fusion (G)	**Definition:** Joining together portions of an articular body part rendering the articular body part immobile
Insertion (H)	**Definition:** Putting in a nonbiological appliance that monitors, assists, performs, or prevents a physiological function bust does not physically take the place of a body part.
Inspection (J)	**Definition:** Visually and/or manually exploring a body part
Introduction (0)	**Definition:** Putting in or on a therapeutic, diagnostic, nutritional, physiological, or prophylactic substance except blood or blood products
Irrigation (P)	**Definition:** Putting in or on a cleansing substance
Measurement (E)	**Definition:** Determining the level of a physiological or physical function at a point in time
Monitoring (2)	**Definition:** Determining the level of a physiological or physical function repetitively over a period of time
Other Procedures (Z)	**Definition:** Methodologies which attempt to remediate or cure a disorder or disease
Replacement (R)	**Definition:** Putting in or on biological or synthetic material that physically takes the place and/or function of all or a portion of a body part
Reposition (S)	**Definition:** Moving to its normal location, or other suitable location, all or a portion of a body part **Explanation:** The body part is moved to a new location from an abnormal location, or from a normal location where it is not functioning correctly. The body part may or may not be cut out or off to be moved to the new location. **Includes/Examples:** Reposition of undescended testicle, fracture reduction
Restriction (V)	**Definition:** Partially closing an orifice or the lumen of a tubular body part
Supplement (U)	**Definition:** Putting in or on biological or synthetic material that physically reinforces and/or augments the function of a portion of a body part
Transfusion (1&2)	**Definition:** Putting in blood or blood products

Appendix B: Type and Qualifier Definitions

Section B - Imaging — Character 3 - Root Type

Computerized Tomography (CT Scan) (2)	**Definition:** Computer reformatted digital display of multiplanar images developed from the capture of multiple exposures of external ionizing radiation
Fluoroscopy (1)	**Definition:** Single plane or bi-plane real time display of an image developed from the capture of external ionizing radiation on a fluorescent screen. The image may also be stored by either digital or analog means
Magnetic Resonance Imaging (MRI) (3)	**Definition:** Computer reformatted digital display of multiplanar images developed from the capture of radiofrequency signals emitted by nuclei in a body site excited within a magnetic field
Other Imaging (5)	**Definition:** Other specified modality for visualizing a body part
Plain Radiography (0)	**Definition:** Planar display of an image developed from the capture of external ionizing radiation on photographic or photoconductive plate
Ultrasonography (4)	**Definition:** Real time display of images of anatomy or flow information developed from the capture of reflected and attenuated high frequency sound waves

Section C - Nuclear Medicine — Character 3 - Root Type

Nonimaging Nuclear Medicine Assay (6)	**Definition:** Introduction of radioactive materials into the body for the study of body fluids and blood elements, by the detection of radioactive emissions
Nonimaging Nuclear Medicine Probe (5)	**Definition:** Introduction of radioactive materials into the body for the study of distribution and fate of certain substances by the detection of radioactive emissions; or, alternatively, measurement of absorption of radioactive emissions from an external source
Nonimaging Nuclear Medicine Uptake (4)	**Definition:** Introduction of radioactive materials into the body for measurements of organ function, from the detection of radioactive emissions
Planar Nuclear Medicine Imaging (1)	**Definition:** Introduction of radioactive materials into the body for single plane display of images developed from the capture of radioactive emissions
Positron Emission Tomographic (PET) Imaging (3)	**Definition:** Introduction of radioactive materials into the body for three dimensional display of images developed from the simultaneous capture, 180 degrees apart, of radioactive emissions
Systemic Nuclear Medicine Therapy (7)	**Definition:** Introduction of unsealed radioactive materials into the body for treatment
Tomographic (Tomo) Nuclear Medicine Imaging (2)	**Definition:** Introduction of radioactive materials into the body for three dimensional display of images developed from the capture of radioactive emissions

Section F - Physical Rehabilitation and Diagnostic Audiology — Character 3 - Root Type

Activities of Daily Living Assessment	**Definition:** Measurement of functional level for activities of daily living
Activities of Daily Living Treatment	**Definition:** Exercise or activities to facilitate functional competence for activities of daily living
Caregiver Training	**Definition:** Training in activities to support patient's optimal level of function
Cochlear Implant Treatment	**Definition:** Application of techniques to improve the communication abilities of individuals with cochlear implant
Device Fitting	**Definition:** Fitting of a device designed to facilitate or support achievement of a higher level of function
Hearing Aid Assessment	**Definition:** Measurement of the appropriateness and/or effectiveness of a hearing device
Hearing Assessment	**Definition:** Measurement of hearing and related functions
Hearing Treatment	**Definition:** Application of techniques to improve, augment, or compensate for hearing and related functional impairment
Motor and/or Nerve Function Assessment	**Definition:** Measurement of motor, nerve, and related functions
Motor Treatment	**Definition:** Exercise or activities to increase or facilitate motor function
Speech Assessment	**Definition:** Measurement of speech and related functions
Speech Treatment	**Definition:** Application of techniques to improve, augment, or compensate for speech and related functional impairment
Vestibular Assessment	**Definition:** Measurement of the vestibular system and related functions
Vestibular Treatment	**Definition:** Application of techniques to improve, augment, or compensate for vestibular and related functional impairment

Section F - Physical Rehabilitation and Diagnostic Audiology — Character 5 - Type Qualifier

Acoustic Reflex Decay	**Definition:** Measures reduction in size/strength of acoustic reflex over time **Includes/Examples:** Includes site of lesion test
Acoustic Reflex Patterns	**Definition:** Defines site of lesion based upon presence/absence of acoustic reflexes with ipsilateral vs. contralateral stimulation
Acoustic Reflex Threshold	**Definition:** Determines minimal intensity that acoustic reflex occurs with ipsilateral and/or contralateral stimulation
Aerobic Capacity and Endurance	**Definition:** Measures autonomic responses to positional changes; perceived exertion, dyspnea or angina during activity; performance during exercise protocols; standard vital signs; and blood gas analysis or oxygen consumption
Alternate Binaural or Monaural Loudness Balance	**Definition:** Determines auditory stimulus parameter that yields the same objective sensation **Includes/Examples:** Sound intensities that yield same loudness perception
Anthropometric Characteristics	**Definition:** Measures edema, body fat composition, height, weight, length and girth
Aphasia (Assessment)	**Definition:** Measures expressive and receptive speech and language function including reading and writing
Aphasia (Treatment)	**Definition:** Applying techniques to improve, augment, or compensate for receptive/expressive language impairments
Articulation/Phonology (Assessment)	**Definition:** Measures speech production
Articulation/Phonology (Treatment)	**Definition:** Applying techniques to correct, improve, or compensate for speech productive impairment
Assistive Listening Device	**Definition:** Assists in use of effective and appropriate assistive listening device/system
Assistive Listening System/Device Selection	**Definition:** Measures the effectiveness and appropriateness of assistive listening systems/devices
Assistive, Adaptive, Supportive or Protective Devices	**Explanation:** Devices to facilitate or support achievement of a higher level of function in wheelchair mobility; bed mobility; transfer or ambulation ability; bath and showering ability; dressing; grooming; personal hygiene; play or leisure
Auditory Evoked Potentials	**Definition:** Measures electric responses produced by the VIIIth cranial nerve and brainstem following auditory stimulation
Auditory Processing (Assessment)	**Definition:** Evaluates ability to receive and process auditory information and comprehension of spoken language
Auditory Processing (Treatment)	**Definition:** Applying techniques to improve the receiving and processing of auditory information and comprehension of spoken language
Augmentative/Alternative Communication System (Assessment)	**Definition:** Determines the appropriateness of aids, techniques, symbols, and/or strategies to augment or replace speech and enhance communication **Includes/Examples:** Includes the use of telephones, writing equipment, emergency equipment, and TDD
Augmentative/Alternative Communication System (Treatment)	**Includes/Examples:** Includes augmentative communication devices and aids
Aural Rehabilitation	**Definition:** Applying techniques to improve the communication abilities associated with hearing loss
Aural Rehabilitation Status	**Definition:** Measures impact of a hearing loss including evaluation of receptive and expressive communication skills
Bathing/Showering	**Includes/Examples:** Includes obtaining and using supplies; soaping, rinsing, and drying body parts; maintaining bathing position; and transferring to and from bathing positions
Bathing/Showering Techniques	**Definition:** Activities to facilitate obtaining and using supplies, soaping, rinsing and drying body parts, maintaining bathing position, and transferring to and from bathing positions
Bed Mobility (Assessment)	**Definition:** Transitional movement within bed
Bed Mobility (Treatment)	**Definition:** Exercise or activities to facilitate transitional movements within bed
Bedside Swallowing and Oral Function	**Includes/Examples:** Bedside swallowing includes assessment of sucking, masticating, coughing, and swallowing. Oral function includes assessment of musculature for controlled movements, structures and functions to determine coordination and phonation
Bekesy Audiometry	**Definition:** Uses an instrument that provides a choice of discrete or continuously varying pure tones; choice of pulsed or continuous signal
Binaural Electroacoustic Hearing Aid Check	**Definition:** Determines mechanical and electroacoustic function of bilateral hearing aids using hearing aid test box
Binaural Hearing Aid (Assessment)	**Definition:** Measures the candidacy, effectiveness, and appropriateness of a hearing aids **Explanation:** Measures bilateral fit

Continued →

Section F - Physical Rehabilitation and Diagnostic Audiology — Character 5 - Type Qualifier

Binaural Hearing Aid (Treatment)	**Explanation:** Assists in achieving maximum understanding and performance
Bithermal, Binaural Caloric Irrigation	**Definition:** Measures the rhythmic eye movements stimulated by changing the temperature of the vestibular system
Bithermal, Monaural Caloric Irrigation	**Definition:** Measures the rhythmic eye movements stimulated by changing the temperature of the vestibular system in one ear
Brief Tone Stimuli	**Definition:** Measures specific central auditory process
Cerumen Management	**Definition:** Includes examination of external auditory canal and tympanic membrane and removal of cerumen from external ear canal
Cochlear Implant	**Definition:** Measures candidacy for cochlear implant
Cochlear Implant Rehabilitation	**Definition:** Applying techniques to improve the communication abilities of individuals with cochlear implant; includes programming the device, providing patients/families with information
Communicative/Cognitive Integration Skills (Assessment)	**Definition:** Measures ability to use higher cortical functions **Includes/Examples:** Includes orientation, recognition, attention span, initiation and termination of activity, memory, sequencing, categorizing, concept formation, spatial operations, judgment, problem solving, generalization and pragmatic communication
Communicative/Cognitive Integration Skills (Treatment)	**Definition:** Activities to facilitate the use of higher cortical functions **Includes/Examples:** Includes level of arousal, orientation, recognition, attention span, initiation and termination of activity, memory sequencing, judgment and problem solving, learning and generalization, and pragmatic communication
Computerized Dynamic Posturography	**Definition:** Measures the status of the peripheral and central vestibular system and the sensory/motor component of balance; evaluates the efficacy of vestibular rehabilitation
Conditioned Play Audiometry	**Definition:** Behavioral measures using nonspeech and speech stimuli to obtain frequency-specific and ear-specific information on auditory status from the patient **Explanation:** Obtains speech reception threshold by having patient point to pictures of spondaic words
Coordination/Dexterity (Assessment)	**Definition:** Measures large and small muscle groups for controlled goal-directed movements **Explanation:** Dexterity includes object manipulation
Coordination/Dexterity (Treatment)	**Definition:** Exercise or activities to facilitate gross coordination and fine coordination
Cranial Nerve Integrity	**Definition:** Measures cranial nerve sensory and motor functions, including tastes, smell and facial expression
Dichotic Stimuli	**Definition:** Measures specific central auditory process
Distorted Speech	**Definition:** Measures specific central auditory process
Dix-Hallpike Dynamic	**Definition:** Measures nystagmus following Dix-Hallpike maneuver
Dressing	**Includes/Examples:** Includes selecting clothing and accessories, obtaining clothing from storage, dressing, fastening and adjusting clothing and shoes, and applying and removing personal devices, prosthesis or orthosis
Dressing Techniques	**Definition:** Activities to facilitate selecting clothing and accessories, dressing and undressing, adjusting clothing and shoes, applying and removing devices, prostheses or orthoses
Dynamic Orthosis	**Includes/Examples:** Includes customized and prefabricated splints, inhibitory casts, spinal and other braces, and protective devices; allows motion through transfer of movement from other body parts or by use of outside forces
Ear Canal Probe Microphone	**Definition:** Real ear measures
Ear Protector Attentuation	**Definition:** Measures ear protector fit and effectiveness
Electrocochleography	**Definition:** Measures the VIIIth cranial nerve action potential
Environmental, Home and Work Barriers	**Definition:** Measures current and potential barriers to optimal function, including safety hazards, access problems and home or office design
Ergonomics and Body Mechanics	**Definition:** Ergonomic measurement of job tasks, work hardening or work conditioning needs; functional capacity; and body mechanics
Eustachian Tube Function	**Definition:** Measures eustachian tube function and patency of eustachian tube
Evoked Otoacoustic Emissions, Diagnostic	**Definition:** Measures auditory evoked potentials in a diagnostic format
Evoked Otoacoustic Emissions, Screening	**Definition:** Measures auditory evoked potentials in a screening format
Facial Nerve Function	**Definition:** Measures electrical activity of the VIIth cranial nerve (facial nerve)
Feeding/Eating (Assessment)	**Includes/Examples:** Includes setting up food, selecting and using utensils and tableware, bringing food or drink to mouth, cleaning face, hands, and clothing, and management of alternative methods of nourishment

Continued →

Section F - Physical Rehabilitation and Diagnostic Audiology — Character 5 - Type Qualifier

Feeding/Eating (Treatment)	**Definition:** Exercise or activities to facilitate setting up food, selecting and using utensils and tableware, bringing food or drink to mouth, cleaning face, hands, and clothing, and management of alternative methods of nourishment
Filtered Speech	**Definition:** Uses high or low pass filtered speech stimuli to assess central auditory processing disorders, site of lesion testing
Fluency (Assessment)	**Definition:** Measures speech fluency or stuttering
Fluency (Treatment)	**Definition:** Applying techniques to improve and augment fluent speech
Gait and/or Balance	**Definition:** Measures biomechanical, arthrokinematic and other spatial and temporal characteristics of gait and balance
Gait Training/Functional Ambulation	**Definition:** Exercise or activities to facilitate ambulation on a variety of surfaces and in a variety of environments
Grooming/Personal Hygiene (Assessment)	**Includes/Examples:** Includes ability to obtain and use supplies in a sequential fashion, general grooming, oral hygiene, toilet hygiene, personal care devices, including care for artificial airways
Grooming/Personal Hygiene (Treatment)	**Definition:** Activities to facilitate obtaining and using supplies in a sequential fashion: general grooming, oral hygiene, toilet hygiene, cleaning body, and personal care devices, including artificial airways
Hearing and Related Disorders Counseling	**Definition:** Provides patients/families/caregivers with information, support, referrals to facilitate recovery from a communication disorder **Includes/Examples:** Includes strategies for psychosocial adjustment to hearing loss for clients and families/caregivers
Hearing and Related Disorders Prevention	**Definition:** Provides patients/families/caregivers with information and support to prevent communication disorders
Hearing Screening	**Definition:** Pass/refer measures designed to identify need for further audiologic assessment
Home Management (Assessment)	**Definition:** Obtaining and maintaining personal and household possessions and environment **Includes/Examples:** Includes clothing care, cleaning, meal preparation and cleanup, shopping, money management, household maintenance, safety procedures, and childcare/parenting
Home Management (Treatment)	**Definition:** Activities to facilitate obtaining and maintaining personal household possessions and environment **Includes/Examples:** Includes clothing care, cleaning, meal preparation and clean-up, shopping, money management, household maintenance, safety procedures, childcare/parenting
Instrumental Swallowing and Oral Function	**Definition:** Measures swallowing function using instrumental diagnostic procedures **Explanation:** Methods include videofluoroscopy, ultrasound, manometry, endoscopy
Integumentary Integrity	**Includes/Examples:** Includes burns, skin conditions, ecchymosis, bleeding, blisters, scar tissue, wounds and other traumas, tissue mobility, turgor and texture
Manual Therapy Techniques	**Definition:** Techniques in which the therapist uses his/her hands to administer skilled movements **Includes/Examples:** Includes connective tissue massage, joint mobilization and manipulation, manual lymph drainage, manual traction, soft tissue mobilization and manipulation
Masking Patterns	**Definition:** Measures central auditory processing status
Monaural Electroacoustic Hearing Aid Check	**Definition:** Determines mechanical and electroacoustic function of one hearing aid using hearing aid test box
Monaural Hearing Aid (Assessment)	**Definition:** Measures the candidacy, effectiveness, and appropriateness of a hearing aid **Explanation:** Measures unilateral fit
Monaural Hearing Aid (Treatment)	**Explanation:** Assists in achieving maximum understanding and performance
Motor Function (Assessment)	**Definition:** Measures the body's functional and versatile movement patterns **Includes/Examples:** Includes motor assessment scales, analysis of head, trunk and limb movement, and assessment of motor learning
Motor Function (Treatment)	**Definition:** Exercise or activities to facilitate crossing midline, laterality, bilateral integration, praxis, neuromuscular relaxation, inhibition, facilitation, motor function and motor learning
Motor Speech (Assessment)	**Definition:** Measures neurological motor aspects of speech production
Motor Speech (Treatment)	**Definition:** Applying techniques to improve and augment the impaired neurological motor aspects of speech production
Muscle Performance (Assessment)	**Definition:** Measures muscle strength, power and endurance using manual testing, dynamometry or computer-assisted electromechanical muscle test; functional muscle strength, power and endurance; muscle pain, tone, or soreness; or pelvic-floor musculature **Explanation:** Muscle endurance refers to the ability to contract a muscle repeatedly over time

Continued →

Section F - Physical Rehabilitation and Diagnostic Audiology — Character 5 - Type Qualifier

Muscle Performance (Treatment)	**Definition:** Exercise or activities to increase the capacity of a muscle to do work in terms of strength, power, and/or endurance **Explanation:** Muscle strength is the force exerted to overcome resistance in one maximal effort. Muscle power is work produced per unit of time, or the product of strength and speed. Muscle endurance is the ability to contract a muscle repeatedly over time
Neuromotor Development	**Definition:** Measures motor development, righting and equilibrium reactions, and reflex and equilibrium reactions
Non-invasive Instrumental Status	**Definition:** Instrumental measures of oral, nasal, vocal, and velopharyngeal functions as they pertain to speech production
Nonspoken Language (Assessment)	**Definition:** Measures nonspoken language (print, sign, symbols) for communication
Nonspoken Language (Treatment)	**Definition:** Applying techniques that improve, augment, or compensate spoken communication
Oral Peripheral Mechanism	**Definition:** Structural measures of face, jaw, lips, tongue, teeth, hard and soft palate, pharynx as related to speech production
Orofacial Myofunctional (Assessment)	**Definition:** Measures orofacial myofunctional patterns for speech and related functions
Orofacial Myofunctional (Treatment)	**Definition:** Applying techniques to improve, alter, or augment impaired orofacial myofunctional patterns and related speech production errors
Oscillating Tracking	**Definition:** Measures ability to visually track
Pain	**Definition:** Measures muscle soreness, pain and soreness with joint movement, and pain perception **Includes/Examples:** Includes questionnaires, graphs, symptom magnification scales or visual analog scales
Perceptual Processing (Assessment)	**Definition:** Measures stereognosis, kinesthesia, body schema, right-left discrimination, form constancy, position in space, visual closure, figure-ground, depth perception, spatial relations and topographical orientation
Perceptual Processing (Treatment)	**Definition:** Exercise and activities to facilitate perceptual processing **Explanation:** Includes stereognosis, kinesthesia, body schema, right-left discrimination, form constancy, position in space, visual closure, figure-ground, depth perception, spatial relations, and topographical orientation **Includes/Examples:** Includes stereognosis, kinesthesia, body schema, right-left discrimination, form constancy, position in space, visual closure, figure-ground, depth perception, spatial relations, and topographical orientation
Performance Intensity Phonetically Balanced Speech Discrimination	**Definition:** Measures word recognition over varying intensity levels
Postural Control	**Definition:** Exercise or activities to increase postural alignment and control
Prosthesis	**Definition:** Artificial substitutes for missing body parts that augment performance or function **Includes/Examples:** Limb prosthesis, ocular prosthesis
Psychosocial Skills (Assessment)	**Definition:** The ability to interact in society and to process emotions **Includes/Examples:** Includes psychological (values, interests, self-concept); social (role performance, social conduct, interpersonal skills, self expression); self-management (coping skills, time management, self-control)
Psychosocial Skills (Treatment)	**Definition:** The ability to interact in society and to process emotions **Includes/Examples:** Includes psychological (values, interests, self-concept); social (role performance, social conduct, interpersonal skills, self expression); self-management (coping skills, time management, self-control)
Pure Tone Audiometry, Air	**Definition:** Air-conduction pure tone threshold measures with appropriate masking
Pure Tone Audiometry, Air and Bone	**Definition:** Air-conduction and bone-conduction pure tone threshold measures with appropriate masking
Pure Tone Stenger	**Definition:** Measures unilateral nonorganic hearing loss based on simultaneous presentation of pure tones of differing volume
Range of Motion and Joint Integrity	**Definition:** Measures quantity, quality, grade, and classification of joint movement and/or mobility **Explanation:** Range of Motion is the space, distance or angle through which movement occurs at a joint or series of joints. Joint integrity is the conformance of joints to expected anatomic, biomechanical and kinematic norms
Range of Motion and Joint Mobility	**Definition:** Exercise or activities to increase muscle length and joint mobility
Receptive/Expressive Language (Assessment)	**Definition:** Measures receptive and expressive language
Receptive/Expressive Language (Treatment)	**Definition:** Applying techniques to improve and augment receptive/expressive language

Section F - Physical Rehabilitation and Diagnostic Audiology — Character 5 - Type Qualifier

Reflex Integrity	**Definition:** Measures the presence, absence, or exaggeration of developmentally appropriate, pathologic or normal reflexes
Select Picture Audiometry	**Definition:** Establishes hearing threshold levels for speech using pictures
Sensorineural Acuity Level	**Definition:** Measures sensorineural acuity masking presented via bone conduction
Sensory Aids	**Definition:** Determines the appropriateness of a sensory prosthetic device, other than a hearing aid or assistive listening system/device
Sensory Awareness/Processing/Integrity	**Includes/Examples:** Includes light touch, pressure, temperature, pain, sharp/dull, proprioception, vestibular, visual, auditory, gustatory, and olfactory
Short Increment Sensitivity Index	**Definition:** Measures the ear's ability to detect small intensity changes; site of lesion test requiring a behavioral response
Sinusoidal Vertical Axis Rotational	**Definition:** Measures nystagmus following rotation
Somatosensory Evoked Potentials	**Definition:** Measures neural activity from sites throughout the body
Speech and/or Language Screening	**Definition:** Identifies need for further speech and/or language evaluation
Speech Threshold	**Definition:** Measures minimal intensity needed to repeat spondaic words
Speech-Language Pathology and Related Disorders Counseling	**Definition:** Provides patients/families with information, support, referrals to facilitate recovery from a communication disorder
Speech-Language Pathology and Related Disorders Prevention	**Definition:** Applying techniques to avoid or minimize onset and/or development of a communication disorder
Speech/Word Recognition	**Definition:** Measures ability to repeat/identify single syllable words; scores given as a percentage; includes word recognition/speech discrimination
Staggered Spondaic Word	**Definition:** Measures central auditory processing site of lesion based upon dichotic presentation of spondaic words
Static Orthosis	**Includes/Examples:** Includes customized and prefabricated splints, inhibitory casts, spinal and other braces, and protective devices; has no moving parts, maintains joint(s) in desired position
Stenger	**Definition:** Measures unilateral nonorganic hearing loss based on simultaneous presentation of signals of differing volume
Swallowing Dysfunction	**Definition:** Activities to improve swallowing function in coordination with respiratory function **Includes/Examples:** Includes function and coordination of sucking, mastication, coughing, swallowing
Synthetic Sentence Identification	**Definition:** Measures central auditory dysfunction using identification of third order approximations of sentences and competing messages
Temporal Ordering of Stimuli	**Definition:** Measures specific central auditory process
Therapeutic Exercise	**Definition:** Exercise or activities to facilitate sensory awareness, sensory processing, sensory integration, balance training, conditioning, reconditioning **Includes/Examples:** Includes developmental activities, breathing exercises, aerobic endurance activities, aquatic exercises, stretching and ventilatory muscle training
Tinnitus Masker (Assessment)	**Definition:** Determines candidacy for tinnitus masker
Tinnitus Masker (Treatment)	**Explanation:** Used to verify physical fit, acoustic appropriateness, and benefit; assists in achieving maximum benefit
Tone Decay	**Definition:** Measures decrease in hearing sensitivity to a tone; site of lesion test requiring a behavioral response
Transfer	**Definition:** Transitional movement from one surface to another
Transfer Training	**Definition:** Exercise or activities to facilitate movement from one surface to another
Tympanometry	**Definition:** Measures the integrity of the middle ear; measures ease at which sound flows through the tympanic membrane while air pressure against the membrane is varied
Unithermal Binaural Screen	**Definition:** Measures the rhythmic eye movements stimulated by changing the temperature of the vestibular system in both ears using warm water, screening format
Ventilation, Respiration and Circulation	**Definition:** Measures ventilatory muscle strength, power and endurance, pulmonary function and ventilatory mechanics **Includes/Examples:** Includes ability to clear airway, activities that aggravate or relieve edema, pain, dyspnea or other symptoms, chest wall mobility, cardiopulmonary response to performance of ADL and IAD, cough and sputum, standard vital signs
Vestibular	**Definition:** Applying techniques to compensate for balance disorders; includes habituation, exercise therapy, and balance retraining

Continued →

Section F - Physical Rehabilitation and Diagnostic Audiology — Character 5 - Type Qualifier

Visual Motor Integration (Assessment)	**Definition:** Coordinating the interaction of information from the eyes with body movement during activity
Visual Motor Integration (Treatment)	**Definition:** Exercise or activities to facilitate coordinating the interaction of information from eyes with body movement during activity
Visual Reinforcement Audiometry	**Definition:** Behavioral measures using nonspeech and speech stimuli to obtain frequency/ear-specific information on auditory status **Includes/Examples:** Includes a conditioned response of looking toward a visual reinforcer (e.g., lights, animated toy) every time auditory stimuli are heard
Vocational Activities and Functional Community or Work Reintegration Skills (Assessment)	**Definition:** Measures environmental, home, work (job/school/play) barriers that keep patients from functioning optimally in their environment **Includes/Examples:** Includes assessment of vocational skill and interests, environment of work (job/school/play), injury potential and injury prevention or reduction, ergonomic stressors, transportation skills, and ability to access and use community resources
Vocational Activities and Functional Community or Work Reintegration Skills (Treatment)	**Definition:** Activities to facilitate vocational exploration, body mechanics training, job acquisition, and environmental or work (job/school/play) task adaptation **Includes/Examples:** Includes injury prevention and reduction, ergonomic stressor reduction, job coaching and simulation, work hardening and conditioning, driving training, transportation skills, and use of community resources
Voice (Assessment)	**Definition:** Measures vocal structure, function and production
Voice (Treatment)	**Definition:** Applying techniques to improve voice and vocal function
Voice Prosthetic (Assessment)	**Definition:** Determines the appropriateness of voice prosthetic/adaptive device to enhance or facilitate communication
Voice Prosthetic (Treatment)	**Includes/Examples:** Includes electrolarynx, and other assistive, adaptive, supportive devices
Wheelchair Mobility (Assessment)	**Definition:** Measures fit and functional abilities within wheelchair in a variety of environments
Wheelchair Mobility (Treatment)	**Definition:** Management, maintenance and controlled operation of a wheelchair, scooter or other device, in and on a variety of surfaces and environments
Wound Management	**Includes/Examples:** Includes non-selective and selective debridement (enzymes, autolysis, sharp debridement), dressings (wound coverings, hydrogel, vacuum-assisted closure), topical agents, etc.

Section G - Mental Health — Character 3 - Root Type

Biofeedback	**Definition:** Provision of information from the monitoring and regulating of physiological processes in conjunction with cognitive-behavioral techniques to improve patient functioning or well-being **Includes/Examples:** Includes EEG, blood pressure, skin temperature or peripheral blood flow, ECG, electrooculogram, EMG, respirometry or capnometry, GSR/EDR, perineometry to monitor/regulate bowel/bladder activity, electrogastrogram to monitor/regulate gastric motility
Counseling	**Definition:** The application of psychological methods to treat an individual with normal developmental issues and psychological problems in order to increase function, improve well-being, alleviate distress, maladjustment or resolve crises
Crisis Intervention	**Definition:** Treatment of a traumatized, acutely disturbed or distressed individual for the purpose of short-term stabilization **Includes/Examples:** Includes defusing, debriefing, counseling, psychotherapy and/or coordination of care with other providers or agencies
Electroconvulsive Therapy	**Definition:** The application of controlled electrical voltages to treat a mental health disorder **Includes/Examples:** Includes appropriate sedation and other preparation of the individual
Family Psychotherapy	**Definition:** Treatment that includes one or more family members of an individual with a mental health disorder by behavioral, cognitive, psychoanalytic, psychodynamic or psychophysiological means to improve functioning or well-being **Explanation:** Remediation of emotional or behavioral problems presented by one or more family members in cases where psychotherapy with more than one family member is indicated
Group Psychotherapy	**Definition:** Treatment of two or more individuals with a mental health disorder by behavioral, cognitive, psychoanalytic, psychodynamic or psychophysiological means to improve functioning or well-being
Hypnosis	**Definition:** Induction of a state of heightened suggestibility by auditory, visual and tactile techniques to elicit an emotional or behavioral response
Individual Psychotherapy	**Definition:** Treatment of an individual with a mental health disorder by behavioral, cognitive, psychoanalytic, psychodynamic or psychophysiological means to improve functioning or well-being
Light Therapy	**Definition:** Application of specialized light treatments to improve functioning or well-being

Continued

Section G - Mental Health — Character 3 - Root Type

Medication Management	**Definition:** Monitoring and adjusting the use of medications for the treatment of a mental health disorder
Narcosynthesis	**Definition:** Administration of intravenous barbiturates in order to release suppressed or repressed thoughts
Psychological Tests	**Definition:** The administration and interpretation of standardized psychological tests and measurement instruments for the assessment of psychological function

Section G - Mental Health — Character 4 - Type Qualifier

Behavioral	**Definition:** Primarily to modify behavior **Includes/Examples:** Includes modeling and role playing, positive reinforcement of target behaviors, response cost, and training of self-management skills
Cognitive	**Definition:** Primarily to correct cognitive distortions and errors
Cognitive-Behavioral	**Definition:** Combining cognitive and behavioral treatment strategies to improve functioning **Explanation:** Maladaptive responses are examined to determine how cognitions relate to behavior patterns in response to an event. Uses learning principles and information-processing models
Developmental	**Definition:** Age-normed developmental status of cognitive, social and adaptive behavior skills
Intellectual and Psychoeducational	**Definition:** Intellectual abilities, academic achievement and learning capabilities (including behaviors and emotional factors affecting learning)
Interactive	**Definition:** Uses primarily physical aids and other forms of non-oral interaction with a patient who is physically, psychologically or developmentally unable to use ordinary language for communication **Includes/Examples:** Includes the use of toys in symbolic play
Interpersonal	**Definition:** Helps an individual make changes in interpersonal behaviors to reduce psychological dysfunction **Includes/Examples:** Includes exploratory techniques, encouragement of affective expression, clarification of patient statements, analysis of communication patterns, use of therapy relationship and behavior change techniques
Neurobehavioral and Cognitive Status	**Definition:** Includes neurobehavioral status exam, interview(s), and observation for the clinical assessment of thinking, reasoning and judgment, acquired knowledge, attention, memory, visual spatial abilities, language functions, and planning
Neuropsychological	**Definition:** Thinking, reasoning and judgment, acquired knowledge, attention, memory, visual spatial abilities, language functions, planning
Personality and Behavioral	**Definition:** Mood, emotion, behavior, social functioning, psychopathological conditions, personality traits and characteristics
Psychoanalysis	**Definition:** Methods of obtaining a detailed account of past and present mental and emotional experiences to determine the source and eliminate or diminish the undesirable effects of unconscious conflicts **Explanation:** Accomplished by making the individual aware of their existence, origin, and inappropriate expression in emotions and behavior
Psychodynamic	**Definition:** Exploration of past and present emotional experiences to understand motives and drives using insight-oriented techniques to reduce the undesirable effects of internal conflicts on emotions and behavior **Explanation:** Techniques include empathetic listening, clarifying self-defeating behavior patterns, and exploring adaptive alternatives
Psychophysiological	**Definition:** Monitoring and alteration of physiological processes to help the individual associate physiological reactions combined with cognitive and behavioral strategies to gain improved control of these processes to help the individual cope more effectively
Supportive	**Definition:** Formation of therapeutic relationship primarily for providing emotional support to prevent further deterioration in functioning during periods of particular stress **Explanation:** Often used in conjunction with other therapeutic approaches
Vocational	**Definition:** Exploration of vocational interests, aptitudes and required adaptive behavior skills to develop and carry out a plan for achieving a successful vocational placement **Includes/Examples:** Includes enhancing work related adjustment and/or pursuing viable options in training education or preparation

Section H - Substance Abuse Treatment — Character 3 - Root Type

Detoxification Services	**Definition:** Detoxification from alcohol and/or drugs **Explanation:** Not a treatment modality, but helps the patient stabilize physically and psychologically until the body becomes free of drugs and the effects of alcohol
Family Counseling	**Definition:** The application of psychological methods that includes one or more family members to treat an individual with addictive behavior **Explanation:** Provides support and education for family members of addicted individuals. Family member participation is seen as a critical area of substance abuse treatment

Section H - Substance Abuse Treatment — Character 3 - Root Type	
Group Counseling	**Definition:** The application of psychological methods to treat two or more individuals with addictive behavior **Explanation:** Provides structured group counseling sessions and healing power through the connection with others
Individual Counseling	**Definition:** The application of psychological methods to treat an individual with addictive behavior **Explanation:** Comprised of several different techniques, which apply various strategies to address drug addiction
Individual Psychotherapy	**Definition:** Treatment of an individual with addictive behavior by behavioral, cognitive, psychoanalytic, psychodynamic or psychophysiological means
Medication Management	**Definition:** Monitoring and adjusting the use of replacement medications for the treatment of addiction
Pharmacotherapy	**Definition:** The use of replacement medications for the treatment of addiction

Appendix C: Approach Definitions

Section 0 - Medical and Surgical — Character 5 - Approach	
External (X)	**Definition:** Procedures performed directly on the skin or mucous membrane and procedures performed indirectly by the application of external force through the skin or mucous membrane
Open (0)	**Definition:** Cutting through the skin or mucous membrane and any other body layers necessary to expose the site of the procedure
Percutaneous (3)	**Definition:** Entry, by puncture or minor incision, of instrumentation through the skin or mucous membrane and any other body layers necessary to reach the site of the procedure
Percutaneous Endoscopic (4)	**Definition:** Entry, by puncture or minor incision, of instrumentation through the skin or mucous membrane and any other body layers necessary to reach and visualize the site of the procedure
Via Natural or Artificial Opening (7)	**Definition:** Entry of instrumentation through a natural or artificial external opening to reach the site of the procedure
Via Natural or Artificial Opening Endoscopic (8)	**Definition:** Entry of instrumentation through a natural or artificial external opening to reach and visualize the site of the procedure
Via Natural or Artificial Opening With Percutaneous Endoscopic Assistance (F)	**Definition:** Entry of instrumentation through a natural or artificial external opening and entry, by puncture or minor incision, of instrumentation through the skin or mucous membrane and any other body layers necessary to aid in the performance of the procedure

Section 1 - Obstetrics — Character 5 - Approach	
External (X)	**Definition:** Procedures performed directly on the skin or mucous membrane and procedures performed indirectly by the application of external force through the skin or mucous membrane
Open (0)	**Definition:** Cutting through the skin or mucous membrane and any other body layers necessary to expose the site of the procedure
Percutaneous (3)	**Definition:** Entry, by puncture or minor incision, of instrumentation through the skin or mucous membrane and any other body layers necessary to reach the site of the procedure
Percutaneous Endoscopic (4)	**Definition:** Entry, by puncture or minor incision, of instrumentation through the skin or mucous membrane and any other body layers necessary to reach and visualize the site of the procedure
Via Natural or Artificial Opening (7)	**Definition:** Entry of instrumentation through a natural or artificial external opening to reach the site of the procedure
Via Natural or Artificial Opening Endoscopic (8)	**Definition:** Entry of instrumentation through a natural or artificial external opening to reach and visualize the site of the procedure

Section 2 - Placement — Character 5 - Approach	
External (X)	**Definition:** Procedures performed directly on the skin or mucous membrane and procedures performed indirectly by the application of external force through the skin or mucous membrane

Section 3 - Administration — Character 5 - Approach	
External (X)	**Definition:** Procedures performed directly on the skin or mucous membrane and procedures performed indirectly by the application of external force through the skin or mucous membrane
Open (0)	**Definition:** Cutting through the skin or mucous membrane and any other body layers necessary to expose the site of the procedure

Continued →

Section 3 - Administration — Character 5 - Approach

Percutaneous (3)	**Definition:** Entry, by puncture or minor incision, of instrumentation through the skin or mucous membrane and any other body layers necessary to reach the site of the procedure
Percutaneous Endoscopic (4)	**Definition:** Entry, by puncture or minor incision, of instrumentation through the skin or mucous membrane and any other body layers necessary to reach and visualize the site of the procedure
Via Natural or Artificial Opening (7)	**Definition:** Entry of instrumentation through a natural or artificial external opening to reach the site of the procedure
Via Natural or Artificial Opening Endoscopic (8)	**Definition:** Entry of instrumentation through a natural or artificial external opening to reach and visualize the site of the procedure

Section 4 - Measurement and Monitoring — Character 5 - Approach

External (X)	**Definition:** Procedures performed directly on the skin or mucous membrane and procedures performed indirectly by the application of external force through the skin or mucous membrane
Open (0)	**Definition:** Cutting through the skin or mucous membrane and any other body layers necessary to expose the site of the procedure
Percutaneous (3)	**Definition:** Entry, by puncture or minor incision, of instrumentation through the skin or mucous membrane and any other body layers necessary to reach the site of the procedure
Percutaneous Endoscopic (4)	**Definition:** Entry, by puncture or minor incision, of instrumentation through the skin or mucous membrane and any other body layers necessary to reach and visualize the site of the procedure
Via Natural or Artificial Opening (7)	**Definition:** Entry of instrumentation through a natural or artificial external opening to reach the site of the procedure
Via Natural or Artificial Opening Endoscopic (8)	**Definition:** Entry of instrumentation through a natural or artificial external opening to reach and visualize the site of the procedure

Section 7 - Osteopathic — Character 5 - Approach

External (X)	**Definition:** Procedures performed directly on the skin or mucous membrane and procedures performed indirectly by the application of external force through the skin or mucous membrane

Section 8 - Other Procedures — Character 5 - Approach

External (X)	**Definition:** Procedures performed directly on the skin or mucous membrane and procedures performed indirectly by the application of external force through the skin or mucous membrane
Open (0)	**Definition:** Cutting through the skin or mucous membrane and any other body layers necessary to expose the site of the procedure
Percutaneous (3)	**Definition:** Entry, by puncture or minor incision, of instrumentation through the skin or mucous membrane and any other body layers necessary to reach the site of the procedure
Percutaneous Endoscopic (4)	**Definition:** Entry, by puncture or minor incision, of instrumentation through the skin or mucous membrane and any other body layers necessary to reach and visualize the site of the procedure
Via Natural or Artificial Opening (7)	**Definition:** Entry of instrumentation through a natural or artificial external opening to reach the site of the procedure
Via Natural or Artificial Opening Endoscopic (8)	**Definition:** Entry of instrumentation through a natural or artificial external opening to reach and visualize the site of the procedure

Section 9 - Chiropractic — Character 5 - Approach

External (X)	**Definition:** Procedures performed directly on the skin or mucous membrane and procedures performed indirectly by the application of external force through the skin or mucous membrane

Section X - New Technology — Character 5 - Approach

External (X)	**Definition:** Procedures performed directly on the skin or mucous membrane and procedures performed indirectly by the application of external force through the skin or mucous membrane
Open (0)	**Definition:** Cutting through the skin or mucous membrane and any other body layers necessary to expose the site of the procedure
Percutaneous (3)	**Definition:** Entry, by puncture or minor incision, of instrumentation through the skin or mucous membrane and any other body layers necessary to reach the site of the procedure
Percutaneous Endoscopic (4)	**Definition:** Entry, by puncture or minor incision, of instrumentation through the skin or mucous membrane and any other body layers necessary to reach and visualize the site of the procedure
Via Natural or Artificial Opening (7)	**Definition:** Entry of instrumentation through a natural or artificial external opening to reach the site of the procedure
Via Natural or Artificial Opening Endoscopic (8)	**Definition:** Entry of instrumentation through a natural or artificial external opening to reach and visualize the site of the procedure

Appendix D: Medical and Surgical Body Parts

Appendices D–F are structured to assist coders with confirming character selections within the Tables. For example, if the coder is considering the body part of Abdomen Muscle, appendix D can be referenced to identify all of the muscles that are included in the body part Abdomen Muscle (see row 2 in the table below). After reviewing the information, the coder can determine if the body part under consideration is correct or if another body part should be reviewed. The same process can be followed for devices which are included in appendix E and substances which are included in appendix F.

Section 0 - Medical and Surgical — Character 4 - Body Part	
1st Toe, Left **1st** Toe, Right	**Includes:** Hallux
Abdomen Muscle, Left **Abdomen** Muscle, Right	**Includes:** External oblique muscle Internal oblique muscle Pyramidalis muscle Rectus abdominis muscle Transversus abdominis muscle
Abdominal Aorta	**Includes:** Inferior phrenic artery Lumbar artery Median sacral artery Middle suprarenal artery Ovarian artery Testicular artery
Abdominal Sympathetic Nerve	**Includes:** Abdominal aortic plexus Auerbach's (myenteric) plexus Celiac (solar) plexus Celiac ganglion Gastric plexus Hepatic plexus Inferior hypogastric plexus Inferior mesenteric ganglion Inferior mesenteric plexus Meissner's (submucous) plexus Myenteric (Auerbach's) plexus Pancreatic plexus Pelvic splanchnic nerve Renal nerve Renal plexus Solar (celiac) plexus Splenic plexus Submucous (Meissner's) plexus Superior hypogastric plexus Superior mesenteric ganglion Superior mesenteric plexus Suprarenal plexus
Abducens Nerve	**Includes:** Sixth cranial nerve
Accessory Nerve	**Includes:** Eleventh cranial nerve
Acoustic Nerve	**Includes:** Cochlear nerve Eighth cranial nerve Scarpa's (vestibular) ganglion Spiral ganglion Vestibular (Scarpa's) ganglion Vestibular nerve Vestibulocochlear nerve
Adenoids	**Includes:** Pharyngeal tonsil

Section 0 - Medical and Surgical — Character 4 - Body Part	
Adrenal Gland **Adrenal** Gland, Left **Adrenal** Gland, Right **Adrenal** Glands, Bilateral	**Includes:** Suprarenal gland
Ampulla of Vater	**Includes:** Duodenal ampulla Hepatopancreatic ampulla
Anal Sphincter	**Includes:** External anal sphincter Internal anal sphincter
Ankle Bursa and Ligament, Left **Ankle** Bursa and Ligament, Right	**Includes:** Calcaneofibular ligament Deltoid ligament Ligament of the lateral malleolus Talofibular ligament
Ankle Joint, Left **Ankle** Joint, Right	**Includes:** Inferior tibiofibular joint Talocrural joint
Anterior Chamber, Left **Anterior** Chamber, Right	**Includes:** Aqueous humour
Anterior Tibial Artery, Left **Anterior** Tibial Artery, Right	**Includes:** Anterior lateral malleolar artery Anterior medial malleolar artery Anterior tibial recurrent artery Dorsalis pedis artery Posterior tibial recurrent artery
Anus	**Includes:** Anal orifice
Aortic Valve	**Includes:** Aortic annulus
Appendix	**Includes:** Appendiceal orifice Vermiform appendix
Atrial Septum	**Includes:** Interatrial septum
Atrium, Left	**Includes:** Atrium pulmonale Left auricular appendix
Atrium, Right	**Includes:** Atrium dextrum cordis Right auricular appendix Sinus venosus
Auditory Ossicle, Left **Auditory** Ossicle, Right	**Includes:** Incus Malleus Stapes

Section 0 - Medical and Surgical — Character 4 - Body Part

Body Part	Includes
Axillary Artery, Left **Axillary** Artery, Right	**Includes:** Anterior circumflex humeral artery Lateral thoracic artery Posterior circumflex humeral artery Subscapular artery Superior thoracic artery Thoracoacromial artery
Azygos Vein	**Includes:** Right ascending lumbar vein Right subcostal vein
Basal Ganglia	**Includes:** Basal nuclei Claustrum Corpus striatum Globus pallidus Substantia nigra Subthalamic nucleus
Basilic Vein, Left **Basilic** Vein, Right	**Includes:** Median antebrachial vein Median cubital vein
Bladder	**Includes:** Trigone of bladder
Brachial Artery, Left **Brachial** Artery, Right	**Includes:** Inferior ulnar collateral artery Profunda brachii Superior ulnar collateral artery
Brachial Plexus	**Includes:** Axillary nerve Dorsal scapular nerve First intercostal nerve Long thoracic nerve Musculocutaneous nerve Subclavius nerve Suprascapular nerve
Brachial Vein, Left **Brachial** Vein, Right	**Includes:** Radial vein Ulnar vein
Brain	**Includes:** Cerebrum Corpus callosum Encephalon
Breast, Bilateral **Breast,** Left **Breast,** Right	**Includes:** Mammary duct Mammary gland
Buccal Mucosa	**Includes:** Buccal gland Molar gland Palatine gland
Carotid Bodies, Bilateral **Carotid** Body, Left **Carotid** Body, Right	**Includes:** Carotid glomus
Carpal Joint, Left **Carpal** Joint, Right	**Includes:** Intercarpal joint Midcarpal joint
Carpal, Left **Carpal,** Right	**Includes:** Capitate bone Hamate bone Lunate bone Pisiform bone Scaphoid bone Trapezium bone Trapezoid bone Triquetral bone
Celiac Artery	**Includes:** Celiac trunk
Cephalic Vein, Left **Cephalic** Vein, Right	**Includes:** Accessory cephalic vein
Cerebellum	**Includes:** Culmen
Cerebral Hemisphere	**Includes:** Frontal lobe Occipital lobe Parietal lobe Temporal lobe
Cerebral Meninges	**Includes:** Arachnoid mater, intracranial Leptomeninges, intracranial Pia mater, intracranial
Cerebral Ventricle	**Includes:** Aqueduct of Sylvius Cerebral aqueduct (Sylvius) Choroid plexus Ependyma Foramen of Monro (intraventricular) Fourth ventricle Interventricular foramen (Monro) Left lateral ventricle Right lateral ventricle Third ventricle
Cervical Nerve	**Includes:** Greater occipital nerve Spinal nerve, cervical Suboccipital nerve Third occipital nerve
Cervical Plexus	**Includes:** Ansa cervicalis Cutaneous (transverse) cervical nerve Great auricular nerve Lesser occipital nerve Supraclavicular nerve Transverse (cutaneous) cervical nerve
Cervical Spinal Cord	Dorsal root ganglion
Cervical Vertebra	**Includes:** Dens Odontoid process Spinous process Transverse foramen Transverse process Vertebral arch Vertebral body Vertebral foramen Vertebral lamina Vertebral pedicle

Continued →

Section 0 - Medical and Surgical — Character 4 - Body Part

Cervical Vertebral Joint	**Includes:** Atlantoaxial joint Cervical facet joint
Cervical Vertebral Joints, 2 or more	**Includes:** Cervical facet joint
Cervicothoracic Vertebral Joint	**Includes:** Cervicothoracic facet joint
Cisterna Chyli	**Includes:** Intestinal lymphatic trunk Lumbar lymphatic trunk
Coccygeal Glomus	**Includes:** Coccygeal body
Colic Vein	**Includes:** Ileocolic vein Left colic vein Middle colic vein Right colic vein
Conduction Mechanism	**Includes:** Atrioventricular node Bundle of His Bundle of Kent Sinoatrial node
Conjunctiva, Left **Conjunctiva,** Right	**Includes:** Plica semilunaris
Dura Mater	**Includes:** Diaphragma sellae Dura mater, intracranial Falx cerebri Tentorium cerebelli
Elbow Bursa and Ligament, Left **Elbow** Bursa and Ligament, Right	**Includes:** Annular ligament Olecranon bursa Radial collateral ligament Ulnar collateral ligament
Elbow Joint, Left **Elbow** Joint, Right	**Includes:** Distal humerus, involving joint Humeroradial joint Humeroulnar joint Proximal radioulnar joint
Epidural Space, Intracranial	**Includes:** Extradural space, intracranial
Epiglottis	**Includes:** Glossoepiglottic fold
Esophagogastric Junction	**Includes:** Cardia Cardioesophageal junction Gastroesophageal (GE) junction
Esophagus, Lower	**Includes:** Abdominal esophagus
Esophagus, Middle	**Includes:** Thoracic esophagus
Esophagus, Upper	**Includes:** Cervical esophagus
Ethmoid Bone, Left **Ethmoid** Bone, Right	**Includes:** Cribriform plate
Ethmoid Sinus, Left **Ethmoid** Sinus, Right	**Includes:** Ethmoidal air cell

Eustachian Tube, Left **Eustachian** Tube, Right	**Includes:** Auditory tube Pharyngotympanic tube
External Auditory Canal, Left **External** Auditory Canal, Right	**Includes:** External auditory meatus
External Carotid Artery, Left **External** Carotid Artery, Right	**Includes:** Ascending pharyngeal artery Internal maxillary artery Lingual artery Maxillary artery Occipital artery Posterior auricular artery Superior thyroid artery
External Ear, Bilateral **External** Ear, Left **External** Ear, Right	**Includes:** Antihelix Antitragus Auricle Earlobe Helix Pinna Tragus
External Iliac Artery, Left **External** Iliac Artery, Right	**Includes:** Deep circumflex iliac artery Inferior epigastric artery
External Jugular Vein, Left **External** Jugular Vein, Right	**Includes:** Posterior auricular vein
Extraocular Muscle, Left **Extraocular** Muscle, Right	**Includes:** Inferior oblique muscle Inferior rectus muscle Lateral rectus muscle Medial rectus muscle Superior oblique muscle Superior rectus muscle
Eye, Left **Eye,** Right	**Includes:** Ciliary body Posterior chamber
Face Artery	**Includes:** Angular artery Ascending palatine artery External maxillary artery Facial artery Inferior labial artery Submental artery Superior labial artery
Face Vein, Left **Face** Vein, Right	**Includes:** Angular vein Anterior facial vein Common facial vein Deep facial vein Frontal vein Posterior facial (retromandibular) vein Supraorbital vein
Facial Muscle	**Includes:** Buccinator muscle Corrugator supercilii muscle Depressor anguli oris muscle Depressor labii inferioris muscle

Section 0 - Medical and Surgical — Character 4 - Body Part

	Depressor septi nasi muscle Depressor supercilii muscle Levator anguli oris muscle Levator labii superioris alaeque nasi Levator labii superioris alaeque nasi Levator labii superioris alaeque nasi Levator labii superioris muscle Mentalis muscle Nasalis muscle Occipitofrontalis muscle Orbicularis oris muscle Procerus muscle Risorius muscle Zygomaticus muscle
Facial Nerve	**Includes:** Chorda tympani Geniculate ganglion Greater superficial petrosal nerve Nerve to the stapedius Parotid plexus Posterior auricular nerve Seventh cranial nerve Submandibular ganglion
Fallopian Tube, Left **Fallopian** Tube, Right	**Includes:** Oviduct Salpinx Uterine tube
Femoral Artery, Left **Femoral** Artery, Right	**Includes:** Circumflex iliac artery Deep femoral artery Descending genicular artery External pudendal artery Superficial epigastric artery
Femoral Nerve	**Includes:** Anterior crural nerve Saphenous nerve
Femoral Shaft, Left **Femoral** Shaft, Right	**Includes:** Body of femur
Femoral Vein, Left **Femoral** Vein, Right	**Includes:** Deep femoral (profunda femoris) vein Popliteal vein Profunda femoris (deep femoral) vein
Fibula, Left **Fibula,** Right	**Includes:** Body of fibula Head of fibula Lateral malleolus
Finger Nail	**Includes:** Nail bed Nail plate
Finger Phalangeal Joint, Left **Finger** Phalangeal Joint, Right	**Includes:** Interphalangeal (IP) joint
Foot Artery, Left **Foot** Artery, Right	**Includes:** Arcuate artery Dorsal metatarsal artery Lateral plantar artery Lateral tarsal artery Medial plantar artery

Foot Bursa and Ligament, Left **Foot** Bursa and Ligament, Right	**Includes:** Calcaneocuboid ligament Cuneonavicular ligament Intercuneiform ligament Interphalangeal ligament Metatarsal ligament Metatarsophalangeal ligament Subtalar ligament Talocalcaneal ligament Talocalcaneonavicular ligament Tarsometatarsal ligament
Foot Muscle, Left **Foot** Muscle, Right	**Includes:** Abductor hallucis muscle Adductor hallucis muscle Extensor digitorum brevis muscle Extensor hallucis brevis muscle Flexor digitorum brevis muscle Flexor hallucis brevis muscle Quadratus plantae muscle
Foot Vein, Left **Foot** Vein, Right	**Includes:** Common digital vein Dorsal metatarsal vein Dorsal venous arch Plantar digital vein Plantar metatarsal vein Plantar venous arch
Frontal Bone	**Includes:** Zygomatic process of frontal bone
Gastric Artery	**Includes:** Left gastric artery Right gastric artery
Glenoid Cavity, Left **Glenoid** Cavity, Right	**Includes:** Glenoid fossa (of scapula)
Glomus Jugulare	**Includes:** Jugular body
Glossopharyngeal Nerve	**Includes:** Carotid sinus nerve Ninth cranial nerve Tympanic nerve
Hand Artery, Left **Hand** Artery, Right	**Includes:** Deep palmar arch Princeps pollicis artery Radialis indicis Superficial palmar arch
Hand Bursa and Ligament, Left **Hand** Bursa and Ligament, Right	**Includes:** Carpometacarpal ligament Intercarpal ligament Interphalangeal ligament Lunotriquetral ligament Metacarpal ligament Metacarpophalangeal ligament Pisohamate ligament Pisometacarpal ligament Scaphotrapezium ligament
Hand Muscle, Left **Hand** Muscle, Right	**Includes:** Hypothenar muscle Palmar interosseous muscle Thenar muscle

Continued →

Section 0 - Medical and Surgical — Character 4 - Body Part		Section 0 - Medical and Surgical — Character 4 - Body Part	
Hand Vein, Left **Hand** Vein, Right	**Includes:** Dorsal metacarpal vein Palmar (volar) digital vein Palmar (volar) metacarpal vein Superficial palmar venous arch Volar (palmar) digital vein Volar (palmar) metacarpal vein	**Hip** Muscle, Left **Hip** Muscle, Right	**Includes:** Gemellus muscle Gluteus maximus muscle Gluteus medius muscle Gluteus minimus muscle Iliacus muscle Obturator muscle Piriformis muscle Psoas muscle Quadratus femoris muscle Tensor fasciae latae muscle
Head and Neck Bursa and Ligament	**Includes:** Alar ligament of axis Cervical interspinous ligament Cervical intertransverse ligament Cervical ligamentum flavum Interspinous ligament cervical Intertransverse ligament, cervical Lateral temporomandibular ligament Ligamentum flavum, cervical Sphenomandibular ligament Stylomandibular ligament Transverse ligament of atlas	**Humeral** Head, Left **Humeral** Head, Right	**Includes:** Greater tuberosity Lesser tuberosity Neck of humerus (anatomical) (surgical)
		Humeral Shaft, Left **Humeral** Shaft, Right	**Includes:** Distal humerus Humerus, distal Lateral epicondyle of humerus Medial epicondyle of humerus
Head and Neck Sympathetic Nerve	**Includes:** Cavernous plexus Cervical ganglion Ciliary ganglion Internal carotid plexus Otic ganglion Pterygopalatine (sphenopalatine) ganglion Sphenopalatine (pterygopalatine) ganglion Stellate ganglion Submandibular ganglion Submaxillary ganglion	**Hypogastric** Vein, Left **Hypogastric** Vein, Right	**Includes:** Gluteal vein Internal iliac vein Internal pudendal vein Lateral sacral vein Middle hemorrhoidal vein Obturator vein Uterine vein Vaginal vein Vesical vein
		Hypoglossal Nerve	**Includes:** Twelfth cranial nerve
		Hypothalamus	**Includes:** Mammillary body
		Inferior Mesenteric Artery	**Includes:** Sigmoid artery Superior rectal artery
Head Muscle	**Includes:** Auricularis muscle Masseter muscle Pterygoid muscle Splenius capitis muscle Temporalis muscle Temporoparietalis muscle	**Inferior** Mesenteric Vein	**Includes:** Sigmoid vein Superior rectal vein
Heart, Left	**Includes:** Left coronary sulcus Obtuse margin	**Inferior** Vena Cava	**Includes:** Postcava Right inferior phrenic vein Right ovarian vein Right second lumbar vein Right suprarenal vein Right testicular vein
Heart, Right	**Includes:** Right coronary sulcus		
Hemiazygos Vein	**Includes:** Left ascending lumbar vein Left subcostal vein		
Hepatic Artery	**Includes:** Common hepatic artery Gastroduodenal artery Hepatic artery proper	**Inguinal** Region, Bilateral **Inguinal** Region, Left **Inguinal** Region, Right	**Includes:** Inguinal canal Inguinal triangle
Hip Bursa and Ligament, Left **Hip** Bursa and Ligament, Right	**Includes:** Iliofemoral ligament Ischiofemoral ligament Pubofemoral ligament Transverse acetabular ligament Trochanteric bursa	**Inner** Ear, Left **Inner** Ear, Right	**Includes:** Bony labyrinth Bony vestibule Cochlea Round window Semicircular canal
Hip Joint, Left **Hip** Joint, Right	**Includes:** Acetabulofemoral joint		

Section 0 - Medical and Surgical — Character 4 - Body Part		**Section 0 - Medical and Surgical — Character 4 - Body Part**	
Innominate Artery	Includes: Brachiocephalic artery Brachiocephalic trunk	**Jejunum**	Includes: Duodenojejunal flexure
Innominate Vein, Left **Innominate** Vein, Right	Includes: Brachiocephalic vein Inferior thyroid vein	**Kidney**	Includes: Renal calyx Renal capsule Renal cortex Renal segment
Internal Carotid Artery, Left **Internal** Carotid Artery, Right	Includes: Caroticotympanic artery Carotid sinus	**Kidney** Pelvis, Left **Kidney** Pelvis, Right	Includes: Ureteropelvic junction (UPJ)
Internal Iliac Artery, Left **Internal** Iliac Artery, Right	Includes: Deferential artery Hypogastric artery Iliolumbar artery Inferior gluteal artery Inferior vesical artery Internal pudendal artery Lateral sacral artery Middle rectal artery Obturator artery Prostatic artery Superior gluteal artery Superior vesical artery Umbilical artery Uterine artery Vaginal artery	**Kidney**, Left **Kidney**, Right **Kidneys**, Bilateral	Includes: Renal calyx Renal capsule Renal cortex Renal segment
		Knee Bursa and Ligament, Left **Knee** Bursa and Ligament, Right	Includes: Anterior cruciate ligament (ACL) Lateral collateral ligament (LCL) Ligament of head of fibula Medial collateral ligament (MCL) Patellar ligament Popliteal ligament Posterior cruciate ligament (PCL) Prepatellar bursa
		Knee Joint, Femoral Surface, Left **Knee** Joint, Femoral Surface, Right	Includes: Femoropatellar joint Patellofemoral joint
		Knee Joint, Left **Knee** Joint, Right	Includes: Femoropatellar joint Femorotibial joint Lateral meniscus Medial meniscus Patellofemoral joint Tibiofemoral joint
Internal Mammary Artery, Left **Internal** Mammary Artery, Right	Includes: Anterior intercostal artery Internal thoracic artery Musculophrenic artery Pericardiophrenic artery Superior epigastric artery		
Intracranial Artery	Includes: Anterior cerebral artery Anterior choroidal artery Anterior communicating artery Basilar artery Circle of Willis Internal carotid artery, intracranial portion Middle cerebral artery Middle meningeal artery, intracranial portion Ophthalmic artery Posterior cerebral artery Posterior communicating artery Posterior inferior cerebellar artery (PICA) Vertebral artery, intracranial portion	**Knee** Joint, Tibial Surface, Left **Knee** Joint, Tibial Surface, Right	Includes: Femorotibial joint Tibiofemoral joint
		Knee Tendon, Left **Knee** Tendon, Right	Includes: Patellar tendon
		Lacrimal Duct, Left **Lacrimal** Duct, Right	Includes: Lacrimal canaliculus Lacrimal punctum Lacrimal sac Nasolacrimal duct
		Larynx	Includes: Aryepiglottic fold Arytenoid cartilage Corniculate cartilage Cuneiform cartilage False vocal cord Glottis Rima glottidis Thyroid cartilage Ventricular fold
Intracranial Vein	Includes: Anterior cerebral vein Basal (internal) cerebral vein Dural venous sinus Great cerebral vein Inferior cerebellar vein Inferior cerebral vein Internal (basal) cerebral vein Middle cerebral vein Ophthalmic vein Superior cerebellar vein Superior cerebral vein		
		Lens, Left **Lens**, Right	Includes: Zonule of Zinn
		Liver	Includes: Quadrate lobe

Section 0 - Medical and Surgical — Character 4 - Body Part

Body Part	Includes
Lower Arm and Wrist Muscle, Left **Lower** Arm and Wrist Muscle, Right	**Includes:** Anatomical snuffbox Brachioradialis muscle Extensor carpi radialis muscle Extensor carpi ulnaris muscle Flexor carpi radialis muscle Flexor carpi ulnaris muscle Flexor pollicis longus muscle Palmaris longus muscle Pronator quadratus muscle Pronator teres muscle
Lower Artery	Umbilical artery
Lower Eyelid, Left **Lower** Eyelid, Right	**Includes:** Inferior tarsal plate Medial canthus
Lower Femur, Left **Lower** Femur, Right	**Includes:** Lateral condyle of femur Lateral epicondyle of femur Medial condyle of femur Medial epicondyle of femur
Lower Leg Muscle, Left **Lower** Leg Muscle, Right	**Includes:** Extensor digitorum longus muscle Extensor hallucis longus muscle Fibularis brevis muscle Fibularis longus muscle Flexor digitorum longus muscle Flexor hallucis longus muscle Gastrocnemius muscle Peroneus brevis muscle Peroneus longus muscle Popliteus muscle Soleus muscle Tibialis anterior muscle Tibialis posterior muscle
Lower Leg Tendon, Left **Lower** Leg Tendon, Right	**Includes:** Achilles tendon
Lower Lip	**Includes:** Frenulum labii inferioris Labial gland Vermilion border
Lower Spine Bursa and Ligament	Iliolumbar ligament Interspinous ligament, lumbar Intertransverse ligament, lumbar Ligamentum flavum, lumbar Sacrococcygeal ligament Sacroiliac ligament Sacrospinous ligament Sacrotuberous ligament Supraspinous ligament
Lumbar Nerve	**Includes:** Lumbosacral trunk Spinal nerve, lumbar Superior clunic (cluneal) nerve
Lumbar Plexus	**Includes:** Accessory obturator nerve Genitofemoral nerve Iliohypogastric nerve Ilioinguinal nerve Lateral femoral cutaneous nerve Obturator nerve Superior gluteal nerve
Lumbar Spinal Cord	**Includes:** Cauda equina Conus medullaris Dorsal root ganglion
Lumbar Sympathetic Nerve	**Includes:** Lumbar ganglion Lumbar splanchnic nerve
Lumbar Vertebra	**Includes:** Spinous process Transverse process Vertebral arch Vertebral body Vertebral foramen Vertebral lamina Vertebral pedicle
Lumbar Vertebral Joint	**Includes:** Lumbar facet joint
Lumbosacral Joint	**Includes:** Lumbosacral facet joint
Lymphatic, Aortic	**Includes:** Celiac lymph node Gastric lymph node Hepatic lymph node Lumbar lymph node Pancreaticosplenic lymph node Paraaortic lymph node Retroperitoneal lymph node
Lymphatic, Head	**Includes:** Buccinator lymph node Infraauricular lymph node Infraparotid lymph node Parotid lymph node Preauricular lymph node Submandibular lymph node Submaxillary lymph node Submental lymph node Subparotid lymph node Suprahyoid lymph node
Lymphatic, Left Axillary	**Includes:** Anterior (pectoral) lymph node Apical (subclavicular) lymph node Brachial (lateral) lymph node Central axillary lymph node Lateral (brachial) lymph node Pectoral (anterior) lymph node Posterior (subscapular) lymph node Subclavicular (apical) lymph node Subscapular (posterior) lymph node
Lymphatic, Left Lower Extremity	**Includes:** Femoral lymph node Popliteal lymph node
Lymphatic, Left Neck	**Includes:** Cervical lymph node Jugular lymph node Mastoid (postauricular) lymph node Occipital lymph node Postauricular (mastoid) lymph node Retropharyngeal lymph node Supraclavicular (Virchow's) lymph node Virchow's (supraclavicular) lymph node

Continued →

Section 0 - Medical and Surgical — Character 4 - Body Part

Lymphatic, Left Upper Extremity	**Includes:** Cubital lymph node Deltopectoral (infraclavicular) lymph node Epitrochlear lymph node Infraclavicular (deltopectoral) lymph node Supratrochlear lymph node
Lymphatic, Mesenteric	**Includes:** Inferior mesenteric lymph node Pararectal lymph node Superior mesenteric lymph node
Lymphatic, Pelvis	**Includes:** Common iliac (subaortic) lymph node Gluteal lymph node Iliac lymph node Inferior epigastric lymph node Obturator lymph node Sacral lymph node Subaortic (common iliac) lymph node Suprainguinal lymph node
Lymphatic, Right Axillary	**Includes:** Anterior (pectoral) lymph node Apical (subclavicular) lymph node Brachial (lateral) lymph node Central axillary lymph node Lateral (brachial) lymph node Pectoral (anterior) lymph node Posterior (subscapular) lymph node Subclavicular (apical) lymph node Subscapular (posterior) lymph node
Lymphatic, Right Lower Extremity	**Includes:** Femoral lymph node Popliteal lymph node
Lymphatic, Right Neck	**Includes:** Cervical lymph node Jugular lymph node Mastoid (postauricular) lymph node Occipital lymph node Postauricular (mastoid) lymph node Retropharyngeal lymph node Right jugular trunk Right lymphatic duct Right subclavian trunk Supraclavicular (Virchow's) lymph node Virchow's (supraclavicular) lymph node
Lymphatic, Right Upper Extremity	**Includes:** Cubital lymph node Deltopectoral (infraclavicular) lymph node Epitrochlear lymph node Infraclavicular (deltopectoral) lymph node Supratrochlear lymph node
Lymphatic, Thorax	**Includes:** Intercostal lymph node Mediastinal lymph node Parasternal lymph node Paratracheal lymph node Tracheobronchial lymph node

Section 0 - Medical and Surgical — Character 4 - Body Part

Main Bronchus, Right	**Includes:** Bronchus Intermedius Intermediate bronchus
Mandible, Left **Mandible,** Right	**Includes:** Alveolar process of mandible Condyloid process Mandibular notch Mental foramen
Mastoid Sinus, Left **Mastoid** Sinus, Right	**Includes:** Mastoid air cells
Maxilla	**Includes:** Alveolar process of maxilla
Maxillary Sinus, Left **Maxillary** Sinus, Right	**Includes:** Antrum of Highmore
Median Nerve	**Includes:** Anterior interosseous nerve Palmar cutaneous nerve
Mediastinum	Mediastinal cavity Mediastinal space
Medulla Oblongata	**Includes:** Myelencephalon
Mesentery	**Includes:** Mesoappendix Mesocolon
Metatarsal, Left **Metatarsal,** Right	Fibular sesamoid Tibial sesamoid
Metatarsal-Phalangeal Joint, Left **Metatarsal-Phalangeal** Joint, Right	**Includes:** Metatarsophalangeal (MTP) joint
Middle Ear, Left **Middle** Ear, Right	**Includes:** Oval window Tympanic cavity
Minor Salivary Gland	**Includes:** Anterior lingual gland
Mitral Valve	**Includes:** Bicuspid valve Left atrioventricular valve Mitral annulus
Nasal Bone	**Includes:** Vomer of nasal septum
Nasal Mucosa and Soft Tissue	Columella External naris Greater alar cartilage Internal naris Lateral nasal cartilage Lesser alar cartilage Nasal cavity Nostril
Nasal Septum	**Includes:** Quadrangular cartilage Septal cartilage Vomer bone
Nasal Turbinate	**Includes:** Inferior turbinate Middle turbinate Nasal concha Superior turbinate

Continued →

Section 0 - Medical and Surgical — Character 4 - Body Part

Nasopharynx	**Includes:** Choana Fossa of Rosenmuller Pharyngeal recess Rhinopharynx
Neck	Parapharyngeal space Retropharyngeal space
Neck Muscle, Left **Neck** Muscle, Right	**Includes:** Anterior vertebral muscle Arytenoid muscle Cricothyroid muscle Infrahyoid muscle Levator scapulae muscle Platysma muscle Scalene muscle Splenius cervicis muscle Sternocleidomastoid muscle Suprahyoid muscle Thyroarytenoid muscle
Nipple, Left **Nipple,** Right	**Includes:** Areola
Occipital Bone	**Includes:** Foramen magnum
Oculomotor Nerve	**Includes:** Third cranial nerve
Olfactory Nerve	**Includes:** First cranial nerve Olfactory bulb
Omentum	Gastrocolic ligament Gastrocolic omentum Gastrohepatic omentum Gastrophrenic ligament Gastrosplenic ligament Greater Omentum Hepatogastric liagment Lesser Omentum
Optic Nerve	**Includes:** Optic chiasma Second cranial nerve
Orbit, Left **Orbit,** Right	**Includes:** Bony orbit Orbital portion of ethmoid bone Orbital portion of frontal bone Orbital portion of lacrimal bone Orbital portion of maxilla Orbital portion of palatine bone Orbital portion of sphenoid bone Orbital portion of zygomatic bone
Pancreatic Duct	**Includes:** Duct of Wirsung
Pancreatic Duct, Accessory	**Includes:** Duct of Santorini
Parotid Duct, Left **Parotid** Duct, Right	**Includes:** Stensen's duct
Pelvic Bone, Left **Pelvic** Bone, Right	**Includes:** Iliac crest Ilium Ischium Pubis

Section 0 - Medical and Surgical — Character 4 - Body Part

Pelvic Cavity	**Includes:** Retropubic space Space of Retzius
Penis	**Includes:** Corpus cavernosum Corpus spongiosum
Perineum Muscle	**Includes:** Bulbospongiosus muscle Cremaster muscle Deep transverse perineal muscle Ischiocavernosus muscle Levator ani muscle Superficial transverse perineal muscle
Peritoneal Cavity	Abdominal cavity
Peritoneum	**Includes:** Epiploic foramen
Peroneal Artery, Left **Peroneal** Artery, Right	**Includes:** Fibular artery
Peroneal Nerve	**Includes:** Common fibular nerve Common peroneal nerve External popliteal nerve Lateral sural cutaneous nerve
Pharynx	**Includes:** Base of Tongue Hypopharynx Laryngopharynx Lignual tonsil Oropharynx Piriform recess (sinus) Tongue, base of
Phrenic Nerve	**Includes:** Accessory phrenic nerve
Pituitary Gland	**Includes:** Adenohypophysis Hypophysis Neurohypophysis
Pons	**Includes:** Apneustic center Basis pontis Locus ceruleus Pneumotaxic center Pontine tegmentum Superior olivary nucleus
Popliteal Artery, Left **Popliteal** Artery, Right	**Includes:** Inferior genicular artery Middle genicular artery Superior genicular artery Sural artery Tibioperoneal trunk
Portal Vein	**Includes:** Hepatic portal vein
Prepuce	**Includes:** Foreskin Glans penis
Pudendal Nerve	**Includes:** Posterior labial nerve Posterior scrotal nerve
Pulmonary Artery, Left	**Includes:** Arterial canal (duct) Botallo's duct Pulmoaortic canal

Continued →

Section 0 - Medical and Surgical — Character 4 - Body Part

Pulmonary Valve	**Includes:** Pulmonary annulus Pulmonic valve
Pulmonary Vein, Left	**Includes:** Left inferior pulmonary vein Left superior pulmonary vein
Pulmonary Vein, Right	**Includes:** Right inferior pulmonary vein Right superior pulmonary vein
Radial Artery, Left **Radial** Artery, Right	**Includes:** Radial recurrent artery
Radial Nerve	**Includes:** Dorsal digital nerve Musculospiral nerve Palmar cutaneous nerve Posterior interosseous nerve
Radius, Left **Radius,** Right	**Includes:** Ulnar notch
Rectum	**Includes:** Anorectal junction
Renal Artery, Left **Renal** Artery, Right	**Includes:** Inferior suprarenal artery Renal segmental artery
Renal Vein, Left	**Includes:** Left inferior phrenic vein Left ovarian vein Left second lumbar vein Left suprarenal vein Left testicular vein
Retina, Left **Retina,** Right	**Includes:** Fovea Macula Optic disc
Retroperitoneum	**Includes:** Retroperitoneal cavity Retroperitoneal space
Rib(s) Bursa and Ligament	Costotransverse ligament
Sacral Nerve	**Includes:** Spinal nerve, sacral
Sacral Plexus	**Includes:** Inferior gluteal nerve Posterior femoral cutaneous nerve Pudendal nerve
Sacral Sympathetic Nerve	**Includes:** Ganglion impar (ganglion of Walther) Pelvic splanchnic nerve Sacral ganglion Sacral splanchnic nerve
Sacrococcygeal Joint	**Includes:** Sacrococcygeal symphysis
Saphenous Vein, Left **Saphenous** Vein, Right	External pudendal vein Great(er) saphenous vein Lesser saphenous vein Small saphenous vein Superficial circumflex iliac vein Superficial epigastric vein
Scapula, Left **Scapula,** Right	**Includes:** Acromion (process) Coracoid process
Sciatic Nerve	**Includes:** Ischiatic nerve

Section 0 - Medical and Surgical — Character 4 - Body Part

Shoulder Bursa and Ligament, Left **Shoulder** Bursa and Ligament, Right	**Includes:** Acromioclavicular ligament Coracoacromial ligament Coracoclavicular ligament Coracohumeral ligament
	Costoclavicular ligament Glenohumeral ligament Interclavicular ligament Sternoclavicular ligament Subacromial bursa Transverse humeral ligament Transverse scapular ligament
Shoulder Joint, Left **Shoulder** Joint, Right	**Includes:** Glenohumeral joint Glenoid ligament (labrum)
Shoulder Muscle, Left **Shoulder** Muscle, Right	**Includes:** Deltoid muscle Infraspinatus muscle Subscapularis muscle Supraspinatus muscle Teres major muscle Teres minor muscle
Sigmoid Colon	**Includes:** Rectosigmoid junction Sigmoid flexure
Skin	**Includes:** Dermis Epidermis Sebaceous gland Sweat gland
Skin, Chest	Breast procedures, skin only
Skin, Perineum	Perianal skin
Sphenoid Bone	**Includes:** Greater wing Lesser wing Optic foramen Pterygoid process Sella turcica
Spinal Canal	**Includes:** Epidural space, spinal Extradural space, spinal Subarachnoid space, spinal Subdural space, spinal Vertebral canal
Spinal Cord	Dorsal root ganglion
Spinal Meninges	**Includes:** Arachnoid mater, spinal Denticulate (dentate) ligament Dura mater, spinal Filum terminale Leptomeninges, spinal Pia mater, spinal
Spleen	**Includes:** Accessory spleen
Splenic Artery	**Includes:** Left gastroepiploic artery Pancreatic artery Short gastric artery
Splenic Vein	**Includes:** Left gastroepiploic vein Pancreatic vein

Continued →

Section 0 - Medical and Surgical — Character 4 - Body Part

Sternum	**Includes:** Manubrium Suprasternal notch Xiphoid process
Sternum Bursa and Ligament	Costotransverse ligament Costoxiphoid ligament Sternocostal ligament
Stomach, Pylorus	**Includes:** Pyloric antrum Pyloric canal Pyloric sphincter
Subclavian Artery, Left **Subclavian** Artery, Right	**Includes:** Costocervical trunk Dorsal scapular artery Internal thoracic artery
Subcutaneous Tissue and Fascia, Chest	**Includes:** Pectoral fascia
Subcutaneous Tissue and Fascia, Face	**Includes:** Chin Masseteric fascia Orbital fascia Submandibular space
Subcutaneous Tissue and Fascia, Left Foot	**Includes:** Plantar fascia (aponeurosis)
Subcutaneous Tissue and Fascia, Left Hand	**Includes:** Palmar fascia (aponeurosis)
Subcutaneous Tissue and Fascia, Left Lower Arm	**Includes:** Antebrachial fascia Bicipital aponeurosis
Subcutaneous Tissue and Fascia, Left Neck	Deep cervical fascia Pretracheal fascia Prevertebral fascia
Subcutaneous Tissue and Fascia, Left Upper Arm	**Includes:** Axillary fascia Deltoid fascia Infraspinatus fascia Subscapular aponeurosis Supraspinatus fascia
Subcutaneous Tissue and Fascia, Left Upper Leg	**Includes:** Crural fascia Fascia lata Iliac fascia Iliotibial tract (band)
Subcutaneous Tissue and Fascia, Right Foot	**Includes:** Plantar fascia (aponeurosis)
Subcutaneous Tissue and Fascia, Right Hand	**Includes:** Palmar fascia (aponeurosis)
Subcutaneous Tissue and Fascia, Right Lower Arm	**Includes:** Antebrachial fascia Bicipital aponeurosis
Subcutaneous Tissue and Fascia, Right Neck	Deep cervical fascia Pretracheal fascia Prevertebral fascia
Subcutaneous Tissue and Fascia, Right Upper Arm	**Includes:** Axillary fascia Deltoid fascia Infraspinatus fascia Subscapular aponeurosis Supraspinatus fascia

Section 0 - Medical and Surgical — Character 4 - Body Part

Subcutaneous Tissue and Fascia, Right Upper Leg	**Includes:** Crural fascia Fascia lata Iliac fascia Iliotibial tract (band)
Subcutaneous Tissue and Fascia, Scalp	**Includes:** Galea aponeurotica
Subcutaneous Tissue and Fascia, Trunk	**Includes:** External oblique aponeurosis Transversalis fascia
Submaxillary Gland, Left **Submaxillary** Gland, Right	**Includes:** Submandibular gland
Superior Mesenteric Artery	**Includes:** Ileal artery Ileocolic artery Inferior pancreaticoduodenal artery Jejunal artery
Superior Mesenteric Vein	**Includes:** Right gastroepiploic vein
Superior Vena Cava	**Includes:** Cavoatrial junction Precava
Tarsal Joint, Left **Tarsal** Joint, Right	**Includes:** Calcaneocuboid joint Cuboideonavicular joint Cuneonavicular joint Intercuneiform joint Subtalar (talocalcaneal) joint Talocalcaneal (subtalar) joint Talocalcaneonavicular joint
Tarsal, Left **Tarsal,** Right	**Includes:** Calcaneus Cuboid bone Intermediate cuneiform bone Lateral cuneiform bone Medial cuneiform bone Navicular bone Talus bone
Temporal Artery, Left **Temporal** Artery, Right	**Includes:** Middle temporal artery Superficial temporal artery Transverse facial artery
Temporal Bone, Left **Temporal** Bone, Right	**Includes:** Mastoid process Petrous part of temoporal bone Tympanic part of temoporal bone Zygomatic process of temporal bone
Thalamus	**Includes:** Epithalamus Geniculate nucleus Metathalamus Pulvinar
Thoracic Aorta Ascending/Arch	**Includes:** Aortic arch Ascending aorta

Continued →

Section 0 - Medical and Surgical — Character 4 - Body Part

Thoracic Duct	**Includes:** Left jugular trunk Left subclavian trunk
Thoracic Nerve	**Includes:** Intercostal nerve Intercostobrachial nerve Spinal nerve, thoracic Subcostal nerve
Thoracic Spinal Cord	Dorsal root ganglion
Thoracic Sympathetic Nerve	**Includes:** Cardiac plexus Esophageal plexus Greater splanchnic nerve Inferior cardiac nerve Least splanchnic nerve Lesser splanchnic nerve Middle cardiac nerve Pulmonary plexus Superior cardiac nerve Thoracic aortic plexus Thoracic ganglion
Thoracic Vertebra	**Includes:** Spinous process Transverse process Vertebral arch Vertebral body Vertebral foramen Vertebral lamina Vertebral pedicle
Thoracic Vertebral Joint	**Includes:** Costotransverse joint Costovertebral joint Thoracic facet joint
Thoracolumbar Vertebral Joint	**Includes:** Thoracolumbar facet joint
Thorax Muscle, Left **Thorax** Muscle, Right	**Includes:** Intercostal muscle Levatores costarum muscle Pectoralis major muscle Pectoralis minor muscle Serratus anterior muscle Subclavius muscle Subcostal muscle Transverse thoracis muscle
Thymus	**Includes:** Thymus gland
Thyroid Artery, Left **Thyroid** Artery, Right	**Includes:** Cricothyroid artery Hyoid artery Sternocleidomastoid artery Superior laryngeal artery Superior thyroid artery Thyrocervical trunk
Tibia, Left **Tibia,** Right	**Includes:** Lateral condyle of tibia Medial condyle of tibia Medial malleolus
Tibial Nerve	**Includes:** Lateral plantar nerve Medial plantar nerve Medial popliteal nerve Medial sural cutaneous nerve

Section 0 - Medical and Surgical — Character 4 - Body Part

Toe Nail	**Includes:** Nail bed Nail plate
Toe Phalangeal Joint, Left **Toe** Phalangeal Joint, Right	**Includes:** Interphalangeal (IP) joint
Tongue	**Includes:** Frenulum linguae
Tongue, Palate, Pharynx Muscle	**Includes:** Chondroglossus muscle Genioglossus muscle Hyoglossus muscle Inferior longitudinal muscle Levator veli palatini muscle Palatoglossal muscle Palatopharyngeal muscle Pharyngeal constrictor muscle Salpingopharyngeus muscle Styloglossus muscle Stylopharyngeus muscle Superior longitudinal muscle Tensor veli palatini muscle
Tonsils	**Includes:** Palatine tonsil
Trachea	**Includes:** Cricoid cartilage
Transverse Colon	**Includes:** Hepatic flexure Splenic flexure
Tricuspid Valve	**Includes:** Right atrioventricular valve Tricuspid annulus
Trigeminal Nerve	**Includes:** Fifth cranial nerve Gasserian ganglion Mandibular nerve Maxillary nerve Ophthalmic nerve Trifacial nerve
Trochlear Nerve	**Includes:** Fourth cranial nerve
Trunk Muscle, Left **Trunk** Muscle, Right	**Includes:** Coccygeus muscle Erector spinae muscle Interspinalis muscle Intertransversarius muscle Latissimus dorsi muscle Quadratus lumborum muscle Rhomboid major muscle Rhomboid minor muscle Serratus posterior muscle Transversospinalis muscle Trapezius muscle
Tympanic Membrane, Left **Tympanic** Membrane, Right	**Includes:** Pars flaccida
Ulna, Left **Ulna,** Right	**Includes:** Olecranon process Radial notch

Continued →

Section 0 - Medical and Surgical — Character 4 - Body Part

Ulnar Artery, Left **Ulnar** Artery, Right	**Includes:** Anterior ulnar recurrent artery Common interosseous artery Posterior ulnar recurrent artery
Ulnar Nerve	**Includes:** Cubital nerve
Upper Arm Muscle, Left **Upper** Arm Muscle, Right	**Includes:** Biceps brachii muscle Brachialis muscle Coracobrachialis muscle Triceps brachii muscle
Upper Artery	**Includes:** Aortic intercostal artery Bronchial artery Esophageal artery Subcostal artery
Upper Eyelid, Left **Upper** Eyelid, Right	**Includes:** Lateral canthus Levator palpebrae superioris muscle Orbicularis oculi muscle Superior tarsal plate
Upper Femur, Left **Upper** Femur, Right	**Includes:** Femoral head Greater trochanter Lesser trochanter Neck of femur
Upper Leg Muscle, Left **Upper** Leg Muscle, Right	**Includes:** Adductor brevis muscle Adductor longus muscle Adductor magnus muscle Biceps femoris muscle Gracilis muscle Pectineus muscle Quadriceps (femoris) Rectus femoris muscle Sartorius muscle Semimembranosus muscle Semitendinosus muscle Vastus intermedius muscle Vastus lateralis muscle Vastus medialis muscle
Upper Lip	**Includes:** Frenulum labii superioris Labial gland Vermilion border
Upper Spine Bursa and Ligament	Interspinous ligament, thoracic Intertransverse ligament, thoracic Ligamentum flavum, thoracic Supraspinous ligament
Ureter **Ureter,** Left **Ureter,** Right **Ureters,** Bilateral	**Includes:** Ureteral orifice Ureterovesical orifice
Urethra	**Includes:** Bulbourethral (Cowper's) gland Cowper's (bulbourethral) gland External urethral sphincter Internal urethral sphincter Membranous urethra Penile urethra Prostatic urethra

Uterine Supporting Structure	**Includes:** Broad ligament Infundibulopelvic ligament Ovarian ligament Round ligament of uterus
Uterus	**Includes:** Fundus uteri Myometrium Perimetrium Uterine cornu
Uvula	**Includes:** Palatine uvula
Vagus Nerve	**Includes:** Anterior vagal trunk Pharyngeal plexus Pneumogastric nerve Posterior vagal trunk Pulmonary plexus Recurrent laryngeal nerve Superior laryngeal nerve Tenth cranial nerve
Vas Deferens **Vas** Deferens, Bilateral **Vas** Deferens, Left **Vas** Deferens, Right	**Includes:** Ductus deferens Ejaculatory duct
Ventricle, Right	**Includes:** Conus arteriosus
Ventricular Septum	**Includes:** Interventricular septum
Vertebral Artery, Left **Vertebral** Artery, Right	**Includes:** Anterior spinal artery Posterior spinal artery
Vertebral Vein, Left **Vertebral** Vein, Right	**Includes:** Deep cervical vein Suboccipital venous plexus
Vestibular Gland	**Includes:** Bartholin's (greater vestibular) gland Greater vestibular (Bartholin's) gland Paraurethral (Skene's) gland Skene's (paraurethral) gland
Vitreous, Left **Vitreous,** Right	**Includes:** Vitreous body
Vocal Cord, Left **Vocal** Cord, Right	**Includes:** Vocal fold
Vulva	**Includes:** Labia majora Labia minora
Wrist Bursa and Ligament, Left **Wrist** Bursa and Ligament, Right	**Includes:** Palmar ulnocarpal ligament Radial collateral carpal ligament Radiocarpal ligament Radioulnar ligament Scapholunate ligament Ulnar collateral carpal ligament
Wrist Joint, Left **Wrist** Joint, Right	**Includes:** Distal radioulnar joint Radiocarpal joint

Appendix D

Appendix E: Medical and Surgical Device Table (Device Key) and Device Aggregation Table

Section 0 - Medical and Surgical — Character 6 - Device

Articulating Spacer in Lower Joints	**Includes:** Articulating Spacer (Antibiotic) Spacer, Articulating (Antibiotic)
Artificial Sphincter in Gastrointestinal System	**Includes:** Artificial anal sphincter (AAS) Artificial bowel sphincter (neosphincter)
Artificial Sphincter in Urinary System	**Includes:** AMS 800® Urinary Control System Artificial urinary sphincter (AUS)
Autologous Arterial Tissue in Heart and Great Vessels	**Includes:** Autologous artery graft
Autologous Arterial Tissue in Lower Arteries	**Includes:** Autologous artery graft
Autologous Arterial Tissue in Lower Veins	**Includes:** Autologous artery graft
Autologous Arterial Tissue in Upper Arteries	**Includes:** Autologous artery graft
Autologous Arterial Tissue in Upper Veins	**Includes:** Autologous artery graft
Autologous Tissue Substitute	**Includes:** Autograft Cultured epidermal cell autograft Epicel® cultured epidermal autograft
Autologous Venous Tissue in Heart and Great Vessels	**Includes:** Autologous vein graft
Autologous Venous Tissue in Lower Arteries	**Includes:** Autologous vein graft
Autologous Venous Tissue in Lower Veins	**Includes:** Autologous vein graft
Autologous Venous Tissue in Upper Arteries	**Includes:** Autologous vein graft
Autologous Venous Tissue in Upper Veins	**Includes:** Autologous vein graft
Biologic with Synthetic Substitute, Autoregulated Electrohydraulic for Replacement in Heart and Great Vessels	**Includes:** Carmat total artificial heart (TAH)
Bone Growth Stimulator in Head and Facial Bones	**Includes:** **Electrical** bone growth stimulator (EBGS) Ultrasonic osteogenic stimulator Ultrasound bone healing system
Bone Growth Stimulator in Lower Bones	**Includes:** **Electrical** bone growth stimulator (EBGS) Ultrasonic osteogenic stimulator Ultrasound bone healing system
Bone Growth Stimulator in Upper Bones	**Includes:** Electrical bone growth stimulator (EBGS) Ultrasonic osteogenic stimulator Ultrasound bone healing system

Section 0 - Medical and Surgical — Character 6 - Device

Cardiac Lead in Heart and Great Vessels	**Includes:** Cardiac contractility modulation lead
Cardiac Lead, Defibrillator for Insertion in Heart and Great Vessels	**Includes:** ACUITY™ Steerable Lead Attain Ability® lead Attain StarFix® (OTW) lead Cardiac resynchronization therapy (CRT) lead Corox (OTW) Bipolar Lead Durata® Defibrillation Lead ENDOTAK RELIANCE® (G) Defibrillation Lead
Cardiac Lead, Pacemaker for Insertion in Heart and Great Vessels	**Includes:** ACUITY™ Steerable Lead Attain Ability® lead Attain StarFix® (OTW) lead Cardiac resynchronization therapy (CRT) lead Corox (OTW) Bipolar Lead
Cardiac Resynchronization Defibrillator Pulse Generator for Insertion in Subcutaneous Tissue and Fascia	**Includes:** COGNIS® CRT-D Concerto II CRT-D Consulta CRT-D CONTAK RENEWAL® 3 RF (HE) CRT-D LIVIAN™ CRT-D Maximo II DR CRT-D Ovatio™ CRT-D Protecta XT CRT-D Viva (XT)(S)
Cardiac Resynchronization Pacemaker Pulse Generator for Insertion in Subcutaneous Tissue and Fascia	**Includes:** Consulta CRT-P Stratos LV Synchra CRT-P
Contraceptive Device in Female Reproductive System	**Includes:** Intrauterine device (IUD)
Contraceptive Device in Subcutaneous Tissue and Fascia	**Includes:** Subdermal progesterone implant
Contractility Modulation Device for Insertion in Subcutaneous Tissue and Fascia	**Includes:** Optimizer™ III implantable pulse generator
Defibrillator Generator for Insertion in Subcutaneous Tissue and Fascia	**Includes:** Evera (XT)(S)(DR/VR) Implantable cardioverter-defibrillator (ICD) Maximo II DR (VR) Protecta XT DR (XT VR) Secura (DR) (VR) Virtuoso (II) (DR) (VR)
Defibrillator Lead in Anatomical Regions, General	EV ICD System (Extravascular implantable defibrillator lead)
Diaphragmatic Pacemaker Lead in Respiratory System	**Includes:** Phrenic nerve stimulator lead

Section 0 - Medical and Surgical — Character 6 - Device

Drainage Device	**Includes:** Cystostomy tube Foley catheter Percutaneous nephrostomy catheter Thoracostomy tube
External Fixation Device in Head and Facial Bones	**Includes:** External fixator
External Fixation Device in Lower Bones	**Includes:** External fixator
External Fixation Device in Lower Joints	**Includes:** External fixator
External Fixation Device in Upper Bones	**Includes:** External fixator
External Fixation Device in Upper Joints	**Includes:** External fixator
External Fixation Device, Hybrid for Insertion in Upper Bones	**Includes:** Delta frame external fixator Sheffield hybrid external fixator
External Fixation Device, Hybrid for Insertion in Lower Bones	**Includes:** Delta frame external fixator Sheffield hybrid external fixator
External Fixation Device, Hybrid for Reposition in Upper Bones	**Includes:** Delta frame external fixator Sheffield hybrid external fixator
External Fixation Device, Hybrid for Reposition in Lower Bones	**Includes:** Delta frame external fixator Sheffield hybrid external fixator
External Fixation Device, Limb Lengthening for Insertion in Upper Bones	**Includes:** Ilizarov-Vecklich device
External Fixation Device, Limb Lengthening for Insertion in Lower Bones	**Includes:** Ilizarov-Vecklich device
External Fixation Device, Monoplanar for Insertion in Upper Bones	**Includes:** Uniplanar external fixator
External Fixation Device, Monoplanar for Insertion in Lower Bones	**Includes:** Uniplanar external fixator
External Fixation Device, Monoplanar for Reposition in Upper Bones	**Includes:** Uniplanar external fixator
External Fixation Device, Monoplanar for Reposition in Lower Bones	**Includes:** Uniplanar external fixator
External Fixation Device, Ring for Insertion in Upper Bones	**Includes:** Ilizarov external fixator Sheffield ring external fixator
External Fixation Device, Ring for Insertion in Lower Bones	**Includes:** Ilizarov external fixator Sheffield ring external fixator
External Fixation Device, Ring for Reposition in Upper Bones	**Includes:** Ilizarov external fixator Sheffield ring external fixator

Section 0 - Medical and Surgical — Character 6 - Device

External Fixation Device, Ring for Reposition in Lower Bones	**Includes:** Ilizarov external fixator Sheffield ring external fixator
Extraluminal Device	**Includes:** AtriClip LAA Exclusion System LAP-BAND® adjustable gastric banding system REALIZE® Adjustable Gastric Band
Feeding Device in Gastrointestinal System	**Includes:** Percutaneous endoscopic gastrojejunostomy (PEG/J) tube Percutaneous endoscopic gastrostomy (PEG) tube
Hearing Device in Ear, Nose, Sinus	**Includes:** Esteem® implantable hearing system
Hearing Device in Head and Facial Bones	**Includes:** Bone anchored hearing device
Hearing Device, Bone Conduction for Insertion in Ear, Nose, Sinus	**Includes:** Bone anchored hearing device
Hearing Device, Multiple Channel Cochlear Prosthesis for Insertion in Ear, Nose, Sinus	**Includes:** Cochlear implant (CI), multiple channel (electrode)
Hearing Device, Single Channel Cochlear Prosthesis for Insertion in Ear, Nose, Sinus	**Includes:** Cochlear implant (CI), single channel (electrode)
Implantable Heart Assist System in Heart and Great Vessels	**Includes:** Berlin Heart Ventricular Assist Device DeBakey Left Ventricular Assist Device DuraHeart Left Ventricular Assist System HeartMate II® Left Ventricular Assist Device (LVAD) HeartMate 3® LVAS HeartMate XVE® Left Ventricular Assist Device (LVAD) MicroMed HeartAssist Novacor Left Ventricular Assist Device Thoratec IVAD (Implantable Ventricular Assist Device)
Infusion Device	**Includes:** Ascenda Intrathecal Catheter InDura, intrathecal catheter (1P) (spinal) Non-tunneled central venous catheter Peripherally inserted central catheter (PICC) Tunneled spinal (intrathecal) catheter
Infusion Device, Pump in Subcutaneous Tissue and Fascia	**Includes:** Implantable drug infusion pump (anti-spasmodic)(chemotherapy)(pain) Injection reservoir, pump Pump reservoir Subcutaneous injection reservoir, pump SynchroMed pump

Section 0 - Medical and Surgical — Character 6 - Device	
Interbody Fusion Device in Lower Joints	**Includes:** Axial Lumbar Interbody Fusion System AxiaLIF® System COALESCE® radiolucent interbody fusion device COHERE® radiolucent interbody fusion device CoRoent® XL Direct Lateral Interbody Fusion (DLIF) device EXtreme Lateral Interbody Fusion (XLIF) device Interbody fusion (spine) cage nanoLOCK™ interbody fusion device Titan Endoskeleton™ XLIF® System
Interbody Fusion Device in Upper Joints	**Includes:** BAK/C® Interbody Cervical Fusion System COALESCE® radiolucent interbody fusion device COHERE® radiolucent interbody fusion device Interbody fusion (spine) cage nanoLOCK™ interbody fusion device Titan Endoskeleton™
Internal Fixation Device in Head and Facial Bones	**Includes:** Bone screw (interlocking)(lag)(pedicle)(recessed) Kirschner wire (K-wire) Neutralization plate
Internal Fixation Device in Lower Bones	**Includes:** Bone screw (interlocking)(lag)(pedicle)(recessed) Clamp and rod internal fixation system (CRIF) Kirschner wire (K-wire) Neutralization plate
Internal Fixation Device in Lower Joints	**Includes:** Fusion screw (compression)(lag)(locking) Joint fixation plate Kirschner wire (K-wire)
Internal Fixation Device in Upper Bones	**Includes:** Bone screw (interlocking)(lag)(pedicle)(recessed) Clamp and rod internal fixation system (CRIF) Kirschner wire (K-wire) Neutralization plate
Internal Fixation Device in Upper Joints	**Includes:** Fusion screw (compression)(lag)(locking) Joint fixation plate Kirschner wire (K-wire)
Internal Fixation Device, Intramedullary in Lower Bones	**Includes:** Intramedullary (IM) rod (nail) Intramedullary skeletal kinetic distractor (ISKD) Kuntscher nail
Internal Fixation Device, Intramedullary in Upper Bones	**Includes:** Intramedullary (IM) rod (nail) Intramedullary skeletal kinetic distractor (ISKD) Kuntscher nail

Section 0 - Medical and Surgical — Character 6 - Device	
Internal Fixation Device, Intramedullary Limb Lengthening for Insertion in Lower Bones	**Includes:** PRECICE intramedullary limb lengthening system
Internal Fixation Device, Intramedullary Limb Lengthening for Insertion in Upper Bones	**Includes:** PRECICE intramedullary limb lengthening system
Internal Fixation Device, Rigid Plate for Insertion in Upper Bones	**Includes:** **Titanium** Sternal Fixation System (TSFS)
Internal Fixation Device, Rigid Plate for Reposition in Upper Bones	**Includes:** **Titanium** Sternal Fixation System (TSFS)
Internal Fixation Device, Sustained Compression for Fusion in Lower Joints	**Includes:** DynaClip® (Forte) DynaNail® (Helix)(Hybrid)(Mini)
Internal Fixation Device, Sustained Compression for Fusion in Upper Joints	**Includes:** DynaClip® (Forte) DynaNail® (Helix)(Hybrid)(Mini)
Intracardiac Pacemaker in Heart and Great Vessels	Aveir™ VR, as single chamber
Intraluminal Device	**Includes:** Absolute Pro Vascular (OTW) Self-Expanding Stent System Acculink (RX) Carotid Stent System AFX® Endovascular AAA System AneuRx® AAA Advantage® Assurant (Cobalt) stent Carotid WALLSTENT® Monorail® Endoprosthesis CoAxia NeuroFlo catheter Colonic Z-Stent® Complete (SE) stent Cook Zenith AAA Endovascular Graft Driver stent (RX) (OTW) E-Luminexx™ (Biliary)(Vascular) Stent Embolization coil(s) Endologix AFX® Endovascular AAA System Endurant® II AAA stent graft system Endurant® Endovascular Stent Graft EXCLUDER® AAA Endoprosthesis Express® (LD) Premounted Stent System Express® Biliary SD Monorail® Premounted Stent System Express® SD Renal Monorail® Premounted Stent System FLAIR® Endovascular Stent Graft Formula™ Balloon-Expandable Renal Stent System GORE EXCLUDER® AAA Endoprosthesis GORE TAG® Thoracic Endoprosthesis Herculink (RX) Elite Renal Stent System LifeStent® (Flexstar)(XL) Vascular Stent System Medtronic Endurant® II AAA stent graft system Micro-Driver stent (RX) (OTW) MULTI-LINK (VISION)(MINI-VISION)(ULTRA) Coronary Stent System

Continued →

Section 0 - Medical and Surgical — Character 6 - Device

Intraluminal Device (*continued*)	Omnilink Elite Vascular Balloon Expandable Stent System Protégé® RX Carotid Stent System Stent, intraluminal (cardiovascular) (gastrointestinal)(hepatobiliary) (urinary) Talent® Converter Talent® Occluder Talent® Stent Graft (abdominal) (thoracic) Therapeutic occlusion coil(s) Ultraflex™ Precision Colonic Stent System Valiant Thoracic Stent Graft WALLSTENT® Endoprosthesis Xact Carotid Stent System Zenith AAA Endovascular Graft Zenith Flex® AAA Endovascular Graft Zenith Renu™ AAA Ancillary Graft Zenith TX2® TAA Endovascular Graft
Intraluminal Device, Airway in Ear, Nose, Sinus	**Includes:** Nasopharyngeal airway (NPA)
Intraluminal Device, Airway in Gastrointestinal System	**Includes:** Esophageal obturator airway (EOA)
Intraluminal Device, Airway in Mouth and Throat	**Includes:** Guedel airway Oropharyngeal airway (OPA)
Intraluminal Device, Bioactive in Upper Arteries	**Includes:** Bioactive embolization coil(s) Micrus CERECYTE microcoil
Intraluminal Device, Branched or Fenestrated, One or Two Arteries for Restriction in Lower Arteries	**Includes:** Cook Zenith® Fenestrated AAA Endovascular Graft EXCLUDER® AAA Endoprosthesis EXCLUDER® IBE Endoprosthesis GORE EXCLUDER® AAA Endoprosthesis GORE EXCLUDER® IBE Endoprosthesis Zenith® Fenestrated AAA Endovascular Graft
Intraluminal Device, Branched or Fenestrated, Three or More Arteries for Restriction in Lower Arteries	**Includes:** Cook Zenith® Fenestrated AAA Endovascular Graft EXCLUDER® AAA Endoprosthesis GORE EXCLUDER® AAA Endoprosthesis Zenith® Fenestrated AAA Endovascular Graft
Intraluminal Device, Drug-eluting in Heart and Great Vessels	**Includes:** CYPHER® Stent Endeavor® (III)(IV) (Sprint) Zotarolimus-eluting Coronary Stent System Everolimus-eluting coronary stent Paclitaxel-eluting coronary stent Sirolimus-eluting coronary stent TAXUS® Liberté® Paclitaxel-eluting Coronary Stent System XIENCE Everolimus Eluting Coronary Stent System Zotarolimus-eluting coronary stent

Section 0 - Medical and Surgical — Character 6 - Device

Intraluminal Device, Drug-eluting in Lower Arteries	**Includes:** Paclitaxel-eluting peripheral stent Zilver® PTX® (paclitaxel) Drug-Eluting Peripheral Stent
Intraluminal Device, Drug-eluting in Upper Arteries	**Includes:** Paclitaxel-eluting peripheral stent Zilver® PTX® (paclitaxel) Drug-Eluting Peripheral Stent
Intraluminal Device, Endobronchial Valve in Respiratory System	**Includes:** Spiration IBV™ Valve System
Intraluminal Device, Flow Diverter for Restriction in Upper Arteries	**Includes:** Flow Diverter embolization device Pipeline™ (Flex) embolization device Surpass Streamline™ Flow Diverter
Intraluminal Device, Pessary in Female Reproductive System	**Includes:** Pessary ring Vaginal pessary
Intraluminal Device, Endotracheal Airway in Respiratory System	**Includes:** Endotracheal tube (cuffed)(double-lumen)
Liner in Lower Joints	**Includes:** Acetabular cup Hip (joint) liner Joint liner (insert) Knee (implant) insert Tibial insert
Magnetic Lengthening Device in Gastrointestinal System	Flourish® Pediatric Esophageal Atresia Device
Monitoring Device	**Includes:** Blood glucose monitoring system Cardiac event recorder Continuous Glucose Monitoring (CGM) device Implantable glucose monitoring device Loop recorder, implantable Reveal (LINQ)(DX)(XT)
Monitoring Device, Hemodynamic for Insertion in Subcutaneous Tissue and Fascia	**Includes:** Implantable hemodynamic monitor (IHM) Implantable hemodynamic monitoring system (IHMS)
Monitoring Device, Pressure Sensor for Insertion in Heart and Great Vessels	**Includes:** CardioMEMS® pressure sensor EndoSure® sensor
Neurostimulator Lead in Central Nervous System and Cranial Nerves	**Includes:** Cortical strip neurostimulator lead DBS lead Deep brain neurostimulator lead RNS System lead Spinal cord neurostimulator lead
Neurostimulator Lead in Peripheral Nervous System	**Includes:** InterStim® Therapy lead
Neurostimulator Generator in Head and Facial Bones	**Includes:** RNS system neurostimulator generator
Nonautologous Tissue Substitute	**Includes:** Acellular Hydrated Dermis Bone bank bone graft Cook Biodesign® Fistula Plug(s) Cook Biodesign® Hernia Graft(s) Cook Biodesign® Layered Graft(s) Cook Zenapro™ Layered Grafts(s) MIRODERM™ Biologic Wound Matrix Tissue bank graft

Continued

Section 0 - Medical and Surgical — Character 6 - Device

Other Device	**Includes:** Alfapump® system
Pacemaker, Dual Chamber for Insertion in Subcutaneous Tissue and Fascia	**Includes:** Advisa (MRI) EnRhythm Kappa Revo MRI™ SureScan® pacemaker Two lead pacemaker Versa
Pacemaker, Single Chamber for Insertion in Subcutaneous Tissue and Fascia	**Includes:** Single lead pacemaker (atrium) (ventricle)
Pacemaker, Single Chamber Rate Responsive for Insertion in Subcutaneous Tissue and Fascia	**Includes:** Single lead rate responsive pacemaker (atrium)(ventricle)
Radioactive Element	**Includes:** Brachytherapy seeds CivaSheet®
Radioactive Element, Cesium-131 Collagen Implant for Insertion in Central Nervous System and Cranial Nerves	Cesium-131 Collagen Implant GammaTile™
Resurfacing Device in Lower Joints	**Includes:** CONSERVE® PLUS Total Resurfacing Hip System Cormet Hip Resurfacing System
Short-term External Heart Assist System in Heart and Great Vessels	Aortix™ System Biventricular external heart assist system BVS 5000 Ventricular Assist Device Centrimag® Blood Pump Impella® heart pump TandemHeart® System Thoratec Paracorporeal Ventricular Assist Device
Spacer in Lower Joints	**Includes:** Joint spacer (antibiotic) Spacer, Static (Antibiotic) Static Spacer (Antibiotic)
Spacer in Upper Joints	**Includes:** Joint spacer (antibiotic)
Spinal Stabilization Device, Facet Replacement for Insertion in Upper Joints	**Includes:** Facet replacement spinal stabilization device
Spinal Stabilization Device, Facet Replacement for Insertion in Lower Joints	**Includes:** Facet replacement spinal stabilization device
Spinal Stabilization Device, Interspinous Process for Insertion in Upper Joints	**Includes:** Interspinous process spinal stabilization device X-Spine Axle Cage X-STOP® Spacer
Spinal Stabilization Device, Interspinous Process for Insertion in Lower Joints	**Includes:** Interspinous process spinal stabilization device X-Spine Axle Cage X-STOP® Spacer
Spinal Stabilization Device, Pedicle-Based for Insertion in Upper Joints	**Includes:** Dynesys® Dynamic Stabilization System Pedicle-based dynamic stabilization device

Section 0 - Medical and Surgical — Character 6 - Device

Spinal Stabilization Device, Pedicle-Based for Insertion in Lower Joints	**Includes:** Dynesys® Dynamic Stabilization System Pedicle-based dynamic stabilization device
Stimulator Generator in Subcutaneous Tissue and Fascia	**Includes:** Baroreflex Activation Therapy® (BAT®) Diaphragmatic pacemaker generator Mark IV Breathing Pacemaker System Phrenic nerve stimulator generator Rheos® System device
Stimulator Generator, Multiple Array for Insertion in Subcutaneous Tissue and Fascia	**Includes:** Activa PC neurostimulator Enterra gastric neurostimulator Neurostimulator generator, multiple channel PERCEPT™ PC neurostimulator PrimeAdvanced neurostimulator (SureScan)(MRI Safe) Vanta™ PC neurostimulator
Stimulator Generator, Multiple Array Rechargeable for Insertion in Subcutaneous Tissue and Fascia	**Includes:** Activa RC neurostimulator Intellis™ neurostimulator Neurostimulator generator, multiple channel rechargeable RestoreAdvanced neurostimulator (SureScan)(MRI Safe) RestoreSensor neurostimulator (SureScan)(MRI Safe) RestoreUltra neurostimulator (SureScan)(MRI Safe)
Stimulator Generator, Single Array for Insertion in Subcutaneous Tissue and Fascia	**Includes:** Activa SC neurostimulator InterStim™ II Therapy neurostimulator Itrel (3)(4) neurostimulator Neurostimulator generator, single channel
Stimulator Generator, Single Array Rechargeable for Insertion in Subcutaneous Tissue and Fascia	**Includes:** InterStim™ Micro Therapy neurostimulator Neurostimulator generator, single channel rechargeable
Stimulator Lead in Gastrointestinal System	**Includes:** Gastric electrical stimulation (GES) lead Gastric pacemaker lead
Stimulator Lead in Muscles	**Includes:** Electrical muscle stimulation (EMS) lead Electronic muscle stimulator lead Neuromuscular electrical stimulation (NEMS) lead
Stimulator Lead in Upper Arteries	**Includes:** Baroreflex Activation Therapy® (BAT®) Carotid (artery) sinus (baroreceptor) lead Rheos® System lead
Stimulator Lead in Urinary System	**Includes:** Sacral nerve modulation (SNM) lead Sacral neuromodulation lead Urinary incontinence stimulator lead
Subcutaneous Defibrillator Lead in Subcutaneous Tissue and Fascia	**Includes:** S-ICD™ lead

Continued →

Appendix E

Section 0 - Medical and Surgical — Character 6 - Device	
Synthetic Substitute	**Includes:** AbioCor® Total Replacement Heart AMPLATZER® Muscular VSD Occluder Annuloplasty ring Bard® Composix® (E/X)(LP) mesh Bard® Composix® Kugel® patch Bard® Dulex™ mesh Bard® Ventralex™ hernia patch Barricaid® Annular Closure Device (ACD) BRYAN® Cervical Disc System Corvia IASD® Ex-PRESS™ mini glaucoma shunt Flexible Composite Mesh GORE® DUALMESH® Holter valve ventricular shunt IASD® (InterAtrial Shunt Device), Corvia InterAtrial Shunt Device IASD®, Corvia MitraClip valve repair system Nitinol framed polymer mesh Open Pivot Aortic Valve Graft (AVG) Open Pivot (mechanical) valve Partially absorbable mesh PHYSIOMESH™ Flexible Composite Mesh Polymethylmethacrylate (PMMA) Polypropylene mesh PRESTIGE® Cervical Disc PROCEED™ Ventral Patch Prodisc-C Prodisc-L PROLENE Polypropylene Hernia System (PHS) Rebound HRD® (Hernia Repair Device) SynCardia Total Artificial Heart Total artificial (replacement) heart ULTRAPRO Hernia System (UHS) ULTRAPRO Partially Absorbable Lightweight Mesh ULTRAPRO Plug V-WAVE Interatrial Shunt System Ventrio™ Hernia Patch Zimmer® NexGen® LPS Mobile Bearing Knee Zimmer® NexGen® LPS-Flex Mobile Knee
Synthetic Substitute, Ceramic for Replacement in Lower Joints	**Includes:** Ceramic on ceramic bearing surface Novation® Ceramic AHS® (Articulation Hip System)
Synthetic Substitute, Intraocular Telescope for Replacement in Eye	**Includes:** Implantable Miniature Telescope™ (IMT)
Synthetic Substitute, Metal for Replacement in Lower Joints	**Includes:** Cobalt/chromium head and socket Metal on metal bearing surface

Section 0 - Medical and Surgical — Character 6 - Device	
Synthetic Substitute, Metal on Polyethylene for Replacement in Lower Joints	**Includes:** Cobalt/chromium head and polyethylene socket
Synthetic Substitute, Oxidized Zirconium on Polyethylene for Replacement in Lower Joints	OXINIUM
Synthetic Substitute, Pneumatic for Replacement in Heart and Great Vessels	**Includes:** SynCardia (temporary) total artificial heart (TAH)
Synthetic Substitute, Polyethylene for Replacement in Lower Joints	**Includes:** Polyethylene socket
Synthetic Substitute, Reverse Ball and Socket for Replacement in Upper Joints	**Includes:** Delta III Reverse shoulder prosthesis Reverse® Shoulder Prosthesis
Tissue Expander in Skin and Breast	**Includes:** Tissue expander (inflatable) (injectable)
Tissue Expander in Subcutaneous Tissue and Fascia	**Includes:** Tissue expander (inflatable) (injectable)
Tracheostomy Device in Respiratory System	**Includes:** Tracheostomy tube
Vascular Access Device, Totally Implantable in Subcutaneous Tissue and Fascia	**Includes:** Implanted (venous)(access) port Injection reservoir, port Subcutaneous injection reservoir, port
Vascular Access Device, Tunneled in Subcutaneous Tissue and Fascia	Tunneled central venous catheter Vectra® Vascular Access Graft
Zooplastic Tissue in Heart and Great Vessels	**Includes:** 3f (Aortic) Bioprosthesis valve Bovine pericardial valve Bovine pericardium graft Contegra Pulmonary Valved Conduit CoreValve transcatheter aortic valve Epic™ Stented Tissue Valve (aortic) Freestyle (Stentless) Aortic Root Bioprosthesis Hancock Bioprosthesis (aortic) (mitral) valve Hancock Bioprosthetic Valved Conduit Melody® transcatheter pulmonary valve Mitroflow® Aortic Pericardial Heart Valve Mosaic Bioprosthesis (aortic) (mitral) valve Porcine (bioprosthetic) valve SAPIEN transcatheter aortic valve SJM Biocor® Stented Valve System Stented tissue valve Trifecta™ Valve (aortic) Xenograft

Appendix E

714

Device Aggregation Table

Specific Device	for Operation	in Body System	General Device
Autologous Arterial Tissue	All applicable	Heart and Great Vessels Lower Arteries Lower Veins Upper Arteries Upper Veins	7 Autologous Tissue Substitute
Autologous Venous Tissue	All applicable	Heart and Great Vessels Lower Arteries Lower Veins Upper Arteries Upper Veins	7 Autologous Tissue Substitute
Cardiac Lead, Defibrillator	Insertion	Heart and Great Vessels	M Cardiac Lead
Cardiac Lead, Pacemaker	Insertion	Heart and Great Vessels	M Cardiac Lead
Cardiac Resynchronization Defibrillator Pulse Generator	Insertion	Subcutaneous Tissue and Fascia	P Cardiac Rhythm Related Device
Cardiac Resynchronization Pacemaker Pulse Generator	Insertion	Subcutaneous Tissue and Fascia	P Cardiac Rhythm Related Device
Contractility Modulation Device	Insertion	Subcutaneous Tissue and Fascia	P Cardiac Rhythm Related Device
Defibrillator Generator	Insertion	Subcutaneous Tissue and Fascia	P Cardiac Rhythm Related Device
Epiretinal Visual Prosthesis	All applicable	Eye	J Synthetic Substitute
External Fixation Device, Hybrid	Insertion	Lower Bones Upper Bones	5 External Fixation Device
External Fixation Device, Hybrid	Reposition	Lower Bones Upper Bones	5 External Fixation Device
External Fixation Device, Limb Lengthening	Insertion	Lower Bones Upper Bones	5 External Fixation Device
External Fixation Device, Monoplanar	Insertion	Lower Bones Upper Bones	5 External Fixation Device
External Fixation Device, Monoplanar	Reposition	Lower Bones Upper Bones	5 External Fixation Device
External Fixation Device, Ring	Insertion	Lower Bones Upper Bones	5 External Fixation Device
External Fixation Device, Ring	Reposition	Lower Bones Upper Bones	5 External Fixation Device
Hearing Device, Bone Conduction	Insertion	Ear, Nose, Sinus	S Hearing Device
Hearing Device, Multiple Channel Cochlear Prosthesis	Insertion	Ear, Nose, Sinus	S Hearing Device
Hearing Device, Single Channel Cochlear Prosthesis	Insertion	Ear, Nose, Sinus	S Hearing Device
Internal Fixation Device, Intramedullary	All applicable	Lower Bones Upper Bones	4 Internal Fixation Device
Internal Fixation Device, Intramedullary Limb Lengthening	Insertion	Lower Bones Upper Bones	6 Internal Fixation Device Intramedullary
Internal Fixation Device, Rigid Plate	Insertion	Upper Bones	4 Internal Fixation Device
Internal Fixation Device, Rigid Plate	Reposition	Upper Bones	4 Internal Fixation Device

Continued →

Specific Device	for Operation	in Body System	General Device	
Intraluminal Device, Airway	All applicable	Ear, Nose, Sinus Gastrointestinal System Mouth and Throat	D	Intraluminal Device
Intraluminal Device, Bioactive	All applicable	Upper Arteries	D	Intraluminal Device
Intraluminal Device, Branched or Fenestrated, One or Two Arteries	Restriction	Heart and Great Vessels Lower Arteries	D	Intraluminal Device
Intraluminal Device, Branched or Fenestrated, Three or More Arteries	Restriction	Heart and Great Vessels Lower Arteries	D	Intraluminal Device
Intraluminal Device, Drug-eluting	All applicable	Heart and Great Vessels Lower Arteries Upper Arteries	D	Intraluminal Device
Intraluminal Device, Drug-eluting, Four or More	All applicable	Heart and Great Vessels Lower Arteries Upper Arteries	D	Intraluminal Device
Intraluminal Device, Drug-eluting, Three	All applicable	Heart and Great Vessels Lower Arteries Upper Arteries	D	Intraluminal Device
Intraluminal Device, Drug-eluting, Two	All applicable	Heart and Great Vessels Lower Arteries Upper Arteries	D	Intraluminal Device
Intraluminal Device, Endobronchial Valve	All applicable	Respiratory System	D	Intraluminal Device
Intraluminal Device, Endotracheal Airway	All applicable	Respiratory System	D	Intraluminal Device
Intraluminal Device, Flow Diverter	Restriction	Upper Arteries	D	Intraluminal Device
Intraluminal Device, Four or More	All applicable	Heart and Great Vessels Lower Arteries Upper Arteries	D	Intraluminal Device
Intraluminal Device, Pessary	All applicable	Female Reproductive System	D	Intraluminal Device
Intraluminal Device, Radioactive	All applicable	Heart and Great Vessels	D	Intraluminal Device
Intraluminal Device, Three	All applicable	Heart and Great Vessels Lower Arteries Upper Arteries	D	Intraluminal Device
Intraluminal Device, Two	All applicable	Heart and Great Vessels Lower Arteries Upper Arteries	D	Intraluminal Device
Monitoring Device, Hemodynamic	Insertion	Subcutaneous Tissue and Fascia	2	Monitoring Device
Monitoring Device, Pressure Sensor	Insertion	Heart and Great Vessels	2	Monitoring Device
Pacemaker, Dual Chamber	Insertion	Subcutaneous Tissue and Fascia	P	Cardiac Rhythm Related Device
Pacemaker, Single Chamber	Insertion	Subcutaneous Tissue and Fascia	P	Cardiac Rhythm Related Device
Pacemaker, Single Chamber Rate Responsive	Insertion	Subcutaneous Tissue and Fascia	P	Cardiac Rhythm Related Device
Spinal Stabilization Device, Facet Replacement	Insertion	Lower Joints Upper Joints	4	Internal Fixation Device
Spinal Stabilization Device, Interspinous Process	Insertion	Lower Joints Upper Joints	4	Internal Fixation Device

Continued

Specific Device	for Operation	in Body System	General Device
Spinal Stabilization Device, Pedicle-Based	Insertion	Lower Joints Upper Joints	4 Internal Fixation Device
Spinal Stabilization Device, Vertebral Body Tether	Reposition	Lower Bones Upper Bones	4 Internal Fixation Device
Stimulator Generator, Multiple Array	Insertion	Subcutaneous Tissue and Fascia	M Stimulator Generator
Stimulator Generator, Multiple Array Rechargeable	Insertion	Subcutaneous Tissue and Fascia	M Stimulator Generator
Stimulator Generator, Single Array	Insertion	Subcutaneous Tissue and Fascia	M Stimulator Generator
Stimulator Generator, Single Array Rechargeable	Insertion	Subcutaneous Tissue and Fascia	M Stimulator Generator
Synthetic Substitute, Ceramic	Replacement	Lower Joints	J Synthetic Substitute
Synthetic Substitute, Ceramic on Polyethylene	Replacement	Lower Joints	J Synthetic Substitute
Synthetic Substitute, Intraocular Telescope	Replacement	Eye	J Synthetic Substitute
Synthetic Substitute, Metal	Replacement	Lower Joints	J Synthetic Substitute
Synthetic Substitute, Metal on Polyethylene	Replacement	Lower Joints	J Synthetic Substitute
Synthetic Substitute, Oxidized Zirconium on Polyethylene	Replacement	Lower Joints	J Synthetic Substitute
Synthetic Substitute, Polyethylene	Replacement	Lower Joints	J Synthetic Substitute
Synthetic Substitute, Reverse Ball and Socket	Replacement	Upper Joints	J Synthetic Substitute

Appendix E

Appendix F: Substance Qualifier Table (Key)

Section 3 – Administration Character 6 – Substance

4-Factor Prothrombin Complex Concentrate	**Includes:** Kcentra
Adhesion Barrier	**Includes:** Seprafilm
Anti-Infective Envelope	**Includes:** AIGISRx Antibacterial Envelope Antibacterial Envelope (TYRX) (AIGISRx) Antimicrobial envelope TYRX Antibacterial Envelope
Clofarabine	**Includes:** Clolar
Globulin	**Includes:** Gammaglobulin Hyperimmune globulin Immunoglobulin Polyclonal hyperimmune globulin
Glucarpidase	**Includes:** Voraxaze
Hematopoietic Stem/Progenitor Cells, Genetically Modified	**Includes:** OTL-101
Human B-type Natriuretic Peptide	**Includes:** Nesiritide
Other Anti-infective	**Includes:** AVYCAZ® (ceftazidime-avibactam) Ceftazidime-avibactam CRESEMBA® (isavuconazonium sulfate) Isavuconazole (isavuconazonium sulfate) Plazomicin
Other Antineoplastic	**Includes:** Blinatumomab BLINCYTO® (blinatumomab)
Other Substance	CBMA (Concentrated Bone Marrow Aspirate) Defitelio MarrowStim™ PAD Kit for CBMA (Concentrated Bone Marrow Aspirate)
Other Therapeutic Substance	**Includes:** Idarucizumab, Pradaxa® (dabigatran) reversal agent Praxbind® (idarucizumab), Pradaxa® (dabigatran) reversal agent
Other Thrombolytic	**Includes:** Tissue Plasinogen Activator (tPA)(r-tPA)
Oxazolidinones	**Includes:** Zyvox
Pathogen Reduced Cryoprecipitated Fibrinogen Complex	**Includes:** INTERCEPT Blood System for Plasma Pathogen Reduced Cryoprecipitated Fibrinogen Complex INTERCEPT Fibrinogen Complex
Recombinant Bone Morphogenetic Protein	**Includes:** Bone morphogenetic protein 2 (BMP 2) rhBMP-2
Vasopressor	Angiotensin II GIAPREZA™ Human angiotensin II, synthetic

Section X - New Technology - Character 6 - Device/Substance/Technology

Afamitresgene Autoleucel Immunotherapy	afami-cel
Amivantamab Monoclonal Antibody	RYBREVANT™
Anacaulase-bcdb	Bromelain-enriched Proteolytic Enzyme NexoBrid™
Antibiotic-eluting Bone Void Filler	CERAMENT® G
Apalutamide Antineoplastic	ERLEADA™
Atezolizumab Antineoplastic	TECENTRIQ®
Axicabtagene Ciloleucel Immunotherapy	Axicabtagene Ciloleucel Yescarta®
Betibeglogene Autotemcel	beti-cel ZYNTEGLO®
Bioengineered Allogeneic Construct	StrataGraft®
Branched Synthetic Substitute with Intraluminal Device in New Technology	Thoraflex™ Hybrid device
Brexanolone	ZULRESSO™
Brexucabtagene Autoleucel Immunotherapy	Tecartus™
Broad Consortium Microbiota-based Live Biotherapeutic Suspension	REBYOTA®
Cefiderocol Anti-infective	FETROJA®
Ceftolozane/Tazobactam Anti-infective	ZERBAXA®
Ciltacabtagene Autoleucel	CARVYKTI™ cilta-cel
Coagulation Factor Xa, Inactivated	Andexanet Alfa, Factor Xa Inhibitor Reversal Agent Andexxa Coagulation Factor Xa, (Recombinant) Inactivated Factor Xa Inhibitor Reversal Agent, Andexanet Alfa
Conduit through Femoral Vein to Popliteal Artery in New Technology	DETOUR® System
Conduit through Femoral Vein to Superficial Femoral Artery in New Technology	DETOUR® System
Conduit to Short-term External Heart Assist System in New Technology	Impella® 5.5 with SmartAssist® System
COVID-19 Vaccine COVID-19 Vaccine Booster COVID-19 Vaccine Dose 1 COVID-19 Vaccine Dose 2 COVID-19 Vaccine Dose 3	COMIRNATY® SPIKEVAX™
Cytarabine and Daunorubicin Liposome Antineoplastic	VYXEOS™
Daratumumab and Hyaluronidase-fihj	Darzalex Faspro®
Durvalumab Antineoplastic	IMFINZI®

Continued →

718

Section X - New Technology - Character 6 - Device/Substance/Technology

culizumab	Soliris®
Engineered Allogeneic Thymus Tissue	RETHYMIC®
Endothelial Damage Inhibitor	DuraGraft® Endothelial Damage Inhibitor
Esketamine Hydrochloride	SPRAVATO™
Exagamglogene Autotemcel	CTX001™
Fosfomycin Anti-infective	CONTEPO™ Fosfomycin injection
Gilteritinib Antineoplastic	XOSPATA®
High-Dose Intravenous Immune Globulin	GAMUNEX-C, for COVID-19 treatment hdIVIG (high-dose intravenous immunoglobulin), for COVID-19 treatment High-dose intravenous immunoglobulin (hdIVIG), for COVID-19 treatment Octagam 10%, for COVID-19 treatment
Hyperimmune Globulin	Anti-SARS-CoV-2 hyperimmune globulin HIG (hyperimmune intravenous immunoglobulin), for COVID-19 treatment hIVIG (hyperimmune intravenous immunoglobulin), for COVID-19 treatment Hyperimmune intravenous immunoglobulin (hIVIG), for COVID-19 treatment IGIV-C, for COVID-19 treatment
Idecabtagene Vicleucel Immunotherapy	ABECMA® Ide-cel Idecabtagene Vicleucel
Imipenem-cilastatin-relebactam Anti-infective	IMI/REL
Inebilizumab-cdon	UPLIZNA®
Interbody Fusion Device, Custom-Made Anatomically Designed in New Technology	aprevo™
Internal Fixation Device, Open-truss Design in New Technology	Ankle Truss System™ (ATS)
Internal Fixation Device with Tulip Connector in New Technology	iFuse Bedrock™ Granite Implant System
Intraluminal Device, Sustained Release Drug-eluting in New Technology	Eluvia™ Drug-Eluting Vascular Stent System SAVAL below-the-knee (BTK) drug-eluting stent system
Intracardiac Pacemaker, Dual-Chamber in New Technology	Aveir™ AR, as dual chamber Aveir™ DR, as dual chamber
Intraluminal Device, Bioprosthetic Valve in New Technology	TricValve® Transcatheter Bicaval Valve System VenoValve®
Intraluminal Device, Sustained Release Drug-eluting, Four or more in New Technology	Eluvia™ Drug-Eluting Vascular Stent System SAVAL below-the-knee (BTK) drug-eluting stent system
Intraluminal Device, Sustained Release Drug-eluting, Three in New Technology	Eluvia™ Drug-Eluting Vascular Stent System SAVAL below-the-knee (BTK) drug-eluting stent system

Section X - New Technology - Character 6 - Device/Substance/Technology

Intraluminal Device, Sustained Release Drug-eluting, Two in New Technology	Eluvia™ Drug-Eluting Vascular Stent System SAVAL below-the-knee (BTK) drug-eluting stent system
Iobenguane I-131 Antineoplastic	AZEDRA® Iobenguane I-131, High Specific Activity (HSA)
Lefamulin Anti-Infective	XENLETA™
Lifileucel Immunotherapy	Lifileucel
Lisocabtagene Maraleucel Immunotherapy	Breyanzi® Lisocabtagene Maraleucel
Lurbinectedin	ZEPZELCA™
Magnetically Controlled Growth Rod(s) in New Technology	MAGEC® Spinal Bracing and Distraction System Spinal growth rods, magnetically controlled
Maribavir Anti-Infective	LIVTENCITY™
Melphalan Hydrochloride Antineoplastic	HEPZATO™ KIT (melphalan hydrochloride Hepatic Delivery System)
Meropenem-vaborbactam Anti-infective	Vabomere™
Mineral-based Topical Hemostatic Agent	Hemospray® Endoscopic Hemostat
Mosunetuzumab Antineoplastic	LUNSUMIO™
Nafamostat Anticoagulant	LTX Regional Anticoagulant Niyad™
Nerinitide	NA-1 (Nerinitide)
Neurostimulator Lead in New Technology	Ischemic Stroke System (ISS500) ISS500 (Ischemic Stroke System)
Neurostimulator Lead with Paired Stimulation System in New Technology	Vivistim® Paired VNS System Lead
Omadacycline Anti-infective	NUZYRA™
Other New Technology Therapeutic Substance	STELARA® Ustekinumab
Posterior (Dynamic) Distraction Device in New Technology	ApiFix® Minimally Invasive Deformity Correction (MID-C) System
Posterior Spinal Motion Preservation Device in New Technology	TOPS™ System
Posterior Vertebral Tether in New Technology	LigaPASS 2.0™ PJK Prevention System
Reduction Device in New Technology	Neovasc Reducer™ Reducer™ System
REGN-COV2 Monoclonal Antibody	Casirivimab (REGN10933) and Imdevimab (REGN10987) Imdevimab (REGN10987) and Casirivimab (REGN10933)
Remdesivir Anti-infective	GS-5734 Veklury
Ruxolitinib	Jakafi®
Sarilumab	KEVZARA®
Satralizumab-mwge	ENSPRYNG™
Sulbactam-Durlobactam	SUL-DUR

Continued →

Section X - New Technology - Character 6 - Device/Substance/Technology

Synthetic Substitute, Extraluminal Support Device in New Technology	VasQ™ External Support Device
Synthetic Substitute, Lateral Meniscus in New Technology	NUsurface® Meniscus Implant
Synthetic Substitute, Mechanically Expandable (Paired) in New Technology	SpineJack® system
Synthetic Substitute, Medial Meniscus in New Technology	NUsurface® Meniscus Implant
Synthetic Substitute, Talar Prosthesis in New Technology	Total Ankle Talar Replacement™ (TATR)
Synthetic Substitute, Ultrasound Penetrable in New Technology	Longeviti ClearFit® Cranial Implant Longeviti ClearFit® OTS Cranial Implant
Tabelecleucel Immunotherapy	tab-cel®
Tagraxofusp-erzs Antineoplastic	ELZONRIS™

Section X - New Technology - Character 6 - Device/Substance/Technology

Taurolidine Anti-infective and Heparin Anticoagulant	DefenCath™
Terlipressin	TERLIVAZ®
Tibial Extension with Motion Sensors in New Technology	Canturio™ te (Tibial Extension)
Tisagenlecleucel Immunotherapy	KYMRIAH® Tisagenlecleucel
Tixagevimab and Cilgavimab Monoclonal Antibody	EVUSHELD™
Tocilizumab	ACTEMRA®
Trilaciclib	COSELA™
Uridine Triacetate	Vistogard®
Vein Graft Extraluminal Support Device(s) in New Technology	VEST™ Venous External Support device
Venetoclax Antineoplastic	Venclexta®

Appendix G: New ICD-10-PCS Codes FY2024

Appendix G is provided online in a format suitable for spreadsheet and/or database use. Go to https://my.ahima.org/learningcenter and follow the directions listed on the inside front cover of this textbook to download the files.